# DIAGNOSTIC TESTING IN NEUROLOGY

# DIAGNOSTIC TESTING IN NEUROLOGY

**Randolph W. Evans, MD**

Chief of Neurology Section
Park Plaza Hospital
Clinical Associate Professor
Department of Neurology
University of Texas
Medical School at Houston
Houston, Texas

**W.B. SAUNDERS COMPANY**
*A Division of Harcourt Brace & Company*
Philadelphia  London  Toronto  Montreal  Sydney  Tokyo

**W.B. SAUNDERS COMPANY**

*A Division of Harcourt Brace & Company*

The Curtis Center
Independence Square West
Philadelphia, Pennsylvania 19106

**Library of Congress Cataloging-in-Publication Data**

Diagnostic testing in neurology / [edited by] Randolph W. Evans. — 1st ed.

     p.   cm.

    Includes bibliographical references.

    ISBN 0-7216-7603-0

    1. Neurologic examination.   2. Nervous system—Diseases—Diagnosis.   I. Evans, Randolph W.

    [DNLM: 1. Nervous System Diseases—diagnosis.   2. Diagnostic Techniques, Neurological.   3. Neuropsychological Tests.

WL 141 D5355 1999]

RC348.D52  1999

616.8'0475—dc21

DNLM/DLC

                             99-25745

DIAGNOSTIC TESTING IN NEUROLOGY          ISBN 0-7216-7603-0

Printed in the United States of America

Last digit is the print number:    9   8   7   6   5   4   3   2   1

**To my family with love**
My parents, Dr. Richard I. Evans and the late Zena A. Evans
My wife, Marilyn, and my children, Elliott, Rochelle, and Jonathan

# Contributors

**JAMES W. ALBERS, MD, PhD**
Professor of Neurology, University of Michigan Medical School, Ann Arbor, Michigan
*Neurotoxicology*

**ROBERT W. BALOH, MD**
Professor of Neurology and Surgery (Head and Neck), University of California Los Angeles School of Medicine, Los Angeles, California
*Neuro-otology*

**GEORGE D. BAQUIS, MD**
Assistant Professor of Neurology, Tufts University School of Medicine, Boston, Massachusetts; Director, Electromyography Laboratory, Baystate Medical Center, Springfield, Massachusetts
*Micturition and Sexual Disorders*

**RUSSELL BARTT, MD**
Assistant Professor, Department of Neurological Sciences, Rush Medical College; Attending Physician, Cook County Hospital, Chicago, Illinois
*Rheumatologic Disorders*

**DAVID G. BENDITT, MD**
Professor of Medicine, University of Minnesota Medical School, Minneapolis, Minnesota
*Syncope*

**STANLEY BERENT, PhD**
Professor of Psychology, University of Michigan Medical School, Ann Arbor, Michigan
*Neurotoxicology*

**H. RICHARD BERESFORD, MD, JD**
Professor of Neurology, University of Rochester School of Medicine, Rochester, New York; Adjunct Professor of Law, Cornell Law School, Ithaca, New York
*Medicolegal Aspects*

**MARIA E. CARLINI, MD**
Clinical Instructor, Department of Medicine, Baylor College of Medicine; Infectious Diseases/Internal Medicine Staff Physician, Memorial Hermann Hospital Southwest, Houston, Texas
*Central Nervous System Infections*

**PIERRE COMBREMONT, MD**
Neurology Resident, University of Massachusetts Medical School, Worcester, Massachusetts
*Cerebrovascular Disease*

**D. R. CORNBLATH, MD**
Professor of Neurology, Johns Hopkins University School of Medicine, Baltimore, Maryland
*Peripheral Nerve Disease*

**RANDOLPH W. EVANS, MD**
Chief of Neurology Section, Park Plaza Hospital; Clinical Associate Professor, Department of Neurology, University of Texas Medical School at Houston, Houston, Texas
*Headaches*

**DANIEL M. FEINBERG, MD**
Clinical Assistant Professor of Neurology, University of Pennsylvania School of Medicine; Attending Physician, Pennsylvania Hospital and Hospital of the University of Pennsylvania, Philadelphia, Pennsylvania
*Mononeuropathies*

**BRUCE J. FISCH, MD**
Professor of Neurology, Department of Neurology, Louisiana State University Medical Center; Director, Louisiana State University/Baptist Memorial Comprehensive Medical and Surgical Epilepsy Program, Memorial Medical Center, Baptist Campus, New Orleans, Louisiana
*Metabolic Encephalopathies and Brain Death*

**MARC FISHER, MD**
Professor of Neurology, University of Massachusetts Medical School, Worcester, Massachusetts
*Cerebrovascular Disease*

**GARY M. FRANKLIN, MD, MPH**
Research Professor, University of Washington, Seattle, Washington; Attending Physician, Memorial Clinic, St. Peter Hospital, Olympia, Washington
*Practice Parameters*

**STEVEN L. GALETTA, MD**
Van Meter Professor of Neurology and Ophthalmology, University of Pennsylvania School of Medicine; Director, Neuro-ophthalmology, University of Pennsylvania Medical Center, Philadelphia, Pennsylvania
*Neuro-ophthalmology*

**DAVID R. GIFFORD, MD, MPH**

Assistant Professor of Medicine and Community Health, Brown University, Providence, Rhode Island

*Decision Making and Diagnostic Reasoning*

**FRANK GILLIAM, MD**

Assistant Professor, University of Alabama Birmingham Epilepsy Center, Department of Neurology, University of Alabama at Birmingham, Birmingham, Alabama

*Seizure Disorders*

**JOHN C. GODERSKY, MD**

Anchorage Neurosurgical Associates, Anchorage, Alaska

*Normal Pressure Hydrocephalus*

**BARRY GORDON, MD, PhD**

Professor of Neurology and Cognitive Science and Director, Division of Cognitive Neurology/Neuropsychology, Department of Neurology, Johns Hopkins University School of Medicine, Baltimore, Maryland

*Neuropsychologic Testing*

**NEILL R. GRAFF-RADFORD, MBBCh, MRCP (UK)**

Professor of Neurology, Mayo Medical School, Rochester, Minnesota; Chair of Neurology, Mayo Clinic Jacksonville, Jacksonville, Florida

*Normal Pressure Hydrocephalus*

**MICHAEL K. GREENBERG, MD**

Associate Professor of Neurology, Uniformed Services University of the Health Sciences, Bethesda, Maryland

*Practice Parameters*

**JOHN W. GRIFFIN, MD**

Professor of Neurology and Neuroscience, Johns Hopkins University School of Medicine; Director, Department of Neurology, and Neurologist-in-Chief, Johns Hopkins Hospital, Baltimore, Maryland

*Peripheral Nerve Disease*

**SCOTT HALDEMAN, MD, PhD, FRCP(C)**

Clinical Professor, Department of Neurology, University of California Irvine, Irvine, California

*Neck and Back Pain*

**SETH HAPLEA, MD**

Instructor, Department of Neurology, Hospital of the University of Pennsylvania, Philadelphia, Pennsylvania

*Molecular Diagnostic Testing*

**RICHARD L. HARRIS, MD**

Associate Professor of Medicine and Associate Dean, Graduate Medical Education, Baylor College of Medicine; Hospital Epidemiologist, The Methodist Hospital, Houston, Texas

*Central Nervous System Infections*

**EDWARD F. JACKSON, PhD**

Assistant Professor, University of Texas M.D. Anderson Cancer Center, Houston, Texas

*Neuroimaging of Brain Tumors*

**KATHLEEN M. JACOBSON, BA**

Staff Research Associate, University of California Los Angeles School of Medicine, Los Angeles, California

*Neuro-otology*

**WILLIAM C. KOLLER, MD, PhD**

Professor of Neurology and Director of Movement Disorders, University of Kansas and Kansas University Medical Center, Kansas City, Kansas

*Movement Disorders*

**ASHOK J. KUMAR, MD**

Professor of Radiology, University of Texas M.D. Anderson Cancer Center, Houston, Texas

*Neuroimaging of Brain Tumors*

**NORMAN E. LEEDS, MD**

Professor of Radiology and Kennedy Chair, University of Texas M.D. Anderson Cancer Center, Houston, Texas

*Neuroimaging of Brain Tumors*

**GRANT T. LIU, MD**

Associate Professor of Neurology and Ophthalmology, University of Pennsylvania School of Medicine; Neuro-ophthalmologist, Hospital of the University of Pennsylvania, Scheie Eye Institute, and Children's Hospital of Philadelphia, Philadelphia, Pennsylvania

*Neuro-opthalmology*

**DAVID R. LYNCH, MD, PhD**

Assistant Professor, Department of Neurology, University of Pennsylvania School of Medicine; Attending Neurologist, Hospital of the University of Pennsylvania, Philadelphia, Pennsylvania

*Molecular Diagnostic Testing*

**MARK W. MAHOWALD, MD**

Professor of Neurology, University of Minnesota Medical School; Senior Associate Physician in Neurology and Director, Minnesota Regional Sleep Disorders Center, Hennepin County Medical Center, Minneapolis, Minnesota

*Sleep Medicine*

**JOSEPH C. MASDEU, MD, PhD**

Professor and Chairman of Neurology, New York Medical College, New York, New York

*Gait Disorders*

**JUSTIN C. McARTHUR, MBBS, MPH**

Professor of Neurology and Epidemiology, Johns Hopkins University School of Medicine and Johns Hopkins Hospital, Baltimore, Maryland

*Peripheral Nerve Disease*

**BRIAN S. MITTMAN, PhD**

Senior Social Scientist, Center for the Study of Healthcare Provider Behavior, Veterans Administration Greater Los Angeles Healthcare System, Los Angeles, California; Senior Social Scientist, RAND Health Sciences Program, Santa Monica, California

*Decision Making and Diagnostic Reasoning*

**PIOTR OLEJNICZAK, MD, PhD**

Assistant Professor of Neurology, Department of Neurology, Louisiana State University Medical Center; Director of Neuroimaging, Louisiana State University and Memorial Comprehensive Epilepsy Program; Staff Physician, Medical Center of Louisiana at New Orleans and Memorial Medical Center, New Orleans, Louisiana

*Metabolic Encephalopathies and Brain Death*

**VICTORIA S. PELAK, MD**

Neuro-Ophthalmology Fellow, Hospital of the University of Pennsylvania, Philadelphia, Pennsylvania

*Molecular Diagnostic Testing*

**A. BERNARD PLEET, MD, FACP**

Professor of Neurology, Tufts University School of Medicine, Boston, Massachusetts; Chief, Neurology Division, Baystate Medical Center, Springfield, Massachusetts

*Neuroendocrine Disorders*

**DAVID C. PRESTON, MD**

Associate Professor of Neurology, Case Western Reserve University; Director, Neuromuscular Service, University Hospitals of Cleveland, Cleveland, Ohio

*Mononeuropathies; Electromyography Waveform Analysis*

**BRUCE H. PRICE, MD**

Assistant Professor of Neurology, Harvard Medical School; Chief, Department of Neurology, McLean Hospital; Assistant in Neurology, Massachusetts General Hospital, Boston, Massachusetts

*Alzheimer's Disease*

**LOREN A. ROLAK, MD**

Clinical Associate Professor of Neurology, University of Wisconsin, Madison, Wisconsin; Director, Marshfield Multiple Sclerosis Center, The Marshfield Clinic, Marshfield, Wisconsin

*Multiple Sclerosis*

**DAVID B. ROSENFIELD, MD**

Professor, Department of Neurology and Department of Otorhinolaryngology and Communication Sciences, and Director, Stuttering Center Speech Motor Control Laboratory, Baylor College of Medicine; Attending Physician, The Methodist Hospital, Houston, Texas

*Neurolaryngology*

**THOMAS A. SANDSON, MD**

Assistant Professor of Neurology, Harvard Medical School; Senior Associate in Neurology, Beth Israel Deaconess Medical Center, Boston, Massachusetts

*Alzheimer's Disease*

**WOLF-RUEDIGER SCHAEBITZ, MD**

Neurology Resident, University of Heidelberg, Heidelberg, Germany

*Cerebrovascular Disease*

**OLA A. SELNES, PhD**

Associate Professor, Division of Cognitive Neurology, Department of Neurology, Johns Hopkins University School of Medicine, Baltimore, Maryland

*Neuropsychologic Testing*

**KATHLEEN M. SHANNON, MD**

Associate Professor, Department of Neurological Sciences, Rush Medical College; Associate Attending Physician, Rush-Presbyterian-St. Luke's Medical Center, Chicago, Illinois

*Rheumatologic Disorders*

**BARBARA E. SHAPIRO, MD, PhD**

Associate Professor of Neurology, Case Western Reserve University School of Medicine; Director, Neuromuscular Research, University Hospitals of Cleveland, Cleveland, Ohio

*Electromyography Waveform Analysis*

**BARBARA G. VICKREY, MD, MPH**

Associate Professor, Department of Neurology, University of California Los Angeles, Los Angeles, California

*Decision Making and Diagnostic Reasoning*

**NAGALAPURA S. VISWANATH, PhD**

Assistant Professor, Department of Neurology, Stuttering Center Speech Motor Control Laboratory, Baylor College of Medicine, Houston, Texas

*Neurolaryngology*

**NICHOLAS J. VOLPE, MD**

Assistant Professor of Ophthalmology and Neurology, Departments of Neurology and Ophthalmology, and Residency Program Director, Department of Ophthalmology, University of Pennsylvania School of Medicine; Attending Physician, Scheie Eye Institute, Philadelphia, Pennsylvania

*Neuro-ophthalmology*

**PAUL G. WASIELEWSKI, MD**

Fellow, Department of Neurology, University of Kansas Medical Center, Kansas City, Missouri

*Movement Disorders*

**LOUIS H. WEIMER, MD**

Assistant Professor of Neurology, College of Physicians and Surgeons, Columbia University; Assistant Professor of Neurology, Neurological Institute of New York, New York Presbyterian Hospital, New York, New York

*Autonomic Function*

**ELAINE WYLLIE, MD**

Pediatric Epilepsy Program, The Cleveland Clinic Foundation, Cleveland, Ohio

*Seizure Disorders*

**DAVID S. YOUNGER, MD**

Clinical Associate Professor of Neurology, New York University School of Medicine; Director of Neuromuscular Diseases, New York University Medical Center; Chief of Neuromuscular Diseases, Lenox Hill Hospital, New York, New York

*Neuromuscular Diseases*

# Preface

Although many neurologic disorders can be diagnosed with a complete history and neurologic examination, others require diagnostic testing. The judicious use of testing distinguishes the unknowledgeable physician who takes a shotgun approach from the expert sharpshooter. The sharpshooter physician is aware of the differential diagnosis of various neurologic disorders as well as the range of tests available to make the diagnosis including their indications, sensitivity, specificity, cost, and risk/benefit. The aim of this book is to improve the acumen of neurologists as well as the many other physicians who see patients with neurologic disorders including primary care physicians, neurosurgeons, and physiatrists. The information in this evidence-based volume often is not presented in general neurology textbooks and to find it may require looking through numerous subspecialty books or literature searches.

Our reasons for recommending diagnostic testing may vary from patient to patient. We consider factors such as diagnostic precision and reducing diagnostic uncertainty, reassuring anxious patients and family members, and medicolegal aspects. The once familiar concerns about financial incentives for overutilization are now being reversed in a managed care environment. Legitimate fears are growing about underutilization because of the rules of the new game, which can include arbitrary utilization review, deselection, capitation, and at-risk financial arrangements. The information in this volume will be useful in helping the physician practice high-quality, cost-effective medicine.

The impetus for this book is the well-received February, 1996, issue of *Neurologic Clinics,* which I edited, *Diagnostic Testing in Neurology.* The original 13 articles have been revised and updated, and 18 new chapters have been added. The book is divided into seven sections: Pain Disorders; Central Nervous System Disorders; Neuro-ophthalmology, Neuro-otology, and Neurotoxicology; Neuromuscular Disorders; Neuromedical Disorders; Molecular Genetic Testing; and Diagnostic Reasoning, Medicolegal Aspects, and Practice Parameters. Coverage includes all the common neurologic disorders as well as many of the uncommon ones. I hope that the use of this book will increase the number of "sharpshooter" physicians.

I thank our outstanding contributors for their superb chapters. I appreciate the encouragement and advice of our editor at W.B. Saunders Company, Allan Ross, and the fine work of the entire Saunders production team.

Randolph W. Evans, MD
February, 1999
Houston, Texas

# Contents

# Color Plate

# Color Plate

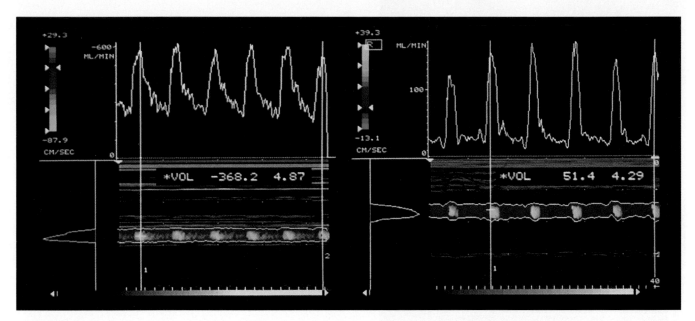

**FIGURE 5—8.** Volume flow rate measurements of the right and left common carotid artery (*CCA*) in right internal carotid artery (*ICA*) occlusion. Color motion mode (M-mode) display of four cardiac cycles on either side is shown below. Volume flow rate estimates in the CCA contralateral to occlusion on the ICA reveal normal to high normal values (368 ml/min). Ipsilateral to occlusion, the volume flow rate is greatly decreased since only the flow directed into the external carotid artery is carried by the CCA (51 ml/min). (From Fisher M, ed. *Stroke Therapy.* Boston: Butterworth-Heinemann; 1995.)

**FIGURE 5—9.** Subclavian steal syndrome assessed by color duplex sonography. In this longitudinal color-flow image, direction of vertebral vein and vertebral artery are both caudal (encoded in blue). The vertebral artery is supplying the brachial artery via subclavian artery on left side. Duplex Doppler spectral waveform at lower left shows flow reversal and total loss of diastolic flow. (From Fisher M, ed. *Stroke Therapy.* Boston: Butterworth-Heinemann; 1995.)

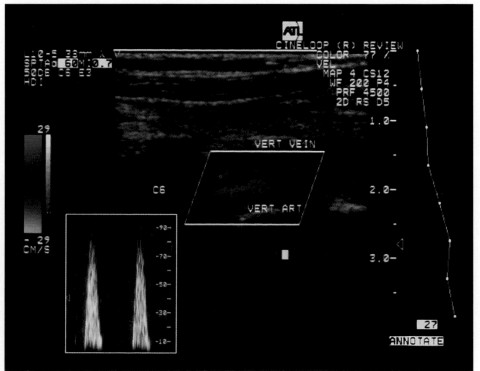

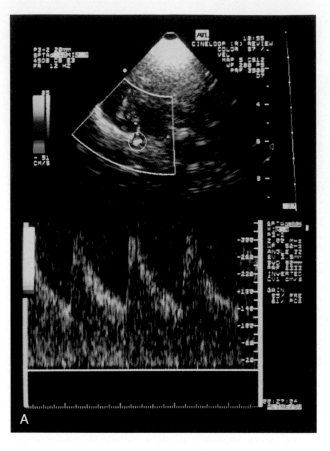

A

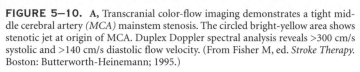

**FIGURE 5—10.** **A,** Transcranial color-flow imaging demonstrates a tight middle cerebral artery *(MCA)* mainstem stenosis. The circled bright-yellow area shows stenotic jet at origin of MCA. Duplex Doppler spectral analysis reveals >300 cm/s systolic and >140 cm/s diastolic flow velocity. (From Fisher M, ed. *Stroke Therapy.* Boston: Butterworth-Heinemann; 1995.)

**FIGURE 5—11.** Patent foramen ovale assessed by transesophageal echocardiography. Color-coded shunt between right and left atrium indicates a patent foramen ovale.

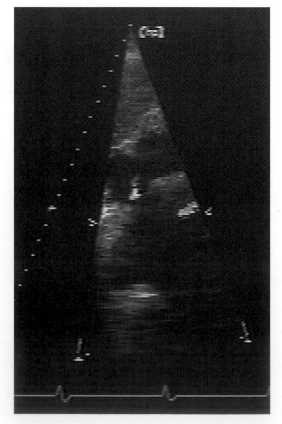

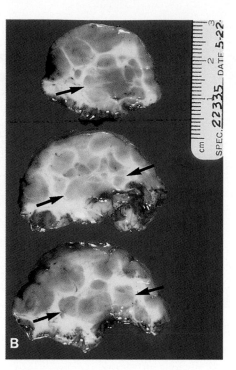

**FIGURE 12–31.** Heterotopic gray matter mimicking primary tumor. **A,** Precontrast axial T1-weighted MR image. **B,** Surgical specimen of the temporal lobe. Abnormal right temporal lobe white matter (*large arrow* in **A**), with loss of gray-white matter differentiation, is seen. The left temporal lobe white matter (*open arrow* in **A**) is normal. Temporal lobe resection revealed islands of heterotopic gray matter (*arrows* in **B**).

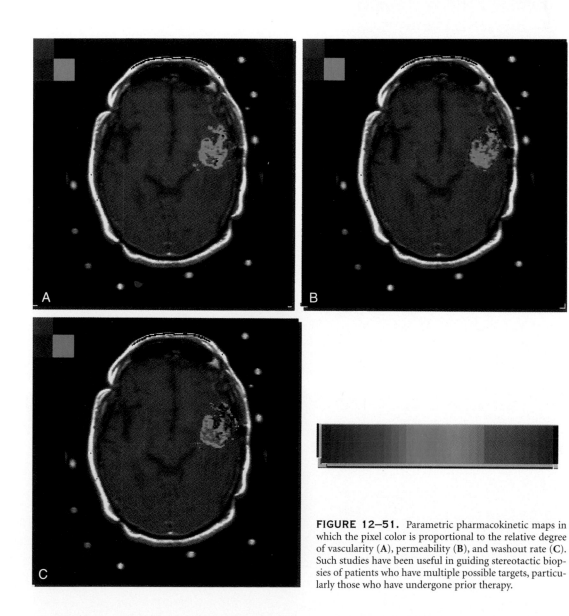

**FIGURE 12–51.** Parametric pharmacokinetic maps in which the pixel color is proportional to the relative degree of vascularity (**A**), permeability (**B**), and washout rate (**C**). Such studies have been useful in guiding stereotactic biopsies of patients who have multiple possible targets, particularly those who have undergone prior therapy.

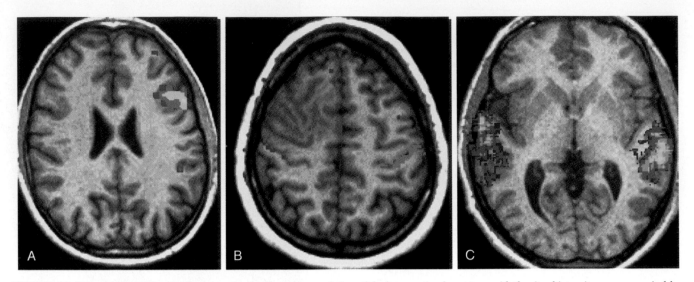

**FIGURE 12–54.** BOLD fMRI activation maps obtained by cross-correlation of the known stimulus pattern with the signal intensity curve on a pixel-by-pixel basis. **A,** Expressive speech task. **B,** Bilateral hand mapping, with *blue* corresponding to a left-hand task and *yellow* corresponding to a right-hand task. **C,** Auditory stimulation.

# Section I

# PAIN DISORDERS

# Headaches

*Randolph W. Evans*

Headaches are one of the most common symptoms that neurologists evaluate. Although most are due to primary headache disorders, the differential diagnosis is one of the longest in all of medicine, with more than 300 different types and causes (Table 1–1).[164] The cause or type of most headaches can be determined by a careful history supplemented by a general and neurologic examination. The classification system of the International Headache Society (IHS)[72] is helpful in providing standardized diagnostic criteria, which may be more reliable and valid than prior formal or informal criteria.[147,176]

## REASONS FOR DIAGNOSTIC TESTING

Authorities differ over general indications for diagnostic testing. Saper et al[164] state: "In general, we believe that most patients with headache will require neurodiagnostic testing. A CT scan or MRI should be performed in most patients with headaches severe enough to prompt medical evaluation and treatment." Lance[100] counters: "Only a small proportion of headache patients require investigation, other than a careful history and physical examination."

Although practice guidelines are being developed,[157] the indications for diagnostic testing are variable and the neurologist must make decisions on a case by case basis. Clinical situations in which neurologists consider diagnostic testing are listed in Table 1–2.[60,167,168]

There are many other reasons why neurologists recommend diagnostic testing: "our stubborn quest for diagnostic certainty"[94]; faulty cognitive reasoning; the medical decision rule that holds that it is better to impute disease than to risk overlooking it; busy practice conditions in which tests are ordered as a shortcut; patient expectations; financial incen-

tives; professional peer pressure in which recommendations for routine and esoteric tests are expected as a demonstration of competence; and medicolegal issues.[209] The attitudes and demands of patients and families and the practice of defensive medicine are especially important reasons in the case of headaches. In this era of managed care, equally compelling reasons for not ordering diagnostic studies include a physician's fear of deselection and at-risk capitation. In some cases, appropriate CT and MRI scans may be denied by managed care companies as not indicated. Lack of funds and underinsurance continue to be barriers for appropriate diagnostic testing for many patients.

This chapter reviews diagnostic testing in the following settings: headaches and a normal neurologic examination; migraine; cluster headaches; trigeminal neuralgia; acute severe new-onset headaches ("first or worst"); cough, exertional, and sexual headaches; low cerebrospinal fluid (CSF) pressure headaches; headaches after mild head injury; and new-onset headaches in patients older than 50.

## HEADACHES AND A NORMAL NEUROLOGIC EXAMINATION

Most scans in patients with headaches and a normal neurologic examination are performed to rule out brain tumors. Patients with headaches often have fears that they have an undetected brain tumor. Although neurologists realize that primary and metastatic neoplasms account for an extremely small percentage of all headaches, concern about missing a neoplasm in a patient with a normal neurologic examination is great. Many neurologists can provide chilling anecdotes of missed or nearly missed diagnoses in this setting. Before discussing the yield of neuroimaging stud-

## TABLE 1–1. IHS Major Categories of Headache Disorders

Migraine
Tension-type headache
Cluster headache and chronic paroxysmal hemicrania
Miscellaneous headaches unassociated with structural lesion
  Idiopathic stabbing, external compression, cold stimulus, benign cough, benign exertional, associated with sexual activity
Headache associated with head trauma
Headache associated with vascular disorders
  Acute ischemic cerebrovascular disorder, intracranial hematoma, subarachnoid hemorrhage, unruptured vascular malformation, arteritis, carotid or vertebral artery pain, venous thrombosis, arterial hypertension, associated with other vascular disorder
Headache associated with nonvascular intracranial disorder
  High and low cerebrospinal fluid pressure, intracranial infection, intracranial sarcoidosis and other noninfectious inflammatory disease, related to intrathecal injections, intracranial neoplasm, associated with other intracranial disorder
Headache associated with substances or their withdrawal
  Acute and chronic substance use or exposure, withdrawal after acute and chronic use, associated with substances with uncertain mechanism
Headache associated with noncephalic infection
  Viral infection, bacterial infection, other infection
Headache associated with metabolic disorder
  Hypoxia, hypercapnia, mixed hypoxia and hypercapnia, hypoglycemia, dialysis, other metabolic abnormality
Headache or facial pain associated with disorder of cranium, neck, eyes, ears, nose, sinuses, teeth, mouth, or other facial or cranial structures
Cranial neuralgias, nerve trunk pain, and deafferentation pain
  Persistent pain of cranial nerve origin, trigeminal neuralgia, glossopharyngeal neuralgia, nervus intermedius neuralgia, superior laryngeal neuralgia, occipital neuralgia, central causes of head and facial pain other than tic douloureux

Data from Headache Classification Committee of the International Headache Society. Classification and diagnostic criteria for headache disorders, cranial neuralgia, and facial pain. *Cephalalgia.* 1988;8(suppl 7):1-96.

ies, it may be helpful to review the characteristics of patients with headaches due to primary and metastatic brain tumors.

## HEADACHES AND BRAIN TUMORS

The prevalence of adults with primary and metastatic brain tumors who complain of headaches at the time of diagnosis has been reported as 31%,[193] 48%,[58] and 71%.[181] The median duration of headache at the time of diagnosis has been reported as 3.5 weeks in a study from New York[58] and 15.7 months in a study from Bangkok.[181] Headaches have been reported as equally frequent with primary and metastatic tumors[58] and more frequent with primary compared to metastatic tumors.[181,193]

In a series from Spain,[193] 8% of patients with headaches and brain tumors had a normal neurologic examination. Papilledema, which is usually associated with headaches, was present in 40% of patients with brain tumors in another series.[181] The presence of headache is related to the size of the tumor and the amount of midline shift. Patients with previous headaches were more likely to have a headache with a brain tumor. The brain tumor headache may have characteristics identical to the prior headaches, but it is more severe or more frequent than the patient's prior headache and is usually associated with other problems, such as seizure, confusion, prolonged nausea, hemiparesis, or other focal findings.[58]

The most common location of headaches is bifrontal, although patients may complain of pain in other locations of the head and neck. Unilateral headaches are usually on the same side as the neoplasm.[58,181] Although the quality of the headache is usually similar to that of the tension type, occasionally patients have headaches similar to migraine without aura and, rarely, migraine with aura[58,181] and cluster headaches.[182] Most of the headaches are intermittent with moderate to severe intensity, but a significant minority of patients report only mild headaches relieved by simple analgesics. The "classic" brain tumor headache—severe, worse in the morning, and associated with nausea and vomiting—occurs in a minority of patients with brain tumors.[58,181]

## NEUROIMAGING STUDIES IN ADULTS

The yield of abnormal neuroimaging studies performed in studies of patients with headaches as the only neurologic symptom and normal neurologic examinations depends on a number of factors, including the duration of the headache, study design (prospective vs. retrospective), who orders the scan, and the type of scan performed.[59] The percentage of abnormal scans is higher when ordered by a neurologist[8] or a tertiary care center[99] compared with a primary care physician, and this finding represents case selection bias. In reported computed tomography (CT scan) series, the yield may vary depending on the generation of scanner and whether iodinated contrast was used. Magnetic resonance imaging (MRI) is more sensitive than CT scanning, with the exception of acute subarachnoid hemorrhage and abnormalities of bone.[2] The yield of MRI may vary depending on the field strength of the magnet, the use of paramagnetic contrast, the selection of acquisition sequences, and the use of magnetic resonance (MR) angiography.

Frishberg[59] reviewed eight CT scan studies, reported between 1977 and 1993, of 1825 patients with unspecified headache type and varying duration.[8,21,99,101,127,160,165,200] The summarized findings from these studies is combined with four additional studies[3,37,45,178] of 1566 CT scans in patients with headache and normal neurologic examinations for a total of 3389 scans. The overall percentages of various patho-

## TABLE 1–2. Reasons to Consider Use of Neuroimaging for Headaches

**Temporal and Headache Features**
1. "First or worst" headache
2. Subacute headaches with increasing frequency or severity
3. Progressive or new daily persistent headache
4. Chronic daily headache
5. Headaches always on same side
6. Headaches not responding to treatment

**Demographics**
7. New-onset headaches in patients who have cancer or who test positive for HIV infection
8. New-onset headaches after age 50
9. Patients with headaches and seizures

**Associated Symptoms and Signs**
10. Headaches associated with symptoms and signs such as fever, stiff neck, nausea, and vomiting
11. Headaches other than migraine with aura associated with focal neurologic symptoms or signs
12. Headaches associated with papilledema, cognitive impairment, or personality change

logic categories are as follows: brain tumors, 1%; arteriovenous malformations, 0.2%; hydrocephalus, 0.3%; aneurysms, 0.1%; subdural hematoma, 0.2%; and strokes (including chronic ischemic process), 1.1%. The studies cited do not give information about the detection of paranasal sinus disease, which may be the cause of some headaches.

Four studies of patients with chronic headaches and a normal neurologic examination have been performed. When three of these studies were combined for a total of 1282 patients, the only clinically significant pathologic conditions were one low-grade glioma and one saccular aneurysm.[3,45,200] However, a fourth study from Belgium of 363 consecutive CT scans found significant pathologic evidence in 11 patients (3%), including two with intraventricular cysts, four with meningiomas, and five with malignant neoplasms.[37]

Weingarten et al[200] extrapolated various types of data from a health maintenance organization of 100,800 adult patients. The estimated prevalence (in patients with chronic headache and a normal neurologic examination) of a CT scan demonstrating an abnormality requiring neurosurgical intervention may have been as low as 0.01%. It is not certain whether detection of additional pathologic evidence on MRI scan would change this percentage. Numerous types of pathology can be missed on a routine CT scan of the head (Table 1–3). For example, complaints of headache with a normal neurologic examination may be noted in patients with type I Arnold-Chiari malformation, which is easily detected on MRI but not on CT scans.[95] Pituitary hemorrhage can produce a migrainelike acute headache with a normal neurologic examination.[49] Pituitary infarction, with severe headache, photophobia, and CSF pleocytosis, initially can be similar to aseptic meningitis or meningoencephalitis.[47] Pituitary pathologic findings are more likely to be detected through routine MRI than by CT scanning.

## NEUROIMAGING STUDIES IN CHILDREN

Children commonly have headaches. Bille[14] reported that 59% of pediatric patients studied had headaches, being

---

### TABLE 1–3. Causes of Headache That Can Be Missed on Routine CT Scan of the Head

**Vascular Disease**
Saccular aneurysms
Arteriovenous malformations (especially posterior fossa)
Subarachnoid hemorrhage
Carotid or vertebral artery dissections
Infarcts
Cerebral venous thrombosis
Vasculitis (white matter abnormalities)
Subdural and epidural hematomas

**Neoplastic Disease**
Neoplasms (especially in the posterior fossa)
Meningeal carcinomatosis
Pituitary tumor and hemorrhage

**Cervicomedullary Lesions**
Chiari malformations
Foramen magnum meningioma

**Infections**
Paranasal sinusitis
Meningoencephalitis
Cerebritis and brain abscess

---

### TABLE 1–4. Reasons to Consider Use of Neuroimaging for Children With Headaches

1. Persistent headaches of less than 6 months' duration that do not respond to medical treatment
2. Headache associated with abnormal neurologic findings, especially if accompanied by papilledema, nystagmus, or gait or motor abnormalities
3. Persistent headaches associated with absence of family history of migraine
4. Persistent headache associated with substantial episodes of confusion, disorientation, or emesis
5. Headaches that awaken a child repeatedly from sleep or occur immediately on awakening
6. Family history or medical history of disorders that may predispose one to central nervous system lesions and clinical or laboratory findings suggestive of central nervous system involvement

Data from Medina LS, Pinter JD, Zurakowski D, et al. Children with headache: clinical predictors of surgical space-occupying lesions and the role of neuroimaging. *Radiology.* 1997;202:819-824.

---

frequent in 10% and of the migraine type in 4%. In a study of adolescents, the prevalence of any headache and migraine, respectively, was as follows: boys, 56%, 3.8%; and girls, 74%, 6.6%.[106]

Five studies have investigated the findings of neuroimaging in children with headaches. Dooley et al[42] reported the retrospective findings on CT scans of 41 children with headaches and normal neurologic examinations referred to a secondary or tertiary care facility. Only one scan was abnormal, demonstrating a choroid plexus papilloma. Chu and Shinnar[24] obtained brain imaging studies in 30 children ages 7 years or younger with headaches who were referred to pediatric neurologists. The studies were normal except for five patients with incidental findings. Maytal et al[118] obtained MRI or CT scans or both in 78 children ages 3 to 18 years with headaches. With the exception of six patients, the neurologic examinations were normal. The studies were normal except for incidental cerebral abnormalities in four patients and mucoperiosteal thickening of the paranasal sinuses in seven patients.

Wöber-Bingöl et al[206] prospectively obtained MRI scans in 96 children ages 5 to 18 years who had headaches and normal neurologic examinations and were referred to an outpatient headache clinic. The studies were normal except for 17 patients (17.7%) with incidental findings. Finally, Medina et al[121] retrospectively reported MRI findings in 315 children ages 3 to 20 years (mean, 11 years) with headaches. The neurologic examinations were abnormal in 89 patients. Thirteen patients (4%) had surgical space-occupying lesions. After analyzing the risk factors for these lesions and the prior literature, Medina and colleagues suggested guidelines for neuroimaging in children with headache (Table 1–4).

## AMERICAN ACADEMY OF NEUROLOGY PRACTICE GUIDELINE

A report of the Quality Standards Subcommittee of the American Academy of Neurology (AAN)[5] in 1994 stated the following: "At this time, there is insufficient evidence to define the role of CT and MRI in the evaluation of patients with headaches that are not consistent with migraine." Recommendations by the AAN for future research include: "1. Large prospective studies to define the clinical characteristics of chronic headaches which would help identify those

**TABLE 1–5. Balance Sheet: CT or MRI in Patients with Headache and Normal Neurologic Examination**

|  | CT (%) | MRI (%) | No Test (%) |
|---|---|---|---|
| **Benefits** | | | |
| Discovery of potentially treatable lesions | | | |
|     (1) Migraine | 0.3 | 0.4 | 0 |
|     (2) Any headache | 2.4 | 2.4 | 0 |
| Relief of anxiety | 30 | 30 | 0 |
| **Risks** | | | |
| Iodine reaction | | | |
|   Mild | 10 | | |
|   Moderate | 1 | | |
|   Severe | 0.01 | | |
|   Death | 0.002 | | |
| Claustrophobia | | | |
|   Mild | 5 | 15 | 0 |
|   Moderate (needs sedation) | 1 | 5–10 | 0 |
|   Severe (unable to comply) | | 1–2 | |
| False-positive studies | No data | No data | |
| Cost (charges) | ———————— Varies widely depending on payor ———————— | | |

Technology: CT with intravenous contrast or MRI without contrast; indications: (1) migraine and (2) any headache.
    Modified from Frishberg BM. The utility of neuroimaging in the evaluation of headache in patients with normal neurologic examination. *Neurology.* 1994;44:1196.

patients at higher risk for intracranial disease. 2. Evaluating the role of repeated neuroimaging in patients with previously negative studies."[5]

### RISK/BENEFIT AND COST/BENEFIT OF NEUROIMAGING

Table 1–5 summarizes the estimated risks and benefits of neuroimaging in patients with headaches and normal neurologic examinations. Although for many patients the scan helps to relieve anxiety, for others it may produce anxiety if nonspecific abnormalities are found, such as incidental anatomic variants or white matter lesions. I suspect that many neurologists have seen patients with isolated headaches who were referred by primary care physicians with a request to rule out multiple sclerosis when white matter lesions were detected.

Although the cost of finding significant pathology is quite high, this cost is decreasing significantly under some managed care contracts. Reimbursement of $400 for a MRI scan of the brain without contrast, including technical and professional components, is not uncommon. Cost/benefit estimates should also include the cost to the physician of malpractice suits filed when patients with significant pathologic evidence do not undergo neuroimaging and the cost to the patient and society of premature death and disability of undetected treatable lesions.

### ELECTROENCEPHALOGRAPHY IN EVALUATION OF HEADACHES

For many years the electroencephalogram (EEG) was a standard test for the evaluation of headaches, especially in the pre–CT scan era. Gronseth and Greenberg[67] reviewed the literature from 1941 to 1994 on the utility of EEG in the evaluation of patients with headache. Most of the articles had serious methodologic flaws. In studies with a relatively nonflawed design the only significant abnormality reported was prominent driving in response to photic stimulation (H-response) in migraineurs with a sensitivity ranging from 26%[154] to 100%[166] with a specificity from 80%[173] to 91%.[171] This finding, while interesting, is not necessary for the clinical diagnosis of migraine. If the purpose of the EEG is to ex-

clude an underlying structural lesion such as a neoplasm, CT or MRI is far superior.

The report of the Quality Standards Subcommittee of the AAN suggests the following practice parameter:

> The electroencephalogram (EEG) is not useful in the routine evaluation of patients with headache. This does not exclude the use of EEG to evaluate headache patients with associated symptoms suggesting a seizure disorder such as atypical migrainous aura or episodic loss of consciousness. Assuming head imaging capabilities are readily available, EEG is not recommended to exclude a structural cause for headache.[6]

## NEUROIMAGING IN MIGRAINE

### INCIDENCE OF PATHOLOGY

Frishberg[57] reviewed four CT scan studies,[20,27,80,115] four MRI scan studies,[82,86,137,175] and one combined MRI and CT scan study,[96] reported from 1976 to 1991, of 897 scans of patients with migraine. These findings can be combined with more recent reports of one CT scan study of 284 patients[45] and five studies of MRI scans of 342 patients[26,35,51,143,156,214] for a total of 1625 scans of patients with various types of migraine. Other than white matter abnormalities, the studies showed no significant pathologic evidence except for four brain tumors (three of which were incidental findings) and one arteriovenous malformation (in a patient with migraine and a seizure disorder).

### WHITE MATTER ABNORMALITIES

Twelve MRI studies have investigated white matter abnormalities (WMAs) on scans of migraine patients (Table 1–6). WMAs are foci of hyperintensity on both proton density and T2-weighted images in the deep and periventricular white matter due to either interstitial edema or perivascular demyelination. WMAs are easily detected on MRI but are not seen on CT scan.[96]

The percentages of WMAs for all types of migraine range from 12%[137] to 46%.[175] WMAs have been reported as both more frequent in the frontal region of the centrum semiovale[35,82] and no more frequent[143] than in the white matter of the parietal, temporal, and occipital lobes. Five of the six studies using controls found a higher incidence of WMAs in migraineurs. The incidence of WMAs in controls ranged from 2%[143] to 14%.[51] One small study reported a similar incidence of WMAs in patients with tension-type headaches (34.3%) as those with migraine (32.1%) and greater than the 7.4% in controls.[35]

Four studies found similar percentages of WMAs comparing migraine with aura to migraine without,[26,35,143,146] whereas two reported a higher percentage in migraine with aura.[51,82] Three small studies of basilar migraine found WMAs in 17%[26,86] and 38%.[51] WMAs are variably reported as more often present in adult migraineurs who are more than 40 years old and less than 60[26,146] and equally present (39% vs. 40%)[51] compared to those 40 or younger. Cooney et al[26] found an increased frequency of WMAs associated with age over 50 and with medical risk factors (hypertension, atherosclerotic heart disease, diabetic mellitus, autoimmune disorder, or demyelinating disease) but not with gender, migraine subtype, or duration of migraine symptoms.

Although the cause of WMAs in migraine is not certain, various hypotheses have been advanced, including increased platelet aggregability with microemboli, abnormal cerebrovascular regulation, and repeated attacks of hypoperfusion during the aura.[35,82,143] The presence of antiphospholipid antibodies might be another risk factor for WMAs in migraine.[184] The reported incidence of antiphospholipid antibodies in migraine ranges from 0%[74] to 24%.[155] In one MRI study, however, the presence of WMAs showed no correlation with the presence of anticardiolipin antibodies.[82] The presence of anticardiolipin antibodies is not an additional risk factor for stroke in migraineurs.[31] In one study, Tietjen et al[185] found that, compared to control subjects, there was no increase in frequency of anticardiolipin positivity in adults younger than 60 years of age with transient focal neurologic events or in those with migraine with or without aura.

## CEREBRAL ATROPHY

Diffuse cerebral atrophy with widening of the lateral ventricles and cerebral sulci is equally well detected by MRI and CT scanning.[96] The incidence of cerebral atrophy in migraineurs on CT and MRI scans has been variably reported as 4%,[20] 26%,[80] 28%,[146] 35%,[96] and 58%.[43] The studies describe most cases of atrophy as mild to moderate. The cause of the atrophy, which can be a nonspecific finding based on often subjective criteria, is not certain.[146,214] Two more recent studies have found the incidence of atrophy in migraineurs to be no greater than in controls.[35,214]

**TABLE 1–6. White Matter Abnormalities (WMAs) Reported on MRI of Migraine Patients**

| STUDY | MIGRAINE TYPE(S) (N) | PATIENT AGES (Y) | % WMA | % WMA IN CONTROLS (N) |
|---|---|---|---|---|
| Soges et al[175] (1988) | Total, 24 | Mean 36.8 | 46 | — |
| | Classic and common, 17 | Range 15–55 | 41 | |
| | Complicated, 7 | | 57 | |
| Jacome & Leborgne[86] (1990) | Basilar, 18 | Avg 30<br>Range 17–57 | 17 | — |
| Kuhn & Shekar[96] (1990) | Classic, 74 | Mean 28<br>Range 9–39 | 26 | — |
| Igarashi et al[82] (1991) | Without aura, 33 | Mean 36.7 | 33.3 | |
| | With aura, 53 | Mean 33.2 | 43.4 | |
| | Prolonged aura, 5 | Mean 24.8 | 40 | |
| | Total, 51 | <40 | 29.4 | 11.2 (98) |
| Osborn et al[137] (1991) | Total, 31 | Avg 29.8<br>Range 18–66 | 12 | — |
| Prager et al[146] (1991) | Without aura, 58 | Mean 41 | 47 | — |
| | With aura, 19 | Mean 40 | 44 | |
| Ziegler et al[214] (1991) | With aura, 18 | Range 27–64 | 17 | 13 (15) |
| Fazekas et al[51] (1992) | Total, 38 | Mean 37.5 | 39 | |
| | Without aura, 11 | Mean 37.9 | 18 | |
| | With aura, 19 | Mean 36.9 | 53 | |
| | Basilar, 8 | Mean 38.4 | 38 | |
| | Total, 24 | <50 | 33 | 14 (14) |
| Robbins & Friedman[156] (1992) | Not specified, 46 | Range 17–55 | 13.6 | 4.3 (69) |
| Pavese et al[143] (1994) | Without aura, 83 | Mean 36.1 | 18 | |
| | With aura, 46 | Mean 34.2 | 21.7 | |
| | Both, 129 | Mean ~35 | 19.3 | 2 (50) |
| De Benedittis et al[35] (1995) | Total, 28 | Mean 40.1 | 32.1 | |
| | Without aura, 19 | — | 31.6 | 7.4 (54) |
| | With aura, 9 | — | 33.3 | |
| Cooney et al[26] (1996) | Total, 185 | Median 38 | 16 | — |
| | Common, 78 | — | 14 | |
| | Classic, 55 | — | 13 | |
| | Basilar, 6 | — | 17 | |
| | Hemiplegic, 8 | — | 12 | |
| | Acephalgic, 38 | — | 26 | |

## ARTERIOVENOUS MALFORMATIONS AND MIGRAINE

The prevalence of arteriovenous malformations (AVMs) is approximately 0.5% in postmortem studies.[17] In contrast to saccular aneurysms, up to 50% present with symptoms or signs other than hemorrhage. Migrainelike headaches with and without visual symptoms can be associated with AVMs, especially those in the occipital lobe, which is the predominant location of about 20% of parenchymal AVMs.[60,98] Although headaches that always occur on the same side (side-locked) are present in 95% of patients with AVMs,[18] 17% of those with migraine without aura and 15% of patients with migraine with aura have side-locked headaches.[104] Typical migraine due to an AVM is the exception, and there are usually distinguishing features. Bruyn[18] reported the following features in patients with migrainelike symptoms and AVMs: unusual associated signs (papilledema, field cut, bruit), 65%; short duration of headache attacks, 20%; brief scintillating scotoma, 10%; absent family history, 15%; atypical sequence of aura, headache, and vomiting, 10%; and seizures, 25%.

## AMERICAN ACADEMY OF NEUROLOGY PRACTICE GUIDELINE

The report of the Quality Standards Subcommittee of the AAN suggests the following guideline for the use of neuroimaging in the evaluation of migraine:

> In adult patients with recurrent headaches defined as migraine, including those with visual aura, with no recent change in headache pattern, no history of seizures, and no other focal neurologic signs or symptoms, the routine use of neuroimaging is not warranted. In patients with atypical headache patterns, a history of seizures, or focal neurologic signs or symptoms, CT or MRI may be indicated.[5]

## CLUSTER HEADACHES

Cluster headaches usually can be diagnosed without the need for neuroimaging studies by using the IHS diagnostic features: at least five attacks of severe unilateral orbital, supraorbital, or temporal pain lasting 156 to 180 minutes untreated and associated with at least one of the following signs, which must be present on the pain side: conjunctival injection, lacrimation, nasal congestion, rhinorrhea, forehead and facial sweating, miosis, ptosis, and eyelid edema. The frequency of attacks is from one every other day to eight per day.[72]

Frishberg[60] reviewed 21 reports of patients with cluster-like headaches from 1975 to 1996. Of these, seven met IHS criteria for cluster headaches and were found to have two AVMs, sinusitis, an impacted wisdom tooth, a midline calcified inoperable mass, a left cerebellopontine angle epidermoid, and an intracavernous carotid pseudoaneurysm. Since then, three additional causes of secondary cluster headache meeting IHS criteria have been reported: middle cerebral artery–dependent AVMs,[132] temporal arteritis presenting as cluster headache,[88a] and a clusterlike headache in a patient with multiple cerebral metastases of pulmonary origin.[182]

Based on these reports, Frishberg[60] recommends neuroimaging, preferably MRI, for patients with the following:

1. A pattern of clusterlike headache that does not conform to the IHS criteria
2. Onset of cluster headaches after age 40
3. A pattern of cluster headaches that is progressive in nature
4. Chronic cluster headache
5. Any focal neurologic deficit other than Horner's syndrome

## TRIGEMINAL NEURALGIA

According to the IHS diagnostic criteria, trigeminal neuralgia is defined by paroxysmal attacks of facial or frontal pain that last a few seconds to less than 2 minutes. The pain has at least four of the following characteristics: distribution along one or more divisions of the trigeminal nerve; sudden, intense, sharp, superficial, stabbing, or burning quality; severe pain intensity; precipitation from trigger areas or by certain daily activities such as eating, talking, washing the face, or cleaning the teeth; and between paroxysms the patient is entirely asymptomatic. In addition, there is no neurologic deficit, attacks are stereotyped in the individual patient, and exclusion of other causes of facial pain is done by history, physical examination, and special investigations.[72] The pain is usually unilateral (involving the second, third, or, occasionally, first division of the trigeminal nerve) but can be bilateral (4%). A sustained, deep, dull ache may be present between paroxysms of pain.

In patients with trigeminal neuralgia and decreased facial sensation, considerations include intracranial aneurysms, temporal arteritis, intracranial tumors, dental mandibular malignancy, and cranial malignancy. In those with normal facial sensation, possible causes include idiopathic trigeminal neuralgia (often with vascular compression), multiple sclerosis (especially in the presentation of younger patients), dental pathology, and dental procedures.[168]

The vast majority of patients with trigeminal neuralgia have an idiopathic type. Of these, perhaps 80% can be found to have vascular compression of the trigeminal nerve at the root entry zone, most commonly by a branch of the superior cerebellar artery. Frequently, the vascular compression can be seen on MRI scan with MR angiography.[188] Fast inflow with steady-state precession (FISP) and contrast material–enhanced magnetization-prepared rapid acquisition gradient echo (MP-RAGE) MRI are useful in demonstrating the vascular contact.[112] A variety of tumors, such as trigeminal schwannomas, meningiomas, lymphomas, lipomas, epidermoid tumors, acoustic schwannomas, metastases, and tumors of the skull base, occasionally can cause trigeminal neuralgia.[113] CT scans are also useful but less sensitive than MRI.

The yield of neuroimaging in older patients with typical trigeminal neuralgia is low. One series of 206 patients with trigeminal neuralgia found 4% with multiple sclerosis and 5% with tumors. However, most of the abnormalities were found in patients with atypical features, less than 40 years of age, and with pain in more than one trigeminal division.[211]

## ACUTE SEVERE NEW-ONSET HEADACHES ("FIRST OR WORST")

### DIFFERENTIAL DIAGNOSIS

Perhaps 1% of patients presenting to the emergency department have headache of acute onset as their chief complaint.[57] The differential diagnosis of the acute severe new-

**TABLE 1–7. Differential Diagnosis of Acute Severe New-Onset Headache ("First or Worst")**

Crash migraine[54]
Cluster headache
Miscellaneous
    Benign exertional headache
    Benign orgasmic cephalgia
Posttraumatic headache
Associated with vascular disorders
    Acute ischemic cerebrovascular disease
    Subdural and epidural hematomas
    Parenchymal hemorrhage
    Unruptured saccular aneurysm
    Subarachnoid hemorrhage
    Systemic lupus erythematosus
    Temporal arteritis
    Internal carotid and vertebral artery dissection[129]
    Cerebral venous thrombosis
    Acute hypertension
        Pressor response
        Pheochromocytoma
        Preeclampsia
Associated with nonvascular intracranial disorders
    Intermittent hydrocephalus
    Benign intracranial hypertension
    Post–lumbar puncture[50]
    Related to intrathecal injections
    Intracranial neoplasm
    Pituitary apoplexy[47,49]
Acute intoxications
Associated with noncephalic infection
    Acute febrile illness
    Acute pyelonephritis
Associated with cephalic infection
    Meningoencephalitis
    Acute sinusitis
Acute mountain sickness
Disorders of eyes
    Acute optic neuritis
    Acute glaucoma
Cervicogenic
    Greater occipital neuralgia[142]
    Cervical myositis
Trigeminal neuralgia

onset headache ("first or worst") is extensive (Table 1–7).[30,167] A prospective study of 148 patients with acute severe headaches seen by general practitioners in the Netherlands found subarachnoid hemorrhage (SAH) to be the cause in 25%.[107]

There are numerous causes of SAH (Table 1–8). About 80% of SAH are due to ruptured intracranial aneurysms[205]; 5% are due to rupture of intracranial AVMs. In about 15% of cases an arteriogram does not reveal the cause of the bleeding. In about 50% of these arteriogram-negative cases the CT scan demonstrates blood confined to the cisterns around the midbrain, perimesencephalic hemorrhage, which may be caused by a ruptured prepontine or interpeduncular cistern dilated vein or venous malformation. Other causes of SAH with a negative arteriogram include occult aneurysm, vertebral or carotid artery dissection, dural AVM, spinal AVM, mycotic aneurysm, pituitary hemorrhage, sickle cell anemia, coagulation disorders, drug abuse (methamphetamine and cocaine use), primary or metastatic intracranial or cervical tumors, infections (e.g., herpes encephalitis), and vasculitis.[94a]

More than 30,000 people per year in the United States have an SAH from a ruptured saccular aneurysm, resulting in more than 18,000 deaths.[148] Estimates of the prevalence of intracranial saccular aneurysms in the general population range from 0.5% to 1%[117] to 1% to 2%[119] to 5%.[76] Based on metaanalysis, the prevalence is about 2%, with 93% of aneurysms ≤10 mm.[152] Perhaps 50% of patients with SAHs will present with Hunt and Hess grade I (no symptoms or minimal headache, slight nuchal rigidity) or II (moderate to severe headache, no neurologic deficit other than cranial nerve palsy). In patients with acute severe headache of new onset, especially with a normal neurologic examination, when and how you should exclude aneurysmal SAH is an important issue.

### HEADACHES FROM SUBARACHNOID HEMORRHAGE

The classic headache following SAH is acute, severe, continuous, and generalized and is often associated with nausea, vomiting, meningismus, focal neurologic symptoms, and loss of consciousness.[201] In a series of 192 patients with SAH, 10% described no headache at the onset and 8% described a mild, gradually increasing headache.[198] The various sites of the headache at onset were as follows: occipital, 32%; frontal, 17%; back of neck, 11%; generalized, 10%; temporal, 6%; and other, 21%. In patients with mild or no headache at the onset, complaints of neck and back pain due to meningeal irritation may lead to misdiagnosis. A supple neck does not exclude SAH; on examination, a stiff neck is absent in 36% of patients.[93]

### SENTINEL HEADACHES

A sentinel headache[9] (a retrospective diagnosis), due to a small SAH or warning leak,[63,64] has been reported as occurring in 15% to 59% of patients before a major rupture of a saccular aneurysm.[11,70] Many of these patients do not seek medical attention or are given an incorrect diagnosis, such as migraine or sinusitis.[92] Proper diagnosis can be lifesaving since major SAH has a morbidity and mortality of 50% to 70% and occurs in 30% to 50% of patients in the days or weeks after the sentinel headache.[11,103,205] Sentinel headaches occasionally may be fleeting but usually persist for several hours or days.[138,205]

In the Danish Aneurysm Study the time interval between the warning leak and the major aneurysmal rupture

**TABLE 1–8. Causes of Nontraumatic Subarachnoid Hemorrhage**

80%  Intracranial saccular aneurysm
  5%  Intracranial arteriovenous malformation
15%  Negative arteriogram
     50%  Benign perimesencephalic hemorrhage
     50%  Other causes
          Occult aneurysm
          Mycotic aneurysm
          Vertebral or carotid artery dissection
          Dural arteriovenous malformation
          Spinal arteriovenous malformation
          Sickle cell anemia
          Coagulation disorders
          Drug abuse (especially cocaine)
          Primary or metastatic intracranial tumors
          Primary or metastatic cervical tumors
          CNS infection
          CNS vasculitides

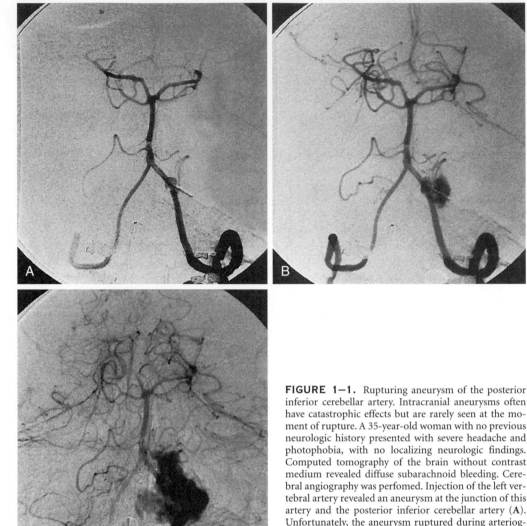

**FIGURE 1–1.** Rupturing aneurysm of the posterior inferior cerebellar artery. Intracranial aneurysms often have catastrophic effects but are rarely seen at the moment of rupture. A 35-year-old woman with no previous neurologic history presented with severe headache and photophobia, with no localizing neurologic findings. Computed tomography of the brain without contrast medium revealed diffuse subarachnoid bleeding. Cerebral angiography was perfomed. Injection of the left vertebral artery revealed an aneurysm at the junction of this artery and the posterior inferior cerebellar artery (**A**). Unfortunately, the aneurysm ruptured during arteriography (**B** and **C**). The patient's condition deteriorated rapidly and could not be stabilized, and she died a few hours later. (From Stockinger Z. N Engl J Med 1998;339:1758. © 1998, Massachusetts Medical Society.)

was less than 1 week in 18.1% of patients (Fig. 1–1) and less than 1 month in 61.4%.[70] Ninety-nine patients (59.6%) with sentinel headaches were evaluated by a physician (including 31 examined by a neurologist and 15 by a neurosurgeon) but misdiagnosed. At 2-year follow-up, 30 patients had a normal mental outcome and 43 patients were dead. With proper early diagnosis, there could have been 66 patients with a normal mental outcome and 25 dead. Headache was present in 83.7% of the patients, with sudden headache the only complaint in 28%. In 56.6% of the patients the headache was followed by nuchal rigidity and pain and/or nausea and vomiting and/or transient loss of consciousness. (Beware of new-onset "migraine" with syncope.) In an Italian series of 73 patients with misdiagnosed warning leaks, sudden, severe and unusual headache was the only symptom in 32.4% and was associated with nausea or vomiting in 28.4%.[11] (Beware of new-onset "migraine" without syncope.)

In a retrospective Canadian report of 34 patients with headaches caused by a "premonitory minor leak," the onset of the headache was sudden, usually unremitting, and persisted until a major aneurysmal rupture occurred or up to 2 weeks.[103] In 17 patients with a posterior communicating artery or internal carotid artery aneurysm, 53% described an ipsilateral periorbital, hemicranial, or hemifacial headache and 18% described a diffuse headache. Anterior communicating aneurysms in 10 patients were associated with an ipsilateral headache in 33%, frontal and bifrontal headache in 40%, bioccipital headache in 40%, bitemporal headache in 10%, and diffuse headache in 10%. Transient nausea, vomiting, and neck pain were reported in 60%. (Beware of new-onset hemicranial "migraine.") Therefore, in patients presenting with sudden onset of the worst headache of their life, it is not possible to distinguish between SAH and benign types of headache without appropriate diagnostic testing.[69]

In a Dutch study of 13 patients with a sentinel headache, the onset was within 1 second in 10 patients and within a few minutes in the other 3 patients.[196] Three of the patients had the onset during sexual intercourse. The duration of the headache was usually several hours to a few days. In most patients the headache was unilateral or occipital, with radiation to the neck in half of those affected. There was no association between the location of the headache at onset and the site of the aneurysm. Only half of the patients visited a physician because of the sentinel headache. Explanations offered by family physicians for the headaches included exertion, influenza, and hypertension.

## CT AND MRI SCANS AND ANEURYSMAL SUBARACHNOID HEMORRHAGE

A CT scan without contrast is the neuroimaging study of choice in the detection of acute SAH with a high initial sensitivity (Table 1–9). In a cooperative series of 3521 patients, findings on the first CT scan after rupture of a saccular aneurysm were as follows: normal, 8.3%; decreased density, 1.1%; mass effect, 6.1%; aneurysm, 5%; hydrocephalus, 15.2%; intraventricular hematoma, 16.7%; intracerebral hematoma, 17.4%; subdural hematoma, 1.3%; and SAH, 85.2%.[93] CT scanning detected aneurysmal SAH in 92% of patients on day 0, decreasing to 58% on day 5. The percentage of scans that were normal on day 0 was 3.3%; on day 1, 7.2%; and on day 5, 27.3%.

Van der Wee et al[190] performed a prospective series of 175 consecutive patients with sudden headache and a normal neurologic examination. CT scans performed within the first 12 hours detected SAH in 117 patients for a detection rate of 98%. In the remaining 58 patients, lumbar puncture was performed 12 or more hours after the onset of the headache. Of the 58 patients, 2 were found to have xanthochromic CSF by spectrophotometric analysis. Both of these patients were found to have aneurysms.

Based on a prospective study of 100 patients, the probability of recognizing an aneurysmal hemorrhage on CT scan is 50% after 1 week, 30% after 2 weeks (mostly patients with hematomas), and almost nil after 3 weeks.[192] The increased attenuation values in the basal cisterns and fissures usually disappeared by day 5 to 9. Most hematomas resolved between days 14 and 22.

The pattern of hemorrhage in the absence of an intracerebral hematoma helps to suggest the location of the ruptured saccular aneurysm (Table 1–10).[83,199] SAH present only in the prepontine cistern or the interpeduncular fossa usually indicates a venous or capillary rupture,[153,213] although approximately 5% of the time a basilar artery aneurysm is responsible.[154]

In the acute stage, CT scan without contrast is preferred over MRI for the evaluation of possible SAH because of the wide availability of CT scans, lower expense, and faster scanning time. Ogawa et al[135] compared MRI at 0.5 tesla and CT scans in the detection of aneurysmal SAH. Acute SAH was detected as an area of high signal intensity relative to that of normal CSF and the surrounding brain

**TABLE 1–10. Aneurysm Sites Suggested by Location of Subarachnoid Hemorrhage**

| SITE OF ANEURYSM | PREDOMINANT LOCATION OF SAH |
| --- | --- |
| Anterior communicating artery | Interhemispheric fissure or septum pellucidum or both |
| Middle cerebral artery | Sylvian fissure cistern |
| Posterior communicating artery | Suprasellar cistern |
| Infratentorial arteries | Posterior fossa cistern |
| Unknown origin | Diffuse symmetric cisterns |

parenchyma on a moderately T2-weighted SE sequence. For the detection of SAH, MRI was almost equal to CT scan in the first 24 hours and was slightly superior in the acute stage (up to 72 hours). More than 3 to 14 days after the ictus, MRI was definitely superior to CT scan in the identification and delineation of SAH.

## LUMBAR PUNCTURE AND SAH

A lumbar puncture should be performed in all patients with a new-onset headache that suggests SAH but who have normal CT scans. Since lumbar puncture can result in clinical deterioration and death after SAH, a CT scan should be performed first, with the exception of certain cases in which acute meningitis is suspected.[44,191]

## CSF EXAMINATION

Red blood cells (RBCs) are present in the CSF in virtually all cases of SAH and clear in a variable period of time from about 6 to 30 days.[186] When the CSF obtained from the first lumbar puncture is bloody, the only certain way to distinguish SAH from a traumatic tap is the presence of a xanthochromic supernatant. Although a decrease in RBCs from the first to the third test tube can be seen after a traumatic tap,[55] a similar decrease can be seen after a previous bleed.[19] Conversely, after a traumatic tap, the number of RBCs may stay constant in all three tubes.[194] Since crenation occurs very soon after RBCs enter the CSF, the presence of crenated RBCs is not a reliable sign of SAH.[195]

When RBCs break down in the CSF, they release oxyhemoglobin, which is degraded by macrophages and other cells in the leptomeninges to bilirubin by the third to fourth day.[10] These two pigments are responsible for xanthochromia (literally "yellow color" but refers to a colored supernatant) after SAH. The CSF supernatant is pink or pink-orange due to oxyhemoglobin, yellow due to bilirubin, and an intermediate color if both are present. Methemoglobin, a reduction product of hemoglobin, is found in encapsulated subdural hematomas and in old loculated intracerebral hemorrhages.[55] Although oxyhemoglobin can be detected as early as 2 hours after entry of RBCs into the CSF, xanthochromia is not present in all cases until after 12 hours.[194,198] Therefore, to avoid confusing blood-stained CSF from a traumatic lumbar puncture with a SAH, the lumbar puncture might best be delayed until 12 hours after the ictus.[195]

Xanthochromia is best detected by spectrophotometry since the naked eye can detect xanthochromia only about half the time.[174,195] Absorption spectrophotometry, which is a measurement of the light intensity in different regions of the visible spectrum (400 to 700 nm) after its transmission through an absorbing medium, can detect oxyhemoglobin

**TABLE 1–9. Approximate Probability of Recognizing Aneurysmal Hemorrhage on CT Scan After Initial Event**

| TIME | PROBABILITY (%) |
| --- | --- |
| Day 0 | 95[1] |
| Day 3 | 74[1] |
| 1 wk | 50[192] |
| 2 wk | 30[192] |
| 3 wk | Almost 0[192] |

**TABLE 1–11. Probability of Detecting Xanthochromia With Spectrophotometry in Cerebrospinal Fluid at Various Times After Subarachnoid Hemorrhage**

| Time | Probability (%) |
|---|---|
| 12 h | 100[194,198] |
| 1 wk | 100[194] |
| 2 wk | 100[194] |
| 3 wk | >70[194] |
| 4 wk | >40[194] |

and bilirubin by their characteristic maximum absorption bands of 415 and 455 nm, respectively.[195,201]

The probability of detecting xanthochromia by spectrophotometry at various times after SAH is shown in Table 1–11.[194] Other causes of xanthochromia include the following: jaundice, usually with a total plasma bilirubin of 10 to 15 mg/dl; CSF protein >150 mg/dl; dietary hypercarotenemia; malignant melanomatosis; oral intake of rifampin[55]; and traumatic lumbar punctures. A recent article raises the possibility of false-positives for SAH. False-positives for SAH can occur from traumatic taps with even a small number of RBCs because oxyhemoglobin can form in vivo.[12,131a] Only bilirubin and methemoglobin can be formed in vitro.

### Cerebral Arteriography, Magnetic Resonance Angiography, and Spiral CT Angiography

After SAH a four-vessel cerebral arteriogram should be performed since about 20% of patients have multiple aneurysms. Although saccular aneurysms are usually detected on the initial arteriogram, false-negatives can occur in 6%[189] to 16%,[85] with an anterior communicating artery aneurysm often missed. Potential reasons for false-negatives include vasospasm, thrombosis of the aneurysm, observer error, and technical factors such as inadequate oblique views.[85,207] A repeat arteriogram should be done after 2 weeks in the following circumstances: findings of vasospasm; an incomplete or inadequate study; an aneurysmal pattern of blood on the initial CT scan[153]; and when a CT scan performed within 4 days after the SAH shows thin or thick subarachnoid blood, particularly with a great deal of blood in the basal frontal interhemispheric fissure.[85] Occasionally, a third arteriogram may be necessary to demonstrate an aneurysm.[122]

Neurologic complications occasionally occur as a result of cerebral arteriography. A prospective study of 1000 consecutive cerebral arteriograms from the Barrow Neurological Institute reported a 1% overall incidence of neurologic deficit and a 0.5% incidence of persistent deficit. All the complications occurred in patients being evaluated for a history of stroke, transient ischemic event, or carotid bruit; the average patient age was 73 years.[73] Although there were no complications associated with vasospasm in the 137 studies performed for SAH, they can certainly occur. A higher incidence of complications may occur with a low volume of studies or when the studies are performed by inexperienced physicians.[61]

Although MR angiography has not yet supplanted cerebral arteriography, the study is useful in some cases (such as thunderclap headaches with normal CT scan and CSF examinations or when a patient declines undergoing arteriography) as a screening procedure.[109] Huston et al[81] compared

aneurysms detected on cerebral arteriograms with time-of-flight and phase-contrast MR angiography and conventional MRI. The sensitivities of the sequences for detecting aneurysms ≥5 mm were as follows: T1-weighted, 37.5%; T2-weighted, 62.5%; phase-contrast, 75%; and time-of-flight, 87.5%. Retrospectively, aneurysms ≥3 mm could be identified. In another MR angiography study of 51 patients with recent SAH, false-positives were reported in 2% and false-negatives in 5.9%.[163]

Recently, spiral (helical) CT angiography has been used to detect intracranial aneurysms. Strayle-Batra et al[180] recently reported a series of 20 aneurysms found in 16 patients. With an examination time of 5 to 7 minutes, the sensitivity of spiral CT angiography as compared to digital subtraction angiography was 85%, with detection of aneurysms ranging from 3 to 20 mm (mean, 8.9 mm). There were no false-positives. The posterior communicating artery was difficult to assess because of its close relationship to bony structures. Spiral CT offers an important addition and an alternative for patients with contraindications to MR angiography, including pacemakers and claustrophobia.

### Thunderclap Headaches

In 1986 Day and Raskin[33] described a 42-year-old woman with three episodes of intense headache of sudden onset. Although the CT scan was normal and lumbar puncture revealed bloodless clear CSF, an arteriogram demonstrated an unruptured right internal carotid artery saccular aneurysm. These authors postulated that hemorrhage into the wall of the aneurysm could be the cause of her "thunderclap headaches." After spending 4 hours reviewing dictionary definitions to find the best adjective, Day and Raskin coined the term *thunderclap headache* to describe an intense acute headache with peak intensity at onset (N. Raskin, personal communication, 1995). This study raised the disturbing prospect that a normal CT scan and CSF examination were not enough to totally exclude an aneurysmal cause of thunderclap headache. Since then, a commonly used definition of thunderclap headache is the sudden onset of a severe headache that reaches maximum intensity within 1 minute without evidence of SAH.[168] Table 1–12 lists the causes of thunderclap headache.

Wijdicks et al[204] performed a long-term follow-up study (average, 3.3 years) of 71 patients who presented with a thunderclap headache and were found to have normal CT scan and CSF examinations. In this group, 17% had identical recurrences without evidence of SAH, and 44% devel-

**TABLE 1–12. Causes of Thunderclap Headache**

**Primary Causes**
Migraine
Benign thunderclap headache
Benign orgasmic headache

**Secondary Causes**
Unruptured intracranial saccular aneurysm
Cerebral vasospasm
Cerebral venous thrombosis
Carotid artery or vertebral artery dissection
Pituitary apoplexy
Occipital neuralgia
Erve virus

oped regular episodes of tension or migraine headaches after the thunderclap headache. The authors suggested that the finding of an unruptured aneurysm, as described by Day and Raskin, was merely incidental and did not justify performing cerebral arteriograms in patients with a thunderclap headache who have a normal CT scan and CSF examination. If cerebral vasospasm is seen, this effect could be attributed to migraine.[203]

Based on two patients with thunderclap headaches with normal neurologic and CT scan examination who were found to have unruptured saccular aneurysms, Hughes[77] suggests that aneurysmal expansion could be responsible for the headache. Based on a retrospective series of 111 patients with unruptured aneurysms, Raps et al[149] postulate that aneurysmal mechanisms of thunderclap headache include aneurysmal expansion, thrombosis, and intramural hemorrhage.

Slivka and Philbrook[172] described four patients with thunderclap headaches without evidence of SAH who were found to have diffuse segmental cerebral vasoconstriction on cerebral arteriography. They suggest that thunderclap headache is a distinct headache category that may present with neurologic signs or symptoms and that may be associated with SAH and unruptured cerebral aneurysm. The significance of the cerebral vasospasm in patients without aneurysms or SAH described in these various studies is still not certain. Migraine and vasculitis are possibilities.

Linn et al[107a] described 37 patients (13 female) with a mean age of 36 years with benign thunderclap headache and negative diagnostic testing. However, they did not limit their definition to maximum intensity within 1 minute. The onset was almost instantaneous in 68% and took 20 to 60 seconds in 5%, 1 to 5 minutes in 19%, and more than 5 minutes in 3%. Benign thunderclap headaches had the following features: exertion or Valsalva-like maneuver at onset, 22%; feeling of a "burst," 14%; nausea, 76%; vomiting, 43%; transient loss or clouding of consciousness, 16%; and transient focal symptoms, 22%. By comparison, a group of 42 patients with aneurysmal SAH reported the onset of headache as follows: almost instantaneous, 50%; 2 to 60 seconds, 24%; and 1 to 5 minutes, 19%. With the exception of seizures (7%) and double vision there were no other features that distinguished aneurysmal SAH headaches from those in the benign thunderclap headache group. Additionally, the characteristics of 23 patients with perimesencephalic hemorrhage were rather similar to those with benign thunderclap headache.

Cerebral venous sinus thrombosis and carotid and vertebral artery dissections can also cause thunderclap headaches. De Bruijn et al[36] reported on 10 patients who presented with thunderclap headache due to cerebral venous sinus thrombosis. The CT scan of the brain was abnormal in five patients. Evidence of SAH was seen in two of the six lumbar punctures performed, and the opening pressure was elevated in one. Thunderclap headaches can also occur in 14% of internal carotid artery and 22% of vertebral artery dissections.[129] For internal carotid artery dissections, the pain in the head, face, or neck is typically ipsilateral to the dissection and usually a constant (aching, pressing, or sharp in quality) rather than a pulsating pain. The pain associated with vertebral artery dissections is typically distributed over the posterior head and neck, can be unilateral or bilateral, and is constant slightly more often than pulsating.[169] Thun-

derclap headache can also be due to pituitary apoplexy (a hemorrhagic pituitary tumor),[41] greater occipital neuralgia,[142] and possibly Erve virus.[187]

The current evidence suggests that only a small percentage of patients with thunderclap headache and a normal neurologic examination, CT scan, and CSF examination will have a secondary cause. In these cases the clinician may wish to consider obtaining an MR angiogram and perhaps a venogram or spiral CT angiogram as a noninvasive alternative to a cerebral arteriogram.[148,149,172]

## COUGH, EXERTIONAL, AND SEXUAL HEADACHES

Headaches can be triggered by coughing, exertion, and sexual activity,[150] and these types have been defined by the IHS.[72] Benign cough headache is a bilateral headache of sudden onset, lasting less than 1 minute, and precipitated by coughing. It may be prevented by avoiding coughing and may be diagnosed only after structural lesions such as posterior fossa tumor have been excluded by neuroimaging. The term *cough headache* also includes headache precipitated by sneezing, weightlifting, bending, stooping, or straining with a bowel movement.

Benign exertional headache is specifically brought on by physical exercise and lasts from 5 minutes to 24 hours. It is bilateral, throbbing in nature at onset, and may develop migrainous features in patients susceptible to migraine. This type of headache is prevented by avoiding excessive exertion, particularly in hot weather or at high altitude, and is not associated with any systemic or intracranial disorder.

There are three types of headache precipitated by sexual excitement (masturbation or coitus). They are all bilateral at onset, can be prevented or eased by ceasing sexual activity before orgasm, and are not associated with any intracranial disorder such as aneurysm. The dull type is characterized by a dull ache in the head and neck that intensifies as sexual excitement increases. The explosive type is a sudden severe headache that occurs at orgasm. The postural type resembles the effect of low CSF pressure developing after coitus. In one study, 40% of patients with the explosive type also had exertional headache.[169]

In 1991, Sands et al[162] reviewed 219 previously reported cases of cough and exertional headaches, most from before the CT-scan era. From the two combined headache types, 78% were benign. The following were found in the 22% with structural lesions: posterior fossa space–occupying lesions, 37.5%; after trauma or after craniotomy, 27%; supratentorial space–occupying lesions, 18.7%; basilar impression/platybasia, 12.5%; and syrinx, 4.2%.

In 1996, Pascual et al[141] reported on 72 benign and symptomatic cases of cough, exertional, and sexual headaches that they had evaluated over a 15-year period. Their findings are summarized in Table 1–13. The sexual headache reported is the explosive type. The one patient with a SAH had only a single headache; those with the benign type had multiple sexual headaches. Pascual and colleagues state that neuroradiologic studies can be avoided in cases with clinically typical benign sexual or exertional headaches (men around the third decade of life; with short-duration, multiple episodes of pulsating pain; response to ergotamine or to preventive beta-blockers); the remaining patients must have brain CT scan and CSF examination if the CT scan is normal. They recommend MRI in all patients with cough headache and mandate the scan when there is no response to indomethacin, in those with posterior fossa signs, or in those younger than age 50.

## LOW CEREBROSPINAL FLUID PRESSURE HEADACHE

Low CSF pressure headaches are most often due to the following: lumbar puncture (most common cause), spontaneous, and CSF shunt overdrainage. Infrequent causes include trauma, postoperative effect (following craniotomy or spinal surgery), and association with other medical conditions (severe dehydration, diabetic coma, uremia, hyperpnea, meningoencephalitis, and severe systemic infection).[102]

A repeat lumbar puncture usually demonstrates an opening pressure from 0 to 70 cm $H_2O$, although the pressure can be in the normal range, especially if the procedure is performed after a period of bedrest.[102] The CSF analysis may be normal, or it can demonstrate a moderate, primarily lymphocytic pleocytosis; the presence of RBCs; and elevated protein level, which can exceed 500 mg/dl.[130]

An MRI scan of the brain may reveal diffuse meningeal enhancement with gadolinium and, in some cases, subdural fluid collections, which return to normal with resolution of the headache.[16,130] The diffuse meningeal enhancement on MRI may be explained by dural vasodilation and a greater concentration of gadolinium in the dural microvasculature and the interstitial fluid of the dura.[56] (Before the characteristic picture of the postural headache and diffuse meningeal enhancement on MRI was recognized, some patients underwent extensive testing, including meningeal biopsy, to exclude other conditions such as meningeal carcinomatosis and neurosarcoidosis.) The pleocytosis and elevated protein level in the CSF and the subdural fluid collections are probably due to decreased CSF volume and hydrostatic pressure changes, resulting in meningeal vasodilation and vascular leak.[130] Lumbar MRI may also be abnormal following lumbar puncture. In one study of 11 patients, all had evidence of CSF leakage, ranging from 1 to 460 ml.[84]

## HEADACHES AFTER MILD HEAD INJURY

Headaches have been estimated to occur in about 30% to 90% of patients who are symptomatic after mild head injury.[38,126] Headaches may occur more often and with longer duration in patients who undergo mild head injury as compared to more severe degrees of trauma.[161,210]

A variety of primary and secondary headache types can occur after mild head injury (Table 1–14).[48,139] Muscle contraction headaches, often associated with greater occipital neuralgia, account for perhaps 85% of all posttraumatic headaches.[48,114] Such headaches may be due to cranial myofascial injury. Cervicogenic causes include cervical myofascial injury, cervical intervertebral disk disease, cervical spondylosis, and injury to the C2-3 facet joint (third occipital headache).[111] Mild head injury can trigger acute migraine episodes, known as "footballer's migraine."[116] Recurring attacks of migraine with and without aura can develop after mild head injury with or without loss of consciousness.[202] Supraorbital and infraorbital neuralgia, dysesthesias over scalp lacerations, and pain due to local trauma may cause other headaches. Rare types of posttraumatic headaches include cluster headache, dysautonomic cephalgia, new-onset orgasmic cephalgia, and headaches resulting from carotid and vertebral artery dissections.[48]

### HEADACHES AND SUBDURAL AND EPIDURAL HEMATOMAS

Headache frequently occurs in patients with posttraumatic subdural hematomas.[65] In McKissock's series from 1960,[120] headache occurred in 11% of patients with acute hematoma, 53% with subacute hematoma, and 81% with chronic subdural hematoma. Since many of the patients with acute subdural hematoma had alteration of consciousness, headache may have been underreported. The headaches due to subdural hematomas are nonspecific and range from mild to severe and paroxysmal to constant.[65] Patients with unilateral headaches usually have the subdural hematoma on the same side.[120] One rare type of headache caused by a subdural hematoma is roller-coaster headache.[15,52] The acceleration-deceleration forces of riding on a roller coaster without experiencing direct head trauma can tear the bridging veins and lead to a subdural hematoma.

---

**TABLE 1–13. Cough, Exertional, and Sexual Headache**

| PARAMETER | COUGH HEADACHE | | EXERTIONAL HEADACHE | | SEXUAL HEADACHE | |
|---|---|---|---|---|---|---|
| | BENIGN | SYMPTOMATIC | BENIGN | SYMPTOMATIC | BENIGN | SYMPTOMATIC |
| Patients (N) | 13 | 17 | 16 | 12 | 13 | 1 |
| Age, range (y) | 67 ± 11, 44–81 | 39 ± 14, 15–63 | 24 ± 11, 10–48 | 42 ± 14, 18–61 | 41 ± 9, 24–57 | 60 |
| Sex (% men) | 77 | 59 | 88 | 43 | 85 | 100 |
| Duration | Seconds to 30 min | Seconds to days | Minutes to 2 d | 1 d to 1 mo | 1 min to 3 h | 10 d |
| Bilateral localization | 92% | 94% | 56% | 100% | 77% | Yes |
| Quality | Sharp, stabbing | Bursting, stabbing | Pulsating | Explosive, pulsating | Explosive + pulsating | Explosive + pulsating |
| Other manifestations | No | Posterior fossa signs | Nausea, photophobia | Nausea, vomiting, double vision, neck rigidity | None | Vomiting, neck rigidity |
| Diagnosis | Idiopathic | Chiari type I malformation | Idiopathic | Subarachnoid hemorrhage, sinusitis, brain metastases | Idiopathic | Subarachnoid hemorrhage |

Modified from Pascual J, Iglesias F, Oterino A, et al. Cough, exertional, and sexual headaches: an analysis of 72 benign and symptomatic cases. *Neurology.* 1996;46:1520-1524.

**TABLE 1–14. Types and Causes of Headaches After Mild Head Injury**

Muscle contraction or tension type
    Cranial myofascial injury
    Secondary to neck injury (cervicogenic)
        Myofascial injury
        Intervertebral disks
        Cervical spondylosis
        C2-3 facet joint (third occipital headache)
    Secondary to temporomandibular joint injury
Migraine
    Without and with aura
    Footballer's migraine
Greater and lesser occipital neuralgia
Mixed type
Cluster type
Supraorbital and infraorbital neuralgia
Due to scalp lacerations or local trauma
Dysautonomic cephalgia
Orgasmic cephalgia
Carotid or vertebral artery dissection
Subdural or epidural hematomas
Hemorrhagic cortical contusions

The classic picture of an acute epidural hematoma is a patient who sustains what may be a minor head injury without loss of consciousness followed by a lucid interval and then deterioration into coma, usually within 12 hours of the injury.[110] However, from 4% to 30% of all epidural hematomas are of the chronic type.[125] The patient is often a child or a young adult who sustains what appears to be a trivial head injury often without loss of consciousness.[13] A persistent headache then develops and is often associated with nausea, vomiting, and memory impairment consistent with a postconcussion syndrome. After the passage of days to weeks, focal findings develop and the correct diagnosis is finally made.

For adults affected by mild head injury and having an initial Glasgow Coma Scale score of 13 to 15, three studies in the United States have reported the incidence of subdural hematomas as 0.5%,[29] 0.8%,[179] and 1%,[88] respectively, and epidural hematomas as 0.2%,[29] 0.3%,[88] and 1%.[179] The incidence of neurosurgical complications after mild head injury has been estimated to be between 1% and 3%.[28,29]

### NEUROIMAGING FOR PATIENTS WITH HEADACHE AFTER MILD HEAD INJURY

#### Skull Radiographs

Skull radiographs are frequently obtained after mild head injury.[87] However, in settings where neurosurgeons and CT scanners are available, routine skull radiographs are probably not justified.[53,158]

#### CT Scans

The indications for CT scanning for patients with headache and an initial Glasgow Coma Scale score of 15 after mild head injury are not certain. On the conservative side, Feuerman et al,[53] based on a retrospective review of 236 adults (68% with loss of consciousness), recommended that patients with a Glasgow Coma Scale score of 15, normal mental status, and no hemispheric neurologic deficit be discharged for observation without a CT scan.

However, two other studies suggest more liberal indications for obtaining a CT scan. Stein and Ross[179] reported a

13% risk of an abnormal CT scan in 1117 patients with a Glasgow Coma Scale score of 15 and no focal neurologic deficits. The number of these patients who required neurosurgical intervention was not reported. Stein and Ross recommended a routine CT scan in all head injury patients who have lost consciousness or are amnesic, even if all other physical findings are normal. Jeret et al,[88] in a prospective study of 712 adults with a Glasgow Coma Scale score of 15, found significant CT scan abnormalities in 9.4% of the patients, including two with epidural hematomas, nine with subdural hematomas, and seven with intracerebral hematomas. Only two patients (0.3%) required neurosurgical intervention, and one died. Risk factors for an abnormal CT scan included older age, white race, signs of basilar skull fracture, and being either a pedestrian hit by a motor vehicle or a victim of an assault.

#### MRI Scans

MRI is more sensitive than CT scanning in evaluation of head injury, including findings of brain contusions and abnormalities compatible with diffuse axonal injury.[75,128,212] Occasionally, MRI will detect isodense subdural[32,34] and vertex epidural hematomas[144] that may not be evident on CT scan. MRI with the fluid-attenuated inversion recovery (FLAIR) sequence nullifies or greatly reduces signal from the CSF, resulting in heavy T2-weighting without high signal and potential CSF artifacts. Since most traumatic lesions, including those associated with diffuse axonal injury, cortical contusion, or brainstem injury, and epidural and subdural hematomas are close to CSF, FLAIR sensitivity is equal to or superior to that of conventional spin-echo sequences.[7]

Delayed subdural and epidural hematomas can develop even after an initially normal CT or MRI scan.[125] The clinician needs to be vigilant to recognize these rare complications.

### NEW-ONSET HEADACHES IN PATIENTS OLDER THAN 50

When new-onset headaches begin in patients older than 50, the physician should consider the various primary disorders as well as the multiplicity of secondary headaches (Table 1–15). Although new-onset tension-type headaches are

**TABLE 1–15. Common Causes of Headache Beginning in Late Life**

**Secondary Headache Disorders**
Mass lesions
Temporal arteritis
Medication-related headache
Trigeminal neuralgia
Postherpetic neuralgia
Systemic disease
Disease of cranium, neck, eyes, ears, and nose
Cerebrovascular disease
Parkinson's disease

**Primary Headache Disorders**
Migraine
Tension-type headache
Cluster headache
Hypnic headache

From Lipton RB, Pfeffer D, Newman LC, Solomon S. Headaches in the elderly. *J Pain Symptom Manage.* 1993;8:88. Copyright 1993 by the US Cancer Pain Relief Committee.

rather common, migraine and cluster-type headaches uncommonly begin after age 50. Hypnic headaches, as originally described, had an age at onset of 65 to 84 years, with presentation as diffuse, often throbbing headaches that awaken the patient from sleep at the same time every night and last from 15 to 60 minutes.[108] Recent reports expand the definition to include headaches that exclusively awaken the patient from sleep at a consistent time in those age 40 or older. The pain, which has a duration of 15 minutes to 6 hours, can be unilateral or bilateral and throbbing or nonthrobbing.[40,66,131] The headache may respond to lithium carbonate, caffeine,[40] and flunarizine.[131] The diagnosis is one of exclusion since secondary causes of nocturnal headaches include drug withdrawal, temporal arteritis, sleep apnea, oxygen desaturation, pheochromocytomas, primary and secondary neoplasms, communicating hydrocephalus, subdural hematomas, and vascular lesions.[66]

The common causes of secondary headache disorders beginning in later life include the following: mass lesions such as subdural hematomas and neoplasms; temporal arteritis; medication-related headaches, including those caused by specific medications and medication rebound (withdrawal headaches); trigeminal neuralgia; postherpetic neuralgia; systemic disease such as infections, acute hypertension, hypoxia or hypercarbia, and other metabolic abnormalities such as hypercalcemia or severe anemia; headaches associated with disorders of the cranium, neck, eyes, ears, and nose, including cervicogenic headache, glaucoma, otitis, sinusitis, and dental infections; cerebrovascular disease; and the one third of patients with Parkinson's disease who report headaches.[46,108]

Pascual and Berciano[140] performed a study of 193 patients age 65 and over who were seen by the neurology service in the past 15 years and had de novo headache as their initial and main symptom. The most frequent diagnoses were tension-type headaches (43%) and trigeminal neuralgia (19%). Only one patient met migraine criteria. Fifteen percent had a secondary headache disorder due to conditions such as stroke, temporal arteritis, or intracranial neoplasm. Although the incidence of patients with de novo headaches attending a general hospital decreased with age, the risk of headache due to serious conditions increased 10 times after age 65.

## TEMPORAL ARTERITIS

Temporal (giant cell) arteritis (TA) is a systemic panarteritis that selectively involves arterial walls with significant amounts of elastin.[151] Approximately 50% of patients with TA have polymyalgia rheumatica, and about 15% of patients with polymyalgia rheumatica have temporal arteritis. Both conditions occur almost exclusively in patients over the age of 50, with a mean age at onset of about 70.[78] The estimated prevalence in this age population is 0.13%.[91]

According to the American College of Rheumatology 1990 criteria,[78] the diagnosis of TA can be established by fulfilling three of the following five criteria:

1. Age at least 50 years
2. New onset of localized headache
3. Temporal artery tenderness or decreased pulse
4. Erythrocyte sedimentation rate of at least 50 mm/h
5. Positive histology

The presence of three or more of the five criteria is associated with a sensitivity of 93.5% and a specificity of 91.2%.

## NEUROLOGIC MANIFESTATIONS OF TEMPORAL ARTERITIS

Neurologic manifestations of TA are rather common.[123,151] In a series of 166 patients with biopsy-proven temporal arteritis, Caselli et al[22] found evidence of neurologic disease in 31% of the patients, including ophthalmologic findings, 20%; mononeuropathies and peripheral neuropathies, 14%; carotid distribution transient ischemic events or stroke, 7%; vertebrobasilar distribution transient ischemic events or stroke, 2%; otologic findings, 7%; tremor, 4%; psychiatric findings, 3%; tongue numbness, 2%; and transverse myelopathy, <1%.[22] Russell[156] reported that depression occurred in 35% of patients seen with TA and confusion in 11%. Occasionally, the extradural vertebral and internal carotid arteries may be involved.[183]

The spectrum of neuroophthalmologic manifestations caused by TA is broad.[123,151] Visual loss may occur because of anterior and posterior ischemic optic neuropathy; central and branch retinal artery occlusion; anterior segment ischemia; and prechiasmal, perichiasmal, and postchiasmal field defects. Ophthalmoparesis can be due to the following: oculomotor, abducens, and trochlear nerve palsies; orbital constriction resulting from orbital cellulitis and cavernous sinus thrombosis; and oculomotor synkinesis. Autonomic dysfunction may be caused by Horner's syndrome and parasympathetic pupillary light dysfunction/near-dissociation. Rarely, complex visual hallucinations occur after infarction of the tertiary visual association cortex.

### Headaches of Temporal Arteritis

Headaches are the most common symptom of TA, reported by 60% to 90% of patients.[133,151] The pain is most often described as throbbing, although many patients describe a sharp, dull, burning, or lancinating type of pain.[151,177] The pain, which may be intermittent or continuous, is more often severe than moderate or slight.[177] For some patients the pain may be worse at night when lying on a pillow, while combing the hair, or when washing the face.[151] Tenderness or decreased pulsation of the superficial temporal arteries on physical examination is present in about half of the patients with TA.[79]

The location of the headache is variable and, contrary to popular misconception, is not just over the temple. In a biopsy-proven series of 124 patients by Jonasson et al,[89] 65% presented with temporofrontal headache. Solomon and Cappa[177] described the headaches from a series of 24 patients with biopsy-proven TA. The following percentages of patients reported the distribution of pain in these categories: 25%, only the temple; 54%, the temple either exclusively or inclusively; 29%, not involving the temple at all; 8%, generalized; and 8%, no headache. When headaches were limited to or included the temple, the headaches were bilateral in 50% of the patients. Intermittent jaw claudication was reported by 38%. The pain may be one-sided in 2% or may affect the face and neck in 8%, according to various reported studies.[177]

In another series of 46 patients with biopsy-proven TA, Jundt and Mock[90] described 17% of patients whose initial presentation was occipital pain (unilateral in 38%). Two of the patients with unilateral pain exactly similar to greater occipital neuralgia had normal sedimentation rates but abnormal temporal artery biopsy results. Tenderness over the greater occipital nerve can be explained by inflammation of the occipital artery, which is adjacent to the greater occipital nerve in the suboccipital region. TA should be considered in patients older than 50 who present with new-onset "occipital neuralgia," even with a normal sedimentation rate, especially when they do not respond to the usual treatments, such as nerve block and administration of nonsteroidal anti-inflammatory medications.

**Diagnostic Testing**

The diagnosis of TA is based upon a large index of clinical suspicion that is usually, but not always, confirmed by laboratory testing. The three best tests are the Westergren erythrocyte sedimentation rate (ESR), the C-reactive protein (CRP), and temporal artery biopsy. Elevation of plasma viscosity has a sensitivity and specificity similar to that of the ESR.[136] Mild normochromic normocytic anemia, elevation of hepatic enzymes (especially alkaline phosphatase), and decreased alpha$_2$-globulin levels are fairly common. These findings, however, lack adequate sensitivity and specificity to help make the diagnosis.[91]

For elderly patients the ESR range of normal may vary from <20 mm/h to 40 mm/h.[97] Based on a study of 27,912 persons age 20 to 65 years, Miller et al[124] derived a formula that included 98% of healthy persons: age in years divided by 2 for men; age in years plus 10 divided by 2 for women. Elevation of the ESR is certainly not specific for TA since any infectious, inflammatory, or rheumatic disease can cause an increase. The level can also be affected by the length of time between the venipuncture and the laboratory testing.[71] TA with a normal ESR has been reported in 10% to 36% of patients.[25,90,208] Repeating the ESR may be helpful in some cases in which the initial ESR is normal and then rises.[68] When abnormal, the ESR averages 70 to 80 and may reach 120 or even 130 mm/h. When the ESR is elevated at the time of diagnosis of TA, it can be followed to help guide the dosage of corticosteroid medication.[79]

CRP is an acute-phase plasma protein from the liver. The CRP, like the ESR, is nonspecific because the level can be elevated with tissue necrosis, inflammatory and infectious diseases, rheumatic disease, surgical tissue injury, myocardial infarction, transplantation, and other conditions.

Since the CRP is not influenced by various hematologic factors or age, it is more sensitive than the ESR. Hayreh et al[71] found the CRP to be more sensitive (100%) than the ESR (92%) for detection of TA. The ESR and CRP combined gave the best specificity (97%). Similarly, Myklebust and Gran[133] reported that both the ESR and the CRP were increased in 93.4% of cases; the ESR was normal and the CRP was elevated in 1.6%; the CRP was normal and the ESR was increased in 3.7%; and a normal ESR and a normal CRP were found in 1.2% of the patients.

Recently, Schmidt et al[166] reported a prospective study of 30 patients with TA that involved the use of color duplex ultrasonography. In 73% of the patients, ultrasonography showed a dark halo around the lumen of the superficial temporal arteries, which may have been caused by edema of the artery wall. The dark halo disappeared after a mean of 16 days of treatment with corticosteroids. Eighty percent of the patients had stenoses or occlusions of temporal artery segments, and 93% had stenoses, occlusions, or a halo. Schmidt

and colleagues concluded: "In patients with typical clinical signs and a halo on ultrasonography, it may be possible to make a diagnosis of temporal arteritis and begin treatment without performing a temporal-artery biopsy."

The diagnosis is made with certainty when the temporal artery biopsy demonstrates necrotizing arteritis characterized by a predominance of mononuclear cell infiltrates or a granulomatous process with multinucleated giant cells.[78] The false-negative rate of temporal artery biopsies in various series ranges from 5% to 44%.[83,134]

Possible reasons for negative temporal artery biopsies include noncontinuous pathologic findings or skip lesions, choice of site and length of the biopsy, examination of an incomplete number of sections, involvement of other vascular territories, and initiation of corticosteroid therapy prior to the biopsy.[91,197] When the biopsy is negative, taking a biopsy of the contralateral temporal artery increases the positive yield by 5% to 15%.[79,145] Pathologic evidence of TA persists for at least 4 to 5 days after the start of corticosteroid treatment.[79] Allison and Gallagher[4] found a decrease in the positive rate from 60% to 20% in patients treated for more than 1 week. Chmelewski et al[23] noted a positive yield of 37% when biopsy was performed after 2 weeks.

Since temporal artery biopsy is a simple, low-risk procedure, a case can be made for obtaining a biopsy in every suspected case of TA. However, when three or four of the American College of Rheumatology criteria are met, a strong argument can be made for treatment without biopsy. The results of color duplex ultrasonography could also influence the decision. In cases in which the clinical presentation is somewhat suspicious or when there is a very high probability of corticosteroid side effects, a biopsy should be obtained.[134] In the occasional patient with a normal or only slightly elevated ESR and a negative biopsy, the same considerations may apply in a decision to biopsy the contralateral artery. In patients with questionable laboratory support for the diagnosis, the usually rapid clinical response to corticosteroid treatment, often within 72 hours,[39] can serve as an empirical measure.

## CONCLUSION

As the era of managed care of medicine evolves, payors may increasingly question the benefit of diagnostic testing for the evaluation of headaches. A careful and complete history and physical examination will enable the astute physician to make the proper diagnosis in most cases without testing. In some cases, however, the nonspecific nature of some headaches in patients with a normal physical examination demand diagnostic testing even though the yield may be low. It is hoped that the gatekeeper model and insurance company review will not prevent patients with troublesome headaches from obtaining appropriate diagnostic testing and neurologic consultation.

**REFERENCES**

1. Adams HP, Kassell NF, Torner JC, Sahs AL. CT and clinical correlations in recent aneurysmal subarachnoid hemorrhage: a preliminary report of the cooperative aneurysm study. *Neurology.* 1983;33:981-988.
2. Adelman JU. Headache and other craniofacial pains. In: Greenberg JO, ed. *Neuroimaging.* New York: McGraw-Hill; 1995: chap 4.
3. Akpek S, Arac M, Atilla S, Onal B, Yucel C, Isik S. Cost-effectiveness of computed tomography in the evaluation of patients with headache. *Headache.* 1995;35:228-230.

4. Allison MC, Gallagher PJ. Temporal artery biopsy and corticosteroid treatment. *Ann Rheum Dis.* 1984;43:416-417.
5. American Academy of Neurology. The utility of neuroimaging in the evaluation of headache in patients with normal neurologic examinations. *Neurology.* 1994;44:1353-1354.
6. American Academy of Neurology. Practice parameter: the electroencephalogram in the evaluation of headache. *Neurology.* 1995;45:1411-1413.
7. Ashikaga R, Araki Y, Ishida O. MRI of head injury using FLAIR. *Neuroradiology.* 1997;39:239-242.
8. Baker H. Cranial CT in the investigation of headache: cost-effectiveness for brain tumors. *J Neuroradiol.* 1983;10:112-116.
9. Ball MJ. Pathogenesis of the "sentinel headache" preceding berry aneurysm rupture. *Can Med Assoc J.* 1975;112:78-79.
10. Barrows LJ, Hunter FT, Banker BQ. The nature and clinical significance of pigments in the cerebrospinal fluid. *Brain.* 1955;78:59-80.
11. Bassi P, Bandera R, Loiero M, Tognoni G, Mangoni A. Warning signs in subarachnoid hemorrhage: a cooperative study. *Acta Neurol Scand.* 1991;84:277-281.
12. Beetham R, Fahie-Wilson MN, Park D. What is the role of spectrophotometry in the diagnosis of subarachnoid haemorrhage? *Ann Clin Biochem.* 1998;35:1-4.
13. Benoit BG, Russell NA, Richard MT, Hugenholtz H, Ventureyra ECG, Choo SH. Epidural hematoma: report of seven cases with delayed evolution of symptoms. *Can J Neurol Sci.* 1982;9:321-324.
14. Bille B. Migraine in school children. *Acta Paediatr.* 1962;51(suppl 136): 1-151.
15. Bo-Abbas Y, Bolton CF. Roller-coaster headache. *N Engl J Med.* 1995;332:1585.
16. Bourekas EC, Jonathan SL, Lanzieri CF. Postcontrast meningeal MR enhancement secondary to intracranial hypotension caused by lumbar puncture. *J Comput Assist Tomogr.* 1995;19:299.
17. Brown RD, Wiebers DO, Forbes G, et al. The natural history of unruptured intracranial arteriovenous malformations. *J Neurosurg.* 1988;68: 352-357.
18. Bruyn GW. Intracranial arteriovenous malformation and migraine. *Cephalalgia.* 1984;4:191-207.
19. Buruma OJS, Janson HLF, Den Bergh FAJTM, Bots GTHAM. Blood-stained cerebrospinal fluid: traumatic puncture or haemorrhage? *J Neurol Neurosurg Psychiatry.* 1981;44:144-147.
20. Cala L, Mastaglia F. Computerized axial tomography findings in a group of patients with migrainous headaches. *Proc Aust Acad Neurol.* 1976;13:35-41.
21. Carrera G, Gerson D, Schnur J, McNeil B. Computerized tomography of the brain in patients with headache or temporal lobe epilepsy: findings and cost-effectiveness. *J Comput Assist Tomogr.* 1977;1:200-203.
22. Caselli RJ, Hunder GG, Whisnant JP. Neurologic disease in biopsy-proven giant cell (temporal) arteritis. *Neurology.* 1988;38:352-359.
23. Chmelewski WL, McKnight KM, Agudelo CA, Wise CM. Presenting features and outcomes in patients undergoing temporal artery biopsy: a review of 98 patients. *Arch Intern Med.* 1992;152:1690-1695.
24. Chu ML, Shinnar S. Headaches in children younger than 7 years of age. *Arch Neurol.* 1992;49:79-82.
25. Cohen DN. Temporal arteritis: improvement in visual prognosis and management with repeat biopsies. *Trans Am Acad Opthalmol Otolaryngol.* 1973;77:74-85.
26. Cooney BS, Grossman RI, Farber RE, et al. Frequency of magnetic resonance imaging abnormalities in patients with migraine. *Headache.* 1996;36:616-621.
27. Cuetter A, Aita J. CT scanning in classic migraine [letter]. *Headache.* 1983;23:195.
28. Dacey RG. Complications after apparently mild head injury and strategies of neurosurgical management. In: Levin HS, Eisenberg HM, Benton AL, eds. *Mild Head Injury.* Oxford: Oxford University Press; 1989:83-101.
29. Dacey RG, Alves WM, Rimel RW, et al. Neurosurgical complications after apparently minor head injury. *J Neurosurg.* 1986;65:203-210.
30. Dalessio DJ. Diagnosing the severe headache. *Neurology.* 1994; 44(suppl 3):S6-S12.
31. Daras M, Koppel B, Leyfermann M, Samkoff L, Tuchman A. Anticardiolipin antibodies in migraine patients: an additional risk factor for stroke? *Neurology.* 1995;45(suppl 4):A367-A368.
32. Davenport RJ, Statham PFX, Warlow CP. Detection of bilateral isodense subdural haematomas. *BMJ.* 1994;309:792-794.
33. Day JW, Raskin NH. Thunderclap headache: symptom of unruptured cerebral aneurysm. *Lancet.* 1986;2:1247-1248.
34. D'Costa DF, Abbott RJ. Bilateral subdural haematomas and normal CT brain scans. *Br J Clin Pract.* 1990;44:666-667.
35. De Benedittis G, Lorenzetti A, Sina C, Bernasconi V. Magnetic resonance imaging in migraine and tension-type headache. *Headache.* 1995;35:264-268.
36. de Bruijn SFTM, Stam J, Kappelle LJ. Thunderclap headache as first symptom of cerebral venous sinus thrombosis. *Lancet.* 1996;348:1623-1625.
37. Demaerel P, Boelaert I, Wilms G, Baert AL. The role of cranial computed tomography in the diagnostic work-up of headache. *Headache.* 1996;36:347-348.
38. Denker PG. The postconcussion syndrome: prognosis and evaluation of the organic factors. *N Y State J Med.* 1944;44:379-384.
39. DiBartolomeo AG, Brick JE. Giant cell arteritis and polymyalgia rheumatica. *Postgrad Med.* 1992;91:107-112.
40. Dodick DW, Mosek AC, Campbell JK. The hypnic ("alarm clock") headache syndrome. *Cephalalgia.* 1998;18:152-156.
41. Dodick DW, Wijdicks EFM. Pituitary apoplexy presenting as a thunderclap headache. *Neurology.* 1998;50:1510-1511.
42. Dooley JM, Camfield PR, O'Neill M, Vohra A. The value of CT scans for children with headaches. *Can J Neurol Sci.* 1990;17:309-310.
43. du Boulay GH, Ruiz JS. CT changes associated with migraine. *AJNR.* 1983;4:472-473.
44. Duffy GP. Lumbar puncture in spontaneous subarachnoid haemorrhage. *BMJ.* 1982;285:1163-1164.
45. Dumas MD, Pexman W, Kreeft JH. Computed tomography evaluation of patients with chronic headache. *Can Med Assoc J.* 1994;151:1447-1452.
46. Edmeads J. Headaches in older people: how are they different in this age-group? *Postgrad Med.* 1997;101:91-94.
47. Embil JM, Kramer M, Kinnear S, Light RB. A blinding headache. *Lancet.* 1997;349:182.
48. Evans RW. The postconcussion syndrome and the sequelae of mild head injury. In: Evans RW, ed. *Neurology and Trauma.* Philadelphia: WB Saunders; 1996:91-116.
49. Evans RW. Migrainelike headaches in pituitary apoplexy. *Headache.* 1997;37:455-456.
50. Evans RW. Complications of lumbar puncture. *Neurol Clin.* 1998; 16:83-105.
51. Fazekas F, Koch M, Schmidt R, et al. The prevalence of cerebral damage varies with migraine type: a MRI study. *Headache.* 1992;32:287-291.
52. Fernandes CMB, Daya MR. A roller coaster headache: case report. *J Trauma.* 1994;37:1007-1010.
53. Feuerman T, Wackym PA, Gade GF, et al. Value of skull radiography, head computed tomographic scanning, and admission for observation in cases of minor head injury. *Neurosurgery.* 1988;22:449-453.
54. Fisher CM. Painful states: a neurological commentary. *Clin Neurosurg.* 1984;31:32-53.
55. Fishman RA. Examination of the cerebrospinal fluid: techniques and complications. In: *Cerebrospinal Fluid in Diseases of the Nervous System.* Philadelphia: WB Saunders; 1992:183-252.
56. Fishman RA, Dillon WP. Dural enhancement and cerebral displacement secondary to intracranial hypotension. *Neurology.* 1993;43:609-611.
57. Fodden DI, Peatfield RC, Milsom PL. Beware the patient with a headache in the accident and emergency department. *Arch Emerg Med.* 1989;6:7-12.
58. Forsyth PA, Posner JB. Headaches in patients with brain tumors: a study of 111 patients. *Neurology.* 1993;43:1678-1683.
59. Frishberg BM. The utility of neuroimaging in the evaluation of headache in patients with normal neurologic examination. *Neurology.* 1994;44:1191-1197.
60. Frishberg BM. Neuroimaging in presumed primary headache disorders. *Semin Neurol.* 1997;17:373-382.
61. Gabrielsen TO. Neurologic complications of cerebral angiography. *AJNR.* 1994;15:1408-1411.
62. Ghoshhajra K, Scotti L, Marasco J, et al. CT detection of intracranial aneurysm in subarachnoid hemorrhage. *AJR.* 1979;132:613-616.
63. Gillingham FJ. The management of ruptured intracranial aneurysm. *Ann R Coll Surg Engl.* 1958;23:89-117.
64. Gillingham FJ. The management of ruptured intracranial aneurysms. *Scot Med J.* 1967;12:377-383.
65. Gorelick PB. Ischemic stroke and intracranial hematoma. In: Olesen J, Tfelt-Hansen P, Welch KMA, eds. *The Headaches.* New York: Raven; 1993:639-645.
66. Gould JD, Silberstein SD. Unilateral hypnic headache: a case study. *Neurology.* 1997;49:1749-1751.

67. Gronseth GS, Greenberg MK. The utility of electroencephalogram in the evaluation of patients presenting with headache: a review of the literature. *Neurology.* 1995;45:1263-1267.

68. Hall S, Lie JT, Kurland LT, et al. The therapeutic impact of temporal artery biopsy. *Lancet.* 1983;2:1217-1220.

69. Harling DW, Peatfield RC, Van Hille PT, Abbott RJ. Thunderclap headache: is it migraine? *Cephalalgia.* 1989;9:87-90.

70. Hauerberg J, Anderssen BB, Eskesen V, Rosenorn J, Schmidt K. Importance of the recognition of a warning leak as a sign of a ruptured intracranial aneurysm. *Acta Neurol Scand.* 1991;83:61-64.

71. Hayreh SS, Podhajsky PA, Raman R, Zimmerman B. Giant cell arteritis: validity and reliability of various diagnostic criteria. *Am J Ophthalmol.* 1997;123:285-296.

72. Headache Classification Committee of the International Headache Society. Classification and diagnostic criteria for headache disorders, cranial neuralgia, and facial pain. *Cephalalgia.* 1988;8(suppl 7):1-96.

73. Heiserman JE, Dean BL, Hodak JA, et al. Neurologic complications of cerebral angiography. *AJNR.* 1994;15:1401-1407.

74. Hering R, Couturier EGM, Steiner TJ, Asherson RA, Rose CF. Anticardiolipin antibodies in migraine. *Cephalalgia.* 1991;11:19-21.

75. Hesselink JR, Dowd CF, Healy ME, et al. MR imaging of brain contusions: a comparative study with CT. *AJR.* 1988;150:1133-1142.

76. Houspian EM, Pool JL. A systematic analysis of intracranial aneurysms from the autopsy file of Presbyterian Hospital, 1914-1956. *J Neuropathol Exp Neurol.* 1958;17:409-423.

77. Hughes RL. Identification and treatment of cerebral aneurysms after sentinel headache. *Neurology.* 1992;42:1118.

78. Hunder GG, Bloch DA, Beat AM, et al. The American College of Rheumatology 1990 criteria for the classification of giant cell arteritis. *Arthritis Rheum.* 1990;33:1122-1128.

79. Hunder GG, Davis JS. Giant cell arteritis and polymyalgia rheumatica. *Hosp Pract.* 1992;27:75-93.

80. Hungerford G, duBoulay G, Zilkha K. Computerized axial tomography in patients with severe migraine: a preliminary report. *J Neurol Neurosurg Psychiatry.* 1976;39:990-994.

81. Huston J, Nichols DA, Luetmer PH, et al. Blinded prospective evaluation of sensitivity of MR angiography to known intracranial aneurysms: importance of aneurysm size. *AJNR.* 1994;15:1607-1614.

82. Igarashi H, Sakai F, Kan S, Okada J, Tazaki Y. Magnetic resonance imaging of the brain in patients with migraine. *Cephalalgia.* 1991;11:69-74.

83. Ikard RW. Clinical efficacy of temporal artery biopsy in Nashville, Tennessee. *South Med J.* 1988;81:1222-1224.

84. Iqbal J, Davis LE, Orrison WW. An MRI study of lumbar puncture headaches. *Headache.* 1995;35:420-422.

85. Iwanaga H, Wakai S, Ochiai C, Narita J, Inoh S, Nagai M. Ruptured cerebral aneurysms missed by initial angiographic study. *Neurosurgery.* 1990;27:45-51.

86. Jacome DE, Leborgne J. MRI studies in basilar artery migraine. *Headache.* 1990;30:88-90.

87. Jennett B. Skull x-rays after mild head injuries. *Arch Emerg Med.* 1987;4:133-135.

88. Jeret JS, Mandell M, Anziska B, et al. Clinical predictors of abnormality disclosed by computed tomography after mild head trauma. *Neurosurgery.* 1993;32:9-16.

88a. Jiménez-Jiménez FJ, Garcia-Albea E, Zurdo M, et al. Giant cell arteritis presenting as cluster headache. *Neurology.* 1998;51:1767-1768.

89. Jonasson F, Cullen JF, Elton RA. Temporal arteritis: a 14-year epidemiological, clinical and prognostic study. *Scot Med J.* 1979;24:111-117.

90. Jundt JW, Mock D. Temporal arteritis with normal erythrocyte sedimentation rates presenting as occipital neuralgia. *Arthritis Rheum.* 1991;34:217-219.

91. Kantor SM. Temporal arteritis. In: Panzer RJ, et al, eds. *Diagnostic Strategies for Common Medical Problems.* Philadelphia: American College of Physicians; 1991:347-354.

92. Kassell NF, Kongable GL, Torner JC, Adams HP, Mazuz H. Delay in referral of patients with ruptured aneurysms to neurosurgical attention. *Stroke.* 1985;16:587-590.

93. Kassell NF, Torner JC, Haley EC, Jane JA, Adams HP, Kongable GL. The International Cooperative Study on the Timing of Aneurysm Surgery. Part I: Overall management results. *J Neurosurg.* 1990;73:18-36.

94. Kassirer JP. Our stubborn quest for diagnostic certainty: a cause of excessive testing. *N Engl J Med.* 1989;320:1489-1491.

94a. Khajavi K, Chyatte D. Subarachnoid hemorrhage. In: Gilman S, Goldstein GW, Waxman SG, eds. *Neurobase.* San Diego: Arbor Publishing; 1999.

95. Khurana RK. Headache spectrum in Arnold-Chiari malformation. *Headache.* 1991;31:151-155.

96. Kuhn MJ, Shekar PC. A comparative study of magnetic resonance imaging and computed tomography in the evaluation of migraine. *Comput Med Imaging Graph.* 1990;14:149-152.

97. Kulvin S. Erythrocyte sedimentation rates in the elderly. *Arch Ophthalmol.* 1972;88:617-618.

98. Kupersmith MJ, Vargas ME, Yashar A, et al. Occipital arteriovenous malformations: visual disturbances and presentation. *Neurology.* 1996;46:953-957.

99. Laffey P, Oaks W, Sawmi R, Teplick J, Haskin M. *Computerized Tomography in Clinical Medicine: Data Supplement.* Philadelphia: Medical Directions; 1978.

100. Lance JW. *Mechanism and Management of Headache.* Oxford: Butterworth-Heinemann; 1993:268.

101. Larson E, Omenn G, Lewis H. Diagnostic evaluation of headache: impact of computerized tomography and cost effectiveness. *JAMA.* 1980;243:359-362.

102. Lay CL, Campbell JK, Mokri B. Low cerebrospinal fluid pressure headache. In: Goadsby PJ, Silberstein SD, eds. *Headache.* Boston: Butterworth-Heinemann; 1997:355-367.

103. LeBlanc R. The minor leak preceding subarachnoid hemorrhage. *J Neurosurg.* 1987;66:35-39.

104. Leone M, D'Amico D, Frediani F, et al. Clinical considerations on sidelocked unilaterality in long-lasting primary headaches. *Headache.* 1993;33:381-384.

105. Lesoin F, Viaud C, Pruvo J, et al. Traumatic and alternating delayed intracranial hematomas. *Neuroradiology.* 1984;26:515-516.

106. Linet MS, Stewart WF, Celentano DD, et al. An epidemiologic study of headache among adolescents and young adults. *JAMA.* 1989;261: 2211-2216.

107. Linn FHH, Wijdicks EFM, van der Graaf Y, Weerdesteyn-van Viiet FAC, Bartelds AIM, van Gijn J. Prospective study of sentinel headache in aneurysmal subarachnoid haemorrhage. *Lancet.* 1994;344: 590-593.

107a. Linn FHH, Rinkel GJE, Algra A, van Gijn J. Headache characteristics in subarachnoid haemorrhage and benign thunderclap headache. *J Neurol Neurosurg Psychiatry.* 1998;65:791-793.

108. Lipton RB, Pfeffer D, Newman LC, Solomon S. Headaches in the elderly. *J Pain Symptom Manage.* 1993;8:87-97.

109. Litt AW. MR angiography of intracranial aneurysms: proceed, but with caution. *AJNR.* 1994;15:1615-1616.

110. Lobato RD, Rivas JJ, Gomez PA, et al. Head-injured patients who talk and deteriorate into coma: analysis of 211 cases studied with computerized tomography. *J Neurosurg.* 1991;75:256-261.

111. Lord SM, Barnsley L, Wallis BJ, Bogduk N. Third occipital headache: a prevalence study. *J Neurol Neurosurg Psychiatry.* 1994;57:1187-1190.

112. Majoie CBLM, Hulsmans FJH, Verbeeten B, et al. Trigeminal neuralgia: comparison of two MR imaging techniques in the demonstration of neurovascular contact. *Radiology.* 1997;204:455-460.

113. Majoie CBLM, Verbeeten B, Dol JA, Peeters FLM. Trigeminal neuropathy: evaluation with MR imaging. *Radiographics.* 1995;15:795-811.

114. Mandel S. Minor head injury may not be "minor." *Postgrad Med.* 1989;85(6):213-225.

115. Masland W, Friedman A, Buchsbaum H. Computerized axial tomography of migraine. *Res Clin Stud Headache.* 1978;6:136-140.

116. Matthews WB. Footballer's migraine. *BMJ.* 1972;2:326-327.

117. Mayberg MR. Management of subarachnoid hemorrhage. *Stroke: Clin Updates.* 1995;6(1):1-4.

118. Maytal J, Bienkowski RS, Patel M, Eviatar L. The value of brain imaging in children with headaches. *Pediatrics.* 1996;96:413-416.

119. McCormick WF, Nofzinger JD. Saccular intracranial aneurysms: an autopsy study. *J Neurosurg.* 1965;22:155-159.

120. McKissock W. Subdural hæmatoma: a review of 389 cases. *Lancet.* 1960;1:1365-1370.

121. Medina LS, Pinter JD, Zurakowski D, et al. Children with headache: clinical predictors of surgical space-occupying lesions and the role of neuroimaging. *Radiology.* 1997;202:819-824.

122. Mehdorn HM, Dietrich V, Kalff R, Hoffman B, Rauhut KF, Grote W. Subarachnoid hemorrhage of unknown etiology: long-term prognosis. *Neurosurg Rev.* 1992;15:27-31.

123. Mehler MR, Rabinowich L. The clinical neuro-ophthalmologic spectrum of temporal arteritis. *Am J Med.* 1988;85:839-844.

124. Miller A, Green M, Robinson D. Simple rule for calculating normal erythrocyte sedimentation rate. *BMJ.* 1983;286:266.

125. Milo R, Razon N, Schiffer J. Delayed epidural hematoma: a review. *Acta Neurochir (Wien).* 1987;84:13-23.

126. Minderhoud JM, Boelens MEM, Huizenga J, et al. Treatment of minor head injuries. *Clin Neurol Neurosurg.* 1980;82:127-140.

127. Mitchell C, Osborn R, Grosskreutz S. Computerized tomography in the headache patient: is routine evaluation really necessary? *Headache.* 1993;33:82-86.

128. Mittl RL, Grossman RI, Hiehle JF, et al. Prevalence of MR evidence of diffuse axonal injury in patients with mild head injury and normal head CT findings. *Am J Neuroradiol.* 1994;15:1583-1589.

129. Mokri B. Headache in spontaneous carotid and vertebral artery dissections. In: Goadsby PJ, Silberstein SD, eds. *Headache.* Boston: Butterworth-Heinemann; 1997:327-353.

130. Mokri B, Piepgras DG, Miller GM. Syndrome of orthostatic headaches and diffuse pachymeningeal gadolinium enhancement. *Mayo Clin Proc.* 1997;72:400-413.

131. Morales-Asín F, Mauri JA, Iñiguez C, et al. The hypnic headache syndrome: report of three new cases. *Cephalalgia.* 1998;18:157-158.

131a. Morgenstern LB, Luna-Gonzales H, Huber JC, et al. Worst headache and subarachnoid hemorrhage: prospective, modern computed tomography and spinal fluid analysis. *Ann Emerg Med.* 1998;32:297-304.

132. Muñoz C, Díez-Tejedor E, Frank A, Barreiro P. Cluster headache syndrome associated with middle cerebral artery arteriovenous malformation. *Cephalalgia.* 1996;16:202-205.

133. Myklebust G, Gran JT. A prospective study of 287 patients with polymyalgia rheumatica and temporal arteritis: clinical and laboratory manifestations at onset of disease and at the time of diagnosis. *Br J Rheumatol.* 1996;35:1161-1168.

134. Nadeau SE. Temporal arteritis: a decision-analytic approach to temporal artery biopsy. *Acta Neurol Scand.* 1988;78:90-100.

135. Ogawa T, Inugami A, Shimosegawa E, et al. Subarachnoid hemorrhage: evaluation with MR imaging. *Radiology.* 1993;186:345-351.

136. Orrell RW, Johnson MH. Plasma viscosity and the diagnosis of giant cell arteritis. *Br J Clin Pract.* 1993;47:71-72.

137. Osborn RE, Alder DC, Mitchell CS. MR imaging of the brain in patients with migraine headaches. *AJNR.* 1991;12:521-524.

138. Østergaard JR. Warning leak in subarachnoid haemorrhage. *BMJ.* 1990;301:190-191.

139. Packard RC. Posttraumatic headache. *Semin Neurol.* 1994;14:40-45.

140. Pascual J, Berciano J. Experience in the diagnosis of headaches that start in elderly people. *J Neurol Neurosurg Psychiatry.* 1994;57:1255-1257.

141. Pascual J, Iglesias F, Oterino A, et al. Cough, exertional, and sexual headaches: an analysis of 72 benign and symptomatic cases. *Neurology.* 1996;46:1520-1524.

142. Pascual-Leone A, Pascual APL. Occipital neuralgia: another benign cause of "thunderclap headache." *J Neurol Neurosurg Psychiatry.* 1992;55:411.

143. Pavese N, Canapicchi R, Nuti A, et al. White matter MRI hyperintensities in a hundred and twenty-nine consecutive migraine patients. *Cephalalgia.* 1994;14:342-345.

144. Plotkin FR, Burke TF. Vertex epidural hematoma: a diagnostic challenge. *Ann Emerg Med.* 1994;24:312-315.

145. Ponge T, Barrier JH, Grolleau JY, Ponge A, Vlasak AM, Cottin S. The efficacy of selective unilateral temporal artery biopsy versus bilateral biopsies for diagnosis of giant cell arteritis. *J Rheumatol.* 1988;15:997-1000.

146. Prager JM, Rosenblum J, Mikulis DJ, Diamond S, Freitag, FG. Evaluation of headache patients by MRI. *Headache Q.* 1991;2:192-196.

147. Rapoport AM. The diagnosis of migraine and tension-type headache, then and now. *Neurology.* 1992;42(suppl 2):11-15.

148. Raps EC, Galetta SL, Rogers J, et al. Unruptured aneurysms and headache. *Arch Neurol.* 1994;51:447-448.

149. Raps EC, Rogers JD, Galetta SL, et al. The clinical spectrum of unruptured intracranial aneurysms. *Arch Neurol.* 1993;50:265-268.

150. Raskin NH. Short-lived head pains. *Neurol Clin.* 1997;15:143-152.

151. Reich KA, Giansiracusa DF, Strongwater SL. Neurologic manifestations of giant cell arteritis. *Am J Med.* 1990;89:67-72.

152. Rinkel GJE, Djibuti M, Algra A, van Gijn J. Prevalence and risk of rupture of intracranial aneurysms: a systematic review. *Stroke.* 1998;29:251-256.

153. Rinkel GJE, Wijdicks EFM, Hasan D, et al. Outcome in patients with subarachnoid haemorrhage and negative angiography according to pattern of haemorrhage on computed tomography. *Lancet.* 1991;338:964-968.

154. Rinkel GJE, Wijdicks EFM, Vermeulen M, et al. Nonaneurysmal perimesencephalic subarachnoid hemorrhage: CT and MR patterns that differ from aneurysmal rupture. *Am J Neuroradiol.* 1991;12:829-834.

155. Robbins L. Migraine and anticardiolipin antibodies: case reports of 13 patients and the prevalence of antiphospholipid antibodies in migraineurs. *Headache.* 1991;31:537-539.

156. Robbins L, Friedman H. MRI in migraineurs. *Headache.* 1992;32:507-508.

157. Rosenberg J, Greenberg MK. Practice parameters: strategies for survival into the nineties. *Neurology.* 1992;42:1110-1115.

158. Rosenborn J, Duus B, Nielsen K, et al. Is a skull x-ray necessary after milder head trauma? *Br J Neurosurg.* 1991;5:135-139.

159. Rowan AJ. The electroencephalographic characteristics of migraine. *Arch Neurol.* 1974;37:95-99.

160. Russell D, Nakstad P, Sjaastad O. Cluster headache: pneumoencephalographic and cerebral computerized axial tomographic findings. *Headache.* 1978;18:272-273.

161. Russell RWR. Giant-cell arteritis: a review of 35 cases. *Q J Med.* 1959;28:471-489.

162. Sands GH, Newman L, Lipton R. Cough, exertional, and other miscellaneous headaches. *Med Clin North Am.* 1991;75:733-743.

163. Sankhla SK, Gunawardena WJ, Coutinho CMA, et al. Magnetic resonance angiography in the management of aneurysmal subarachnoid haemorrhage: a study of 51 cases. *Neuroradiology.* 1996;38:724-729.

164. Saper JR, Silberstein S, Gordon CD, Hamel RL, eds. *Handbook of Headache Management.* Baltimore: Williams & Wilkins; 1993:8, 23.

165. Sargent J, Lawson C, Solbach P, Coyne L. Use of CT scans in an outpatient headache population: an evaluation. *Headache.* 1979;19:388-390.

166. Schmidt WA, Kraft HE, Volker L, Vorpahl K, et al. Color duplex ultrasonography in the diagnosis of temporal arteritis. *N Engl J Med.* 1997;337:1336-1342.

167. Silberstein SD. Evaluation and emergency treatment of headache. *Headache.* 1992;32:396-407.

168. Silberstein SD, Lipton RB, Goadsby PJ. *Headache in Clinical Practice.* Oxford, England: Isis Medical Media; 1998.

169. Silbert PL, Edis RH, Stewart-Wynne EG, Gubbay SS. Benign vascular sexual headache and exertional headache: interrelationships and long-term prognosis. *J Neurol Neurosurg Psychiatry.* 1991;54:417-421.

170. Silbert PL, Mokri B, Schievink WI. Headache and neck pain in spontaneous internal carotid and vertebral artery dissections. *Neurology.* 1995;45:1517-1522.

171. Simon RH, Zimmerman AW, Tasman A, Hale MS. Spectral analysis of photic stimulation in migraine. *Electroenceph Clin Neurophysiol.* 1982;53:270-276.

172. Slivka A, Philbrook B. Clinical and angiographic features of thunderclap headache. *Headache.* 1995;35:1-6.

173. Smyth VOG, Winter AL. The EEG in migraine. *Electroenceph Clin Neurophysiol.* 1964;16:194.

174. Söderström CE. Diagnostic significance of CSF spectrophotometry and computer tomography in cerebrovascular disease: a comparative study in 231 cases. *Stroke.* 1977;5:606-612.

175. Soges LJ, Cacayorin ED, Petro GR, Ramachandran TS. Migraine: evaluation by MR. *AJNR.* 1988;9:425-429.

176. Solomon S. Diagnosis of primary headache disorders: validity of the International Headache Society criteria in clinical practice. *Neurol Clin.* 1997;15:15-26.

177. Solomon S, Cappa KG. The headache of temporal arteritis. *J Am Geriatr Soc.* 1987;35:163-165.

178. Sotaniemi KA, Rantala M, Pyhtinen J, Myllyla VV. Clinical and CT correlates in the diagnosis of intracranial tumours. *J Neurol Neurosurg Psychiatry.* 1991;54:645-647.

179. Stein SC, Ross SE. Mild head injury: a plea for routine early CT scanning. *J Trauma.* 1992;33:11-33.

180. Strayle-Batra M, Skalej M, Wakhloo AK, et al. Three-dimensional spiral CT angiography in the detection of cerebral aneurysm. *Acta Radiologica.* 1998;39:233-238.

181. Suwanwela N, Phanthumchinda K, Kaoropthum S. Headache in brain tumor: a cross-sectional study. *Headache.* 1994;34:435-438.

182. Tajti J, Sas K, Szok D, et al. Clusterlike headache as a first sign of brain metastases of lung cancer. *Headache.* 1996;36:259-260.

183. Thielen KR, Wijdicks EFM, Nichols DA. Giant cell (temporal) arteritis: involvement of the vertebral and internal carotid arteries. *Mayo Clin Proc.* 1998;73:444-446.

184. Tietjen GE. Migraine and antiphospholipid antibodies. *Cephalalgia.* 1992;12:69-74.

185. Tietjen GE, Day M, Norris L, et al: Role of anticardiolipin antibodies

in young persons with migraine and transient focal neurologic events: a prospective study. *Neurology.* 1998;50:1433-1440.

186. Tourtellotte WW, Metz LN, Bryan ER, DeJong RN. Spontaneous subarachnoid hemorrhage: factors affecting the rate of clearing of the cerebrospinal fluid. *Neurology.* 1964;14:301-306.

187. Treib J, Dobler G, Haass A, et al. Thunderclap headache cause by Erve virus? *Neurology.* 1998;50:509-511.

188. Umehara F, Kamishima K, Kashio N, et al. Magnetic resonance tomographic angiography: diagnostic value in trigeminal neuralgia. *Neuroradiology.* 1995;37:353-355.

189. Urbach H, Zentner J, Solymosi L. The need for repeat angiography in subarachnoid haemorrhage. *Neuroradiology.* 1998;40:6-10.

190. Van der Wee N, Rinkel GJE, Hasan D, van Gijn J. Detection of subarachnoid haemorrhage on early CT: is lumbar puncture still needed after a negative scan? *J Neurol Neurosurg Psychiatry.* 1995;58:357-359.

191. van Gijn J. Subarachnoid hemorrhage. *Lancet.* 1992;339:653-655.

192. van Gijn J, Van Dongen KJ. The time course of aneurysmal haemorrhage on computed tomograms. *Neuroradiology.* 1982;23:153-156.

193. Vazquez-Barquero A, Ibanex FJ, Herrera S, et al. Isolated headache as the presenting clinical manifestation of intracranial tumors: a prospective study. *Cephalalgia.* 1994;14:270-272.

194. Vermeulen M, Hasan D, Blijenberg BG, Hijdra A, van Gijn J. Xanthochromia after subarachnoid haemorrhage needs no revisitation. *J Neurol Neurosurg Psychiatry.* 1989;52:826-828.

195. Vermeulen M, van Gijn J. The diagnosis of subarachnoid haemorrhage. *J Neurol Neurosurg Psychiatry.* 1990;53:365-372.

196. Verweij RD, Wijdicks EFJ, van Gijn J. Warning headache in aneurysmal subarachnoid hemorrhage: a case-control study. *Arch Neurol.* 1988;45:1019-1020.

197. Vilaseca J, Gonzalez A, Cid MC, Lopez-Vivancos J, Ortega A. Clinical usefulness of temporal artery biopsy. *Ann Rheumat Dis.* 1987;46:282-285.

198. Walton JN. *Subarachnoid Hemorrhage.* Edinburgh: E & S Livingstone; 1956.

199. Wang AM, Bisese JH, Jackson CTL. Computed tomography of cerebrovascular disease. In: Rumbaugh CL, Wang AM, Tsai FY, eds. *Cerebrovascular Disease. Imaging and Interventional Treatment Options.* New York: Igaku-Shoin; 1995:153-187.

200. Weingarten S, Kleinman M, Elperin L, Larson E. The effectiveness of cerebral imaging in the diagnosis of chronic headache: a reappraisal. *Arch Intern Med.* 1992;152:2457-2462.

201. Weir B. Headaches from aneurysms. *Cephalalgia.* 1994;14:79-87.

202. Weiss HD, Stern BJ, Goldberg J. Post-traumatic migraine: chronic migraine precipitated by minor head or neck trauma. *Headache.* 1991;31:451-456.

203. Wijdicks EFM, Kerkhoff H, van Gijn J. Cerebral vasospasm and unruptured aneurysm in thunderclap headache. *Lancet.* 1988;2:1020.

204. Wijdicks EFM, Kerkhoff H, van Gijn J. Long-term follow-up of 71 patients with thunderclap headache mimicking subarachnoid haemorrhage. *Lancet.* 1988;2:68-70.

205. Wilterdink JL. Sentinel headaches and aneurysmal subarachnoid hemorrhage. In: Feldmann E, ed. *Current Diagnosis in Neurology.* St Louis: Mosby; 1994:62-67.

206. Wöber-Bingöl C, Wöber C, Prayer D, et al. Magnetic resonance imaging for recurrent headache in childhood and adolescence. *Headache.* 1996;36:83-90.

207. Wolpert SM, Caplan LR. Current role of cerebral angiography in the diagnosis of cerebrovascular diseases. *AJR.* 1992;159:191-197.

208. Wong RL, Korn JH. Temporal arteritis without an elevated erythrocyte sedimentation rate. *Am J Med.* 1986;80:959-964.

209. Woolf SH, Kamerow DB. Testing for uncommon conditions: the heroic search for positive test results. *Arch Intern Med.* 1990;15:2451-2458.

210. Yamaguchi M. Incidence of headache and severity of head injury. *Headache.* 1992;32:427-431.

211. Yang J, Simonson TM, Ruprecht A, et al. Magnetic resonance imaging used to assess patients with trigeminal neuralgia. *Oral Surg Oral Med Oral Pathol Oral Radiol Endod.* 1996;81:343-350.

212. Yokota H, Kurokawa A, Otsuka T, et al. Significance of magnetic resonance imaging in acute head injury. *J Trauma.* 1991;31:351-357.

213. Yuichi I, Shigeo S, Takeshi M, et al. Postcontrast computed tomography in subarachnoid hemorrhage from ruptured aneurysms. *J Comput Assist Tomogr.* 1981;5:341-344.

214. Ziegler DK, Batnitzky S, Barter R, McMillan JH. Magnetic resonance image abnormality in migraine with aura. *Cephalalgia.* 1991;11:147-150.

# 2

# Neck and Back Pain

*Scott Haldeman*

The number and cost of available diagnostic tests for patients with back and neck pain have grown dramatically over the past two decades. The impact of managed care and an increased understanding of the natural history of these conditions has led to close evaluation of the sensitivity and specificity of these tests and their effect on patient outcomes. Within the first month of patient management, advanced anatomic and physiologic tests should be reserved for patients with "red flags" for serious pathology on clinical examination. Specific criteria are being developed for each electrodiagnostic and imaging test used in the evaluation of patients who do not recover within 1 month. Guidelines for the testing of patients with chronic back and neck pain have yet to be developed. Stronger emphasis on psychosocial issues and the assurance that progressive pathology has not been missed without the use of repetitive testing form the mainstay of diagnostic protocols in this population.

The past two decades have seen a proliferation of tests and treatment methods for the management of patients with back and neck pain. Many of these tests are for the evaluation of neurologic deficits or lesions that potentially could compress neural structures. Treatments such as surgery, steroid injections, and even certain exercises have been designed specifically to remove or ease neural compressive lesions. This approach has led to an increase in the referral of patients with back and neck pain to neurologists, sometimes for electrodiagnostic testing only but more often for a complete evaluation and opinion regarding diagnosis, treatment, prognosis, and disability or impairment. The neurologist is often being placed in the position of the primary care physician or spine specialist for these patients and is responsible for the management of nonneurologic as well as neurologic causes of back and neck pain.

Back and neck pain has become increasingly important as the costs for health care have become the focus of attention in the nineties. Grazier et al[29] estimated the total direct costs for treatment of patients with spinal disorders in 1981 to be $12,922,740,000. Cats-Baril and Frymoyer[17] extrapolated these direct medical costs to be $23,536,153,000 by 1990. The figures for x-rays alone were estimated by Scavone

et al[49] to be $600 million in 1981, which, when extrapolated to 1990, reaches a figure of $1.79 billion.[17] Furthermore, the 1981 figures do not include such testing as magnetic resonance imaging (MRI), evoked potentials, high-technology thermography, computerized strength testing, and multiple other technologic advances. More recent estimates of the costs related to back pain done by Frymoyer and Durett[23] suggest that the cost to society is currently in the range of $38 to $50 billion.

Despite advances in knowledge and the proliferation of diagnostic tests and treatment methods, there is no evidence of a decrease in the frequency or severity of back or neck pain. The yearly prevalence of this disorder remains at 15% to 20%,[4] and surveys of working-age individuals note that 50% admit to symptoms each year.[54,58] Back pain remains the most common cause of disability for persons younger than age 45,[19] and at any given time 2% of the population is undergoing some form of chronic or temporary disability.[4]

The increasing use and cost of diagnostic and treatment methods for back and neck pain without a corresponding change in morbidity has let to more intense investigation of all the medical procedures used in the treatment of this disorder. Increasingly, it is becoming necessary to document the reliability of each procedure, and each test is being examined in regard to the frequency of abnormalities in the asymptomatic population, sensitivity and specificity, and effect on patient outcomes. The *Clinical Practice Guideline on Acute Low Back Problems in Adults* published by the Agency for Health Care Policy and Research (AHCPR)[10] illustrates how these tests are being evaluated. Similarly, a Task Force on Whiplash-Associated Disorders has been commissioned by the Quebec government.[16]

Diagnostic testing for back and neck pain can be addressed through a detailed analysis of the strengths and weaknesses of each testing method. Such an analysis, however, would fill a textbook and would often create confusion. A more practical approach is to define groups of patients according to their most common presentations and to discuss current opinions about the best methods of evaluating such patients.

## ACUTE UNCOMPLICATED BACK AND NECK PAIN

This condition can be defined as back or neck pain of recent origin without clinical signs or symptoms (red flags) of a destructive pathologic condition or neurologic deficits. The word *acute* has been defined as less than 7 days by the Quebec Task Force on Spinal Disorders[53] but more often refers to the first month following onset of symptoms.[10]

The history and physical examination remain the primary basis for screening patients with acute low back pain. Estimates of the sensitivity and specificity of the basic clinical evaluation have been published in the AHCPR low back pain guidelines (Tables 2–1 and 2–2). These figures have been derived from the literature and suggest that a very brief history and a few physical examination techniques can essentially screen out any serious pathologic condition in patients with acute low back pain. These guidelines specifically state that "plain x-rays are not recommended for routine evaluation of patients with acute low back problems within the first month of symptoms unless a red flag is noted on clinical examination."[10] The data supporting this position were taken mainly from preemployment x-ray examinations, which were commonly performed in the 1970s and early 1980s. Structural abnormalities such as lordosis, degenerative changes (including disk narrowing and osteophytic spurs in both the cervical and lumbar spine), and even spondylolisthesis at the L5–S1 level on routine x-ray films do not predict the presence of back pain and are seen in almost equal numbers in both asymptomatic and symptomatic patients.[8,11,24,26,27] The Quebec Task Force on Whiplash-Associated Disorders[16] does,

however, recommend baseline studies in patients who have neck pain with findings of decreased range of motion, tenderness, or neurologic signs (grade II, III, or IV) but not in patients who present with neck pain or stiffness without physical signs (grade I).

Electrodiagnostic evaluation would not be appropriate in this group of patients since by definition they have no clinical evidence of neural deficits. Imaging studies are unlikely to be of value because surgery is never an issue in this situation. A substantial school of thought suggests that imaging studies such as computed tomography (CT) and MRI may actually be detrimental to this group of patients. MRI, CT, or diskography shows changes commonly described as abnormal in 30% to 40% of the population (depending mostly on age). The perception of an abnormality suggesting fragility may lead the physician or patient to unnecessarily perceive the presence of an illness or disability and may precipitate nonbeneficial treatment or surgery, which could lead to increased disability.

## RED FLAGS FOR FRACTURE OR DISLOCATION

Certain patients present with an acute history that raises the possibility of bony fracture or dislocation. Grazier et al[29] estimate that 162,000 patients present to a physician in the United States with some form of spinal fracture. There are two situations in which this is likely to occur: (1) major trauma in a healthy young individual or (2) minor trauma in an elderly patient or a patient with risk factors for osteo-

---

**TABLE 2–1. Estimated Accuracy of Medical History in Diagnosis of Spine Diseases Causing Low Back Problems**

| REFERENCES | DISEASE TO BE DETECTED | MEDICAL HISTORY RED FLAGS | TRUE-POSITIVE RATE (SENSITIVITY) | TRUE-NEGATIVE RATE (SPECIFICITY) |
|---|---|---|---|---|
| Deyo and Diehl*[26] | Cancer | Age ≥50 y | 0.77 | 0.71 |
| | | Previous cancer history | 0.31 | 0.98 |
| | | Unexplained weight loss | 0.15 | 0.94 |
| | | Failure to improve with 1 mo of therapy | 0.31 | 0.9 |
| | | Bedrest no relief | >0.9 | 0.46 |
| | | Duration of pain >1 mo | 0.5 | 0.81 |
| | | Age ≥50 y or history of cancer or unexplained weight loss or failure of conservative therapy | 1 | 0.6 |
| Waldvogel and Vasey[61] | Spinal osteomyelitis | Intravenous drug abuse, urinary tract infection, or skin infection | 0.4 | NA |
| Unpublished data† | Compression fracture | Age ≥50 y | 0.84 | 0.61 |
| | | Age ≥70 y | 0.22 | 0.96 |
| | | Trauma | 0.3 | 0.85 |
| | | Corticosteroid use | 0.06 | 0.995 |
| Deyo and Tsui-Wu[22]; Spangfort[50] | Herniated disk | Sciatica | 0.95 | 0.88 |
| Turner, Ersek, Herron, et al[57] | Spinal stenosis | Pseudoclaudication | 0.6 | NA |
| | | Age ≥50 y | 0.9† | 0.7 |
| Gran[28] | Ankylosing spondylitis | Positive responses Four out of five | 0.23 | 0.82 |
| | | Age at onset ≤40 y | 1 | 0.07 |
| | | Pain not relieved in supine position | 0.8 | 0.49 |
| | | Morning back stiffness | 0.64 | 0.59 |
| | | Duration of pain ≥3 mo | 0.71 | 0.54 |

From Bigos SJ, Bowyer O, Braen G, et al. *Acute Low Back Problems in Adults.* Clinical Practice Guideline No 14. Washington DC: US Department of Health and Human Services, Agency for Health Care Policy and Research, December 1994.

*From 833 patients with back pain at a walk-in clinic as reported in Deyo, Rainville, and Kent (*JAMA.* 1992;268(6):760-765). All received plain lumbar roentgenograms.

†Author's estimate.

**TABLE 2–2. Estimated Accuracy of Physical Examination for Lumbar Disk Herniation Among Patients with Sciatica**

| REFERENCES | TEST | TRUE-POSITIVE RATE (SENSITIVITY)* | TRUE-NEGATIVE RATE (SPECIFICITY)* | COMMENTS |
|---|---|---|---|---|
| Hakelius and Hindmarsh[30]; Kosteljanetz, Epersen, Halaburt, et al[44] | Ipsilateral SLR | 0.8 | 0.4 | Positive result: Leg pain at <60° |
| Hakelius and Hindmarsh[30]; Spangfort[50] | Crossed SLR | 0.25 | 0.9 | Positive result: Reproduction of contralateral pain |
| Hakelius and Hindmarsh[30]; Spangfort[50] | Ankle dorsiflexion weakness | 0.35 | 0.7 | HNP, usually at L4–L5 (80%) |
| Hakelius and Hindmarsh[30]; Kortelainen, Puranen, Koivisto, et al[43] | Great toe extensor weakness | 0.5 | 0.7 | HNP, usually at L5–S1 (60%) or L4–L5 (30%) |
| Hakelius and Hindmarsh[30]; Spangfort[50] | Impaired ankle reflex | 0.5 | 0.6 | HNP, usually at L5–S1; absent reflex increases specificity |
| Kortelainen, Puranen, Koivisto, et al[43]; Kosteljanetz, Espersen, Halaburt, et al[44] | Sensory loss | 0.5 | 0.5 | Area of loss poor predictor of HNP level |
| Aronson and Dunsmore[5] | Patellar reflex | 0.5 | NA | For upper lumbar HNP only |
| Hakelius and Hindmarsh[30] | Ankle plantar flexion weakness | 0.06 | 0.95 | — |
| Hakelius and Hindmarsh[30] | Quadriceps weakness | <0.01 | 0.99 | — |

From Bigos SJ, Bowyer O, Braen G, et al. *Acute Low Back Problems in Adults.* Clinical Practice Guideline No 14. Washington DC: US Department of Health and Human Services, Agency for Health Care Policy and Research, December 1994.

*Sensitivity and specificity were calculated by Deyo, Rainville, and Kent (*JAMA.* 1992;268(6):760-765). Values represent rounded averages where multiple references were available. All results are from surgical case series.

HNP, herniated nucleus pulposus; SLR, straight leg raising.

porosis or other bone-softening diseases or with a congenital anomaly.

Major trauma that is likely to injure the neck tends to be either forced flexion or extension movements, such as in a motor vehicle accident or from sports such as skiing, wrestling, surfing, or football. Vertebral fractures may also be the result of a compression force on top of the head, which can occur, for example, on a construction site where heavy objects may fall from heights. In these situations the possibility of fracture or dislocation may be obvious on clinical examination in which angulation of the spine or myelopathy is detectable. Many patients, however, may present with neck pain only and no neurologic deficits. When fracture is suspected, a detailed x-ray series may be indicated. A cross-table lateral view should show both the anterior and posterior elements down to C7; a swimmer's view may be required to delineate the C7-T1 junction. These are followed by anteroposterior and oblique views and an open-mouth view to visualize the odontoid or C1-C2 relationship. Additional views, such as pillar views for facet fractures or basilar views to study the ring of the atlas for a Jefferson's (burst) fracture of C1, may be indicated. If a fracture is documented or still suspected at a particular level, a detailed CT evaluation may be necessary to localize the position of fragments of bone prior to treatment or to visualize a bony structure in greater detail. Contrast CT scans or MRI scans may be necessary to visualize any compression on the spinal cord or nerve roots.

The thoracolumbar area is the predominant site for spinal fractures; thoracolumbar fractures, if severe, may end in paraplegia.[45] The initial evaluation is radiographic, consisting of anteroposterior and lateral radiographs. In 70% to 90% of cases a cross-table lateral view will show the fracture.[7,20] Oblique views may be necessary to define a facet fracture. Conventional tomography or CT scanning, how-

ever, is usually necessary to evaluate the nature of the fracture and the location of fragments. Patients at greater risk of complications from fractures are those with diseases such as ankylosing spondylitis, diffuse idiopathic skeletal hyperostosis (DISH), and preexisting spinal stenosis (as in achondroplasia).

Fractures may also occur in disorders of the spine associated with weakening of bony structures such as osteoporosis, osteomalacia, or Paget's disease. In these disorders fractures can occur with minor injuries or even spontaneously. The diagnosis begins by identifying the patient at risk; for example, the patient who is taking steroids has a major metabolic disorder or is elderly. The diagnosis of compression fracture is usually radiographic, but under certain circumstances it may be necessary to order a technetium bone scan to determine if a fracture is recent or old. Additional studies such as densitometry, dual photon absorptiometry, and metabolic tests are not commonly considered part of the back and neck pain evaluation but rather a search for the metabolic disorder that is the underlying factor.

## RED FLAGS FOR NEOPLASTIC OR INFECTIOUS DISEASES

On occasion a patient presents with pure back or neck pain and a history that raises the specter of a neoplastic or infectious destructive process. Painful neoplastic spinal tumors (as opposed to primary spinal cord tumors and neurofibromas, which are often nonpainful) can be primary or metastatic. Nonneurogenic spinal neoplasms occur in patients older than 50 or younger than 20 and may or may not be associated with neurologic deficits in the early or, sometimes, advanced stages. Since almost any solid tumor in the body may metastasize to the spinal column, a history of prior cancer should be considered a major red flag. The pain associated with neoplasm also has specific characteristics. Unlike mechanical back pain, this type of pain tends to be worse when the patient is supine and is more severe at night, often waking the patient. It tends to follow a relentless progressive course, and the patient is unable to find any comfortable position.

Spinal infections may occur as osteomyelitis, diskitis, meningitis, or perivertebral abscess. The risk factors are similar to those of any local or systemic infection. Infection is most likely to occur in patients who are immunosuppressed. Thus the patient with human immunodeficiency virus (HIV) infection, the patient taking corticosteroids, or the patient undergoing immune suppression therapy who has an unexplained onset of back or neck pain should be evaluated for a possible infectious cause of the pain, especially if there is associated fever. Infections can also spread hematologically from other organs, for example, in patients with urinary tract infections. Intravenous drug abusers have a relatively high incidence of spinal infection, often due to *Pseudomonas*. Patients who have undergone spinal surgery or other invasive procedures such as diskography or who have had a penetrating wound such as a gunshot or stab injury are at risk for localized abscess formation. Finally, spinal infections are found more often in association with diabetes mellitus, sickle cell disease, and paraplegia. The patient presents with an insidious, slowly progressing back pain that initially may ease with rest and therefore may be ignored by the patient. Systemic symptoms of fever, chills, weight loss, or dysuria may be the factor that first triggers the suspicion of infection in physician and patient.

When a patient presents with risk factors for either a neoplastic or infectious cause of back pain, the assessment is relatively straightforward. Often a destructive lesion will be seen on routine x-ray films with loss of bone structure, blurring of bony margins, or bone reactivity. The sedimentation rate should show significant elevation in spinal infections, although the complete blood count (CBC) may not be markedly abnormal. A technetium bone scan is probably the most sensitive screening tool for both bony tumors and infections; however, it is nonspecific in assessment of inflammation, and it is also positive in one third of older patients, who are at highest risk for these diseases but also have a high incidence of osteoarthritis.[18] CT scanning of an area of uptake on bone scan helps to isolate bony destruction, whereas MRI scanning aids in detailing the spread of the infection or tumor in soft tissue. Further investigation of the nature and extent of the tumor or infection falls outside the scope of this chapter.

## RED FLAGS FOR MYELOPATHY OR CAUDA EQUINA SYNDROME

Patients can present to a physician with either mild or severe back or neck pain in which the primary danger is progressive loss of neurologic function. Initially symptoms may be minimal—episodes of impotence, changes in bladder or bowel habits, or unsteadiness in gait—and easy to miss in a brief history. The condition of these patients, however, can progress rapidly to paraplegia and incontinence.

Acute cauda equina syndrome is most likely to occur after spinal trauma, either by lumbosacral fractures or

massive disk herniations, or following spinal surgery. This condition is rare, however, accounting for approximately 1% to 3% of patients who undergo spinal surgery.[47] Common presenting symptoms are bilateral sciatica with saddle anesthesia and recent onset of bladder dysfunction in the form of urinary retention, increased frequency, or overflow incontinence. Loss of strength in the lower extremities, bladder incontinence, laxity of anal sphincter tone, and perianal sensory loss confirm the clinical diagnosis. The evaluation is primarily a search for an acute surgical lesion. X-ray films may reveal a fracture or dislocation but are usually unremarkable in patients with large disk herniations. Increasingly, MRI is becoming the imaging test of choice for disk herniation, but many physicians still think that the only way to distinguish cauda equina syndrome from other compressive lesions is by myelography and postmyelogram CT scanning.

Acute cervicothoracic myelopathy has a considerably broader differential diagnosis than does acute cauda equina syndrome. Severe trauma, including whiplash injuries, falls and blows to the head or spine, and penetrating stab or bullet wounds, is the most common cause of paraplegia through bony fracture, massive disk herniation, or spinal cord contusion. Many patients with an acute onset of myelopathy, however, have a much more subtle history. Minor trauma in a patient with ligamentous instability as seen in rheumatoid arthritis, congenital stenosis as in achondroplasia, or acquired spinal stenosis as in severe degenerative spondylosis or ossification of the posterior longitudinal ligament (OPLL) may cause decompensation and often can lead to myelopathic symptoms. Affected patients may present with only minor neck pain and unsteadiness. Acute transverse myelitis in multiple sclerosis may present as sudden onset of myelopathy and may include concomitant neck or back pain symptoms, often with Lhermitte's sign. Syringomyelia, spinal infections, and neoplasms may also present primarily as myelopathy.

The presentation of acute or progressive paresis in the lower extremities (possibly including the upper extremities), sensory loss to a spinal level or in a Brown-Séquard pattern, urinary urgency, urinary frequency, stress incontinence, impotence, and incoordination with signs of spasticity in a patient with back or neck pain requires an immediate evaluation. The initial search is for a surgically treatable lesion. MRI of the cervical or thoracic spine, depending on the suspected level of the lesion, has the greatest ability to differentiate a primary disorder of the spinal cord from a compressive extradural defect. MRI is often the only test necessary to diagnose a large disk herniation or tumor. If the primary lesion is bony or ligamentous stenosis or a fracture or dislocation, a myelogram with postmyelogram CT scanning may be the test of choice. With multiple sclerosis, infection, tumor, metastatic infiltration, or carcinomatous meningitis, a spinal tap may be essential to make the initial diagnosis. Further differentiation is beyond the realm of investigation for back or neck pain.

## ACUTE BACK AND NECK PAIN WITH RADIATION TO ARMS OR LEGS

When a patient presents with back or neck pain radiating to the extremities but without the risk factors described in the preceding discussion, the assessment should be much less aggressive. The algorithm suggested by the AHCPR panel (Fig. 2–1) presents a reasonable outline of testing in these patients to rule out the red flags for a serious pathologic condition. The majority of patients with sciatica or cervicobrachial neuralgia, even those with minor sensory, motor, or reflex changes, will recover spontaneously within the first month with only activity modification and symptomatic control. Extensive diagnostic evaluation in this group of patients is unlikely to change the outcome, and surgery is not indicated in the first 1 to 3 months.[10] If the symptoms persist for longer than 1 month, and especially if signs of significant or progressive neurologic deficit are present, testing may become necessary.

Under these circumstances diagnostic testing can be divided into two categories: (1) testing for evidence of physiologic dysfunction and (2) testing for anatomic lesions (Table 2–3). The argument that extensive pathologic evidence can be observed through imaging of the asymptomatic population[13,38,62] has lead to increasing reliance on electrodiagnostic testing in the surgical decision-making process.[51,52] Increasingly, the combination of imaging and electrodiagnostic studies is being advocated to reach an accurate diagnosis.[11,32]

Electromyography (EMG) remains the primary tool for the documentation of radiculopathy but is by no means infallible. When judged against compressive lesions noted through imaging or surgery, there is a relatively strong correlation between the level of the lesion and EMG findings. Young et al[65] noted that EMG correctly predicted the level of radiculopathy in 84% of patients with positive surgical findings, but in seven patients the wrong level was predicted and in nine patients only one abnormal root was detected (when two were involved). Aiello et al[2] found similar results but noted that they varied with the level of involvement. At the L4-L5 level there was a 96% true-positive rate and a 38% true-negative rate, whereas at the L5-S1 level the results were 75% true positive and 79% true negative. Khatri et al[42] further noted that the combination of EMG and imaging tests

## A1. Initial assessment of acute low back symptoms

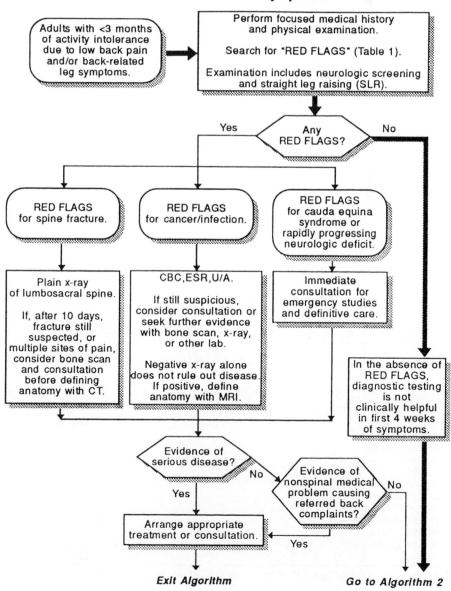

**FIGURE 2–1.** Initial assessment of acute low back pain symptoms. (For algorithms 2–5 and additional information please see the following source from which this algorithm was borrowed: Bigos SJ, Bowyer O, Braen G, et al. *Acute Low Back Problems in Adults.* Clinical Practice Guideline No 14. Washington DC: US Department of Health and Human Services, Agency for Health Care Policy and Research, December 1994.)

**TABLE 2–3. Ability of Different Techniques to Identify and Define Pathology**

| Technique | Identify Physiologic Unit[‡] | Define Anatomic Effect[‡] |
|---|---|---|
| History | + | + |
| Physical examination | | |
|   Circumference measurements | + | + |
|   Reflexes | ++ | ++ |
|   Straight leg raising | ++ | + |
|   Crossed straight leg raising | +++ | ++ |
|   Motor | ++ | ++ |
|   Sensory | ++ | ++ |
| Laboratory studies (ESR, CBC, UA) | ++ | 0 |
| Bone scan* | +++ | ++ |
| EMG/SEP | +++ | ++ |
| Radiography | 0 | + |
| CT* | 0 | ++++[†] |
| MRI | 0 | ++++[†] |
| Myelo-CT* | 0 | ++++[†] |
| Myelography* | 0 | ++++[†] |

From Bigos SJ, Bowyer O, Braen G, et al. *Acute Low Back Problems in Adults*. Clinical Practice Guideline No 14. Washington DC: US Department of Health and Human Services, Agency for Health Care Policy and Research, December 1994.

*Risk of complications (radiation, infection—highest for myelo-CT, second highest for myelography, and relatively less risk for bone scan, radiography, and CT).

[†]False-positive diagnostic findings in up to 30% of people without symptoms at age 30 years.

[‡]Number of plus signs indicates relative ability to identify or define.

ESR, erythrocyte sedimentation rate; CBC, complete blood count; UA, urine analysis; EMG, electromyography; SEP, sensory evoked potential; CT, computed tomography; MRI, magnetic resonance imaging.

could predict outcome at 1 year in the absence of surgery. EMG, however, is of no significant value in the first 3 to 4 weeks before the onset of acute denervation spontaneous activity and tends to normalize over time in many patients.

The reason for the lack of sensitivity of EMG in detecting the involved nerve root can be extrapolated from the data presented by Levin et al.[46] These authors correlated the preoperative EMG findings in 50 patients who had surgically proven solitary-root lesions. Table 2–4 is derived from their data and demonstrates the wide distribution of denervation potentials from isolated nerve root lesions. Even with extensive sampling of muscles, there is sufficient overlap to miss a nerve root by one level. The pattern, however, is accurate enough to obtain a diagnosis within two levels. Similar tables can be drawn for the lumbar spine. However, as Wilbourn and Aminoff[63] point out, it is virtually impossible to differentiate between L2, L3, and L4 radiculopathies because of overlap of the myotomes. An L5 radiculopathy is defined by abnormalities in the tibialis posterior, internal hamstring, and gluteus medius muscles. An S1 and S2 radiculopathy is defined by abnormalities in the lateral gastrocnemius, external hamstring, and gluteus maximus muscles.

Reflex studies (H-reflexes and F-responses) have the advantage of showing abnormal results immediately after the onset of a neuropathy. H-reflex testing is of particular value because it has a high (90% to 100%) true-positive rate for S1 radiculopathies with a low false-positive rate.[2,15] The evaluation of H-reflex response has become almost routine, com-

**TABLE 2–4. Correlation Between Positive Electromyography and Surgically Defined Root Level of Involvement**

| Muscle | C5 (N = 7) | C6 (N = 9) | C7 (N = 28) | C8 (N = 6) |
|---|---|---|---|---|
| Supraspinatus | 28% | 22% | | |
| Infraspinatus | 71% | 33% | | |
| Deltoid | 78% | 33% | | |
| Brachioradialis | 71% | 55% | | |
| Biceps brachii | 71% | 44% | | |
| Pronator teres | | 77% | 60% | |
| Flexor carpi radialis | | 44% | 89% | |
| Triceps brachii | | 55% | 96% | 16% |
| Anconeus | | 44% | 53% | |
| Extensor digitorum communis | | 11% | 10% | 16% |
| Extensor indicis proprius | | | 3.5% | 100% |
| Flexor pollicis longus | | | | 66% |
| Abductor pollicis brevis | | | | 50% |
| First dorsal interosseous | | | 3.5% | 91% |
| Abductor digiti minimi | | | | 91% |
| Paraspinals | 71% | 55% | 28% | 66% |

Derived from Levin KH, Maggiano HJ, Wilbourn AJ. Cervical radiculopathies: comparison of surgical and EMG localization of single root lesions. *Neurology*. 1996;46:1123.

bined with EMG when an S1 radiculopathy is suspected. Its usefulness, however, is diminished in patients with peripheral neuropathy or in elderly patients in whom the response may be difficult to elicit. F-responses are more controversial and have a poorer correlation with imaging studies.

Somatosensory evoked potentials (SEPs) have been proposed for the evaluation of sensory radiculopathies, neurogenic claudication, and myelopathy. The most convincing studies have dealt with myelopathies due to multiple sclerosis, cervical spondylosis, or tumors. The AHCPR panel recommendation for the use of SEPs for diagnosis of spinal stenosis was based in part on a paper by Stolov and Slimp[55] that demonstrated a 94% correlation with surgical results. The use of dermatomal SEPs or small sensory nerve SEPs for measurement of sensory radiculopathy has led to variable results.

The combination of thermography and surface EMG has been proposed as a means of documenting radiculopathy, but this approach has been hampered by variability in reported sensitivity and specificity, excessive claims, and lack of demonstration that these methods assist the physician in treatment decisions or in changing patient outcomes. Most reviews of these tests by independent agencies have resulted in negative recommendations for their use.[3,10]

The value of imaging studies (CT, MRI, myelography, and CT myelography) has been strengthened by an abundance of research documenting the ability of these tests to define anatomy. The primary weaknesses of these tests are a high false-positive rate and high cost. These factors have led to increasingly stringent criteria for ordering the tests. If no red flags are present, testing is generally not recommended within the first month.[10] After 1 month the primary criteria for ordering these tests is the documentation of a surgically amenable lesion. The other issue that is a source of debate is determination of the preferable test to order. Sensitivity and specificity varies somewhat among tests. For myelography the true-positive rate has been reported to be between 75% and 94%, with a true-negative rate of 55% to 100%.[1,36,37,43] CT scanning has been described as having a true-positive rate for lumbar disk herniation that varies from 60% to 91% and a true-negative rate that ranges from 57% to 100%. Bosacco et al,[14] Gillström et al,[25] and Haughton et al[35] noted that combining CT and myelography greatly increased the true-positive rate and diminished the false-positive rate. Other studies, however, have not shown significant differences between MRI scanning, CT, and CT myelography in terms of false-positive and false-negative rates.[40,56] Since MRI is noninvasive, does not involve radiation, covers a large area of the spine, and images soft tissues other than disk, it has become the imaging test of choice, when available, in the diagnosis of structural causes of radiculopathy.

Since CT scanning is superior to MRI in imaging of bony structures, CT has been perceived as the test of choice for spinal stenosis, either with or without contrast.[6,59] However, a detailed review of the literature and an attempted meta-analysis by Kent et al[41] failed to demonstrate that CT scanning was significantly more sensitive or specific than MRI in the diagnosis of stenosis.

Diskography with and without CT scanning was reviewed in depth by the AHCPR panel, which concluded that the potential complications and the invasive nature of the test could not be justified by the limited evidence that it would help select patients for surgery.[10]

## CHRONIC NONSPECIFIC LOW BACK PAIN

The data supporting the use of different tests for patients with back pain within the first 3 to 6 months are often inconclusive, variable in quality, and difficult to analyze. These data, however, are considerably better than the data on the value of testing in patients with back or neck pain of more than 6 months' duration. Many of the assumptions made for acute back pain (e.g., a direct correlation between symptoms, disability, and pathologic condition) seem to break down in management of the patient with chronic pain.[31] The close correlation between the clinical examination, EMG, and imaging studies reported in patients with acute pain is not as clear in patients with chronic disability, especially in the workers' compensation arena.[34] It can be assumed that the red flags for serious and progressive pathologic diseases have been ruled out in the evaluation of acute back pain.

The greatest predictors of disability associated with back pain appear to be psychosocial rather than physical.[9,60] Multiple factors, such as litigation, workers' compensation, loneliness, and coping skills, have been considered significant in the prediction of chronic disability in patients with back pain. These studies suggest that testing for psychosocial factors may be more productive than testing for pathology. Simple tests such as pain drawings and the Minnesota Multiphasic Personality Inventory (MMPI) have helped to determine the likelihood of success following surgery[48,64] and should be considered in such patients. Other psychological tests, however, have yet to be demonstrated to influence the outcome of patients with chronic back pain.

## CHRONIC BACK AND NECK PAIN WITH NEUROLOGIC SYMPTOMS

The most challenging patients to evaluate are the individual with chronic back or neck pain who complains of increasing pain or disability or the person who presents with new onset of numbness, weakness, and bowel, bladder, or sexual dysfunction. These patients have commonly undergone one or more surgical procedures, often with residual permanent neurologic deficits. The new symptoms or progressive complaints are often presented in vague terms, and the examination findings can be extremely variable and unreliable. To make matters more difficult, managed care monitors often insist on definitive justification for each test and refuse to authorize testing based on vague (rule-out) diagnoses. Furthermore, none of the agencies or associations have felt capable of addressing this issue, thus leaving physicians and patients in a vacuum.

It is no longer acceptable to order repeat imaging studies every time a patient presents with minor changes in symptoms or states that he or she feels worse. It is becoming increasingly necessary to assess such patients in a stepwise fashion with a well-defined anticipated conclusion and outcome. When there is a major change in the form of a new red flag (e.g., fever, newly discovered neoplasm, major trauma, new-onset paresis, or incontinence), the patient's condition is no longer considered chronic, and it can be managed as an acute condition. When the new or progressive symptoms are vague or generalized, the problem is more difficult.

Vague symptoms of bladder urgency, constipation, decreased sexual function, or loss of balance and coordination raise the specter of progressive cauda equina symptoms or myelopathy. These symptoms, however, can be due to a wide variety of nonneurologic or unrelated neurologic conditions. Metabolic disturbances such as diabetes can cause these symptoms through peripheral neuropathy, whereas central nervous system disorders such as multiple sclerosis may have similar presenting symptoms. There is no reason why patients with back or neck pain could not have these diseases. In fact, back pain has a greater incidence in these patients than in the general population.[8,39]

The patient with back or neck pain and subacute or chronic changes in bladder or bowel function is particularly challenging. In this patient population the primary goal is to differentiate neurogenic from nonneurogenic causes. Results of cystometry and penile tumescence studies, when normal, may reduce the likelihood of a neurologic cause of these symptoms. When the results are abnormal, however, it becomes necessary to do further testing to isolate the cause. Peripheral nerve conduction testing should be able to isolate the presence or absence of a peripheral neuropathy. SEPs from lower extremity nerves may help to determine the presence of a myelopathy or brainstem lesion. SEPs from the pu-

dendal nerve combined with bulbocavernosus reflex studies can further help differentiate cauda equina or pudendal nerve lesions from spinal cord lesions affecting the lower sacral centers.[33] Needle EMG can demonstrate acute denervation in a progressive radiculopathy.

When a neurologic deficit is determined to be new or progressive on physical examination or electrodiagnostic testing, imaging can be justified and directed at the source of a potential treatable lesion. In postsurgical patients the test of choice to differentiate epidural scarring from recurrent disk herniation is gadolinium-enhanced MRI. Arachnoiditis often is best viewed by water-soluble myelography.

## CONCLUSION

The use of expensive, often invasive testing in the management of patients with back and neck pain is undergoing intense scrutiny for sensitivity, specificity, and effect on patient outcomes. Figure 2–2, which reflects the conclusion from the Quebec Task Force on Whiplash-Associated Disorders, illustrates the vagueness of consensus guidelines for the use of diagnostic testing.

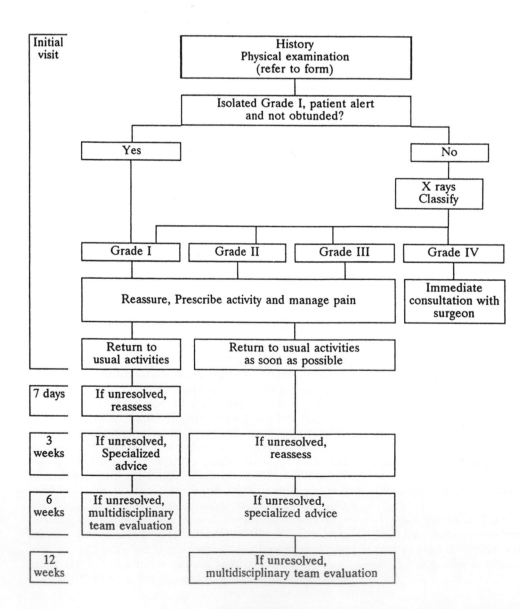

**FIGURE 2–2.** Recommendations from Quebec Task Force on Whiplash-Associated Disorders. (From Cassidy JD, ed. Scientific monograph of the Quebec Task Force on Whiplash-Associated Disorders. *Spine*. 1995;20(suppl 85):375.

The majority of patients with acute uncomplicated back and neck pain recover spontaneously without the necessity of testing. Red flags for fracture or dislocation require specific x-ray studies or CT scanning, or MRI. Red flags for neoplastic or infectious diseases require a determination of sedimentation rate, a complete blood count, x-rays or other imaging studies, and possibly a technetium bone scan. Red flags for myelopathy or cauda equina syndrome require imaging studies with or without myelography.

In patients with acute back or neck pain radiating to the extremities without progressive neurologic deficits, the symptoms often resolve spontaneously. When symptoms persist for longer than 1 month or become worse, the search for a surgical lesion by means of physiologic tests (EMG, H-reflexes, and SEPs) and anatomic studies (x-ray, CT, MRI, myelography) may be necessary with specific indications for each test.

Chronic nonspecific back and neck pain may not correlate well with standard diagnostic testing. The strong association of chronic disability with psychosocial issues suggests the potential value of pain drawings, MMPI, and other psychologic tests, but the effect of such tests on patient outcomes remains unknown. Patients with chronic pain complaints with or without prior surgery or persistent neurologic deficits may develop new or progressive symptoms, which can be analyzed only through the use of specific testing of bladder and sexual dysfunction, epidural scarring, recurrent disk herniation, or stenosis.

## REFERENCES

1. Aejmelaeus R, Hiltunen H, Härkönen M, et al. Myelographic versus clinical diagnostics in lumbar disc disease. *Arch Orthop Trauma Surg.* 1984;103(1):18-25.
2. Aiello I, Serra G, Tugnoli V, et al. Electrophysiological findings in patients with lumbar disc prolapse. *Electromyogr Clin Neurophysiol.* 1984;24(4):313-320.
3. American Academy of Neurology (AAN) Therapeutics and Technology Assessment Subcommittee. Assessment: thermography in neurologic practice. *Neurology.* 1990;40:523-525.
4. Andersson GBJ. The epidemiology of spinal disorders. In: Frymoyer JW, ed. *The Adult Spine: Principles and Practice.* New York: Raven Press; 1991:107-146.
5. Aronson HA, Dunsmore RH. Herniated upper lumbar discs. *J Bone Joint Surg.* 1963;45:311-317.
6. Bell GR, Rothman RH, Booth RE, et al. A study of computer-assisted tomography. II. Comparison of metrizamide myelography and computed tomography in the diagnosis of herniated lumbar disc and spinal stenosis. *Spine.* 1984;9(6):552-556.
7. Berquist T. *Imaging of Orthopedic Trauma and Surgery.* Philadelphia: WB Saunders; 1986.
8. Biering-Sorensen F, Hansen FR, Schrull M, Runeborg O. The relation of spinal x-ray to low back pain and physical activity among 60-year-old men and women. *Spine.* 1985;10(5):445-451.
9. Bigos SJ, Battie M, et al. *A Longitudinal, Prospective Study of Acute Industrial Back Problems: The Influence of Physical and Non-physical Factors.* Kyoto, Japan: Proceedings, International Society for the Study of the Lumbar Spine, 1989:19.
10. Bigos SJ, Bowyer O, Braen G, et al. *Acute Low Back Problems in Adults.* Clinical Practice Guideline No 14. Washington, DC: US Department of Health and Human Services, Agency for Health Care Policy and Research, December 1994.
11. Bigos SJ, Hansson T, Castillo RN, et al. The value of preemployment roentgenographs for predicting acute back injury claims and chronic back pain disability. *Clin Orthop.* 1992;283:124-129.
12. Bischoff C, Meyer BU, Machetanz J, Conrad B. The value of magnetic stimulation in the diagnosis of radiculopathies. *Muscle Nerve.* 1993;16:154-161.
13. Boden SD, Davis DO, Dina TS, et al. Abnormal magnetic resonance scans of the lumbar spine in asymptomatic subjects. *J Bone Joint Surg Am.* 1990;72(3):403-408.
14. Bosacco SJ, Berman AT, Garbarino JL, et al. A comparison of CT scanning and myelography in the diagnosis of lumbar disc herniation. *Clin Orthop.* 1984;190:124-128.
15. Braddom RI, Johnson EW. Standardization of H reflex and diagnostic use in S1 radiculopathy. *Arch Phys Med Rehabil.* 1974;55:161-166.
16. Cassidy JD, ed. Scientific monograph of the Quebec Task Force on Whiplash-Associated Disorders. *Spine.* 1994;20(suppl 85):1S-73S.
17. Cats-Baril WL, Frymoyer JW. The economics of spinal disorders. In: Frymoyer JW, ed. *The Adult Spine: Principles and Practice.* New York: Raven Press; 1991.
18. Corcoran RJ, Thrall JH, Kyle RW, et al. Solitary abnormalities in bone scans of patients with extraosseous malignancies. *Radiology.* 1976;121:663-667.
19. Cunningham LS, Kelsey JL. Epidemiology of musculoskeletal impairments and associated disability. *Am J Public Health.* 1984;74:574-579.
20. Dalinka M, Boorstein J, Zlatkin M. Computed tomography of musculoskeletal trauma. *Radiol Clin North Am.* 1989;27:933-944.
21. Deyo RA, Diehl AK. Cancer as a cause of back pain: frequency, clinical presentation, and diagnostic strategies. *J Gen Intern Med.* 1988;3(3):230-238.
22. Deyo RA, Tsui-Wu YJ. Descriptive epidemiology of low-back pain and its related medical care in the United States. *Spine.* 1987;12(3):264-268.
23. Frymoyer JW, Durett CI. The economics of spinal disorders. In: Frymoyer JW, ed. *The Adult Spine.* Philadelphia: Lippincott-Raven; 1997:143-150.
24. Fullenlove TM, Williams AJ. Comparative roentgen findings in symptomatic and asymptomatic backs. *Radiology.* 1957;68:572-574.
25. Gillström P, Ericsson K, Hindmarsh T. A comparison of computed tomography and myelography in the diagnosis of lumbar disc herniation. *Arch Orthop Trauma Surg.* 1986;106(1):12-14.
26. Gore DR, Sepic SB, Gardner GM. Roentgenographic findings of the cervical spine in asymptomatic people. *Spine.* 1986;11:521-524.
27. Gore DR, Sepic SB, Gardner GM, Murray MP. Neck pain: a long-term follow-up of 205 patients. *Spine.* 1987;12:1-5.
28. Gran JT. An epidemiological survey of the signs and symptoms of ankylosing spondylitis. *Clin Rheumatol.* 1985;4(2):161-169.
29. Grazier KL, Holbrook TL, et al, eds. *The Frequency of Occurrence, Impact, and Cost of Musculoskeletal Conditions in the United States.* Chicago: American Academy of Orthopedic Surgeons; 1984.
30. Hakelius A, Hindmarsh J. The comparative reliability of preoperative diagnostic methods in lumbar disc surgery. *Acta Orthop Scand.* 1972;43:234-238.
31. Haldeman S. Failure of the pathology model to predict back pain. Presidential Address, North American Spine Society. *Spine.* 1990;15(7):718-724.
32. Haldeman S. The neurodiagnostic evaluation of spinal stenosis. In: Andersson GBJ, McNeil TW, eds. *Lumbar Spinal Stenosis.* St Louis: Mosby; 1992.
33. Haldeman S, Bradley WE, Bhatia NN. Evoked responses from the pudendal nerve. *J Urol.* 1982;128:974-980.
34. Haldeman S, Shouka M, Robboy S. Computed tomography, electrodiagnostic and clinical findings in chronic workers' compensation patients with back and leg pain. *Spine.* 1988;13:345-350.
35. Haughton VM, Eldevik OP, Magnaes B, Amundsen P. A prospective comparison of computed tomography and myelography in the diagnosis of herniated lumbar discs. *Radiology.* 1982;142(1):103-110.
36. Herron LD, Turner J. Patient selection for lumbar laminectomy and discectomy with a revised objective rating system. *Clin Orthop.* 1985;199:145-152.
37. Hirsch C, Nachemson A. The reliability of lumber disc surgery. *Clin Orthop.* 1963;29-189.
38. Hitselberger WD, Witten RM. Abnormal myelograms in asymptomatic patients. *J Neurosurg.* 1968;28:204-208.
39. Holm S. Does diabetes induce degenerative processes in the lumbar intervertebral disc? Kyoto, Japan: Proceedings, International Society for the Study of the Lumber Spine; 1989:8.
40. Jackson RP, Cain JE, Jacobs RR, et al. The neuroradiographic diagnosis of lumbar herniated nucleus pulposus. II: a comparison of computed tomography (CT), myelography, CT-myelography, and magnetic resonance imaging. *Spine.* 1989;14(12):1362-1367.
41. Kent DL, Haynor DR, et al. Diagnosis of lumbar spine stenosis in adults: a metaanalysis of the accuracy of CT, MR, and myelography. *AJR.* 1994;158:1135-1144.
42. Khatri BO, Baruah J, McQuillen MP. Correlation of electromyography with computed tomography in evaluation of lower back pain. *Arch Neurol.* 1984;41(6):594-597.

43. Kortelainen P, Puranen J, Koivisto E, Lähde S. Symptoms and signs of sciatica and their relation to the localization of the lumbar disc herniation. *Spine*. 1985;10(1):88-92.

44. Kosteljanetz M, Espersen JO, Halaburt H, Miletic T. Predictive value of clinical and surgical findings in patients with lumbago-sciatica: a prospective study (Part I). *Acta Neurochir (Wien)*. 1984;73(1-2):67-76.

45. Kostuik JP, Huler RJ, et al. Thoracolumbar spine fracture. In: Frymoyer JW, ed. *The Adult Spine: Principles and Practice*. New York: Raven Press; 1991.

46. Levin KH, Maggiano HJ, Wilbourn AJ. Cervical radiculopathies: comparison of surgical and EMG localization of single root lesions. *Neurology*. 1996;46:1021-1025.

47. Mooney V. Differential diagnosis of low back disorders: principles of classification. In: Frymoyer JW, ed. *The Adult Spine: Principles and Practice*. New York: Raven Press, 1991.

48. Rausford AO, Cairns D, Mooney V. The pain drawing as an aid to the psychological evaluation of patients with low back pain. *Spine*. 1976;1:127-134.

49. Scavone JG, Latshaw RF, Rohrer GV. Use of lumbar spine films: statistical evaluation at a university teaching hospital. *JAMA*. 1981;246:1105-1108.

50. Spangfort EV. The lumbar disc herniation. *Acta Orth Scand*. 1972;142(suppl):1-95.

51. Spengler DM, Freeman CW. Patient selection for lumbar discectomy: an objective approach. *Spine*. 1979;4(2):129-134.

52. Spengler DM, Ouellette EA, Battie M, Zeh J. Elective discectomy for herniation of a lumbar disc: additional experience with an objective method. *J Bone Joint Surg Am*. 1990;72(2):230-237.

53. Spitzer WO, et al [Quebec Task Force on Spinal Disorders]. Scientific approach to the assessment and management of activity-related spinal disorders: a monograph for clinicians. Report of the Quebec Task Force on Spinal Disorders. *Spine*. 1987;12:S1-S59.

54. Sternbach RA. Survey of pain in the United States: the Nuprin pain report. *Clin J Pain*. 1986;2(1):49-53.

55. Stolov WC, Slimp JC. Dermatomal somatosensory evoked potentials in lumbar spinal stenosis. *Am Assoc Electromyograph Electrodiagn, Am Electroencephalograph Soc Joint Symp*. 1988:17-22.

56. Szypryt EP, Twining P, Wilde GP, et al. Diagnosis of lumbar disc protrusion: a comparison between magnetic resonance imaging and radiculopathy. *J Bone Joint Surg Br*. 1988;70(5):717-722.

57. Turner JA, Ersek M, Herron L, Deyo R. Surgery for lumbar spinal stenosis: attempted meta-analysis of the literature. *Spine*. 1992;17(1):1-8.

58. Vällfors B. Acute, subacute and chronic low back pain: clinical symptoms, absenteeism and working environment. *Scand J Rehab Med*. 1985;11(suppl):1-98.

59. Voelker JL, Mealey J Jr, Eskridge JM, Gilmor RL. Metrizamide-enhanced computed tomography as an adjunct to metrizamide myelography in the evaluation of lumbar disc herniation and spondylosis. *Neurosurgery*. 1987;20(3):379-384.

60. Waddell G. Biopsychosocial analysis of low back pain. *Baillieres Clin Rheumatol*. 1992;6(3):523-557.

61. Waldvogel FA, Vasey H. Osteomyelitis: the past decade. *N Engl J Med*. 1980;303(7):360-370.

62. Wiesel SW, Tsourmas N, Feffer HL, et al. A study of computer-assisted tomography. I. The incidence of positive CAT scans in an asymptomatic group of patients. *Spine*. 1984;9(6):549-551.

63. Wilbourn AJ, Aminoff MJ. The electrophysiologic examination in patients with radiculopathy. *Muscle Nerve*. 1988;11:1099-1114.

64. Wiltse LL, Rocchio PD. Preoperative psychological tests as predictors of success of chemonucleolysis in the treatment of the low back syndrome. *J Bone Joint Surg Am*. 1975;57A:478-483.

65. Young A, Getty J, Jackson A, et al. Variations in the pattern of muscle innervation by the L1 and S1 nerve roots. *Spine*. 1983;8(6):616-624.

# Section II

# CENTRAL NERVOUS SYSTEM DISORDERS

# Alzheimer's Disease

*Thomas A. Sandson and Bruce H. Price*

In recent years, dramatic progress has been made in understanding the neurogenetics and pathophysiologic bases of Alzheimer's disease (AD).[50] Four different genes have been associated with AD, and transgenic mice have been produced that develop memory deficits and many of the pathologic features of AD. Furthermore, the mechanisms by which amyloid deposition, cytoskeletal destabilization, inflammation, oxidative stress, and hormonal changes may produce neuronal degeneration in AD are being delineated. Rationale pharmacologic interventions based on these discoveries are developing rapidly. Therefore the clinical diagnosis of AD has become increasingly important. However, the accurate diagnosis of AD, especially in the early stages and in atypical cases, remains a difficult challenge. The differential diagnosis of Alzheimer's disease is extensive (Table 3–1), and there are few established biologic markers to use in reliably differentiating the specific causes of dementia. Although sound clinical decision making remains the cornerstone of diagnosis, a number of promising ancillary tests have recently become available. This chapter reviews the potential role of various diagnostic modalities in the evaluation of patients with dementia.

Many standard textbooks contain formidable lists of the causes of dementia, including many systemic and psychiatric illnesses and almost every disease process that can affect the brain. The diagnosis of AD is often said to be made by a process of exclusion. Improved understanding of the clinical features of AD is changing the focus from one of exclusion to one of inclusion. Nonetheless, it is still necessary to consider the broad differential diagnosis of conditions that can cause dementia. As noted elsewhere,[143] a careful history, past medical history, and family history should be taken from both the patient and family or associates whenever a patient presents with cognitive or behavioral decline. A thorough physical and neurologic examination also needs to be performed. Table 3–1 reviews abnormalities found on the neurologic examination that may suggest particular etiologic bases of dementia.

The laboratory workup of a patient with suspected dementia should be individualized according to the clinical situation. The Quality Standards Subcommittee of the American Academy of Neurology (AAN) recommends the following blood work: complete blood cell count, serum electrolyte levels, calcium level, glucose level, blood urea nitrogen concentration, creatinine level, liver function, thyroid-stimulating hormone level, free thyroid index, serum vitamin $B_{12}$ level, and syphilis serologic value.[135] A recent retrospective study[25] found that these laboratory studies were pertinent to patient management in 13% of cases and changed the diagnosis in 9% of cases. In addition to these laboratory tests, we often obtain a urinalysis and an erythrocyte sedimentation rate. Other tests, such as human immunodeficiency virus (HIV), toxicology screen, antinuclear antibody, Lyme titer, heavy metals, arterial blood gas, and anti-Hu antibody, may be useful in selected cases. A number of pediatric neurodegenerative conditions, some treatable, can cause dementia in adults and can be diagnosed with special studies.[29] A chest x-ray examination and ECG should also be considered if they have not been done recently, especially if there is a history of cardiac or pulmonary disease or tobacco use.

The structural neuroimaging studies most commonly used today are computed tomography (CT) and magnetic

| TABLE 3–1. Neurologic Findings and Associated Dementias | |
|---|---|
| FINDING | ASSOCIATED DEMENTING ILLNESS |
| Ataxia | AzD, cerebellar degenerations, GM$_2$ gangliosidosis, Med, MS, prion disease, PML, WK, WD |
| Dysarthria | AzD, dementia pugilistica, dialysis dementia, HS, MND, MS, PML, PSP, WD |
| Dystonic or choreoathetotic movements | AzD, HS, HD, ICBG, PD, WD |
| Extrapyramidal signs | AD, ALSPDG, AzD, dementia pugilistica, DLBD, GM$_1$ gangliosidosis type III, HS, HD, ICBG, Med, MID, multiple systems atrophy, neuroacanthocytosis, NPH, PD, postencephalitic parkinsonism, PSP, striatonigral degeneration, SSPE, WD |
| Extraocular movements | Gaucher's disease type 1, Kearns-Sayre syndrome, MID, MS, Niemann-Pick disease type IIc, PSP, WK |
| Gait disorder | AMN, AzD, dementia pugilistica, MID, MS, NPH, PD, PSP, syphilis, WK |
| Neuropathy | AMN, ADC, B$_{12}$ deficiency, MLD, porphyria, Med, thyroid disease, uremia |
| Myoclonus | Dialysis dementia, HS, Kufs' disease, Lafora's disease, MERRF, prion disease, SSPE |
| Pyramidal tract signs | AMN, ADC, B$_{12}$ deficiency, GM$_2$ gangliosidosis, HS, Kufs' disease, MLD, MND, MID, MS, PML, syphilis, spinocerebellar degenerations |

From Sandson TA, Price BH. Diagnostic testing and dementia. *Neurol Clin.* 1996;14:47.

AD, Alzheimer's disease; ADC, AIDS dementia complex; ALSPDG, amyotrophic lateral sclerosis–parkinsonism–dementia complex; AMN, adrenomyeloneuropathy; AzD, Azorean disease; DLBD, diffuse Lewy body disease; HD, Huntington's disease; HS, Hallervorden-Spatz disease; ICBG, idiopathic calcification of basal ganglia; Med, medications and toxins; MERRF, myopathy and encephalopathy with ragged red fibers; MID, multiinfarct dementia; MLD, metachromatic leukodystrophy; MND, motor neuron disease; MS, multiple sclerosis; NPH, normal pressure hydrocephalus; PD, Parkinson's disease; PML, progressive multifocal leukoencephalopathy; PSP, progressive supranuclear palsy; SSPE, subacute sclerosing panencephalitis; WD, Wilson's disease; WK, Wernicke-Korsakoff syndrome.

resonance imaging (MRI). Both modalities provide remarkable neuroanatomic detail and can reliably detect potentially treatable conditions, such as tumors, abscesses, subdural hematomas, and hydrocephalus, that may produce dementia. MRI provides spatial resolution and contrast sensitivity superior to those of CT and offers the advantage of multiplanar display. In particular, MRI is much more sensitive than CT in detecting white matter hyperintensity (WMH).[44,84] However, this increased sensitivity comes at the cost of diminished specificity, and the clinical significance of WMH noted on MRI is often unclear.

Controversy exists as to whether an imaging study should be done routinely in the evaluation of patients with dementia.[26,90] Bradshaw et al[19] performed CT scans on 500 consecutive patients diagnosed with dementia and found a potentially treatable lesion, including tumor, hydrocephalus or subdural hematoma, in 10%. Half of these patients had no signs or symptoms except dementia. Similarly, structural neuroimaging studies altered patient management in 15% of the 119 cases reviewed by Chui and Zhang.[25] They found that clinical indicators such as early onset, noninsidious course, focal signs, and gait disturbance were only 67% sensitive in detecting surgically treatable lesions. Therefore these authors concluded that the "selective use of neuroimaging studies remains an elusive challenge." On the other hand, Engel and Gelber[42] detected CT findings "of possible clinical significance" in 5% of patients meeting strict clinical criteria for AD and in 34% of dementia patients not meeting these clinical criteria. No patients in the AD group and 9% of patients in the non-AD group had "potentially treatable lesions." Therefore Engel and Gelber suggested that CT should be done selectively based on clinical criteria.

The yield of lumbar puncture in unselected patients with dementia is low.[5] However, a lumbar puncture should be done whenever infection, vasculitis, inflammatory disease, carcinomatous meningitis, or transmissible spongiform encephalopathy is being considered. Removal of a large volume of cerebrospinal fluid (CSF) or measuring CSF outflow resistance via a lumbar or ventricular infusion test may be helpful in determining which patients with normal pressure hydro-

cephalus (NPH) will respond to shunting.[63,70,171] However, the sensitivity and specificity of these tests remains unknown. An electroencephalogram (EEG) is of limited specificity in the evaluation of patients with dementia because of overlap with normal age-related changes. Reduction of EEG amplitude and slowing of the posterior alpha rhythm are commonly seen in early AD, but these signs are not specific. Focal slow activity may be seen in vascular dementia (VaD). Widespread slow-wave activity suggests a toxic-metabolic encephalopathy. Periodic sharp-wave complexes are important in the diagnosis of Creutzfeldt-Jakob disease, although their absence does not exclude the diagnosis. Computer-assisted spectral analysis of EEG activity is probably not significantly more useful than a conventional EEG.[4]

## TESTING THE TESTS

Before a discussion of diagnostic modalities that may help with the inclusionary diagnosis of AD, it is useful to consider how diagnostic tests for AD are assessed. The accuracy of a diagnostic test is frequently measured by its sensitivity, specificity, and predictive values. The sensitivity of a test for AD is the probability that a patient with AD will test positive, whereas its specificity is the probability that a patient without AD will test negative. In addition, it is necessary to consider the prevalence of the disease in the population being tested. For example, if a disease is common in a particular population, a screening test must be highly sensitive to be useful. Otherwise, a negative test result will often be a false-negative. Based on age alone, the prior probability of AD in a person older than 85 may be as high as 47%.[46] The negative predictive value of a test is the probability that a person with a negative result does not have the disease. This value represents the likelihood of having a true-negative test result divided by the chance of either a true-negative or a false-negative test result. Similarly, the positive predictive value of a test is the probability that a person with a positive result actually has the disease. It represents the likelihood of having a true-positive test result divided by the chance of either a true-positive or a false-positive result.

To determine a test's sensitivity, specificity, and predictive values, a "gold standard" for diagnosing AD is needed. Neuropathology has traditionally been considered the gold standard by which diagnostic tests for AD are compared. However, as we learn more about the neurogenetic and neurobiologic aspects of AD, the limitations of even neuropathologic diagnosis are become increasingly apparent. For example, not all patients who meet pathologic criteria for AD are demented. In fact, 43% of patients in the Nun Study who met neuropathologic criteria for AD were not considered to be demented based on a battery of neuropsychologic tests.[158] On the other hand, Roses[140] described a nice example of a patient with AD who did not meet neuropathologic criteria for AD. The patient and her sister had the same mutation in the amyloid precursor protein gene. Both sisters developed early-onset dementia. Despite having the same age of onset, the same disease course, and the same apolipoprotein E (apo E) genotype, one sister met the neuropathologic criteria for AD but the other did not. Most studies done to assess diagnostic tests for AD have used clinical rather than pathologic criteria to determine the sensitivity and specificity of the test. The control groups are usually age-matched "normals" or patients who have been diagnosed clinically with other forms of dementia, such as vascular or frontotemporal dementia. These studies are limited by inadequacies in clinical diagnosis that create the need for the diagnostic test in the first place.

Finally, the clinical utility of a diagnostic test depends on its ability to improve the diagnostic accuracy of the clinical evaluation. The diagnostic accuracy for a clinical diagnosis of AD is usually quite high. However, it is significantly lower in the early stages of the disease and in patients with atypical presentations.[20,136] It is in such situations that ancillary diagnostic tests will likely prove most useful.

## CLINICAL CRITERIA AND NEUROPSYCHOLOGICAL PROFILE

The most commonly used diagnostic criteria for AD are those established by the National Institute of Neurological and Communicative Disorders and Stroke–Alzheimer's Disease and Related Disorders Association (NINCDS-ADRDA) in 1984.[113] A diagnosis of probable AD (PRAD) requires dementia, progressive memory loss, deficits in two or more areas of cognition, and the absence of any other disorder that could account for the progressive deficits. From 81% to 92% of patients who meet NINCDS-ADRDA criteria for PRAD also meet pathologic criteria for AD.[9,12,95,164] Interrater reliability is quite high for experienced clinicians.[9,94] However, the specificity of NINCDS-ADRDA and other clinical criteria for a diagnosis of AD is relatively low,[110] and approximately one third of those patients with a clinical diagnosis of PRAD and neuropathologic findings of AD will have additional pathologic changes such as infarcts or cortical Lewy bodies.[60,61] Hachinski's ischemic score is useful in differentiating patients with AD from those with VaD and is frequently used as an exclusion criterion in clinical trials of medications for AD.[117,139,168] However, the ischemic score cannot reliably distinguish patients with pathologic features of AD from patients with both pathologic features of AD and infarcts.[107] Diagnostic criteria have been proposed for VaD by the National Institute for Neurological Disorders and Stroke with the Association Internationale pour la Recherche et l'Enseignement en Neurosciences (NINDS-AIREN), but the related research awaits validity and reliability studies.[138] One recent retrospective clinicopathologic study found a sensitivity of 58% and a specificity of 80% for the NINDS-AIREN criteria.[65] Twenty-nine percent of cases with mixed dementia were misclassified as having VaD.

The pattern of cognitive dysfunction determined by neuropsychologic testing or careful bedside mental status testing by the physician usually corresponds to the predominant site of neuropathologic evidence and can greatly aid in the diagnosis of AD. Early pathologic changes in AD preferentially affect the temporolimbic regions (hippocampus and adjacent parahippocampal, entorhinal, and perirhinal cortexes) and the cholinergic systems.[10,132] Because these structures are believed to perform a central role in memory,[160] it is not surprising that episodic memory deficits are often the earliest manifestation of AD and may help predict the onset of dementia in elderly individuals with mild cognitive impairment.[14,80,108,165] Price et al[131] described 39 patients with dementia characterized by salient progressive memory loss noted at autopsy. Only one patient did not meet neuropathologic criteria for AD. Therefore demented patients with a typical clinical and neuropsychologic presentation for AD have a very high likelihood of meeting neuropathologic criteria for AD.

## STRUCTURAL NEUROIMAGING STUDIES

Involutional changes, including sulcal enlargement and ventricular dilatation, occur in normal aging and in dementing illnesses such as AD and VaD.[28,163] Various techniques, such as qualitative ratings, linear measures, planimetry, and volumetric measures, have been used to assess for atrophy by CT and MRI.[33] Some studies have found that these measures of atrophy, especially volumetric measures, can differentiate patients with AD from age-matched controls[2,59,62,82,159,163] and that these measures correlate with the degree of cognitive dysfunction.[37,62,159] Other studies have revealed significant overlap in the degree of atrophy between AD patients and controls.[33,48,172] Measures of atrophy appear to lack sensitivity and specificity on account of marked intersubject variability, which increases with age.[32,48,172] Longitudinal studies of the rate of atrophy on serial CTs and MRIs control for intersubject variability and appear to better differentiate AD patients from controls.[32,55,106] The rate of volume loss on serial MRIs may also predict the onset of AD in asymptomatic patients at risk for AD.[55]

A number of studies have found that regional atrophy of temporal lobe structures, particularly the enterorhinal cortex, temporal neocortex, amygdala, and hippocampus, may distinguish patients with AD from age-matched controls better than measures of global atrophy.[45,78,83,92,101,102,151,153] In addition, memory loss appears to correlate well with the degree of hippocampal atrophy in patients with AD.[47] AD patients who are homozygous for the apo E4 allele have more severe medial temporal atrophy than do AD patients with other apolipoprotein genotypes.[100] Hippocampal atrophy appears to be a sensitive marker of early AD,[79] and a recent longitudinal study of patients at risk for familial AD revealed hippocampal formation atrophy prior to the onset of symptoms.[56] However, the specificity of hippocampal atrophy remains uncertain because it has also been described in patients with VaD and Parkinson's disease.[97] One study of amygdala atrophy did find that it could be used to distinguish patients with AD from patients with other forms of dementia.[109]

The relationship between dementia and periventricular lucencies, or leuko-araiosis, on CT (or WMH on MRI) remains unclear. These lesions are commonly seen in elderly subjects without dementia; they are related to age and possibly to hypertension.[36,75,105] Steingart et al[162] looked at leuko-araiosis on CT in "normal" elderly volunteers and found that those with leuko-araiosis performed worse on a neuropsychologic test battery. Most studies have not found an association between WMH on MRI and neuropsychologic performance in healthy subjects unless the lesions are extensive.[3,17,49,133,166] Leuko-araiosis on CT or WMH on MRI is seen in about one third of patients with AD[1,44,162] and in at least 90% of patients with a clinical diagnosis of VaD.[1,44] The severity of these changes is greater in patients with VaD than in those with AD.[3,91] Dementia severity does appear to correlate with the degree of periventricular white matter abnormalities.[13,84] MRI reveals more infarctions and white matter abnormalities than does CT in patients with a clinical diagnosis of VaD.[44] Studies comparing patients with multiple infarcts with and without dementia have found a greater number of infarcts, especially bilateral and left-sided infarcts, in patients with VaD.[99,105] AD patients with leukoariosis may be more apathetic and may have more extrapyramidal signs than AD patients without leukoariosis.[161]

## FUNCTIONAL NEUROIMAGING STUDIES

Both positron emission tomography (PET) and single photon emission computed tomography (SPECT) use radioactive tracers to provide information about cerebral function. Commonly used PET isotopes include $^{18}$F-2-fluoro-2-deoxy-D-glucose (FDG) to measure glucose metabolism and $^{15}$O-O$_2$ and $^{15}$O-water to measure oxygen metabolism and blood flow, respectively. SPECT studies commonly use $^{133}$Xenon, N-isopropyl-p-$^{123}$I-iodoamphetamine (IMP) and $^{99m}$Tc hexamethyl-propyleneamine oxime (HM-PAO) to measure cerebral blood flow. Although SPECT is easier, less expensive, and more readily available, PET offers quantitation and greater spatial resolution. The in vivo distribution and activity of neurotransmitters are being studied with the use of PET and SPECT ligands.

AD causes a global decline in cortical metabolism and superimposed hypometabolism in association cortexes, especially in the temporoparietal regions.[53,57] Frontal association cortex tends to be involved later in the course of the disease. Dementia severity correlates with the degree of hypometabolism,[31] and specific cognitive deficits correlate with the topography of hypometabolism.[21,52] Similar findings are noted for hypoperfusion with SPECT, as would be expected since blood flow and glucose metabolism are normally coupled.[81,86,126] Abnormalities may be seen on functional neuroimaging studies before atrophy is seen on CT or MRI.[39,48] When PET and SPECT data are corrected for atrophy, group differences in perfusion persist but are reduced.[88,98,163] Reiman et al[134] found reduced temporoparietal metabolism in cognitively normal subjects at high risk for AD.

The diagnostic value of SPECT and PET in the diagnosis of patients with dementia remains unclear. Bilateral temporoparietal abnormalities are not specific for AD and have also been described in patients with VaD, Lewy body disease, Parkinson's disease, NPH, hepatic encephalopathy, acquired immunodeficiency syndrome (AIDS), depression, and Creutzfeldt-Jakob disease.[15,149] Controlled studies have found sensitivities of 21% to 95% and specificities of 52% to 98% in the diagnosis of AD.[7,38,72,85,170] This wide variability is probably related to differences in (1) methodology and equipment, (2) diagnostic criteria (clinical vs. pathologic), (3) dementia severity, and (4) control groups used (normal vs. patients with other causes of dementia). In the largest study with histopathologic correlation, Bonte et al[16] found a sensitivity of 86% (37 of 43) and a specificity of 73% (8 of 11). However, several authors have concluded that the sensitivity, specificity, and predictive value of PET and SPECT are too low for them to be useful diagnostic tests for AD.[27,127,130]

PET and SPECT abnormalities have been described in many non-AD types of dementia. Multiple asymmetric patchy areas of hypometabolism have been described in VaD.[114,115] Both frontal and parietal abnormalities have been seen in patients with Parkinson's disease who have dementia.[128,148] Patients with Lewy body dementia may have temporoparietal and occipital hypoperfusion.[35] Progressive supranuclear palsy causes extensive subcortical and frontal hypometabolism,[11,54] whereas patients with Huntington's disease demonstrate caudate and putamenal hypometabolism.[93,173] Patients with Pick's disease, amyotrophic lateral sclerosis with dementia, and dementia of the frontal lobe type demonstrate frontal lobe abnormalities.[89,125] Patients with primary progressive aphasia have left temporal and parietal hypometabolism.[22] The sensitivity, specificity, and predictive value of PET and SPECT in diagnosing non-AD types of dementia remain unknown.

A number of functional MRI techniques have been developed that can also measure cerebral perfusion.[40,41] One potential advantage of these techniques over other functional neuroimaging modalities is that the functional MRI scan can be performed during the same scanning session as a structural MRI study. Preliminary studies have found significant correlation between perfusion MRI and PET and SPECT in patients with AD, non-AD dementia, and controls.[66,87] As expected, patients with AD have demonstrated significantly reduced temporoparietal perfusion indexes.[71,144]

## CEREBROSPINAL FLUID MARKERS

A number of older studies have focused on various potential CSF markers of AD, including neurotransmitters, neuropeptides, immunoglobulins, and trace elements without success.[167] More recently, CSF markers directly related to the neurodegenerative process in AD have been investigated. There appears to be substantial overlap in CSF β-amyloid and CSF tau concentrations between patients with AD and normal and demented control subjects. However, the ratio of tau to β-amyloid 42 peptide in the CSF has been found to have high specificity (but relatively low sensitivity) in the diagnosis of AD.[118] Recently, de la Monte et al[34] studied the CSF concentration of AD7c-NTP, which causes neuritic sprouting and apoptotic cell death, in patients with AD, normal controls, and controls with neurologic disease. Levels of AD7c-NTP >2 ng/ml were found in 89% of patients with AD and in 11% of age-matched controls.

# GENETIC TESTING

A great deal of progress has been made in understanding the neurogenetics of AD over the past decade. A number of kindreds with autosomal dominant early-onset AD have been found to have amino acid substitutions in the amyloid precursor protein (APP), which is encoded by a gene on chromosome 21.[64,121] Mutations of APP appear to have a very high penetrance. From 50% to 70% of autosomal dominant, early-onset AD cases appear to be associated with a locus (AD3) mapped by genetic linkage to the long arm of chromosome 14 (14q24.3).[147,150] Numerous missense mutations have been identified on a strong candidate gene, called presenilin 1.[142,154] Another autosomal dominant locus responsible for autosomal dominant, early-onset AD is chromosome 1.[104] Two mutations have been identified on a candidate gene, designated presenilin 2.[103,137] Autosomal dominant early-onset AD cases represent a small minority of AD cases, and the prevalence of APP and presenilin mutations in patients with sporadic early-onset AD or familial late-onset AD appears to be low.[58] Therefore testing for presenilin or APP mutations should be restricted to patients with early-onset dementia and very strong family histories.

In 1993 Chorder et al[24] and Saunders et al[146] reported an association between late-onset sporadic and familial AD and apolipoprotein E (apo E) genotype. Apo E is inherited as an autosomal codominant trait with three alleles. Apo E3 is the most common allele (75% to 85%), followed by apo E4 (10% to 15%) and apo E2 (5% to 10%), although the reported prevalence varies somewhat among ethnic groups.[74,111,141] Apo E4 gene dose is correlated with increased risk and earlier onset of AD.[24] The odds ratio of AD for an E4 allele is approximately 15.[123] On the other hand, the apo E2 allele may confer a protective effect.[23,77] The apo E4 gene appears to exert its maximal affect on risk of developing AD by the age of 70.[169] Apo E4 status may help predict which patients with mild cognitive impairment will progress to AD.[129] Although apo E genotype allele does not appear to affect the rate of deterioration on global measures of dementia severity,[5,96,120] there is disagreement as to whether apo E4 status influences specific cognitive realms.[69,157]

Saunders et al[145] followed up to autopsy 67 patients who met NINCDS-ADRDA criteria for probable AD. Similarly to prior reports, 57 (85%) of the patients who met NINCDS-ADRDA criteria for probable AD also met pathologic criteria for AD. Of the 57 patients who met pathologic criteria for AD, 43 had an E4 allele, for a sensitivity of 75%. None of the 10 patients who did not meet pathologic criteria for AD had an E4 allele, for a specificity of 100%. However, among 52 patients who met NINCDS-ADRDA criteria for possible rather than probable AD and who went to autopsy, Smith et al[156] found a sensitivity of 70% and a specificity of only 60% for an E4 allele. In the largest study to date, Mayeux et al[110] performed apo E genotyping in 2188 patients with dementia who went to autopsy. The presence of an apo E4 allele had a sensitivity of 65% and a specificity of 68%. For the 1833 patients who met clinical criteria for AD, the sensitivity was 61% and the specificity 84%. Therefore an E4 allele may add some certainty to a clinical diagnosis of PRAD. However, the specificity of an E4 allele appears to be substantially lower for patients with more ambiguous clinical presentations.

The use of apo E genotyping in the diagnosis of AD remains controversial.[8,76,140] The presence of an apo E4 allele acts as a strong biologic risk factor for AD, especially before the age of 70, and increases the likelihood that a patient with dementia has AD. Therefore Roses[141] has argued that apo E genotyping might be helpful in guiding the subsequent clinical evaluation of patients with dementia. However, the presence of an apo E4 allele does not predict AD or appear to alter the course of AD. Many patients with AD do not have an E4 allele, and apo E4 carriers may not develop AD.[77,122] Other forms of dementia, including VaD, Creutzfeldt-Jakob disease, Lewy body disease, and frontal lobe dementia, have also been associated with the E4 allele. Several groups have made consensus statements regarding the use of apo E genotyping in AD. There is unanimous agreement that apo E genotyping should not be used to predict future risk of AD in asymptomatic individuals. Only one organization, the National Institute on Aging/Alzheimer's Association Working Group, has yet to recommend the discretionary use of apo E genotyping as an adjunctive diagnostic test in patients with dementia.[124]

# MISCELLANEOUS

Magnetic resonance spectroscopy (MRS) allows for the in vivo measurement of neuronal and energy metabolites. Hydrogen-1 MRS studies have revealed reduced N-acetylaspartate (NAA), a putative neuronal marker, and increased myo-inositol in AD.[112,116] Shonk et al[155] found that patients with other forms of dementia have reduced levels of NAA but normal levels of myo-inositol. Some reports have described abnormal phospholipid metabolism in AD by using phosphorus 31 MRS,[30,67] whereas other studies have not found significant differences between patients with AD and controls.[18,119] Currently, the clinical utility of MRS appears to be limited by low interrater, intermeasurement, and test-retest reliabilities.[173]

Scinto et al[152] reported that eye drops containing a 0.01% concentration of the cholinergic antagonist tropicamide resulted in an exaggerated mydriatic response in clinically diagnosed AD patients but not in controls and demented patients without AD. It is notable that almost all subjects without a diagnosis of AD but with memory dysfunction had an abnormal pupillary response on neuropsychologic screening. Other groups have not been able to replicate these finding and have found the test-retest reliability to be low.[51,68]

# CONCLUSION

AD is a major public health problem that is expected to intensify as our population ages. It has been estimated that the cost of evaluating new patients with dementia is $2.5 to $3.2 billion each year in the United States.[25] However, the expense of evaluating patients with dementia must be weighed against the personal and financial cost of misdiagnosis. There is no "dementia workup" that is appropriate for all patients. Patients with a history, neuropsychologic profile, and physical examination that are typical for AD have a high likelihood of meeting pathologic criteria for AD. Nonetheless, laboratory studies and structural neuroimaging studies often affect diagnosis and management. Newer ancillary diagnostic tests such as functional neuroimaging studies, genetic testing, and CSF assays may eventually prove most useful in atypical cases or by enabling early diagnosis. It is only through the combination of a skilled clinician and the appropriate use of diagnostic tests that patients can be diagnosed both accurately and efficiently.

## REFERENCES

1. Aharon-Peretz J, Cummings JL, Hill MA. Vascular dementia and dementia of the Alzheimer's type: cognition, ventricular size, and leukoaraiosis. *Arch Neurol.* 1988;45:719-721.
2. Albert M, Naeser MA, Levine HL, et al. Ventricular size in patients with presenile dementia of the Alzheimer's type. *Arch Neurol.* 1984; 41:1258-1263.
3. Almkvist O, Wahlund LO, Andersson-Lundman, et al. White matter hyperintensity and neuropsychological functions in dementia and healthy aging. *Arch Neurol.* 1992;49:626-632.
4. American Academy of Neurology, Therapeutics and Technology Assessment Subcommittee. Assessment: EEG brain mapping. *Neurology.* 1989;39:1100-1101.
5. Asada T, Kariya T, Yamagata Z, et al. ApoE ε4 allele and cognitive decline in patients with Alzheimer's disease. *Neurology.* 1996;47:603.
6. Becker PM, Feussner JR, Mulrow CD, et al. The role of lumbar puncture in the evaluation of dementia: the Durham Veterans Administration/Duke University study. *J Am Geriatr Soc.* 1985;33:392-396.
7. Bergman H, Chertkow H, Wolfson C, et al. HM-PAO (CERETEC) SPECT brain scanning in the diagnosis of Alzheimer's disease. *J Am Geriatr Soc.* 1997;45:15-20.
8. Bird TD. Apolipoprotein E genotyping in the diagnosis of Alzheimer's disease: a cautionary view. *Ann Neurol.* 1995;38:2-4.
9. Blacker D, Abert MS, Bassett SS, et al. Reliability and validity of NINCDS-ADRDA criteria for Alzheimer's disease. The National Institute of Health Genetics Initiative. *Arch Neurol.* 1994;51:1198-1204.
10. Blessed G, Tomlinson BE, Roth M. The association between quantitative measures of dementia and of change in the cerebral grey matter of elderly subjects. *Br J Psychiatry.* 1968;114:797-881.
11. Blin J, Baron JC, Dubois B, et al. Positron emission tomography study in progressive supranuclear palsy: brain hypometabolism pattern and clinicometabolic correlations. *Arch Neurol.* 1990;47:747-752.
12. Boller F, Lopez OL, Moossy J. Diagnosis of dementia: clinicopathologic correlations. *Neurology.* 1989;39:76-79.
13. Bondareff W, Raval J, Woo B, et al. Magnetic resonance imaging and the severity of dementia in older adults. *Arch Gen Psychiatry.* 1990;47: 47-51.
14. Bondi MW, Salmon DP, Butters N. Neuropsychological features of memory disorders in Alzheimer disease. In: Terry RD, Katzman R, Bick KL, eds. *Alzheimer Disease.* New York: Raven Press; 1994:41-63.
15. Bonte FJ, Tinter R, Weiner MF, et al. Brain blood flow in the dementias: SPECT with histopathologic correlation. *Radiology.* 1993;186: 361-365.
16. Bonte FJ, Weiner MF, Bigio EH, et al. Brain blood flow in the dementias: SPECT with histopathologic correlation in 54 patients. *Radiology.* 1997;202:793-797.
17. Boone KB, Miller BL, Lesser, et al. Neuropsychological correlates of white-matter lesions in healthy elderly subjects: a threshold effect. *Arch Neurol.* 1992;49:549-554.
18. Bottomley PA, Cousins JP, Pendrey DL. Alzheimer dementia: quantification of energy metabolism and mobile phosphesters with P-31 NMR spectroscopy. *Radiology.* 1992;183:695-699.
19. Bradshaw JR, Thomson JLG, Campbell MJ. Computed tomography in the investigation of dementia. *BMJ.* 1983;286:277-280.
20. Burns A, Luthert P, Levy R, et al. Accuracy of clinical diagnosis of Alzheimer's disease. *BMJ.* 1990;301:1026.
21. Chase TN, Foster NL, Brooks FP, et al. Regional cortical dysfunction in Alzheimer's disease as determined by positron emission tomography. *Ann Neurol.* 1984;15(suppl):S170-S174.
22. Chawluk JB, Mesulam MM, Hurtig H, et al. Slowly progressive aphasia without generalized dementia: studies with positron emission tomography. *Ann Neurol.* 1986;19:68-74.
23. Chorder EH, Saunders AM, Risch NH, et al. Protective effect of apolipoprotein E type 2 allele for late onset Alzheimer's disease. *Nat Genet.* 1994;7:180-184.
24. Chorder EH, Saunders AM, Strittmatter WJ, et al. Gene dose of apolipoprotein E type 4 and risk of Alzheimer's disease in late onset families. *Science.* 1993;261:921-923.
25. Chui H, Zhang Q. Evaluation of dementia: a systematic study of the usefulness of the American Academy of Neurology's Practice Parameters. *Neurology.* 1997;49:925-935.
26. Clarfield AM, Larson EB. An opposing view. *J Fam.* 1990;31:405-410.
27. Claus JJ, Van Horskamp F, Breteler MB, et al. The diagnostic value of SPECT with Tc 99m HMPAO in Alzheimer's disease: a population based study. *Neurology.* 1994;44:454-461.
28. Coffey CE, Wilkinson WE, Parashos IA, et al. Quantitative cerebral anatomy of the aging human brain: a cross-sectional study using magnetic resonance imaging. *Neurology.* 1992;42:527-536.
29. Coker SB. The diagnosis of childhood neurodegenerative disorders presenting as dementia in adults. *Neurology.* 1991;41:794-798.
30. Cuenod CA, Kaplan DB, Michot JL, et al. Phospholipid abnormalities in early Alzheimer's disease: in vivo phosphorus 31 magnetic resonance spectroscopy. *Arch Neurol.* 1995;52:89-94.
31. Cutler NR, Haxby JV, Duara R, et al. Clinical history, brain metabolism, and neuropsychological function in Alzheimer's disease. *Neurology.* 1985;18:298-309.
32. DeCarli C, Haxby JV, Gillette JA, et al. Longitudinal changes in lateral ventricular volume of the Alzheimer type. *Neurology.* 1992;42:2029-2036.
33. DeCarli C, Kaye JA, Horwitz B, et al. Critical analysis of the use of computer-assisted transverse axial tomography to study human brain in aging and dementia of the Alzheimer type. *Neurology.* 1990;40:872-883.
34. de la Monte SM, Ghanbari K, Frey WH, et al. Characterization of the AD7C-NTP cDNA in Alzheimer's disease and measurement of a 41-kD protein in cerebrospinal fluid. *J Clin Invest.* 1997;100:3093-3104.
35. Donnemiller E, Heilmann J, Wenning GK, et al. Brain perfusion scintigraphy with 99m Tc-HMPAO or 99m Tc-ECD and 123I-beta-CIT single-photon emission tomography in dementia of the Alzheimer-type and diffuse Lewy body disease. *Eur J Nucl Med.* 1997; 24:320-325.
36. Drayer BP. Imaging of the aging brain. I. Normal findings. *Radiology.* 1988;166:785-796.
37. Drayer BP, Heyman A, Wilkinson W, et al. Early-onset Alzheimer's disease: an analysis of CT findings. *Ann Neurol.* 1985;17:407.
38. Duara R, Barker W, Loewenstein D, et al. Sensitivity and specificity of positron emission tomography and magnetic resonance imaging studies in Alzheimer's disease and multi-infarct dementia. *Eur Neurol.* 1989;29(suppl 3):9-15.
39. Duara R, Grady C, Haxby J, et al. Positron emission tomography in Alzheimer's disease. *Neurology.* 1986;36:879-887.
40. Edelman RR, Mattle HP, Atkinson DJ, et al. Cerebral blood flow: assessment with dynamic contrast-enhanced t2*-weighted MR imaging at 1.5 T. *Radiology.* 1990;176:211-220.
41. Edelman RR, Siewert B, Darby DG, et al. Qualitative mapping of cerebral blood flow and functional localization with echo-planar MR imaging and signal targeting with alternating radio frequency. *Radiology.* 1994;192:513-520.
42. Engel PA, Gelber J. Does computed tomographic brain imaging have a place in the diagnosis of dementia? *Arch Intern Med.* 1992;152:1437-1440.
43. Erkinjuntti T, Ketonen L, Sulkava R, et al. CT in the differential diagnosis between Alzheimer's disease and vascular dementia. *Acta Neurol Scand.* 1987;75:262-270.
44. Erkinjuntti T, Ketonen L, Sulkava R, et al. Do white matter changes on MRI and CT differentiate vascular dementia from Alzheimer's disease? *J Neurol Neurosurg Psychiatry.* 1987;50:37-42.
45. Erkinjuntti T, Lee DH, Gao F, et al. Temporal lobe atrophy on magnetic resonance imaging in the diagnosis of early Alzheimer's disease. *Arch Neurol.* 1993;50:305-310.
46. Evans DA, Funkenstein HH, Albert MS, et al. Prevalence of Alzheimer's disease in a community population of older persons: higher than previously reported. *JAMA.* 1989;262:2551-2556.
47. Fama R, Sullivan EV, Shear PK, et al. Selective cortical and hippocampal volume correlates of Mattis Dementia Rating Scale in Alzheimer's disease. *Arch Neurol.* 1997;54:719-728.
48. Fazekas F, Alavi A, Chawluk JB, et al. Comparison of CT, MR, and PET in Alzheimer's dementia and normal aging. *J Nucl Med.* 1989;30:1607-1615.
49. Fein G, Van Dyke C, Davenport L, et al. Preservation of normal cognitive functioning in elderly subjects with extensive white-matter lesions of long duration. *Arch Gen Psychiatry.* 1990;47:220-223.
50. Felician O, Sandson TA. Recent developments in the pathophysiology

and pharmacotherapy of Alzheimer's disease (pt 1). *Drugs of Today.* 1997;33:555-562.

51. Fitz Simon JS, Waring SC, Kokmen E, et al. Response of the pupil to tropicamide is not a reliable test for Alzheimer's disease. *Arch Neurol.* 1997;54:155-159.

52. Foster NL, Chase TN, Fedio P, et al. Alzheimer's disease: focal cortical changes shown by positron emission tomography. *Neurology.* 1983;33:961-965.

53. Foster NL, Chase TN, Mansi L, et al. Cortical abnormalities in Alzheimer's disease. *Ann Neurol.* 1984;16:649-654.

54. Foster NL, Gilman S, Berent S, et al. Cerebral hypometabolism in progressive supranuclear palsy studied with positron emission tomography. *Ann Neurol.* 1988;24:399-406.

55. Fox NC, Freeborough PA, Rossor MN. Visualisation and quantification of rates of atrophy in Alzheimer's disease. *Lancet.* 1996;348:94-97.

56. Fox NC, Warrington EK, Freeborough PA, et al. Presymptomatic hippocampal atrophy in Alzheimer's disease: a longitudinal MRI study. *Brain.* 1996;119(pt 6):2001-2007.

57. Frackowiak RSJ, Pozzilli C, Legg NJ, et al. Regional cerebral oxygen supply and utilization in dementia: a clinical and physiological study with oxygen-15 and positron tomography. *Brain.* 1981;104:753-778.

58. Frisoni GB, Trabucchi M. Clinical rationale of genetic testing in dementia. *J Neurol Neurosurg Psychiatry.* 1997;62:217-221.

59. Gado M, Hughes CP, Danziger W, et al. Volumetric measurements of the cerebrospinal fluid spaces in demented subjects and controls. *Radiology.* 1982;144:535-538.

60. Galasko D, Hansen LA, Katzman R, et al. Clinical-neuropathological correlations in Alzheimer's disease and related dementias. *Arch Neurol.* 1994;51:888-895.

61. Gearing M, Mirra SS, Hedreen JC, et al. The consortium to establish a registry for Alzheimer's disease (CERAD), X: neuropathology confirmation of the clinical diagnosis of Alzheimer's disease. *Neurology.* 1995;45:461-466.

62. George AE, de Leon MJ, Rosenbloom S, et al. Ventricular volume and cognitive deficit: a computed tomographic study. *Radiology.* 1983;149:493-498.

63. Gjerris F, Borgensen SE, Sorensen PS, eds. *Outflow of cerebrospinal fluid.* Alfred Benzon Symposium 27. Copenhagen: Munksgaard; 1989. As quoted in *Lancet.* 1990;335:22.

64. Goate A, Chartier-Harlin MC, Mullan M, et al. Segregation of a missense mutation in the amyloid precursor protein gene with familial Alzheimer's disease. *Nature.* 1991;349:704-706.

65. Gold G, Giannakopoulos P, Montes-Paixao C, et al. Sensitivity and specificity of newly proposed clinical criteria for possible vascular dementia. *Neurology.* 1997;49:690-694.

66. Gonzalez RG, Fischman AJ, Guimaraes AR, et al. Functional MR in the evaluation of dementia: correlation of abnormal dynamic cerebral blood volume measurements with changes in cerebral metabolism on positron emission tomography with fludeoxyglucose F 18. *Am J Neuroradiol.* 1995;16:1763-1770.

67. Gonzalez RG, Guimaraes AR, Moore GJ, et al. Quantitative in vivo 31P magnetic resonance spectroscopy of Alzheimer's disease. *Alzheimer Dis Assoc Disord.* 1996;10:46-52.

68. Graff-Radford NR, Lin SC, Brazis PW, et al. Tropicamide eyedrops cannot be used for reliable diagnosis of Alzheimer's disease. *Mayo Clin Proc.* 1997;72:495-504.

69. Growdon JH, Locascio JJ, Corkin S, et al. Apolipoprotein E genotype does not influence rates of cognitive decline in Alzheimer's disease. *Neurology.* 1996;47:444-448.

70. Haan J, Thomeer RTWM. Predictive value of temporary external lumbar drainage in normal pressure hydrocephalus. *Neurosurgery.* 1988;22:388-391.

71. Harris GJ, Lewis RF, Satlin A, et al. Dynamic susceptibility contrast MRI of regional cerebral blood volume in Alzheimer's disease. *Am J Psychiatry.* 1996;153:721-724.

72. Herholz K, Perani D, Salmon E, et al. Comparability of FDG PET studies in probable Alzheimer's disease. *J Nucl Med.* 1993;34:1460-1466.

73. Heun R, Schlegel S, Graf-Morgenstern M, et al. Proton magnetic resonance spectroscopy in dementia of Alzheimer type. *Int J Geriatr Psychiatry.* 1997;12:349-359.

74. Hill JS, Pritchard PH. Improved phenotyping of apolipoprotein E: application to population frequency distribution. *Clin Chem.* 1990;36:1871-1874.

75. Hunt AL, Orrison WW, Yeo RA, et al. Clinical significance of MRI white matter lesions in the elderly. *Neurology.* 1989;39:1470-1474.

76. Hyman BT. Apolipoprotein E genotype: utility in clinical practice in Alzheimer's disease. *J Am Geriatr Soc.* 1996;44:1469-1471.

77. Hyman BT, Gomez-Isla T, Briggs M, et al. Apolipoprotein E and cognitive change in an elderly population. *Ann Neurol.* 1996;40:55-66.

78. Jack CR, Peterson RC, O'Brien PC, et al. MR based hippocampal volumetry in the diagnosis of Alzheimer's disease. *Neurology.* 1992;42:183-188.

79. Jack CR, Petersen RC, Xu YC, et al. Medial temporal atrophy on MRI in normal aging and very mild Alzheimer's disease. *Neurology.* 1997;49:786-794.

80. Jacobs DM, Sano M, Dooneief G. Neuropsychological detection and characterization of preclinical Alzheimer's disease. *Neurology.* 1995;45:657-662.

81. Jagust WJ, Budinger TF, Reed BR. The diagnosis of dementia with single photon emission computed tomography. *Arch Neurol.* 1987;44:258-262.

82. Jernigan TL, Achibald SL, Berhow MT, et al. Cerebral structure on MRI, II: specific changes in Alzheimer's and Huntington's diseases. *Biol Psychiatry.* 1991;29:68-81.

83. Jobst KA, Smith AD, Szatmari M, et al. Detection in life of confirmed Alzheimer's disease using a simple measurement of medial temporal lobe atrophy by computed tomography. *Lancet.* 1992;340:1179-1183.

84. Johnson KA, Davis KR, Buonanno, et al. Comparison of magnetic resonance and roentgen ray computed tomography in dementia. *Arch Neurol.* 1987;44:1075-1080.

85. Johnson KA, Holman L, Rosen TJ, et al. Iofetamine I 123 single photon emission computed tomography is accurate in the diagnosis of Alzheimer's disease. *Arch Intern Med.* 1990;150:752-756.

86. Johnson KA, Mueller ST, Walshe TM, et al. Cerebral perfusion imaging in Alzheimer's disease: use of single photon emission computed tomography and iofetamine hydrochloride I 123. *Arch Neurol.* 1987;44:165-168.

87. Johnson KA, Renshaw JA, Becker A, et al. Comparison of functional MRI and SPECT in Alzheimer's disease. *Neurology.* 1995;45:A405-A406.

88. Johnson KA, Sperling RA, Becker JA, et al. Atrophy-corrected SPECT cerebral perfusion in Alzheimer's disease. *Neurology.* 1994;44(suppl 2):A179.

89. Kamo H, McGeer PL, Harrop R, et al. Positron emission tomography and histopathology in Pick's disease. *Neurology.* 1987;37:439-445.

90. Katzman R. Should a major imaging procedure (CT or MRI) be required in the workup of dementia? An affirmative view. *J Fam.* 1990;31:401-405.

91. Kertesz A, Polk M, Carr T. Cognition and white matter changes on magnetic resonance imaging in dementia. *Arch Neurol.* 1990;47:387-391.

92. Kesslak JP, Nalcioglu O, Cotman CW. Quantification of magnetic resonance scans for hippocampal and parahippocampal atrophy in Alzheimer's disease. *Neurology.* 1991;41:51-54.

93. Kuhl DE, Phelps ME, Markham CH, et al. Cerebral metabolism and atrophy in Huntington's disease determined by 18FDG and computed tomographic scan. *Ann Neurol.* 1982;12:425-434.

94. Kukull WA, Larson EB, Reifler BV. Interrater reliability of Alzheimer's disease diagnosis. *Neurology.* 1990;40:257-260.

95. Kukull WA, Larson EB, Reifler BV. The validity of clinical diagnostic criteria for Alzheimer's disease. *Neurology.* 1990;40:1364-1369.

96. Kurz A, Egensperger R, Haupt M, et al. Apolipoprotein E ε4 allele, cognitive decline, and deterioration of everyday performance in Alzheimer's disease. *Neurology.* 1996;47:440-443.

97. Laakso MP, Partanen K, Riekkinen P, et al. Hippocampal volumes in Alzheimer's disease, Parkinson's disease with and without dementia, and in vascular dementia: an MRI study. *Neurology.* 1996;46:678-681.

98. Labbe C, Froment JC, Kennedy A, et al. Positron emission tomography metabolic data corrected for cortical atrophy using magnetic resonance imaging. *Alzheimer Dis Assoc Disord.* 1996;10:141-170.

99. Ladurner G, Iliff LD, Lechner H. Clinical factors with dementia in ischaemic stroke. *J Neurol Neurosurg Psychiatry.* 1982;45:97-101.

100. Lehtovirta M, Soininen H, Laakso MP, et al. SPECT and MRI analysis in Alzheimer's disease: relation to apolipoprotein E epsilon 4 allele. *J Neurol Neurosurg Psychiatry.* 1996;60:644-649.

101. LeMay M. CT changes in dementing diseases: a review. *AJR.* 1986;147:963-975.

102. LeMay M, Stafford JL, Sandor T, et al. Statistical assessment of perceptual CT scan ratings in patients with Alzheimer type dementia. *J Comput Assist Tomograph.* 1986;10:802-809.

103. Levy-Lahad E, Wasco W, Poorkaj P, et al. Candidate gene for the chromosome 1 familial Alzheimer's disease locus. *Science*. 1995;269:973-977.

104. Levy-Lahad E, Wijsman EM, Nemens E, et al. A familial Alzheimer's disease locus on chromosome 1. *Science*. 1995;269:970-973.

105. London E, de Leon MJ, George AE, et al. Periventricular lucencies in the CT scans of aged and demented patients. *Biol Psychiatry*. 1986;21:960-962.

106. Luxenberg JS, Haxby JV, Creasey H, et al. Rate of ventricular enlargement in dementia of the Alzheimer type correlates with rate of neuropsychological deterioration. *Neurology*. 1987;37:1135-1140.

107. Maroney JT, Bagiella E, Desmond DW, et al. Meta-analysis of the Hachinski Ischemic Score in pathology verified dementias. *Neurology*. 1997;49:1096-1105.

108. Masur D, Sliwinsky M, Lipton R, et al. Neuropsychological prediction of dementia and the absence of dementia in healthy elderly persons. *Neurology*. 1994;44:1427-1431.

109. Maunoury C, Michot JL, Caillet H, et al. Specificity of temporal amygdala atrophy in Alzheimer's disease: quantitative assessment with magnetic resonance imaging. *Dementia*. 1996;7:10-14.

110. Mayeux R, Saunders AM, Shea S, et al. Utility of the apolipoprotein E genotype in the diagnosis of Alzheimer's disease. *N Engl J Med*. 1998;338:506-511.

111. Mayeux R, Stern Y, Ottman R, et al. The apolipoprotein E4 allele in patients with Alzheimer's disease. *Ann Neurol*. 1993;34:752-754.

112. McClure RJ, Kanfer JN, Panchalingam K, et al. Magnetic resonance spectroscopy and its application to aging and Alzheimer's disease. *Neuroimaging Clin North Am*. 1995;5:69-83.

113. McKhan G, Drachman D, Folstein M, et al. Clinical diagnosis of Alzheimer's disease: report of the NINCDS-ADRDA Work Group under the auspices of Department of Health and Human Services Task Force on Alzheimer's Disease. *Neurology*. 1984;34:939-944.

114. Metter JE, Mazziotta JC, Itabashi HH, et al. Comparison of glucose metabolism, x-ray CT, and postmortem data in a patient with multiple cerebral infarcts. *Neurology*. 1985;35:1695-1701.

115. Mielke R, Herholz K, Grond M, et al. Severity of vascular dementia is related to volume of metabolically impaired tissue. *Arch Neurol*. 1992;49:909-913.

116. Miller BL, Moates RA, Shonk T, et al. Alzheimer disease: depiction of increased cerebral *myo*-inositol with proton MR spectroscopy. *Radiology*. 1993;187:433-437.

117. Molsa PK, Paljarvi L, Rinne JO, et al. Validity of clinical diagnosis in dementia: a prospective clinicopathologic study. *J Neurol Neurosurg Psychiatry*. 1985;48:1085-1090.

118. Motter R, Vigo-Pelfrey C, Kholodenko D, et al. Reduction of β-amyloid peptide 42 in the cerebrospinal fluid of patients with Alzheimer's disease. *Ann Neurol*. 1995;38:643-648.

119. Murphy DGM, Bottomley PA, Salerno JA, et al. An in vivo study of phosphorus and glucose metabolism in Alzheimer's disease using magnetic resonance spectroscopy and PET. *Arch Gen Psychiatry*. 1993;50:341-349.

120. Murphy GM, Taylor J, Kraemer HC, et al. No association between apolipoprotein E epsilon 4 allele and rate of decline in Alzheimer's disease. *Am J Psychiatry*. 1997;154:603-608.

121. Murrell J, Farlow M, Ghetti B. A mutation in the amyloid precursor protein associated with hereditary Alzheimer's disease. *Science*. 1991;254:97-99.

122. Myers RH, Schaefer EJ, Wilson PWF, et al. Apolipoprotein E ε4 association with dementia in a population-based study: the Framingham study. *Neurology*. 1996;46:673-677.

123. Nalbantoglu J, Gilfix BM, Bertrand P, et al. Predictive value of apolipoprotein E genotyping in Alzheimer's disease: results of an autopsy series and an analysis of several combined studies. *Ann Neurol*. 1994;35:889-895.

124. National Institute on Aging/Alzheimer's Association Working Group. Apolipoprotein E genotyping in Alzheimer's disease. *Lancet*. 1996;347:1091-1095.

125. Neary D, Snowden JS, Mann DMA, et al. Frontal lobe dementia and motor neuron disease. *J Neurol Neurosurg Psychiatry*. 1990;53:23-32.

126. O'Brien JT, Eagger S, Syed GMS, et al. A study of regional cerebral blood flow and cognitive performance in Alzheimer's disease. *J Neurol Neurosurg Psychiatry*. 1992;55:1182-1187.

127. Pasquier F, Lavenu I, Lebert F, et al. The use of SPECT in a multidisciplinary memory clinic. *Dement Geriatr Cogn Disord*. 1997;8:85-91.

128. Peppard RF, Martin WRW, Carr GD, et al. Cerebral glucose metabolism in Parkinson's disease with and without dementia. *Arch Neurol*. 1992;49:1262-1268.

129. Petersen RC, Smith GE, Ivnik RJ, et al. Apolipoprotein E status as a predictor of the development of Alzheimer's disease in memory-impaired individuals. *JAMA*. 1995;273:1274-1278.

130. Powers WJ, Perlmutter JS, Videen TO, et al. Blinded clinical evaluation of positron emission tomography for diagnosis of probable Alzheimer's disease. *Neurology*. 1992;42:765-770.

131. Price BH, Gurvit H, Weintraub S, et al. Neuropsychological patterns and language deficits in 20 consecutive cases of autopsy-confirmed Alzheimer's disease. *Arch Neurol*. 1993;50:931-937.

132. Price JL, Davis PB, Morris JC, et al. The distribution of tangles, plaques and related immunohistochemical markers in healthy aging and Alzheimer's disease. *Neurobiol Aging*. 1991;12:295-312.

133. Rao SM, Mittenberg W, Bernardin L, et al. Neuropsychological test findings in subjects with leukoariosis. *Arch Neurol*. 1989;46:40-44.

134. Reiman EM, Caselli RJ, Yun LS, et al. Preclinical evidence of Alzheimer's disease in persons homozygous for the epsilon 4 allele for apolipoprotein E. *N Engl J Med*. 1996;334:752-758.

135. Report of the Quality Standards Subcommittee of the American Academy of Neurology. Practice parameter for diagnosis and evaluation of dementia (summary statement). *Neurology*. 1994;44:2203-2206.

136. Risse SC, Raskind MA, Nochlin D, et al. Neuropathological findings in patients with clinical diagnosis of probable Alzheimer's disease. *Am J Psychiatry*. 1990;147:168-172.

137. Rogaev EI, Sherrington R, Rogaeva EA, et al. Familial Alzheimer disease in kindreds with missense mutations in a gene on chromosome 1 related to the Alzheimer disease type 3 gene. *Nature*. 1995;376:775-778.

138. Roman GC, Tatemichi TK, Erkinjuntti TE, et al. Vascular dementia: diagnostic criteria for research studies. Report of the NINDS-AIREN International Workshop. *Neurology*. 1993;43:250-260.

139. Rosen WG, Terry RD, Fuld PA, et al. Pathologic verification of ischemic score in differentiation of dementias. *Ann Neurol*. 1980;7:486-488.

140. Roses AD. Apolipoprotein E genotyping in the differential diagnosis, not prediction, of Alzheimer's disease. *Ann Neurol*. 1995;38:6-14.

141. Roses AD. Genetic testing for Alzheimer's disease: practical and ethical issues. *Arch Neurol*. 1997;54:1226-1229.

142. Sandbrink R, Zhang D, Schaeffer S, et al. Missense mutations of the *PS-1/S182* gene in German early-onset Alzheimer's disease patients. *Ann Neurol*. 1996;2:265-266.

143. Sandson TA, Price BH. Diagnostic testing and dementia. *Neurol Clin*. 1996;14:45-59.

144. Sandson TA, O'Connor M, Sperling RA, et al. Perfusion MRI with EPISTAR in Alzheimer's disease: preliminary results. *Neurology*. 1996;47:1339-1342.

145. Saunders AM, Hulette C, Welsh-Bohmer KA, et al. Specificity, sensitivity, and predictive value of apolipoprotein-E genotyping for sporadic Alzheimer's disease. *Lancet*. 1996;348:90-93.

146. Saunders AM, Strittmatter WJ, Schmechel D, et al. Association of apolipoprotein E allele E4 with late onset familial and sporadic Alzheimer's disease. *Neurology*. 1993;43:1467-1472.

147. St. George-Hyslop P, Haines J, Rogaev E, et al. Genetic evidence for a novel familial Alzheimer's disease locus on chromosome 14. *Nat Genet*. 1992;2:330-334.

148. Sawada H, Udaka F, Kameyama M, et al. SPECT findings in Parkinson's disease associated with dementia. *J Neurol Neurosurg Psychiatry*. 1992;55:960-963.

149. Schapiro MB, Pietrini P, Grady CL, et al. Reductions in parietal and temporal cerebral metabolic rates for glucose are not specific for Alzheimer's disease. *J Neurol Neurosurg Psychiatry*. 1993;56:859-864.

150. Schellenberg GD, Bird TD, Wijsman EM, et al. Genetic linkage evidence for a familial Alzheimer's disease locus on chromosome 14. *Science*. 1992;258:668-671.

151. Scheltens P, Leys D, Barkhof F, et al. Hippocampal atrophy on magnetic resonance imaging in Alzheimer's disease and normal aging. *Neurology*. 1991;41(suppl 1):341-342.

152. Scinto LFM, Daffner KR, Dressler D, et al. A potential noninvasive neurobiologic test for Alzheimer's disease. *Science*. 1994;266:1051-1054.

153. Seab JP, Jagust WJ, Wong STS, et al. Quantitative NMR measurements of hippocampal atrophy in Alzheimer's disease. *Magn Reson Med*. 1988;8:200-208.

154. Sherrington R, Rogaev EI, Liang Y, et al. Cloning of a gene bearing missense mutations in early-onset familial Alzheimer's disease. *Nature*. 1995;375:754-760.

155. Shonk TK, Moats RA, Gifford P, et al. Probable Alzheimer's disease: diagnosis with proton MR spectroscopy. *Radiology.* 1995;195:65-72.

156. Smith AD, Jobst KA, Johnston C, et al. Apolipoprotein-E genotyping in diagnosis of Alzheimer's disease. *Lancet.* 1996;348:483-484.

157. Smith GE, Bohac DL, Waring SC, et al. Apolipoprotein E genotype influences cognitive "phenotype" in patients with Alzheimer's disease but not in healthy control subjects. *Neurology.* 1998;50:355-362.

158. Snowdon DA, Greiner LH, Mortimer JA, et al. Brain infarction and the clinical expression of Alzheimer disease. *JAMA.* 1997;277:813-817.

159. Soininen H, Puranen M, Riekkinen PJ. Computed tomography findings in senile dementia and normal aging. *J Neurol Neurosurg Psychiatry.* 1982;45:50-54.

160. Squire LR, Zola-Morgan S. The medial temporal lobe memory system. *Science.* 1991;20:1380-1386.

161. Starkstein SE, Sabe L, Vazquez S, et al. Neuropsychological, psychiatric, and cerebral perfusion correlates of leukoariosis in Alzheimer's disease. *J Neurol Neurosurg Psychiatry.* 1997;63:66-73.

162. Steingart A, Hachinski VC, Lau C. Cognitive and neurologic findings in subjects with diffuse white matter lucencies on computed tomographic scan (leuko-araiosis). *Arch Neurol.* 1987;44:32-35.

163. Tanna NK, Kohn MI, Horwich DN, et al. Analysis of brain and cerebrospinal fluid volumes with MR imaging: impact on PET data correction for atrophy. II: aging and Alzheimer dementia. *Radiology.* 1991;178:123-130.

164. Tierney MC, Fisher RH, Lewis AL, et al. The NINCDS-ADRDA Work Group criteria for the clinical diagnosis of probable Alzheimer's disease: a clinicopathologic study of 57 cases. *Neurology.* 1988;38:359-364.

165. Tierney MC, Szalai JP, Snow WG, et al. Prediction of probable Alzheimer's disease in memory-impaired patients: a prospective longitudinal study. *Neurology.* 1996;46:661-665.

166. Tupler LA, Coffey E, Logue P, et al. Neuropsychological importance of subcortical white matter hyperintensity. *Arch Neurol.* 1992;49:1248-1252.

167. Van Gool WA, Bolhuis PA. Cerebrospinal fluid markers of Alzheimer's disease. *J Am Geriatr Soc.* 1991;39:1025-1039.

168. Wade JP, Mirsen TR, Hachinski VC, et al. The clinical diagnosis of Alzheimer's disease. *Arch Neurol.* 1987;44:24-29.

169. Waring SC, Rocca WA, Schaid DJ, et al. Apolipoprotein E and Alzheimer's disease: trends in risk by age of onset. *Ann Neurol.* 1995;38:324.

170. Wasterman DL, Mendez MF, Fairbanks LA, et al. Sensitivity, specificity, and positive predictive value of technetium 99-HMPAO SPECT in discriminating Alzheimer's disease from other dementias. *J Geriatr Psychiatry Neurol.* 1997;10:15-21.

171. Wikkelso C, Andersson H, Blomstrand C, et al. The clinical effect of lumbar puncture in normal pressure hydrocephalus. *J Neurol Neurosurg Psychiatry.* 1982;45:64-69.

172. Wippold FJ, Gado MH, Morris JC, et al. Senile dementia and healthy aging: a longitudinal CT study. *Radiology.* 1991;179:215-219.

173. Young AB, Penney JB, Starosta-Rubinstein S, et al. PET scan investigation of Huntington's disease: cerebral metabolic correlates of neurological features and functional decline. *Ann Neurol.* 1986;20:296-303.

# 4

# Seizure Disorders

*Frank Gilliam and Elaine Wyllie*

Epilepsy is a common paroxysmal neurologic disorder. The cumulative incidence of epilepsy, or recurrent unprovoked seizures, is estimated to be 3%. The lifetime incidence of at least one seizure may be as high as 9%.[47] The variety of clinical presentations of seizures often makes accurate diagnosis problematic, but most patients can be appropriately diagnosed following a well-organized, deliberate evaluation. This chapter reviews the current diagnostic techniques that are useful in the assessment of patients with the possible diagnosis of seizures. Emphasis is placed on exclusion of treatable causes, appropriate classification, and accurate localization. Common electroencephalographic (EEG) and magnetic resonance imaging (MRI) findings are described, as well as other adjunctive neuroimaging techniques. Specific clinical situations, such as the first seizure, febrile convulsions, intractable epilepsy, and psychogenic seizures, are discussed. To place the diagnostic evaluation in clinical context, the classification and etiologic basis of seizures are briefly summarized.

## SEIZURE CLASSIFICATION AND ETIOLOGY

The Commission on Classification and Terminology of the International League Against Epilepsy (ILAE) devised a widely accepted classification system based on a review of videotaped seizures at commission workshops.[23] This classification system categorizes seizures in a format that facilitates diagnosis, treatment, and communication between medical professionals through standardized nomenclature. Seizures are conveniently divided into two major categories, partial and generalized. Tables 4–1 and 4–2 summarize the ILAE classification system for seizures and epileptic syndromes.

Partial seizures are defined as "those in which the first clinical and electrographic changes indicate initial activation of a system of neurons in one hemisphere" and are subclassified according to the presence or absence of impairment of consciousness.[23] Simple partial seizures involve minimal change in awareness, usually indicated clinically by the patient's complete recollection of the event. Complex partial seizures are associated with alteration of awareness and amnesia for at least a portion of the seizure. Partial seizures may involve signs or symptoms correlating with activation of any

brain region, specifically motor, autonomic, somatosensory or special sensory, or psychic.[91] Both simple and complex partial seizures can propagate throughout the brain to become secondarily generalized seizures, often with tonic and clonic features.

Generalized seizures are defined as "those in which the first clinical changes indicate initial involvement of both hemispheres."[23] The subclassification of generalized seizures includes absence, tonic-clonic, myoclonic, clonic, tonic, and atonic seizures. The generalized epilepsies, as opposed to seizures, are often divided into idiopathic (primary) and symptomatic (secondary).[22] This distinction is useful because seizures in idiopathic generalized epilepsy are often

---

**TABLE 4–1. International Classification of Epileptic Seizures**

I. Partial (focal, local) seizures
  A. Simple partial seizures
    1. With motor signs
    2. With somatosensory or special sensory symptoms
    3. With autonomic symptoms or signs
    4. With psychic symptoms
  B. Complex partial seizures
    1. Simple partial onset followed by impairment of consciousness
    2. With impairment of consciousness at onset
  C. Partial seizures evolving to secondarily generalized seizures
    1. Simple partial seizures evolving to generalized seizures
    2. Complex partial seizures evolving to generalized seizures
    3. Simple partial seizures evolving to complex partial seizures evolving to generalized seizures
II. Generalized seizures (convulsive or nonconvulsive)
  A. Absence seizures
    1. Typical absences
    2. Atypical absences
  B. Myoclonic seizures
  C. Clonic seizures
  D. Tonic seizures
  E. Tonic-clonic seizures
  F. Atonic seizures (astatic seizures)
III. Unclassified epileptic seizures

Adapted from Commission on Classification and Terminology of the International League Against Epilepsy. Proposal for revised clinical and electroencephalographic classification of epileptic seizures. *Epilepsia.* 1981;22: 489-501.

---

**TABLE 4–2. International Classification of Epilepsy and Epileptic Syndromes**

1. Localization-related (focal, local, partial) epilepsies and syndromes
   1.1 Idiopathic with age-related onset
   At present, two syndromes are established, but more may be identified in the future:
   - Benign childhood epilepsy with centrotemporal spikes
   - Childhood epilepsy with occipital paroxysms
   1.2 Symptomatic
   This category comprises syndromes of great individual variability, which will mainly be based on anatomic localization, clinical features, seizure types, and etiologic factors (if known)
2. Generalized epilepsies and syndromes
   2.1 Idiopathic, with age-related onset, listed in order of age
   - Benign neonatal familial convulsions
   - Benign neonatal convulsions
   - Benign myoclonic epilepsy in infancy
   - Childhood absence epilepsy (pyknoepilepsy)
   - Juvenile absence epilepsy
   - Juvenile myoclonic epilepsy (impulsive petit mal)
   - Epilepsy with grand mal seizures on awakening
   Other generalized idiopathic epilepsies, if they do not belong to one of the above syndromes, can still be classified as generalized idiopathic epilepsies
   2.2 Idiopathic and/or symptomatic, in order of age of appearance
   - West syndrome (infantile spasms, Blitz-Nick, and Salaam Krämpfe)
   - Lennox-Gastaut syndrome
   - Epilepsy with myoclonic-astatic seizures
   - Epilepsy with myoclonic absences

2.3 Symptomatic
   2.3.a Nonspecific etiology
   - Early myoclonic encephalopathy
   2.3.b Specific syndromes
   Epileptic seizures may complicate many disease states
   Included under this heading are those diseases in which seizures are a presenting or predominant feature
3. Epilepsies and syndromes undetermined as to whether they are focal or generalized
   3.1 With both generalized and focal seizures
   - Neonatal seizures
   - Severe myoclonic epilepsy in infancy
   - Epilepsy with continuous spike waves during slow-wave sleep
   - Acquired epileptic aphasia (Landau-Kleffner syndrome)
   3.2 Without unequivocal generalized or focal features
   This heading covers all cases where clinical and EEG findings do not permit classification as clearly generalized or localization-related, such as in many cases of sleep grand mal
4. Special syndromes
   4.1 Situation-related seizures
   - Febrile convulsions
   - Seizures related to other identifiable situations, such as stress, hormonal changes, drugs, alcohol or sleep deprivation
   4.2 Isolated, apparently unprovoked epileptic events
   4.3 Epilepsies characterized by specific modes of seizure precipitation
   4.4 Chronic progressive epilepsia partialis continua of childhood

Adapted from Commission on Classification and Terminology of the International League Against Epilepsy. Proposal for revised classifications of epilepsies and epileptic syndromes. *Epilepsia.* 1989;30:389-399.

hereditary,[27,116,123] limited to childhood or adolescence, and readily respond to certain anticonvulsant medications.[59,92]

Knowledge of the frequency of the common causes of epilepsy is necessary when assessing the seizure patient. As presented in Figure 4–1, cerebrovascular disease is the most frequently identified cause of epilepsy, followed by developmental disorders, head trauma, brain tumor, infection, and

degenerative disorders.[8,48] The proportional incidence of the etiology of seizures varies considerably with age, with cerebrovascular disease predominating in senior adults, head trauma and brain tumors most common in adolescents and adults, and developmental and infectious disorders proportionally most common in neonates and young children.[8] The most common type of epilepsy at all ages is idiopathic, how-

## EPILEPSY ETIOLOGY
## ROCHESTER, MN 1935-1984, INCIDENCE

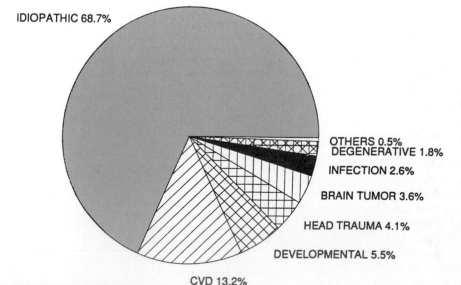

IDIOPATHIC 68.7%

OTHERS 0.5%
DEGENERATIVE 1.8%

INFECTION 2.6%

BRAIN TUMOR 3.6%

HEAD TRAUMA 4.1%

DEVELOPMENTAL 5.5%

CVD 13.2%

PRESUMED PREDISPOSING CAUSE N=888

**FIGURE 4–1.** Presumed predisposing cause of epilepsy. Incidence in Rochester, Minn., 1935–1984. (From Annegers JF. The epidemiology of epilepsy. In: Wyllie E, ed. *The Treatment of Epilepsy: Principles and Practice.* Philadelphia: Lea & Febiger; 1993: 161.)

# REMOTE SYMPTOMATIC EPILEPSY PROPORTIONAL INCIDENCE BY AGE AND ETIOLOGY

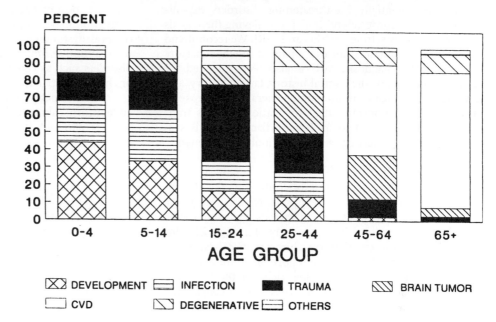

**FIGURE 4–2.** Proportional incidence of remote symptomatic epilepsy by age and cause. (From Annegers JF. The epidemiology of epilepsy. In: Wyllie E, ed. *The Treatment of Epilepsy: Principles and Practice.* Philadelphia: Lea & Febiger; 1993:161.)

ever. Figure 4–2 summarizes the proportional frequencies of the causes of epilepsy by age.

## DIAGNOSTIC APPROACH TO THE FIRST SEIZURE

### ACUTE ASSESSMENT

The patient presenting with normal mental status and neurologic examination after a seizure does not typically represent an emergency (this clinical situation is discussed in the next section). If the mental status and neurologic examination have not quickly normalized, however, two questions must be answered as rapidly as possible. First, is there an underlying medical or neurologic condition that requires immediate treatment? Second, has the seizure ended? These two questions must be addressed whether the patient is in an emergency room, intensive care unit, or ambulatory setting.

The urgent evaluation includes serum glucose, sodium, urea nitrogen, creatinine, calcium, hepatic enzyme concentrations, and complete blood count. Arterial blood pH, oxygen, and carbon dioxide should be measured. A toxicology screen should be obtained if no other etiology is readily identified, especially screening for ethyl alcohol, cocaine, amphetamines, benzodiazepines, opioids, phencyclidine, tricyclic antidepressants, and antipsychotic drugs.[5] Hypothyroidism with myxedema coma has been associated with seizures in rare cases.[31]

Brain imaging, preferably computed tomography (CT) because of its rapid availability at most centers, is necessary to exclude a structural cerebral injury such as hemorrhage, tumor, abscess, or contusion. If significant temperature elevation, nuchal rigidity, leukocytosis, or other sign of possible central nervous system (CNS) inflammation is present, a lumbar puncture is required to exclude infection or subarachnoid hemorrhage. If the patient has a possible history of seizures, the anticonvulsant medications taken should be identified and the serum concentrations determined.

Decreased responsiveness or unusual behavior may be the only indication of persistent seizure.[14,93] An EEG therefore is recommended for any patient whose mentation does not recover soon after a seizure. Furthermore, an EEG should be considered for any patient without a clearly defined cause of altered mental status. If "subclinical" seizures are believed to be a possible cause of confusion or abnormal behavior and the EEG is not diagnostic, a short-acting intravenous benzodiazepine (e.g., lorazepam) may clarify the diagnosis if clinical improvement is observed soon after its administration.[84]

### SEIZURE EVALUATION IN THE AMBULATORY SETTING

The patient presenting in an ambulatory setting with a history of a possible seizure is a common clinical situation. Often, an acute evaluation as described above already has been performed in the emergency room prior to referral. If the metabolic assessment has not been obtained, the serum studies previously described should be considered. The subsequent evaluation aims at answering four questions:

1. Was the paroxysmal behavior a change or a symptom of a seizure?
2. What is the classification of the seizure?
3. Is there an etiology that requires specific treatment?
4. What is the probability of another seizure?

A thorough history of the event, taken from both the patient and a witness, often is the most helpful diagnostic tool. An epigastric, olfactory, or experiential (psychic) aura suggests a partial seizure of temporal lobe onset,[63] for example, whereas generalized clonic activity immediately preceding the tonic-clonic phase may indicate an idiopathic generalized epilepsy. The clinical history may be ambiguous or suggest multiple possible diagnoses, including cardiac syncope, dysautonomia, conversion disorder, or panic attacks. In this situation the physician must use diagnostic tests judiciously to make a definitive diagnosis and to exclude progressive or potentially life-threatening disorders expeditiously. The two most helpful tests for achieving these goals in the ambulatory setting are EEG and MRI. We recommend that an EEG be obtained for every patient in whom seizure is a reasonable diagnosis. MRI is also recommended for these patients, unless the clinical history, family history, and EEG strongly indicate an idiopathic generalized epilepsy or unless a definite nontraumatic provocation, such as transient hypoglycemia, is known. If a cardiac etiology is suspected, appropriate testing or referral should be obtained.

## ELECTROENCEPHALOGRAPHY

EEG is an indispensable test for confirming the diagnosis of seizures as well as classifying seizures accurately. The typical EEG abnormalities seen in various seizure types are described in this section. The sensitivity of a single EEG for identifying specific epileptiform abnormalities is approximately 50%, increasing in some reports to more than 90% with the third recording.[4] The specificity of the EEG to a large extent depends on the interpreter; utmost care should always be taken not to misinterpret normal variants as epileptiform abnormalities.[62]

### Technical Considerations

Since Hans Berger[11] described abnormalities in the EEGs of patients with convulsions in 1933, EEG has been the single most important test used to confirm and define the diagnosis of epilepsy. In the 1950s Herbert Jasper[57] proposed the ten-twenty electrode system for standardization of electrode position on the scalp. Sharbrough et al expanded this system in the "modified combinatorial nomenclature" to include electrodes at 10% spacing and additional anterior and inferior temporal electrodes, as shown in Figure 4–3.[6] The "closely spaced" electrode array has demonstrated improved localization and increased sensitivity for identifying epileptiform abnormalities.[79,100] The American Electroencephalography Society has published guidelines to ensure technical adequacy of the recording; these should be followed as the minimum standard of EEG practice.[7] Although eight-channel recordings are acceptable, we recommend 18-21 channels with additional anterior temporal electrodes for routine EEG. At least three montages, both bipolar and referential, should be employed during the recording of at least 20 minutes. A channel dedicated to the electrocardiogram (ECG) is also useful practice to identify potentially symptomatic dysrhythmias. Digital EEG has improved over recent years and currently offers high-fidelity recording and presentation, with the advantage of the capability to reformat montages for optimal review.[7,74]

### Activation Procedures

Activation procedures should be used routinely in the EEG of patients with the possible diagnosis of epilepsy.[28] Hyperventilation activates generalized 3 Hz spike-wave discharges in at least 80% of patients with absence seizures.[24] Adams and Lüders[3] found that hyperventilation was a more reliable indicator of the frequency of absence seizures than a 6-hour recording. Focal spikes may also be activated, especially if the hyperventilation is vigorous and prolonged. One

study of 255 patients with complex partial seizures found that 4.4% had hyperventilation-activated clinical seizures, and another 6.6% had striking activation of interictal spikes.[77] Focal or lateralized slowing during or after hyperventilation may signify a region of potentially epileptogenic cerebral dysfunction. Hyperventilation should be induced with caution or omitted in patients with a history of medical disorders such as cerebrovascular disease, cardiac ischemia, or chronic obstructive pulmonary disease.

Intermittent photic stimulation (IPS) most often elicits epileptiform abnormalities in patients with generalized seizures, although it may cause spike and slow-wave bursts in 1% to 3% of normal subjects. The photoparoxysmal response is the hallmark finding, consisting of a reproducible short burst of generalized polyspike or spike and slow-wave activity,[121] as shown in Figure 4–4. Such a response typically occurs at the middle flash frequencies of 10 to 20 Hz and are not time-locked to the stimulation rate. In a video/EEG study of 1062 epilepsy patients, Wolf and Goosses[128] found that 91 of 103 patients with a photoparoxysmal response had generalized epilepsy, 31% had juvenile myoclonic epilepsy, 18% had childhood absence seizure, 17% had secondary generalized epilepsy, and 8% had juvenile absence seizure. When a photoparoxysmal response occurs in an EEG with focal interictal epileptiform abnormalities, however, the patient usually has partial seizures.[42] Care should always be taken to distinguish nonepileptic findings, such as a photomyogenic or photoelectric response, from a photoparoxysmal response.

Many types of progressive myoclonic epilepsies, a subtype of secondary generalized epilepsy, demonstrate a high rate of photoparoxysmal responses.[28] A photoparoxysmal response in an adult with dementia may suggest the diagnosis of the adult form of neuronal ceroid lipofuscinosis (Kufs'

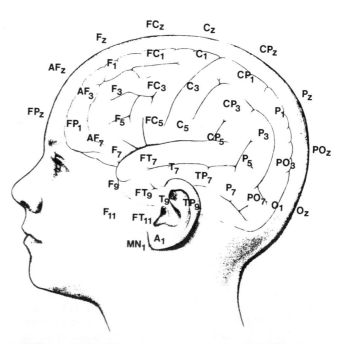

**FIGURE 4–3.** Modified combinatorial nomenclature and electrode position proposed by the American Electroencephalographic Society. (From Noachtar S, Wyllie E. EEG atlas of epileptiform abnormalities. In: Wyllie E, ed. *The Treatment of Epilepsy: Principles and Practice.* Philadelphia: Lea & Febiger; 1993:299.)

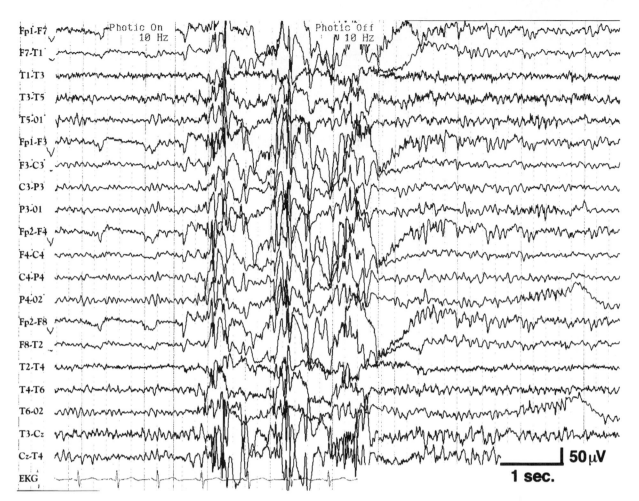

**FIGURE 4–4.** Example of a photoparoxysmal response to photic strobe stimulation at rate of 10 Hz.

disease). In the late childhood form of neuronal ceroid lipo-fuscinosis, high-amplitude occipital evoked responses are seen with slow IPS rates.

In 1947 Gibbs and Gibbs[38] reported markedly increased rates of interictal epileptiform discharges during sleep. Controversy has arisen over the significance of the sleep EEG, however, especially regarding the method of sleep induction. There appears to be no consensus on the effect of sleep deprivation on interictal discharges.[29,119] Nevertheless, non-REM sleep increases the rate of epileptiform abnormalities in certain epilepsies; 3 Hz spike-wave bursts of absence epilepsy, slow spike-wave activity of Lennox-Gastaut syndrome, and centrotemporal sharp waves of benign childhood epilepsy increase as sleep deepens, whereas generalized spike-wave bursts of juvenile myoclonic epilepsy decrease during stage II and deeper sleep.[28]

Drowsiness and sleep activate benign epileptiform variants that may be confused with truly epileptogenic abnormalities. Although typically <50 μV and brief, small sporadic sleep spikes (small sharp spikes or benign epileptiform transients of sleep) may have a broad morphologic range and amplitude up to 100 μV, mimicking true temporal spikes, as shown in Figure 4–5.[125] The phantom spike-wave pattern can be mistaken for atypical spike-wave discharges, and slow rhythmic temporal theta activity of drowsiness (psychomotor variant) may closely resemble temporal intermittent rhythmic delta activity (TIRDA). The review by Klass and Westmoreland[62] is recommended for a more complete discussion of normal variants.

### EEG in Patients With Partial Seizures

Spike discharges and sharp waves are the epileptiform abnormalities typically seen in patients with partial seizures. Spike discharges are predominantly negative waveforms of 20 to 70 ms duration with characteristic steep ascending and descending phases.[4,17,25,82,124] Sharp waves have a duration of 70 to 200 ms with a similar morphology of steep climbs. The localization and morphology of interictal epileptiform patterns usually provide useful information about the site of the primary epileptogenic zone. Interictal focal epileptiform abnormalities may be present at a significant distance from the region of seizure onset, however. Jayakar et al[58] have published an excellent review of EEG localization of seizure foci.

The most common epileptiform abnormality seen in patients with partial seizures is the anterior temporal spike or sharp wave.[25,82] Most patients with partial seizures have temporal lobe epilepsy, most commonly arising in the mesial temporal structures.[127] The negative field of the discharge is characteristically maximal in the sphenoidal or anterior/inferior temporal electrodes (FT9, FT10, T9, or T10), as demonstrated in Figure 4–6. Seventy to 80% of patients will have anterior temporal sharp wave localized to a single temporal

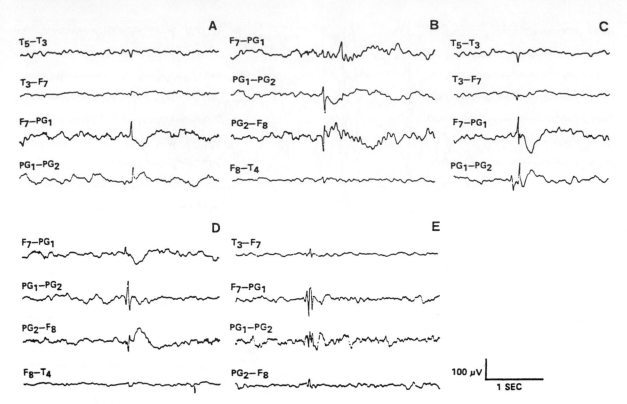

**FIGURE 4–5.** Examples of variability of benign epileptiform transients recorded from several normal volunteers during sleep (small sporadic sleep spikes). (From White JC, Langston JW, Pedley TA. Benign epileptiform transient of sleep. *Neurology.* 1977;27:1063.)

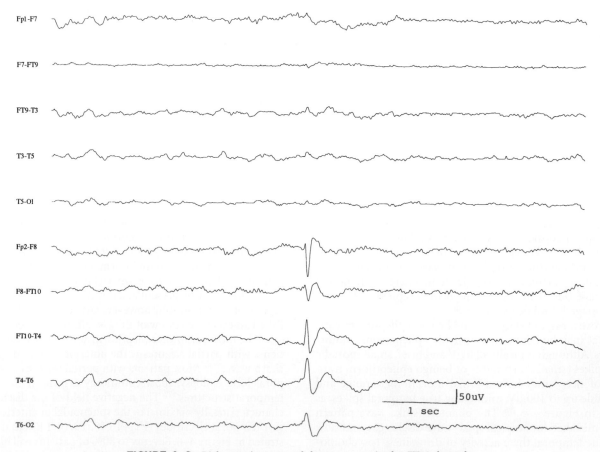

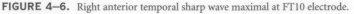

**FIGURE 4–6.** Right anterior temporal sharp wave maximal at FT10 electrode.

lobe, with the remainder exhibiting independent bitemporal discharges. Most patients with bitemporal discharges will have all seizures beginning in a single temporal lobe, however, and therefore should not be rejected from potential surgical candidacy based on the bitemporal interictal findings.[105] Closely spaced electrodes may aid in delineating the topography of temporal spikes.[79] Sphenoidal electrodes increase the sensitivity of EEG for both identifying and defining mesial temporal epilepsy, but to what extent is not clear.[13,60,64,100,107] In addition, anterior temporal sharp waves may occur in patients with extratemporal epileptogenic lesions.

Frontal sharp waves have been associated with epileptogenic lesions in the various areas of the frontal lobes, such as supplementary motor, dorsolateral, orbitofrontal, cingulate, and frontal pole.[97,111,126] A typical frontal sharp wave is demonstrated in Figure 4–7. The sensitivity and reliability for specific localization of frontal lobe sharp waves are less than with anterior temporal sharp waves.[97] A recent study of 34 patients who remained free of seizures following frontal corticectomy identified a specific localized EEG pattern in only 9% of the patients.[95] A lateralized multilobar interictal abnormality was observed in 59% of patients. The interictal EEG demonstrated no epileptiform abnormalities in 12% of those studied.

Central sharp waves generated in the dorsolateral posterior frontal or anterior parietal region may be seen in both symptomatic and idiopathic epilepsies but may not be associated with seizures in up to 50% of patients.[39,124] The characteristic central midtemporal sharp waves of benign childhood

epilepsy with centrotemporal spikes is a high-voltage diphasic or polyphasic discharge of 200 to 300 ms duration in the C3/C4 and T7/T8 electrodes. The sharp waves may be unilateral or bilateral and are typically most frequent during drowsiness or sleep. A tangential dipole may be present, with a negative polarity in the central and midtemporal regions and positive polarity in the ipsilateral anterior frontal region. As many as 40% of patients with these centrotemporal sharp waves will not have seizures. Similarly, not all children with "classic" central midtemporal discharges have a benign childhood epilepsy. Midline or vertex spikes are sometimes seen in children with generalized tonic-clonic seizures[80] and with supplementary motor seizures.[87] The distribution of these spikes necessitates adequate sampling with midline electrodes.

Occipital spikes are the least epileptogenic interictal epileptiform abnormality, with only 40% to 50% of patients with these findings having seizures.[61,124] They are most commonly seen in children. Gastaut[35] described an idiopathic childhood epilepsy in which seizures frequently begin with visual phenomena and end with headache. The characteristic interictal EEG abnormality is repetitive occipital spike and slow-wave complexes that attenuate with eye opening. This constellation of findings may also be seen in children with posterior cerebral structural abnormalities and intractable epilepsy.[43] Occipital "needle-sharp spikes" are sometimes seen in congenitally blind individuals without seizures.[25]

Interictal TIRDA, as shown in Figure 4–8, is described in patients with complex partial seizures of temporal lobe

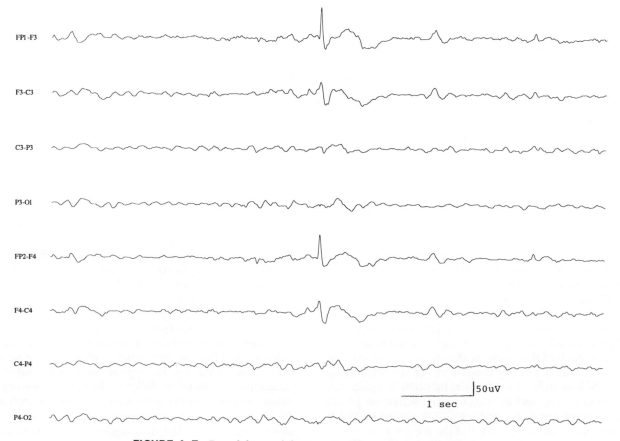

**FIGURE 4–7.** Frontal sharp and slow-wave complex maximal at Fp1 electrode.

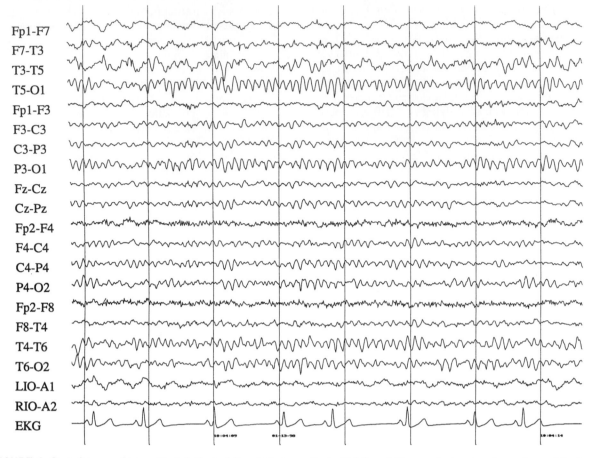

**FIGURE 4–8.** Left temporal intermittent rhythmic delta activity in a patient with left mesial temporal sclerosis and complex partial seizures.

origin.[34,37,98] The discharge consists of runs of moderate-amplitude rhythmic delta activity in the temporal region. The runs are most prominent during drowsiness and non-REM sleep. They have epileptogenic significance similar to that of temporal sharp waves.

Interictal generalized (typically bilateral frontal) spike and slow-wave activity may be seen in patients with partial seizures, as shown in Figure 4–9. This finding is often associated with inferior and mesial frontal epileptogenic regions, suggesting rapid propagation of discharges through interhemispheric pathways. Tukel and Jasper[117] proposed the term *secondary bilateral* synchrony to differentiate this phenomenon from *primary bilateral synchrony* in patients with idiopathic generalized epilepsy. Focal epileptiform activity should consistently precede generalized discharges to be reliably diagnosed as secondary bilateral synchrony rapidly propagated from a focal onset.

Although periodic lateralized epileptiform discharges (PLEDs) are typically seen in acute cerebral injuries, they are discussed in this section with other epileptiform abnormalities. PLEDs usually are biphasic or triphasic spikes or sharp waves followed by a slow wave, as shown in Figure 4–10. The discharges occur at a rate of about once per second, ranging from 0.5 to 5 seconds. The rate varies by <20% in a given patient and does not react to sleep or other activation procedures but may decrease over time.[21,102] A review by Walsh and Brenner[120] indicates that PLEDs are seen most frequently in patients with acute cerebral infarctions and ma-

lignant neoplasms but may also be seen in other disorders, such as brain abscess or herpes simplex encephalitis. These authors also found PLEDs to be highly epileptogenic, with 36 of 39 (92%) patients experiencing seizures during the hospitalization in which PLEDs were identified.

## EEG in Patients with Generalized Seizures

Several diffuse, paroxysmal EEG patterns have been described in patients with either idiopathic or symptomatic generalized epilepsies. Although these patterns are helpful for classification, the clinician should be aware that there is overlap between syndromes.[81] The 3 Hz generalized spike and slow-wave and atypical faster (3.5 to 6 Hz) spike and slow-wave patterns are typical for childhood and juvenile absence epilepsy, whereas generalized slow spike and wave discharges, diffuse paroxysmal fast activity, and hypsarrhythmia are more common in the secondary or symptomatic generalized epilepsies.

The "classic" description of the 3 Hz spike and slow-wave paroxysm as a surface negative spike followed by a negative slow wave is probably an oversimplification. After reviewing the EEGs of 200 patients with absence seizures, Weir[122] concluded that the typical complex consisted of a surface-positive transient followed by two surface-negative spikes and a slow wave. Furthermore, small differences in the discharge onset can be measured between hemispheres by using digital EEG.[99] The discharges may be potentiated by drowsiness, hyperventilation, or eye closure. The morphology may change during sleep into fragmented spike and slow-wave bursts. The 3 Hz spike and slow-wave pattern is considered highly epileptogenic, typically recorded in children and adolescents with absence seizures, as shown in Figure 4–8.

Generalized spike and slow-wave activity may be described as "atypical" when it is faster than 3 Hz (3.5 to 6 Hz) or varies in morphology.[25] These faster frequency spike or polyspike and slow-wave discharges usually indicate an age-related idiopathic generalized epilepsy when the background EEG is normal. This pattern may increase during non-REM sleep, although attenuation has been reported in stage II and deeper sleep in patients with juvenile myoclonic epilepsy.[28]

Gibbs et al[40] initially distinguished the 3 Hz spike and slow-wave pattern from slower patterns. Lennox and Davis[73] and later Gastaut et al[36] correlated spike and slow-wave activity of <3 Hz with patients experiencing multiple seizure types (often including tonic) and mental retardation. The spikes are less sharply contoured, and the complexes are more variable in frequency and distribution. The bursts of slow spike and wave activity may be prolonged, sometimes potentiated by drowsiness or sleep. Hyperventilation has less effect on slow spike and wave activity than on typical 3 Hz discharges. Focal or generalized slow activity may be present in the background EEG.

Generalized paroxysmal fast activity has been called the "grand mal discharge" because of the association with the tonic phase of tonic-clonic seizures.[39,124] The generalized discharges are usually low- to moderate-amplitude repetitive spike activity at 10 to 20 Hz. This pattern is often during tonic, atonic, and generalized tonic-clonic seizures,[32] but it is also present interictally in some children and adults with secondary generalized epilepsies.

Hypsarrhythmia refers to generalized high-amplitude (>300 µV) irregular slow-wave activity with admixed multifocal spikes or sharp waves.[50] Hypsarrhythmia is typically seen in children between 4 months and 5 years of age with infantile spasms. However, not all children with hypsarrhythmia have infantile spasms, and children with infantile spasms do not necessarily have hypsarrhythmia.[50] The EEG does not differentiate between symptomatic, cryptogenic, and idiopathic infantile spasms, although focal or lateralized features are more commonly seen in cases with identified cerebral injury. An electrodecrement may be seen during the spasms, and the hypsarrhythmia pattern may become discontinuous during non-REM sleep.[49]

### Ambulatory EEG Monitoring

For patients with unclear paroxysmal clinical events and a normal or nondiagnostic EEG, ambulatory EEG monitoring has been shown to be a useful tool. A common clinical situation involves events that cannot be reliable classified as epileptic seizure, psychogenic seizure, or cardiac/vasovagal syncope. Morris et al[78] reported the results of computer-assisted ambulatory 16-channel EEG in 191 patients with a normal or nonspecific routine EEG; interictal epileptiform abnormalities or electrographic seizures were recorded in 48 patients (25.1%), whereas "normal" push-button events were recorded in 81 patients (42.4%). They concluded that clinically useful recordings were obtained in 129 patients

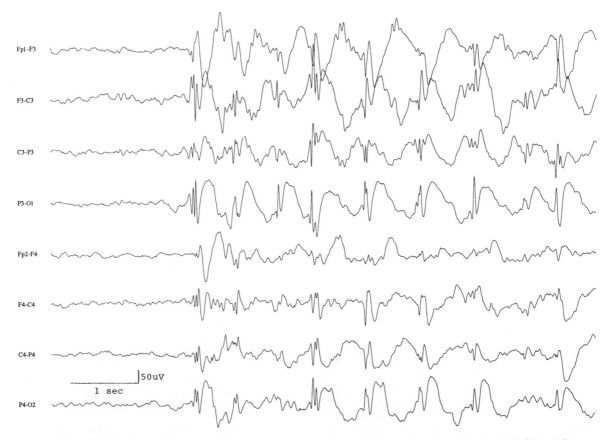

**FIGURE 4–9.** Example of rapid bilateral synchrony of polyspike and slow-wave complexes most prominent in left hemisphere.

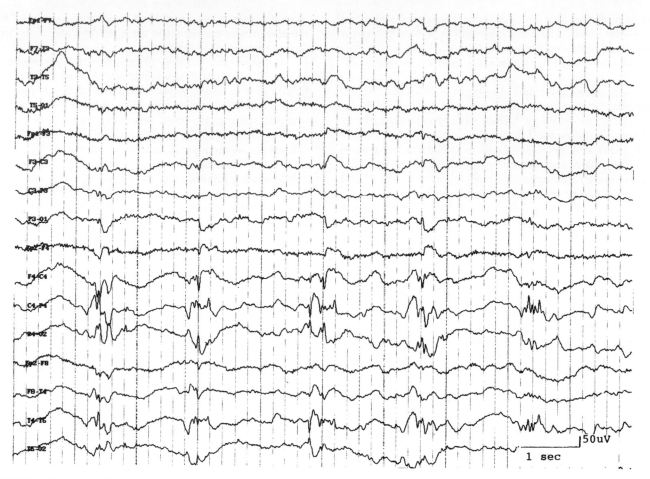

**FIGURE 4–10.** Periodic lateralized epileptiform discharges in a patient with recent right middle cerebral artery distribution stroke and subsequent secondarily generalized seizures.

(67.5%). The yield of epileptiform abnormalities of 25.1% was greater than that previously reported by Bridgers and Ebersole,[15] who used 8-channel ambulatory EEG (17.4%), presumably because of the increased spatial sampling.

## MAGNETIC RESONANCE IMAGING

MRI has dramatically improved the imaging of normal and pathologic brain structures. Although CT remains a useful tool, especially for imaging calcified structures, the limited resolution and bone artifact are problematic in assessing patients with focal seizures. The first goal of neuroimaging of seizure patients is to exclude a progressive or dangerous lesion such as a tumor or vascular malformation. Several studies have shown MRI to be superior to CT for identifying small lesions.[68,109,114] Therefore we recommend that MRI, when available, be performed in all patients with suspected partial seizures.

### Technical Considerations

MRI is a dynamic technology that is rapidly improving. Thus the definition of the optimal MRI method for evaluating patients with seizures is constantly changing. In general, T1-weighted short-repetition time/echo time (TR/TE) scans demonstrate anatomic relationships with superior resolution, whereas T2-weighted long TR/TE sequences are more sensitive for revealing focal pathology. New strategies such as "short flip angle" scans have been suggested to identify small

calcifications or hemorrhages.[112] Reviews of optimal acquisition sequences and methods of MRI evaluation of various types of epileptogenic lesions are available.[18,70]

Although broad anatomic coverage is necessary to maximize sensitivity in most MRI screening examinations, more detailed and specific imaging is useful in certain situations. In particular, since the temporal lobe is the most common site of onset in patients with partial seizures, attention to the mesial temporal region is advantageous. Kuzniecky et al[66,67] proposed the following protocol to aid in detection of epileptogenic abnormalities in the hippocampus and temporal lobe:

1. T1-weighted coronal images, 1.5 mm or 3 mm thick, gap 0.5 mm, perpendicular to the long axis of the hippocampus.
2. T2-weighted and T1-weighted coronal images 3 mm thick, gap 2.5 mm, in the same plane using short (TE, 20 to 30 ms) and long (TE, 80 to 100 ms) echo and motion-compensation techniques.
3. Axial T2-weighted and T1-weighted, 5 mm thick, parallel to the temporal lobe axis.
4. Coronal inversion recovery images in the coronal plane (TE, 26 ms; TI, 300 to 400; TR, 3600 ms) using 5 mm slice thickness every 7.5 mm.

In addition, FLAIR (fluid-attenuated inversion recovery) has emerged as a useful technique for the evaluation of mesial

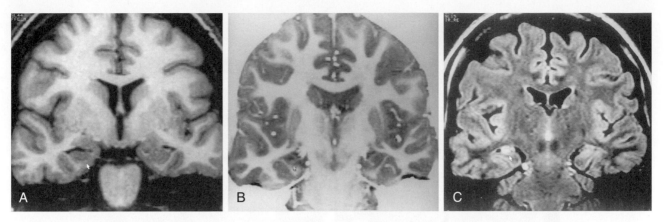

**FIGURE 4–11.** **A,** Atrophy of right hippocampus on T1-weighted image in a patient with seizures arising from right temporal lobe. **B,** Hypointense signal in right hippocampus on inversion recovery image in same patient. **C,** Hyperintense signal in right hippocampus on FLAIR image in same patient.

temporal sclerosis and other pathologic entities. The attenuation of water signal by FLAIR allows differentiation of the increased signal intensity of the sclerotic hippocampus from the cerebrospinal fluid signal in the temporal horn of the lateral ventricle.[12,53]

## COMMON EPILEPTOGENIC LESIONS

Mesial temporal sclerosis (MTS) is the most common pathologic substrate found in patients with temporal lobe epilepsy. The amygdala appears to be variably involved. When atrophy on T1-weighted images and increased signal intensity on T2-weighted images of the hippocampus are used to identify MTS, the sensitivity ranges from 80% to 93% with a specificity between 86% and 93%.[54,68] Quantitative T2 relaxometry also appears to be a useful technique.[55] The sensitivity and interobserver reliability is high when these criteria are determined by visual inspection, but quantitative volumetric analysis remains valuable for identifying bilateral MTS and for research studies.[19,51,52] High-resolution MRI may also demonstrate loss of definition of the internal morphologic structure of the sclerotic hippocampus.[56] Figure 4–11A demonstrates right hippocampal atrophy on a T1-weighted image; Figure 4–11B shows hypointense signal in the right hippocampus on an inversion recovery image; and Figure 4–11C shows increased signal in the hippocampus on FLAIR image.

As described earlier, a variety of structural abnormalities have been associated with epilepsy. Because of the frequent association of these abnormalities with seizures, the MRI characteristics of certain cerebral neoplasms, vascular malformations, and developmental malformations are reviewed in the remainder of this section.

Fibrillary astrocytomas comprise about 75% of hemispheric astrocytic neoplasms in adults.[16] They typically have a homogeneous hypointense signal on T1-weighted images and high signal on T2-weighted images, but increased signal intensity on T1-weighted images may occur. Enhancement with gadolinium contrast is variable. Higher grade anaplastic tumors or glioblastomas tend to have a more heterogeneous signal and commonly enhance with contrast. Pilocystic astrocytomas are usually well demarcated, with hypointense signal on T1 images and highly hyperintense T2 sequences, displaying contrast enhancement; these tumors

are most common in children, typically located in the diencephalon. Gangliogliomas typically appear as an inhomogeneous signal in the mesial temporal area, having a cystic component in 25% of cases.[110] Oligodendrogliomas are less common than astrocytic tumors, but they often have a characteristic heterogeneous signal from calcifications, vascularity, and mixed glial components.[72] Oligodendrogliomas are often located in the mesial temporal and superficial frontal regions. Dysembryoplastic neuroepithelial tumors (DNT) constitute about 10% of all tumors removed from patients with intractable epilepsy.[26] Characteristic MRI findings of DNT are well-localized hypointensity on T1 images and hyperintensity to gray matter on T2 images; although the tumors lack edema and may resemble benign cysts, their increased signal intensity on proton-density images suggests a more complex lesion.

The most common vascular abnormality reported in patients with intractable epilepsy is the cavernous angioma, shown in Figure 4–12.[9,45] The MRI features are characteris-

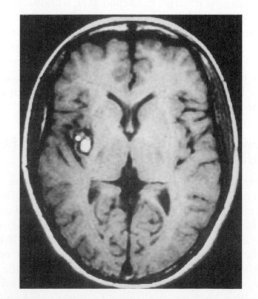

**FIGURE 4–12.** Cavernous angioma in right insular region on T1-weighted image in a 45-year-old woman. Another angioma was found in left frontal lobe. Patient recently began having EEG-confirmed simple partial seizures consisting of unusual sensation in pharynx and upper neck.

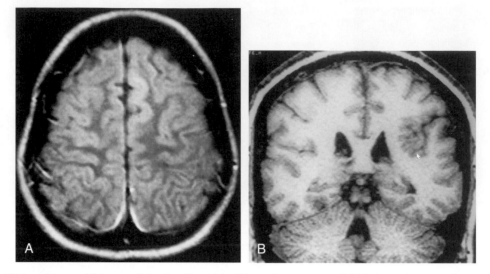

**FIGURE 4–13.** **A,** Thickened gyrus with increased signal on T2-weighted image in superior medial left frontal lobe in a patient with intractable partial seizures. Pathology showed cortical dysplasia. **B,** Thickened gyrus in left posterior insular region on T1-weighted image, probably representing focal polymicrogyria or cortical dysplasia.

tic, with a reticulated central core of mixed signals indicating blood by-products of different ages. Methemoglobin in the core typically appears as a high-signal image, surrounded by a rim of hypointense signal on both short and long echo images. There is no mass effect, vascular flow void, or surrounding edema. Venous angiomas are probably more common, but they are much less frequently associated with seizures. The typical dilated vascular structures of arteriovenous malformations usually allow unambiguous diagnosis with MRI, although small lesions may present more difficulty.

Regional developmental malformations, such as focal cortical dysplasia, hamartomas, and focal macrogyria and polymicrogyria, are much more readily identified by MRI than by CT.[84,85] The MRI appearance of these lesions frequently consists of large, thickened gyri, with increased signal on T2-weighted images, as shown in Figure 4–13.[70] More extensive hemispheric pathology may occur, such as in unilateral megalencephaly; the findings may range from mild polymicrogyria to lissencephaly. Other diffuse neuronal migration disorders, such as the "double cortex" syndrome[83] and the bilateral perisylvian syndrome,[65] have been clearly identified by MRI.

## PREDICTIVE VALUE OF EEG AND MRI FOR SEIZURE RECURRENCE

Berg and Shinnar[10] performed a meta-analysis of 17 studies of the risk of seizure recurrence following a first unprovoked seizure. Three studies in children focused on specific EEG abnormalities; the pooled risk of recurrence at 2 years was 58% with epileptiform abnormalities, 37% with nonepileptiform abnormalities, and 27% with a normal EEG. Although MRI was not considered in any of the studies, the pooled risk of recurrence at 2 years was 57% for patients with a known cause (remote symptomatic) and 32% for patients with idiopathic first seizures.

Shinnar et al[104] found similar results in a prospective study of EEG abnormalities following a first unprovoked seizure. Of 321 children less than 19 years of age, 59% with an epileptiform abnormality had recurrence, compared to 35% with a nonepileptiform abnormality and 25% with a normal EEG. In a prospective study of adults following an isolated idiopathic seizure, van Donselaar et al[118] had strikingly similar findings; 64% with epileptiform abnormalities had recurrence, compared to 41% with nonepileptiform abnormalities and 22% with a normal EEG.

## SPECIAL CLINICAL SITUATIONS

### INTRACTABLE EPILEPSY

Although medically intractable epilepsy cannot be defined in absolute terms, many centers consider alternative nonmedical treatment after three or more drugs have failed over a period of at least 2 years. Less stringent criteria are sometimes applied to young children with catastrophic epilepsy. Other than MRI and routine EEG, continuous video/EEG monitoring may be the most helpful test for evaluating intractable epilepsy, since up to 20% of referrals to specialized epilepsy centers have psychogenic seizures. Also, one study reclassified 47% of evaluated patients based on video/EEG results.[108] Antiepileptic medications were reduced in 60% of patients, whereas 60% of patients had a reduction in seizure frequency. Video/EEG has been considered a standard component of the evaluation of patients for possible epilepsy surgery.[94] The combination of EEG monitoring and MRI has been shown to be a powerful predictor of outcome from temporal lobectomy.[41] The American Electroencephalographic Society has published specific guidelines for long-term monitoring in epilepsy.[7]

Functional neuroimaging with interictal fluorodeoxyglucose positron emission tomography (PET) and ictal single photon emission computed tomography (SPECT) has proven to be useful for presurgical evaluation of the primary epileptogenic zone.[106] Unilateral interictal hypometabolism is found in 70% to 80% of patients with complex partial seizures, usually of temporal lobe origin.[2,30,113] Asymmetry of the mesial temporal region may be a specific predictor of good outcome following anterior temporal lobectomy.[75] PET appears to be complementary to focal MRI or EEG abnormalities in extratemporal lobe epilepsy, although the region of abnormality is often larger with PET.[1] Although interictal and postictal SPECT have inadequate specificity to be used for presurgical localization, Harvey et al[46] reported localization by ictal SPECT in 91% of patients with frontal lobe epilepsy. Ictal SPECT may be more technically feasible with the recent availability of a more stable technetium-binding agent lasting up to 6 hours. Further studies are required to determine the value of ictal SPECT without concordant EEG and MRI abnormalities. Magnetic resonance spectroscopy is a promising technology that can measure specific substances in the epileptogenic brain region.[20,69–71] It offers not only the possibility of gaining additional localizing information in individual patients but also important biochemical aspects of epileptogenicity in general.

## FEBRILE CONVULSIONS

Febrile convulsions are classified as either simple or complex.[33] The simple febrile seizure is a single generalized tonic-clonic convulsion lasting less than 15 minutes. A complex febrile seizure is defined by focal features, prolongation more than 15 minutes, or recurrence within 24 to 48 hours. Shinnar[103] has suggested a rational approach to the assessment of the first febrile convulsion, emphasizing exclusion of meningitis or encephalitis. A lumbar puncture is recommended for any patient with a focal seizure, abnormal neurologic examination, seizure after arrival at the emergency department, or prior treatment within 48 hours.[103] Meningismus is not reliably present in young children, so lumbar puncture is indicated in every child younger than 12 months with a first febrile convulsion. When in doubt, it is judicious to err on the side of lumbar puncture. EEG is of limited value in this setting. A CT scan is also recommended for any child with a focal febrile seizure or persistent new neurologic deficit, but it should not delay a lumbar puncture or treatment in patients with suspected meningitis.

## PSYCHOGENIC SEIZURES AND NONEPILEPTIC PAROXYSMAL DISORDERS

Confirmation of the diagnosis of nonepileptic events presents a significant problem for many neurologists, psychiatrists, pediatricians, and epilepsy centers. Several excellent reviews of the topic are available,[86] the most recent of which are by Gumnit[44] and Pellock.[88] Although a discussion of the wide variety of disorders and normal variants that may mimic epileptic seizures is beyond the scope of this chapter, several techniques may facilitate the diagnosis. Video/EEG monitoring to record a typical event is the single most useful test.[130] Caution should be used in attempting to distinguish psychogenic from frontal lobe seizures because the clinical characteristics can be similar and frontal lobe seizures often have no EEG accompaniment.[101] Various provocation techniques have been used, but injection of a placebo has been reported to have excessive false-positive results.[44] In cases with definite ictal EEG changes, ambulatory EEG monitoring may be adequate.[78] The serum prolactin level increases over the initial 10 minutes following 90% of generalized tonic-clonic seizures but only about 60% of complex partial seizures.[129] Rao et al[96] suggested that pro-

lactin levels measured 10 minutes after a seizure be compared to the levels 2 hours later. Wyllie et al[131] reported that serum creatine kinase elevations occur later following generalized tonic-clonic seizures and may be more useful in outpatients.

## DIAGNOSING ANTIEPILEPTIC MEDICATION-INDUCED TOXICITY

Some degree of toxicity is experienced by most patients taking antiepileptic drugs (AEDs). Most adverse effects involve the CNS and are easily alleviated by slowing the rate of titration or reducing the stable dose. Some side effects, however, require specific testing to determine the cause. For example, carbamazepine may cause hyponatremia, inducing fatigue and cognitive symptoms easily mistaken for direct CNS drug effects. Valproic acid has been associated with elevated ammonia levels without other evidence of hepatic dysfunction, also causing fatigue and mental status changes. The topic of all adverse AED effects is beyond the scope of this chapter, but comprehensive reviews are available for additional information.[115]

Pellock and Willmore[90] have reviewed the literature on severe idiosyncratic AED reactions and offered recommendations regarding routine serum testing. Although some prior studies suggested a need for serial serum testing for most AEDs, Pellock and Willmore concluded that "routine monitoring rarely identifies or protects patients at risk for AED-associated life-threatening reactions." Other than baseline hematologic, serum chemistry, and coagulation assessment before initiating AED treatment, no routine laboratory testing was recommended in otherwise healthy patients. Although more vigilant clinical monitoring may be necessary with felbamate because of the increased risk of aplastic anemia and hepatotoxicity, recent recommendations for routine serum testing were similar to those for other AEDs.[89]

Routine evaluation of medication levels does not seem warranted for most patients, despite the fact that this is common practice.[76] Three scenarios cover the presentation of patients in most clinic visits: (1) no seizures and no AED-induced toxic symptoms; (2) recurrent seizures but no symptoms of toxicity; and (3) recurrent seizures and toxicity. The first presentation requires no medication change, the second requires an increase in dosage, and the third probably warrants consideration of another medication. None of these situations requires serum drug concentrations to guide the clinical decision. Questions of noncompliance and hypermetabolic or hypometabolic states may be answered by assessing the serum AED concentration, which yields clinically useful information.

## ACKNOWLEDGMENTS

The authors thank Ruben Kuzniecky, M.D., for review of the imaging section and Mary Jo Sewell for assistance with manuscript preparation. Supported by National Institutes of Health grant NS01794-01.

## REFERENCES

1. Abou-Khalil B, Kuzniecky RI, Kessler RM, et al. Positron emission tomography in extratemporal lobe epilepsy. *Epilepsia.* 1993;34:121.
2. Abou-Khalil BW, Siegel GJ, Sackellares JC, et al. Positron emission tomography studies of cerebral glucose metabolism in chronic partial epilepsy. *Ann Neurol.* 1987;22:480-486.

3. Adams DJ, Lüders H. Hyperventilation and six-hour EEG recording in evaluation of absence seizures. *Neurology.* 1981;31:1175-1177.

4. Ajmone-Marsan C, Zivin LS. Factors related to the occurrence of typical paroxysmal abnormalities in the EEG records of epileptic patients. *Epilepsia.* 1970;11:361-381.

5. Alldredge BK, Lowenstein DH, Simon RP. Seizures associated with recreational drug abuse. *Neurology.* 1989;39:1037-1039.

6. American Electroencephalographic Society. Guideline thirteen: guideline for standard electrode position nomenclature. *J Clin Neurophysiol.* 1994;11:111-113.

7. American Electroencephalographic Society. Guidelines in EEG, evoked potentials, and polysomnography. *J Clin Neurophysiol.* 1994; 11:1-147.

8. Annegers JF. The epidemiology of epilepsy. In: Wyllie E, ed. *The Treatment of Epilepsy: Principles and Practices.* Philadelphia: Lea & Febiger; 1993:157-164.

9. Awad IA, Robinson JR. Cavernous malformations and epilepsy. In: Awad IA, Barrow DL, eds. *Cavernous Malformations.* Park Ridge, Ill: American Association of Neurological Surgeons; 1993:49-64.

10. Berg AT, Shinnar S. The risk of seizure recurrence following a first unprovoked seizure: a quantitative review. *Neurology.* 1991;41:965-972.

11. Berger H. Uber das elektrenkephalogram des menschen. *Arch Psychiatr Nervenkr.* 1929;87:527-570.

12. Bergin P, Fish D, Shorvon S, et al. Magnetic resonance imaging in partial epilepsy: additional abnormalities shown with the FLAIR pulse sequence. *J Neurol Neurosurg Psychiatry.* 1995;58:439-443.

13. Binnie CD, Marston D, Polkey CE, et al. Distribution of temporal spikes in relation to the sphenoidal electrode. *Electroencephalogr Clin Neurophysiol.* 1989;73:403-409.

14. Boggs JG, Towne AR, Smith J, et al. Frequency of potentially ictal patterns in comatose ICU patients. *Epilepsia.* 1994;35:135.

15. Bridgers SL, Ebersole JS. Ambulatory cassette EEG in clinical practice: experience with 500 patients. *Neurology.* 1985;35:1767-1768.

16. Burger PC. Malignant astrocytic neoplasms: classification, pathologic anatomy and response to treatment. *Semin Oncol.* 1986;13:16.

17. Cascino GD, Herkes GK. Interpretation of interictal EEG. In: Wyllie E, ed. *The Treatment of Epilepsy: Principles and Practices.* Philadelphia: Lea & Febiger; 1993:249-260.

18. Cascino GD, Jack CR. *Neuroimaging in Epilepsy: Principles and Practice.* Boston: Butterworth-Heinemann; 1996.

19. Cascino GD, Jack CR, Parisi JE, et al. Magnetic resonance imaging–based volume studies in temporal lobe epilepsy: pathological correlations. *Ann Neurol.* 1991;30:31-36.

20. Cendes F, Andermann F, Preul PC, et al. Proton MR spectroscopic imaging in temporal lobe epilepsy. *Neurology.* 1993;43(suppl):A223.

21. Chatrian GE, Shaw CM, Leffman H. The significance of periodic, lateralized epileptiform discharges in EEG: an electrographic, clinical and pathological study. *Electroencephalogr Clin Neurophysiol.* 1964;17: 177-193.

22. Commission on Classification and Terminology of the International League Against Epilepsy. A revised proposal for the classification of epilepsy and epileptic syndromes. *Epilepsia.* 1989;30:268-278.

23. Commission on Classification and Terminology of the International League Against Epilepsy. Proposal for revised clinical and electroencephalographic classification of epileptic seizures. *Epilepsia.* 1981;22: 489-501.

24. Dalby MA. Epilepsy and three per second spike and wave rhythms: a clinical, electroencephalographic and prognostic analysis of 346 patients. *Acta Neurol Scand.* 1969;40:1983.

25. Daly DD. Epilepsy and syncope. In: Daly DD, Pedley TA, eds. *Current Practice of Clinical Electroencephalography.* New York: Raven Press; 1990:269-334.

26. Daumas-Duport C. Dysembryoplastic neuroepithelial tumours. *Brain Pathol.* 1993;3:283-295.

27. Delgado-Escueta AV, Greenberg D, Weissbecker K, et al. Gene mapping in the idiopathic generalized epilepsies: juvenile myoclonic epilepsy, childhood absence epilepsy, epilepsy with grand mal seizures on awakening, and early childhood myoclonic epilepsy. *Epilepsia.* 1990;31:S19-S29.

28. Drury I. Activation procedures. In: Wyllie E, ed. *The Treatment of Epilepsy: Principles and Practices.* Philadelphia: Lea & Febiger; 1993:234-248.

29. Ellingson RJ, Wilken K, Bennet DR. Efficacy of sleep deprivation as an activation procedure in epilepsy patients. *J Clin Neurophysiol.* 1984;2: 83-101.

30. Engel J Jr, Kuhl DE, Phelps ME, et al. Interictal cerebral glucose metabolism in partial epilepsy and its relation to EEG changes. *Ann Neurol.* 1982;12:510-517.

31. Evans EC. Neurologic complications of myxedema: convulsions. *Ann Intern Med.* 1960;52:434-444.

32. Farrell K. Generalized tonic and atonic seizures. In: Wyllie E, ed. *The Treatment of Epilepsy: Principles and Practice.* Philadelphia: Lea & Febiger; 1993:443-450.

33. Febrile seizures: Consensus development conference summary. *Natl Inst Health.* 1980;3(2).

34. Gambardella A, Gotman J, Cendes F, et al. Focal intermittent delta activity in patients with mesiotemporal atrophy: a reliable marker of the epileptogenic focus. *Epilepsia.* 1995;36:122-129.

35. Gastaut H. A new type of epilepsy: benign partial epilepsy of childhood with occipital spike-waves. *Clin Electroencephalogr.* 1982;13:13-22.

36. Gastaut H, Roger J, Soulayrol R, et al. Childhood epileptic encephalopathy with diffuse slow spike-waves (otherwise known as "petit mal variant") or Lennox syndrome. *Epilepsia.* 1966;7:139-179.

37. Geyer JD, Bilir E, Faught RE, Kuzniecky R, Gilliam F. Significance of interictal temporal lobe delta activity for localization of the primary epileptogenic region. *Neurology.* 1999;52:202-205.

38. Gibbs EL, Gibbs FA. Diagnostic and localizing value of electroencephalographic studies in sleep. *Res Publ Assoc Res Nerv Ment Dis.* 1947;23:366-376.

39. Gibbs FA, Gibbs EL. Grand mal. In: *Atlas of Electroencephalography.* Cambridge, Mass: Addison-Wesley; 1952;2:109-161.

40. Gibbs FA, Gibbs EL, Lennox WG. Influence of the blood sugar level on the wave and spike formation in petit mal epilepsy. *Arch Neurol Psychiatry.* 1939;41:1111-1116.

41. Gilliam F, Bowling S, Bilir E, et al. Association of combined MRI, interictal EEG, and ictal EEG results with outcome and pathology after temporal lobectomy. *Epilepsia.* 1997;38:1315-1320.

42. Gilliam FG, Chiappa KH. Significance of spontaneous epileptiform abnormalities associated with a photoparoxysmal response. *Neurology.* 1995;45:453-456.

43. Gilliam F, Wyllie E. Ictal amaurosis: magnetic resonance imaging, electroencephalographic, and clinical features. *Neurology.* 1995.

44. Gumnit RJ. The differential diagnosis of epilepsy: nonepileptic paroxysmal disorders. In: Wyllie E, ed. *The Treatment of Epilepsy: Principles and Practice.* Philadelphia: Lea & Febiger; 1993:692-696.

45. Hardjasudarma M. Cavernous and venous angiomas of the CNS. *J Neuroimaging.* 1991;1:191-196.

46. Harvey AS, Hopkins IJ, Bowe JM, et al. Frontal lobe epilepsy: clinical seizure characteristics and localization with ictal 99mTc-HMPAO SPECT. *Neurology.* 1993;43:1966-1980.

47. Hauser WA, Hesdorffer DS. Incidence and prevalence. In: *Epilepsy: Frequency, Causes and Consequences.* New York: Demos Publications; 1990:1-51.

48. Hauser WA, Kurland LT. The epidemiology of epilepsy in Rochester, Minnesota, 1935 through 1967. *Epilepsia.* 1975;16:1-66.

49. Hrachovy RA, Frost JD, Kellaway P. Sleep characteristics in infantile spasms. *Neurology.* 1981;31:688-694.

50. Hrachovy RA, Frost JD, Kellaway P. Hypsarrhythmia: variations on a theme. *Epilepsia.* 1984;35:317-325.

51. Jack JC. MRI-based hippocampal volume measurements in epilepsy. *Epilepsia.* 1994;35:S21-S29.

52. Jack CJ, Gehring DG, Sharbrough FW, et al. Temporal lobe volume measurement from MR images: accuracy and left-right asymmetry in normal persons. *J Comput Assist Tomogr.* 1988;12:21-29.

53. Jack C, Rydberg C, Krecke K. Mesial temporal sclerosis: diagnosis with FLAIR versus spin-echo MR imaging. *Radiology.* 1996;199:367-373.

54. Jackson GD, Berkovic SF, Tress BM, et al. Hippocampal sclerosis can be reliably detected by magnetic resonance imaging. *Neurology.* 1990;40: 1869-1875.

55. Jackson GD, Duncan JS, Connelly A, et al. Increased signal in the mesial temporal region on T2-weighted MRI: a quantitative study of hippocampal sclerosis. *Neurology.* 1991;41(suppl 1):170-171.

56. Jackson GD, Kuzniecky RI, Cascino GD. Hippocampal sclerosis without detectable hippocampal atrophy. *Neurology.* 1993;44:42-46.

57. Jasper HH. The ten-twenty electrode system of the international federation. *Electroencephalogr Clin Neurophysiol.* 1958;10:371-375.

58. Jayakar P, Duchowny M, Trevor R, et al. Localization of seizure foci: pitfalls and caveats. *J Clin Neurophysiol.* 1991;8:414-431.

59. Jeavons PM, Clerk JE, Maheshwari MC. Treatment of generalized epilepsies of childhood and adolescence with sodium valproate ("Epilim"). *Dev Med Child Neurol.* 1977;19:9-25.

60. Kanner AM, Ramirez L, Jones JC. The utility of placing sphenoidal electrodes under the foramen ovale with fluoroscopic guidance. *J Clin Neurophysiol.* 1995;12:72-81.

61. Kellaway P. The incidence, significance and natural history of spike foci in children. In: Henry CE, ed. *Course in Clinical Electroencephalography: Current Clinical Neurophysiology: Update on EEG and Evoked Potentials.* New York: Elsevier/North-Holland; 1980:151-175.

62. Klass DW, Westmoreland BF. Nonepileptogenic epileptiform electroencephalographic activity. *Ann Neurol.* 1985;18:627-635.

63. Kotagal P. Seizure symptomatology of temporal lobe epilepsy. In: Luders H, ed. *Epilepsy Surgery.* New York: Raven Press; 1991:143-156.

64. Krauss GL, Lesser RP, Fisher RS, et al. Anterior "cheek" electrodes are comparable to sphenoidal electrodes for the identification of ictal activity. *Electroencephalogr Clin Neurophysiol.* 1992;83:333-338.

65. Kuzniecky R, Andermann F, Guerrini R. Congenital bilateral perisylvian syndrome: study of 31 patients. *Lancet.* 1993;341:608-612.

66. Kuzniecky R, Bilir E, Gilliam F, et al. Multimodality MRI in mesial temporal sclerosis: relative sensitivity and specificity. *Neurology.* 1997; 49:774-778.

67. Kuzniecky R, Cascino GD, Palmini A, et al. Structural imaging. In: Engel J Jr, ed. *Surgical Treatment of the Epilepsies.* 2nd ed. New York: Raven Press; 1993:197-200.

68. Kuzniecky R, De La Sayette V, Ethier R, et al. Magnetic resonance imaging in temporal lobe epilepsy: pathological correlations. *Ann Neurol.* 1987;22:341-347.

69. Kuzniecky R, El Gavish GA, Hetherington HP, et al. In vivo 31P nuclear magnetic resonance spectroscopy of human temporal lobe epilepsy. *Neurology.* 1992;42:1586-1590.

70. Kuzniecky R, Jackson GD. Neuroimaging in epilepsy. In: *Magnetic Resonance in Epilepsy.* New York: Raven Press; 1995:27-48.

71. Laxer KD, Hubesch B, Sappey-Marinier D, et al. Increased pH and inorganic phosphate in temporal seizure foci, demonstrated by (31P) MRS. *Epilepsia.* 1992;33:618-623.

72. Lee Y, Tassel PV. Intracranial oligodendrogliomas: imaging findings in 35 untreated cases. *AJNR.* 1989;10:119-127.

73. Lennox WG, Davis JP. Clinical correlates of the fast and slow spike-wave electroencephalogram. *Pediatrics.* 1950;5:626-644.

74. Levy SR, Berg AT, Testa FM, et al. Comparison of digital and conventional electroencephalogram (EEG) interpretation. *Epilepsia.* 1994;35:127.

75. Manno EM, Sperling MR, Ding X, et al. Predictors of outcome after anterior temporal lobectomy: positron emission tomography. *Neurology.* 1994;44:2331-2336.

76. McKee JW, Brodie MJ. Therapeutic drug monitoring. In: Engel J Jr, Pedley TA. *Epilepsy: A Comprehensive Textbook.* Philadelphia: Lippincott-Raven; 1997:1181-1194.

77. Miley CE, Forster FM. Activation of partial complex seizures by hyperventilation. *Arch Neurol.* 1977;34:371-373.

78. Morris GL, Galezowska J, Leroy R, et al. The results of computer-assisted ambulatory 16-channel EEG. *Electroencephalogr Clin Neurophysiol.* 1994;91:229-231.

79. Morris H, Luders H, Lesser RP, et al. The value of closely spaced scalp electrodes in the localization of epileptiform foci: a study of 26 patients with complex partial seizures. *Electroencephalogr Clin Neurophysiol.* 1986;63:107-111.

80. Nelson KR, Brenner RP, de la Paz D. Midline spikes: EEG and clinical features. *Arch Neurol.* 1983;40:473-476.

81. Niedermeyer E. *The Generalized Epilepsies.* Springfield, Ill: Charles C Thomas; 1972.

82. Niedermeyer E, da Silva FL. Abnormal EEG patterns (epileptic and paroxysmal). In: *Electroencephalography: Basic Principles, Clinical Applications and Related Fields.* Baltimore: Urban & Schwarzenberg; 1987: 183-207.

83. Palmini A, Andermann F, Aicardi J, et al. Diffuse cortical dysplasia, or the 'double cortex' syndrome: the clinical and epileptic spectrum in 10 patients. *Neurology.* 1991;41:1656-1662.

84. Palmini A, Andermann F, Olivier A, et al. Focal neuronal migration disorders and intractable partial epilepsy: a study of 30 patients. *Ann Neurol.* 1991;30:741-749.

85. Palmini A, Andermann F, Olivier A, et al. Neuronal migration disorders: a contribution of modern neuroimaging to the etiologic diagnosis of epilepsy. *Can J Neurol Sci.* 1991;18:580-587.

86. Pedley TA. Differential diagnosis of episodic symptoms. *Epilepsia.* 1983;24:S31-S44.

87. Pedley TA, Tharp BR, Herman KR. Clinical and electroencephalographic characteristics of midline parasagittal foci. *Ann Neurol.* 1981; 9:142-149.

88. Pellock JM. The differential diagnosis of epilepsy: nonepileptic paroxysmal disorders. In: Wyllie E, ed. *The Treatment of Epilepsy: Principles and Practice.* Philadelphia: Lea & Febiger; 1993:697-706.

89. Pellock JM, Brodie MJ. Felbamate: 1997 update. *Epilepsia.* 1997;38:1261-1264.

90. Pellock JM, Willmore LJ. A rational guide to routine blood monitoring in patients receiving antiepileptic drugs. *Neurology.* 1991;41:961-964.

91. Penfield W, Jasper H. Functional localization in the cerebral cortex. In: *Epilepsy and the Functional Anatomy of the Human Brain.* Boston: Little, Brown; 1954:41-155.

92. Penry JK, Dean JC, Riela AR. Juvenile myoclonic epilepsy: long-term response to therapy. *Epilepsia.* 1989;30:S19-S23.

93. Privitera M, Hoffman M, Moore JL, et al. EEG detection of nontonic-clonic status epilepticus in patients with altered consciousness. *Epilepsy Res.* 1994;18:155-166.

94. Quesney LF. Extracranial EEG evaluation. In: Engel J Jr, ed. *Surgical Treatment of the Epilepsies.* 2nd ed. New York: Raven Press; 1993:129-166.

95. Quesney LF, Constain M, Fish DR, et al. Frontal lobe epilepsy: a field of recent emphasis. *Am J EEG Technol.* 1990;30:177-193.

96. Rao ML, Stefan H, Bauer J. Epileptic but not psychogenic seizures are accompanied by simultaneous elevation of serum pituitary hormones and cortisol levels. *Neuroendocrinology.* 1989;49:33-39.

97. Rasmussen T. Characteristics of a pure culture of frontal lobe epilepsy. *Epilepsia.* 1983;24:482-493.

98. Reiher J, Beaudry M, Leduc CP. Temporal intermittent rhythmic delta activity (TIRDA) in the diagnosis of complex partial epilepsy: sensitivity, specificity and predictive value. *Can J Neurol Sci.* 1989;16:398-401.

99. Rodin E, Ancheta O. Cerebral electrical fields during petit mal absences. *Electroencephalogr Clin Neurophysiol.* 1987;66:457-466.

100. Sadler RM, Goodwin J. Multiple electrodes for detecting spikes in partial complex seizures. *Can J Neurol Sci.* 1989;16:326-329.

101. Saygi S, Katz A, Marks DA, et al. Frontal lobe partial seizures and psychogenic seizures: comparison of clinical and ictal characteristics. *Neurology.* 1992;42:1274-1277.

102. Schwartz MD, Prior PF, Scott DF. The occurrence and evolution in the EEG of a lateralized periodic phenomenon. *Brain.* 1973;96:613-622.

103. Shinnar S. Febrile seizures. In: *Current Therapy in Neurologic Therapy.* Philadelphia: B.C. Decker; 1990;3:29-32.

104. Shinnar S, Kang H, Berg AT, et al. EEG abnormalities in children with a first unprovoked seizure. *Epilepsia.* 1994;35:471-476.

105. So N, Gloor P, Quesney LF, et al. Depth electrode investigations in patients with bitemporal epileptiform abnormalities. *Ann Neurol.* 1989; 25:423-431.

106. Spencer SS. The relative contributions of MRI, SPECT, and PET imaging in epilepsy. *Epilepsia.* 1994;35:S72-S89.

107. Sperling MR, Mendius JR, Engel J Jr. Mesial temporal spikes: a simultaneous comparison of sphenoidal, nasopharyngeal, and ear electrodes. *Epilepsia.* 1986;27:81-86.

108. Sutula TP, Sackellares JC, Miller JQ, et al. Intensive monitoring in refractory epilepsy. *Neurology.* 1981;31:243-247.

109. Swartz BE, Halgren E, Delgado-Escueta AV, et al. Neuroimaging in patients with seizures of probable frontal lobe origin. *Epilepsia.* 1989;30: 547-558.

110. Tampieri D, Moumdjian R, Melanson D, et al. Intracerebral gangliogliomas in patients with complex partial seizures: CT and MR imaging findings. *AJNR.* 1991;12:749-755.

111. Tharp BR. Orbital frontal seizures: a unique electroencephalographic and clinical syndrome. *Epilepsia.* 1972;13:627-642.

112. Theodore WH. Neuroimaging in the evaluation of patients for focal resection. In: Wyllie E, ed. *The Treatment of Epilepsy: Principles and Practices.* Philadelphia: Lea & Febiger; 1993:1039-1050.

113. Theodore WH, Brooks R, Sato S, et al. The role of positron emission tomography in the evaluation of seizure disorders. *Ann Neurol.* 1984.

114. Theodore WH, Dorwart R, Holmes M, et al. Neuroimaging in refractory partial seizures: comparison of PET, CT, and MRI. *Neurology.* 1986;36:750-759.

115. Timmings P. Toxicity of antiepileptic drugs. In: Engel J Jr, Pedley TA. *Epilepsy: A Comprehensive Textbook.* Philadelphia: Lippincott-Raven; 1997:1165-1173.

116. Treiman LJ, Treiman DM. Genetic aspects of epilepsy. In: Wyllie E, ed. *The Treatment of Epilepsy: Principles and Practice.* Philadelphia: Lea & Febiger; 1993:145-156.

117. Tukel K, Jasper H. The electroencephalogram in parasagittal lesions. *Electroencephalogr Clin Neurophysiol.* 1952;4:481-494.

118. van Donselaar CA, Schimsheimer RJ, Geerts AT, et al. Value of the electroencephalogram in adult patients with untreated idiopathic first seizures. *Arch Neurol.* 1992;49:231-237.

119. Veldhuizen R, Binnie CD, Beintema DJ. The effect of sleep deprivation on the EEG in epilepsy. *Electroencephalogr Clin Neurophysiol.* 1983;55:505-512.

120. Walsh JM, Brenner RP. Periodic lateralized epileptiform discharges: long-term outcome in adults. *Epilepsia.* 1987;28:533-536.

121. Waltz S, Christen HJ, Doose H. The different patterns of the photoparoxysmal response: a genetic study. *Electroencephalogr Clin Neurophysiol.* 1992;83:138-145.

122. Weir B. The morphology of the spike-wave complex. *Electroencephalagr Clin Neurophysiol.* 1965;19:284-290.

123. Weissbecker KA, Durner M, Janz D, et al. Confirmation of linkage between the juvenile myoclonic epilepsy locus and the HLA region of chromosome 6. *Am J Med Genet.* 1991;38:32-36.

124. Westmoreland BW. The electroencephalogram in patients with epilepsy. In: Aminoff MJ, ed. *Neurologic Clinics.* Philadelphia: WB Saunders; 1985:599-613.

125. White JC, Langston JW, Pedley TA. Benign epileptiform transients of sleep. *Neurology.* 1977;27:1061-1068.

126. Williamson PD, Spencer DD, Spencer SS, et al. Complex partial seizures of frontal lobe origin. *Ann Neurol.* 1985;18:497-504.

127. Williamson PD, Wieser H-G, Delgado-Escueta AV. Clinical characteristics of partial seizures. In: Engel J Jr, ed. *Surgical Treatment of the Epilepsies.* New York: Raven Press; 1987:101-120.

128. Wolf P, Goosses R. Relation of photosensitivity to epileptic syndromes. *J Neurol Neurosurg Psychiatry.* 1986;49:1386-1391.

129. Wroe SJ, Henley R, John R, et al. The clinical value of serum prolactin measurement in the differential diagnosis of complex partial seizures. *Epilepsy Res.* 1989;3:248-252.

130. Wyllie E, Friedman D, Rothner AD, et al. Psychogenic seizures in children and adolescents: outcome after diagnosis by ictal video and electroencephalographic recording. *Pediatrics.* 1990;85:480-484.

131. Wyllie E, Luders H, Pippenger C, et al. Postictal serum creatine kinase in the diagnosis of seizure disorders. *Arch Neurol.* 1985;42:123-126.

# 5

# Cerebrovascular Disease

*Wolf-Ruediger Schaebitz, Pierre Combremont, and Marc Fisher*

Since being introduced to clinical medicine almost two decades ago, computed tomography (CT) and magnetic resonance imaging (MRI) have provided a new understanding of cerebrovascular diseases. The formerly used time course–dependent and clinically derived classification of transient ischemic attack (TIA), progressive stroke, and completed stroke were modified. A more pathophysiologically oriented classification evolved that categorizes ischemic lesions into small and large vessel disease and differentiates among the affected vascular territories. This approach has become the clinical routine and is currently part of the training of medical students and residents. In the meantime a second generation of imaging techniques, including diffusion- and perfusion-weighted imaging, as well as positron emission tomography (PET) and single photon emission computed tomography (SPECT) were developed. These modalities also gave new insights, especially into the acute phase of cerebral ischemia, and acute stroke became an emergency with a limited time window for therapeutic opportunities. As with recombinant tissue plasminogen activator (rt-PA) for the treatment of acute stroke, these new imaging techniques are beginning to enter clinical practice. Their great promise includes not only improved diagnosis of acute stroke but also better patient management and the development of new treatment strategies. Since special equipment and training are required, however, these newer techniques will be available in the near future only at larger medical centers. More available at small centers and even in practice settings are ultrasound techniques for the diagnosis of abnormalities of the cervical and transcranial arteries and the heart. Ultrasonography has become standard for the neurologic assessment of patients with cerebrovascular disorders. Noninvasiveness, availability, and relative economy combined with high sensitivity and specificity make ultrasonography a good diagnostic tool to detect treatable risk factors of stroke such as artery-artery or cardiac embolic sources. Cerebral angiography is an invasive procedure that is reserved for specific diagnostic situations (e.g., endarterectomy for carotid stenosis) and provides the possibility for interventional procedures such as intraarterial embolization of vascular malformations. This chapter provides an overview of the principles and findings of the major diagnostic tools for the assessment of patients with cerebrovascular disorders. Practice-oriented paradigms offer strategies for the diagnostic workup of specific stroke patients.

## NEUROIMAGING

### HEAD COMPUTED TOMOGRAPHY

Brain imaging is one of the most important diagnostic tools for cerebrovascular diseases. Twenty percent of head CT studies are performed to evaluate patients with stroke.[140] CT plays a role in every step of the evaluation of patients who have had ischemic strokes: (1) establishment of the diagnosis, (2) differential diagnosis of the stroke subtype and of its etiologic complex, (3) selection of the best treatment, and (4) estimation of the prognosis.

The diagnosis of ischemic stroke requires a clinical evaluation of the symptoms and signs presented by the patient. One must exclude other conditions that may be associated with a neurologic deficit mimicking a stroke: postictal Todd's paralysis, brain abscess,[122] encephalitis, metabolic imbalance, or toxicity. Although the clinical examination is the first step in the assessment of a patient with a cerebral infarct, an imaging study is frequently necessary to diagnose it accurately. A head CT is strongly recommended as the initial evaluation.[1,66] It is also helpful to determine the stroke subtype (Fig. 5–1), and treatment is dependent on the results. A head CT or MRI is frequently the only way to determine the diagnosis with certainty.[10] In most trials of new acute stroke treatment, particularly thrombolysis,[64,102] brain imaging is required. Finally, it has been established that head CT and MRI are useful in evaluating the outcome after brain infarction.[120] This chapter reviews the use of different brain imaging techniques in ischemic stroke, namely CT and MRI, and briefly discusses PET and SPECT.

### Principles of Computed Tomography

In CT an x-ray source rotates around the target, namely the brain, which absorbs a portion of the x-ray beam. The absorption is directly related to the electron density in the target. Therefore attenuation of the beam occurs in correlation with the tissue density and structure. A computerized

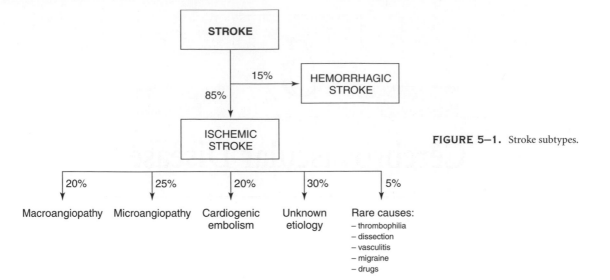

**FIGURE 5–1.** Stroke subtypes.

analysis of the beam's attenuation leads to the establishment of a tissue density map, which permits reconstruction of the tissue's architecture and an image of it.

During an acute cerebral infarction, cellular edema occurs.[80] This edema produces a change in tissue density that is the basis for the detection of a stroke in the acute phase. During the first hours, these changes in density are subtle. This points to the main sensitivity limitation of head CT: in 30% to 50% of patients with an acute ischemic stroke, the CT shows no abnormality.[52] The other major limitations are visualization of the posterior fossa and movement of the patient.

### Head Computed Tomography During Different Phases of Ischemic Stroke

*Acute Phase.* Density change is one of the early signs of brain infarction. The ischemic tissue becomes hypodense, often in the first few hours after the onset of symptoms. The hypodensity appears as decreased cortical gray matter–white matter differentiation, loss of distinction of the insular ribbon cortex, and blurring of the clarity of the internal capsule (Fig. 5–2).[136,137]

Another early sign is the demonstration of thrombosis of a major intracranial vessel, such as the middle cerebral artery or the basilar artery.[109] The "dense MCA sign" for example, is present in about 50% of head CT scans within 4 hours after the beginning of symptoms.[54,92] This sign usually is noted in situations in which other early signs are seen, such as hypodensity changes. The CT scan can also demonstrate vasogenic edema, sometimes associated with mass effect in early phase of stroke. This edema can occur after 3 to 6 hours and is proportional to the size of the infarction.[139] It is more likely to occur with prolonged occlusion of a vessel followed by reperfusion. In the acute phase of stroke, the use of contrast material is of limited value. It can mask the hypodense area, and its use has been found to be associated with a poor outcome.[81,143] That negative effect is probably due to the neurotoxicity of contrast agents. These agents can extravasate through the altered blood-brain barrier and affect borderline viable neurons located in the periphery of the infarct.

*Subacute Phase.* After 24 hours the infarct is usually well demonstrated by hypodensity, located in a specific vas-

cular territory (Fig. 5–3). During this phase, edema may be seen, and it can be differentiated from edema surrounding a tumor by the involvement of the cortex (in the case of an infarct).[98] The edema is maximal between days 3 and 5. Subsequently, the hypodensity tends to decrease and can sometimes completely disappear. This phenomenon is known as the "fogging effect." This effect is probably related to the breakdown of infarcted tissue, the proliferation of capillaries and macrophages, and, sometimes, the presence of focal petechial hemorrhages.[16]

During the subacute period the use of contrast has two indications. First, it helps to differentiate between old and

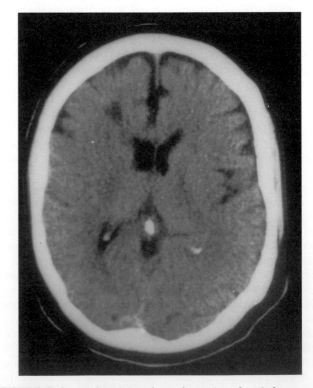

**FIGURE 5–2.** Head CT image shows obscuration of cortical gray matter–white matter differentiation and loss of distinction of insular ribbon cortex localized in territory of right middle cerebral artery.

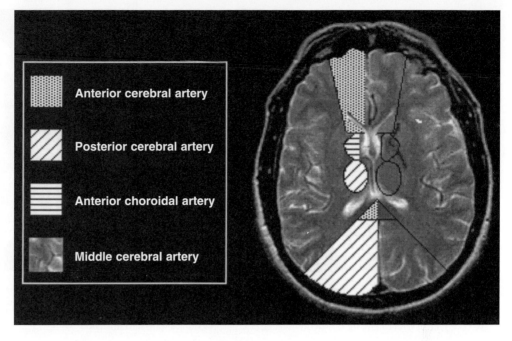

**FIGURE 5–3.** Vascular territories of major cerebral arteries.

subacute infarcts. Subacute infarcts show enhancement that is due to leakage of new permeable capillaries.[76] Second, a contrast agent can also demonstrate an infarct that would not be seen because of the fogging effect.

*Chronic Phase.* Old ischemic infarcts are hypodense and well demarcated. They may be associated with tissue atrophy. Such infarcts do not enhance with contrast material.

### Appearance of Ischemic Infarcts on Computed Tomography

The appearance of the infarct on CT can be an indication of the mechanism of the stroke. It helps the clinician to select the most appropriate additional tests in evaluating the etiologic basis of stroke, which is the key to selecting the best treatment for secondary stroke prevention.

A large infarct that extends to the cortex and has a triangular shape or an extensive lenticular infarct is consistent with an embolism. In either case investigation should be directed toward a cardiac or artery-to-artery source of embolism (Fig. 5–4A).

Lacunar infarcts appear as small areas of hypodensity, with sharp margins and sometimes enhancement through contrast on CT (Fig. 5–4B). These findings on CT are consistent with small artery occlusive disease. The same is true for leukoencephalopathy, which is best seen through MRI. In such situations, ultrasonography, angiography, or cardiac tests may not be helpful because none of these tests can demonstrate microvascular disease.

A hemodynamic infarct must be considered when the hypodensity lies in a watershed area (Fig. 5–4C).[21] There are two typical sites for a watershed infarct. One is between two main cerebral arteries (i.e., between the middle cerebral artery [MCA] and the anterior cerebral artery [ACA] or the posterior cerebral artery [PCA]). The other is in the corona radiata or the centrum semiovale (i.e., between the medullary arteries in the superficial pial plexus and the deep pen-

etrating arteries). A unilateral watershed infarct likely indicates severe stenosis of the carotid artery on that side.

### Hemorrhagic Infarct on Computed Tomography

A hemorrhage can appear in ischemic brain tissue, usually within 24 hours after the onset of the infarct. CT shows a hyperdense region within the hypodense area of the infarcted brain tissue (Fig. 5–5). The exact location is difficult to determine. If the head CT is done after hemorrhagic transformation of the infarct, the lesion may resemble a primary brain hemorrhage.[24] Hemorrhage should be suspected when the localized area is consistent with an embolic infarct (which more frequently has hemorrhagic transformation). It should also be considered when there are potential sources of cardioembolism, especially endocarditis, when there was a prior transient ischemic attack (TIA) or when the CT shows "silent" infarct.

### MAGNETIC RESONANCE IMAGING

For many, MRI has become the preferred imaging technique for the human brain, particularly because of its capability of demonstrating both vivo anatomic structures and pathologic phenomena. MRI can accurately diagnose cerebrovascular disorders, including subacute and chronic stroke, venous sinus thrombosis, and arteriovenous malformations. However, standard MRI findings during the critical acute phase of stroke are disappointing. The newer magnetic resonance (MR) technologies, such as diffusion-weighted imaging (DWI) and perfusion imaging (PI), can visualize the lesion in acute stroke and can follow the evolution of the lesion over time. Another MRI technique, magnetic resonance spectroscopy (MRS), provides information about in vivo biochemical parameters from the acute stroke patient to improve our understanding of the pathophysiologic basis of the disease. MR angiography is an elegant technique that noninvasively allows construction of an arteriogram to detect vascular stenoses and malformations. The following discussion explains the basic principles of these techniques

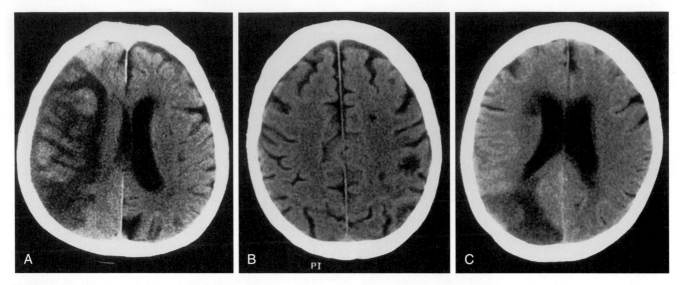

**FIGURE 5–4.** **A,** Head CT with hypointensity in distribution of right middle cerebral artery consistent with subacute infarction. Note displacement of lateral ventricle as a result of mass effect. **B,** Head CT with two small, round hypodensities in the white matter of the left hemisphere representing lacunar infarcts. Note large hypodensity in left parietal cortex–white matter junction consistent with an old infarct. **C,** Head CT with wedgelike hypointensity at the border of right middle cerebral and right posterior cerebral artery representing a watershed infarction.

and their usefulness for the diagnosis of cerebrovascular diseases.

## Techniques

MRI is performed by placing the patient in a strong magnetic field. Certain nuclei of the body tissues, such as water and fat protons, become susceptible to excitation by intermittent radiofrequency pulses. The energy released from the excited protons over a period of time is defined by two relaxation constants, T1 and T2, that determine the contrast on MRI studies. Applied radiofrequency pulses and receiver coils generate and detect different signals from tissue on the basis of the number of protons per unit volume of different substances (i.e., spin density). For routine clinical use, three types of images are generated: T1-weighted, T2-weighted, and spin-density-weighted images.[70] In T1-weighted images cerebrospinal fluid (CSF) has a low-signal intensity relative to the brain, whereas fat has a high-signal intensity. T1-weighted images provide good anatomic definition and are useful for detection of hemorrhage or vascular thrombosis. In addition, gyral swelling often can be appreciated. In T2-weighted imaging, CSF has an increased signal relative to the brain, whereas fat has almost no signal. T2-weighted images are best suited for demonstration of ischemic cerebral parenchymal damage and increases in tissue water content. This pulse sequence is also useful for distinguishing the normal signal void from arteries and veins and often allows the identification of occluded or stenotic vessels. On spin-density-weighted images the brain and CSF are comparable in signal intensity. The image contrast is primarily dependent on the abundance of protons in a given pixel. Spin-density-weighted images help to identify infarctions close to the ventricles and are best suited to detecting the hyperacute ischemic changes of stroke. Gradient echo images emphasize the T2* effect of paramagnetic blood products and are useful for the evaluation of intraparenchymal hemorrhage.

DWI is based on the natural translational motion of water molecules, brownian motion.[86] Application of a mag-

netic field gradient causes a phase shift of the transverse magnetization of protons carried by water molecules, thus attenuating the signal. The intensity of the attenuation depends directly on the amplitude of the molecular phase shift and the applied magnetic field gradient. DWI is a sensitive detector of acute stroke because presumably it can visualize the movement of water from the extracellular into the intracellular space that occurs during the formation of cytotoxic edema in the acute phase of stroke. Structures with slow diffusion and less attenuation are hyperintense on DWI. Structures with fast diffusion are darker and hypointense on DWI. Adding a pair of dephasing and rephasing magnetic field

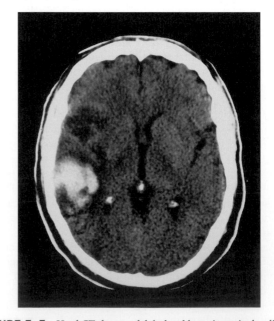

**FIGURE 5–5.** Head CT shows polylobulated hyperintensity localized in an area of hypodensity that represents a hemorrhagic infarction in distribution of the right middle cerebral artery.

gradients to the standard spin-echo sequence can sensitize the MRI for diffusion.[87] DWI requires fast imaging techniques, such as echo planar imaging (EPI), to avoid motion artifacts; these techniques can generate an image in less than 1 second.[46] Diffusion can be quantified by calculating the apparent diffusion coefficient (ADC), and this value can be used to define the severity of the lesion.

PI enables one to evaluate the microcirculation of the brain and can provide quantitative information about localized changes in cerebral blood flow (CBF) and cerebral blood volume (CBV). Two perfusion strategies are applicable to clinical problems; they are based on either the magnetic susceptibility effect of gadolinium-containing agents or noninvasive magnetic labeling of arterial blood. For "contrast agent bolus tracking," ultrafast MR images are obtained after the intravenous injection of a gadolinium-containing contrast agent.[19] The contrast agent transits through the brain, interferes with the acquisition of T2* signal intensity in perfused regions, and consequently induces a strong localized magnetic field. Therefore perfused areas on PI become dark. In nonperfused or hypoperfused regions, less or no reduction in signal intensity occurs because the contrast agent induces a smaller reduction of T2* acquisition.[19] For magnetic-labeling PI, arterial blood protons (spins) in arterial water are labeled with a radiofrequency pulse, and the label is followed through the arterial circulation of the brain.[118] Both techniques enable qualitative and quantitative analysis of CBF and are able to demonstrate varying degrees of perfusion deficits within the ischemic lesion from the core to the penumbra of the ischemic region.[45,114,118]

Another MR-based technique, MRS, provides biochemical information about normal and ischemic brain tissue. Hydrogen ($^1$H) and phosphorus ($^{31}$P) are the two atomic nuclei most commonly evaluated by MRS. Carbon, fluorine, and sodium can be also measured by MRS, although such studies are more difficult because of a lower signal-to-noise ratio. $^1$H MRS yields information about lactate, N-acetylaspartate, creatinine, and choline. $^{31}$P MRS studies display high-energy phosphates, such as adenosine triphosphate (ATP), phosphocreatine, inorganic phosphates, and phosphomonoesters and diesters.[12,72]

## Stroke

The pattern of cerebral infarctions is largely dependent on the vascular anatomy involved. A single intracranial major-vessel occlusion, particularly after thromboembolism, causes imaging abnormalities in the region supplied by that vessel. Acute changes on both conventional MRI and CT fall into one of these two categories: those related to gyral changes and those related to the affected vasculature itself. The gyral changes are thought to reflect the development of vasogenic edema and include sulcal effacement and gyral hyperintensity on proton-density and T2-weighted images. Subtle gyral hypointensity can be appreciated on T1-weighted images. Changes involving the affected vasculature are related to slow or absent flow. The normal signal void of rapidly flowing blood is not observed. After paramagnetic contrast administration, abnormal enhancement within the affected artery can be seen. This intravascular enhancement sign is thought to result from sluggish flow within the vessel and can be seen in 77% of cortical infarcts that are 1 to 3 days old.[47] Another sign observed on standard MRI within

acute cerebral infarction is the meningeal enhancement sign.[47] This MRI sign is seen in 35% of cortical infarctions that are 1 to 3 days old. It involves the dura mater overlying large cortical infarcts and is thought to be caused either by the recruitment of collateral vessels or by irritation and reactive hyperemia from the underlying infarction. Vascular and meningeal enhancement typically disappear 2 to 4 days after stroke. Furthermore, MR angiography can be crucial for the diagnosis of an acute ischemic event and may directly show embolic occlusion of the arteries that supply the intracerebral brain, consequently leading to therapeutic intervention such as rt-PA lysis.

For visual demonstration of subacute and chronic changes of stroke, CT and MRI are almost equally effective. Changes in the intensity of the parenchyma of the infarcted brain occur in 90% of stroke patients by 24 hours.[29,145] These changes are usually visible as bright hyperintensities, particularly on the proton-density and T2-weighted images (Fig. 5–6). In contrast, T1-weighted images are not highly sensitive and show only faint changes at the same site. These hyperintense abnormalities are thought to reflect the development of vasogenic edema, which results from damage to the blood-brain barrier. The region of the hyperintensity on the T2-weighted image typically enlarges between the first and second day after stroke, probably as a result of conversion of penumbral tissue into infarcted tissue, which then contributes to the final infarct size.

Hemorrhagic infarction occurs when an area of infarcted tissue becomes revascularized before the affected endothelium and the disrupted blood-brain barrier are sufficiently repaired. Hemorrhagic transformation is more common in embolic and cortical infarctions and typically occurs 24 to 48 hours after reperfusion at the margin of the infarction.[71,144] Disruption of the vasculature causes either punctate or gyral petechial hemorrhage or, more rarely, larger multifocal hematomas, which are often hard to distinguish from cerebral hematomas without an ischemic insult.[51] Findings on MRI include an increased signal on T1-weighted images (especially 24 to 48 hours after stroke onset), a decreased signal on T2-weighted images, and a decreased signal on the gradient echo images in comparison to those seen in white matter. Primary hematomas are more homogeneous in density, round to oval in shape, and more sharply defined than hemorrhagic infarcts. The MRI is sensitive to deoxyhemoglobin, methemoglobin, and hemosiderin, and the presence of these blood products characterizes the acute (1 to 2 days), subacute (2 to 7 days), and chronic phase of a hematoma. The acute phase is characterized by a slightly hypointense region at the site of the bleeding in T1-weighted imaging and a clearly hypointense signal on T2-weighted imaging. The subacute stage is typically visible on T2-weighted imaging as a bright, central hyperintense signal with a hypointense ring and a hyperintense rim of edema. During the transition toward more chronic stages, the hematoma becomes homogeneously hyperintense on both T1- and T2-weighted imaging, whereas in very late stages, beyond 1 month, the hematoma is typically hypointense on T1- and T2-weighted imaging.[40,58,59]

Contrast enhancement studies are useful for determining the age of an ischemic stroke, since contrast enhancement usually is not seen prior to 6 days after stroke and persists for 2 to 3 months.[33] The enhancement pattern is often

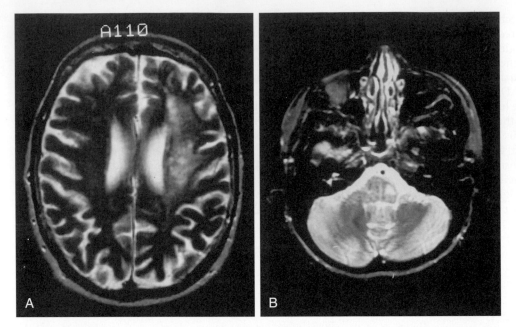

**FIGURE 5–6. A,** Hyperintensity in the vessel territory of the left middle cerebral artery assessed by T2-weighted imaging demonstrates a subacute ischemic infarct. **B,** Hyperintensity in the left pons on T2-weighted imaging representing an ischemic brainstem infarct. For detection of infarction in posterior circulation, MRI is superior to CT.

peripheral, ringlike or gyroform. During the second week after stroke onset the once prominent and clearly visible infarction often is absent from the image. This so-called fogging occurs with both CT and MRI.[11] Fogging is due to either small petechial hemorrhages or to macrophage ingestion of lipidlike substances and gliosis. In the fogging phase of cerebral infarction, dramatic contrast enhancement often can be seen. The chronic stage of infarction (3 to 4 weeks) is characterized by restoration of the integrity of the blood-brain barrier, resorption of edema, and necrotic tissue. On MRI, mass effect and enhancement are usually absent. Cortical calcification or hemorrhage can be seen as increased signal on T1-weighted images and as decreased signal on T2-weighted images, often in a gyroform pattern.

Infarction of the deep white matter and the capsular and ganglionic areas is thought to be due to progressive occlusion and hypoperfusion rather than embolization of deep perforating end arterioles. These lacunar infarcts are difficult to distinguish in the acute phase and usually appear on MRI 2 to 3 days after onset as small areas of high signal on T2- and spin-density-weighted images. Typical locations include the lentiform nucleus, the cauda, the pons, and the internal capsule. Watershed infarctions appear as a hypoperfusion pattern in the boundary zones between the distribution of the adjacent major vessels. Typical findings on MRI are hyperintense wedge like lesions, for example, between the middle and posterior cerebral arteries on T2-weighted imaging after chronic internal carotid narrowing.

Despite the capabilities of MRI in subacute and chronic stroke, conventional MR techniques are usually unable to visualize cerebral infarction during the initial hours. The new imaging techniques of DWI and PI allow visualization of the acute ischemic lesion within minutes of stroke onset. In both experimental and human stroke, ADC values rapidly decline after occlusion.[67,99,141] The ischemic region is visualized as a hyperintense area in comparison to the surrounding normal brain tissue (Fig. 5–7A). In stroke patients, focal ischemic lesions, with diameters as small as 4 mm (i.e., lacunar lesions), have been detected within 2 hours of the onset of ische-

mia.[141] The location and the extent of the ischemic lesion in animals can be defined, and the evolution of the lesion can be followed in time and space.[113] Potentially salvageable areas of the lesion might be distinguished from irreversibly injured tissue, and monitoring of therapeutic intervention can be appreciated.[67] Recent studies in humans suggest that lesion volumes determined by DWI in the acute phase can be used to predict clinical severity and outcome of stroke.[94] Furthermore, experimental and clinical studies have shown that the ADC recovers and becomes elevated after 1 week and allows for determination of the age of the lesion.[95]

PI allows qualitative and quantitative measurements of CBF in acute stroke. The perfusion deficit caused by an acute stroke in experimental studies is clearly visible within seconds after the onset of the occlusion and within 2 hours after onset of ischemia in humans (Fig. 5–7B).[124,142] The combination of early DWI and PI may provide prognostic information capable of distinguishing stroke patients who will respond to therapy, such as rt-PA lysis and future neuroprotective agents, from those who will not. Furthermore, PI can demonstrate the efficacy of therapy by documenting reperfusion after thrombolysis.

The strength and promise of MRS in stroke comes from its unique ability to measure aspects of biochemistry in vivo and noninvasively in the human brain subject to ischemia. Combined with the anatomic images of structural pathology and measurements of the biophysical status of water by the MRI methods previously described, the specific biochemical information supplied by MRS can expand understanding of stroke pathophysiology. Several biochemical abnormalities caused by human stroke have been detected by MRS since studies of acutely ill patients became feasible. The $^{31}P$ spectrum of the brain contains information about energy metabolites such as phosphocreatine and adenosine triphosphate and demonstrates an overall loss of signal but normal metabolite ratios in chronic phases of stroke, which is consistent with replacement of infarcted tissue by interstitial fluid.[25,90] Lactate elevation as an indicator of metabolic failure can be studied by $^{1}H$ MRS in both the acute and chronic phases of stroke and was correlated with clinical outcome.[20,28,61] Neuronal loss may be indicated by a decrease in signal of *N*-acetyl groups, mainly *N*-acetylaspartate, measured by [1]H MRS several days after stroke.[60] Elevation of choline-containing compounds may reflect a breakdown of the myelin.[13] Combining the [1]H and the [31]P spectra to multinuclear MRS studies, which can be obtained from the same subject in a single recording session, enables faster and more efficient studies of the biochemical nature of the human stroke.

## Dural Sinus Thrombosis

MRI is the best method for diagnosis of venous sinus thrombosis, even when clinical symptoms are absent or non-

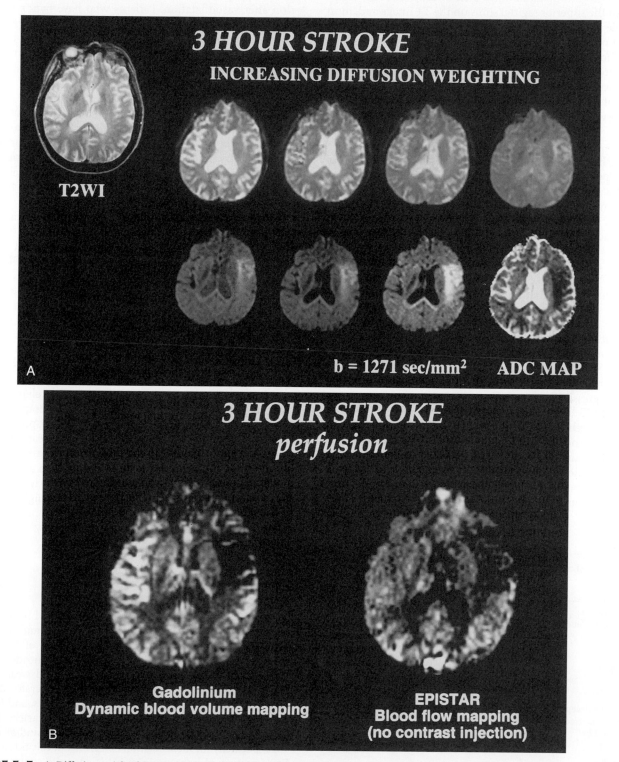

**FIGURE 5–7.** **A,** Diffusion-weighted imaging 3 hours after onset of symptoms (hemiparesis) demonstrates hyperintensity in the territory of the left middle cerebral artery, whereas T2-weighted imaging appears to be normal. **B,** Perfusion imaging 3 hours after stroke shows a perfusion deficit as a region of hypointensity in the territory of the left middle cerebral artery. (From Fisher M, ed. *Stroke Therapy.* Boston: Butterworth-Heinemann; 1995.)

specific.[135] Superior sagittal sinus thrombosis may cause bilateral or unilateral parasagittal hemorrhagic infarctions. These infarctions are not limited to vascular territories and tend to occur at the gray matter–white matter junction. Hemorrhagic transformation within the infarction is seen as increased signal on the T1-weighted image or a signal void on the T2-weighted image, depending on the age of the hemorrhage. Additional findings include absence of the signal void in the superior sagittal sinus on the T1 image and, most reliable, the hyperintensity of the sinus on T1 image because of the methemoglobin phase.[96,132] The T2-weighted images may show a signal void in the sinus that is due to the paramagnetic effect of blood products such as methemoglobin or deoxyhemoglobin.[125,132] The diagnosis can be difficult in cases of partial thrombosis of the sinus or recanalization of the previously occluded sinus.[134]

### SINGLE PHOTON EMISSION TOMOGRAPHY

SPECT is a simple technique of increasing interest in neurology. It has several clinical applications, such as cerebrovascular diseases, epilepsy, dementia, and extrapyramidal syndromes.[128] Its principle is based on the use of a gamma camera that is sensitive to the radiation emitted by tracers. The tracers can be classified as intravascular tracers, perfusion tracers, ligands of specific receptors, and metabolic tracers, all of which have specific uses (Table 5–1).

In the setting of acute ischemic stroke, SPECT shows perfusion abnormalities (hypofixation of tracers) with greater sensitivity than does CT. The use of SPECT in acute stroke has become especially interesting since the availability of acute cerebral infarction therapy (e.g., rt-PA) because it can be a useful test to screen out candidates for such treatment.[6] SPECT also shows incomplete infarction after ischemic stroke and can be useful in determining the need for more aggressive treatment.[55]

SPECT also has some applications in subacute and chronic cerebral infarction. Coupled with CT, it is a good prognostic tool for long-term recovery.[100] It can also demonstrate alterations of CBF that are not directly correlated to the localization of a lesion on CT or MRI but that are clinically significant, SPECT also shows alteration of CBF related to a deafferentation mechanism: the diaschisis.[111] This phenomenon explains how clinical deficits can occur at a distance from a cerebral infarct.

In addition, SPECT is used in the evaluation of arterial stenosis. By giving acetazolamide (a carbonic anhydrase inhibitor that produces cerebral vasodilatation by increasing carbon dioxide), one can evaluate the cerebral flow reserve. For example, if an arterial stenosis is significant, SPECT shows hypoperfusion or worsening of previous hypoperfusion after vasodilatation. Patients who have hypoperfusion ipsilateral to a carotid artery stenosis before endarterectomy have normal perfusion after surgery. In contrast, patients who have bilateral or contralateral hypoperfusion before surgery show no improvement after endarterectomy.

### POSITRON EMISSION TOMOGRAPHY

PET is an interesting technique, but its clinical use is restricted, mainly because of its technical complexity and limited availability. It is the most complete technique for studying ischemic stroke since it provides information about CBF, CBV, cerebrovascular mean transit time (t), cerebral metabolic rate of oxygen ($CMRO_2$), oxygen extraction fraction (OEF), and cerebral glucose use.

PET can be especially useful in acute stroke for targeting the population most likely to benefit from therapy (thrombolysis or neuroprotective agents) with a minimal risk of side effects.[50] By combining information about CBF, CBV, OEF, and $CMRO_2$, one can differentiate among three types of acute cerebral infarct.[15] These types are (1) a hyperperfusion state with nearly normal metabolism, which accounts for one third of patients between 5 and 8 hours after onset[97]; (2) hypoperfusion with increased OEF and moderately decreased $CMRO_2$, which corresponds to the situation described as penumbra with minimal infarction; and (3) marked hypoperfusion associated with hypometabolism, which corresponds to infarction. With such a characterization of patients, one can select the best therapeutic approach. Patients with a PET pattern corresponding to penumbra are likely to benefit most from a treatment such as thrombolysis. In these patients, one should avoid aggressive reduction of blood pressure. Patients with a pattern of complete infarction are likely to respond poorly to thrombolysis and to be at risk for side effects. They might be good candidates for reduction of blood pressure to minimize the risk of hemorrhagic transformation, and they also might benefit from treatment of edema.

## CERVICAL AND TRANSCRANIAL ULTRASOUND

Doppler sonography of the extracranial and transcranial arteries is an easily available, cost-effective, safe, and relatively fast technique that allows in vivo monitoring of CBF and imaging of the vascular anatomy. As with all diagnostic modalities, ultrasound techniques have strengths and weaknesses. Doppler sonography of the cranial vessels is operator dependent and requires knowledge of anatomy, physics, and hemodynamics as well as experience. However, carotid artery duplex scanning can achieve a 90% to 95% sensitivity and at least a 90% specificity for identification of significant carotid stenosis. For detection of intracranial stenosis, Doppler sonography is usually as specific as for extracranial vessels (although less sensitive). We recommend performing Doppler sonography, if

---

### TABLE 5–1. Types of Tracers

| TRACER TYPE | SPECIFICITY |
|---|---|
| **Intravascular** | |
| Erythrocytes labeled with technetium 99m | Strictly intravascular<br>Cerebral blood volume evaluation<br>Blood vessels visualization |
| **Perfusion** | |
| Xenon 133 | Quantitative cerebral blood flow evaluation |
| Microspheres | Cerebral blood flow evaluation |
| **Ligands of Receptors** | |
| Molecules labeled with iodine 123 | Visualization of specific receptors sites (e.g., gamma-aminobutyric acid, muscarinic acetylcholine receptor) |
| **Metabolic** | |
| Amino acids radioactively labeled | Tumor metabolism |

possible, as a screening method in the initial workup of every stroke patient. The most important findings include extracranial carotid artery atherosclerosis, one of the most treatable causes of ischemic stroke, as well as cerebral embolism, intracranial stenosis, cervical artery dissection, steal syndrome, and arterial vasospasm.

## PRINCIPLES

The key components of ultrasound techniques used for cardiac and cerebral imaging are Doppler ultrasonography and B-mode imaging. Duplex scanning and color-flow imaging represent further developments of these ultrasound principles. Doppler sonography is used to evaluate the velocity, pattern, or characteristics of blood flow.[69] The Doppler principle basically involves a shift in frequency when a sound source or scatterer and a receiver are moving relative to one another. The sound is shifted to a higher frequency when the two are moving toward each other and to a lower frequency when they are moving relatively apart. The unit of measure for this Doppler shift is hertz (Hz), and since it is in the audible range (20 to 20,000 Hz), it can be appreciated as a pitch in the shift of a sound.[7,69]

A transducer converts electrical energy to high frequency sound waves (usually 2 to 10 MHz) that are transmitted into the soft tissue and reflected or scattered by moving blood particles, causing a shift in frequency to the scattered sound. From the portion of the scattered sound that returns to the transducer, the magnitude of the Doppler shift can be quantified. Knowledge of the direction of the flow relative to the path of the sound beam allows the calculation of the flow velocity, a uniform and comparable diagnostic parameter. Since sound travels through soft tissue at a virtually constant speed, the depth of sampling (or depth and size of sample volume) can be determined.[85] The Doppler shift is then processed by the use of a fast Fourier transformation technique to analyze the velocity spectrum.[26] Parameters used for spectral analysis include flow direction, peak systolic velocity, diastolic velocity, shape, width, and appearance of the velocity spectrum. Primarily peak systolic and diastolic velocities are used to evaluate vascular hemodynamics and stenosis. Normal vessels, for instance, have an expected range of flow velocities and a compact, narrow-velocity spectrum. Disturbed or turbulent flow broadens the velocity spectrum, even to the point of flow reversal. Stenosis or vasospasm increases flow velocity. Ranges of stenosis assessed by velocity changes in Doppler sonography correlate well with diagnosis made by arteriography and pathologic findings and can be used to predict clinical outcome.[4,27,73,127]

The second type of ultrasound technique is the B-mode, or brightness-mode, image that provides a two-dimensional gray-scale image of the soft tissue and the vessels. The B-mode principle is based on the part of the sound energy that is scattered or reflected back to the transducer to create an acoustic picture. Since sound travels at constant speeds in soft tissue, the time from transmission to return can be used to localize the point along the path of the sound beam from which a scattered signal returns. Strong signals are coded bright gray or white, whereas weak signals are coded darker gray to black. To create a two-dimensional gray-scale image, multiple B-mode scan lines are obtained by sweeping the ultrasound beam across the field of interest. These are then put together to create an acoustic picture of the slice of the tissue that provides anatomic information in vivo.[69,133]

The combination of Doppler sonography and B-mode imaging overcomes many of the shortcomings of one technique alone. Duplex scanning enables the investigator to obtain a Doppler sample of a specific location visually guided by the two-dimensional gray-scale image. In addition, flow velocity information can be coded with a red or blue color, depending on the direction of flow (toward or away from the transducer) and superimposed on the B-mode image. The resulting color-flow image provides both anatomic and hemodynamic information simultaneously in a real-time visual display. Advantages of color-flow imaging include rapid documentation of the presence and direction of flow, greater accuracy of estimation of the angle of insonation and location of the region of highest flow velocity, better identification of surface structures, improved detection of hypoechoic plaques through a color void, and better detection of nearly complete occlusion.[7,82,123,127]

## CAROTID ARTERY ULTRASONOGRAPHY

### Carotid Artery Stenosis and Occlusion

Before an analysis of the velocity data is begun, listening to the arterial pulsation may be useful for vessel identification and detection of stenotic changes. The common carotid, external carotid, and internal carotid arteries all have distinct sounds. The common carotid artery is elastic, the external carotid artery supplies a high-resistance vascular bed, and the internal carotid artery delivers blood to a low-resistance system. In general, vessel narrowing causes a local increase of flow velocity; however, a narrowing of less than 40% of the lumen of the vessel frequently remains undetectable. Flow velocities with peak frequencies ranging above 4 kHz are typical with mild stenosis (40% to 60%). A moderate degree of stenosis (60% to 80%) is characterized by distortion of the normal pulsatile flow and increased flow velocities with peak frequencies between 4 and 8 MHz. Peak systolic flow deceleration is found in the poststenotic segment. A severe stenosis (>80%) produces drastically increased local peak flow velocities (>8 kHz) and reduced prestenotic and poststenotic spectra. Flow in the ophthalmic artery may be retrograde. A subtotal stenosis (>95%) is characterized by a small signal of variable frequencies that decreases once a stenosis becomes pseudoocclusive. With internal carotid artery occlusion the local ultrasound signal is absent, whereas the spectra of the common carotid artery are reduced and ophthalmic flow may be retrograde (Fig. 5–8). Severe intracranial stenosis within the carotid siphon or the middle cerebral artery may reduce spectra in the ipsilateral extracranial carotid artery and alter direction of flow and signal frequency in the ophthalmic artery.[69,73,116]

Application of duplex or color-flow imaging in patients with cervical artery disease enables not only visual guidance for accurate placement of the Doppler sample but also visualization of typical mechanisms of stenosis such as plaques. Characterization of plaque with ultrasonography includes location and distribution, surface features (smooth, irregular, crater, or ulcer), echodensity or calcification, texture (homogenous, heterogeneous, intraplaque hemorrhage), and pulsation pattern (normal, radial, or longitudinal). Heterogeneous plaque configuration with intraplaque hemorrhage and surface ulcerations are correlated with a higher risk for stroke.[17,53,56] Ultrasonography provides a noninvasive means of detecting patients who can be treated through endarterectomy. However, confirmation of significant stenosis by standard angiography or MR angiography is recommended.

Since arterial dissection creates a second false lumen between the intima and the media or the media and the adventitia, it is possible, although sometimes difficult, to differentiate the true from the false lumen with Doppler sonography. On B-mode ultrasonography the loosened intima flutters back and forth during each cardiac cycle or duplicated carotid lumen is found. Distal internal carotid artery dissection may mimic subtotal stenosis or occlusion of the artery.[69]

### Vertebral Artery Stenosis and Occlusion

The same techniques described in the preceding section can be used to detect stenoses in the vertebral artery. The criteria for classification of the extent of the lesion basically are the same as for the carotid arteries, although Doppler velocity criteria are less reliable for the diagnosis of vertebral stenosis. The use of duplex or color-flow imaging makes differentiation between obstructive lesions and anatomic variations such as hypoplasia easier. Doppler sonography of the vertebral arteries can also be helpful in evaluating collateral pathways, vertebral dissection, or a vertebral source of embolism. Flow direction in the vertebral arteries is important for detecting a subclavian steal syndrome (Fig. 5–9).

## TRANSCRANIAL DOPPLER SONOGRAPHY

### Intracranial Stenosis and Occlusion

Transcranial Doppler sonography (TCD) uses a sound emitted at a 2 MHz frequency that allows deeper tissue penetration through the acoustic windows of the skull to obtain flow velocity information about the intracranial arteries. The transtemporal acoustic window provides access to hemodynamic data from the middle, anterior, and posterior cerebral arteries. A suboccipital approach, with insonation through the foramen magnum, provides access to the intracranial and basilar arteries, whereas a transorbital approach can be used to insonate the ophthalmic artery and the carotid siphon via the optic foramen.[117] Identification of vessels relies on the acoustic window used, the depth of sampling, the flow direction, the direction of the transducer, the flow velocity, and the characteristics of the Doppler spectral pattern, in light of knowledge of the normal anatomic and hemodynamic relationships.[103]

Pathologic conditions result in a narrowing, constriction, stenosis, or occlusion of the affected vessel. This change leads to an increase of the blood flow velocity (BFV) (commonly >80 cm/s for mean flow velocity). Additional findings include side-to-side asymmetry of the mean flow velocity (MFV) of >30 cm/s and turbulence of flow at the site of the stenosis (Fig. 5–10A). Distal to the stenosis, upstroke and BFV usually are reduced, carbon dioxide reactivity is decreased, and collateral blood flow may be induced.[34] Intracranial atherosclerosis (tandem lesions), intracranial dissection, vasospasm or vasoconstriction, and cerebral embolism can be identified by such changes.[5,79,146]

### Detection of Microemboli

Platelet thrombi, air emboli, or atheromatous materials are detected during TCD monitoring by a characteristic "chirping" sound of at least 15 dB as they pass near the recording ultrasound probe during the cardiac cycle (Fig. 5–10B).[34] Detection of these high-intensity transient signals (HITS) helps to identify the source of embolization as the heart and aorta vs. the carotid artery and to distinguish subgroups of patients with symptomatic and asymptomatic high-grade carotid artery stenosis.[130] It furthermore enables detection of an intracardiac right-to-left shunt (e.g., patent foramen ovale) by transcranial identification of microbubbles after intravenous injection of agitated saline or contrast agent.[43,77]

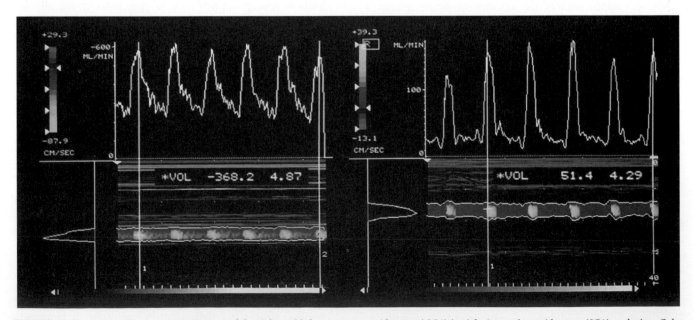

**FIGURE 5–8.** Volume flow rate measurements of the right and left common carotid artery (*CCA*) in right internal carotid artery (*ICA*) occlusion. Color motion mode (M-mode) display of four cardiac cycles on either side is shown below. Volume flow rate estimates in the CCA contralateral to occlusion on the ICA reveal normal to high normal values (368 ml/min). Ipsilateral to occlusion, the volume flow rate is greatly decreased since only the flow directed into the external carotid artery is carried by the CCA (51 ml/min). (See Color Plate.) (From Fisher M, ed. *Stroke Therapy.* Boston: Butterworth-Heinemann; 1995.)

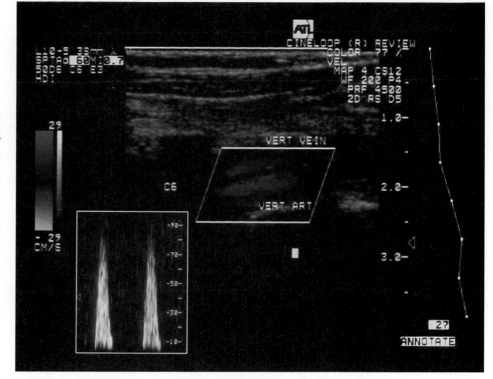

**FIGURE 5–9.** Subclavian steal syndrome assessed by color duplex sonography. In this longitudinal color-flow image, direction of vertebral vein and vertebral artery are both caudal (encoded in blue). The vertebral artery is supplying the brachial artery via subclavian artery on left side. Duplex Doppler spectral waveform at lower left shows flow reversal and total loss of diastolic flow. (See Color Plate.) (From Fisher M, ed. *Stroke Therapy.* Boston: Butterworth-Heinemann; 1995.)

### Arteriovenous Malformations

TCD noninvasively enables detection of arteriovenous malformations. Increased BFVs, decreased pulsatility index, and a lack of carbon dioxide reactivity characterize the feeding vessel. Pulsatile flow characterizes draining veins.[93,121] Furthermore, TCD is useful for the follow-up of patients with and without treatment (e.g., surgery, radiation) and as a monitoring tool during therapeutic intravascular embolization procedures.[107]

### Vasospasm After Subarachnoid Hemorrhage

TCD is an excellent instrument for monitoring vasospasm following subarachnoid hemorrhage (SAH). Vasospasm occurs after SAH, usually between days 3 and 10, and is indicated by a rapid increase of flow velocities and an increased risk of ischemic injury. Maximum flow velocities usually can be seen between day 11 and day 18. Flow velocities normalize 3 to 4 weeks after SAH. The method is reliable for detection of vasospasm in the middle cerebral artery but problematic for spasms in the anterior cerebral, basilar, and vertebral arteries.[37,62,63]

## CARDIAC IMAGING

The goal of the cardiac examination in stroke patients is the detection of a potential source of cardiac emboli (Table 5–2), which cause 15% to 20% of ischemic strokes.[30,108] Although some potential sources of cardioembolization can be diagnosed at the bedside by routine cardiac examination or electrocardiography (e.g., mitral stenosis, atrial fibrillation, myocardial infarction), modern cardiac imaging techniques give more reliable information. Such techniques include CT, MRI, transesophageal echocardiography (TEE), and transthoracic echocardiography (TTE). For practical reasons of availability, safety, and economy, echocardiography is for clin-

icians the most relevant cardiac imaging technique. It is able to detect most of the abnormalities listed in Table 5–2. Echocardiography should be considered in patients with large subcortical (>1.5 cm) or cortical infarcts with normal cerebrovascular imaging studies. Patients with proven noncardiac disease, such as carotid stenosis, large vessel intracranial occlusive disease, or small vessel disease with lacunar infarction (<1.5 cm), probably should not have electrocardiographic studies. The following discussion focuses on the indications and findings of TTE and TEE when used to search for an embolic source of ischemic stroke.

### TRANSTHORACIC ECHOCARDIOGRAPHY

TTE is performed by placing an ultrasound probe on the chest wall and evaluating cardiac structures through the intervening tissue, using the spaces between or under the ribs. In general, TTE accurately images the anterior structures of the heart and easily assesses atrial and ventricular dimensions, wall motion abnormalities, stenotic or regurgitant valvular lesions, and pericardial disease. TTE is a relatively insensitive technique for imaging intracardiac

| TABLE 5–2. **Potential Source of Cardiac Embolism** | |
| --- | --- |
| **HIGH-RISK SOURCES** | **LOW-RISK SOURCES** |
| Atrial fibrillation | Patent foramen ovale |
| Prosthetic heart valves | Atrial septal defect |
| Rheumatic mitral stenosis | Atrial septal aneurysm |
| Recent myocardial infarction | Ventricular septal defect |
| Left ventricular aneurysm | Hypercoagulable status |
| Intraluminal thrombus | Mitral valve prolapse |
| Left atrial spontaneous echo contrast | |
| Dilated cardiomyopathy | |
| Valvular vegetations | |
| Sick sinus syndrome | |

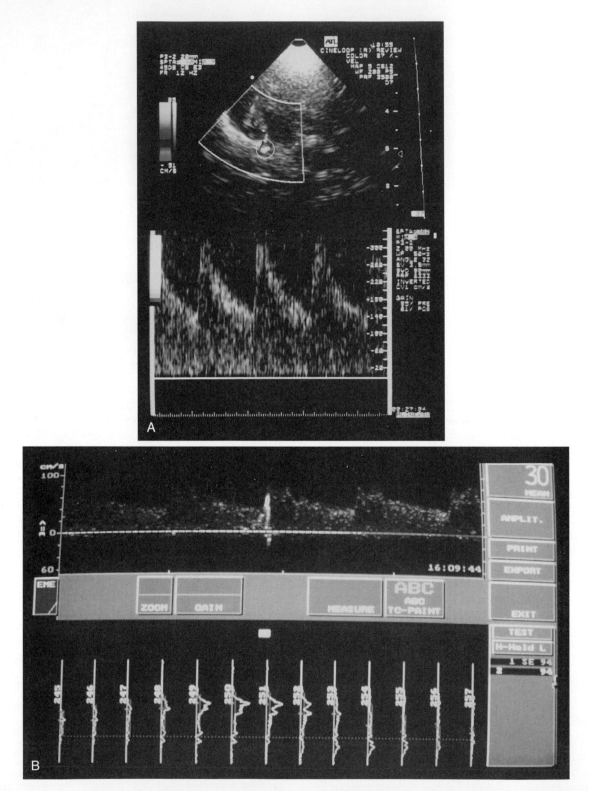

**FIGURE 5–10.** **A,** Transcranial color-flow imaging demonstrates a tight middle cerebral artery (*MCA*) mainstem stenosis. The circled bright-yellow area shows stenotic jet at origin of MCA. Duplex Doppler spectral analysis reveals >300 cm/s systolic and >140 cm/s diastolic flow velocity. **B,** High-intensity transient signal assessed by transcranial Doppler sonography of MCA in center of spectral display. Signal intensity is displayed by color-encoded dB scale. Cold colors depict low intensity and warm colors indicate higher intensity. Amplitude and relative intensity of signal are displayed below. White bar denotes area of analysis. Highest intensity is reached in line 251. Air bubbles or formed matter emboli are much stronger scatterers and reflectors than surrounding blood. (See Color Plate.) (From Fisher M, ed. *Stroke Therapy.* Boston: Butterworth-Heinemann; 1995.)

masses, the left atrium, the left atrial appendage, and certain parts of the left ventricle. A normal TTE often does not rule out a source of cardiac embolization, but the technique is widely available, relatively inexpensive, and noninvasive. A typical scenario for the use of TTE is a stroke that occurs after an acute anterior wall myocardial infarction in which a left ventricular mural thrombus is the suspected cause of the stroke.

## TRANSESOPHAGEAL ECHOCARDIOGRAPHY

TEE uses an ultrasound probe at the tip of a flexible endoscope that is inserted into the esophagus and positioned directly behind the left atrium. TEE not only is superior to TTE for imaging left-sided structures of the heart (atrium, atrial appendages, intraatrial septum, parts of the ventricle, atrial surfaces of the mitral and tricuspid valves) but also provides better images of cardiac chambers and valvular structures, intracardiac thrombi and masses, and valvular vegetations and offers much better spontaneous echocardiographic contrast. TEE also is an excellent technique for imaging the descending aorta, which is posterior to and to the left of the esophagus at the level of the left atrium. Typical indications for TEE are (1) stroke and coexistent mitral stenosis, (2) atrial fibrillation, (3) presence of a prosthetic valve, or (4) fever and a newly detected cardiac murmur (i.e., suspected endocarditis). Patients with stroke of undetermined cause without clinical evidence of cardiac disease are better suited for TEE than TTE because TEE is more accurate for detecting asymptomatic but potentially embolic lesions, such as patent foramen ovale, atrial septal aneurysm, aortic atherosclerosis, and small cardiac tumors.

## Patent Foramen Ovale

One source of cardiac embolization that is reliably detectable with TEE is patent foramen ovale, which usually is identified during TEE when microbubbles cross from the right atrium into the left atrium following the intravenous injection of agitated saline contrast (Fig. 5–11). A diagnosis can be made when two or more microbubbles are seen in the left atrium within three cardiac cycles of contrast appearance in the right atrium, although less strict criteria are also acceptable.[3] Paradoxical embolism is presumably the cause of stroke in patients with patent foramen ovale when no other etiologic factors have been identified.[42,88]

## Atrial Septal Aneurysm

TEE also reliably detects atrial septal aneurysm, which consists of a local bulging of the septum primum through the fossa ovalis into the right atrium, the left atrium, or both. Atrial septal aneurysm is associated with other cardiac abnormalities, including mitral and tricuspid valve prolapse, patent foramen ovale, and a right or left shunt. Atrial septal aneurysm must be distinguished from atrial myxoma, the eustachian valve (valve of the inferior vena cava) and its extension, Chiari's network, and the thebesian valve (a valve of the coronary sinus; or bulging of the entire atrial septum).[18] Mechanisms for stroke related to atrial septal aneurysm include paradoxical embolization (in cases associated with patent foramen ovale) and direct embolization from thrombi in the aneurysm.[106] It is interesting to note that atrial septal aneurysm is significantly associated with lacunar infarction.[3]

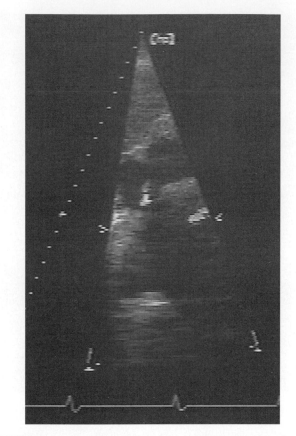

**FIGURE 5–11.** Patent foramen ovale assessed by transesophageal echocardiography. Color-coded shunt between right and left atrium indicates a patent foramen ovale. (See Color Plate.)

## Aortic Atheromatous Changes

TEE is a sensitive technique for detecting atheromatous changes in the aorta. It provides excellent cross-sectional images of the aorta from the level of transverse arch to the more distal portions of the descending thoracic aorta.[22] Several studies have documented an association between the existence, dimension, and mobility of aortic plaques and increased risk of embolic stroke.[8,9,78]

## Spontaneous Echo Contrast

Another finding on TEE includes spontaneous echo contrast, a dynamic smokelike signal caused by stasis of blood, most commonly located in the left atrium but also in the left ventricle, the aorta, and occasionally, the right atrium and right ventricle.[38] Left atrial spontaneous echo contrast is most commonly associated with atrial fibrillation and mitral valve stenosis. Several studies demonstrated an association of left atrial spontaneous echo contrast and cardioembolic stroke.[32] Furthermore, some studies indicate an increased cardioembolic risk for patients with left atrial spontaneous echo contrast and nonvalvular atrial fibrillation.[89]

## Intracardiac Thrombi

A major advantage of echocardiography is the detection of intracardiac thrombi, which occur in all heart chambers and usually lead clinicians to recommend systemic anticoagulation. TEE is clearly superior to TTE for identifying left atrial thrombi. The two techniques are almost equal in detecting ventricular thrombi. Left atrial thrombi usually are

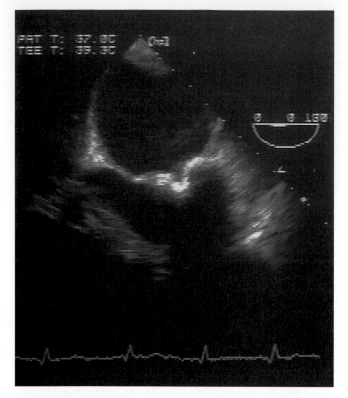

**FIGURE 5–12.** Intracardiac thrombus assessed by transesophageal echocardiography. Hyperdensity in the upper part of the image indicates a left atrial thrombus located in the atrial appendage.

located in the atrial appendage in patients with atrial fibrillation or mitral stenosis (Fig. 5–12). Thrombi within the left atrial cavity most commonly are seen in patients with rheumatic atrial fibrillation. Ventricular thrombi most commonly occur in patients with left ventricular dysfunction and either a dyskinetic or akinetic left ventricular segment. These thrombi most commonly are seen in the acute phase following myocardial infarction.[44,101,112]

### Other Abnormalities

Other abnormalities associated with an increased risk of cardioembolic stroke that can be identified with echocardiography include mitral annular calcification, intracardiac tumors such as atrial myxomas, bacterial and nonbacterial endocarditis with valvular vegetations, and abnormalities on prosthetic cardiac valves.[2,23,35]

## ANGIOGRAPHY

The evaluation of blood vessels in cerebrovascular diseases is an important step in primary or secondary stroke prevention. The use of the different tests available is currently subject to intense debate.[14] Several techniques are routinely used that can be classified as invasive ("conventional" angiography) or noninvasive (Doppler ultrasonography, MRI, and CT). Conventional angiography is still considered the gold standard. However, angiography is not an absolute gold standard when compared to pathologic specimens.[129] The technologic problems associated with the noninvasive tests are constantly improving, and these tests have the advantage of safety. These reasons might explain the declining use of conventional angiography observed in the United States.[31]

### CONVENTIONAL ANGIOGRAPHY

The safety of angiography is one of the main concerns limiting its use. When it was first introduced in the 1920s, angiography was performed by direct puncture of the carotid artery. This technique was used until the 1950s, when Seldinger introduced the technique of percutaneous angiography by puncture of distant vessels. To perform this technique, it is necessary to use a flexible metal guidewire. Currently, the average complication rate is estimated to be approximately 1%. A study conducted in 68 American teaching hospitals showed a global complication rate of 0.6%.[31] The rate is higher when patients with a previous history of stroke or transient ischemic attack are included. Heiserman et al.[68] studied the complication rate of 1000 consecutive cerebral angiographies. The risk of a neurologic deficit was 1%, with half of the deficits being permanent. All the complications occurred in patients with a history of stroke. The complication rate can reach 10% in patients with proven symptomatic carotid stenosis and seems to be related to the degree of stenosis.[36] Complications are probably related to microemboli, which can be seen in almost every patient undergoing cerebral angiography.[57] The nature of these microemboli is air or small atherosclerotic plaques. The safety of cerebral angiography is related to the duration of the procedure, the total volume of contrast material, the patient's age, and the presence of cerebrovascular disease. Some of these factors can be controlled, but when a patient has several nonmodifiable risk factors (e.g., longstanding hypertension, diabetes), the indication for conventional angiography must be compelling.

### Atherosclerosis

In the context of cerebral ischemia, atherosclerosis of cerebral vessels is the most common finding. It involves the carotid arteries, the vertebral arteries, and the intracranial arteries in decreasing frequency. The patterns of atherosclerosis are stenosis, ulceration of a plaque, plaque hemorrhage, intraluminal thrombus, and occlusion.[126] Stenosis is the most frequent finding in clinical practice (Fig. 5–13). The estimation of its severity differs among carotid stenosis protocols. The European Carotid Surgery Trial evaluated the degree of stenosis by measuring the point of the greatest stenosis compared to the size of the bulb of the carotid artery.[48] The North American Symptomatic Carotid Endarterectomy Trial protocol considered the point of the greatest stenosis compared to the point of the distal cervical internal carotid artery where the vessel walls are parallel again.[104]

### Embolism

Embolism is frequently seen in the intracranial arteries. These arteries are more often occluded by embolism than by local atherosclerosis. The source of emboli can be cardiac or arterial (proximal atherosclerosis). It can be difficult to distinguish between occlusion due to embolism and occlusion due to local atherosclerosis. Typically, the latter is described as having a convex proximal edge. An embolus is indicated by an abrupt arrest of contrast flow.

## Other Findings

Dissection of cerebral arteries, most commonly the carotid, vertebral, and basilar arteries, is a frequent cause of stroke in young patients. On angiography, it appears as an irregular stenosis, beginning with a tapered, flamelike narrowing in 75% of cases. When the dissection involves the carotid artery, it starts after the bulb (in contrast to atheromatous stenosis). A definitive diagnosis on angiography is made by visualization of a false lumen. Arterial dissection can also be associated with an aneurysm, an intimal flap, or an occlusion. Vasculitis is characterized by "beadlike" vascular narrowing, which is not specific but occurs principally in the intracranial arteries. Fibromuscular dysplasia can be associated with ischemic stroke by causing artery-to-artery embolism.[131] The lesion appears as a multifocal stenosis alternating with dilatation in 80% to 90% of cases. It can also appear as a longitudinal stenosis of mild severity in 10% to 20% of cases.

### NONINVASIVE ANGIOGRAPHIC METHODS

This discussion focuses on MR angiography and computed tomography angiography (CTA).

MR angiography, as opposed to conventional MRI, in which normal flow is demonstrated as "signal voids," uses gradient echo pulse sequences that produce increased in-travascular signal intensity with normal flow. An image similar to that of a conventional arteriogram can be reconstructed from the intravascular signals. This technique is sensitive for detecting large cerebral vessel occlusion or narrowing and vascular malformations. It has limited use in evaluating smaller peripheral vessels. There are two methods of MR angiography: the time-of-flight method and the phase-contrast method. The time-of-flight method requires a single acquisition and is quicker than the phase-contrast method.

In the evaluation of the brachiocephalic vessels and the carotid arteries, MR angiography is widely used. Compared to conventional angiography, it tends to overestimate the degree of carotid stenosis.[39,74] Globally, its accuracy is 94%, its sensitivity reaches 100%, and its specificity is 93% for evaluating carotid artery stenosis.[138] When combined with the results of ultrasonography, MR angiography can reduce the need for conventional angiography if the two procedures are concordant.[115] It can accurately diagnose arterial dissection (Fig. 5–14), especially in correlation with ultrasonography. MR angiography is also useful in fibromuscular dysplasia and for diagnosis of lesions in the wall of the carotid artery, such as a thrombosed aneurysm. As in the carotid artery circulation, MR angiography tends to overestimate stenosis in the vertebrobasilar circulation system, and high-grade

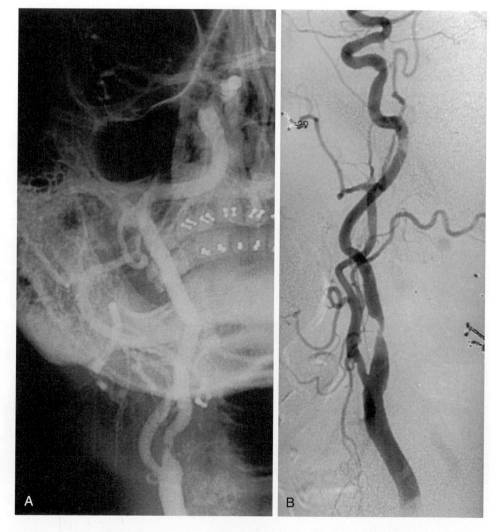

**FIGURE 5–13.** **A,** There is a reduction of the internal carotid artery lumen representing atherosclerotic stenosis of <70%. **B,** Arteriogram shows >70% stenosis of the internal carotid artery.

stenosis can be mistaken for occlusion. For intracranial circulation, the sensitivity and specificity of MR angiography is 96% and 97%, respectively.[83] It also tends to overestimate the degree of stenosis.

MR angiography also provides the ability to detect arteriovenous malformations noninvasively. The great advantage of MRI or MR angiography over conventional arteriography is not only the possibility to detect evidence of prior hemorrhage and its source but also to visualize the surrounding brain parenchyma. MRI or MR angiography regularly shows the size of the nidus and the source of flow to the lesion and the draining veins.[75,105] The MRI findings of arteriovenous and cavernous malformations often include a distinctive central focus of high signal surrounded by hypointensity that differentiates tumors and hematomas.[75,110] MRI or MR angiography is also useful for the diagnosis of large compressive intracranial lesions, such as cavernous aneurysms, dolichoectatic basilar arteries, and large basilar aneurysms.

With the arrival of spiral CT, it became possible to construct images of vessels. Unlike conventional CT, in spiral CT the x-ray source rotates continuously and the patient progresses forward at a constant velocity during the acquisition of data. Because of the recent availability of spiral CT, only a few studies have compared its accuracy with that of conventional angiography. Globally, CTA tends to overestimate stenosis, as does MR angiography.[119]

In conclusion, noninvasive testing should be the first choice for investigation of a patient with cerebrovascular disease. For routine use, both MR angiography and CTA are more expensive than duplex scanning. However, when used in conjunction with a routine head scan, they can be cost-effective. MR angiography or CTA could be used as a secondary tool after initial evaluation with ultrasonography, when the results are abnormal. Conventional angiography would be reserved for the situation in which duplex scanning and MR angiography or CTA shows discrepancies. CTA may be a good alternative for the patient suffering from claustrophobia or one who is unable to have an MR angiography study for any other reason. In acute stroke, CT combined with CTA can be very useful. This combination is not as sensitive as MR angiography and provides less information, but it is more readily available.

## DIAGNOSTIC STRATEGIES IN ACUTE STROKE

Since the time window for implementation of specific treatment strategies in acute stroke is short, as reflected by the inclusion threshold of 3 hours for the use of rt-PA, acute stroke should be treated as an emergency. When the patient is admitted to the hospital, a straightforward program of primary diagnostic and medical procedures should be performed to save time for further advanced diagnostics and to provide optimum therapy. The recent establishment of stroke units in large medical centers exemplifies this concept. However, the concept of a stroke unit with an efficient organization of diagnostic evaluation and medical therapy is also potentially available in smaller hospitals.

After admission to the hospital, physical and neurologic examinations and CT or MRI scanning should be performed in almost every patient, regardless of the acuteness

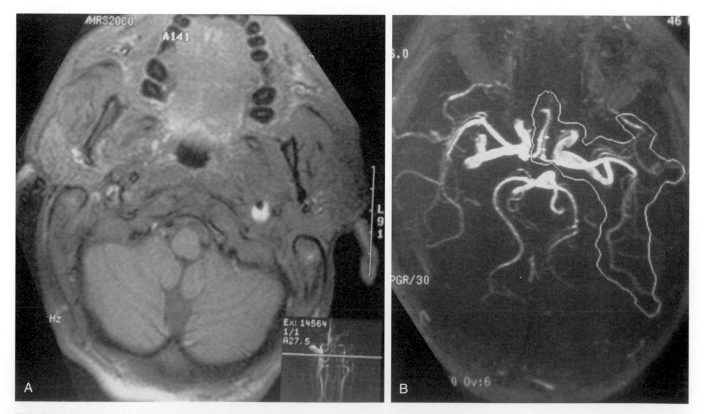

**FIGURE 5–14.** **A,** Axial MRI image demonstrating a false lumen without flow tract of the left internal carotid artery (*black dot*), characteristic of a spontaneous dissection. **B,** Same left internal carotid artery dissection is seen as an irregular reduction of the lumen of the vessel.

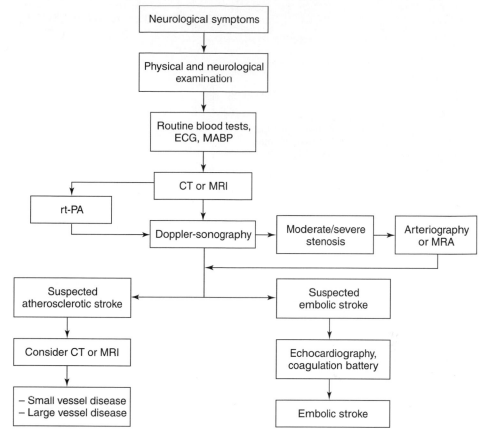

**FIGURE 5–15.** Evaluation of acute stroke.

of the disease. The major possible findings in the hyperacute stage are early signs of infarction and exclusion of cerebral hemorrhage. The initial CT or MRI should be performed as soon as possible since rt-PA use depends on exclusion of cerebral hemorrhage within 3 hours. The next diagnostic step that we recommend for all patients as a screening method is the investigation of extracranial and intracranial vessels through Doppler sonography. Findings may include stenosis or occlusion and dissection of the artery. Transcranial Doppler detection of microembolization or $CO_2$ reactivity and detection of intracranial stenosis usually can be performed later. CT or MRI scanning and Doppler sonography represent the benchmark for the initial acute stroke workup. Correlated with the medical history, physical and neurologic examinations, routine blood tests, and electrocardiography, these scanning methods can be used to make a diagnosis (Fig. 5–15). This diagnostic evaluation paradigm is relatively cost-effective, and we recommend it for almost every stroke patient.

When the initial workup provides no conclusive diagnosis about the source of the stroke, further diagnostic testing must be considered, particularly in patients younger than 60. A second imaging study of the brain made 24 hours after the onset of symptoms is recommended and will usually demonstrate the infarcted area. A CT should be sufficient to confirm the location of the infarct. Younger patients without a history of atherosclerosis and patients with possible small vessel disease may require an MRI. When a cardioembolic mechanism is suspected, TEE is useful, and we recommend performing it in all younger patients with no obvious cause of stroke. A 24-hour Holter monitor can be

useful in patients with suspected intermittent atrial fibrillation. In younger patients with an unknown cause or in patients with prior thrombotic events, coagulation studies are indicated. Our battery includes measurements of antithrombin III, protein S, protein C, prothrombin time, lupus anticoagulant, and anticardiolipin antibodies. If a patient is APC-resistant, a factor V point mutation analysis must be considered. When the initial Doppler sonogram of the carotid arteries reveals a moderate or severe stenosis, standard arteriography or MR arteriography is usually necessary before an endarterectomy. Arteriography is also useful, though not mandatory, in younger patients with suspected arterial dissection (Fig. 5–15).

## EVALUATION OF TRANSIENT ISCHEMIC ATTACK

A transient ischemic attack (TIA) is defined as a neurologic deficit due to cerebral ischemia that is completely reversible within 24 hours. The arbitrary limit of 24 hours was defined in an era before brain imaging techniques were used routinely. Therefore this definition is not always useful in clinical practice. Most TIAs last less than 1 hour. The median duration of a TIA in the carotid circulation is 14 minutes; in the vertebrobasilary circulation, 8 minutes. Two thirds of TIAs resolve in less than 1 hour. If the symptoms last longer than 1 hour, only 14% of patients have complete resolution of symptoms after 24 hours (and have a TIA by definition).[91] Since the introduction of CT and MRI, significant brain lesions have been shown in patients who would have had a TIA based only on the time criteria.

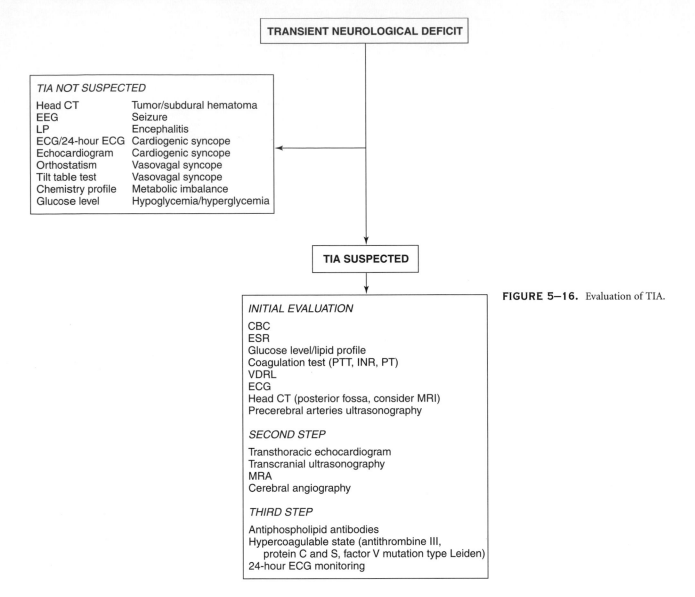

**FIGURE 5—16.** Evaluation of TIA.

The main consequence of a TIA is its prognosis for future stroke. Longitudinal studies of patients with TIA have shown variations of prognosis. There are several reasons to explain these differences, namely, differences in the definition of a TIA, selection bias (hospital vs. community based), study design, composition of the groups (inclusion of patients with amaurosis fugax, who have a better prognosis). Globally, the 5-year risk of stroke after a TIA is 24% to 29%.[41] The risk is highest during the first month after the event. Therefore diagnosis of a TIA must be followed by prompt investigations to determine its cause and to limit the risk of stroke.

There are a number of conditions in which transient focal neurologic deficits are presenting symptoms. These include TIA, migraine with aura, partial seizure, subdural hematoma, demyelinating diseases, brain tumor, focal encephalitis, hyperglycemia, and hypoglycemia. The history and physical examination, basic blood tests, and a head CT should be the initial investigational step.

Typically, symptoms develop in about 2 minutes (shorter development suggests seizure, and longer suggests migraine). Amaurosis fugax is a disorder of vision usually described as "blurring vision" that descends like a curtain over the eyes. Hemispheric TIAs are often first noted by weakness or numbness of the face or limbs. Speech disorders or neuropsychologic symptoms can occur. Brainstem TIAs most often begin with vertigo, ataxia, dysarthria, diplopia, or cranial nerve dysfunction. These different symptoms are frequently associated with limb weakness or numbness. Isolated vertigo, amnesia, confusion, or loss of consciousness rarely represent TIA. The clinical examination is frequently normal. The variability of the symptoms, the broad differential diagnosis, and the minimal help given by the physical examination explain why even experienced clinicians sometimes disagree about the diagnosis of TIA.[84]

Blood tests should include a complete blood count and erythrocyte sedimentation rate (ESR; to detect polycythemia, thrombocythemia, and evidence of infectious or inflammatory state), chemistry profile (to check for electrolyte imbalance), glucose level (to detect diabetes or hypoglycemia), Venereal Disease Research Laboratory (VDRL) test (to screen for syphilis and indirectly for anticardiolipin antibodies), lipid profile, and routine coagulation tests. An electrocardiogram (ECG) is also necessary (to detect arrhythmia and myocardial infarction). A head CT is useful to exclude nonvascular disorders. It may show a nonvascular disorder, with significant treatment and prognosis differences in 1% of patients who have a presumed diagnosis of TIA.[65] The routine use of head CT in TIA is not accepted by everyone. Finally, ultrasonography is recommended in the initial investigation of a patient with a carotid artery territory TIA.[49] It is a noninvasive test with low cost and good sensitivity that can demonstrate pathologic findings having important therapeutic consequences (e.g., significant carotid artery stenosis to be treated by endarterectomy).

The approach we propose for the investigation in TIAs is presented in Fig. 5–16. Such an approach is subject to variations and should be adapted to the specific presentation of individual patients.

## REFERENCES

1. Adams HP Jr, Brott TG, Crowell RM, et al. Guidelines for the management of patients with acute ischemic stroke: a statement for healthcare professionals from a special writing group of the Stroke Council, American Heart Association. *Circulation.* 1994;90:1588-1601.
2. Alam M, Sun I, Smith S. Transesophageal echocardiographic evaluation of right atrial mass lesion. *J Am Soc Echocardiogr.* 1991;4:331-337.
3. Albers GW, Comess KA, DeRook FA, et al. Transesophageal echocardiographic findings in stroke subtypes. *Stroke.* 1994;25:23-28.
4. Alexandrov AV, Bladin CF, Maggisano R, et al. Measuring carotid stenosis: time for a reappraisal. *Stroke.* 1993;24:1292-1296.
5. Alexandrov AV, Bladin CF, Norris JW. Intracranial blood flow velocities in acute ischemic stroke. *Stroke.* 1994;25:1378-1383.
6. Alexandrov AV, Masdeu JC, Devous MD Sr, et al. Brain single-photon emission CT with HMPAO and safety of thrombolytic therapy in acute ischemic stroke. Proceedings of the meeting of the SPECT Safe Thrombolysis Study Collaborators and the members of the Brain Imaging Council of the Society of Nuclear Medicine. *Stroke.* 1997;28(9);1830-1834.
7. Alexandrov AV, Norris JW. Cervical ultrasound. In: Welch KMA, Reis DJ, Caplan LR, Siesjoe BK, Weir B, eds. *Primer on Cerebrovascular Diseases.* New York: Academic Press; 1997:614-620.
8. Amarenco P, Cohen A, Baudrimont M, et al. Transesophageal echocardiographic detection of aortic arch disease in patients with cerebral infarction. *Stroke.* 1992;23:1005-1009.
9. Amarenco P, Cohen A, Tzourio C, et al. Atherosclerotic disease of the aortic arch and the risk of ischemic stroke. *N Engl J Med.* 1994;331: 1474-1479.
10. Argentino C, De Michele M, Florelli M, et al. Posterior circulation infarcts simulating anterior circulation stroke: perspective of the acute phase. *Stroke.* 1996;27:1306-1309.
11. Asato R, Okumura R, Konishi J. Fogging effect in MR of cerebral infarct. *J Comput Assist Tomogr.* 1991;15:160-162.
12. Barker PB. Magnetic resonance spectroscopy and spectroscopic imaging. In: Welch KMA, Reis DJ, Caplan LR, Siesjoe BK, Weir B, eds. *Primer on Cerebrovascular Diseases.* New York: Academic Press; 1997:650-659.
13. Barker PB, Gillard JH, vanZijl PC, et al. Acute stroke: evaluation with serial proton MR spectroscopic imaging. *Radiology.* 1994;92:723-732.
14. Barnes RW. The non-invasive vascular laboratory: who needs it? *Cardiovasc Surg.* 1995;3:261-264.
15. Baron JC. Clinical use of positron emission tomography in cerebrovascular diseases. *Neurosurg Clin North Am.* 1996;7(4):653-664.
16. Becker H, Desch H, Hacker H, Pencz A. CT fogging effect with ischemic cerebral infarcts. *Neuroradiology.* 1976;18:185-192.
17. Belcaro G, Laurora G, Cesarone MR, et al. Ultrasonic classification of carotid plaques causing less than 60% stenosis according to ultrasound morphology and events. *J Cardiovasc Surg.* 1993;34:287-294.
18. Belkin RN, Kisslo J. Atrial septum aneurysm: recognition and clinical relevance. *Am Heart J.* 1990;120:948-957.
19. Belliveau JW, Rosen BR, Kantor HL, et al. Functional cerebral imaging by susceptibility-contrast NMR. *Magn Reson Med.* 1990;14:538-546.
20. Berkelbach van der Sprenkel JW, Luyten PR, van Rijen PC, et al. Cerebral lactate detected by regional proton magnetic resonance spectroscopy in a patient with cerebral infarction. *Stroke.* 1988;19:1556-1560.
21. Bladin CF, Chambers BR. Clinical features, pathogenesis, and computed tomographic characteristics of internal watershed infarction. *Stroke.* 1993;24:1925-1932.
22. Blanchard DG, Kimura BJ, Dittrich HC, et al. Transesophageal echocardiography of the aorta. *JAMA.* 1994;272:546-551.
23. Blanchard DG, Ross RS, Dittrich HC. Nonbacterial thrombotic endocarditis: assessment by transesophageal echocardiography. *Chest.* 1992;102:954-956.
24. Bogousslavsky J, Regli F, Uske A, Maeder P. Early spontaneous hematoma in cerebral infarct: is primary cerebral hemorrhage overdiagnosed? *Neurology.* 1991;41:837-840.
25. Bottomley PA, Drayer BP, Smith LS. Chronic adult cerebral infarction studied by phosphorus NMR spectroscopy. *Radiology.* 1986;160:763-766.
26. Bracewell RE. *The Fourier Transform and Its Application.* New York: McGraw-Hill; 1978:112-115.
27. Bricheaux JC. Color Doppler imaging of the supraaortic arterial systems. *J Neuroradiol.* 1993;20:162-167.
28. Bruhn H, Frahm J, Gyngell ML, et al. Cerebral metabolism in men after acute stroke: new observation using localized NMR spectroscopy. *Magn Reson Med.* 1989;9:126-131.
29. Bryan RN, Levy LM, Whitlow WD, et al. Diagnosis of acute cerebral infarction: comparison of CT and MR imaging. *AJNR.* 1991;12:611-620.
30. Cerebral Embolism Task Force. Cardiogenic brain embolism: the second report of the Cerebral Embolism Task Force. *Arch Neurol.* 1989; 46:727-743.
31. Chaturvedi S, Policheria PN, Femino L. Cerebral angiography practices at U. S. teaching hospitals: implications for carotid endarterectomy. *Stroke.* 1997;28:1895-1897.
32. Chimnowitz MI, DeGeorgia MA, Poole RM, et al. Left atrial spontaneous echo contrast is highly associated with previous stroke in patients with atrial fibrillation or mitral stenosis. *Stroke.* 1993;24:1015-1019.
33. Crain MR, Yuh WTC, Greene GM, et al. Cerebral ischemia: evaluation with contrast enhanced MR imaging. *AJNR.* 1991;12:631-640.
34. Dafer RM, Ramadan NM. Transcranial Doppler sonography and stroke. In: Welch KMA, Reis DJ, Caplan LR, Siesjo BK, Weir B, eds. *Primer on Cerebrovascular Diseases.* New York: Academic Press; 1997: 620-634.
35. Daniel WG, Muegge A, Grote J, et al. Comparison of transthoracic and transesophageal echocardiography for detection of abnormalities of prosthetic and bioprosthetic valves in the mitral and aortic positions. *Am J Cardiol.* 1993;71:210-215.
36. Davies KN, Humphrey PR. Complications of cerebral angiography in patients with symptomatic carotid territory ischaemia screening by carotid ultrasound. *J Neurol Neurosurg Psychiatry.* 1993;56:967-972.
37. Davis SM, Andrews JT, Lichtenstein M, et al. Correlation between cerebral arterial velocities, blood flow, and delayed ischemia after subarachnoid hemorrhage. *Stroke.* 1992;23:10-18.
38. DeGeorgia MA, Chimnowitz MI, Heppner A, et al. Right atrial spontaneous contrast: echocardiographic and clinical features. *Int J Card Imaging.* 1994;10:227-232.
39. De Marco JK, Nesbit GM, Wesbey GE, Richardson D. Prospective evaluation of extracranial carotid stenosis: MR angiography with maximum-intensity projections and multiplanar reformation compared with conventional angiography. *AJR.* 1994;163:1205-1212.
40. Demearel P, Van Hecke P, Marchal G, et al. MRI of intraparenchymal hematoma: responsible mechanisms. *J Belge Radiol.* 1990;73:279-288.
41. Dennis M, Bamford J, Sandercock P, Warlow C. Prognosis of transient ischemic attacks in the Oxfordshire Community Stroke Project. *Stroke.* 1990;21:848-853.
42. Di Tullio M, Sacco RL, Gopal A, et al. Patent foramen ovale as a risk factor for cryptogenic stroke. *Ann Intern Med.* 1992;117:461-465.
43. Di Tullio M, Sacco RL, Venketasubramanian N, et al. Comparison of diagnostic techniques for the detection of a patent foramen ovale. *Stroke.* 1993;24:120-124.
44. Dressler FA, Labovitz AJ. Systemic arterial emboli and cardial masses: assessment with transesophageal echocardiography. *Cardiol Clin.* 1993;11:447-460.
45. Edelman RR, Siewert B, Darby DG, et al. Qualitative mapping of cerebral blood flow and functional localization with echo-planar MR

imaging and signal targeting with alternating radio frequency. *Radiology.* 1994;192:513-520.

46. Edelman RR, Wielpolski O, Schmitt F. Echoplanar MR imaging. *Radiology.* 1994;192:600-612.

47. Elster AD, Moody DM. Early cerebral infarction: gadopentate dimeglumine enhancement. *Radiology.* 1990;177:627-632.

48. European Carotid Surgery Trialists' Collaborative Group. MRC European Carotid Surgery Trial: interim results for symptomatic patients with severe (70-99%) or with mild (0-29%) carotid stenosis. *Lancet.* 1991;337:1235-1243.

49. Feinberg WM, Albers GW, Barnett HJ, et al. Guidelines for the management of transient ischemic attacks. (From the Ad Hoc Committee on Guidelines for the Management of Transient Ischemic Attacks of the Stroke Council of the American Heart Association.) *Circulation.* 1994;89:2950-2965.

50. Fisher M. Characterizing the target of acute stroke therapy. *Stroke.* 1997;28:866-872.

51. Fisher M, Zito JL, Siva A, et al. Hemorrhagic infarction: a clinical and CT study. *Stroke.* 1994;15:192-197.

52. Foulkes MA, Wolf PA, Price TR, et al. The Stroke Data Bank: design, methods, and baseline characteristics. *Stroke.* 1988;19:547-554.

53. Furst H, Hartl WH, Jansen I, et al. Color-flow Doppler sonography in the identification of ulcerative plaques in patients with high-grade carotid artery stenosis. *AJNR.* 1992;13:1581-1587.

54. Gacs G, Fox AJ, Barnett HJ, Vinuela F. Title CT visualization of intracranial arterial thromboembolism. *Stroke.* 1993;14:756-762.

55. Garcia JH, Lassen NA, Weiller C, et al. Ischemic stroke and incomplete infarction. *Stroke.* 1996;27:761-765.

56. Geroulakos G, Ramaswami G, Nicolaides A, et al. Characterization of symptomatic and asymptomatic carotic plaques using high-resolution real-time ultrasonography. *Br J Surg.* 1993;80:1274-1277.

57. Gerraty RP, Bowser DN, Infeld B, et al. Microemboli during carotid angiography: association with stroke risk factors or subsequent magnetic resonance imaging changes? *Stroke.* 1996;27:1543-1547.

58. Gomori JM, Grossman RI, Goldberg HI, et al. Intracranial hematomas: imaging by high field MR. *Radiology.* 1985;157:87-94.

59. Gomori JM, Grossman RI, Hackney DB, et al. Variable appearances of subacute intracranial hematomas on high field spin echo MR. *AJR.* 1988;150:171-179.

60. Graham GD, Blamire AM, Rothman DL, et al. Early temporal variation of cerebral metabolites after human stroke: a proton magnetic resonance spectroscopic study. *Stroke.* 1993;24:1891-1896.

61. Graham GD, Kalvach P, Blamire AM, et al. Clinical correlates of proton magnetic resonance spectroscopy findings after acute cerebral infarction. *Stroke.* 1995;26:225-229.

62. Grosset DG, Straiton J, duTrevou M, et al. Prediction of symptomatic vasospasm after subarachnoid hemorrhage by rapidly increasing transcranial Doppler velocity and cerebral blood flow changes. *Stroke.* 1992;23:674-679.

63. Grosset DG, Straiton J, McDonald I, et al. Angiographic and Doppler diagnosis of cerebral artery vasospasm following subarachnoid hemorrhage. *Br J Neurosurg.* 1993;7:79-85.

64. Hacke W, Kaste M, Fieschi C, et al. Intravenous thrombolysis with recombinant tissue plasminogen activator for acute hemispheric stroke: the European Cooperative Acute Stroke Study (ECASS). *JAMA.* 1995; 274:1017-1025.

65. Hankey GJ, Warlow CP. Cost-effective investigation of patients with suspected transient ischaemic attacks. *J Neurol Neurosurg Psychiatry.* 1992;55:171-176.

66. Hankey GJ, Warlow CP. The role of imaging in the management of cerebral and ocular ischaemia. *Neuroradiology.* 1991;33:381-390.

67. Hasegawa Y, Fisher M, Latour LL, et al. MRI diffusion mapping of reversible and irreversible ischemic injury in focal brain ischemia. *Neurology.* 1994;44:1484-1490.

68. Heiserman JE, Dean BL, Hodak JA, et al. Neurologic complications of cerebral angiography. *AJNR.* 1994;15:1401-1411.

69. Hennerici M. Ultrasound imaging and Doppler sonography in the diagnosis of cerebrovascular diseases. In: Barnett HJM, Mohr JP, Stein BM, Yatsu FM, eds. *Stroke.* New York: Churchill Livingstone; 1992: 241-270.

70. Hilal SK, Mohr JP. Magnetic resonance scanning. In: Barnett HJPM, Mohr JP, Stein B, Yatsu FM. *Stroke.* New York: Churchill Livingstone; 1992:189-214.

71. Hornig CR, Domdorf W, Agnoli AL. Hemorrhagic cerebral infarction: a prospective study. *Stroke.* 1986;17:179-184.

72. Hoult D, Busby S, Gadian D, et al. Observation of tissue metabolites using 31P nuclear magnetic resonance spectroscopy. *Nature.* 1974; 252:285-287.

73. Hunink MG, Polak JF, Barlan MM, et al. Detection and quantification of carotid artery stenosis: efficacy of various Doppler velocity parameters. *AJR.* 1993;160:619-625.

74. Huston J III, Lewis BD, Wiebers DO, et al. Carotid artery: prospective blinded comparison of two-dimensional time-of-flight MR angiography with conventional angiography and duplex US. *Radiology.* 1993; 186:339-344.

75. Imakita S, Nishimura T, Yamada N, et al. Cerebro-vascular malformations: application of magnetic resonance imaging to differential diagnosis. *Neuroradiology.* 1989;31:320-325.

76. Inoue Y, Takemoto K, Miyamoto T, et al. Sequential computed tomography scans in acute cerebral infarction. *Radiology.* 1980;135:655-662.

77. Jauss M, Kaps M, Keberle M, et al. A comparison of transesophageal echocardiography and transcranial Doppler sonography with contrast medium for detection of patent foramen ovale. *Stroke.* 1994;25:1265-1267.

78. Jones EF, Kalman JM, Tonkin AM, et al. Proximal aortic atheroma: an independent risk factor for cerebral ischemia. *Stroke.* 1994;25:259.

79. Kaps M, Damian MS, Teschendorf U, Dorndorf W. Transcranial Doppler ultrasound findings in middle cerebral artery occlusion. *Stroke.* 1990;21:532-537.

80. Kempski O. Cell swelling mechanism in the brain. In: Baethmann A, Go KG, Unterberg A, eds. *Mechanisms of Secondary Brain Damage.* NATO ASI Series A, Vol 115. New York: Plenum; 1986:203-220.

81. Kendall BE, Pullicino P. Intravascular contrast injection in ischaemic lesions. II: effect on prognosis. *Neuroradiology.* 1980;19:241-243.

82. Kirsch JD, Wagner LR, James EM, et al. Carotid artery occlusion: positive predictive value of duplex sonography compared with arteriography. *J Vasc Surg.* 1994;19:642-649.

83. Korogi Y, Takahashi M, Mabuchi N, et al. Intracranial vascular stenosis and occlusion: diagnostic accuracy of three-dimensional, Fourier transform, time-of-flight MR angiography. *Radiology.* 1994;193:187-193.

84. Kraaijeveld CL, van Gijn J, Schouten HJ, Staal A. Interobserver agreement for the diagnosis of transient ischemic attacks. *Stroke.* 1984;15: 723-725.

85. Kremkau FW. *Diagnostic Ultrasound: Principles and Instruments.* Philadelphia: WB Saunders; 1993.

86. LeBihan D. Molecular diffusion nuclear resonance imaging. *Magn Reson O.* 1991;7:1-30

87. LeBihan D, Turner R, Douek P, Patronas N. Diffusion MR imaging: clinical applications. *AJR.* 1992;159:591-599.

88. Lechat P, Mas JL, Lascult G, et al. Prevalence of patent foramen ovale in patients with stroke. *N Engl J Med.* 1988;318:1148-1152.

89. Leung DY, Black IW, Cranney GB, et al. Prognostic implications of spontaneous echo contrast in nonvalvular atrial fibrillation. *J Am Coll Cardiol.* 1994;24:755-762.

90. Levine SR, Helpern JA, Welch KM, et al. Human focal cerebral ischemia: evaluation of brain pH and energy metabolism with P-31 NMR spectroscopy. *Radiology.* 1992;185:537-544.

91. Levy DE. How transient are transient ischemic attacks? *Neurology.* 1988;38:674-677.

92. Leys D, Pruvo JP, Godefroy O, et al. Prevalence and significance of hyperdense middle cerebral artery in acute stroke. *Stroke.* 1992;23:317-324.

93. Lindegaard KF, Grolimund P, Aaslid R, et al. Evaluation of cerebral AVM's using transcranial Doppler ultrasound. *J Neurosurg.* 1986;65: 335.

94. Lovblad KO, Baird AE, Schlaug G, et al. Ischemic lesion volumes in acute stroke by diffusion-weighted magnetic resonance imaging correlate with clinical outcome. *Ann Neurol.* 1997;42:164-170.

95. Lutsep HL, Albers GW, DeCrispigny A, et al. Clinical utility of diffusion-weighted resonance imaging in the assessment of ischemic stroke. *Ann Neurol.* 1997;41:574-580.

96. Macchi PJ, Grossman RI, Gomori JM, et al. High field MR imaging of cerebral venous thrombosis. *J Comput Assist Tomogr.* 1986;10:10-18.

97. Marchal G, Serrati C, Rioux P, et al. PET imaging of cerebral perfusion and oxygen consumption in acute ischaemic stroke: relation to outcome. *Lancet.* 1993;341:925-927.

98. Monajati A, Heggeness L. Patterns of edema in tumors vs. infarcts: visualization of white matter pathways. *AJR.* 1982;3;251-255.

99. Moseley ME, Cohen Y, Mintorovitch J, et al. Early detection of re-

gional cerebral ischemia in cats: comparison of diffusion and T2-weighted MRI and spectroscopy. *Magn Reson Med.* 1990;14:330-346.

100. Mountz JM, Modell JG, Foster NL, et al. Prognostication of recovery following stroke using the comparison of CT and technetium-99m HM-PAO SPECT. *J Nucl Med.* 1990;31(1):61-66.

101. Muegge A, Daniel WG, Haverich A, et al. Diagnosis of noninfective cardiac mass lesions by two-dimensional echocardiography. *Circulation.* 1991;83:70-78.

102. National Institute of Neurological Disorders and Stroke (NINDS) rt-PA Stroke Study Group. Tissue plasminogen activator for acute ischemic stroke. *N Engl J Med.* 1995;333:1581-1587.

103. Niederkorn K, Meyers LG, Nunn CL, et al. Three-dimensional transcranial Doppler flow mapping in patients with cerebrovascular disorders. *Stroke.* 1988;19:1335-1344.

104. North American Symptomatic Carotid Endarterectomy Trial Collaborators. Beneficial effect of carotid endarterectomy in symptomatic patients with high-grade carotid stenosis. *N Engl J Med.* 1991;325:445-453.

105. Nussel F, Wegmueller H, Huber P. Comparison of magnetic resonance angiography, magnetic resonance imaging and conventional angiography in arteriovenous malformation. *Neuroradiology.* 1991;33:56-64.

106. Pearson AC, Nagelhout D, Castello R, et al. Atrial septal aneurysm and stroke: a transesophageal echocardiographic study. *J Am Coll Cardiol.* 1991;18:1223-1229.

107. Petty GW, Massaro AR, Tatemichi TK, et al. Transcranial Doppler ultrasonographic changes after treatment of arteriovenous malformations. *Stroke.* 1990;21:260.

108. Poole RM, Chimnowitz MI. Cardiac imaging for stroke diagnosis. In: Fisher M, Bogousslavsky J, eds. *Current Review of Cerebrovascular Disease. Current Medicine Series.* Philadelphia: 1996:189-203.

109. Pressman BD, Tourje EJ, Thompson JR. An early CT sign of ischemic infarction: increased density in a cerebral artery. *AJR.* 1987;149:583-586.

110. Rapacki TF, Brently MJ, Furlow TW, et al. Heterogeneity of cerebral cavernous hemangiomas diagnosed by MR imaging. *J Comput Assist Tomogr.* 1990;14:18-24.

111. Rapin PA, Bogousslavsky J, Regli F, et al. Subcortical cerebrovascular accidents: correlation between clinical aspects, topography and flow measurements using single photon emission tomography. *Schweiz Med Wochenschr.* 1993;123:1829-1836.

112. Reeder GS, Khandheria BK, Seward JB, et al. Transesophageal echocardiography and cardiac masses. *Mayo Clin Proc.* 1992;66:1101-1109.

113. Reith W, Hasegawa Y, Latour LL, et al. Multislice diffusion mapping for 3-D evolution of cerebral ischemia in rat stroke model. *Neurology.* 1995;45:172-177.

114. Reith W, Heiland S, Forsting M. Magnetic resonance angiography. In: Fisher M, Bogousslavsky J, eds. *Current Review of Cerebrovascular Disease. Current Medicine Series.* Philadelphia: 1996:147-158.

115. Riles TS, Eidelman EM, Litt AW, et al. Comparison of magnetic resonance angiography, conventional angiography, and duplex scanning. *Stroke.* 1992;23:341-346.

116. Ringelstein EB. Scepticism toward carotid ultrasonography: a virtue, an attitude, or fanaticism? *Stroke.* 1995;26:1743-1746.

117. Ringelstein EB, Kahlscheuer B, Niggemeyer E, et al. Transcranial Doppler sonography: anatomical landmarks and abnormal velocity values. *Ultrasound Med Biol.* 1990;16:745-762.

118. Robert DA, Detre JY, Bolinger L, et al. Quantitative magnetic resonance imaging of brain perfusion at 1.5T using steady-state inversion of arterial water. *Proc Natl Acad Sci U S A.* 1994;91:33-37.

119. Rubin GD, Dake MD, Semba CP, et al. Current status of three-dimensional spiral CT scanning for imaging the vasculature. *Radiol Clin North Am.* 1995;33:51-70.

120. Saunders DE, Clifton AG, Brown MM. Measurement of infarct size with MRI predicts prognosis in middle cerebral artery infarction. *Stroke.* 1995;26:2272-2273.

121. Schwartz A, Hennerici M. Non-invasive transcranial Doppler ultrasound in intracranial angiomas. *Neurology.* 1986;36:626.

122. Shintani S, Tsuruoka S, Koumo Y, Shiligai T. Sudden "stroke-like" onset of homonymous hemianopsia due to bacterial brain abscess. *J Neurol Sci.* 1996;143:190-194.

123. Sievers C, Knappertz V, Rothacher G, et al. Correlation of color duplex cross section of carotid artery stenosis with PW-Doppler and angiography. *Stroke.* 1994;24:749.

124. Siewert B, Schlaug G, Edelmenn RR, et al. Comparison of Epistar and T2-weighted gadolinium-enhanced perfusion imaging in patients with acute cerebral ischemia. *Neurology.* 1997;48:673-679.

125. Snyder TC, Sachdev HS. MR imaging of cerebral sinus thrombosis. *J Comput Assist Tomogr.* 1986;10:889-898.

126. Special report from the National Institute of Neurological Disorders and Stroke: classification of cerebrovascular diseases III. *Stroke.* 1990; 21:637-676.

127. Steinke W, Hennerici M, Rautenberg W, et al. Symptomatic and asymptomatic high-grade carotid stenoses in Doppler color-flow imaging. *Neurology.* 1992;42:131-138.

128. Stievenart JL, Vera P, Verstichel P, et al. Neurological applications of single photon emission tomoscintigraphy. *Rev Neurol (Paris).* 1995; 151:619-633.

129. Streifler JY, Eliasziw M, Fox AJ, et al. Angiographic detection of carotid plaque ulceration: comparison with surgical observations in a multicenter study. North American Symptomatic Carotid Endarterectomy Trial. *Stroke.* 1994;25:113-1132.

130. Stump DA, Tegeler CH, Hager R, et al. In vivo emboli detection: CW Doppler monitoring and B-mode imaging of gaseous and solid material. *Stroke.* 192;23:474.

131. Tan AK, Venketasubramanian N, Tan CB, et al. Ischaemic stroke from cerebral embolism in cephalic fibromuscular dysplasia. *Ann Acad Med, Singapore.* 1995;24:891-894.

132. Tasi FY, Wang AM, Matovich VB, et al. MR staging of dural sinus thrombosis: correlation with venous pressure measurements and implications for treatment and prognosis. *AJNR.* 1995;16:1021-1029.

133. Tegeler CH, Knappertz VA, Ultrasound in stroke. In: Fisher M, ed. *Stroke Therapy.* Boston: Butterworth-Heinemann; 1995:81-116.

134. Thron A, Wessel K, Linden D, et al. Superior sagittal sinus thrombosis: neuroradiological evaluation and clinical findings. *J Neurol.* 1986;233: 283-295.

135. Toms SA, Chyatte D. Cerebral venous thrombosis. In: Welch KMA, Reis DJ, Caplan LR, Siesjoe BK, Weir B, eds. *Primer on Cerebrovascular Diseases.* New York: Academic Press; 1997:528-532.

136. Tomura N, Uemura K, Inugami A, et al. Early CT finding in cerebral infarction: obscuration of the lentiform. *Radiology.* 1988;168:463-467.

137. Truwit CL, Barkovich AJ, Gean-Marton A, et al. Loss of the insular ribbon: another early CT sign of acute middle cerebral artery infarction. *Radiology.* 1990;176:801-806.

138. Turnipseed WD, Kennell TW, Turski PA, et al. Combined use of duplex imaging and magnetic resonance angiography for evaluation of patients with symptomatic ipsilateral high-grade carotid stenosis. *J Vasc Surg.* 1993;17:832-839 (discussion 839-840).

139. Viroslav AB, Hoffman JC Jr. The use of computed tomography in the diagnosis of stroke. *Heart Dis Stroke.* 1993;2:299-307.

140. Wang AM, Lin JC, Rumbaugh CL. What is expected of CT in the evaluation of stroke? *Neuroradiology.* 1988;30:54-58.

141. Warach S, Gaa J, Siewart B, et al. Acute human stroke studied by whole echo-planar diffusion-weighted imaging. *Ann Neurol.* 1995;37:231-241.

142. Warach S, Li W, Ronthal M, et al. Acute cerebral ischemia: evaluation with dynamic contrast enhanced MR imaging and MR angiography. *Radiology.* 1992;182:41-47.

143. Wing SD, Norman D, Pollock JA, Newton TH. Contrast enhancement of cerebral infarcts in computed tomography. *Radiology.* 1976;121: 89-92.

144. Wolpert SM, Bruckmann H, Greenlee R, et al. Neuroradiologic evaluation of patients with acute stroke treated with rt-PA. *AJNR.* 1993; 14:3-13.

145. Yuh WTC, Crain MR. Magnetic resonance imaging of acute cerebral ischemia. *Neuroimaging Clin N Am.* 1992;2:421-440.

146. Zanette EM, Fiesche C, Bozzao L, et al. Comparison of cerebral angiography and transcranial Doppler sonography in acute stroke. *Stroke.* 1989;20:899-903.

# 6

# Multiple Sclerosis

*Loren A. Rolak*

Neurologists must often diagnose diseases for which there is no definitive test. Migraines, Parkinson's disease, Alzheimer's disease, and amyotrophic lateral sclerosis (ALS) are a few examples. For patients with such conditions, neurologists can, nevertheless, integrate features of the history, physical examination, and laboratory tests to achieve such accuracy that they rarely doubt their diagnosis. Yet with multiple sclerosis (MS) the same process seems more difficult, the diagnosis is less certain, and the doubt is much greater. The reputation of MS as a puzzling disease to diagnose is a medical axiom.

When given a diagnosis of MS, a patient may lose his or her present job and future employability. It may be impossible to obtain life or health insurance, to donate blood, or to adopt a child. Divorce is a common sequel of the diagnosis, often with loss of child custody. Peace of mind is certainly lost because the diagnosis of a chronic relapsing, often disabling but unpredictable disease can crumble even the sturdiest psychological defenses, especially in young persons.

There are also medical reasons for affirming a diagnosis of MS. Proven therapies are currently available (e.g., beta-interferons and glatiramer), with new ones pending approval in the immediate future. These therapies are capable of altering the natural history of MS by minimizing attacks, decreasing the magnetic resonance imaging (MRI) evidence of MS, and possibly slowing the progression of this condition. They may be most effective when they are initiated as early as possible in the course of the disease. An erroneous diagnosis also has medical consequences; physicians usually attribute any change and every worsening to "MS," greatly delaying an accurate alternative diagnosis.

The three essential pieces of evidence the neurologist should examine when attempting to arrive at a diagnosis are the history, the physical examination, and laboratory evidence. Any one of these may be convincing alone, but all may need scrutiny before a final verdict is rendered.

## THE HISTORY

MS produces symptoms by recurrent episodes of demyelination in the central nervous system (CNS). The evidence that these episodes are autoimmune attacks is strong, although circumstantial. The inflammatory demyelination interrupts nerve conduction and thus nerve function, producing the deficits seen in MS.

Most symptoms develop abruptly, within minutes or hours[21] (Table 6–1). Patients often awaken with symptoms. Such exacerbations of MS generally persist for 6 to 8 weeks from onset to recovery, and they usually involve multiple areas of the CNS simultaneously, producing a polysymptomatic picture. At times the pattern of presentation, like so many features of MS, is atypical, and symptoms fluctuate quickly or even progress with little resolution. Patients may transpose readily from an exacerbating and remitting pattern to a chronic progressive one and back again, with a frequency and variability that defies labels or predictions.

The disease affects women nearly twice as often as men, and it usually appears between the ages of 20 and 40, with a peak occurrence at age 30. Fewer than 10% of patients present with MS after age 50; less than 1% after age 60. Among these older patients, slowly progressing weakness and spasticity are the most common initial symptoms.[26,32] Approximately 5% of patients present in childhood, usually with abrupt symptoms very similar to those seen in typical adult MS. The diagnosis is usually quite apparent clinically.

Caucasians are especially vulnerable, particularly those of Northern European extraction and those living in northern latitudes, where the incidence of the disease is highest. However, the "melting pot" of the United States is so geographically mobile and genetically intermixed that these epidemiologic features provide little useful diagnostic information.

Variability and diversity characterize MS, both in its symptoms and their manner of presentation. Table 6–1 shows the most common initial symptoms of MS. Although there is virtually no neurologic complaint that has not been traced to MS at one time or another, symptoms other than those shown in Table 6–1 seldom prompt a neurologist to consider MS diagnostically. Some symptoms, reflecting primarily gray matter damage, occur so rarely that their appearance casts doubt on the diagnosis of MS (Table 6–1).

Most symptoms of MS are focal, representing the inflammation of a specific tract or pathway within the CNS, such as monocular visual loss from optic neuritis, or weak-

---

**TABLE 6–1. Presenting Symptoms of Multiple Sclerosis**

**Speed of Onset of Presenting Symptoms**
Minutes (20%)
Hours (25%)
Days (30%)
1–8 weeks (15%)
Long-term (10%)

**Most Common Presenting Symptoms\***
1. Weakness in one or more limbs (50%)
2. Numbness in one or more limbs (45%)
3. Optic neuritis (20%)
4. Unsteady gait (15%)
5. Diplopia (10%)
6. Vertigo or "dizziness" (5%)

**Uncommon Presenting Symptoms (Cast Doubt on Diagnosis)†**
1. Loss of consciousness: seizures or syncope
2. Decreased sensorium: lethargy or coma
3. Dementia
4. Aphasia
5. Muscle atrophy or fasciculations
6. Pain
7. Dystonia, chorea, or other involuntary movements

**Isolated Symptoms as Initial Presentation‡**
1. Optic neuritis or Uhthoff's symptom
2. Paresthesias, either in one limb or at a sensory level
3. Limb (especially leg) weakness, particularly after prolonged exertion
4. Diplopia
5. Trigeminal neuralgia
6. Acute urinary retention
7. Vertigo

---

\*Percentages vary greatly among different studies and are only approximate.
  †Although these symptoms do not exclude multiple sclerosis, their rarity should prompt a search for other etiologic evidence.
  ‡In approximately descending order of frequency.

---

ness or numbness in one or more limbs from spinal cord damage. Diffuse nonfocal symptoms occur only rarely, for example, dementia, behavioral changes, or syncope. (One exception is fatigue, an overwhelming sense of lassitude that often accompanies focal symptoms of MS but is sufficiently vague and nonspecific that little diagnostic value can be derived from it.)

Most symptoms are also persistent, and care should be taken not to overemphasize the multitude of transient disturbances that plague all normal people, such as itches, twitches, "falling asleep" limbs, and fleeting visual obscurations. This is particularly true of purely sensory symptoms, and many patients have been wrongly diagnosed with MS because of tingling limbs and a spot or two on their MRI. Numbness is a more compelling sign if it is persistent and progressive (e.g., beginning distally in a limb and spreading proximally or ascending to a sensory level).

The tendency for initial symptoms to disappear and reappear in identical form in subsequent attacks distinctly characterizes MS. Early neurologists, including Charcot and Oppenheim, emphasized such recurring symptoms as highly suggestive of MS.

The 45% of patients in whom the initial symptom of MS is a single lesion pose a greater challenge than do the majority, who present polysymptomatically.[21] Table 6–1 lists (in approximately descending order of frequency) symptoms seen in young people that most frequently prove to be the onset of MS. Note that none of these are pathognomonic for MS. Iso-

lated damage to the optic nerve or to the spinal cord poses particular diagnostic dilemmas, which are discussed later.

In summary, a diagnosis of MS is supported by abrupt symptoms that are focal and persist for weeks, especially if polysymptomatic.

## THE PHYSICAL EXAMINATION

Ideally, only "hard" reproducible abnormal signs should be accepted as evidence of MS. Some signs, such as an afferent pupillary defect or an internuclear ophthalmoplegia (INO), are typical of MS and so are supportive of that diagnosis. Other compelling signs are those that reflect white matter damage, especially in the pyramidal and spinothalamic tracts. Such findings enhance the likelihood that MS is present but remain, in and of themselves, nonspecific. Obviously, the examination may localize a lesion to, for example, the spinal cord (a sensory level, extensor weakness, spasticity, Babinski sign, and sphincter disturbances), but it cannot prove that the myelopathy results from an MS plaque.

Very few neurologic signs are specific for MS, but a few are so characteristic they should always be sought. Optic neuritis, an INO, and Lhermitte's sign are virtually diagnostic of MS.

Much of the danger of misdiagnosis arises from the interpretation of "soft" neurologic findings. Many otherwise healthy young adults have a slightly asymmetric facial movement or smile, a few beats of nystagmus on far lateral gaze, a slight arm drift, or absent abdominal reflexes. The frequently observed tendency of analytic patients to report that pinprick or other sensory changes are not quite the same in one part of the body compared to another can also falsely imply that a true sensory deficit exists.

Obviously, a patient with MS may have a normal neurologic examination, so the absence of physical findings does not exclude the diagnosis. However, without the support of this major piece of evidence, the history and the laboratory tests assume even greater importance and the diagnostic uncertainty almost inevitably increases.

## LABORATORY EVIDENCE

Because no laboratory test can unequivocally prove a diagnosis of MS, many authorities insist that MS remains a clinical diagnosis. This is simply not true. The diagnosis of MS may not be strictly clinical, but in many cases it can depend heavily on laboratory support. A clinician who spurns laboratory studies or refuses to make a definite diagnosis of MS unless all clinical criteria are met resembles the attorney who insists on convicting a suspect by using only clinical evidence (e.g., eyewitness reports) and ignoring laboratory evidence (e.g., fingerprints, ballistics tests, blood and hair analysis). In diagnostic medicine, as in the courtroom, laboratory tests often prove decisive. Currently, virtually no neurologist will diagnose MS without at least an abnormal MRI study or other piece of supporting laboratory data.

However, the interpretation of the tests for MS requires considerable judgment and expertise. The most common reason for misdiagnosing MS is misinterpretation of laboratory tests.[15] The most valuable tests for MS are MRI of the brain, cerebrospinal fluid (CSF) analysis, and evoked potential recordings.[28,31] These tests differ in sensitivity and specificity, and each has pitfalls that limit its usefulness.[40] For example, a young patient with an isolated abnormal physical finding, such as a positive Babinski sign, may have MS or any number of other conditions; similarly, a young patient with an abnormal MRI may have MS or any number of other conditions. An abnormal test is simply one piece of evidence to be considered in determining the diagnosis, and, like the history and physical examination, it must be considered in context and its strengths and limitations must be understood.

## MAGNETIC RESONANCE IMAGING

Since the first publication in 1981 of MRI scans of the brain of a patient with MS, MRI has revolutionized the diagnosis of MS and remains the cornerstone of testing.[11,13,43] Unfortunately, despite its great sensitivity, the lack of specificity and the high rate of false-positives associated with MRI have proven to be major drawbacks and a source of considerable confusion. Punctate lesions in the white matter appear on MRI scans in at least 5% to 10% of normal persons between age 30 and 40 and so require particular caution to interpret.[10,32] Misunderstanding of MRI changes continues to bedevil the physician and complicates the diagnosis (Fig. 6–1).

No MRI findings are specific for MS, but the characteristic features are shown in Table 6–2. The confluent periventricular signal should be sought to differentiate MS from the multitude of other conditions that can produce abnormal white matter changes on the MRI scan. MS also frequently affects the corpus callosum. Involvement of the posterior fossa provides a useful diagnostic "pearl." Hypertension, ischemia, and most other conditions producing "unidentified bright objects" that can mimic MS lesions almost never produce MRI changes in the brainstem or the cerebellum.

MRI is most valuable as a diagnostic test, to simply determine whether the disease is present or not. It is much less helpful as a monitor of clinical activity, a determinant of disease severity, or a surrogate marker for treatment of MS. Nevertheless, the true accuracy of MRI for diagnosing MS remains difficult to determine because various studies have used different populations, various definitions of MS, and different criteria for MRI abnormalities. In a study of 200 patients with definite MS by Paty et al[33] approximately half (98 patients) had abnormal MRIs with typical lesions strongly suggestive of MS, and another 26 patients had other, less characteristic changes on MRI scan. Sixty-nine patients (approximately 35%) had entirely normal scans. However, Ormerod[29] showed that 95% of patients with definite MS had at least some abnormality on their MRI scan. If the special situation of patients with early monosymptomatic disease, whose scans less often show any abnormalities, is excluded, the sensitivity of a brain MRI for diagnosing definite MS probably approaches 90%, with a specificity of 60%.[32]

Gadolinium enhancement implies a breakdown of the blood-brain barrier and typically highlights acute MS plaques. Such enhancement may last from 2 to 6 weeks or

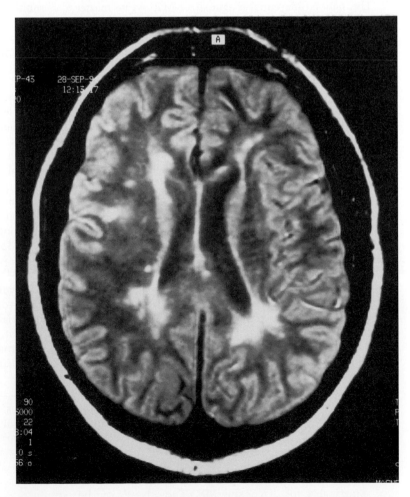

**FIGURE 6–1.** MRI scan in a 37-year-old man with multiple sclerosis, showing typical characteristic features of the disease: confluent, irregular periventricular white matter changes accompanied by scattered focal lesions, with generalized atrophy out of proportion to patient's age.

**TABLE 6–2. Characteristic MRI Features and Differential Diagnosis of White Matter Changes in Multiple Sclerosis**

**Characteristic MRI Features of MS Lesions**
1. Immediate proximity to the ventricles, especially in a confluent, poorly demarcated, "lumpy-bumpy" pattern; vertical (perpendicular) orientation to the ventricles is also common
2. Lesions >6 mm in diameter
3. Infratentorial or corpus callosum lesions

**Differential Diagnosis of MRI White Matter Changes in MS**
Cerebrovascular disease
   Migrainous ischemia
   Vasculitis
   Lacunes
   Binswanger's disease
   Thromboembolic infarcts
   Moyamoya disease
Acute disseminated encephalomyelitis
Progressive multifocal leukoencephalopathy
Inherited white matter diseases
Effects of radiation therapy
Metastatic neoplasm
Primary CNS lymphoma
Lyme disease
HTLV-1 infection
"Normal," especially if elderly or hypertensive

even longer. However, acute MS lesions readily produce abnormalities on T2-weighted scans, so gadolinium is seldom needed for diagnostic purposes.

The major differential diagnosis of MRI white matter lesions is shown in Table 6–2. Cerebrovascular disease is certainly the most common confusing condition. Approximately 35% of individuals age 50 or older have substantial white matter MRI signal abnormalities, and many normal young persons show similar changes.[10] Patients with migraine comprise an especially challenging group because they are often young women with recurrent neurologic symptoms and their MRI scans may closely resemble those of MS patients.

An MRI of the spinal cord is seldom necessary for the diagnosis of MS, but it may be useful (1) when the diagnosis of MS is strongly suspected but the brain MRI study is normal or shows only nonspecific changes or (2) when the diagnosis remains uncertain but the patient has clinical evidence of a spinal cord lesion (this will almost always be in the cervical cord). Although the ability of MRI to visualize MS lesions in the cord is limited, in some patients with clinically definite optic neuritis or cord lesions, MRI scans through the spinal cord can have a high yield.[20,42]

Magnetization transfer imaging and MRI spectroscopy are new techniques that promise greater sensitivity and enhanced understanding of plaque physiologic features, but their value for diagnosis has not been assessed in clinical studies. It is unlikely that these techniques will attain general acceptance as diagnostic tests within the next few years.[12]

Despite the limitations of MRI, in most patients with a history and physical examination that are strongly suggestive of MS, MRI scanning should be the first laboratory test ordered.[12]

## SPINAL FLUID

Oligoclonal bands in the spinal fluid are the most useful CSF abnormality for diagnosing MS.[1] These bands can be

detected by agarose gel electrophoresis or by isoelectric focusing on polyacrylamide, which is more sensitive. The frequency of abnormal oligoclonal bands in various conditions is shown in Table 6–3. When sufficiently powerful techniques are used, the immunoglobulins normally present in CSF can be isolated and separated from their neighbors—in other words, all of us have oligoclonal bands of immunoglobulin G (IgG) in our CSF. However, if the standard commercial kits and diagnostic criteria are used, only 2% of healthy people will meet the requirements for "abnormal oligoclonal bands present." The test is qualitative (i.e., subjective) since it requires a person (ideally, a well-trained pathologist) to examine a stained smear of proteins and make a judgment on whether the stain is abnormally intense in several (oligoclonal) discrete areas (bands). The presence of abnormal oligoclonal bands in healthy patients may be a result of overinterpretation (i.e., laboratory error) or some process other than MS, such as the residual of a previous CNS infection. Even in pathologically proven cases of MS, careful analysis of large volumes of CSF taken at autopsy may not disclose abnormal oligoclonal bands. In some patients with MS the bands are truly absent and not just undetected through laboratory error.[44] Nevertheless, the presence of abnormal oligoclonal banding is an extremely accurate test for MS since the bands appear in some form in nearly 90% of all patients, and other diseases that produce similar banding are seldom mistaken for MS. (The specificity also approaches 90%.) Analysis of CSF is often the most useful test to differentiate MS from other conditions that produce multifocal neurologic disease (or multifocal MRI abnormalities), such as diabetes or infarcts. Indeed, the major drawback to the use of CSF analysis for the diagnosis of MS is the reluctance of patients to undergo lumbar puncture.

Additional CSF tests, such as the IgG synthesis rate and the IgG index, are not superior to oligoclonal bands. Conventional measurements of myelin basic protein are certainly less sensitive and less specific than banding. Other immunologic changes, such as the presence of free kappa light chains, are undergoing analysis as diagnostic tests, but tests based on these changes are not yet ready to enter routine clinical practice.[1]

Arguments against a diagnosis of MS include a significant increase in CSF protein or in white blood cells (especially polymorphonuclear cells), since, apart from the immunologic changes, the CSF is usually normal in patients with MS.

## EVOKED POTENTIALS

Evoked potentials (EPs) are commonly assessed as visual evoked potentials (VEPs), brainstem auditory evoked potentials (BAEPs), and somatosensory evoked potentials (SSEPs). When all three are used together as a battery, some abnormality can be detected in a high percentage of patients with definite MS. Various studies have found abnormalities

**TABLE 6–3. Incidence of Cerebrospinal Fluid Oligoclonal Bands**

| | |
|---|---|
| Clinically definite multiple sclerosis | 90% |
| Isolated optic neuritis | 50% |
| Isolated transverse myelitis | 30% |
| Normal controls | 2% |

in 20% to 80% of suspected MS patients.[20] Most comparative studies of EPs, MRI, and spinal fluid have not been done well, and results differ considerably among them. In addition, comparing a physiologic test (e.g., EPs) to a structural test (e.g., MRI) to an immunologic analysis (e.g., oligoclonal bands) is somewhat like comparing apples to oranges to peaches. Nevertheless, the relatively lower sensitivity and specificity of EPs probably make them less useful than MRI or CSF for the diagnosis of MS.

The purpose of testing EPs should not be forgotten—to detect silent lesions. EPs measure conduction along specific CNS pathways by recording the electroencephalographic response to visual, auditory, or sensory (electrical) stimulation. A slowing in conduction is presumed to reflect inflammation and demyelination in that pathway, indicating an asymptomatic or subclinical MS lesion. There is no diagnostic value to an abnormal VEP in a patient known to have optic neuritis, nor of an SSEP in a patient with known spinal cord disease. One of the most fruitful uses of EPs is to confirm an organic basis for a vague symptom and thereby heighten the probability of MS. It is because they detect lesions disseminated in space that EPs have assumed secondary importance to the MRI, which shows additional lesions more accurately.

VEPs must be interpreted with caution, since normal values vary greatly from laboratory to laboratory, as do variables such as the size of the stimulating squares, the luminance, and the transition time of the pattern. As with most such diagnostic tests, it is better to deemphasize changes and asymmetries rather than to erroneously assume the presence of an abnormality. For instance, changes in amplitude and waveform are much less convincing than delays in latency of conduction.

The SSEP is abnormal in 50% to 70% of patients with definite MS. However, its value in early or suspected MS is less clear. The BAEP may show changes in 50% of patients with definite MS, but some studies have found only approximately 20% abnormal BAEPs, even in patients with clinically definite brainstem lesions, and many authorities have abandoned the use of this method as having too low a yield for diagnostic purposes.[20] Certainly, fewer abnormalities are found with BAEPs than with VEPs or SSEPs.

Magnetic stimulation for measuring motor conduction uses a single, brief high-voltage magnetic stimulus over the scalp to induce contraction of muscles of the opposite limbs, thus measuring the latency of conduction. It is too early to tell if this approach will be a useful diagnostic technique or simply an elaborate method of confirming a positive Babinski sign.

## MONOSYMPTOMATIC PRESENTATIONS

Optic neuritis dominates the monosymptomatic presentation of MS, and it is likely, although not proven, that the two conditions represent the same disease; that is, optic neuritis is simply mild MS. The percentage of patients with isolated "idiopathic" optic neuritis who subsequently develop other signs and symptoms and progress to the clinical picture of typical MS varies widely among studies, but the true incidence probably approaches 50%. Approximately half of the patients who present with isolated optic neuritis will have abnormal MRIs of the brain and oligoclonal bands in the spinal fluid (the two tests closely parallel each other in

this cohort),[39] and these patients have a special risk of developing MS. In the optic neuritis treatment trial (ONTT), 3% of patients with normal MRIs developed MS within 2 years compared to 36% with abnormal scans.[4] In a 5-year study from England, 6% of patients with normal MRIs developed MS compared to 82% with abnormal imaging.[24] It seems reasonable, at least in those patients with suggestive MRI or CSF findings, to discuss MS in the context of their optic neuritis and allow these patients to plan their lives knowing that MS is a possibility.[7,8]

Conversely, acute transverse myelitis seldom heralds MS.[17] Although similar in many ways to acute optic neuritis as a monosymptomatic demyelination, transverse myelitis differs in its prognosis for subsequent CNS lesions and development of clinical MS. No more than 20% of patients with acute transverse myelitis will progress to MS, and in some studies the rate is as low as 3%.[18] As with optic neuritis, MRI abnormalities and oligoclonal banding can identify a group of patients at greatest risk for later development of MS.[30]

## DIFFERENTIAL DIAGNOSIS

Any disease that produces scattered lesions of the CNS can be confused with MS, and thus the catalog of differential diagnosis is extensive (Tables 6–4 and 6–5).[19] Some of these conditions deserve special attention because they so frequently cause diagnostic confusion.

Systemic lupus erythematosus produces overt CNS involvement in approximately 40% of patients, but almost always in a setting of unmistakable evidence of systemic disease. Therefore lupus is actually seldom confused with MS. However, optic neuritis, myelopathies, and INOs occasionally have been reported in patients with lupus, closely mimicking the clinical picture of MS. IgG in CSF is increased in 70% of CNS lupus patients, with oligoclonal bands in perhaps 50%. MRI changes may be indistinguishable from those of MS.[23] Confounding the diagnosis, a positive antinuclear antibody test, at least in low titers, can be seen in up to 81% of patients with MS.[2] Nevertheless, lupus differs from MS because of the presence of systemic symptoms (e.g., joint disease, rashes, and alopecia) and laboratory abnormalities (e.g., markedly elevated sedimentation rate). The CSF also often shows very high protein and polymorphonuclear cell counts, more closely resembling meningitis than MS. What is true of lupus also holds true for many other connective tissue diseases, such as Sjögren's syndrome, Behçet's syndrome, and rheumatoid arthritis.

Sarcoidosis may also produce CNS lesions and abnormal VEPs and otherwise mimic MS. However, patients with neurosarcoidosis often have seizures, dementia, deafness, and other features that are unusual for MS. Their spinal fluid seldom shows increased IgG synthesis or oligoclonal bands, and the MRI frequently indicates a basal meningitis and other changes distinct from MS.

Lyme disease has received considerable attention, at least in the lay press, as a mimicker of MS. Indeed, patients with Lyme disease may have CNS deficits, abnormal MRI scans, and positive oligoclonal bands. However, they also frequently have facial nerve palsies, headaches, peripheral neuropathies and radiculopathies, and markedly elevated white cell counts and CSF protein levels, suggesting a picture of meningitis. The characteristic erythema chronicum migrans rash also differentiates Lyme disease from MS, but antibody

**TABLE 6–4.  Partial Differential Diagnosis of Multiple Sclerosis**

| DISEASE | MRI | CSF BANDS | VEP | DIFFERENTIATING FEATURES |
|---|---|---|---|---|
| Hereditary ataxias | + | No | + | Family history<br>Genetic testing available for some |
| Familial spastic paraplegia | No | No | + | Family history<br>Deficits often confined to cord or pyramidal tract |
| Sarcoidosis | No | No | + | ↑ Angiotensin-converting enzyme<br>Systemic (often pulmonary) signs |
| Vitamin B$_{12}$ deficiency | No | No | + | Low serum levels<br>Slow peripheral nerve conductions |
| Tropical spastic paraparesis | + | + | + | Largely confined to tropics<br>Serology available for HTLV-1<br>Strictly progressive pattern |
| Systemic lupus erythematosus | + | + | + | Systemic symptoms<br>Abnormal serology and sedimentation rate |
| Sjögren's syndrome | + | + | + | Anti-Ro and anti-La antibodies<br>Dry eyes and mouth |
| Behçet's syndrome | + | No | No | Meningitis<br>Oral and genital ulcers |
| Acute disseminated encephalomyelitis | + | + | + | Often a preceding viral infection |
| Lyme disease | + | + | + | Erythema chronicum migrans rash<br>↑ CSF protein and cells<br>Abnormal Lyme serologic evidence |
| Adrenoleukodystrophy | + | No | + | Only in males (X-linked)<br>↑ Very long chain fatty acids |
| Isolated central nervous system vasculitis | + | No | No | Usually presents as encephalopathy without focal findings |

CSF, Cerebrospinal fluid; MRI, magnetic resonance imaging; VEP, visual evoked potential.

NOTE: Abnormal MRI, CSF, or VEP findings have, on occasion, been reported in many diseases, including normal controls. These tests are considered abnormal here only if they are frequently positive in the disease.

titers, polymerase chain reaction studies, and similar specific diagnostic tools may be needed for a definitive differentiation. Some patients with MS also have positive Lyme serologic test results and even anti-Lyme antibodies in the CSF, but these are usually incidental or false-positive findings.[5]

**TABLE 6–5.  Selected Diseases Often Confused With Multiple Sclerosis**

**Lesions Often Disseminated in Time but Not Space**
Cerebellar ataxias
Familial spastic paraparesis
Primary lateral sclerosis
Leukodystrophies
Neoplasms
Arnold-Chiari and skull base malformations
Arteriovenous malformations

**Lesions Often Disseminated in Space but Not Time**
Acute disseminated encephalomyelitis
Shower of emboli
Thrombocytopenic purpura
Sarcoidosis
Lyme disease

**Lesions Often Disseminated in Both Time and Space**
Vascular disease emboli and lacunes
Vasculitis: lupus erythematosus, Behçet's syndrome
Sjögren's syndrome
Lymphoma
Progressive multifocal leukoencephalopathy
Myasthenia gravis
Subacute combined degeneration
Tropical spastic paraparesis (HTLV-1)

Acute disseminated encephalomyelitis (ADEM), following a viral infection or vaccination, is often absolutely indistinguishable from an initial attack of MS. This condition is more common in children than in adults, but it may produce all the clinical and laboratory abnormalities seen in patients with MS. Although definitive studies are lacking, as many as 25% of all patients diagnosed as having an isolated postviral demyelination actually develop MS.[35]

Among patients referred to MS centers for diagnostic opinions who prove not to have MS, the most common cause of their complaints is psychiatric (i.e., depression, anxiety, or a somatization disorder such as conversion reaction or hypochondriasis). Among patients who do have MS but were initially diagnosed as having another condition, the most common misdiagnosis was psychiatric. Therefore psychiatric illness is both the leading reason for erroneously considering MS and the leading reason for erroneously rejecting MS. Diagnosis is particularly puzzling when such patients have a slight EP asymmetry, a dot or two on the MRI, or a "soft" neurologic finding on physical examination. These patients often require time, patience, and reexamination before a conclusive diagnosis can be reached. Nevertheless, most patients who are diagnosed with a nonorganic symptom are diagnosed correctly and never develop any neurologic disease.[6]

In the differential diagnosis of MS, certain features should raise the suspicion that some other condition is responsible for the patient's presenting complaints. Table 6–6 lists some of the "red flags" that militate against MS and should prompt the clinician to reevaluate the diagnosis.[15] Although these features may occur in patients with definite MS, they do so only rarely.

**TABLE 6–6. Features Casting Doubt on Diagnosis of Multiple Sclerosis**

1. Normal neurologic examination
2. Localized progressive disease, with signs or symptoms confined to one area (e.g., spinal cord) and stable or progressing; in other words, no dissemination in time or space
3. Family history of similar neurologic symptoms
4. No eye involvement
5. Abrupt hemiparesis
6. Pain (except trigeminal neuralgia)
7. No immunoglobulin G abnormalities in cerebrospinal fluid
8. Transient, very brief symptoms
9. Age >50 years
10. Symptoms listed in Table 6–1
11. Presence of other diseases that can affect nervous system (e.g., lupus erythematosus, diabetes)

Modified from Herndon RM. The changing pattern of misdiagnosis in multiple sclerosis. In: Herndon RM, Seil FJ, eds. *Multiple Sclerosis: Current Status of Research and Treatment.* New York: Demos Publications; 1994: 149-155.

## DIAGNOSTIC CRITERIA

Many experts have devised diagnostic criteria in an effort to deal with the ambiguity of the diagnosis of MS. Among the better known guidelines are those by McAlpine,[21] Bauer,[3] McDonald and Halliday,[22] Rose et al,[36] and, especially, Schumacher et al[37]; the more recent criteria of Poser et al[34] incorporate laboratory studies to supplement the clinical findings (Table 6–7). All these proposals are based on the demonstration of lesions disseminated in time and space: two separate attacks at two separate times. However, these criteria are far from perfect. The criteria of Poser et al[34] are the most sensitive, correctly identifying 87% of autopsy-proven cases in one series,[16] but only after an average of 8 years of symptoms; however, the specificity (false-positives) could not be determined. These formal diagnostic criteria, designed for use in therapeutic trials rather than in office practice, exclude many true cases of MS (false-negatives) that do not meet all their rigorous requirements. Therefore many patients who suffer from MS, and for whom most clinicians would never doubt the diagnosis, will not be properly counseled or treated if these criteria are rigidly relied on for treatment. Although formal diagnostic criteria may serve as an aid to the practicing neurologist, they should not be considered inviolable rules. The diagnosis of MS is not a laundry list of findings and tests to be checked off, with no conclusion reached unless all items are marked.

## WHAT TO TELL PATIENTS

Although many MS criteria employ terms such as *possible MS* or *probable MS*, these designations should be avoided in clinical practice, as should euphemisms such as *demyelinating disease* or *viral inflammation*. Such labels leave most patients confused and often prompt them to visit other physicians in an attempt to resolve the ambiguities.

Most studies have shown that patients with MS want to know their diagnosis as soon as it is established and want to hear it from the physician who made it, generally the consultant neurologist rather than the primary care practitioner.[9,14,25,27,38] When physicians are vague or evasive, especially if they delay in discussing the diagnosis, patients assume it is because they do not know; they may believe the physician is incompetent.[14] Since MS is a chronic disease that requires life-long rapport with the patient, avoiding communication is a poor way to begin the physician-patient relationship. In general, a prompt, honest discussion is most appropriate. Many clinicians also find it useful to schedule a return visit soon after presenting the diagnosis for the specific purpose of reviewing the diagnosis and discussing the prognosis, the treatment plan, and other issues.

A patient with presenting symptoms of possible MS can be thought of as a defendant in a court of law who is accused of committing a crime. The process a neurologist uses to diagnose MS resembles that which a juror uses to convict a criminal. Because there is no definitive test for MS, the diagnosis must be reached by careful examination of all the evidence in each case, both for and against the disease. Through questioning, examining, and testing, the neurologist must assemble this evidence until it is sufficiently compelling to find the patient "guilty" or "not guilty" of having MS. Even when great care is taken, the diagnosis may be made in error (innocent person found guilty) or inappropriately dismissed (guilty person found innocent), and expert neurologists may disagree among themselves (hung jury).[41] As with all endeavors so heavily dependent on human judgment, some doubt often exists as to whether justice was served. This inability to prove the diagnosis "beyond a shadow of a doubt" (short of autopsy), combined with the many nuances and pitfalls in the history, physical examination, and testing, makes MS one of the most challenging of all diseases to diagnose.

The courtroom analogy is often useful in explaining to patients why the diagnosis does or does not seem correct and why it may be so difficult to prove conclusively ("beyond a shadow of a doubt"). The example of a courtroom is simple to understand and allows most patients to accept the uncertainty often associated with a diagnosis of MS.

**TABLE 6–7. Summary of Poser and Schumacher Criteria for Definite Multiple Sclerosis**

**Summary of Poser Criteria for Diagnosing Definite MS for Research Protocols**

*Clinically Definite MS*
1. Two attacks plus clinical evidence of two lesions
   *or*
2. Two attacks plus clinical evidence of one lesion and test evidence (such as magnetic resonance imaging or evoked potentials) of a second lesion

*Laboratory-Supported Definite MS*
Requires oligoclonal bands or elevated immunoglobulin G in the spinal fluid
   *plus*
1. Two attacks and either clinical or test evidence of one lesion
   *or*
2. One attack with clinical evidence of two lesions
   *or*
3. One attack with clinical evidence of one lesion plus test evidence of a second lesion

**Summary of Schumacher Criteria for Definite MS**
1. Two separate central nervous system lesions
2. Two separate episodes or attacks
3. Abnormal neurologic examination
4. White matter signs and symptoms
5. Age 10 through 50 years
6. No other disease present to account for findings

## RECOMMENDATIONS

There is no algorithm to guide the clinician to the correct diagnosis of MS. Instead, the diagnosis requires assembling and analyzing as much evidence as necessary to permit the conclusion that the disease either is or is not present. Although this evidence includes the history and physical examination, the diagnosis is seldom strictly a clinical one. Usually it requires laboratory tests such as MRI, CSF, and EPs and tests to exclude other diseases (when indicated). Some patients with a typical clinical picture will require no laboratory support, whereas others will remain undiagnosed even after extensive testing. The dogmatic ordering of a battery of "MS tests" for all patients suspected of having MS will, of course, yield a sufficient number of false-positive and false-negative tests to guarantee diagnostic confusion. Tests should be chosen wisely. No invariable battery of investigations can be promulgated or endorsed. Ultimately, the diagnosis of MS depends on the judgment of an experienced neurologist.

## REFERENCES

1. Andersson M, Alvarez-Cermeno J, Bernardi G, et al. Cerebrospinal fluid in the diagnosis of multiple sclerosis: a consensus report. *J Neurol Neurosurg Psychiatry.* 1994;57:897-902.
2. Barned S, Goodman AD, Mattson DH. Frequency of antinuclear antibodies in multiple sclerosis. *Neurology.* 1995;45:384.
3. Bauer HJ. IMAB-Enquete concerning the diagnostic criteria for multiple sclerosis. In: Bauer HJ, Poser S, Ritter G, eds. *Progress in Multiple Sclerosis Research.* Berlin: Springer; 1980:55.
4. Beck RW, Cleary PA, Trobe JD, et al. The effect of corticosteroids for acute optic neuritis on the subsequent development of multiple sclerosis. *N Engl J Med.* 1993;329:1764-1769.
5. Coyle PK, Krupp LB, Doscher C. Significance of reactive Lyme serology in multiple sclerosis. *Ann Neurol.* 1993;34:745-747.
6. Crimlisk HI, Bhatia K, Cope N, et al. Slater revisited: 6 year follow-up study of patients with medically unexplained motor symptoms. *BMJ.* 1998;316:582-586.
7. Dutton JJ, Slamovits TL. What to tell the patient with optic neuritis about multiple sclerosis. *Surv Ophthalmol.* 1991;36:47-50.
8. Ebers GC. Optic neuritis and multiple sclerosis. *Arch Neurol.* 1985;42:702-704.
9. Elian M, Dean E. To tell or not to tell the diagnosis of multiple sclerosis. *Lancet.* 1985;2:27.
10. Fazekas F. Magnetic resonance signal abnormalities in asymptomatic individuals: their incidence and functional correlates. *Eur Neurol.* 1989;29:164.
11. Fazekas F, Offenbacher H, Hartung H-P. What is the role of ancillary investigations in establishing the diagnosis of multiple sclerosis? *Eur Neurol.* 1997;38:255-257.
12. Francis GS, Evans AC, Arnold DL. Neuroimaging in multiple sclerosis. *Neurol Clin.* 1995;13:147-171.
13. Giang DW, Grow VM, Mooney C, et al. Clinical diagnosis of multiple sclerosis: the impact of magnetic resonance imaging and ancillary testing. *Arch Neurol.* 1994;51:61.
14. Gorman E, Rudd A, Ebers GC. Giving the diagnosis of multiple sclerosis. In: Poser C, Paty D, Scheinberg L, McDonald WI, Ebers GC, eds. *The Diagnosis of Multiple Sclerosis.* New York: Thieme-Stratton; 1984:216-224.
15. Herndon RM. The changing pattern of misdiagnosis in multiple sclerosis. In: Herndon RM, Seil FJ, eds. *Multiple Sclerosis: Current Status of Research and Treatment.* New York: Demos; 1994:149.
16. Izquierdo G, Hauw JJ, Lyon-Caen O, et al. Value of multiple sclerosis diagnostic criteria. Seventy autopsy-confirmed cases. *Arch Neurol.* 1985;42:848.
17. Jeffery DR, Mandler RN, Davis LE. Transverse myelitis: retrospective analysis of 33 cases, with differentiation of cases associated with multiple sclerosis and parainfectious events. *Arch Neurol.* 1993;50:532-535.
18. Lipton HL, Teasdale RD. Acute transverse myelopathy in adults. *Arch Neurol.* 1979;28:252-257.
19. Matthews WB. Differential diagnosis. In: Matthews WB, Compston A, Allen IV, Martyn CN. *McAlpine's Multiple Sclerosis.* 2nd ed. Edinburgh: Churchill Livingstone; 1991:165.
20. Matthews WB. Laboratory diagnosis. In: Matthews WB, Compston A, Allen IV, Martyn CN. *McAlpine's Multiple Sclerosis.* 2nd ed. Edinburgh: Churchill Livingstone; 1991:189.
21. McAlpine D. Course and prognosis. In: McAlpine D, Lumsden CE, Acheson ED. *Multiple Sclerosis: A Reappraisal.* Edinburgh: Churchill Livingstone; 1972:202.
22. McDonald WI, Halliday AM. Diagnosis and classification of multiple sclerosis. *Br Med Bull.* 1977;33:4.
23. Miller DH, Ormerod IE, Gibson A, et al. MR brain scanning in patients with vasculitis: differentiation from multiple sclerosis. *Neuroradiology.* 1987;29:226.
24. Morrissey SP, Miller DH, Kendall BE, et al. The significance of brain magnetic resonance imaging abnormalities at presentation with clinically isolated syndromes suggestive of multiple sclerosis. *Brain.* 1993;116:135-146.
25. Mushlin AI, Mooney C, Grow V, Phelps CE, affiliated with the Rochester-Toronto MRI Study Group. The value of diagnostic information to patients with suspected multiple sclerosis. *Arch Neurol.* 1994;51:67.
26. Noseworthy JH, Paty DW, Wonnacott T, et al. Multiple sclerosis after age 50. *Neurology.* 1983;33:1537-1544.
27. O'Connor P, Detsky AS, Tansey C, Kucharczyk W, and the Rochester-Toronto MRI Study Group. Effect of diagnostic testing for multiple sclerosis on patient perceptions. *Arch Neurol.* 1994;51:46.
28. O'Connor PE, Tansey C, Kucharczyk W, Detsky AS, and the Rochester-Toronto MRI Study Group. A randomized trial of test result sequencing in patients with suspected multiple sclerosis. *Arch Neurol.* 1994;51:53.
29. Ormerod IE, Miller DH, McDonald WI, et al. The role of NMR imaging in the assessment of multiple sclerosis and isolated neurologic lesions. *Brain.* 1987;110:1579-1616.
30. Paolino E, Fainardi E, Ruppi P, et al. A prospective study on the predictive value of CSF oligoclonal bands and MRI in acute isolated neurological syndromes for subsequent progression to multiple sclerosis. *J Neurol Neurosurg Psychiatry.* 1996;60:572-575.
31. Paty DW, McFarlin DE, McDonald WI. Magnetic resonance imaging and laboratory aids in the diagnosis of multiple sclerosis. *Ann Neurol.* 1991;29:3.
32. Paty DW, Noseworthy JH, Ebers GC. Diagnosis of multiple sclerosis. In: Paty DW, Ebers GC, eds. *Multiple Sclerosis.* Philadelphia: FA Davis; 1998.
33. Paty DW, Oger JJF, Kastrukoff LF, et al. MRI in the diagnosis of MS: a prospective study with comparison of clinical evaluation, evoked potentials, oligoclonal banding, and CT. *Neurology.* 1988;38:180.
34. Poser CM, Paty DW, Scheinberg L, et al. New diagnostic criteria for multiple sclerosis: guidelines for research protocols. *Ann Neurol.* 1983;13:227.
35. Rolak LA. Acute disseminated encephalomyelitis. In: Rolak LA, Harati Y. *Neuro-immunology for the Clinician.* Boston: Butterworth-Heinemann; 1997:167-176.
36. Rose AS, Ellison GW, Myers LW, Tourtellotte WW. Criteria for the clinical diagnosis of multiple sclerosis. *Neurology.* 1976;26(suppl 20):22.
37. Schumacher GA, Beebe G, Kibler RF, et al. Problems of experimental trials of therapy in multiple sclerosis. *Ann N Y Acad Sci.* 1965;122:552.
38. Sencer W. Suspicion of multiple sclerosis: to tell or not to tell? *Arch Neurol.* 1988;45:441.
39. Sharief MK, Thompson EJ. The predictive value of intrathecal immunoglobulin synthesis and magnetic resonance imaging in acute isolated syndromes for subsequent development of multiple sclerosis. *Ann Neurol.* 1991;29:147.
40. Sola P, Scarpa P, Faglioni P, et al. Diagnostic investigations in MS: which is the most sensitive? *Acta Neurol Scand.* 1989;80:394.
41. Solari A, Filippini G, Gagliardi L, et al. Interobserver agreement in the diagnosis of multiple sclerosis. *Arch Neurol.* 1989;46:289.
42. Thorpe JW, Kidd D, Moseley IF, et al. Spinal MRI in patients with suspected multiple sclerosis and negative brain MRI. *Brain.* 1996;119:709-714.
43. Young JR, Hall AS, Pallis CA, et al. Nuclear magnetic resonance imaging of the brain in multiple sclerosis. *Lancet.* 1981;2:1063-1066.
44. Zeman AZJ, Kidd D, McLean BN, et al. A study of oligoclonal band negative multiple sclerosis. *J Neurol Neurosurg Psychiatry.* 1996;60:27-30.

# 7

# Normal Pressure Hydrocephalus

*Neill R. Graff-Radford and John C. Godersky*

Two diagnostic aspects of hydrocephalus are discussed in this chapter: (1) the factors that are useful in deciding which patients with suspected normal pressure hydrocephalus (NPH), also called symptomatic hydrocephalus, should be referred for shunt surgery and (2) how to evaluate a patient with possible shunt failure. These two aspects were chosen because they are particularly difficult diagnostic dilemmas that are frequently faced by clinicians caring for patients with hydrocephalus.

NPH is an uncommon condition that presents primarily with hydrocephalus and gait difficulty. In addition to gait difficulty, patients may suffer from the other two symptoms in the triad, that is, incontinence of urine and dementia. The dilemma physicians and their patients face is that 30% to 40% of patients who undergo shunt surgery are reported to suffer complications.[2,31] Further, improvement occurs in only 50% to 70% of patients.[17,23] The following sections discuss the factors associated with either a favorable or an unfavorable surgical prognosis.

## USEFUL INFORMATION IN DECISION MAKING FOR SHUNT SURGERY

### HISTORY

There are several important questions that should be asked when taking a history from affected patients and their families.

1. *How long has the patient had dementia?* If the answer is more than 2 years, it is less likely that the patient will respond to surgery.[17,31] Note that the question is not how long the patient has had gait abnormality but how long the patient has had dementia. Refer to Table 7–1 to see how reliable this information was in predicting surgical outcome in our series.[17]

2. *Which started first, gait abnormality or dementia?* If the gait abnormality began before or at the same time as the dementia, there is a better chance for successful surgery. However, if dementia began before gait abnormality, shunting is less likely to help[12,15,17] (Table 7–1).

3. *Is there a history of alcohol abuse?* Alcohol abuse is a poor prognostic indicator.[7]

4. *Is there a secondary cause of hydrocephalus?* Examples of such causes are subarachnoid hemorrhage, meningitis, previous brain surgery, and head injury. If any of these are present, the chances of improvement with surgery are better.[3,4,7,31]

### PHYSICAL EXAMINATION

On physical examination, the following two issues should be addressed:

1. *Measure the head circumference.* If it is greater than 59 cm in males or 57.5 cm in females (i.e., greater than the 98th percentile for head circumference), the patient could have congenital hydrocephalus that has become symptomatic in later life.[16,27]

2. *Exclude diseases that may mimic symptomatic hydrocephalus.* Such diseases or conditions include Parkinson's disease, cervical spondylosis with spinal cord compression, progressive supranuclear palsy, multiple system atrophy, phenothiazine use, Alzheimer's disease with extrapyramidal features, diffuse Lewy body disease, and multiple subcortical infarctions. This differential diagnosis is sometimes easier said than done, but keeping it in mind during the physical examination is helpful.

### NEUROPSYCHOLOGIC FINDINGS

Look for evidence of aphasia. If such evidence is found, for example, anomia, it is a poor prognostic indicator for surgical success[7,17] (see Table 7–1).

### CEREBROSPINAL FLUID DRAINAGE PROCEDURES

If the patient's gait improves after removing a large quantity of cerebrospinal fluid (CSF) by lumbar puncture (30 to 50 ml, which can be repeated daily), this person is a good candidate for shunt surgery.[40,41] A modification of this technique has also been reported; it is continuous CSF drainage via a catheter placed in the lumbar CSF space.[20,21] This method involves placement of a thin subarachnoid catheter in the lumbar CSF space and leading into a drainage bag. The height of the drainage bag is adjusted to allow drainage of 5 to 10 ml/h and yet avoid the hypotensive symptoms of headache. This closed system allows an average of 150 ml/d drainage and helps prevent infection. The thin tube prevents rapid CSF drainage, decreasing the risk of subdural hemor-

**TABLE 7–1. Variables Predicting Surgical Outcome in Symptomatic Hydrocephalus**

| VARIABLE | NO. OF PATIENTS | ODDS RATIO | p VALUE* | 95% CONFIDENCE INTERVAL FOR ODDS RATIO[†] | CORRECT CLASSIFICATION UNIMPROVED | CORRECT CLASSIFICATION IMPROVED |
|---|---|---|---|---|---|---|
| Age | 30 | 1.031 | 0.59 | 0.919–1.157 | | |
| Education | 30 | 0.906 | 0.41 | 0.716–1.146 | | |
| Sex | 30 | 4.615 | 0.215[‡] | 0.423–233.0 | | |
| Gait abnormality (yr) | 30 | 1.133 | 0.51 | 0.789–1.626 | | |
| Incontinence (yr) | 30 | 1.441 | 0.402 | 0.614–3.408 | | |
| Dementia (yr) | 30 | 9.002 | <0.001 | 1.542–52.56 | 5/7 | 21/23 |
| Order of onset (gait vs. dementia) | 30 | 0 | 0.009[‡] | 0–0.425 | 3/7 | 23/23 |
| % time B-waves present | 28 | 0.969 | 0.04 | 0.937–1.001 | 2/6 | 22/22 |
| % time pressure >15 mm Hg | 28 | 0.968 | 0.055 | 0.930–1.006 | 0/6 | 22/22 |
| % time pressure >20 mm Hg | 28 | 0.979 | 0.23 | 0.940–1.020 | | |
| Visual naming test | 25 | 0.941 | 0.093 | 0.875–1.013 | 2/7 | 17/18 |
| Visual naming, pass/fail | 25 | 8.750 | 0.058[‡] | 0.887–113.3 | 5/7 | 14/18 |
| Cerebral blood flow (anterior/posterior ratio slice 4) | 30 | 1.120 | <0.001 | 1.026–1.224 | 5/7 | 22/23 |
| CSF conductance | 23 | 0.254 | 0.956 | 0–infinity | | |
| CSF conductance, 0.08 as cutoff value | 23 | 1.071 | 1.00[‡] | 0.065–67.354 | | |

*p value based on likelihood ratio test.
[†]Based on Wald test (which is slightly different from likelihood ratio test) and on Fisher's exact test when this test was used.
[‡]p value based on Fisher's exact test.
From Graff-Radford NR, Godersky JC. Variables predicting surgical outcome in symptomatic hydrocephalus in the elderly. *Neurology.* 1989;39:1601-1604.

rhage. Another approach was described by Hanley et al,[21] who use a larger (16-gauge) catheter through which CSF pressure can also be monitored. They pay particular attention to the level of the drainage bag, with the goal of draining 240 ml/d. To minimize infection, the drainage system is kept to 2 to 5 days. If symptoms of headache and nausea develop, it is possible that too much CSF is being drained.

There are shortcomings to these diagnostic tests. We have seen patients who eventually responded to shunt surgery but had no obvious improvement for the first post-surgical week. The drainage test could have given a false-negative result in these patients. While this test is being done, the patient may appear improved (the placebo effect), but this initial response may not be maintained, leading to a false-positive result. In addition, meningitis and subdural hematoma are possible complications of the continuous CSF drainage procedures.

## COMPUTED TOMOGRAPHY AND MAGNETIC RESONANCE IMAGING

### Computed Tomography

Since the advent of computed tomography (CT), the documentation of ventriculomegaly has become easier. This situation has had both advantages and disadvantages. There is a clear advantage to not needing to subject the patient to the uncomfortable procedure of air encephalography to diagnose hydrocephalus. However, the physician is often left with the responsibility of knowing that a patient has ventriculomegaly when the scan may have been ordered for an unrelated indication.

A patient has ventriculomegaly (above the 95th percentile) when the modified Evans ratio is >3.2.[19] The Evans ratio can be calculated on the axial CT slice, where the frontal horns are largest. One measures the maximal diameter of the frontal horns and the inner table of the skull at the same level and then calculates the two measurements as a ratio, the inner table of the skull divided by the maximal di-

ameter of the frontal horns. The ventricles normally enlarge with age,[35] a point that should be taken into account in the diagnosis of hydrocephalus. There is slow ventricular enlargement until age 60, and then the rate of enlargement increases. In a study by Barron and Jacobs,[1] the mean ventricular size was 5.2% (percent of intracranial area) in the decade from 50 to 59 years, 6.4% from 60 to 69 years, 11.5% from 70 to 79 years, and 14.1% from 80 to 89 years.

Hydrocephalus without sulcal enlargement is a favorable factor in surgical prognosis. However, hydrocephalus with sulcal enlargement can still be improved with surgery. Borgesen and Gjerris[4] measured the largest sulcus in the high frontal or parietal region and found that if the cortical sulcus was less than 1.9 mm, 17 of 17 patients who were shunted improved; if the sulcus was 1.9 to 5 mm, 17 of 20 shunted patients improved; and if the sulcus was 5 mm or greater, 15 of 27 who were shunted improved.

### Magnetic Resonance Imaging

Magnetic resonance imaging (MRI) is an excellent method for evaluating patients with possible symptomatic hydrocephalus. It has the advantage of allowing visualization of structures in the posterior fossa that may be related to the patient's problem, such as the cerebral aqueduct, the level of the cerebellar tonsils, and infarctions in the brainstem. Further, MRI can be used to obtain volumetric measures of medial temporal lobe structures, a technique that has been shown to be useful in distinguishing patients with Alzheimer's disease from normal elderly controls.[25]

About 10% of elderly patients with symptomatic hydrocephalus may have congenital hydrocephalus that has become symptomatic in later years.[16] The clinical clue to this situation is that the patient has a head circumference above the 98th percentile. On MRI the ventricular enlargement shows no or little associated periventricular increased signal on T2-weighted imaging, indicating a chronic process. In addition, a cause for the congenital hydrocephalus may be found, such as an Arnold-Chiari malformation.

Deep white matter changes noted on MRI have many possible causes and may also be seen on CT as "transependymal flow." Some report that the presence of transependymal flow may be related to a good surgical prognosis. In a study by Borgesen and Gjerris,[4] 16 of 16 patients with periventricular hypodensity on CT improved with surgery, whereas in a study by Bradley et al,[6] MRI studies were rated for deep white matter changes and the presence or extent of these changes did not correlate with outcome. Jack et al[24] retrospectively reviewed the charts of 57 patients, 17 with NPH, 8 with obstructive hydrocephalus, 8 with Alzheimer's disease, and 21 with non-Alzheimer dementia. They considered increased periventricular signal and white matter signal on T2-weighted images, CSF flow void in the aqueduct, and corpus callosum thinning. However, those factors were not useful in distinguishing among the four patient groups. All 17 patients with NPH underwent shunt-surgery, and a better response was noted in patients without increased white matter signal but with increase in periventricular signal. In a postmortem MRI study of fixed brains and the histologic analysis of the same brains, Munoz et al[30] found that the white matter changes seen on MRI are correlated with decreased density of axons and myelinated fibers, diffuse vacuolation of white matter (spongiosis), and decreased density of glia. Infarctions were not common in these areas. Although this study does not necessarily apply to the white matter changes seen in hydrocephalic patients, it does indicate that white matter findings noted on MRI do not necessarily indicate irreversible periventricular infarctions, making it unlikely that shunt surgery would be effective.

We have seen numerous patients, both with and without white matter changes on MRI, improve. In acute hydrocephalus, as might occur after subarachnoid hemorrhage, breakdown of the ependyma and CSF migration at the frontal horn angle occur.[28] Thus the observation of Borgesen and Gjerris[4] that transependymal flow is a good prognostic indicator may be more applicable to patients with secondary hydrocephalus because their series was heavily weighted with such patients. However, patients with chronic hydrocephalus characteristically have little transependymal flow, and these patients often improve with surgery.[16]

Another area where MRI has the potential to aid in prognosis is volumetric measurements of certain structures in the temporal lobe. Jack et al[25] developed a technique for measuring the volume of structures in the anterior temporal lobe and hippocampal formation. The volume of the hippocampal formation has also been shown to correlate with relevant cognitive variables. Occasionally when patients are shunted for symptomatic hydrocephalus and do not respond, they are ultimately found to have Alzheimer's disease. This procedure is being evaluated for its predictive value in this clinical situation. MRI has advanced our knowledge regarding hydrocephalus, and we recommend it as the imaging method of choice in patients with this condition.

## Magnetic Resonance Detection of Cerebrospinal Fluid Flow Through the Aqueduct

In 1991 Bradley et al[6] retrospectively reviewed the MRI scans of 20 patients who had undergone ventriculoperitoneal shunt surgery for NPH. They rated the initial surgical outcome as excellent, good, or poor and correlated this rating with the extent of flow void in the cerebral aqueduct. We should point out that the method of acquiring magnetic resonance (MR) images may affect the flow void appearance. Bradley and colleagues used a 0.35-T MR imaging unit and a 128 by 128 acquisition matrix (1.7 mm spatial resolution), 7 mm section thickness with a 3 mm gap, a repetition time (TR) of 2 seconds, echo-times (TEs) of 28 and 56 ms, and four signal averages (17-minute acquisition time). They scored the extent (not signal loss per se) of flow void extension into the third and fourth ventricles on a 0-4 scale. Grade 0 indicated no signal loss; grade 1 meant signal loss in the aqueduct that did not extend to the middle of the fourth ventricle; and grades 2, 3, and 4 demonstrated progressively more extensive signal loss, with the maximum being flow void extending from the posterior third ventricle through the entire fourth ventricle. Bradley et al[6] found a significant correlation ($p < 0.003$) between the extent of increased aqueduct flow void and the initial surgical outcome. More specifically, 8 of 10 patients with increased CSF flow void scores had an excellent or good response to surgery, whereas only 1 of 9 who had a normal flow void score improved with surgery. They speculate that the increased flow in the aqueduct in hydrocephalus is based on the following mechanism.

A major cause of CSF motion is systolic expansion of the cerebral hemispheres and choroid plexus.[11] Systolic enlargement of the hemispheres normally results in outward expansion (with venting of cortical blood) and inward expansion with venting of CSF. However, in hydrocephalus the brain is positioned tightly against the skull, allowing less outward expansion during systole and resulting in more inward expansion and increased CSF venting. We believe that this is a promising method for predicting surgical prognosis in symptomatic hydrocephalus. Future studies should be prospective, demonstrate better quantitation of flow through the aqueduct, and include more objective measures of surgical outcome.

### Summary of Factors to Be Addressed

1. *Hydrocephalus must be present.* The modified Evans ratio (maximum width of the frontal horns divided by the measurement of the inner table at the same place) should be >3.1.[4]

2. *Is cortical atrophy prominent?* If there is extensive cortical atrophy, this factor reduces, but does not eliminate, the chance of improvement with surgery.[4,22,31]

3. *The pattern of atrophy may be useful diagnostically.* For example, does the atrophy involve the medial temporal lobes, as in Alzheimer's disease? Although data on this point are lacking, prominent medial temporal cortical atrophy may lessen the chance for surgical improvement because these patients may have Alzheimer's disease.[14]

4. *Is there evidence of congenital hydrocephalus?* For example, is there aqueductal stenosis or an Arnold-Chiari malformation?[16,27]

5. *Consider newer MRI techniques.* Cine-MRI, which involves the analysis of a CSF flow void in the aqueduct of Sylvius, may be helpful in predicting who will respond to a shunt.[5,6,10,24]

## REGIONAL CEREBRAL BLOOD FLOW

It has been reported that regional cerebral blood flow (rCBF) is decreased in the frontal areas in hydrocephalus[26] and in the parietotemporal areas in Alzheimer's disease.[13]

On the presumption that many of the nonimproved group have Alzheimer's disease (which we have confirmed in two patients who came to autopsy), we tried to differentiate those who will respond to shunt surgery from those who will not, based on the pattern of preoperative CBF.[18] To do this, we calculated the ratio of frontal to posterior regional blood flow. We expected a lower frontal-posterior ratio in true symptomatic hydrocephalus and a higher ratio in pseudo-symptomatic hydrocephalus patients who have Alzheimer's disease. In fact, this approach has been a good method of predicting surgical outcome: the ratio predicted 5 of 7 unimproved and 22 of 23 improved patients in our series[17] (see Table 7–1).

### CISTERNOGRAPHY

Our experience with cisternography is limited, but the literature suggests that there are numerous patients with positive test results (radioisotope seen within the ventricles 48 to 72 hours after injection in the lumber area) who do not improve with surgery and patients with equivocal or negative tests who do improve. Further, the test itself may be difficult to interpret. Black,[2] in a review of his experience with this test, found the following: of 11 patients who had a positive test, 9 improved and 2 did not; of 6 patients who had mixed results, 3 improved and 3 did not; of 6 who had negative results, 4 improved and 2 did not. Black suggests that a positive test result is helpful but that an equivocal or negative test is not. A study by Vanneste et al[38] reported that "cisternography did not improve the accuracy of combined clinical and computerized tomography in patients with presumed normal-pressure hydrocephalus." We do not use cisternography.

### CEREBROSPINAL FLUID PRESSURE MONITORING

There have been reports of a significant relationship between measures of intracranial CSF pressure monitoring and surgical outcome for symptomatic hydrocephalus. For example, in a study by Borgesen and Gjerris[4] and in our study,[17] the greater the percentage of time B waves were present, the greater the chance of a good outcome. Also, in our series, the longer the pressure was >15 mm Hg, the better the chance of successful surgery (see Table 7–1). These findings imply that increased pressure may be pathogenetic in symptomatic hydrocephalus.

These data raise the issue of what is meant by NPH. Does it mean normal pressure at one spinal tap, or does it imply that the pressure remains normal all the time? We do not know what 24-hour CSF pressure recordings in healthy individuals would show. It follows that we do not know if the pressure is normal or abnormal in those who respond to surgery but have CSF pressures >15 mm Hg for a percentage of time. For this reason, at present, we prefer the term *symptomatic hydrocephalus* to NPH.

A continuous printout over 24 to 72 hours with a paper speed of between 50 and 150 mm/h is needed to assess the overall intracranial pressure (ICP) and the presence of B waves. Sedation may be helpful at night to reduce the frequency of artifact in the recording.

### INFUSION TESTS

Borgesen and Gjerris[4] described the CSF conductance test, in which CSF absorption is measured at different CSF pressures. They reported in their series a greater than 90% accuracy in predicting short-term prognosis following shunt surgery and an approximately 85% accuracy in predicting long-term prognosis. The concept is that the greater the pressure needed to obtain an amount of absorption, the better the chances of that patient's improving with shunt surgery. Absorption is calculated by infusing fluid through an LP (lumber puncture) needle for a given time (5 minutes) while catching the overflow from a ventricular catheter. There is some evidence to show that the amount of CSF produced does not vary much at different CSF pressures and is about 0.4 ml/min. Because how much is infused through the LP needle and how much overflows through the ventricular catheter is known, it is possible to calculate the amount produced in this period. The following equation gives absorption:

$$\text{Absorption} = (\text{Infused} + \text{Produced}) - \text{Overflow}$$

The overflow pressure for the ventricular catheter is then raised, and absorption is calculated at this new pressure. Between six and eight absorption and pressure measures are obtained in this way. Next, absorption is plotted against pressure, and the slope of the line is calculated (i.e., absorption divided by pressure). The slope of this line is called the conductance. Borgesen and Gjerris[4] reported that a conductance of <0.08 predicted a favorable outcome. In our study,[17] we found no significant correlation between CSF conductance and improvement (see Table 7–1). However, we chose our patients based on the conductance result, so this factor was not an independent variable. In addition, most of our patients had idiopathic hydrocephalus, whereas many of Borgesen and Gjerris's patients had secondary hydrocephalus. The conductance test, which relates to CSF absorption, may be a better predictor of outcome in secondary hydrocephalus in which an absorption defect may be causative.

## COMPLICATIONS OF SHUNT INSERTION

It is anticipated that all patients will improve clinically following shunt placement. If there is no improvement, a determination must be made that the shunt is indeed working before the failure is attributed to incorrect patient selection. Shunt malfunction is quite common both in the early and late postoperative periods.[9,32,34,36]

Weiner et al[39] place complications into three major groups: (1) those related to the surgical procedure, (2) mechanical shunt problems, and (3) complications related to the flow characteristic of the shunt system. Surgical complications include infection, intracranial hemorrhage, abdominal viscus injury, and placement of the shunt in an incorrect location. Mechanical shunt problems are often seen later in the patient's course. They include shunt obstruction of the ventricular or peritoneal catheters and fracture of the shunt. Flow characteristics can cause problems with overdrainage or inadequate drainage. Overdrainage leads to the development of subdural fluid collections or subdural hematomas and can cause CSF hypotensive headaches. Inadequate drainage results in failure to resolve the hydrocephalus.

Shunt infections are a common cause of early shunt malfunction.[9,32] They most often result from wound contamination by skin bacteria (staphylococcal species) or from wound contamination from bacteria in the air of the operating suite. The manifestation of the infection depends on its location. Redness or purulent drainage of the incision or along the shunt path, indicates wound infection. Meningitis and ventriculitis can cause shunt malfunction, irritability, fever, headache, or other neurologic dysfunction without external evidence of infection. Intraabdominal infection can result from the transport of infected CSF into the peritoneum with resultant peritonitis or pseudocyst formation.

Late shunt infection can occur as a result of bacteremia or violation of the shunt for testing; such infections are much less common than early infections.[9,32,36] Delayed malfunctions are most commonly mechanical in origin and often involve obstruction of the peritoneal portion of the shunt.

In symptomatic adult hydrocephalus, overdrainage of CSF may be manifest by symptomatic or asymptomatic subdural fluid collections. Raftopoulos et al[34] have studied this problem over time with CT scanning. In their study of 23 adults with idiopathic chronic hydrocephalus, 43% developed subdural fluid collections. Significantly, only the subdural collections seen within the first 9 days of surgery had a risk of evolving into subdural hematomas (4 of 7). Of the three subdural collections noted more than 2 months after shunt placement, none evolved into subdural hematomas.

Since overdrainage is a consequence of shunt design, it would seem that systems that prevent siphoning (development of negative intracranial pressure in the upright position) would resolve this problem. Unfortunately, the solution is not so simple. Weiner et al[39] retrospectively studied this possibility in 37 patients and found that a regulated valve system did not prevent the development of subdural hematomas. This finding raises the issue of which type of shunt system or valve pressure is appropriate for management of symptomatic adult hydrocephalus. This question is not answerable at this time.[35] Investigators in the field have a variety of opinions about the most appropriate shunt system to use. There are supporters of high pressure, medium pressure, and low pressure systems, supporters of programmable systems (pressure can be adjusted externally after shunt placement), and supporters of differential flow systems. This debate is likely to continue for some time. However, a multicenter trial is underway in Japan to address some of these points.[29]

## ASSESSMENT OF SHUNT FUNCTION

There is information to support the observation that the ventricular size need not diminish after shunt placement for improvement to occur.[29,34] This concept suggests that there are factors other than an increase in the ventricular volume that cause neurologic dysfunction—perhaps periodic elevations in ICP (B waves) or alterations in CBF or metabolism that are reversed by shunting. Obviously, reduction in ventricular size does not guarantee improvement if the preoperative diagnosis is incorrect. Responders and nonresponders had equivalent reductions in ventricular size.[42]

Knowing that shunt malfunctions occur frequently, how do we evaluate the adequacy of the shunt function? A time-honored, hands-on approach has been to "pump" the shunt. Unfortunately, this is not a reliable means of determining either the adequacy or the inadequacy of the shunt,[33] even in highly experienced hands. A postoperative CT or MRI scan, when compared with the preoperative imaging study, may

answer the question. If the ventricles are smaller after shunt placement, the shunt is likely to be functional. The shunt may be working well, and the ventricles may not be reduced in size.[34] Furthermore, reduction in ventricular size may be present early in the course of a shunt infection before the shunt becomes occluded. Plain film x-rays of the shunt system are also beneficial for assessing shunt disconnections, migrations, and fractures. These images complement the CT or MRI studies. Removal of CSF from the shunt system is the most accurate means of identifying a ventriculitis. The lumbar CSF may not reflect the presence of intraventricular infection.

Percutaneous assessment of the shunt system, or "tapping" the shunt, risks introducing infection and damaging the shunt with the needle. These risks should be taken into account when the shunt function is assessed. Because of these risks, noninvasive means of assessment of shunt function have been sought. These have included detection of thermal changes along the shunt following cooling, the use of ultrasound to detect flow, and, most recently, the use of color-flow Doppler imaging.[37] Significant limitations exist even with color-flow Doppler imaging, and widespread acceptance and use have not been forthcoming.

Shunt systems vary greatly in design and function. All ventriculoperitoneal shunt systems contain a ventricular catheter, a valve, and a peritoneal catheter. In addition, most contain a reservoir (CSF holding chamber) that is either separate and proximal to the valve or incorporated into the valve device as a separate chamber. This reservoir serves as the access site for "shunt tapping." Knowing the structural components of the shunt system is critical to the safe and successful evaluation of the shunt. Those familiar with the shunt hardware can often identify the components on x-ray.

To tap the shunt, identify the reservoir, shave the hair around it, sterilize the area with a surgical soap, and drape a sterile sticky drape with aperture over the area. Puncture the reservoir using a no. 25 beveled butterfly needle. If the ventricular catheter is patent, the fluid should flow into the butterfly tubing. A manometer can be attached to the butterfly needle tubing to measure intraventricular pressure (IVP). After the pressure is measured, obtain CSF fluid for analysis. If the fluid does not flow into the butterfly tubing and cannot be obtained by gentle aspiration, there is a proximal shunt malfunction.

To test the distal shunt, inject 2 to 3 ml of a low-osmolality iodinated dye (e.g., Isovue 370 or Omnipaque 180 or 240) and visualize the flow of the reagent with fluoroscopy. Alternatively, inject 1 millicurie of technetium 99m followed by 2 to 3 ml of preservative-free sterile saline to flush the material into the shunt, and visualize the flow with a gamma camera. During the injection it is best to occlude the tube proximal to the reservoir with finger pressure, although this is not always possible, depending on the shunt design. The contrast agent should flow readily through the system and diffuse gradually within the abdominal cavity. Sometimes the contrast agent does not flow spontaneously, and the flow needs to be facilitated by pumping on the valve. If flow fails to occur or if the contrast material pools in a small area within the abdomen, the distal shunt is malfunctioning. Although this invasive testing may be necessary to check shunt function, it is important that this testing be done by a professional who is knowledgeable about shunt devices and that the patient be informed of the risks of shunt damage and infection.

The use of MRI to detect flow through the shunt is also being investigated[8]; however, this method has not found wide acceptance.

## CONCLUSION

Shunt complications occur frequently and are often significant and difficult to treat. It is important that the patient and family be informed of this situation before the patient undergoes surgery for NPH.

## REFERENCES

1. Barron SA, Jacobs L, Kinkel WR. Changes in size of normal lateral ventricles during aging determined by computerized tomography. *Neurology.* 1976;26(11):1011-1013.
2. Black PM. Idiopathic normal-pressure hydrocephalus: results of shunting in 62 patients. *J Neurosurg.* 1980;52(3):371-377.
3. Black PM, Ojemann RG, Tzouras A. CSF shunts for dementia, incontinence, and gait disturbance. *Clin Neurosurg.* 1985;32:632-651.
4. Borgesen SE, Gjerris F. The predictive value of conductance to outflow of CSF in normal pressure hydrocephalus. *Brain.* 1982;105(pt 1):65-86.
5. Bradley WG, Kortman KE, Burgoyne B. Flowing cerebrospinal fluid in normal and hydrocephalic states: appearance on MR images. *Radiology.* 1986;159:611-616.
6. Bradley WG Jr, Whittemore AR, Kortman KE, et al. Marked cerebrospinal fluid void: indicator of successful shunt in patients with suspected normal-pressure hydrocephalus. *Radiology.* 1991;178(2):459-466.
7. De Mol J. Prognostic factors for therapeutic outcome in normal-pressure hydrocephalus: review of the literature and personal study. *Acta Neurol Belg.* 1985;85(1):13-29.
8. Drake J, Martin A, Henkelman R. Determination of CSF shunt obstruction with MR phase imaging. *J Neurosurg.* 1991;75:535-540.
9. Drake J, Sainte-Rose C. Shunt complications. In: Drake J, Sainte-Rose C, eds. *The Shunt Book.* Cambridge, Mass: Blackwell Scientific; 1995; vol 1.
10. Enzmann D, Pelc N. Normal flow patterns of intracranial and spinal cerebrospinal fluid defined with phase-contrast CINE-MRI imaging. *Radiology.* 1991;178:467-474.
11. Feinberg D, Mark A. Human brain motion and cerebrospinal fluid circulation demonstrated with MR velocity imaging. *Radiology.* 1987;163: 793-799.
12. Fisher CM. The clinical picture in occult hydrocephalus. *Clin Neurosurg.* 1977;24:270-284.
13. Foster N, Chase T, Fedio P. Alzheimer's disease: focal cortical changes shown by positron emission tomography. *Neurology.* 1983;33:961-965.
14. George A, De Leon M, Kluger A, et al. CT diagnostic features of Alzheimer's disease: importance of the choroidal/hippocampal fissure complex. *AJNR.* 1990;11:101-107.
15. Graff-Radford NR, Godersky JC. Normal-pressure hydrocephalus: onset of gait abnormality before dementia predicts good surgical outcome. *Arch Neurol.* 1986;43(9):940-942.
16. Graff-Radford NR, Godersky JC. Symptomatic congenital hydrocephalus in the elderly simulating normal pressure hydrocephalus. *Neurology.* 1989;39(12):1596-1600.
17. Graff-Radford NR, Godersky JC, Jones MP. Variables predicting surgical outcome in symptomatic hydrocephalus in the elderly. *Neurology.* 1989;39(12):1601-1604.
18. Graff-Radford NR, Rezai K, Godersky J, et al. Regional cerebral blood flow in normal pressure hydrocephalus. *J Neurol Neurosurg Psychiatry.* 1987;50:1589-1596.

19. Gyldensted C. Measurements of the normal ventricular system and hemispheric sulci of 100 adults with computed tomography. *Neuroradiology.* 1977;14:183-192.
20. Haan J, Thomeer RT. Predictive value of temporary external lumbar drainage in normal pressure hydrocephalus. *Neurosurgery.* 1988;22(2): 388-391.
21. Hanley D, Borel CSH. Normal-pressure hydrocephalus. In: Johnson R, ed. *Current Therapy in Neurological Disease,* 3rd ed. Philadelphia: BC Decker; 1990:305-309.
22. Huckman M. Normal pressure hydrocephalus: evaluation of diagnosis and prognostic tests. *AJNR.* 1981;2:385-395.
23. Hughes C, Siegal B, Coxe W, et al. Adult idiopathic communicating hydrocephalus with and without shunting. *J Neurol Neurosurg Psychiatry.* 1978;41:961-971.
24. Jack CR Jr, Mokri B, Laws ER Jr, et al. MR findings in normal-pressure hydrocephalus: significance and comparison with other forms of dementia. *J Comput Assist Tomogr.* 1987;11(6):923-931.
25. Jack CR Jr, Petersen RC, O'Brien PC. MR-based hippocampal volumetry in the diagnosis of Alzheimer's disease. *Neurology.* 1992;42:183-188.
26. Jagust W, Friedland R, Budinger T. Positron emission tomography with (18F)-fluodeoxyglucose differentiates normal pressure hydrocephalus from Alzheimer-type dementia. *J Neurol Neurosurg Psychiatry.* 1985;48: 1091-1096.
27. McHugh P. Occult hydrocephalus. *QJM.* 1964;130:297-308.
28. Mori K, Honda H, Murata T, Nahano Y. Periventricular lucency in computed tomography of hydrocephalus and cerebral atrophy. *J Comput Assist Tomogr.* 1980;4:204-209.
29. Mori K, Mima T. Can we predict the benefit of a shunting operation for suspected normal pressure hydrocephalus? *Crit Rev Neurosurg.* 1997;7: 263-275.
30. Munoz D, Hasak S, Harper B, et al. Pathological correlates of increased signals of the centrum ovale on magnetic resonance imaging. *Arch Neurol.* 1993;50:492-497.
31. Petersen RC, Mokri B, Laws ER Jr. Surgical treatment of idiopathic hydrocephalus in elderly patients. *Neurology.* 1985;35(3):307-311.
32. Piatt J. Cerebrospinal fluid shunt failure: late is different from early. *Pediatr Neurosurg.* 1995;23:133-139.
33. Piatt J. Pumping the shunt revisited: a longitudinal study. *Pediatr Neurosurg.* 1996;25:73-77.
34. Raftopoulos C, Massager N, Baleriaux D, et al. Prospective analysis by computed tomography and long-term outcome of 23 adult patients with chronic idiopathic hydrocephalus. *Neurosurgery.* 1996;38:51-59.
35. Rekate H. Does it matter which shunt is used? *Crit Rev Neurosurg.* 1996; 6:57-63.
36. Sgouros S, John P, Walsh A. The value of colour Doppler imaging in assessing flow through ventricular-peritoneal shunts. *Child Nervous System.* 1996;12:454-459.
37. Sgouros S, Malluci C, Walsh AR, Hockley AD. Long term complications of hydrocephalus. *Pediatr Neurosurg.* 1995;23:127-132.
38. Vanneste J, Augustijn P, Tan WF, Dirven C. Shunting normal pressure hydrocephalus: the predictive value of combined clinical and CT data. *J Neurol Neurosurg Psychiatry.* 1993;56(3):251-256.
39. Weiner HL, Constantini S, Cohen H, Wisoff JH. Current treatment of normal-pressure hydrocephalus: comparison of flow-regulated and differential-pressure shunt valves. *Neurosurgery.* 1995;37:877-884.
40. Wikkelso C, Andersson H, Blomstrand C, Lindqvist G. The clinical effect of lumbar puncture in normal pressure hydrocephalus. *J Neurol Neurosurg Psychiatry.* 1982;45(1):64-69.
41. Wikkelso C, Andersson H, Blomstrand C, et al. Normal pressure hydrocephalus: predictive value of the cerebrospinal fluid tap-test. *Acta Neurol Scand.* 1986;73(6):566-573.
42. Wikkelso C, Andersson H, Blomstrand C, et al. Computed tomography of the brain in the diagnosis of and prognosis in normal pressure hydrocephalus. *Neuroradiology.* 1989;31(2):160-165.

# 8

# Movement Disorders

*Paul G. Wasielewski and William C. Koller*

The field of movement disorders is fascinating. Improvements in neuroimaging, electrophysiology, and molecular biology have increased our knowledge of the pathology, pathophysiology, and etiology of movement disorders, permitting more accurate diagnosis and improved treatment. Movement disorders exist along a spectrum, ranging from slow or decreased movements (e.g., an akinetic-rigid state) to excessive movements (e.g., chorea, athetosis, dystonia, myoclonus, or tremor). The most common movement disorders encountered in clinical practice—essential tremor (ET), Parkinson's disease (PD), and dystonia—are idiopathic. They are easily recognized and typically require no further investigations. Occasionally, however, patients with such "classic" presentations may have an underlying medical or neurologic disorder resulting in the tremor, parkinsonism, or dystonia. In such cases there are often either historical or clinical features present that do not typically accompany the classic presentation. It is for these patients that further investigation is warranted. In patients presenting with a complex neurologic picture highlighted by either a lack of movements or an excess of movements, a thorough diagnostic evaluation is required. In addition, although the majority of movement disorders are idiopathic, the possibility of an underlying cause should be kept in mind, since the condition may be a treatable disorder or may be an inherited disorder and thus have a bearing on future family planning.

The most important diagnostic step in the approach to a patient with a disorder of movement is to identify the abnormal movement correctly. This step can be difficult at times, but careful observation and a thorough history can help delineate accurately the specific type of abnormal movement. This chapter focuses on the most common movement disorders typically encountered—tremor, akinetic-rigid state (parkinsonism), choreoathetosis, dystonia, and myoclonus. For each movement a diagnostic approach is outlined, accompanied by an algorithm. Common denominators in the investigation of virtually all patients with abnormal movements are a medication history, the consideration of Wilson's disease, and the possibility of a psychogenic etiologic basis.

## WILSON'S DISEASE

Wilson's disease (WD) is a rare but interesting disorder. Because WD can appear with any one of several movement disorders, as well as with other neurologic manifestations, it is addressed separately. WD is a genetic disease that is inherited in an autosomal recessive manner. It is a disorder of copper metabolism, resulting in excessive copper (i.e., copper toxicity), with the primary defect being faulty biliary excretion of copper.[3,5] Copper accumulates in the liver, and once storage capacity is exceeded, the copper spills over into other tissues for storage and begins to be excreted in the urine. Hence it is not a disease entirely caused by ceruloplasmin deficiency, since 5% to 15% of patients with WD have normal or only slightly reduced ceruloplasmin levels.[5] Underlying this process is a defect in the WD gene, *Wc1* on chromosome 13q, that encodes for a copper-transporting adenosinetriphosphatase (ATPase), which if impaired, may result in faulty incorporation of copper into ceruloplasmin in the liver and reduced copper biliary excretion from the liver.[1]

Clinically, the presentation of WD is varied because the copper toxicity may involve numerous organ systems. Signs of liver dysfunction remain the most common mode of presentation, being the initial feature in more than 50% of cases. Involvement of the central nervous system (CNS) can also be a common form of initial presentation, with psychiatric manifestations being the initial feature in approximately 20% of cases[2] and neurologic manifestations noted as presenting symptoms in 40% to 50% of patients.[7] The neurologic presentation can be quite varied, but typically the basal ganglia are involved, with a resultant movement disorder. Studies have differed regarding the most common initial neurologic feature. Dysarthria and clumsiness of the hands are often the earliest symptoms.[8] The dysarthria can be either hypokinetic or cerebellar. Tremor, the most characteristic feature, is variable in presentation. It can be resting, postural, or kinetic; fine or coarse; proximal or distal. There may also be a characteristic "wing-beating" tremor when the arms are held in front of the body and flexed at the elbows. Other manifestations include dystonia, rigidity, parkinsonism, chorea, tics, and myoclonus. Cerebellar dysfunction is also common, as are gait abnormalities of a parkinsonian type or a wide-based cerebellar type. Despite the potential for numerous presentations, some are more common than others. In a study of 136 cases, the most common presentation was parkinsonian, followed by "pseudosclerotic," dystonic, and choreic presentations.[8] The parkinsonian presentation was the most common type in both children and adults. *Pseudosclerotic* refers to the severe "wing-beating" tremor sometimes seen in multiple sclerosis. Therefore any adolescent or young adult (up to age 40) who presents with any of the above features should be evaluated for WD. The need for such an evaluation is even more important if these signs occur in the setting of unexplained psychiatric manifestations.[10]

The evaluation of a patient suspected of having WD involves a few simple screening laboratory studies and an examination for Kayser-Fleischer rings (KFRs) of the cornea. Measurement of serum ceruloplasmin level is a good screening test, but as mentioned earlier, levels can be normal or just slightly below normal in 5% to 15% of cases. A 24-hour urine collection to measure copper excretion, which is markedly elevated in WD, should also be performed as part of a screening workup to complement the ceruloplasmin level. Levels of free, not total, serum copper are elevated in WD, and this measurement can be useful in the diagnostic workup.[6] The KFR is formed by the deposition of copper in Descemet's membrane in the cornea. It is best observed by slit-lamp examination, although the ring can be seen unaided in individuals with a light-colored iris. It has been stated that KFRs are always present in cases of WD with neurologic involvement; however, there have been rare case reports of neurologic WD without KFRs.[4,9] The most sensitive test for WD is measurement of hepatic copper content by liver biopsy. However, this test is usually not needed if neurologic symptoms are present.

## TREMOR

Tremor is the most common movement disorder seen by neurologists and nonneurologists. It is defined as an involuntary oscillatory movement of a body part due to alternating or synchronous contractions of reciprocally innervated muscles.[28] Tremor has many presentations and can be classified best by occurrence in relation to activity—at rest or during action.[21] Resting tremor occurs when a limb is fully supported against gravity, requiring no active muscle contraction. Action tremor occurs during any voluntary muscle contraction. There are two subtypes of action tremor: postural and kinetic. Postural tremor becomes apparent during the voluntary maintenance of a particular posture that is opposed by the force of gravity. Kinetic tremor may be noted during any type of movement and may occur as a movement approaches termination (i.e., terminal tremor) or while a specific task is being performed (i.e., task-specific tremor, such as writing tremor). Physiologic tremor is present in everyone, but it is asymptomatic unless tasks that require precision are being performed. However, physiologic tremor can be enhanced by several factors, most notably medications, emotional stress, fatigue, exercise, hypoglycemia, thyrotoxicosis, pheochromocytoma, and alcohol withdrawal. Patients with enhanced physiologic tremor demonstrate a postural or terminal tremor or both on examination.

The most common tremor conditions are PD and ET, both of which are idiopathic. Patients presenting with the classic features of these disorders need few, if any, diagnostic tests performed. However, resting tremor in a patient with signs of parkinsonism plus other neurologic features may require further diagnostic evaluation. (These tests are outlined in the discussion of akinetic-rigid states parkinsonism.) Likewise a patient with a slowly progressive action tremor of both upper extremities, frequently with head and voice involvement, and a family history of tremor does not need a diagnostic workup.

Tremor can be caused by disease afflicting almost any component of the nervous system—cerebral hemispheres, basal ganglia, thalamus, posterior fossa structures, and peripheral nerves. Tremors due to underlying pathologic condition (i.e., secondary or symptomatic tremors) can have variable clinical characteristics and may show no predilection for occurring either at rest or during action. Symptomatic tremors are listed in Table 8–1. Patients with symptomatic tremors often have either historical or clinical features suggestive of an underlying cause for the tremor. If such a suspicion arises, we propose a diagnostic workup, as shown in Figure 8–1.

An inquiry about the patient's current medications and general medical conditions should be the first step. Hyperthyroidism may result in an enhanced physiologic tremor.[48] Medications that cause tremor typically produce a postural or enhanced physiologic tremor, although antidopaminergic agents can also cause rest tremor associated with parkinsonism. There are many implicated tremorogenic medications[36]; the most common include:

- Antidepressants: tricyclic antidepressants, monoamine oxidase inhibitors, lithium[50]
- Antiepileptics: valproic acid[30]
- Stimulants
- Asthma medications: isoproterenol, terbutaline, theophylline
- Immunosuppressants: cyclosporine-A[41]
- Cardiac medications: amiodarone[23]
- Antidopaminergics: antipsychotics, antiemetics[27]

WD should always be considered in a patient presenting with tremor, particularly in an adolescent or a young adult. Tremor is a common feature of WD. Other manifestations of WD and an outline for evaluation are listed in the preceding discussion of WD.

---

**TABLE 8–1. Symptomatic Tremors**

Secondary to medications
Wilson's disease
Cerebellar tremor
Midbrain tremor
Tremor due to stroke
Rest tremor
Orthostatic tremor
Symptomatic palatal tremor
Tremor associated with peripheral neuropathy
Dystonic tremor
Cortical tremor
Psychogenic tremor

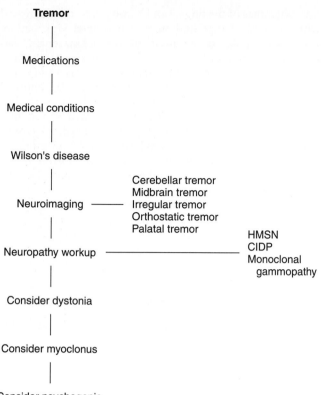

**FIGURE 8–1.** Approach to patient with tremor. See text for details and Table 8–2 for abbreviations and acronyms.

A neuroimaging study should be the next step, particularly for those patients demonstrating cerebellar tremor or midbrain tremor. Cerebellar tremor is characterized by irregular amplitude and frequency and can manifest as terminal tremor only; tremor during an entire movement (e.g., finger-to-nose or heel-to-shin test) with worsening as the target is reached; postural tremor; head or trunk tremor (i.e., titubation); and, rarely, rest tremor. Any disease that damages the cerebellum, the cerebellar nuclei, or the afferent[11] or efferent[39] pathways can result in cerebellar tremor. Typical causes include vascular lesions, multiple sclerosis[39] and neurodegenerative diseases. Neurodegenerative diseases include the spinocerebellar ataxias (types I through VII) and dentatorubropallidoluysian atrophy (DRPLA); these all have other associated neurologic findings, are autosomal dominantly inherited, and are due to the expansion of an unstable CAG trinucleotide repeat in the respective disease gene, which can be tested for by mutational analysis.[51] Neuroimaging should also be done in those patients with midbrain, or "rubral," tremor, which is typically described as a combination of rest, postural, and kinetic tremor[18]; the tremor may be mild at rest but worsens with posture and becomes uncontrollable when movements are being performed. Etiologic factors implicated in midbrain tremor include vascular,[13,20,46] trauma,[44] infection,[34] and multiple sclerosis.

Neuroimaging may also reveal lesions elsewhere in the CNS responsible for tremor. In particular, vascular lesions may cause tremor. Irregular tremors, often with dystonic posturing, may appear after a stroke or at the onset of stroke; lesions typically involve the thalamus.[19] Vascular lesions affecting the caudate nucleus and the thalamus were responsi-

ble for resting hand tremor in three patients following stroke[32] and also after a midbrain hemorrhage.[14] A predominant action and postural tremor was noted ipsilateral to a chronic subdural hematoma.[37] A hemibody resting tremor occurred several months after a lacunar stroke of the contralateral caudate nucleus.[15]

Orthostatic tremor (OT) consists of rapid, irregular, and asynchronous tremors involving the legs and trunk that occur shortly after standing and progressively increase only while standing.[24] It is a rare movement disorder, and the pathophysiologic complex has yet to be fully elucidated. Most cases are idiopathic; however, there are reports of OT due to lesions of the central and peripheral nervous system. Examples are pontine lesions, including a cavernoma and a cerebellopontine angle mass[12]; hydrocephalus due to aqueductal stenosis[22]; chronic relapsing polyradiculoneuropathy[22]; and head trauma.[45] The patients had neurologic manifestations in addition to OT. Thus when there are findings in addition to OT on physical examination, a neuroimaging procedure should be performed. If the results are negative, an investigation for a neuropathy should be pursued (if suggested by signs or symptoms).

Palatal myoclonus is a rare movement disorder. It was reclassified as palatal tremor (PT) at the First International Congress of Movement Disorders in 1990. PT, which consists of rhythmic movements of the soft palate, is classified as essential (idiopathic) or symptomatic (secondary); criteria for this classification have been established.[17] Use of such criteria may be helpful in identifying patients with a possible underlying cause. In particular, patients with symptomatic PT will present with ataxia or oscillopsia, typically acute in

| TABLE 8–2. | **Selected Abbreviations and Acronyms** |
|---|---|
| AD | Autosomal dominant |
| APAS | Antiphospholipid antibody syndrome |
| AR | Autosomal recessive |
| AT | Ataxia-telangiectasia |
| BCP | Birth control pill |
| BHC | Benign hereditary chorea |
| CBC | Complete blood count |
| CBD | Corticobasal degeneration |
| CG | Chorea gravidarum |
| CJD | Creutzfeldt-Jakob disease |
| CIDP | Chronic inflammatory demyelinating polyneuropathy |
| DRD | Dopa-responsive dystonia |
| DRPLA | Dentatorubropallidoluysian atrophy |
| GTC | Generalized tonic-clonic seizures |
| HD | Huntington's disease |
| HMSN | Hereditary motor and sensory neuropathy |
| MERRF | Myoclonic epilepsy and ragged-red fibers |
| MLD | Metachromatic leukodystrophy |
| MRI | Magnetic resonance imaging |
| MS | Multiple sclerosis |
| NA | Neuroacanthocytosis |
| NCL | Neuronal ceroid lipofuscinosis |
| NIID | Neuronal intranuclear inclusion disease |
| PD | Parkinson's disease |
| PMA | Progressive myoclonic ataxia |
| PME | Progressive myoclonic epilepsy |
| RBC | Red blood cell |
| R/O | Rule out |
| SCA I–III | Spinocerebellar ataxia types I–III |
| SLE | Systemic lupus erythematosus |
| ULD | Unverricht-Lundborg disease |
| WD | Wilson's disease |

onset, whereas those with essential PT will complain of ear clicks. Magnetic resonance imaging (MRI) in essential PT is normal, whereas in symptomatic PT it is abnormal, demonstrating hypertrophic olivary degeneration in addition to a possible lesion. Secondary causes have included vascular lesions of the brainstem, brainstem abscess, multiple sclerosis, and cerebellar degeneration.[17] Thus any patient with ataxia and abnormal eye movements who is found to have rhythmic palatal movements on examination should undergo neuroimaging.

Tremor can be a manifestation of peripheral nerve disease and is typically present as a postural tremor or a kinetic tremor, less often as a rest tremor. Neuropathies commonly associated with tremor include hereditary motor and sensory neuropathy (HMSN), chronic inflammatory demyelinating polyneuropathy (CIDP), and chronic demyelinating polyneuropathy with immunoglobulin M (IgM) paraproteinemia (i.e., monoclonal gammopathy),[47] and diabetes and uremia.[43] Investigations include electrodiagnostic studies (electromyogram [EMG] and nerve conduction velocity [NCV]) to delineate demyelinating vs. axonal neuropathies, as well as focal, multifocal, or generalized neuropathies; cerebrospinal fluid (CSF) examination for protein level and white cell count; genetic testing for HMSN; and serum protein electrophoresis (SPEP) followed by immunofixation for detection of paraproteins. SPEP is an important step taken in the investigation of patients with idiopathic neuropathies since approximately 10% of such patients have an associated monoclonal gammopathy.[31] If the SPEP with immunofixation is suggestive of a monoclonal protein, a 24-hour urine collection for Bence Jones protein should be performed, as well as further blood work, including complete blood count (CBC) with differential, quantitative serum immunoglobulins, cryoglobulins, and calcium level. A skeletal survey should also be performed to look for lytic or sclerotic bone lesions seen with multiple myeloma or osteosclerotic myeloma. A bone marrow biopsy and aspirate may be needed to differentiate a plasma cell dyscrasia from monoclonal gammopathy of undetermined significance (MGUS). Finally, a nerve biopsy may be needed, particularly if amyloidosis is a consideration.[35]

Tremor is frequently associated with dystonia.[29,38] There are two primary tremor types: (1) a small amplitude postural tremor, which does not cause significant disability and which physiologically resembles enhanced physiologic tremor more than essential tremor, and (2) "dystonic" tremor, which is an action-induced, localized extremity and head tremor seen in the same topographic region as the dystonia.[16] If the movements associated with the dystonia are irregular and jerking, it is most likely myoclonus, referred to as myoclonic dystonia.[40] Tremor may even precede the dystonia. In such cases a slow tremor may occur initially in the trunk or head, particularly in a "no-no" direction, followed subsequently by the appearance of cervical dystonia.[25,42] The majority of these cases are idiopathic; however, if there are any historical or clinical features suggestive of an underlying cause, an investigation should be pursued (see discussion of dystonia).

The term *cortical tremor* was first introduced in a report describing two patients with essential tremor refractory to standard therapy and found to have electrophysiologic evidence of cortical reflex myoclonus.[26] The tremor consisted of fine twitchings of the fingers and hands at rest that increased with postural change and further worsened with action. Both patients also experienced seizures. Clonazepam, valproate, and primidone were effective in reducing the tremor. It was concluded that "cortical tremor" is a variant of cortical reflex myoclonus. Another report described 10 additional such patients.[49] Of the total of 12 cases, 5 patients were idiopathic, whereas the remainder primarily had action myoclonus, which was due to the typical causes of myoclonus (e.g., Lafora body disease, Baltic myoclonus). The approach to such patients is outlined in the discussion of myoclonus.

The possibility of a tremor being psychogenic should be considered in certain cases. This is, of course, a diagnosis of exclusion. The clinical features of psychogenic tremors have been well delineated: abrupt onset, static course, spontaneous remissions, complex tremors, changing tremor characteristics, increase in tremor with attention, and decrease in tremor with distractibility.[33]

## AKINETIC-RIGID STATES (PARKINSONISM)

A clinical picture of progressive slowness, stiffness, shuffling gait, and resting tremor is a classic in neurology. To the treating physician, it instantly brings to mind a diagnosis of PD. However, it is important to remember that this constellation of clinical features is a syndrome that can have multiple causes. Fortunately, the most common cause of the parkinsonian syndrome is idiopathic (i.e., PD). There is no biologic marker for PD, and hence, no diagnostic test. A patient who manifests unilateral resting tremor along with other signs of parkinsonism and who has a dramatic and sustained response to levodopa (L-dopa) replacement therapy can be accurately diagnosed as having PD. The most important point in reaching the diagnosis of PD is the response to L-dopa therapy. If a patient with suspected PD fails to respond to L-dopa therapy, an alternative diagnosis should be pursued. In our clinic we consider an adequate trial of L-dopa to be a minimum of 1000 mg/d for a few weeks.

The most likely entities to be misdiagnosed as PD are a group of neurodegenerative conditions that have in common parkinsonian features but are relatively distinct from one another by the presence of other neurologic features. These conditions are appropriately grouped together under the rubric of "Parkinson-plus" syndromes. They include multiple system atrophy (MSA), progressive supranuclear palsy (PSP), corticobasal degeneration (CBD), the parkinsonism-dementia-ALS (amyotrophic lateral sclerosis) complex of Guam, and dementia with Lewy bodies. The MSAs consist of four entities with a dominant parkinsonian picture and an additional outstanding feature: autonomic failure in the Shy-Drager syndrome; cerebellar dysfunction in olivopontocerebellar atrophy; lower motor neuron dysfunction in parkinsonism-amyotrophy; and pyramidal features and extrapyramidal features in striatonigral degeneration (SND). PSP is characterized by oculomotor abnormalities, particularly vertical gaze palsy with intact oculocephalic reflex, absent optokinetic nystagmus reflex, and early presence of square wave jerks.[70,75] CBD is characterized by persistent unilateral features, such as myoclonus, alien limb, apraxia, and cortical sensory loss.[71] Like that of PD, the diagnosis is mainly clinical because there is not a diagnostic test for these syndromes. However, they are characterized by a poor response to levodopa therapy. Sophisticated neuroimaging studies, such as positron emission tomography (PET) and single photon emission computed tomography (SPECT), as well as autonomic testing, are not yet practical or specific for routine use in the diagnosis of suspected Parkinson-plus syndromes.

If it is concluded that the patient who presents with parkinsonism does not have PD or a Parkinson-plus syndrome, we propose an investigational workup, as shown in Figure 8–2. It is essential to make a thorough inquiry into the patient's medication history since several medications have been associated with inducing parkinsonism (i.e., drug-induced parkinsonism [DIP]). Most notable are the antipsychotics and the antiemetics. These drugs act by blocking dopamine receptors. Virtually all known types of antipsychotics can induce parkinsonism. However, this effect appears to be less likely with clozapine (an "atypical" antipsychotic), probably because of its strong antagonism of $D_4$ receptors and its relatively weak antagonism of $D_2$ receptors[53] (the typical antipsychotics have strong antagonism of $D_2$ receptors). Prochlorperazine and metoclopramide are dopamine receptor blockers used for treatment of nausea and vomiting and impaired gastric motility; they have both been associated with DIP.[54] At times DIP may be indistinguishable from PD, but some features may be helpful in differentiating between them.[63] In DIP, features develop bilaterally and symmetrically and acutely or subacutely. In contrast, the typical onset of PD is unilateral and insidious. If DIP is suspected yet the patient's history is negative for medication use, a urine screen may detect the presence of

antipsychotics; this was found to be the case in three patients who were being poisoned with haloperidol by their spouses.[52] Suspicion arose in these cases when the victims' features of parkinsonism improved in the hospital but worsened when they returned home.

Parkinsonism that appears in childhood, adolescence, or early adulthood should spark investigation into at least three disorders, two of which are treatable. As mentioned in the preceding discussion of WD, parkinsonism is the most common mode of presentation in both juveniles and adults (the diagnostic workup is outlined in that section). Parkinsonism is also a feature of dopa-responsive dystonia (DRD). DRD is characterized initially by dystonia that affects the lower extremities, resulting in a gait disturbance; the onset varies from age 1 year to the midteens.[68] Features of parkinsonism follow the dystonia. Distinguishing features include a diurnal fluctuation (dystonia worsening throughout the day and following exercise but improving with sleep) and a dramatic response to small doses of levodopa. Childhood-onset Huntington's disease (HD) can manifest features of parkinsonism, particularly rigidity.[55] However, typically associated seizures and cognitive dysfunction are present. Diagnosis is by genetic testing for the unstable CAG trinucleotide repeat expansion in the HD gene on chromosome 4p.[60]

Since parkinsonism is a common presentation of WD in both juveniles and adults, any young adult who is suspected of having PD but who does not respond well to levodopa therapy should undergo investigation for WD.

Neuroimaging, preferably MRI, can be used to identify a variety of cerebral insults that may result in parkinsonism:

**FIGURE 8–2.** Approach to patient with parkinsonism. See text for details and Table 8–2 for abbreviations and acronyms.

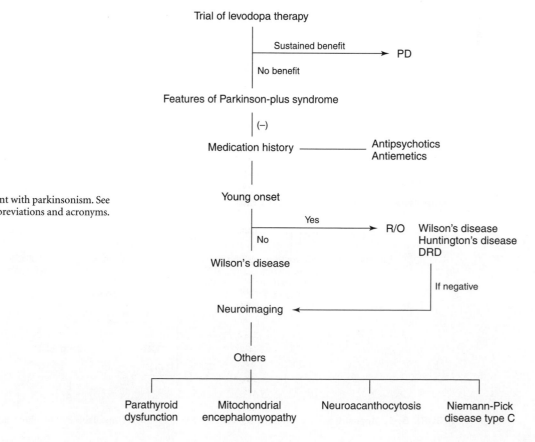

- Hydrocephalus—both communicating and noncommunicating.[56] The cases of communicating hydrocephalus represent normal pressure hydrocephalus and are often associated with dementia or urinary incontinence. Some patients benefit from levodopa therapy.
- Mass lesions—including neoplasms[64,66,67,69] and subdural hematoma.[59]
- Vascular disease. Parkinsonism can be a result of vascular disease caused by either multiple small-vessel infarcts or widespread lesions of the cerebral white matter (i.e., Binswanger's disease).[65] Vascular parkinsonism is characterized by a short-stepped (or frozen) gait, lead-pipe rigidity, absence of resting tremor, poor response to levodopa, and, in a majority, pyramidal tract signs and pseudobulbar palsy.[77]
- Toxic exposure. Carbon monoxide intoxication can result in parkinsonism. Necrotic globus pallidus lesions are seen on computed tomography (CT) or MRI.
- Rare causes of parkinsonism, such as Hallervorden-Spatz disease (HSD) and hemiparkinsonism-hemiatrophy syndrome (HPHAS). HSD is a rare neurodegenerative disease characterized by the deposition of excessive iron in the globus pallidus; it typically presents with dystonia in early life (see discussion of dystonia). However, late-onset cases may result in parkinsonism and dementia.[61] The presence of the iron produces a characteristic "eye of the tiger" appearance on MRI, allowing premortem diagnosis.[72,73] HPHAS is characterized by hemiatrophy and the development of unilateral parkinsonism years later on the same side as the hemiatrophy.[62] Neuroimaging usually reveals contralateral cerebral hemisphere atrophy.[58]

There are other rare causes of parkinsonism. Pseudohypoparathyroidism has been reported as producing parkinsonian features.[57] Other features include short stature, round face, obesity, dental abnormalities, and mental retardation; laboratory data reveal normal or low serum calcium levels, elevated phosphate levels, and markedly elevated parathyroid hormone levels, indicative of end-organ resistance. There

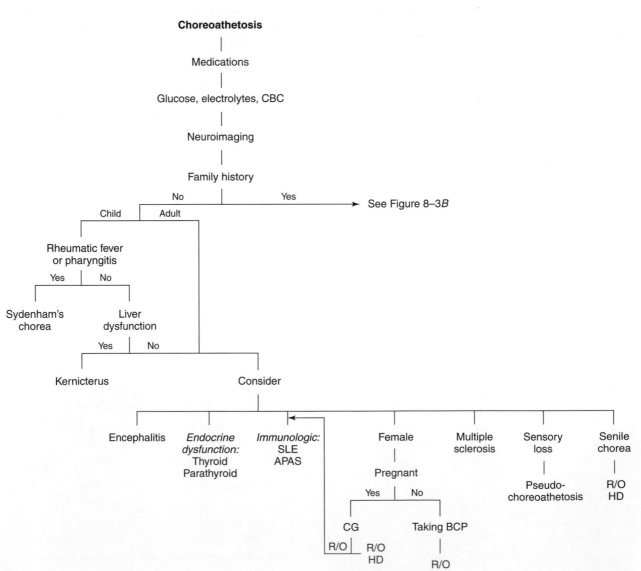

A

**FIGURE 8–3.** Approach to patient with choreoathetosis. See text for details and Table 8–2 for abbreviations and acronyms.

may also be calcification of the basal ganglia on head CT. It is interesting that several of these features—short stature, mental retardation, basal ganglia calcification—are observed in patients with mitochondrial encephalomyopathies; in a report by Evans and Donley,[57] inheritance was maternal through three generations. Movement disorders are rare among the mitochondrial encephalomyopathies; however, akinetic-rigid features have been described, along with dystonia, chorea, and tremor.[76] See also the discussion of dystonia. Investigation for suspected mitochondrial disease is outlined in Figure 8–4. Parkinsonism has been reported to occur in the clinical course of neuroacanthocytosis.[74] Chorea is a typical feature of neurologic syndromes associated with acanthocytes and is described in the following section. Parkinsonian features have been described in Niemann-Pick disease type C; diagnosis is by bone marrow aspirate and demonstration of foamy histiocytes (see discussion of dystonia).

## CHOREA AND ATHETOSIS

Chorea may appear in a wide variety of patient contexts, occurring as a manifestation of a primary neurologic disease or secondary to systemic disease, toxic insults, or medications. An extensive review listed 143 possible etiologic factors, a majority of which are rare.[115] It must be emphasized that chorea can exist along a wide spectrum of excessive movement: the patient may simply appear to be fidgety or restless; the condition may be manifested as quick, nonstereotyped, semipurposeful movements of the distal extremities; or chorea may be noted as large-amplitude flinging movements of the proximal extremities (such movements are ballistic in nature; hence the term *ballism,* which may be unilateral [hemiballism] or bilateral [biballism]). In addition, chorea may be present with other neurologic findings, in particular athetosis, which can be thought of as a slow form of chorea and consists of slow writhing movements. Most patients have both chorea and athetosis, but such movements should be differentiated from motor tics, myoclonus, and dystonia.

Our approach to the patient who presents with chorea is outlined in Figure 8–3. An inquiry into the use of medication or illicit drugs may disclose possible offending agents known to cause chorea. These include the antipsychotics and other dopamine receptor blockers, for example, antiemetics such as metoclopramide; L-dopa; anticonvulsants such as phenytoin[95] and valproic acid,[101] stimulants such as amphetamines,[119,127] theophylline,[128], or cocaine,[85] and others such as lithium[97,118] and oral contraceptives.[114] Obtaining a serum or urine drug screen may be helpful in identifying these agents. Checking routine serum chemistries for any abnormalities in glucose,[96,104] sodium,[126] calcium,[98] and magne-

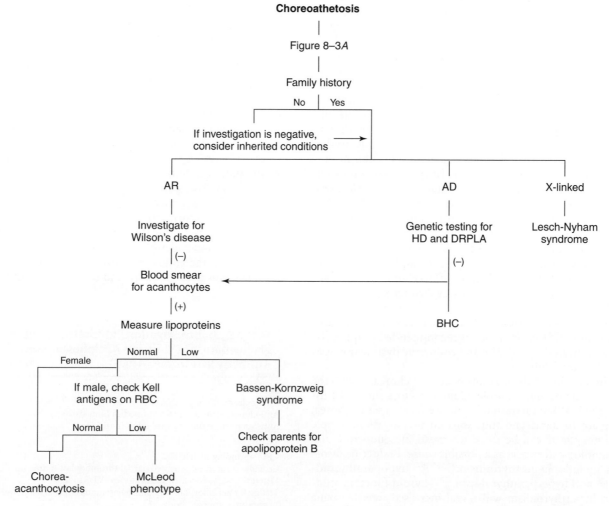

**FIGURE 8–3.** *Continued*

sium may identify a metabolic cause for chorea. A CBC should also be checked to rule out polycythemia vera (PCV), which can be a cause of chorea.[83,111] The CBC in PCV will reveal an elevated red blood cell (RBC) count (>6 million/mm³), elevated hemoglobin level (>18 g/dl in men, >16 g/dl in women), and an elevated hematocrit level (>54% in men, >49% in women).

Since chorea can be caused by focal structural lesions, a neuroimaging study should be obtained to exclude neoplasms, both primary and metastatic, including lymphoma,[117,122] or vascular lesions, including infarctions,[80,86] hemorrhage,[89] or subdural hematoma,[79,90] as a cause of chorea. In the child who develops choreoathetosis, "double athetosis" or dyskinetic cerebral palsy needs to be considered; neuroimaging may reveal lesions within the basal ganglia that are congenital in origin.

Regardless of patient age, inquiring about any family history of excessive movements is the next step. In the child or adolescent with no family history of choreoathetosis, if there is any history of symptoms suggestive of rheumatic fever or streptococcal infection (e.g., pharyngitis) in the recent past, Sydenham's chorea should be suspected. Common through the mid-1900s, Sydenham's chorea is now an uncommon disease, but recurrences can occur.[113] An elevated antistreptolysin O titer and erythrocyte sedimentation rate will help to confirm the diagnosis, as does the presence of beta-hemolytic streptococci from nose or throat cultures. An electrocardiogram (ECG) or echocardiogram may show evidence of cardiac involvement. MRI reveals increased signal on T2-weighted images of the striatum and globus pallidum, which resolved with clinical improvement.[100,131] PET imaging reveals increased glucose metabolism in the striatum, which also resolves with clinical improvement.[91,132]

Other conditions, though uncommon, to investigate for in the child or adolescent with choreoathetosis include bilirubin encephalopathy (i.e., kernicterus, encephalitis, thyroid and parathyroid dysfunction) and systemic lupus erythematosus (SLE). Classic kernicterus, a complication of erythroblastosis fetalis (i.e., hemolytic [Rh] disease), is now uncommon because of current preventative therapy. However, it can still occur in premature infants or those with respiratory distress (i.e., hypoxia). In those infants who survive, athetosis may occur months or longer after the initial insult. There is typically impairment of upward gaze and hearing loss because of the susceptibility of the auditory nerve and pathways to bilirubin. Evaluation of liver function tests, audiometry, and brainstem auditory evoked responses (BAER) can help with the diagnosis and with measuring the response to therapy.[112] Choreoathetosis can also occur in the setting of encephalitis; CSF examination is recommended in appropriate cases. Evaluation for SLE and endocrine dysfunction is as described for adults.

In the adult with no family history of chorea, as with the child or adolescent, multiple etiologic factors should be investigated. Although most of these are rare causes of chorea, some are treatable and thus warrant investigation. Simple laboratory tests can be done to investigate endocrine and immunologic disorders as a possible cause. Endocrine disorders include hyperthyroidism,[88,105,107] hypoparathyroidism,[129] and hyperparathyroidism.[120] Thyroid function studies in hyperthyroidism will reveal increased free thyroxine ($T_4$) and triiodothyronine ($T_3$) and decreased thyroid-stimulating hormone (TSH). In hypoparathyroidism, the serum calcium level is low and the serum phosphate level is elevated, whereas in hyperparathyroidism, the serum calcium level is elevated and the serum phosphate level is low, along with an elevated parathyroid hormone.

SLE may be the most common systemic disease causing chorea. Although chorea occurs in only 2% of patients with SLE, it is the presenting manifestation in 25% of those with chorea.[84] SLE should be looked for in teenage girls and women who present with chorea. Diagnostic tests for SLE include testing for antinuclear antibody (ANA) and antibodies to double-stranded DNA and anti-Sm nuclear antigens, both of which are highly specific for SLE. Another immunologic disorder associated with chorea is the antiphospholipid antibody syndrome (APAS). In this disorder, autoantibodies interfere with phospholipid-dependent coagulation factors, with the result being increased thrombotic tendency. Hence acute ischemic events are the most common neurologic manifestation of APAS, although others, such as migraine, seizures, and chorea, also occur less commonly.[103] Diagnostic tests to detect antiphospholipid antibodies (aPLs) include CBC, which may show thrombocytopenia; a false-positive Venereal Disease Research Laboratories (VDRL) test result; coagulation studies demonstrating prolonged (by at least 5 seconds) activated partial thromboplastin time (aPTT) that does not correct with 1:1 dilution of the patient's plasma with normal or control plasma; and direct testing for the presence of antiphospholipid antibodies, including the lupus anticoagulant and anticardiolipin antibody.[92] Diagnostic tests for SLE and APAS are summarized in Table 8–3.

Chorea can occur during pregnancy (i.e., chorea gravidarum [CG]) and typically resolves following delivery. However, the occurrence of CG may be the initial manifestation of SLE,[87] HD,[81] or APAS.[106] Hence, ruling out these conditions in any pregnant woman who develops chorea is warranted. Similarly, the occurrence of chorea while oral contraceptives are being taken may also be the presenting manifestation of SLE.[99]

Sensory loss, particularly proprioceptive sensory loss, can result in "pseudochoreoathetosis." In a report of seven patients with proprioceptive sensory loss and choreoathetosis, lesions located along the sensory pathways conveying position sense were identified.[124] Lesions included a parietal cortex injury, thalamic infarction, spinal cord lesions, dorsal root ganglion neuronopathy, and ulnar neuropathy.

---

**TABLE 8–3. Investigations for Systemic Lupus Erythematosus (SLE) and Antiphospholipid Antibody Syndrome (APAS)**

**SLE**
Antinuclear antibody (ANA)
Anti–double-stranded DNA antibodies (anti-dsDNA)
Anti-Sm nuclear antigen antibodies (anti-Sm)

**APAS**
CBC (including platelets)
Coagulation studies: activated partial thromboplastin time (aPTT)
Venereal Disease Research Laboratories (VDRL) test
Testing for antiphospholipid antibodies: lupus anticoagulant and anticardiolipin antibody

Although reports of chorea and other movement disorders in multiple sclerosis are infrequent, demyelinating disease should be considered.[78,110] Paroxysmal dyskinesias may be more frequent, which can include chorea.[121] Appropriate diagnostic tests for MS are MRI, CSF analysis, and evoked potentials (EPs).[116]

Chorea that appears in late life without dementia, psychiatric disturbance, or a family history of chorea and no other identifiable cause has been labeled senile chorea. It has been debated whether this condition is actually a separate entity or late-onset HD. Mutational analysis in such patients has demonstrated normal CAG repeat lengths, thus confirming that senile chorea is a distinct entity.[125] However, it must be kept in mind that there are cases of late-onset chorea with no mental disturbance or family history that have been shown to be HD by mutational analysis.[82] Thus, if faced with this situation and if there is any suspicion of HD, testing for the HD mutation may be warranted, particularly regarding subsequent genetic counseling for younger family members.

With inherited choreatic disorders, those that follow an autosomal recessive mode of inheritance may first appear in the absence of a family history of chorea. Therefore, in a child, adolescent, or adult with a negative family history who develops choreoathetosis and whose workup is negative, autosomal recessive conditions should be considered. Investigation for WD should be undertaken first, as outlined earlier. If the test results for WD are normal, proceed with examination of a blood smear for acanthocytes. If acanthocytes are present, proceed to checking serum levels of cholesterol, triglycerides, and lipoproteins. These results help to differentiate among the three different neurologic syndromes associated with acanthocytes[94]:

1. *Bassen-Kornzweig syndrome.* This syndrome is characterized by abetalipoproteinemia, a condition of very low cholesterol (<1.5 mmol/L) and triglycerides (<0.1 mmol/L). Clinically the patient presents with a progressive spinocerebellar syndrome, pigmentary retinopathy, and areflexia. Involuntary movements are typically not part of the clinical picture, although severe position sense loss can result in pseudoathetosis. There is absent apolipoprotein B with resultant fat malabsorption, including the fat-soluble vitamins. It is the absence of vitamin E that is responsible for the clinical features, which are reversible with vitamin E supplementation. The parents of the patient should also be checked for the presence of apolipoprotein B. Its presence is normal in heterozygotes of Bassen-Kornzweig syndrome. If partial deficiency of apolipoprotein B exists in either parent, hypobetalipoproteinemia is the correct diagnosis. This is an autosomal dominant condition but one in which the heterozygotes are usually asymptomatic and acanthocytosis does not occur in vivo.
2. *Chorea-acanthocytosis.* With this condition, there is a normal lipoprotein study in association with acanthocytosis. Clinical features consist of chorea, orofacial dyskinesias with tongue and lip biting, motor tics, peripheral neuropathy, amyotrophy, and vocalizations. The hyperkinetic manifestations may be followed by progressive parkinsonism.[74]
3. *McLeod phenotype.* With this phenotype, the lipoprotein study is normal and acanthocytosis is present with weak expression of the Kell blood group antigens. This X-linked recessive condition occurs only in males. Features consistently noted include elevated creatine kinase level, a slowly progressive myopathy, and evidence of cardiomyopathy. However, there are reports of male patients developing a clinical picture of chorea-acanthocytosis who were found to have the McLeod phenotype.[109,123,130,133] Thus, because of the different modes of inheritance and the implications of genetic counseling, it is extremely important to check all male patients presenting with chorea-acanthocytosis for the McLeod phenotype on red blood cells (RBCs).

Those children, adolescents, or adults presenting with choreoathetosis who have a family history of such movements that follows an autosomal dominant mode of inheritance should be evaluated for HD and DRPLA. Both conditions are due to the unstable expansion of a CAG trinucleotide repeat within the coding region of the gene for the disorder—the "Huntington" gene on 4p and the "atrophin" gene on 12q. Onset of HD in early life may manifest as chorea, but typically it is different from adult-onset HD, with rigidity, seizures, and cognitive decline as prominent features.[55] In atypical cases of suspected HD with normal CAG repeat sizes, checking for acanthocytes is recommended.

If genetic testing is negative for HD and DRPLA, benign hereditary chorea (BHC) may be the ultimate diagnosis. BHC is characterized by chorea in childhood that is nonprogressive through adulthood; in addition, there is no impairment of the intellect in BHC.[93] Although there is no biologic marker for this disorder, its clinical characteristics set it apart from HD; however, one kindred thought to have BHC did have the mutation for HD.[108] Thus genetic testing for HD is recommended in families thought to have BHC.

Choreoathetosis can be seen in Lesch-Nyhan syndrome, which is an X-linked recessive disorder of purine metabolism characterized by hypotonia followed by spasticity, dystonia, mental retardation, developmental delay, self-mutilation, hyperuricemia, and nephrolithiasis.[102] The enzymatic defect is hypoxanthine-guanine phosphoribosyl-transferase. Diagnosis is made by demonstration of absent enzyme activity in fibroblasts or RBCs.

## HEMIBALLISMUS

There is a broad spectrum of chorea, with the most severe form consisting of large-amplitude, violent, flinging movements of the extremities. This type is referred to as ballism, which is typically one-sided (hemiballism) but rarely may be bilateral (biballism or paraballism). Hemiballismus often coexists with hemichorea. The approach to the patient with hemiballismus-hemichorea is similar to the patient presenting with chorea since similar entities are involved.

The conditions that can cause hemiballismus-hemichorea are lesions involving the contralateral subthalamic nucleus and other components of the basal ganglia and thalamus. Neuroimaging, particularly MRI, is quite sensitive for detecting deep subcortical lesions and thus should be the initial step in patient evaluation. Vascular lesions are the most common cause of hemiballismus-hemichorea.[137,139,140,149] These include transient ischemia, infarction, hemorrhage,[134] and vascular malformations.[135,136,147,150] Other less common structural lesions are metastatic cancer,[138,148] cystic glioma of the midbrain, and *Toxoplasma* abscess in patients with acquired immunodeficiency syndrome (AIDS).[137] Other less common lesions should be looked for in young adults who have no stroke risk factors. If a structural lesion is not identified, inquiring about medications and checking blood chemistries may be helpful because there have been scattered reports of medications, particularly oral contraceptives[114] and phenytoin,[143] and serum glucose disturbances as the cause of hemiballismus-hemichorea.[141,145,146] Other nonstructural causes reported[137,149] include Sydenham's chorea, SLE, encephalitis, and MS.[142,144]

## DYSTONIA

Dystonia is defined as an abnormal movement characterized by sustained muscle contractions, which may then cause twisting and repetitive movements or abnormal postures.[175] It can appear in many different ways—inversion of a foot; writer's cramp; rotation, flexion, or extension of the neck; arching and twisting of the back; or excessive blinking of the eyes—to name just a few. Clinically, dystonia is categorized as focal, segmental, multifocal, hemidystonia, or generalized. The etiologic basis of dystonia can be either primary (idiopathic) or secondary (symptomatic), and the condition can be either inherited or sporadic. The majority of dystonias are idiopathic. However, it is important to recognize dystonias that may be secondary and initiate the proper investigation.

In idiopathic dystonia, typically there are no neurologic findings apart from the dystonia. The presence of other neurologic features, such as spasticity, cerebellar signs, abnormal eye movements, or sensory changes, suggests an underlying cause for the dystonia. In addition, certain clinical features are suggestive of a secondary cause; these include onset of dystonia while at rest, early occurrence of sustained postures, early affliction of speech (other than spasmodic dysphonia), oculogyric crises, sudden onset, rapid course, and hemidystonia.[187] Thus a patient with dystonia presenting with any of these historical features or abnormal unexplained findings on examination should be investigated for a possible secondary cause of the dystonia. We propose the approach outlined in Figure 8–4.

As with choreoathetosis, there is a large number of possible secondary causes of dystonia. Most are rare, and extensive lists are available.[162] The first step is an inquiry into the patient's history about the use of antidopaminergic drugs, most notably antipsychotics or antiemetics. Tardive dystonia is the most common cause of symptomatic dystonia and may appear to be identical to idiopathic dystonia.[160] Next in the evaluation is a neuroimaging study, preferably MRI. Focal brain lesions have been found to be a common cause of symptomatic dystonia, particularly hemidystonia, with the most common areas involved being the basal ganglia, thalamus, and brainstem.[197,204,205] The putamen is the most common area of involvement within the basal ganglia and tends to result in hemidystonia or limb dystonia whereas brainstem lesions tend to result in cranial dystonia, such as blepharospasm.[170,183] Any lesion located in these areas may result in dystonia, although vascular lesions are the most common, including infarction,[161,171] hemorrhage,[164] and vascular malformations.[177,195] Patients with vascular lesions may initially have hemiplegia following the vascular insult, only to develop dystonia later (posthemiplegic dystonia). Anoxic insult to the brain at or around the time of birth may be the most common cause of focal lesions resulting in nonprogressive motor dysfunction (i.e., cerebral palsy). This dysfunction may manifest as primarily hemiplegic, ataxic, choreoathetotic, or dystonic. However, in some patients dystonia does not appear

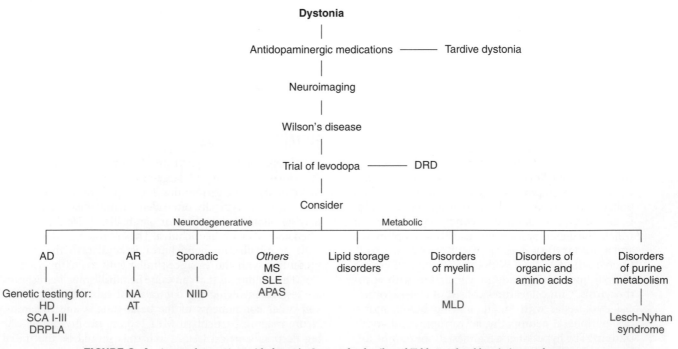

**FIGURE 8–4.** Approach to patient with dystonia. See text for details and Table 8–2 for abbreviations and acronyms.

for up to several years later and is designated "delayed-onset" dystonia.[159] Dystonia, typically a posthemiplegic hemidystonia, can arise several months to years following head injury. Neuroimaging in such patients reveals contralateral basal ganglion lesions.[189] Thus it is important to inquire about birth history and history of head trauma in all individuals and to perform a neuroimaging study before declaring that the patient has idiopathic dystonia.

Systemic diseases that can result in dystonia include SLE[168] and APAS.[152] The reports describe patients with hemidystonia having demonstrable lesions on imaging studies that are most likely secondary to infarction or demyelination. Investigation for these diseases is outlined in Table 8–3.

Other lesions include neoplasms,[117,190,200] subdural hematoma,[173] infection,[210] multiple sclerosis (MS), and structural abnormalities such as syringomyelia. Mass lesions such as a neoplasm or subdural hematoma can indirectly result in dystonia secondary to herniation, which can result in ischemia to the basal ganglia. Dystonia may occur in the course of MS, typically as paroxysmal dystonia. However, it has been reported as the presenting feature of MS.[165] In this report two patients with MS are described. In both the initial feature was writer's cramp, which was a part of hemidystonia in one. Thus, although a rare presentation of MS, focal dystonia in a young adult with features of demyelinating disease found on examination requires neuroimaging followed by lumbar puncture for CSF analysis. In three children with torticollis who were later found to have a syrinx, scoliosis was a common examination finding and spinal cord tumor was an associated pathologic finding.[188]

In addition to identifying focal lesions, MRI may aid in determining etiologic factors based solely on appearance. For example, HSD, which is an autosomal recessive disorder characterized by iron deposition in the pallidum and substantia nigra, has an "eye of the tiger" sign on MRI that is depicted as pallidal hypointensity with a central area of hyperintensity on T2-weighted images; identification of this sign has allowed for the diagnosis of HSD prior to postmortem examination.[72,73] HSD can have a variable presentation, but infantile-onset HSD typically has prominent dystonia, particularly oromandibular dystonia,[151] whereas parkinsonism, or akinetic-rigid state, characterizes the late-onset form in addition to dystonia and other features.[172] Neuroimaging, particularly CT scan, may also reveal calcification throughout the CNS and the basal ganglia, which is variably associated with mental retardation, dysarthria, rigidity, tremor, and choreoathetosis.[158] Dystonia has also been reported to occur in association with basal ganglia calcifications.[163,193] Calcification of the basal ganglia can be idiopathic, secondary to parathyroid dysfunction, or hereditary. Hypoparathyroidism and pseudohypoparathyroidism should be excluded by measurement of serum calcium, phosphate, and parathyroid hormone levels. The mitochondrial encephalomyopathies, which may have diverse neurologic manifestations, may also demonstrate basal ganglia calcification.[174] Movement disorders are rare among patients with mitochondrial encephalomyopathies, except for myoclonus and its association with the syndrome of myoclonic epilepsy and ragged-red fibers.[178] Dystonia, chorea, tremor, and akinetic-rigid states are rarely reported. In one report of 85 patients with mitochondrial myopathies, nine

---

**TABLE 8–4. Investigation for Disorder of Oxidative Phosphorylation**

1. Lactate, pyruvate, alanine levels in blood, urine, cerebrospinal fluid
2. Muscle biopsy:
    Gomori-trichrome stain
    Succinate dehydrogenase stain
    Cytochrome-*c* oxidase stain
    Electron microscopy
3. Mutational analysis of mitochondrial DNA
4. Oxidative phosphorylation enzyme analysis

---

had associated movement disorders and two developed generalized dystonia (one together with an akinetic-rigid state).[76] Dystonia can also be a part of other disorders of impaired mitochondrial function that have demonstrable basal ganglia lesions; such disorders include Leigh disease, bilateral striatal necrosis (BSN), and Leber's hereditary optic neuropathy (LHON). Leigh's syndrome, or subacute necrotizing encephalopathy, is characterized by progressive neurologic decline following normal development within the first few years of life; it has several modes of inheritance, including autosomal recessive, X-linked, and mitochondrial.[206] Dystonia is the most common movement disorder in Leigh disease.[196] Neuroimaging reveals symmetric lesions involving the basal ganglia, thalamus, and brainstem. BSN is similar to Leigh disease but tends to be less severe; neuroimaging in BSN demonstrates lesions within the striatum. BSN has been shown to be due to point mutations in the ATPase 6 gene of the mitochondrial genome.[209]

LHON is characterized by acute or subacute painless loss of vision due to severe bilateral optic atrophy, with onset usually between 12 and 30 years of age.[202] Dystonia has also been seen in families with LHON.[203,208] In such families, children develop a generalized dystonia and optic neuropathy occurs at a typical age (i.e., adolescence or early adulthood); rarely, an individual manifests both dystonia and optic neuropathy. The motor dysfunction in children initially is manifested as rigidity of the lower extremities, which then progresses to generalized dystonia. Neuroimaging in these patients reveals lesions within the putamen and the caudate nuclei. This mitochondrial disease has been shown to be due to a specific mutation within the mitochondrial DNA (mtDNA)—a point mutation at base pair 14459 in the ND6 gene, which encodes for the ND6 polypeptide, a component of complex I.[184] Reduced activity of complex I has also been demonstrated in patients with idiopathic dystonia.[154]

Diagnostic testing for a suspected disorder of oxidative phosphorylation can be extensive, often requiring special laboratory techniques[207] (see Table 8–4). Initial screening for energy-dependent metabolic processes includes checking for elevations of the levels of lactate, pyruvate, and alanine in the blood, urine, or CSF. Since these levels can be normal, a muscle biopsy is often needed. Appropriate histochemical techniques include the modified Gomori-trichrome stain and staining of succinate dehydrogenase and cytochrome-*c* oxidase reactions. These methods can detect evidence of a mitochondrial myopathy. Electron microscopy of the muscle may also reveal abnormal mitochondria. If the preceding measures are suggestive of a disorder of oxidative phosphorylation, the disorder can be confirmed by oxidative phosphorylation enzyme analysis or genetic testing. Although analysis for specific mutations with the mtDNA can be used to identify specific disease entities, enzyme analysis is needed to identify a majority of the cases.

WD should always be considered in any individual who presents with a movement disorder, particularly an adolescent or a young adult. Although dystonia can be an initial feature of WD, it is more likely to occur later during the disease. Making the diagnosis of WD is important for family counseling and for initiating effective treatment. Diagnostic testing for WD was outlined earlier.

Any child presenting with dystonia merits a trial of L-dopa therapy. In a sense this is a diagnostic test because if the child responds dramatically, the diagnosis is dopa-responsive dystonia (DRD). The clinical picture consists of an abnormal, usually stiff-legged, gait that worsens throughout the day and improves with sleep, in addition to dystonia and features of parkinsonism.[68] Small amounts of L-dopa (100 to 200 mg/d) can result in complete resolution of symptoms.

The preceding evaluations are likely to identify the most common causes of symptomatic dystonia. Other, less common causes include entities in which the dystonia is part of a complex neurologic presentation, resulting from either a neurodegenerative condition or a metabolic disturbance. Dystonia can be a part of HD, occurring either late in the disease in the presence of the more distinguishing features of HD or in juvenile-onset HD along with bradykinesia as rigidity.[198] Definitive testing for HD is by mutational analysis for the expanded CAG trinucleotide repeat in the HD gene on chromosome 4p. Dystonia can also be a variable component of spinocerebellar ataxia types I, II, and III, and well as DRPLA. Like HD, these are autosomal dominant neurodegenerative conditions associated with an unstable, expanded CAG repeat in their respective genes, which can be identified by mutational analysis.[51] Dystonia, particularly an orolingual-action dystonia leading to lip and tongue self-mutilation, can be part of the neurologic syndromes that accompany acanthocytosis (discussed in preceding evaluation of choreoathetosis).

Dystonia can also be part of the clinical picture of ataxia-telangiectasia (AT). This autosomal recessive disorder is characterized by progressive ataxia starting in early childhood along with oculocutaneous telangiectasias and increased frequency of infections and malignancies due to immunodeficiency. Dystonia often appears later in the disease, after the ataxia is noted, initially being focal and progressing to generalized dystonia.[179] However, dystonia was the presenting feature in one child, beginning with torticollis with rapid progression over several months to sustained postures following any attempt at movement. Subsequent treatment of the dystonia unmasked the ataxia.[157] Choreoathetosis is also common in AT, which also may mask the ataxia.[213] It is interesting that the oculomotor disturbances seen in AT, such as difficulty initiating voluntary lateral gaze (oculomotor apraxia), are not cerebellar in nature but are similar to those seen in PD and HD.[153] Hence, any child presenting with dystonia, choreoathetosis, or oculomotor disturbances should be examined for oculocutaneous telangiectasias and evaluated for AT. Diagnosis in AT is confirmed by measuring serum immunoglobulin A (IgA) levels, which are low, as well as alphafetoprotein and carcinoembryonic antigen, which are elevated.[156,212]

Dystonia may be part of the presentation of neuronal intranuclear inclusion disease (NIID), which is a rare disorder characterized by cognitive decline, behavioral disturbances, lower motor neuron disease, and extrapyramidal and pyramidal signs. Onset is typically in childhood, but it can also occur in adults. The pathologic hallmark is eosinophilic intranuclear inclusions in the neurons of both the central and the autonomic nervous systems, typically observed at autopsy. However, the diagnosis has been made antemortem by rectal biopsy in a child with initial features of behavioral disturbances, oculogyric crises, and blepharospasm.[181]

Dystonia can be part of numerous medical and neurologic conditions that are due to an inherited metabolic disturbance. These are typically seen in infancy or childhood, although there can be presentations in adulthood. $GM_1$ gangliosidosis is an autosomal recessive disorder of lipid metabolism resulting from a deficiency of beta-galactosidase. There are three designated types of $GM_1$ gangliosidosis, based on age of onset and clinical course; type 3 is manifested in childhood, adolescence, and adulthood and is characterized by prominent dystonia and other extrapyramidal features.[180] MRI has demonstrated bilateral putaminal lesions in these patients.[211] Diagnosis is by demonstration of reduced enzyme activity in fibroblasts. Dystonia can also be the presenting feature in children and adults with $GM_2$ gangliosidosis,[199,201] which is due to a deficiency of hexosaminidase. Diagnosis is by measurement of enzyme activity in white blood cells (WBCs) or fibroblasts. Niemann-Pick disease is a group of disorders that have in common an impairment of sphingomyelin metabolism that results in the accumulation of sphingomyelin within the reticuloendothelial system, including lipid-laden macrophages. There are several types of Niemann-Pick disease: type A is the acute neuropathic form, occurring in early infancy with death usually by 2 years; type B is the chronic visceral form, without CNS involvement; type C is the chronic neuropathic form; and type D is the Nova Scotia form, essentially similar to type C but occurring in families from Nova Scotia, where the condition is common.[167] Types A and B have deficient sphingomyelinase activity, whereas types C and D do not. Type C can have a variable neurologic presentation, including dystonia, ataxia, tremor, akinetic-rigid state, and choreoathetosis, and may occur in childhood, adolescence, or adulthood.[166] Such cases have been labeled juvenile dystonic lipidosis[185] and adult dystonic lipidosis[194] in the past. A characteristic feature is a supranuclear vertical gaze paresis and splenomegaly with normal sphingomyelinase activity. Diagnosis is made by the observation of foamy histiocytes on bone marrow aspirate. Metachromatic leukodystrophy (MLD) is a disorder of central and peripheral myelin metabolism caused by deficient activity of arylsulfatase A. A woman thought to have typical dystonia musculorum deformans was found to have MLD by measurement of enzyme activity in leukocytes and skin fibroblasts, which was markedly reduced; sulfatide content of both urine and serum[192] was also markedly elevated.

Measurement of urine organic acids and serum and urine amino acids may also be helpful in the evaluation of an infant or child with dystonia. Disorders of organic acids, such as glutaric aciduria type I and methylmalonicaciduria, have been associated with generalized dystonia in the first few years of life.[182,191] Dystonia has also been described in association with homocystinuria, an aminoaciduria caused by deficiency of cystathionine beta-synthase.[155,169,182] Although homocystinuria is characterized by spontaneous arterial and venous thrombotic events, the dystonia has been shown to occur in the absence of vascular insults to the striatum; the proposed etiologic basis is neurochemical changes in the striatum associated with the metabolic defect.[169] Diagnosis is made by adding 1 ml of 5% sodium cyanide to l ml of urine; after 5 minutes, 3 to 5 drops of 5% sodium nitroprusside is added; a deep red color results if homocystine is present. Definitive diagnosis is made by demonstration of enzyme deficiency in fibroblasts. Dystonia can be seen in Lesch-Nyhan syndrome, an X-linked recessive disorder of purine metabolism characterized by hypotonia followed by spasticity, choreoathetosis, mental retardation, developmental delay, self-mutilation, hyperuricemia, and nephrolithiasis.[102] The enzymatic defect is hypoxanthine-guanine phosphoribosyltransferase. Diagnosis is made by demonstration of absent enzyme activity in fibroblasts or RBCs.

Although such cases of dystonia associated with neurodegenerative and metabolic disorders are uncommon, they should be pursued in patients with historical and clinical features that suggest a possible secondary cause of the dystonia. Many of these conditions are hereditary, thus carry implications regarding future family planning, and some are treatable. If an investigation has been fruitless and a secondary cause is still suspected, psychogenic dystonia is a possibility. Essentially a diagnosis of exclusion, nonorganic dystonia is suggested by certain historical and clinical features. These include multiple somatic complaints, give-way weakness, sensory complaints of the involved body region, abrupt onset, and atypical movements not seen with dystonia.[176]

## MYOCLONUS

Myoclonus is a brief, shocklike muscle contraction. It is due to abnormal neuronal discharges occurring in the cerebral cortex, brainstem, or spinal cord. The contraction can be random and irregular or rhythmic, occasionally simulating tremor. It must always be distinguished from other hyperkinetic dyskinesias, such as chorea, tics, tremor, and dystonia. Careful observation and history taking typically allow for such distinction. However, it must be remembered that more than one movement disorder can exist in a patient.

Clinically, myoclonus can occur spontaneously during a movement (action myoclonus) or in response to various stimuli (reflex myoclonus). Negative myoclonus occurs only during active muscle contraction and consists of a sudden, brief interruption of ongoing voluntary muscle contraction, resulting in sudden lapses of muscle action.[234] The most common forms are asterixis and postural lapses. The myoclonus may be generalized, segmental, or focal in distribution and can be caused by lesions anywhere along the neuraxis.

There are numerous causes of myoclonus. Myoclonus is rarely an isolated feature. Typically present are other neurologic features that may be more helpful in reaching a diagnosis. However, in some instances the presence of myoclonus may be the most helpful feature in making the correct diagnosis. The approach to the patient with myoclonus is based on the presence of other neurologic features and the distribution of myoclonus and is depicted in Figure 8–5.

Rarely, myoclonus may present as a solitary feature. In essential myoclonus the myoclonus appears in the first two

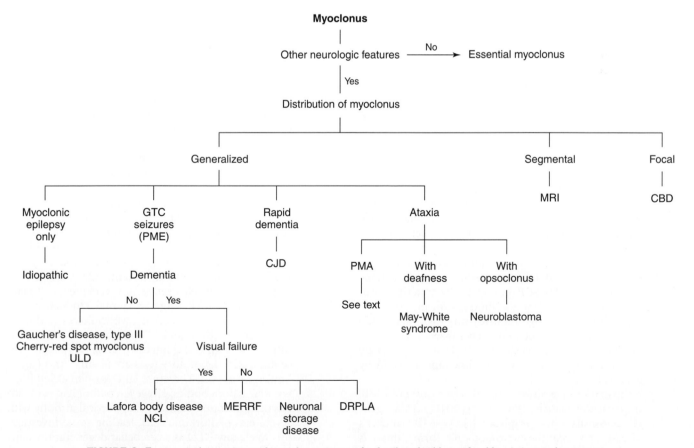

**FIGURE 8–5.** Approach to patient with myoclonus. See text for details and Table 8–2 for abbreviations and acronyms.

decades and is nonprogressive and variable, allowing affected individuals to lead an active life.[230] Although this condition occurs sporadically, typically it is inherited in an autosomal dominant manner, with variable penetrance and expression. Some individuals also have certain components of dystonia, but there are no other neurologic features, and the results of routine laboratory tests, electroencephalography (EEG), and neuroimaging are normal. An interesting feature is a dramatic response to alcohol, which could be considered diagnostic.

### Generalized Myoclonus

Myoclonus can be a main feature of some primary (idiopathic) generalized epilepsies, such as juvenile myoclonic epilepsy, in which there is no other outstanding neurologic feature. However, it can also be present in patients with secondary generalized epilepsies, such as a static or progressive encephalopathy. These conditions are collectively labeled as the progressive myoclonic epilepsies (PMEs). The PMEs are characterized by the presence of myoclonus, tonic-clonic seizures, and progressive neurologic dysfunction (e.g., dementia and ataxia). The conditions that give rise to PME include[215]:

- Lafora body disease is characterized by generalized seizures, rapidly progressive dementia, and myoclonic seizures. Onset is in adolescence following normal development. In about half of the cases there may be focal occipital seizures. Visual hallucinations may be part of the presentation. Later, vision is lost despite normal fundi. Diagnosis is made by skin biopsy to detect the characteristic periodic acid-Schiff-positive cytoplasmic inclusions,[216] which are also present in muscle, liver, and brain.
- Neuronal ceroid lipofuscinosis (NCL), or cerebroretinal degeneration, is characterized by the accumulation of lipopigment in lysosomes. There are several types based on age of onset: infantile, late infantile, juvenile, and adult. All but the infantile form may present with PME. Visual failure may be the initial symptom (except in adults, in whom retinal degeneration does not occur), followed by generalized seizures, myoclonus, and dementia. Estimation of the urine dolichol levels is a good test for diagnosis, although false-positive results approach 15%.[242] Definitive diagnosis is by electron microscopic examination of rectal mucosa, skin, brain, or skeletal muscle and by demonstration of characteristic inclusions.[219]
- The syndrome of myoclonic epilepsy and ragged-red fibers (MERRF) is a mitochondrial encephalomyopathy associated with point mutations in the mitochondrial genome. MERRF is maternally inherited, can occur in childhood or adulthood, with the complete expression consisting of a myopathy with ragged-red fibers on biopsy, myoclonus, generalized seizures, dementia, ataxia, and hearing loss.[236] Diagnosis is made by mutational analysis of the mitochondrial DNA by genetic testing.
- Neuronal storage diseases can also be a cause of PME. In particular, Gaucher's disease type III and $GM_2$ gangliosidosis have been implicated. In type III Gaucher's disease (noninfantile neuronopathic form), onset is in childhood or adolescence and consists of seizures, severe myoclonus, and supranuclear horizontal gaze disorder, with sparing of the intellect. The disease is due to deficiency of glucocerebrosidase. The diagnosis is confirmed by the presence of characteristic Gaucher cells seen in bone marrow aspirate.[241] Childhood onset of $GM_2$ gangliosidosis (Tay-Sachs disease) may present with myoclonus and seizures, along with dementia, ataxia, and spasticity. Diagnosis is by demonstration of low hexosaminidase A activity in leukocytes or cultured fibroblasts.[217]
- PME is a feature of DRPLA, a neurodegenerative disease with autosomal dominant inheritance that is most prevalent in Japan.[223] There are three clinical phenotypes: those with predominant features of ataxia and choreoathetosis, others with a pseudo-Huntington's presentation, and a third group with myoclonic epilepsy.[222] The myoclonic-epilepsy type has its onset in childhood or early adolescence and consists of generalized seizures, myoclonus, and cognitive decline. DRPLA is caused by the expansion of an unstable CAG trinucleotide repeat in the atrophin gene on chromosome 12p.[225,233] Diagnosis is by direct mutational analysis for the expanded repeat. Those patients with myoclonic epilepsy have the largest repeats, and anticipation may be so great that the affected parent is asymptomatic.

Disorders causing PME with relatively little cognitive dysfunction include the following:

- Gaucher's disease type III.
- The cherry-red spot–myoclonus syndrome is characterized by the development of myoclonus, tonic-clonic seizures, visual failure, and macular cherry-red spots, usually occurring in adolescence. Cognition remains relatively normal. This syndrome is one type of sialidosis, which is an autosomal recessively inherited condition caused by a deficiency of neuraminidase. The presence of the cherry-red spots is highly suggestive of the disease, but definitive diagnosis is made by demonstration of enzyme deficiency in leukocytes or cultured fibroblasts.[228,235]
- The first PME to be described was that of Unverricht and Lundborg.[229,239] It consists of progressive myoclonus and generalized tonic-clonic seizures with no (or only mild) cognitive impairment. Unverricht-Lundborg disease (ULD), which shows autosomal recessive inheritance, is most common in Finland and so is called Baltic myoclonus. The diagnosis is clinical, the criteria being (1) onset between 6 and 15 years, following normal development; (2) tonic-clonic seizures; (3) stimulus-sensitive myoclonus; (4) characteristic EEG, including paroxysmal 3 to 5 Hz generalized spike and wave activity, which increases during photic stimulation; and (5) progressive course, with little or no cognitive change.[226] Ataxia is typically present. Routine laboratory tests are normal, and Lafora bodies are absent. Therefore ULD is often called PME without Lafora bodies. However, pathologic evidence has demonstrated pancerebellar cortical atrophy with severe loss of Purkinje cells, leading some investigators to classify ULD as a cerebellar degeneration, clinically compatible with the Ramsay Hunt syndrome.[232]

Generalized myoclonus is virtually a constant feature of the human prion disease Creutzfeldt-Jakob disease (CJD). CJD is characterized by a rapidly progressive dementia and myoclonus, with other variable features such as ataxia and pyramidal or extrapyramidal signs. The majority of cases are sporadic; others are inherited or iatrogenic (i.e., infectious). In the sporadic cases definitive diagnosis is made by brain biopsy and demonstration of spongiform changes and the presence of the pathologic isoform of the prion protein by immunohistochemistry.[227] However, other diagnostic tests may be helpful in a suspected case of CJD before resorting to brain biopsy; these include an EEG to detect periodic sharp wave complexes,[237] CSF analysis, and demonstration of the 14-3-3 protein.[220]

Since the original report by Ramsay Hunt in 1921,[221] the clinical triad of (1) severe myoclonus, (2) progressive ataxia, and (3) only mild epilepsy and cognitive change has been called the Ramsay Hunt syndrome. There has been debate regarding its classification among the PMEs or as a separate neurologic syndrome with more than one cause.[214,232] In a study of 30 patients who fit the criteria for the Ramsay Hunt syndrome, a diagnosis could be made in only 12 patients: 5 patients met the criteria for a mitochondrial encephalomyopathy, 5 met the criteria for ULD, and 2 had celiac disease.[231] This clinical syndrome may be best described by the label progressive myoclonic ataxia (PMA) because the name Ramsay Hunt syndrome has been misinterpreted in the literature as a distinct disease rather than a clinical syndrome with numerous causes.[231] Hence, patients fitting the clinical triad of PMA should undergo the following diagnostic workup[232]:

1. Investigation for an underlying defect in oxidative phosphorylation (discussed in dystonia; see Figure 8–4).
2. If suspected clinically, the conditions listed earlier as causes of PME should be pursued.
3. Celiac disease, as well as Whipple's disease, investigated by jejunal biopsy.[216]
4. Consideration of the spinocerebellar ataxias and DRPLA, particularly if there is a positive family history indicative of autosomal dominant inheritance. These conditions are caused by the expansion of an unstable CAG trinucleotide repeat within the corresponding disease gene. Genetic testing is available.

Myoclonus that occurs with ataxia and deafness along with a positive family history represents the May-White syndrome; it is most likely a mitochondrial encephalomyopathy.[240] Such patients should undergo an appropriate workup, as outlined in Figure 8–5.

Infants or children presenting with myoclonus, ataxia, and chaotic eye movements (opsoclonus) should be investigated intensely for an underlying neuroblastoma. Opsoclonus is similar to myoclonus, but it involves the ocular muscles. It consists of spontaneous, conjugate, irregular movements of the eyes in all directions. Investigations include neuroimaging of the chest and abdomen (preferably MRI) and measurement of homovanillic acid (HVA) and vanillylmandelic acid (VMA) in the urine.[238]

## SEGMENTAL MYOCLONUS

Segmental myoclonus refers to myoclonus that occurs in muscle groups supplied by one or more contiguous segments of the brainstem (branchial myoclonus) or spinal cord (spinal myoclonus).[224] The most common branchial myoclonus is palatal myoclonus (discussed in the section on tremor). Diverse etiologic complexes were found to be associated with spinal myoclonus—trauma, cervical spondylosis with myelopathy, neoplasia, demyelinating disease, and lumbar laminectomy.[224] MRI of the spine is the most logical initial investigation in such patients.

## FOCAL MYOCLONUS

Myoclonus is a typical feature of corticobasal degeneration, a Parkinson-plus syndrome characterized by asymmetric features, such as cortical sensory loss, limb apraxia, or alien limb, combined with slowness and rigidity.[71] The myoclonus is present in the affected limb and is highly stimuli sensitive (i.e., cortical reflex myoclonus). There is no diagnostic test. The diagnosis is clinical, supported by a poor response to L-dopa replacement therapy.

## REFERENCES

### Wilson's Disease

1. Bull PC, Thomas GR, Rommens JM, et al. The Wilson disease gene is a putative copper transporting P-type ATPase similar to the Menkes gene. *Nat Genet.* 1993;5:327-337.
2. Medalia A, Scheinberg IH. Psychopathology in patients with Wilson's disease. *Am J Psychiatry.* 1989;146:662-664.
3. O'Reilly S, Weber PM, Oswald M, Shipley L. Abnormalities of the physiology of copper in Wilson's disease. *Arch Neurol.* 1971;25:28-32.
4. Ross E, Jacobson IM, Dienstag JL, Martin JB. Late onset Wilson's disease with neurologic involvement in the absence of Kayser-Fleischer rings. *Ann Neurol.* 1985;17:411-413.
5. Scheinberg IH, Sternlieb I. *Wilson's Disease.* Philadelphia: WB Saunders; 1984.
6. Stremmel W, Meyerrose K-W, Niederau C, et al. Wilson's disease: clinical presentation, treatment, and survival. *Ann Intern Med.* 1991;115:720-726.
7. Walshe JM. Wilson's disease: the presenting symptoms. *Arch Dis Child.* 1962;37:253-256.
8. Walshe JM, Yealland M. Wilson's disease: the problem of delayed diagnosis. *J Neurol Neurosurg Psychiatry.* 1992;55:692-696.
9. Willeit J, Kiechl SG. Wilson's disease with neurologic impairment but no Kayser-Fleischer rings. *Lancet.* 1991;377:1426.
10. Yarze JC, Martin P, Munoz SJ, Friedman LS. Wilson's disease: current status. *Am J Med.* 1992;92:643-654.

### Tremor

11. Albin R. Cerebellar input tremor. *Neurology.* 1998;50:307-308.
12. Benito-Leon J, Rodriguez J, Orti-Pareja M, et al. Symptomatic orthostatic tremor in pontine lesions. *Neurology.* 1997;49:1439-1441.
13. Berkovic SF, Bladin PF. Rubral tremor: clinical features and treatment of three cases. *Clin Exp Neurol.* 1984;20:119.
14. Defer GL, Remy P, Malapert D, et al. Rest tremor and extrapyramidal symptoms after midbrain haemorrhage: clinical and 18F-dopa PET evaluation. *J Neurol Neurosurg Psychiatry.* 1994;57:987.
15. Dethy S, Luxen A, Bidaut LM, Goldman S. Hemibody tremor related to stroke. *Stroke.* 1993;24:2094-2096.
16. Deuschl G, Heinen F, Guschlbauer B, et al. Hand tremor in patients with spasmodic torticollis. *Mov Disord.* 1997;12:547-552.
17. Deuschl G, Toro C, Valls-Sole J, et al. Symptomatic and essential palatal tremor. 1. Clinical, physiological and MRI analysis. *Brain.* 1994;117:775-788.
18. Elble RJ, Koller WC. *Tremor.* Baltimore: Johns Hopkins University Press; 1990.
19. Ferbert A, Gerwig M. Tremor due to stroke. *Mov Disord.* 1993;8:179-182.
20. Findley LF, Gresty MA. Suppression of "rubral" tremor with levodopa. *BMJ.* 1980;28:1043.
21. Findley LJ, Koller WC, De Witt P, et al. Classification and definition of tremor. In: Royce WL, ed. *Indications for and Clinical Implications of Botulinum Toxin Therapy.* London: Society of Medicine, Ltd; 1993:22-23.

22. Gabellini AS, Martinelli P, Gulli MR, et al. Orthostatic tremor: essential and symptomatic cases. *Acta Neurol Scand.* 1990;81:113-117.

23. Greene HL, Graham EL, Werner JA, et al. Toxic and therapeutic effects of amiodarone in the treatment of cardiac arrhythmias. *J Am Coll Cardiol.* 1983;2:1114.

24. Heilman KM. Orthostatic tremor. *Arch Neurol.* 1984;41:880-881.

25. Hughes AJ, Lees AJ, Marsden CD. Paroxysmal dystonia head tremor. *Mov Disord.* 1991;6:85-86.

26. Ikeda A, Kakigi R, Funai N, et al. Cortical tremor: a variant of cortical reflex myoclonus. *Neurology.* 1990;40:1561-1565.

27. Indo T, Ando K. Metoclopramide-induced parkinsonism: clinical characteristics of ten cases. *Arch Neurol.* 1982;39:494.

28. Jankovic J, Fahn S. Physiological and pathological tremors: diagnosis, mechanisms, and management. *Ann Intern Med.* 1980;93:460-465.

29. Jankovic J, Leder S, Warner D, Schwartz K. Cervical dystonia: clinical findings and associated movement disorders. *Neurology.* 1991;41:1088-1091.

30. Karas BJ, Wilder BJ, Hammond EJ, Bauman AW. Valproate tremors. *Neurology.* 1982;32:428.

31. Kelly JJ Jr, Kyle RA, O'Brien PC, et al. Prevalence of monoclonal protein in peripheral neuropathy. *Neurology.* 1981;31:1480-1483.

32. Kim JS. Delayed onset of hand tremor caused by cerebral infarction. *Stroke.* 1992;23:292.

33. Koller W, Lang A, Vetere-Overfield B, et al. Psychogenic tremors. *Neurology.* 1989;39:1094-1099.

34. Koppel BS, Daras M. "Rubral" tremor due to midbrain toxoplasma abscess. *Mov Disord.* 1990;5:154.

35. Kyle RA. Amyloidosis: clinical and laboratory features in 229 cases. *Mayo Clin Proc.* 1983;58:665-683.

36. Lang AE. *Drug-Induced Movement Disorders.* Mt. Kisco, NY: Futura Publishing; 1992.

37. Lin JJ, Chang DC. Tremor caused by ipsilateral chronic subdural hematoma: case illustration. *J Neurosurg.* 1997;37:474.

38. Marsden CD, Harrison MJG. Idiopathic torsion dystonia (dystonia musculorum deformans): a review of forty-two patients. *Brain.* 1974;97:793-810.

39. Nakamura R, Kamakura K, Tadano Y, et al. MR imaging findings of tremor associated with lesions in cerebellar outflow tracts: report of two cases. *Mov Disord.* 1993;8:209-212.

40. Obeso JA, Rothwell JC, Lang AE, Marsden CD. Myoclonic dystonia. *Neurology.* 1983;33:825-830.

41. Palmer BF, Toto RD. Severe neurologic toxicity induced by cyclosporine A in three renal transplant patients. *Am J Kidney Dis.* 1991;18:116.

42. Rivest J, Marsden CD. Trunk and head tremor as isolated manifestations of dystonia. *Mov Disord.* 1990;5:60-65.

43. Said G, Bathien N, Cesaro P. Peripheral neuropathies and tremor. *Neurology.* 1982;32:480-485.

44. Samie MR, Selhorst JB, Koller WC. Post-traumatic midbrain tremors. *Neurology.* 1990;40:62.

45. Sanitate SS, Meerschaert JR. Orthostatic tremor: delayed onset following head trauma. *Arch Phys Med Rehabil.* 1993;74:886-889.

46. Shepherd GMG, Tauboll E, Bakke SJ, Nyberg-Hansen R. Midbrain tremor and hypertrophic olivary degeneration after pontine hemorrhage. *Mov Disord.* 1997;12:432-437.

47. Smith IS. Tremor in peripheral neuropathy. In: Findley LJ, Koller WC, eds. *Handbook of Tremor Disorders.* New York: Marcel Dekker; 1995:443-454.

48. Swanson JW, Kelly JJ, McConahey WM. Neurologic aspects of thyroid dysfunction. *Mayo Clin Proc.* 1981;56:504-512.

49. Toro C, Pascual-Leone A, Deuschl G, et al. Cortical tremor: a common manifestation of cortical myoclonus. *Neurology.* 1993;43:2346-2353.

50. Vestergaard P. Clinically important side effects of long-term lithium treatment: a review. *Acta Psychiatr Scand.* 1983;67(suppl):1.

51. Wasielewski PG, Scharre DW, Mendell JR. Inherited neurological disorders: relevant considerations and new aspects. In: Joynt RJ, Griggs RC, eds. *Clinical Neurology.* Philadelphia: Lippincott-Raven; 1998:chap 65.

### Akinetic-Rigid State (Parkinsonism)

52. Albanese A, Colosimo C, Bentivoglio AR, Bergonzi P. Unsuspected, surreptitious drug-induced parkinsonism. *Neurology.* 1992;42:459.

53. Baldessarini RJ, Frankenburg FR. Clozapine: a novel antipsychotic agent. *N Engl J Med.* 1991;324:746-754.

54. Bateman DN, Darling WM, Boys R, Rawlins MD. Extrapyramidal reactions to metoclopramide and prochlorperazine. *QJM.* 1989;71:307-311.

55. Bittenbender JB, Quadfasel FA. Rigid akinetic forms of Huntington's chorea. *Arch Neurol.* 1962;7:275-288.

56. Curran T, Lang AE. Parkinsonian syndromes associated with hydrocephalus: case reports, a review of the literature, and pathophysiological hypotheses. *Mov Disord.* 1994;9:508-520.

57. Evans B, Donley D. Pseudohypoparathyroidism, parkinsonism syndrome, with no basal ganglia calcification. *J Neurol Neurosurg Psychiatry.* 1988;51:709-713.

58. Giladi N, Burke RE, Kostic V, et al. Hemiparkinsonism-hemiatrophy syndrome: clinical and neuroradiologic features. *Neurology.* 1990;40:1731-1734.

59. Glatt S, Fine S, Kaplan J. Parkinsonism as a presentation of subdural hematoma. *Neurology.* 1983;33(suppl 2):61.

60. Huntington's Disease Collaborative Research Group. A novel gene containing a trinucleotide repeat that is expanded and unstable on Huntington's disease chromosomes. *Cell.* 1993;72:971-983.

61. Jankovic J, Kirkpatrick JB, Blomquist KA, Langlais PJ, Bird ED. Late-onset Hallervorden-Spatz disease presenting as familial parkinsonism. *Neurology.* 1985;35:227-234.

62. Klawans HL. Hemiparkinsonism as a late complication of hemiatrophy: a new syndrome. *Neurology.* 1981;31:625-628.

63. Klawans HL, Bergen D, Bruyn GW, et al. Prolonged drug-induced parkinsonism. *Cont Neurol.* 1973;35:368-377.

64. Kulali A, Tugtedin M, et al. Ipsilateral hemi-parkinsonism secondary to an astrocytoma. *J Neurol Neurosurg Psychiatry.* 1991;54:655.

65. Mark MH, Sage JI, Walters AS, Duvoisin RC, Miller DC. Binswanger's disease presenting as levodopa-responsive parkinsonism: clinicopathologic study of three cases. *Mov Disord.* 1995;10:450-454.

66. Navarro JA, Exquerro JJR, et al. Parkinsonism due to corpus callosum astrocytoma. *J Neurol Neurosurg Psychiatry.* 1986;49:1457-1458.

67. Nicholson AN, Turner EA. Parkinsonism produced by parasagittal meningiomas. *J Neurosurg.* 1964;21:104-113.

68. Nygaard TG, Marsden CD, Duvoisin RC. Dopa-responsive dystonia. *Adv Neurol.* 1988;50:377-384.

69. Pall HS. 74-year-old lady who developed bilateral parkinsonism secondary to an intrinsic cerebral tumor. *J Neurol Neurosurg Psychiatry.* 1987;50:1386-1387.

70. Rascol O, Sabatini U, Simonetta-Moreau M, et al. Square wave jerks in parkinsonian syndromes. *J Neurol Neurosurg Psychiatry.* 1991;54:599-602.

71. Rinne JO, Lee MS, Thompson PD, Marsden CD. Corticobasal degeneration: a clinical study of 36 cases. *Brain.* 1994;117:1183-1196.

72. Schaffert DA, Johnsen SD, Johnson PC, Drayer BP. Magnetic resonance imaging in pathologically proven Hallervorden-Spatz disease. *Neurology.* 1989;39:440-442.

73. Sethi KD, Adams RJ, Loring DW, El Gamm T. Hallervorden-Spatz syndrome: clinical and magnetic resonance imaging correlations. *Ann Neurol.* 1998;24:692-694.

74. Spitz MC, Jankovic J, Killian JM. Familial tic disorder, parkinsonism, motor neuron disease, and acanthocytosis: a new syndrome. *Neurology.* 1985;35:366-370.

75. Troost BT, Daroff RB. The ocular motor defects in progressive supranuclear palsy. *Ann Neurol.* 1977;2:397-403.

76. Truong DD, Harding AE, Scaravilli F, et al. Movement disorders in mitochondrial myopathies: a study of nine cases with two autopsy studies. *Mov Disord.* 1990;5:109-117.

77. Yamanouchi H, Nagura H. Neurological signs and frontal white matter lesions in vascular parkinsonism. *Stroke.* 1997;28:965-969.

### Chorea and Athetosis

78. Bachman DS, Lao-Velez C, Estanol B. Dystonia and choreoathetosis in multiple sclerosis. *Arch Neurol.* 1976;33:590.

79. Bean S, Ladisch S. Chorea associated with a subdural hematoma. *J Pediatr.* 1977;90:255-256.

80. Bhatia KP, Lera G, Luthert PJ, Marsden CD. Vascular chorea: case report with pathology. *Mov Disord.* 1994;9:447-450.

81. Bolt JM. Abortion and Huntington's chorea. *BMJ.* 1968;1:840.

82. Britton JW, Uitti RJ, Ahlskog JE, Robinson RG, Kremer B, Hayden MR. Hereditary late-onset chorea without significant dementia: genetic evidence for substantial phenotypic variation in Huntington's disease. *Neurology.* 1995;45:443-447.

83. Bruyn GW, Padberg G. Chorea and polycythemia. *Eur Neurol.* 1984;23:26-33.

84. Bruyn GW, Padberg G. Chorea and systemic lupus erythematosus. *Eur Neurol.* 1984;23:278-290.

85. Daras M, Koppel BS, Atos-Radzion E. Cocaine-induced choreoathetoid movements ('crack dancing'). *Neurology.* 1994;44:751-752.
86. Defebvre L, Destee A, Cassim F, Muller JP. Transient hemiballism and striatal infarct. *Stroke.* 1990;21:967-968.
87. Donaldson IM, Espiner EA. Disseminated lupus erythematosus presenting as chorea gravidarum. *Arch Neurol.* 1971;25:240-244.
88. Fidler SM, O'Rourke RA, Buchsbaum HM. Choreoathetosis as a manifestation of thyrotoxicosis. *Neurology.* 1971;21:55-57.
89. Freilich RJ, Chambers BR. Choreoathetosis and thalamic haemorrhage. *Clin Exp Neurol.* 1988;25:115-120.
90. Gilmore PC, Brenner RP. Chorea: a late complication of a subdural hematoma. *Neurology.* 1979;29:1044-1045.
91. Goldman S, Amrom D, Szliwowski HB, et al. Reversible striatal hypermetabolism in a case of Sydenham's chorea. *Mov Disord.* 1993;8:355-358.
92. Green D, Hougie C, Kazmier FJ, et al. Report of the working party on acquired inhibitors of coagulation: studues of the 'lupus anticoagulant.' *Thromb Haemost.* 1983;49:144-146.
93. Haerer AF, Currier RD, Jackson JF. Hereditary nonprogressive chorea of early onset. *N Engl J Med.* 1967;276:1220-1224.
94. Hardie RJ. Acanthocytosis and neurological impairment: a review. *QJM.* 1989;264:291-306.
95. Harrison MB, Lyons GR, Landow ER. Phenytoin and dyskinesias: a report of two cases and review of the literature. *Mov Disord.* 1993;8:19-27.
96. Hefter H, Mayer P, Benecke R. Persistent chorea after recurrent hypoglycemia. *Eur Neurol.* 1993;33:244-247.
97. Helmuth D, Ljaljevic Z, Ramirez L, Meltzer HY. Choreoathetosis induced by verapamil and lithium treatment. *J Clin Psychopharmacol.* 1989;9:454-455.
98. Howdle PD, Bone I, Losowsky MS. Hypocalcemic chorea secondary to malabsorption. *Postgrad Med J.* 1979;55:560-563.
99. Iskander MK, Khan M. Chorea as the initial presentation of oral contraceptive related systemic lupus erythematosus. *J Rheumatol.* 1989;16:850-851.
100. Kienzle GD, Breger RK, Chun RW, et al. Sydenham chorea: MR manifestations in two cases. *AJR.* 1991;12:73-76.
101. Lancman ME, Asconape JJ, Penry JK. Choreiform movements associated with the use of valproate. *Arch Neurol.* 1994;51:702-704.
102. Lesch M, Nyham WL. A familial disorder of uric acid metabolism and central nervous system function. *Am J Med.* 1964;36:561-570.
103. Levine SR, Welch KMA. The spectrum of neurologic disease associated with antiphospholipid antibodies. *Arch Neurol.* 1987;44:876-883.
104. Linazasoro G, Urtasun M, Poza JJ, et al. Generalized chorea induced by nonketotic hyperglycemia. *Mov Disord.* 1993;8:119-120.
105. Logothetic J. Neurologic and muscular manifestations of hyperthyroidism. *Arch Neurol.* 1961;5:533-544.
106. Lubbe WF, Walker EB. Chorea gravidarum associated with circulating lupus anticoagulant: successful outcome of pregnancy with prednisone and aspirin therapy. *Br J Obstet Gynaecol.* 1983;90:487-490.
107. Lucantoni C, Grottoli S, Moretti A. Chorea due to hyperthyroidism in old age: a case report. *Acta Neurol Scand.* 1994;16:129-133.
108. MacMillan JC, Morrison PJ, Nevin NC, et al. Identification of an expanded CAG repeat in the Huntington's disease gene (IT15) in a family reported to have benign hereditary chorea. *J Med Genet.* 1993;30:1012-1013.
109. Malandrini A, Fabrizi GM, Truschi F, et al. Atypical McLeod syndrome manifested as X-linked chorea-acanthocytosis, neuromyopathy, and dilated cardiomyopathy: report of a family. *J Neurol Sci.* 1994;124:89-94.
110. Mao C, Gancher ST, Herndon RM. Movement disorders in multiple sclerosis. *Mov Disord.* 1998;3:109-116.
111. Mas JL, Guergen B, Bouche P, et al. Chorea and polycythaemia. *J Neurol.* 1985;232:168-171.
112. Nakamura H, Takeda S, Shimabuku R, et al. Auditory nerve and brainstem responses in newborns with hyperbilirubinemia. *Pediatrics.* 1985;75:703.
113. Nausieda PA, Grossman BJ, Koller WC, Weiner WJ, Klawans HL. Sydenham chorea: an update. *Neurology.* 1980;30:331-334.
114. Nausieda PA, Koller WC, Weiner WJ, Klawans HL. Chorea induced by oral contraceptives. *Neurology.* 1979;29:1605-1609.
115. Padberg G, Bruyn GW. Chorea: differential diagnosis. In: Vinken PR, Bruyn GW, Klawans HL, eds. *Handbook of Clinical Neurology.* Amsterdam: Elsevier; 1986, vol 49:549-564.
116. Paty DW, McFarlin DE, McDonald WI. Magnetic resonance imaging and laboratory aids in the diagnosis of multiple sclerosis. *Ann Neurol.* 1991;29:3.
117. Poewe WH, Kleedorfer B, Willeit J, Gerstenbrand F. Primary CNS lymphoma presenting as a choreic movement disorder followed by segmental dystonia. *Mov Disord.* 1988;3:320-325.
118. Reed SM, Wise MG, Timmerman I. Choreoathetosis: a sign of lithium toxicity. *J Neuropsychiatry Clin Neurosci.* 1989;1:57-60.
119. Rhee KJ, Albertson TE, Douglas JC. Choreoathetoid disorder associated with amphetamine-like drugs. *Am J Emerg Med.* 1988;6:131-133.
120. Rizzo GN, Olanow CW, Roses AD. Chorea in hyperparathyroidism: report of a case. *AMB Rev Assoc Med Bras.* 1981;27:155-156.
121. Roos RA, Wintzen AR, Vielvoye G, Polder TW. Paroxysmal kinesigenic choreoathetosis as presenting symptom of multiple sclerosis. *J Neurol Neurosurg Psychiatry.* 1991;154:657-658.
122. Sakai M, Hashizume Y, Yamamoto H, Kawakami A. An autopsy case of primary cerebral malignant lymphoma initiated with choreoathetosis. *Clin Neurol.* 1990;30:849-854.
123. Schwartz SA, Marsh WL, Symmans A, et al. New clinical features of McLeod syndrome. *Transfusion.* 1982;22:404.
124. Sharp FR, Rando TA, Greenberg SA, Brown L, Sagar SM. Pseudochoreoathetosis: movements associated with loss of proprioception. *Arch Neurol.* 1994;51:1103-1109.
125. Shinotoh H, Calne DB, Snow B, et al. Normal CAG repeat length in the Huntington's disease gene in senile chorea. *Neurology.* 1994;44:2183-2184.
126. Sparacio RR, Anziska B, Schutta HS. Hypernatremia and chorea. *Neurology.* 1976;26:46-50.
127. Sperling LS, Horowitz JL. Methamphetamine-induced choreoathetosis and rhabdomyolysis. *Ann Intern Med.* 1994;121:986.
128. Stuart AM, Worley LM, Spillane J. Choreiform movements observed in an 8-year-old child following use of an oral theophylline preparation. *Clin Pediatr.* 1992;31:692-694.
129. Tabee-Zadeh MJ, Frame B, Kapphahn K. Kinesiogenic choreoathetosis and idiopathic hypoparathyroidism. *N Engl J Med.* 1972;286:762-763.
130. Takashima H, Sakai T, Iwashita H, et al. A family of McLeod syndrome, masquerading as chorea-acanthocytosis. *J Neurol Sci.* 1994;124:56-60.
131. Traill Z, Pike M, Byrne J. Sydenham's chorea: a case showing reversible striatal abnormalities on CT and MRI. *Dev Med Child Neurol.* 1995;37:270-273.
132. Weindl A, Kuwert T, Leenders KL, et al. Increased striatal glucose consumption in Sydenham's chorea. *Mov Disord.* 1993;8:437-444.
133. Witt T, Danek A, Reiter M, et al. McLeod syndrome: a distinct form of neuroacanthocytosis. *J Neurol.* 1992;239:302-306.

*Hemiballismus*

134. Altafullah I, Pascual-Leone A, Duvall K, Anderson DC, Taylor S. Putaminal hemorrhage accompanied by hemichorea-hemiballism. *Stroke.* 1990;21:1093-1094.
135. Carella F, Caraceni T, Girotti F. Hemichorea due to a cavernous angioma of the caudate: case report of an aged patient. *Ital J Neurol Sci.* 1992;13:783-785.
136. Carpay HA, Arts WF, Kloet A, et al. Hemichorea reversible after operation in a boy with cavernous angioma in the head of the caudate nucleus. *J Neurol Neurosurg Psychiatry.* 1994;57:1547-1548.
137. Dewey RB, Jankovic J. Hemiballism-hemichorea: clinical and pharmacologic findings in 21 patients. *Arch Neurol.* 1989;46:862-867.
138. Glass PJ, Jankovic J, Borit A. Hemiballism and metastatic brain tumour. *Neurology.* 1984;34:204-207.
139. Johnson WG, Fahn S. Treatment of vascular hemiballism and hemichorea. *Neurology.* 1977;27:634-636.
140. Klawans HL, Moses H, Nausieda PA, Bergen D, Wiener WJ. Treatment and prognosis of hemiballismus. *N Engl J Med.* 1976;295:1348-1350.
141. Lin JJ, Chang MK. Hemiballism-hemichorea and non-ketotic hyperglycaemia. *J Neurol Neurosurg Psychiatry.* 1994;57:748-750.
142. Masucci EF, Saini N, Kurtzke JF. Bilateral ballism in multiple sclerosis. *Neurology.* 1989;39:1641-1642.
143. Opida CL, Korthals JK, Somasundaram M. Bilateral ballismus in phenytoin intoxication. *Ann Neurol.* 1978;3:186.
144. Riley D, Lang AE. Hemiballism in multiple sclerosis. *Mov Disord.* 1988;3:88-94.
145. Sethi KD, Allen M, Sethi RK, McCord JW. Chorea in hypoglycemia and hyperglycemia (abstract). *Neurology.* 1990;40(suppl 1):337.
146. Stone LA, Armstrong RM. An unusual presentation of diabetes: hyperglycemia inducing hemiballismus (abstract). *Ann Neurol.* 1989;26:164.
147. Tamaoka A, Sakuta M, Yamada H. Hemichorea-hemiballism caused by arteriovenous malformations in the putamen. *J Neurol.* 1987;234:124-125.

148. Thompson HG, Carpenter MB. Hemichorea due to metastatic lesions in the subthalamic nucleus. *Arch Neurol.* 1960;2:183-187.

149. Vidakovic A, Dragasevic N, Kostic V. Hemiballism: report of 25 cases. *J Neurol Neurosurg Psychiatry.* 1994;57:945-949.

150. Vincent FM. Hyperglycemia-induced hemichoreoathetosis: the presenting manifestation of a vascular malformation of the lenticular nucleus. *Neurosurgery.* 1986;18:787-790.

### Dystonia

151. Angelini L, Nardocci N, Rumi V, et al. Hallervorden-Spatz disease: clinical and MRI study of 11 cases diagnosed in life. *J Neurol.* 1992; 239:417-425.

152. Angelini L, Rumi V, Nardocci N, et al. Hemidystonia symptomatic of primary antiphospholipid syndrome. *Mov Disord.* 1993;8:383-386.

153. Baloh RW, Yee RD, Boder E. Eye movements in ataxia-telangiectasia. *Neurology.* 1978;28:1099-1104.

154. Benecke R, Strumper P, Weiss H. Electron transfer complex I defect in idiopathic dystonia. *Ann Neurol.* 1992;32:683-686.

155. Berardelli A, Thompson PD, Zaccagnini M, et al. Two sisters with generalized dystonia associated with homocystinuria. *Mov Disord.* 1991; 6:163-165.

156. Bigger WD, Good RA. Immunodeficiency in ataxia-telangiectasia. *Birth Defects.* 1975;11:271-273.

157. Bodesteiner JB, Goldblum RM, Goldman AS. Progressive dystonia masking ataxia telangiectasia. *Arch Neurol.* 1980;37:464-465.

158. Boller F, Boller M, Gilbert J. Familial idiopathic cerebral calcifications. *J Neurol Neurosurg Psychiatry.* 1977;40:280-285.

159. Burke RE, Fahn S, Gold A. Delayed onset dystonia in patients with "static" encephalopathy. *J Neurol Neurosurg Psychiatry.* 1980;43:789-797.

160. Burke RE, Fahn S, Jankovic J, et al. Tardive dystonia: late onset and persistent dystonia caused by antipsychotic drugs. *Neurology.* 1982;32: 1335-1346.

161. Burton K, Farrel K, Li D, Calne DB. Lesions of the putamen and dystonia: computed tomography and magnetic resonance imaging. *Neurology.* 1984;34:962-965.

162. Calne DB, Lang AE. Secondary dystonia. *Adv Neurol.* 1988;50:9-34.

163. Caraceni T, Broggi G, Avanzini G. Familial idiopathic basal ganglia calcification exhibiting "dystonia musculorum deformans" features. *Eur Neurol.* 1974;12:351-359.

164. Chiang CY, Lu CS. Delayed-onset posthemiplegic dystonia and imitation synkinesia. *J Neurol Neurosurg Psychiatry.* 1990;53:623.

165. Coleman RJ, Quinn NP, Marsden CD. Multiple sclerosis presenting as adult onset dystonia. *Mov Disord.* 1988;3:329-332.

166. Coleman RJ, Robb SA, Lake BD, Brett EM, Harding AE. The diverse neurological features of Niemann-Pick disease type C: a report of two cases. *Mov Disord.* 1988;3:295-299.

167. Crocker AC. The cerebral defect in Tay-Sachs disease and Niemann-Pick disease. *J Neurochem.* 1961;7:69-80.

168. Daras M, Georgakopoulos T, Avdelidis D. Late onset post-hemiplegic dystonia in systemic lupus erythematosus. *J Neurol Neurosurg Psychiatry.* 1988;51:151-152.

169. Davous P, Rondot P. Homocystinuria and dystonia. *J Neurol Neurosurg Psychiatry.* 1983;46:283-286.

170. Day TJ, Lefroy RB, Mastaglia FL. Meige's syndrome and palatal myoclonus associated to brainstem stroke: a common mechanism? *J Neurol Neurosurg Psychiatry.* 1986;48:1324-1325.

171. Demiere B, Rondot P. Dystonia caused by putamino-capsulo-caudate vascular lesions. *J Neurol Neurosurg Psychiatry.* 1983;46:404-409.

172. Dooling EC, Schoene WC, Richardson EP. Hallervorden-Spatz syndrome. *Arch Neurol.* 1974;30:70-83.

173. Eaton JM. Hemidystonia due to subdural hematoma. *Neurology.* 1988; 38:507.

174. Egger J, Kendall BE. Computed tomography in mitochondrial cytopathy. *Neuroradiology.* 1981;22:73-78.

175. Fahn S. Concept and classification of dystonia. *Adv Neurol.* 1988;50:1.

176. Fahn S, Williams DT. Psychogenic dystonia. *Adv Neurol.* 1988;50:431-455.

177. Friedman DJ, Jankovic J, Rolak LA. Arteriovenous malformation presenting as hemidystonia. *Neurology.* 1986;36:1590-1593.

178. Fukuhara N, Tokiguchi S, Shirakawa K, Tsubaki T. Myoclonus epilepsy associated with ragged red fibers: disease entity or syndrome? *J Neurol Sci.* 1980;47:117-133.

179. Garcia Urra D, Campos J, Garcia Ruiz P, Varela de Seijas E, de Yebenes JG. Movement disorders in ataxia telangiectasia. *Neurology.* 1989; 39(suppl 1): 321.

180. Goldman JE, Katz D, Rapin I, et al. Chronic GM1 gangliosidosis presenting as dystonia. I. Clinical and pathological features. *Ann Neurol.* 1981;9:465-475.

181. Goutieres F, Mikol J, Aicardi J. Neuronal intranuclear inclusion disease in a child: diagnosis by rectal biopsy. *Ann Neurol.* 1990;27:103-106.

182. Heindenreich R, Natowicz M, Hainline BE, et al. Acute extrapyramidal syndrome in methylmalonic acidemia: "metabolic stroke" involving the globus pallidus. *J Pediatr.* 1988;113:1022-1027.

183. Jankovic J, Patel SC. Blepharospasm associated with brainstem lesions. *Neurology.* 1983;33:1237-1240.

184. Jun AS, Brown MD, Wallace DC. A mitochondrial DNA mutation at np14459 of the ND6 gene associated with maternally inherited Leber's hereditary optic neuropathy and dystonia. *Proc Natl Acad Sci U S A.* 1994;91:6206-6210.

185. Karpati G, Carpenter S, Wolfe LS, Andermann F. Juvenile dystonic lipidosis: an unusual form of neurovisceral storage disease. *Neurology.* 1977;27:32-42.

186. Kempster PA, Brenton DP, Gale AN, Stern GM. Dystonia in homocystinuria. *J Neurol Neurosurg Psychiatry.* 1988;51:859-862.

187. Kishore A, Calne DB. Approach to the patient with a movement disorder and overview of movement disorders. In: Watts RL, Koller WC, eds. *Movement Disorders: Neurologic Principles and Practice.* New York: McGraw-Hill; 1997:chap 1.

188. Kiwak KJ, Deray MJ, Shields WD. Torticollis in three children with syringomyelia and spinal cord tumor. *Neurology.* 1983;33:946-948.

189. Krauss JK, Mohadjer M, Braus DF, et al. Dystonia following head trauma: a report of nine patients and review of the literature. *Mov Disord.* 1992;7:263-272.

190. Krauss JK, Mohadjer M, Nobbe F, Scheremet R. Hemidystonia due to a contralateral parieto-occipital metastasis: disappearance after removal of the mass lesion. *Neurology.* 1991;41:1519-1520.

191. Kyllerman M, Skjeldal OH, Lundberg M, et al. Dystonia and dyskinesia in glutaric aciduria type I: clinical heterogeneity and therapeutic considerations. *Mov Disord.* 1994;9:22-30.

192. Lang AE, Clarke JTR, et al. Progressive long-standing "pure" dystonia: a new phenotype of juvenile metachromatic leukodystrophy (MLD). *Neurology.* 1985;35(suppl 1):194.

193. Larsen TA, Dunn HG, Jan JE, Calne DB. Dystonia and calcification of the basal ganglia. *Neurology.* 1985; 35:533-537.

194. Longstreth WT, Daven JR, Farrell DF, Bolen JW, Bird TD. Adult dystonic lipidosis: clinical, histologic, and biochemical findings of a neurovisceral storage disease. *Neurology.* 1982;32:1295-1299.

195. Lorenzana L, Cabezudo JM, Porras LF, et al. Focal dystonia secondary to cavernous angioma of the basal ganglia: case report and review of the literature. *Neurosurgery.* 1992;31:1108-1112.

196. Macaya A, Munell F, Burke RE, De Vivo DC. Disorders of movement in Leigh's syndrome. *Neuropediatrics.* 1993;24:60-67.

197. Marsden CD, Obeso JA, Zarranz JJ. The anatomical basis of symptomatic dystonia. *Brain.* 1985;108:463-483.

198. Marshall FJ, Shoulson I. Clinical features and treatment of Huntington's disease. In: Watts RL, Koller WC, eds. *Movement Disorders: Neurologic Principles and Practice.* New York: McGraw-Hill; 1997:chap 35.

199. Meek D, Wolfe LS, Andermann E, Andermann F. Juvenile progressive dystonia: a new phenotype of GM2 gangliosidosis. *Ann Neurol.* 1984; 15:348-352.

200. Narbona J, Obeso JA, Luguin R, et al. Hemidystonia secondary to localised basal ganglia tumor. *J Neurol Neurosurg Psychiatry.* 1984;47: 704-709.

201. Nardocci N, Bertagnolio B, Rumi V, Angelini L. Progressive dystonia symptomatic of juvenile GM2 gangliosidosis. *Mov Disord.* 1992;7:64-67.

202. Newman NJ, Lott MT, Wallace DC. The clinical characteristics of pedigrees of Leber's hereditary optic neuropathy with the 11,778 mutation. *Am J Ophthalmol.* 1991;111:750-762.

203. Novotny EJ, Singh G, Wallace DC, et al. Leber's disease and dystonia: a mitochondrial disease. *Neurology.* 1986;36:1053-1060.

204. Obeso JA, Gimenez-Roldan S. Clinicopathological correlation in symptomatic dystonia. *Adv Neurol.* 1988;50:113-122.

205. Pettigrew LC, Jankovic J. Hemidystonia: a report of 22 patients and a review of the literature. *J Neurol Neurosurg Psychiatry.* 1985;48:650-657.

206. Rahman S, Blok RB, Dahl H, et al. Leigh syndrome: clinical features and biochemical and DNA abnormalities. *Ann Neurol.* 1996;39:343-351.

207. Shoffner JM. Oxidative phosphorylation diseases and movement disorders. In: Watts RL, Koller WC, eds. *Movement Disorders: Neurologic Principles and Practice.* New York: McGraw-Hill; 1997:chap 4.

208. Shoffner JM, Brown MD, Stugard C, et al. Leber's hereditary optic neuropathy plus dystonia is caused by a mitochondrial DNA point mutation. *Ann Neurol.* 1995;38:163-169.

209. Thyagarajan D, Shanske S, Vasquez-Memije M, et al. A novel mitochondrial ATPase 6 point mutation in familial bilateral striatal necrosis. *Ann Neurol.* 1995;38:468-472.

210. Tolge CF, Factor SA. Focal dystonia secondary to cerebral toxoplasmosis in a patient with acquired immune deficiency syndrome. *Mov Disord.* 1991;6:69-72.

211. Uyama E, Terasaki T, Watanabe S, et al. Type 3 GM1 gangliosidosis: characteristic MRI findings correlated with dystonia. *Acta Neurol Scand.* 1992;86:609-615.

212. Waldman TA, McIntire KR. Serum-alpha-fetoprotein levels in patients with ataxia-telangiectasia. *Lancet.* 1972;2:1112.

213. Wells CE, Shy GM. Progressive familial choreoathetosis with cutaneous telangiectasia. *J Neurol Neurosurg Psychiatry.* 1957;20:98-104.

*Myoclonus*

214. Andermann F, Berkovic S, Carpenter S, Andermann E. Viewpoints on the Ramsay Hunt syndrome. 2. The Ramsay Hunt syndrome is no longer a useful diagnostic category. *Mov Disord.* 1989;4:13-17.

215. Berkovic SF, Andermann F, Carpenter S, Wolfe LS. Progressive myoclonus epilepsies: specific causes and diagnosis. *N Engl J Med.* 1986; 315:296-305.

216. Bhatia KP, Brown P, Gregory R, et al. Progressive myoclonic ataxia associated with coeliac disease. *Brain.* 1995;118:1087-1093.

217. Brett EM, Ellis RB, Haas L, et al. Late onset GM$_2$-gangliosidosis: clinical, pathological, and biochemical studies on 8 patients. *Arch Dis Child.* 1973;48:775-785.

218. Carpenter S, Karpati G. Sweat gland duct cells in Lafora disease: diagnosis by skin biopsy. *Neurology.* 1981;31:1564-1568.

219. Carpenter S, Karpati G, Andermann F, Jacob JC, Andermann E. The ultrastructural characteristics of the abnormal cytosomes in Batten-Kufs disease. *Brain.* 1977;100:137-156.

220. Hsich G, Kenney K, Gibbs CJ Jr, Lee KH, Harrington MG. The 14-3-3 brain protein in cerebrospinal fluid as a marker for transmissible spongiform encephalopathies. *N Engl J Med.* 1996;335:924-930.

221. Hunt JR. Dyssynergia cerebellaris myoclonica-primary atrophy of the dentate system. *Brain.* 1921;44:490-538.

222. Iizuka R, Hirayama K, Maehara K. Dentato-rubro-pallido-luysian atrophy: a clinico-pathological study. *J Neurol Neurosurg Psychiatry.* 1984;47:1288-1298.

223. Ikeuchi T, Koide R, Onodera O, et al. Dentatorubral-pallidoluysian atrophy (DRPLA). *Clin Neurosci.* 1995;3:23-27.

224. Jankovic J, Pardo R. Segmental myoclonus: clinical and pharmacological study. *Arch Neurol.* 1986;43:1025-1031.

225. Koide R, Ikeuchi T, Onodera O, et al. Unstable expansion of CAG repeat in hereditary dentatorubral-pallidoluysian atrophy (DRPLA). *Nat Genet.* 1994;6:9-13.

226. Koskiniemi M, Donner M, Majuri H, Haltia M, Norio R. Progressive myoclonus epilepsy: a clinical and histopathological study. *Acta Neurol Scand.* 1974;50:307-332.

227. Kretzschmar HA, Ironside JW, DeArmond SJ, Tateishi J. Diagnostic criteria for sporadic Creutzfeldt-Jakob disease. *Arch Neurol.* 1996;53: 913-920.

228. Lowden JA, O'Brien JS. Sialidosis: a review of human neuraminidase deficiency. *Am J Hum Genet.* 1979;31:1-18.

229. Lundborg H. *Die progressive myoklonus-epilepsie (Unverricht's Myoklonie).* Uppsala: Almquist and Wiksell; 1903:1-207.

230. Mahloudji M, Pikielny RT. Hereditary essential myoclonus. *Brain.* 1967;90:669-674.

231. Marsden CD, Harding AE, Obeso JA, Lu CS. Progressive myoclonic ataxia (The Ramsay Hunt Syndrome). *Arch Neurol.* 1990;47:1121-1125.

232. Marsden CD, Obeso JA. Viewpoints on the Ramsay Hunt syndrome. 1. The Ramsay Hunt syndrome is a useful clinical entity. *Mov Disord.* 1989;4:6-12.

233. Nagafuchi S, Yanagisawa H, Sato K, et al. Dentatorubral and pallidoluysian atrophy expansion of an unstable CAG trinucleotide on chromosome 12p. *Nat Genet.* 1994;6:14-18.

234. Obeso JA, Artieda J, Burleigh A. Clinical aspects of negative myoclonus. *Adv Neurol.* 1996;67:1-8.

235. Rapin I, Goldfischer S, Katzman R, Engel J Jr, O'Brien JS. The cherry-red spot-myoclonus syndrome. *Ann Neurol.* 1978;3:234-242.

236. Silvestri G, Ciafaloni E, Santorelli FM, et al. Clinical features associated with the A-to-G transition at nucleotide 8344 of mtDNA ("MERRF mutation"). *Neurology.* 1993;43:1200-1206.

237. Steinhoff BJ, Racker S, Herrendorf G, et al. Accuracy and reliability of periodic sharp wave complexes in Creutzfeldt-Jakob disease. *Arch Neurol.* 1996;53:162-166.

238. Tuchman M, Morris CL, Ramnaraine ML, et al. Value of random urinary homovanillic acid and vanillylmandelic acid levels in diagnosis and management of patients with neuroblastoma. *Pediatrics.* 1985;75:324.

239. Unverricht H. *Die Myoclonie.* Leipzig: Franz Deuticke; 1891:1-128.

240. Vaamonde J, Muruzabal J, Tunon T, et al. Abnormal muscle and skin mitochondria in family with myoclonus, ataxia, and deafness (May and White syndrome). *J Neurol Neurosurg Psychiatry.* 1992;55:128-132.

241. Winkelman MD, Banker BQ, Victor M, Moser HW. Noninfantile neuronopathic Gaucher's disease: a clinico-pathologic study. *Neurology.* 1983;33:994.

242. Wolfe LS, Palo J, Santavuori P, et al. Urinary sediment dolichols in the diagnosis of neuronal ceroid-lipofuscinosis. *Ann Neurol.* 1986;19:270-274.

# 9

# Metabolic Encephalopathies and Brain Death

*Piotr Olejniczak and Bruce J. Fisch*

The diffuse encephalopathies are progressive, transient, or static disorders that impair cognition, attention, and arousal. Although they may be associated with obvious multifocal structural abnormalities (e.g., inflammatory or degenerative diseases), more often they are caused by metabolic disorders that do not produce discrete lesions (e.g., anoxia, hypoglycemia, renal or hepatic failure, or drug overdose). Routine laboratory chemistries, electroencephalography (EEG), and neuroimaging are currently the main clinical tests used in the initial evaluation of encephalopathies. The diagnostic value of these tests varies, but because these disorders typically produce profound changes in cerebral function and little change in structure, the EEG is usually abnormal. Indeed, the EEG, which has been used in the investigation of metabolic and degenerative encephalopathies since the earliest studies were performed by Hans Berger in the 1920s,[8,9] continues to be the leading clinical laboratory test for assessing cerebral function in encephalopathic patients.

EEG progressive increases in generalized slowing and attenuation and reduced reactivity to noxious stimulation, all of which can be easily quantified for cerebral monitoring in the intensive care unit (ICU) or the operating room, are direct measures of the severity of an acute or subacute encephalopathy. Generalized slowing and attenuation are common findings that help to rule out the presence of a major localized structural abnormality, a focal epileptic condition, status epilepticus, or a purely psychiatric disorder. In patients with encephalopathy certain findings are etiologically specific, such as the periodic patterns seen in Creutzfeldt-Jakob disease or subacute sclerosing panencephalitis, the excessive beta activity noted in barbiturate or benzodiazepine drug overdose, or the high-amplitude occipital dominant spikes in response to slow photic stimulation in the Bielschowsky-Jansky (late infantile) form of ceroid lipofuscinosis.[30] Alcohol withdrawal is typically associated with a low-voltage fast pattern. Contrary to earlier reports, alcohol withdrawal is not associated with photoconvulsive (photoparoxysmal) responses.[32] In certain clinical settings the specificity of the EEG increases. For example, in patients with encephalopathic changes caused by encephalitis, the finding of pseudoperiodic epileptiform discharges is highly suggestive of herpes encephalitis.

The EEG may also provide important prognostic information for patients in coma. Diffuse beta activity suggests the potential for complete recovery, whereas a burst-suppression pattern found more than several hours after cardiopulmonary arrest in an adult is almost always a sign of impending death. Monitoring EEG responses to photic, auditory, and tactile stimulation during recording and performing repeated or prolonged recordings increase the diagnostic and prognostic value of the EEG. In the absence of severe hypothermia, hypertension, or general anesthesia, failure of the EEG to react to vigorous, noxious stimulation suggests a poor prognosis for recovery of function or survival.

Evoked potentials (EPs), whether somatosensory or brainstem auditory, are less sensitive than EEG, but they are useful for detecting or confirming central neuronal injury in patients with impaired consciousness.[16,59,63] Severe acute metabolic encephalopathies caused by specific systemic disorders often reveal laboratory abnormalities measurable in the blood, urine, or cerebrospinal fluid (CSF) that are important for establishing the diagnosis. However, unless these biochemical or hematologic abnormalities are extreme, their correlation with cerebral dysfunction or prognosis is poor.

## DIAGNOSTIC ASSESSMENT OF HEPATIC ENCEPHALOPATHY

### CLINICAL EVALUATION

The severity of hepatic encephalopathy is initially determined by grading the level of consciousness (Table 9–1).

Once the level of consciousness has been assessed, a complete mental status examination should be performed. Impairments in orientation, memory, affect, perception, attention, judgment, and cognition are often present, but they may be subtle and detectable only by formal neuropsychologic testing.[65,88] A variety of abnormalities may be found on the clinical examination. Asterixis, sometimes referred to as "liver flap," is one of the most useful signs. The postural lapses of asterixis are associated with periods of complete electrical silence in the involved muscles.

**TABLE 9–1. Grading of Hepatic Encephalopathy**

| GRADE | CHARACTERISTIC FEATURES |
|---|---|
| 0 | Normal sensorium |
| 1 | Drowsiness, irritability, short attention span |
| 2 | Lethargy, impaired cognition |
| 3 | Confusion, stupor |
| 4 | Coma, unresponsiveness to external stimuli |

Data from Lockwood[63] and Menkes.[76]

## ELECTROPHYSIOLOGIC DIAGNOSIS

EEG can be used to help establish the diagnosis of hepatic encephalopathy and is a reliable laboratory test for monitoring the effectiveness of therapy. The EEG changes in hepatic failure correlate more closely with clinical status than with laboratory chemistries.[31,88] In the earliest stages only mild background slowing or excessive intermixed theta waveforms are seen. As the encephalopathy becomes more severe, sleep patterns become less well defined, slowing increases and intermittent rhythmic delta activity (IRDA); triphasic waves recur in more than half of all patients. Bickford and Butt[10] described the evolution of EEG abnormalities as beginning with diffuse 4 to 7 Hz waves, followed by the appearance of triphasic waves with surface-positive maximum deflections and random nonrhythmic, asynchronous delta slowing. In the terminal stages of encephalopathy EEG amplitude and waveform complexity decline and periods of diffuse attenuation appear. Quantitative EEG, with the use of spectral analysis, has been shown to be a sensitive method for monitoring hepatic encephalopathy, particularly when mild EEG changes are present.

As the encephalopathy worsens, two distinctive patterns appear, IRDA and triphasic waves. Both of these patterns are also commonly seen in other metabolic and toxic encephalopathies. The first pattern, IRDA, consists of bilaterally symmetric rhythmic waveforms, approximately 2.5 Hz, usually >50µV, that may be either sinusoidal or notched in appearance. They occur in brief (1 to 3 second) runs with greatest amplitude over either the anterior (frontal intermittent rhythmic delta activity [FIRDA] [Fig. 9–1A]) or posterior head regions (occipital intermittent rhythmic delta activity [OIRDA]). FIRDA and OIRDA are frequently seen in association with a variety of diffuse encephalopathies. The earliest clinical change that occurs with IRDA in any acute encephalopathy is a mild impairment of concentration and alerting.[95] IRDA is also more likely to occur during the evolution of a transient or progressive disorder than in a static encephalopathy.[97]

The second distinctive pattern, the triphasic wave pattern, was first recognized by Foley et al[36] in patients with hepatic encephalopathy. However, it was Bickford and Butt[10] who described these waves in detail and named them. They characterized them as blunted-spike and slow-wave complexes consisting of an initial negativity (blunted spike) followed by a longer duration and greater amplitude positive wave ending with a lower amplitude and an even longer negative phase. As noted by subsequent investigators, the total duration of each triphasic wave varies between approximately one-third and one-half second, and amplitudes typically range from 50 to 150 µV in ipsilateral ear reference montages. Triphasic waves may appear sporadically, or they may occur in brief or prolonged periodic runs with a repetition rate of 1.5 to 2.5 Hz. In most cases the triphasic waves are maximal over the anterior head regions (Fig. 9–1B). Triphasic waves also frequently demonstrate an apparent lag of the second positive phase between the anterior and posterior head regions in longitudinal bipolar montages. This delay can occur in either the anterior-to-posterior or the posterior-to-anterior direction and may last more than 150 ms. The pathophysiologic basis of triphasic waves is poorly understood. As with other bisynchronous patterns, thalamic pacing or modulation probably plays an important role. Indeed, unilateral lesions may result in an ipsilateral loss of both sleep spindles and triphasic waves.[31]

Approximately one half of all adults with moderate to severe hepatic encephalopathy and one fourth of those with renal encephalopathy will develop a triphasic wave pattern. It is interesting to note that certain disorders, such as Wilson's disease and Reye's syndrome, which also disrupt hepatic and cerebral function, rarely cause triphasic waves. This may be so partly because triphasic waves are an age-related phenomenon. These waves rarely occur in individuals less than 20 years of age, are infrequent before age 30, and increase in incidence thereafter.[31] The triphasic wave pattern has been reported in numerous disorders, including hyponatremia or hypernatremia, hypercalcemia, hypoglycemia, thyroid disease, stroke, hypertensive encephalopathy, cerebral abscess, encephalitis, congestive heart failure, septic shock, lithium intoxication, and the postictal state. Sporadic triphasic waves are also occasionally seen in awake elderly individuals with clinically advanced dementing disorders, often with greatest amplitude over the posterior head regions[80] (Brenner, personal communication).

Background slowing is a better predictor of the level of consciousness or prognosis than is the presence or absence of triphasic waves. However, when blunted triphasic waves are combined with severely slow, low-amplitude background activity without any activity >4.5 Hz, then the diagnosis is almost always either hepatic, renal, or anoxic encephalopathy.[31] When diffuse nonreactive low-amplitude delta predominates (typically seen late in the course of hepatic encephalopathy), survival is unusual.[30]

## NEUROIMAGING

The diagnostic value of neuroimaging (computed tomography [CT], magnetic resonance imaging [MRI]) in hepatic encephalopathy is mainly the exclusion of structural lesions such as subdural hematomas, which are indirect complications of chronic liver disease. Mild and reversible changes, consisting of pallidal hyperintensity on T1-weighted sequences, have been demonstrated in patients with high blood ammonia levels.[61,65] Magnetic resonance spectroscopy has shown that the areas of pallidal hyperintensity on T1-weighted sequences are associated with an increase in glutamine compounds and a decrease in myoinositol and choline.[87] According to Hauser et al,[49] these changes may be related to hypermagnesemia.

## LABORATORY DIAGNOSIS

Laboratory chemistries can be used to establish the diagnosis of hepatic encephalopathy. The arterial blood ammonia level done in the fasting state correlates well with the depth of coma. The metabolites of ammonia, glutamine, and alpha-ketoglutaramate are elevated in the brain and CSF of patients with hepatic encephalopathy.[22,64,88] Hypoalbuminemia and coagulation factor deficiency are commonly seen as direct consequences of liver failure.

The hypothesis that excessive gamma-aminobutyric acid (GABA) causes hepatic encephalopathy led to trials of the benzodiazepine antagonist flumazenil. Improvement occurred but was mild and transient.[45,86] Groenweg et al,[42] in a double-blind, randomized, placebo-controlled study, also found a mild effect of flumazenil on the EEG of patients with portosystemic encephalopathy. The pathophysiologic significance of abnormalities of the mercaptan, phenols, short-chain fatty acid levels, and false neurotransmitters (e.g., octopamine), is less well established.[65] For example, the mercaptan methanechiol, which is formed in the intestine from methionine, is elevated in hepatic encephalopathy, but elevations in blood methanechiol and dimethyl sulfide concentration in children with congenital hypermethioninemia are not associated with neurologic or EEG signs of hepatic coma.[73]

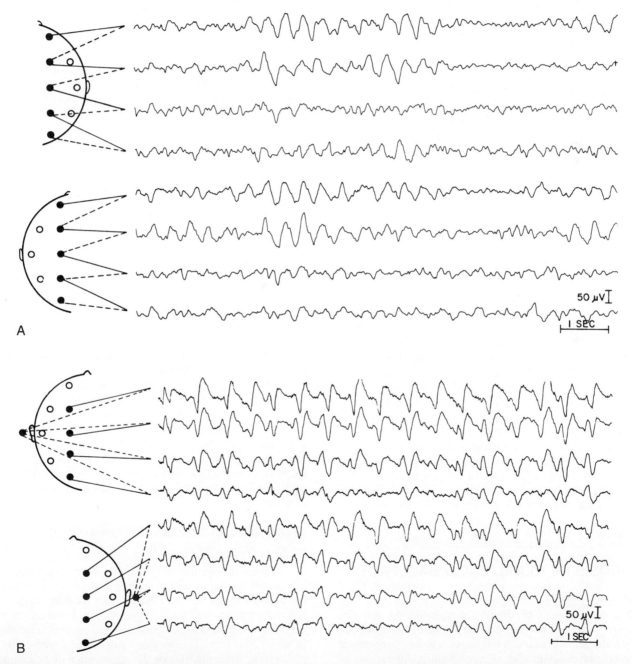

**FIGURE 9–1.  A,** Pattern of frontal intermittent delta activity (FIRDA) in an 18-year-old woman following severe head injury and coma. Patient was oriented and responsive, and neurologic examination was normal at time of recording. EEG shows runs of anteriorly dominant 2 to 3 Hz rhythmic delta on a background of predominantly intermixed delta, theta, and alpha activity. **B,** Pattern of anteriorly dominant triphasic waves in a 68-year-old man in hepatic coma caused by alcoholism. A variety of morphologies (biphasic and quadriphasic waveforms) and phase lags are demonstrated. (Reprinted from Fisch BJ. *Spehlmann's EEG Primer,* 2nd ed, 1991, with permission from Elsevier Science.)

## SPECIFIC CAUSES OF HEPATIC ENCEPHALOPATHIES

### Wilson's Disease

The diagnostic evaluation of Wilson's disease includes a careful ophthalmoscopic slit-lamp examination for the presence of Kayser-Fleischer rings. The serum ceruloplasmin level in this condition is usually low (<20 mg/dl). The concentration of unbound copper is elevated in the blood, with secondary increased copper excretion in the urine (>100 μg/24 h). The diagnosis is confirmed by liver biopsy with quantitative determination of an elevated liver copper content. These findings are consistent with the discovery that the gene for Wilson's disease (localized to the long arm of chromosome 13-13q14.3) encodes a copper-transporting ATPase.[65,76] Gene therapy, however, awaits characterization of the disease-specific mutations and the gene product itself[96] and an efficient method of gene delivery to hepatocytes.

### Urea Cycle Disorders

The presence of elevated blood ammonia levels in neonates and infants suggests a urea cycle or another organic acid disorder. Vomiting and lethargy correlate with plasma ammonia concentrations >200 μg/dl; coma, with concentrations >300 μg/dl; and seizures, with those >500 μg/dl.[29] The initial evaluation should include routine blood chemistries, plasma lactate levels, liver function tests, and a quantitative assay of urine for organic acids and orotic acid.[76] In some instances the fasting blood ammonia level may be normal, but significant elevations occur after protein loading. Determination of a specific enzymatic deficiency confirms the diagnosis.

### Reye's Syndrome

Reye's syndrome is a rapidly progressive and often fatal childhood encephalopathy in which fatty infiltration of the liver is associated with hyperammonemia and hypoglycemia without hyperbilirubinemia. Serial EEGs are useful for assessing prognosis. Aoki and Lombroso[3] found that children with reactive delta and theta slowing usually survived, whereas children with nonreactive, continuous low-amplitude delta or burst-suppression patterns died or suffered severe neurologic impairment. Although 14 and 6 Hz positive spikes may rarely occur in other childhood encephalopathies[26] and adult hepatic encephalopathy,[31] they are commonly seen in Reye's syndrome and, as in other encephalopathies, may be enhanced by auditory or other stimulation.[116] As the patient recovers, the 14 and 6 Hz pattern occurs less frequently and usually disappears. The incidence of Reye's syndrome has declined dramatically with the avoidance of aspirin use for treatment of pediatric patients.

# DIAGNOSIS OF RENAL ENCEPHALOPATHY

## CLINICAL DIAGNOSIS

The pathogenesis of uremic encephalopathy remains unknown. The severity of cerebral symptoms correlates poorly with blood urea levels but appears to be proportional to the rate of development of renal failure. Alterations of alertness and awareness are the most reliable indications of uremic encephalopathy. Clinical studies have suggested that elevated levels of parathyroid hormone can account for some of the symptoms seen in uremia.[77]

The most common symptoms include mental status changes, seizures, myoclonus, tremor, cerebellar dysfunction, and asterixis.[6,18,35,64,109] About one third of patients with renal insufficiency develop epileptic seizures, which are apparently due to water and electrolyte imbalance. In chronic uremia, mental functions stabilize with prolonged dialysis treatment.

## ELECTROPHYSIOLOGIC DIAGNOSIS

The EEG in renal encephalopathy is initially characterized by mild diffuse background slowing. A pattern of generalized theta-alpha slowing with intermittent 1 to 3 Hz epochs of moderate- to high-amplitude anterior dominant delta activity is also frequently seen (sometimes referred to as an "alternating pattern"). As the severity of the encephalopathy increases, EEG changes similar to those of other metabolic encephalopathies occur. In addition, there may be triphasic waves and photoparoxysmal responses.[30]

In acute uremia, bilateral spike discharges may or may not be associated with myoclonic jerking. Exceptionally, the epileptiform activity may be focal.[81]

In chronic uremia, the EEG changes may stabilize, but occasional periods of deterioration may occur with seizures and diffuse delta and theta activity. Hughes[51] reported that EEG changes correlated with the clinical examination and acute blood urea nitrogen fluctuations. Sleep EEGs of chronic uremic patients may show long bursts of high voltage, 12 to 13/s waves with enhanced-vertex sharp activity in drowsiness, lack of spindles in stage 2 sleep, and prolonged high-voltage slow bursts with awakening.[56]

## NEUROIMAGING

Neuroimaging studies of the brain in patients with end-stage uremia show a high incidence of cerebral atrophy in children, suggesting an adverse effect of uremia on brain development.[77,85,109] Other suspected causes of atrophy are malnutrition, aluminum intoxication, and psychosocial deprivation.[27] Renal transplantation has been reported to accelerate head growth and mental development.[23] Renal transplantation itself is associated with a risk of central nervous system (CNS) infections, tumors, central pontine myelinolysis,[70] and encephalopathies related to immunosuppressants (e.g., cyclosporine, FK 506, or OKT3).[77] The causes of posttransplantation encephalopathy are diverse, and the diagnostic evaluation should address treatable disorders such as infection, transplant rejection, and intracranial hemorrhage.

## SPECIFIC CAUSES OF RENAL ENCEPHALOPATHY

### Dialysis Dysequilibrium

Dialysis dysequilibrium is a clinical syndrome that usually occurs during or within several hours after dialysis, but the onset of symptoms occasionally may be delayed up to 24 hours. Symptoms of headache, nausea, and muscle cramps occur in about 50% of patients; delirium, seizures, or coma, in about 5%. The EEG demonstrates either a worsening of preexisting abnormalities or the appearance of new abnormalities. EEG abnormalities may also appear during and shortly after dialysis in asymptomatic patients. Although a variety of generalized changes may occur, frequent bursts of high-amplitude mixed rhythmic or arrhythmic delta and theta waveforms combined with varying degrees of background slowing are characteristic. In some cases spikes or spike and wave complexes may be seen.

### Dialysis Dementia

Dialysis dementia is a fatal disorder characterized clinically by symptoms that include dementia, behavioral changes, myoclonus, seizures, and a stammering and hesitant speech disorder. The typical EEG features, which may precede the onset of symptoms, consist of bursts of high-voltage anterior dominant delta waveforms often with intermixed epileptiform spikes and sharp waves. Triphasic waves, FIRDA, and more randomly distributed localized epileptiform spikes and sharp waves are also commonly seen. Background slowing roughly parallels the onset and progression of dementia. Many of the earlier changes are similar to those seen in dialysis dysequilibrium. However, they persist more than 24 hours after dialysis, and a clear progression of worsening is seen with repeated EEGs. The role of aluminum in the etiologic complex of dialysis-dementia is well established.[38]

### Hypertensive Encephalopathy

Hypertensive encephalopathy is discussed here because it often accompanies renal disease. It is associated with symptoms and signs of increased intracranial pressure with headache, vomiting, disturbance of vision, and papilledema.[77] Such focal findings as seizures and cortical blindness are also common. MRI in patients with transient cortical blindness usually reveals resolving signal abnormalities in the occipital lobes.[24,48,74]

## DIAGNOSIS OF HYPOGLYCEMIC ENCEPHALOPATHY

### CLINICAL DIAGNOSIS

There is an approximate relationship between blood glucose levels and levels of consciousness. Confusion usually occurs at 30 to 40 mg/dl; stupor and seizures, at about 20 mg/dl; and coma, below 10 mg/dl.[115] Malouf and Brust,[71] in a prospective study of consecutive 125 patients evaluated for symptomatic hypoglycemia in the Harlem Hospital Emergency Room, found that 65 patients presented with obtundation, stupor, or coma; 38 had confusion or bizarre behavior; 10 were dizzy or tremulous; 9 had seizures; and 3 had suffered sudden hemiparesis. Diabetes mellitus, alcoholism, and sepsis, alone or in combination, accounted for 90% of predisposing conditions. Average blood glucose levels were lower among comatose than among obtunded persons, but overlap was considerable. Although mortality was 11%, only one death was attributable to hypoglycemia per se, and only four survivors had focal neurologic residua.

### ELECTROPHYSIOLOGIC DIAGNOSIS

The EEG is a highly sensitive tool for detection of hypoglycemia because the brain heavily depends on the supply of carbohydrates for its functioning. A drop in blood sugar levels diminishes oxygen utilization, producing an effect similar to hypoxic-ischemic encephalopathy.[110] Berger[9] was the first to describe EEG alterations during insulin-induced coma for treatment of schizophrenia. Brazier et al[13,14] provided a grading of EEG changes during physiologic hypo-

glycemia. Prominent anteriorly dominant slowing with hyperventilation occurs first. As hypoglycemia progresses, hyperventilation activates FIRDA that persists after the cessation of hyperventilation. With blood glucose levels of 50 to 80 mg/dl, alpha rhythm slows and intermittent theta waves appear. Below the 40 mg/dl, diffuse theta and delta activity appear in addition to IRDA. Some authors[11,108] have noted a topographic maximum of slow frequencies posteriorly during deep hypoglycemia. Loss of consciousness is associated with diffuse delta activity. If focal slowing appears in diabetics, it is likely to be a sign of preexisting focal ischemia or borderline perfusion. Epileptiform activity is rare though hypoglycemic seizures are relatively common. EEG changes reflect absolute levels, the rapidity of the fall in glucose levels, and the duration of hypoglycemia. Although brief episodes can be easily corrected with intravenous or oral glucose administration, the duration of coma increases the likelihood of enduring disability. EEG abnormalities in insulin-dependent individuals should always raise the suspicion of prior episodes of hypoglycemia, which may be nocturnal and go unnoticed by the patient and family. According to Hauser et al[47] there is a correlation between high values of hemoglobin A1c in children and adolescents and decreased relative power of the alpha band. Patients with previous ketoacidotic episodes also have increased relative power of the delta-theta band.

### HYPERGLYCEMIA

Alterations in level of consciousness are more prevalent in nonketotic hyperosmolar hyperglycemia than in diabetic ketoacidosis, reflecting both the higher serum osmolalities (due to glucose and sodium) and the effects of associated medical illness on the encephalopathy.[115] Only high glucose levels (>400 mg/dl) have been associated with EEG changes (a mixture of slow and fast frequencies with sporadic spikes), and those may be due to ketoacidosis, hyperosmolality, or electrolyte imbalance rather than hyperglycemia itself.[40,110] In diabetic ketoacidosis the severity of generalized slowing parallels declining consciousness. Ketosis makes seizures less likely. In contrast, focal seizures with corresponding focal abnormalities, including pseudoperiodic lateralized epileptiform discharges (PLEDs), are common in nonketotic hyperglycemia.[98]

## DIAGNOSIS OF ENCEPHALOPATHY RELATED TO WATER AND ELECTROLYTE IMBALANCE

### HYPOCALCEMIA

Hypocalcemia and hypomagnesemia produce CNS and peripheral nervous system (PNS) irritability, with seizures and tetany being the major clinical manifestations.[92] Hypocalcemia is often associated with hypoparathyroidism. Severe hypocalcemia is very epileptogenic and is associated with prominent EEG diffuse slowing and generalized bursts of spikes.

### HYPERCALCEMIA

In general, hypercalcemia and hypermagnesemia produce CNS and PNS depression with encephalopathy and muscle weakness, respectively.[92] Hypercalcemia occurs in a variety of conditions, including hyperparathyroidism due to parathyroid hyperplasia, renal failure, or skeletal decalcification, vitamin D intoxication, or bony metastases. Clinically the condition manifests itself by a decreased level of consciousness proportional to the blood calcium level and degree of EEG abnormality. EEG findings consist mainly of slowing of the basic rhythm, bursts of 1 to 2/s waves,[81] diffuse theta and delta activity, and, occasionally, triphasic waves.[72] According to Spatz et al,[99] EEG changes may begin to appear at blood calcium levels of approximately 13 mg/dl. With very high calcium levels (>16 mg/dl), focal neurologic deficits appear in association with focal slowing and epileptiform activity (ictal and interictal). Particularly common is a unilateral occipital dysfunction manifested by homonymous hemianopia and seizures.[7,53]

## SODIUM AND OSMOLAR IMBALANCE

Disorders of sodium and osmolality, whether hypernatremia, hyponatremia, hyperosmolality, or hypoosmolality, all produce CNS depression with encephalopathy as the major clinical manifestation.[92] Hyponatremia is associated with mental status changes and severe EEG slowing. Severe hyponatremia and water intoxication may cause generalized status epilepticus—with spike and slow-wave complexes, papilledema, and diffuse EEG slowing in the range of 0.5 to 2/s.[84,119] Hyponatremia is the most common cause of seizures in children with burns.[78] Lithium toxicity is often associated with hyponatremia and diffuse or lateralized epileptiform activity.[102] Rapid correction of lithium toxicity may carry the same risks as rapid correction of hyponatremia (including central pontine myelinolysis). PLEDs and triphasic waves may also occur in patients with hyponatremia.[55]

## DIAGNOSIS OF ISCHEMIC-ANOXIC ENCEPHALOPATHY

### CLINICAL DIAGNOSIS

Ischemic-anoxic encephalopathy occurs in the setting of cardiopulmonary arrest from diverse causes. Rarely, it may result from a failure to provide adequate oxygenation during general anesthesia. The severity and duration of global cerebral ischemia or anoxia is the most important predictor of outcome.

The most important tools for the assessment of ischemic-anoxic encephalopathy remain serial neurologic examinations, which include the Glasgow Coma Scale (Table 9–2), and assessment of brainstem functions.[66]

### ELECTROPHYSIOLOGIC DIAGNOSIS

In the case of cardiac arrest, the cardiac rhythm identified by electrocardiogram (ECG) at the start of resuscitation has a prognostic value. Asystole and electromechanical dissociation usually carry a worse prognosis than does ventricular fibrillation.[12,60] However, the most useful electrophysiologic test in anoxia is the EEG. Indeed, the EEG in anoxia is useful for (1) determining severity and prognosis for recovery; (2) monitoring coma; (3) identifying complicating epileptic, focal (e.g., stroke), or toxic cerebral disorders; and (4) confirming brain death.

The grading of EEG abnormalities for monitoring postanoxic coma and determining the severity and progno-

**TABLE 9–2. Glasgow Coma Scale**

| Eyes | Opens spontaneously | 4 |
|---|---|---|
| | To verbal commands | 3 |
| | To pain | 2 |
| | No response | 1 |
| Best motor response | | |
| To verbal commands | Obeys | 6 |
| To painful stimuli | Localizes pain | 5 |
| | Flexion-withdrawal | 4 |
| | Flexion-abnormal | 3 |
| | Extension | 2 |
| | No response | 1 |
| Best verbal response | Oriented and converses | 5 |
| | Disoriented and converses | 4 |
| | Inappropriate words | 3 |
| | Incomprehensible | 2 |
| | No response | 1 |

Data from Jennett[56] and Teasdale and Jennett.[105]

sis is based on amplitude, spontaneous variability, reactivity to noxious stimuli, the presence of epileptiform activity,[103] and the presence of specific patterns, such as suppression-burst. Electrocerebral inactivity, burst-suppression, and status epilepticus are all associated with a poor prognosis, as are patterns that lack spontaneous variability and reactivity. The prognosis for survival with myoclonic status epilepticus is extremely poor,[66,114] which has led some investigators to conclude that it is an agonal phenomenon associated with irreversible cortical damage. On the other hand, the "frequency and activity-specific" EEG coma patterns such as beta or spindle coma are usually associated with survival and a more favorable prognosis for complete recovery.

The following EEG patterns occur in patients with anoxic encephalopathy but may also be seen in other disorders that affect the brain diffusely or cause multiple bilateral lesions.

### Electrocerebral Inactivity

As defined by the American Electroencephalographic Society,[1] electrocerebral inactivity (ECI) includes the absence of cerebral activity over 2 μV/mm in recordings performed for at least 30 minutes with the use of long inter-electrode distances and periods of vigorous stimulation to test for reactivity. Although used as a supportive measure for the diagnosis of brain death, ECI has certain limitations. The EEG does not actually sample activity from the entire brain. Its prognostic value also depends on the cause of encephalopathy. Patients with drug intoxication or hypothermia who receive aggressive supportive care may occasionally recover completely. However, if these factors are not present, survival is highly unlikely and recovery with independent function does not occur.

### Suppression-Burst Pattern

The suppression-burst pattern consists of moderate to high amplitude, typically 0.5- to 5-second generalized bursts, of mixed frequency activity separated by longer intervals of generalized background suppression or very low amplitude slow activity (Fig. 9–2A). The bursts of activity may contain epileptiform spikes or sharp waves. Myoclonus may or may not be associated with the bursts of activity. Rarely, oral, ocular, or appendicular movements can be asso-

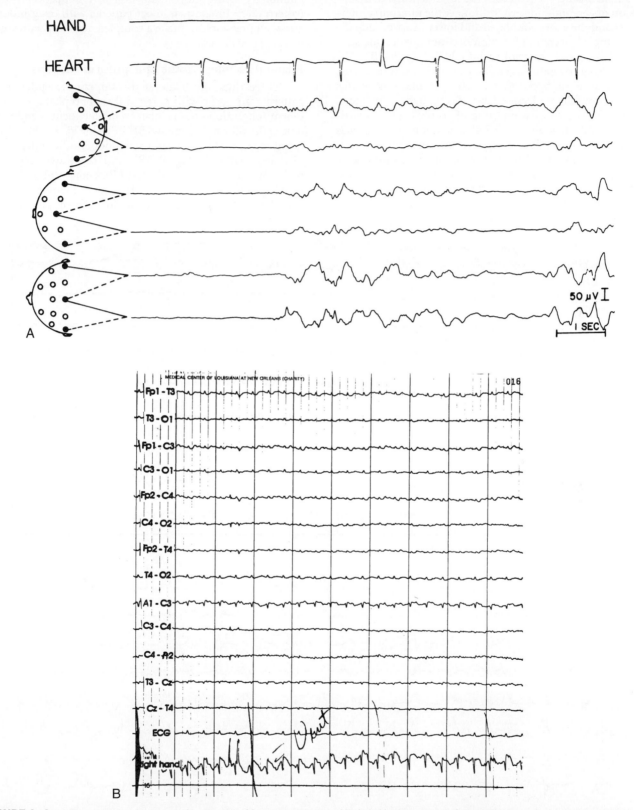

**FIGURE 9–2.** **A,** Burst-suppression pattern in a 60-year-old man in coma caused by lethal barbiturate overdose. **B,** Electrocerebral inactivity (ECI) in a 73-year-old man with left parietal stroke. Thirty-minute stretch of recording was performed with double interelectrode distances of at least 10 cm and sensitivity of 2 μV/mm according to the American Clinical Neurophysiology Society (formerly American EEG Society) guidelines. ECG and ventilator-related artifacts contaminate recording. (*A* reprinted from Fisch BJ. *Spehlmann's EEG Primer,* 2nd ed, 1991, with permission from Elsevier Science.)

ciated with bursts of EEG activity recorded following cerebral anoxic insult.[89] The deeper the level of coma and suppression of cerebral function, the longer the interburst intervals last and the more simplified and lower in amplitude the bursts appear. If cerebral function declines further, the suppression-burst pattern evolves into ECI (Fig. 9–2B). The suppression-burst pattern is usually caused by severe anoxia, drug overdose, or hypothermia. The pathogenesis of this pattern is not fully understood, but it is thought to be due in part to a functional disconnection of cortex from subcortical gray matter structures. Cortical isolation in both animals and humans can produce a suppression-burst pattern. Discrete areas of abnormal human cortex may also produce a localized suppression-burst pattern in response to systemic administration of barbiturates.[100] As with other patterns, etiologic factors play an important role in predicting outcome.[118] Thus, in patients with anoxic coma due to cardiopulmonary arrest, more than 95% with suppression-burst pattern die.[62] In contrast, most patients with drug-induced burst-suppression can make a complete recovery with vigorous supportive care.

## Bilateral Pseudoperiodic Epileptiform Patterns

Three rhythmic bilateral pseudoperiodic epileptiform patterns can occur with either diffuse encephalopathies or bihemispheric lesions: (1) bilateral independent pseudoperiodic epileptiform discharges (BIPLEDs) (Fig. 9–3A); (2) frequent repetitive bisynchronous pseudoperiodic epileptiform discharges (PEDs) (Fig. 9–3B); and (3) slowly repetitive high-amplitude PEDs. Both BIPLEDs and PEDs demonstrate approximately 0.5 to 1.5 Hz single- or multiple-wave complexes that vary in morphology from apiculate to

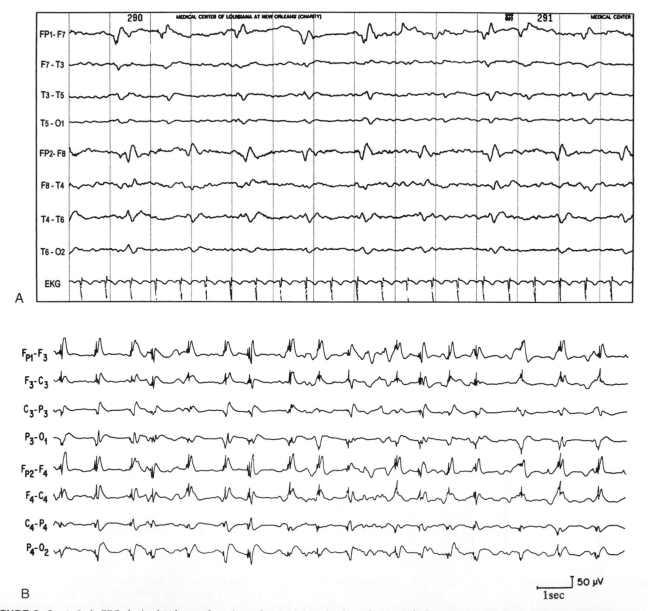

**FIGURE 9–3.** **A,** Scalp EEG obtained 14 hours after seizure showing bilateral independent periodic lateralized epileptiform discharges (BIPLEDs). Recording using Grass Model International 10-20 system. **B,** Pseudoperiodic epileptiform discharges (PEDs) in a 50-year-old woman following cardiac arrest. Discharges are associated with myoclonic jerks (fast components). (*B* from Westmoreland B. In: Vas GA, Cracco JB. *Diffuse Encephalopathies: Current Practice of Clinical Electroencephalography.* New York: Raven Press; 1990.)

blunted and are typically between 50 and 150 μV in amplitude. BIPLEDs are variably asynchronous, with the interhemispheric time difference between waveform complexes usually >200 ms. BIPLEDs typically occur in comatose or obtunded patients with bilateral independent lesions (e.g., bilateral cerebral infarctions, herpes simplex encephalitis) or severe anoxia, often in association with partial or secondarily generalized motor convulsions. PEDs appear as symmetric bisynchronous waveforms with a variety of morphologies, including low-amplitude blunted wave complexes, sharp waves, spikes, and biphasic or multiphasic waves. The intervening background activity is often completely suppressed or consists of very low amplitude theta and delta waveforms. Myoclonus may occur with a variable relationship to the epileptiform discharges. PEDs occur in patients with diffuse encephalopathies mainly because of anoxia, drug intoxication, or disorders associated primarily with myoclonus (e.g., Creutzfeldt-Jakob disease). In coma due to anoxia with PEDs, recovery rarely occurs; when the coma is associated with myoclonus (postanoxic myoclonic status epilepticus), survival is extremely unlikely.[113,114] PEDs caused by drug toxicity have a less certain prognosis. Slowly repetitive high-amplitude PEDs are most commonly seen in the childhood and adolescent disorder of subacute sclerosing panencephalitis (SSPE), rarely in disorders such as tuberous sclerosis,[30] and only exceptionally with lower amplitude anoxia.

The treatment of PEDs and other bisynchronous epileptiform-like patterns (e.g., atypical triphasic waves) in anoxic encephalopathy is controversial. Some regard these patterns as evidence of nonconvulsive status epilepticus, whereas others think they are interictal or are simply a result of cortical injury rather than a cause of continuing coma. Wengs et al[111] reported a case of ifosfamide intoxication in the course of which the patient developed encephalopathy with myoclonus and an EEG pattern with pseudoperiodic atypical triphasic waves. Both alertness and EEG pattern improved after administration of intravenous diazepam. Based on experience, however, even if benzodiazepines attenuate an abnormal EEG pattern, if rapid clinical improvement does not occur, there is little basis to conclude that the encephalopathy is due to nonconvulsive status epilepticus. There has never been a report of clinical improvement in level of consciousness or outcome as a result of anticonvulsant intervention in patients with anoxic coma and PEDs.

## Beta Coma Pattern

Beta coma may appear in postanoxic patients who have received benzodiazepines or barbiturates, but it is usually seen in patients who have overdosed with these substances, either alone or in combination with other drugs. The pattern appears as continuous, prominent, generalized beta activity with variable admixtures of low-amplitude slower theta and delta waveforms. The topography of the beta activity is frontocentral dominant or generalized, similar to that seen in normal drowsiness, but with greater amplitude and persistence. The frequency of drug-induced beta activity is usually in the 15 to 30 Hz range, but, depending on the severity of coma, activity in the lower beta or alpha frequency range may predominate. Because drug-induced beta range activity requires normal cortical function, it is not

surprising that a beta coma pattern predicts substantial recovery if no further cerebral insult occurs and adequate supportive care is given.

## Spindle Coma Pattern

Sleep spindle activity (with or without other EEG features of non-rapid eye movement [NREM sleep]) in comatose or stuporous patients is commonly referred to as the "spindle coma pattern" (Fig. 9–4). Depending on the depth of coma, there may be prominent reactivity with easily evoked K complexes, vertex waves, or background changes. The original descriptions of spindle patterns in coma were in patients with structural abnormalities, particularly head trauma, who were initially unarousable but later regained full consciousness.[20] It was therefore thought that the spindle pattern indicated a reversible arousal disorder caused by direct injury to the brainstem tegmentum. However, subsequent investigators found the pattern to be associated with diverse causes and not consistently associated with a favorable outcome.[52] Hansotia et al[46] found the spindle coma pattern in 6% of 370 consecutive patients evaluated for coma. Only one third of patients with a spindle coma pattern had undergone head trauma. In cases of nontraumatic coma, the most common causes are anoxia and stroke, with only a minority of strokes directly involving the brainstem.[15,46] The likelihood of survival in patients with the spindle coma pattern is intermediate between those with beta coma patterns and with nonreactive background activity.

## Alpha and Theta Coma Patterns

A pattern of sustained, nonreactive, generalized or frontocentral dominant alpha or theta activity with minimal or absent delta or beta activity occurs in patients with coma caused by cardiopulmonary arrest, hypoglycemia, or drug overdose. Depending on which frequency predominates, these patterns are referred to as either "alpha coma"[112] (Fig. 9–5) or "theta coma."[101] Generalized or posterior-dominant alpha patterns that attenuate with passive eye opening or other stimulation suggest a diagnosis of locked-in syndrome, in which the patient may actually be conscious but paralyzed as a result of destruction of the ventral pons. Alpha coma due to drug overdose is often associated with the typical anesthetic pattern of anterior-dominant alpha with intermixed low to moderate delta activity. In contrast, alpha or theta coma due to hypoxia may not be associated with significant admixtures of other frequencies and will appear as a sustained uniform frequency.

The incidence of alpha coma following cardiopulmonary arrest is approximately 5%. The pathogenesis is unclear, but as pointed out by Chatrian,[19] it is not likely to be a distortion of the normal alpha rhythm for the following reasons: (1) it occurs as an inappropriately fast rhythm in infants and children with anoxic coma; (2) it has a different topography from the alpha rhythm; and (3) it is nonreactive. Gurvitch et al[44] have proposed that the amygdala is the pacemaker of the alpha coma pattern because of their observations in dogs recovering from circulatory arrest in which rhythmic alpha activity occurred first in the amygdala and later in the thalamus, basal ganglia, and cortex. Young et al[117] have proposed that the alpha coma pattern is a sign of thalamocortical dysfunction. This theory is supported by the case of a patient with fatal familial insomnia and alpha coma in whom neuronal loss was limited to the anterior and dorsomedial nuclei of the thalamus.[68] Chatrian[19] noted that in some patients in coma there is a combination of alpha and theta waveforms with little or no delta or beta activity. Young et al[117] refer to this effect as the alpha-theta coma pattern. In their study of 50 patients with alpha (10 patients), theta (16 patients), or alpha-theta (24 patients) coma, Young and colleagues found no significant difference with regard to recovery of consciousness. None of their patients suffered from drug overdose, and most had anoxic-ischemic events. Recovery of consciousness occurred in 20% of those with alpha, 25% of those with alpha-theta, and 12.5% of those with theta coma pattern. Their results are similar to those of others and emphasize the importance of considering the etiologic basis. Iraqui and McCutchen[54] found that 10 of 86 (12%) patients with alpha coma survived, whereas 7 of 8 patients (88%) with respiratory arrest survived. Similarly, patients with brainstem strokes usually do not survive, whereas those with drug overdose and the alpha-delta anesthetic pattern recover. Additional important information is obtained through serial recordings. The alpha, theta, and alpha-theta patterns occur transiently and may be succeeded by various reactive patterns, generalized slowing, or more ominous patterns such as suppression-burst or ECI. The progression from alpha to theta coma is currently thought to be a poor prognostic sign. The appearance of increasingly benign patterns, particularly of reactivity to loud auditory or noxious tactile stimulation, predicts a favorable prognosis in most cases and provides encouragement for vigorous supportive care.

## Low-Amplitude EEG

The voltage of alpha rhythm is <20 µV in 10% to 28% of adults[82]; however, a recording in an adult in which no activity exceeds 10 µV (including sleep) or one in an infant or young child in which no activity exceeds 20 µV, is abnormal. As metabolic, toxic, or inflammatory encephalopathies become increasingly severe, the overall amplitude of the EEG declines and periods of flattening or burst-suppression appear prior to ECI.[30]

EPs have been of limited use in the evaluation of anoxic encephalopathy.[63] They are etiologically nonspecific and must be carefully integrated into the clinical situation.[50] Both brainstem auditory evoked potentials (BAEPs) and somatosensory evoked potentials (SSEPs) may indicate brainstem dysfunction and can be used for determination of prognosis.[66] SSEPs are perhaps more useful because they allow for an assessment of thalamocortical function.[37,41,104] Thus the absence of a short latency median nerve N20 response is associated with an extremely poor prognosis for survival.[16,59,69,94]

## Neuroimaging

Classic CT and magnetic resonance (MR) neuroimaging in hypoxic encephalopathy shows a loss of gray-white matter differentiation and cortical edema.

Positron emission tomography (PET)[28] has been used to define whole-brain ischemia and foci of critical ischemic regions (tissue at risk). Diffusion-weighted MRI and advances in MR spectroscopy have enhanced our ability to detect cere-

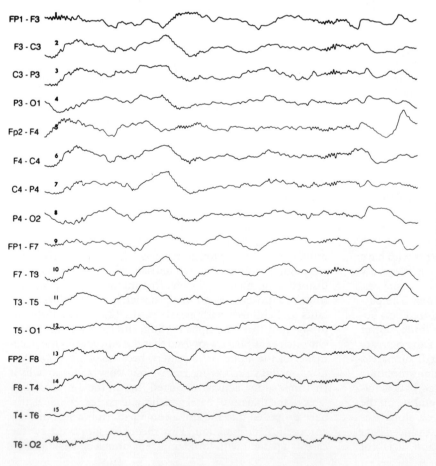

**FIGURE 9–4.** "Spindle coma" pattern in a 29-year-old. Low-voltage (5 Hz and 1 Hz) activity is joined by 14 Hz spindles. Calibration signal is 1 second and 50 µV. (From Blume WT, Kaibara M. *Atlas of Adult Electroencephalography.* New York: Raven Press; 1995.)

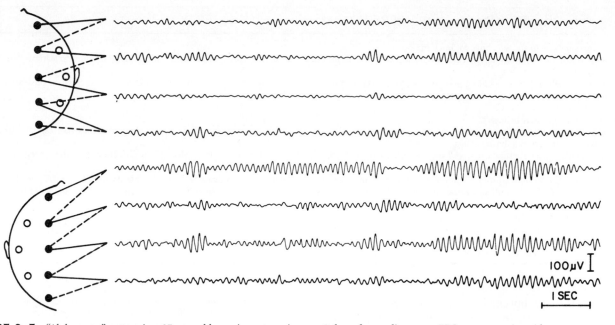

**FIGURE 9–5.** "Alpha coma" pattern in a 27-year-old man in postanoxic coma 2 days after cardiac arrest. EEG was unreactive without spontaneous variability. Follow-up EEG 9 days later showed generalized very low amplitude slow waves. Patient died 3 weeks later without regaining consciousness. (Reprinted from Fisch BJ. *Spehlmann's EEG Primer,* 2nd ed, 1991, with permission from Elsevier Science.)

bral ischemia shortly after onset,[33] guiding diagnosis and potentially helping in the development of acute interventions to improve outcome. Single photon emission computed tomography (SPECT)[79,107] has definite value in the evaluation of cerebrovascular disease and may have a role in the diagnosis of brain death.

## LABORATORY DIAGNOSIS

Except for blood glucose levels on admission, routine laboratory tests are not helpful for prognostication. A high blood glucose level preceding a cardiac arrest is associated with more severe brain injury. Creatine kinase (CK) activity peaks in the CSF 48 to 72 hours following global cerebral ischemia. In one large study the CSF CK activity was significantly higher in subjects who never awakened (mean 120 U/L) than in those who did (mean 10 U/L).[67] Its brain-specific isoenzyme (CK-BB) and neuron-specific enolase (NSE) levels in the CSF are prognostic indicators of hypoxic brain injury when measured 28 to 76 hours after cardiac arrest, whereas blood samples have no prognostic value.[58] Northern hybridization of ribosome-bound RNA revealed a discrete band of messenger RNA (mRNA) for CK-BB in experimentally induced global cerebral ischemia in animals.[25]

## BRAIN DEATH

In 1968 an ad hoc committee of Harvard faculty publicly redefined death as "brain death."[39] In 1995 the American Academy of Neurology (AAN) issued a summary statement on "Practice Parameters for Determining Brain Death in Adults."[90] That statement is reproduced in its entirety in Appendix 9–1. Criteria for determination of brain death are presented in Table 9–3.[17]

Currently, brain death is considered a clinical diagnosis. A repeat clinical evaluation 6 hours following the initial examination is recommended, but this interval is arbitrary.

One of the most important aspects of the diagnostic evaluation of brain death is demonstration of apnea[113] because it is a manifestation of brainstem function loss. The "Guidelines for the Determination of Death" submitted in the "Report of the Medical Consultants on the Diagnosis of Death to the President's Commission for the Study of Ethical Problems in Medicine and Biomedical and Behavioral Research" recommend that apnea testing be performed with partial pressure of carbon dioxide in arterial blood ($PaCO_2$) levels >60 mm Hg for maximal stimulation of the brainstem.[43] The EEG is considered the most readily available and reliable confirmatory test of brain death, but strict technical criteria as defined by the American Electroencephalographic Society must be fulfilled[1] (Figure 9–2B). The main difficulty in EEG interpretation is usually caused by artifact, which readily occurs at the high amplifier gains used during testing. When present, muscle artifact can usually be eliminated with neuromuscular blockers.

Unresponsiveness is judged by a lack of motor responses following painful stimulation (supraorbital and nailbed pressure) with the caveat that some spinal reflexes, such as the "Lazarus sign,"[93] can be precipitated by nonspecific stimuli (e.g., hypoxia) during apnea testing in brain-dead patients. Reflex spinal myoclonus should also be disregarded.[21,83]

Caloric testing should be done with the patient's head elevated to 30 degrees during irrigation of the tympanum with 50 ml of ice water in each ear. Tympanum irrigation can be performed easily by inserting a small catheter into the external auditory canal and connecting it to a 50 ml syringe filled with ice water. Tonic deviation of the eyes toward the cold stimulus is absent in brain death. Up to 1 minute should be allowed after injection, and the time between stimulation on each side should be at least 5 minutes.

There has been considerable variability in the diagnostic approach to brain death in infants and children,[75] although the guidelines are well established.[4] Diagnosis of

**TABLE 9–3. Criteria for Determination of Brain Death**

1. Coma, unresponsive to stimuli above foramen magnum.
2. Apnea off ventilator (with oxygenation) for a duration sufficient to produce hyperbaric respiratory drive (usually 10 to 20 minutes to achieve $Pco_2$ of 50 to 60 mm Hg).
3. Absence of cephalic reflexes, including pupillary, oculocephalic, oculovestibular (caloric), corneal, gag sucking, swallowing, and extensor posturing. Purely spinal reflexes may be present, including tendon reflexes, plantar responses, and limb flexion to noxious stimuli.
4. Body temperature above 34° C.
5. Systemic circulation may be intact.
6. Diagnosis known to be structural disease or irreversible metabolic disturbance; absence of drug intoxication, including ethanol, sedatives, potentially anesthetizing agents, or paralyzing drugs.
7. In adults with known structural cause and without involvement of drugs or ethanol, at least 6 hours of absent brain function; for others, including those with anoxic-ischemic brain damage, at least 24 hours' observation plus negative drug screen.
8. Diagnosis of brain death inappropriate in infants younger than 7 days of age. Observation of at least 48 hours for infants aged 7 days to 2 months, at least 24 hours for those aged 2 months to 1 year, and at least 12 hours for those aged 1 to 5 years (24 hours if anoxic-ischemic brain damage). For older children, adult criteria apply.
9. Optional confirmatory studies include:
   a. EEG isoelectric for 30 minutes at maximal gain
   b. Absent brainstem evoked responses
   c. Absent cerebral circulation demonstrated by radiographic, radioisotope, or magnetic resonance angiography

brain death is inappropriate in infants younger than 7 days. Observation of at least 48 hours is required for infants aged 7 days to 2 months, at least 24 hours for those aged 2 months to 1 year, and at least 12 hours for those aged 1 to 5 years (24 hours with anoxic-ischemic brain damage).[17,105] For older children adult criteria apply. As noted by Fishman,[34] one of the most important factors to consider in irreversible coma and brain death is the cause of coma.

## THE PERSISTENT VEGETATIVE STATE

The persistent vegetative state (PVS) was clinically defined by the American Neurological Association (ANA) Committee on Ethical Affairs in 1993.[2] In 1995 the AAN issued a summary statement entitled "Practice Parameters: Assessment and Management of Patients in the Persistent Vegetative State."[91] The guidelines are based on clinical observations, and the diagnosis of PVS does not require specialized ancillary tests. As noted by Ashwal et al,[5] the PVS parameters developed by the AAN Quality Standards Subcommittee represent the first step in the national consensus toward this goal. The vegetative state is a clinical condition of complete unawareness of the self and the environment accompanied by sleep-wake cycles with either complete or partial preservation of hypothalamic and brainstem autonomic functions. The criteria include (1) no awareness of self or environment (no interaction); (2) no evidence of purposeful behavioral responses to sensory or noxious stimuli; (3) no evidence of language comprehension or expression; (4) intermittent wakefulness with sleep-wake cycles; (5) sufficiently preserved autonomic functions to permit survival with medical and nursing care; (6) bowel and bladder incontinence; and (7) variably preserved cranial and spinal reflexes. The PVS can be diagnosed as persistent at 1 month after a traumatic injury and at 3 months for nontraumatic injury in adults and children after careful, repeated neurologic examinations. Once PVS is considered to be permanent, a "Do not resuscitate" (DNR) order is appropriate.

## REFERENCES

1. American Electroencephalographic Society guidelines in electroencephalography, evoked potentials, and polysomnography. Guideline three: minimum technical standards for EEG recording in suspected cerebral death. J Clin Neurophysiol. 1986;3(suppl 1):12;1995;11:10.
2. ANA Committee on Ethical Affairs. Issues in clinical neuroscience. Persistent vegetative state: report of the American Neurological Association Committee for Ethical Affairs. Ann Neurol. 1993;33(4):386.
3. Aoki Y, Lombroso CT. Prognostic value of electroencephalography in Reye's syndrome. Neurology. 1974;23:333.
4. Ashwal S. Brain death in early infancy. J Heart Lung Transplant. 1993;12(6 pt 2):S176.
5. Ashwal S, Cranford RE, Rosenberg JH. Commentary on the practice parameters for the persistent vegetative state. Neurology. 1995;45:859.
6. Bale JF Jr, Siegler RL, Bray PF. Encephalopathy in young children with moderate chronic renal failure. Am J Dis Child. 1980;134(6):581.
7. Barolin GS, Karbowski K. Okzipitale Krisen im "Grenzland der Epilepsie." Z EEG-EMG. 1973;4:1.
8. Berger H. Das Elektrenkephalogramm des Menschen. 12 Mittlg. Arch Psychiatr Nervenkr. 1937;106:165.
9. Berger H. On the electroencephalogram of man. Electroencephalogr Clin Neurophysiol. 1969;28:267.
10. Bickford RG, Butt HR. Hepatic coma: the electroencephalographic pattern. J Clin Invest. 1955;34:790.
11. Bjorgaas M, Sand T, Gimse R. Quantitative EEG in type 1 diabetic children with and without episodes of severe hypoglycemia: a controlled blind study. Acta Neurol Scand. 1996;93(6):398.
12. Bonnin MJ, Pepe PE, Kimball KJ, Clark PS Jr. Distinct criteria for termination of resuscitation in the out-of-hospital setting. JAMA. 1993;270:1457.
13. Brazier MAB, Finesinger J, Schwab RS. Characteristics of normal electroencephalogram. II. The effect of varying sugar levels on the occipital cortical potentials in adults during quiet breathing. J Clin Invest. 1944;23:313.
14. Brazier MAB, Finesinger J, Schwab RS. Characteristics of normal electroencephalogram. III. The effect of varying sugar levels on the occipital cortical potentials in adults during hyperventilation. J Clin Invest. 1944;23:319.
15. Britt CW. Nontraumatic "spindle coma": clinical, EEG and prognostic features. Neurology. 1981;31:393.
16. Brunko E, Zegers de Beyl D. Prognostic value of early cortical somatosensory evoked potentials after resuscitation from cardiac arrest. Electroencephalogr Clin Neurophysiol. 1987;66:15.
17. Brust JCM. Coma. In: Rowland LP, ed. Merritt's Textbook of Neurology. 9th ed. Baltimore: Williams & Wilkins; 1995:19.
18. Cadilhac J. The EEG in renal insufficiency. In: Remond A, ed. Handbook of Electroencephalography and Clinical Neurophysiology, vol 15C. Amsterdam: Elsevier; 1976:351.
19. Chatrian GE. Coma, other states of altered responsiveness and brain death. In: Daly DD, Pedley TA, eds. Current Practice of Clinical Electroencephalography. 2nd ed. New York: Raven Press; 1990:425.
20. Chatrian GE, White LW, Daly D. Electroencephalographic patterns resembling those of sleep in certain comatose states after injuries to the head. Electroencephalogr Clin Neurophysiol. 1963;15:272.

21. Christie JM, O'Lenic TD, Cane RD. Head turning in brain death. *J Clin Anesth.* 1996;8(2):141.
22. Cooper AJ, Plum F. Biochemistry and physiology of brain ammonia. *Physiol Rev.* 1987;67(2):440.
23. Davis ID, Chang P-N, Nevins TE. Successful renal transplantation accelerates development in young uremic children. *Pediatrics.* 1990;86:594.
24. Dedeoglu IO, Springate JE, Najdzionek JS, Feld LG. Hypertensive encephalopathy and reversible magnetic resonance imaging changes in a renal transplant patient. *Pediatr Nephrol.* 1996;10(6):769.
25. DeGracia DJ, O'Neil BJ, Frisch C, et al. Studies of the protein synthesis system in the brain cortex during global ischemia and reperfusion. *Resuscitation.* 1993;25(2):161.
26. Drury I. 14 and 6 positive bursts in childhood encephalopathies. *Electroencephalogr Clin Neurophysiol.* 1989;72:479.
27. Elzouki A, Carroll J, Butinar D, Moosa A. Improved neurological outcome in children with chronic renal disease from infancy. *Pediatr Nephrol.* 1994;8(2):205.
28. Enblad P, Valtysson J, Andersson J, et al. Simultaneous intracerebral microdialysis and positron emission tomography in th detection of ischemia in patients with subarachnoid hemorrhage. *J Cereb Blood Flow Metab.* 1996;16(4):637.
29. Fenichel GM. Paroxysmal disorders: urea cycle disturbances. In: *Clinical Pediatric Neurology: A Signs and Symptoms Approach.* 3rd ed. Philadelphia: WB Saunders; 1997:10.
30. Fisch BJ. *Spehlmann's EEG Primer.* 2nd ed. Amsterdam: Elsevier; 1991.
31. Fisch BJ, Klass DW. The diagnostic specificity of triphasic wave patterns. *Electroencephalogr Clin Neurophysiol.* 1988;70:1.
32. Fisch BJ, Hauser WA, Brust JCM, et al. The EEG response to diffuse and patterned photic stimulation during acute untreated alcohol withdrawal. *Neurology.* 1989;39:434.
33. Fisher M, Prichard JW, Warach S. New magnetic resonance techniques for acute ischemic stroke. *JAMA.* 1995;274(11):908.
34. Fishman MA. Validity of brain death criteria in infants. *Pediatrics.* 1995;96(3):513. Commentaries.
35. Foley CM, Polinsky MS, Gruskin AB, et al. Encephalopathy in infants and children with chronic renal disease. *Arch Neurol.* 1981;38(10):656.
36. Foley JM, Watson CW, Adams RD. Significance of electroencephalographic changes in hepatic coma. *Trans Am Neurol Assoc.* 1950;75:161.
37. Ganji S, Peters G, Frazier E. Somatosensory and brainstem auditory evoked potential studies in nontraumatic coma. *Clin Electroencephalogr.* 1988;31:248.
38. Geary DF, Fennel RS, Andriola M, et al. Encephalopathy in children with chronic renal failure. *J Pediatr.* 1980;97(1);41.
39. Giacomini M. A change of heart and a change of mind? Technology and the redefinition of death in 1968. *Soc Sci Med.* 1997;44(10):1465.
40. Gibbs FA, Williams D, Gibbs EL. Modification of the cortical frequency spectrum by changes in $CO_2$, blood sugar and $O_2$. *J Neurophysiol.* 1940;3:49.
41. Goldie WD, Chiappa KH, Young RR, Brooks EB. Brainstem auditory and short-latency somatosensory evoked responses in brain death. *Neurology.* 1981;31:248.
42. Groenweg M, Gyr K, Amrein R, et al. Effect of flumazenil on the electroencephalogram of patients with portosystemic encephalopathy: results of a double-blind, randomised, placebo-controlled multicentre trial. *Electroencephalogr Clin Neurophysiol.* 1996;98(1):29.
43. Guidelines for the Determination of Death: Report of the Medical Consultants on the Diagnosis of Death to the President's Commission for the Study of Ethical Problems in Medicine and Biomedical and Behavioral Research. *JAMA.* 1981;246:2184.
44. Gurvitch AM, Zarzhetsky YV, Trush VD, Zonov VM. Experimental data on the nature of postresuscitation alpha frequency activity. *Electroencephalogr Clin Neurophysiol.* 1984;58:426.
45. Gyr K, Meier R, Haussler J, et al. Evaluation of the efficacy and safety of flumazenil in the treatment of portal systemic encephalopathy: a double-blind, randomised, placebo-controlled multicentre study. *Gut.* 1996;39(2):319.
46. Hansotia P, Gottschalk P, Green P, Zais D. Spindle coma: incidence, clinicopathologic correlates, and prognostic value. *Neurology.* 1981;31:83.
47. Hauser E, Strohmayer C, Seidl R, et al. Quantitative EEG in young diabetics. *J Child Neurol.* 1995;10(4):330.
48. Hauser RA, Lacey DM, Knight MR. Hypertensive encephalopathy: magnetic resonance imaging demonstration of reversible cortical and white matter lesions. *Arch Neurol.* 1988;45:1078.
49. Hauser RA, Zesiewicz TA, Martinez C, et al. Blood manganese correlates with brain magnetic resonance imaging changes in patients with liver disease. *Can J Neurol Sci.* 1996;23(2):95.
50. Hill RA, Chiappa KH. Electrophysiologic monitoring in the intensive care unit. *Can J Neurol Sci.* 1994;21(2):S12.
51. Hughes JR. Correlations between EEG and chemical changes in uremia. *Clin Neurophysiol.* 1980;48:583.
52. Hulihan JF, Syna DR. Electroencephalographic sleep patterns in postanoxic stupor and coma. *Neurology.* 1994;44:758.
53. Huott AD, Madison DS, Niedermeyer E. Occipital lobe epilepsy: a clinical and electroencephalographic study. *Eur Neurol.* 1974;11:325.
54. Iraqui VJ, McCutchen CB. Physiologic and prognostic significance of "alpha coma." *J Neurol Neurosurg Psychiatry.* 1983;46:632.
55. Itoh N, Matsui N, Matsui S. Periodic lateralized epileptiform discharges in EEG during recovery from hyponatremia: a case report. *Clin Electroencephalogr.* 1994;25(4):164.
56. Jacob JC, Gloor P, Elwan OH, Dossetor JB, Pateras VR. Electroencephalographic changes in chronic renal failure. *Neurology.* 1965;15:419.
57. Jennett B. Some aspects of prognosis after severe head injury. *Scand J Rehab Med.* 1972;4(1):16.
58. Karkela J, Bock E, Kaukinen S. CSF and serum brain-specific creatine kinase isoenzyme (CK-BB), neuron-specific enolase (NSE) and neural cell adhesion molecule (NCAM) as prognostic markers for hypoxic brain injury after cardiac arrest in man. *J Neurol Sci.* 1993;116(1):100.
59. Karnaze D, Fisher M, Ahmadi J, Gott P. Short latency somatosensory evoked potentials correlate with the severity of the neurological deficit and sensory abnormalities following cerebral ischemia. *Electroencephalogr Clin Neurophysiol.* 1987;67:147.
60. Kellerman AL, Hackman BB, Somos G. Predicting the outcome of unsuccessful prehospital advanced cardiac life support. *JAMA.* 1993;270:1433.
61. Kulisevsky J, Pujol J, Balanzo J, et al. Pallidal hyperintensity on magnetic resonance imaging in cirrhotic patients: clinical correlations. *Hepatology.* 1992;16(6):1382.
62. Kuroiwa Y, Celesia GG, Chung HD. Periodic EEG discharges and status spongiosus of the cerebral cortex in anoxic encephalopathy: a necropsy case report. *J Neurol Neurosurg Psychiatry.* 1982;45(8):740.
63. Ledsome JR, Cole C, Sharp-Kehl JM. Somatosensory evoked potentials during hypoxia and hypocapnia in conscious humans. *Can J Anaesth.* 1996;43(10):1025.
64. Lockwood AH. Neurologic complications of renal disease. *Neurol Clin.* 1989;7:617.
65. Lockwood AH. Hepatic encephalopathy and other neurological disorders associated with gastrointestinal disease. In: Aminoff MJ, ed. *Neurology and General Medicine: The Neurological Aspects of Medical Disorders.* 2nd ed. New York: Churchill Livingstone; 1995:247.
66. Longstreth WT Jr. Neurological complications of cardiac arrest. In: Aminoff, MJ, ed. *Neurology and General Medicine.* 2nd ed. New York: Churchill Livingstone; 1995:159.
67. Longstreth WT Jr, Clayson KJ, Chandler WL, Sumi SM. Cerebrospinal fluid creatine kinase activity and neurologic recovery after cardiac arrest. *Neurology.* 1984;34:834.
68. Lugaresi E, Medori R, Montagna P, et al. Fatal familial insomnia and dysautonomia with selective degeneration of thalamic nuclei. *N Engl J Med.* 1986;315(16):997.
69. Madl C, Grimm G, Kramer L, et al. Early prediction of individual outcome after cardiopulmonary resuscitation. *Lancet.* 1993;341.
70. Mahoney CA, Arieff AI. Uremic encephalopathies: clinical, biochemical, and experimental features. *Am J Kidney Dis.* 1982;2(3):324.
71. Malouf R, Brust JCM. Hypoglycemia: causes, neurological manifestations, and outcome. *Ann Neurol.* 1985;17:421.
72. Marchau MMB. Das Elektroenzephalogramm bei Hyperkalzamie. *Z EEG-EMG.* 1982;13:61.
73. Al Mardini H, Leonard J, Bartlett K, et al. Effect of methionine loading and endogenous hypermethioninemia on blood mercaptans in man. *Clin Chim Acta.* 1988;176(1):83.
74. Marra TR, Shah M, Mikus MA. Transient cortical blindness due to hypertensive encephalopathy: magnetic resonance imaging correlation. *J Clin Neuroophthalmol.* 1993;13(1):35.
75. Mejia RE, Pollack MM. Variability in brain death determination practices in children. *JAMA.* 1995;274(7):550.
76. Menkes JH. Metabolic diseases of the nervous system. In: Menkes JH, ed. *Textbook of Child Neurology.* 5th ed. Baltimore: Williams & Wilkins; 1995:29.

77. Menkes JH, Hurvitz CGH, McDiarmid SV, Williams RG. Neurologic manifestations of systemic disease. In: Menkes JH, ed. *Textbook of Child Neurology.* 5th ed. Baltimore: Williams & Wilkins; 1995:873.

78. Mukhdoni GJ, Desai MH, Herndon DN. Seizure disorder in burned children: a retrospective review. *Burns.* 1996;22(4):316.

79. Mullan BP, O'Connor MK, Hung JC. Single photon emission computed tomography brain imaging. *Neurosurg Clin Am.* 1996;7(4):617.

80. Muller HF, Kral VA. The electroencephalogram in advanced senile dementia. *J Am Geriatr Soc.* 1967;15:415.

81. Niedermeyer E. Metabolic central nervous system disorders. In: Niedermeyer E, da Silva FL, eds. *Electroencephalography: Basic Principles, Clinical Applications, and Related Fields.* 3rd ed. Baltimore: Williams & Wilkins; 1993:405.

82. Niedermeyer E. The normal EEG of the waking adult. In: Niedermeyer E, da Silva FL, eds. *Electroencephalography: Basic Principles, Clinical Applications, and Related Fields.* 3rd ed. Baltimore: Williams & Wilkins; 1993:131.

83. Nokura K, Yamamoto H, Uchida M, Hashizume Y, Inagaki T. Automatic movements of extremities induced in primary massive brain lesion with apneic coma. *Rinsho Shinkeigaku.* 1997;37(3):198. English abstract.

84. Okura M, Nagamine I, Okada K, et al. EEG changes during and after water intoxication. *Electroencephalogr Clin Neurophysiol.* 1990;75: S110. Abstract.

85. Passer JA. Cerebral atrophy in end-stage uremia. *Proc Dialysis Transplant Forum.* 1977;7:91.

86. Peroux JL, Paolini O, Tran A, et al. Encephalopathie hepatique chronique traitee de facon prolongee en ambulatoire par flumazenil intraveineux. [Chronic hepatic encephalopathy treated by long-term intravenous administration of flumazenil in ambulatory care.] *Gastroenterol Clin Biol.* 1996;20(1):106.

87. Pujol J, Kulisevsky J, Moreno A, et al. Neurospectroscopic alterations and globus pallidus hyperintensity as related magnetic resonance markers of reversible hepatic encephalopathy. *Neurology.* 1996;47(6): 1526.

88. Quero JC, Hartmann IJ, Meulstee J, et al. The diagnosis of subclinical hepatic encephalopathy in patients with cirrhosis using neuropsychological testing and automated electroencephalogram analysis. *Hepatology.* 1996;24(3):556.

89. Reeves AL, Westmoreland BF, Klass DW. Clinical accompaniments of the burst-suppression EEG pattern. *J Clin Neurophysiol.* 1997;14(2): 150.

90. Report of the Quality Standards Subcommittee of the American Academy of Neurology. Practice parameters for determining brain death in adults. *Neurology.* 1995;45:1012.

91. Report of the Quality Standards Subcommittee of the American Academy of Neurology. Practice parameters: assessment and management of patients in the persistent vegetative state (summary statement). *Neurology.* 1995;45:1015.

92. Riggs JE. Neurologic manifestations of fluid and electrolyte disturbances. *Neurol Clin.* 1989;7(3):509.

93. Ropper AH. Unusual spontaneous movements in brain-dead patients. *Neurology.* 1984;34:1089.

94. Rothstein TL, Tomas EM, Sumi SM. Predicting outcome in hypoxic ischemic coma: a prospective clinical and electrophysiologic study. *Electroencephalogr Clin Neurophysiol.* 1991;79:101.

95. Schaul N, Gloor P, Gotman J. The EEG in deep midline lesions. *Neurology.* 1981;31:157.

96. Schilsky ML. Wilson disease: genetic basis of copper toxicity and natural history. *Semin Liver Dis.* 1996;16(1):83.

97. Sharbrough F. Nonspecific abnormal EEG patterns. In: Niedermeyer E, da Silva FL, eds. *Electroencephalography: Basic Principles, Clinical Applications, and Related Fields.* 3rd ed. Baltimore: Williams & Wilkins; 1993:197.

98. Singh BM, Gupta DR, Strobos RJ. Nonketotic hyperglycemia and epilepsia partialis continua. *Arch Neurol.* 1973;29:187.

99. Spatz R, Kugler J, Angstwurm H. Zur Bedeutung elektroenzephalographischen Veranderungen beim Hyperkalzamie-Syndrom. *Z EEG-EMG.* 1977;8:70.

100. Sperling MR, Brown WJ, Crandall PH. Focal burst-suppression induced by thiopental. *Electroencephalogr Clin Neurophysiol.* 1986;63(3):203.

101. Suter C. Theta coma. *Neurology.* 1973;23:445.

102. Swartz CM, Dolinar RJ. Encephalopathy associated with rapid decrease of high levels of lithium. *Comment Ann Clin Psychiatry.* 1996; 8(2):111.

103. Synek VM. Value of a revised EEG coma scale for prognosis after cerebral anoxia and diffuse head injury. *Clin Electroencephalogr.* 1990; 21(1):25.

104. Synek VM, Trubuhovich RV. Important abnormalities in recordings of somatosensory evoked potentials in coma. *Clin Electroencephalogr.* 1991;22(2):118.

105. Task Force on Brain Death in Children. Guidelines for the determination of brain death in children. *Pediatrics.* 1987;80:298.

106. Teasdale G, Jennett B. Assessment of coma and impaired consciousness: a practical scale. *Lancet.* 1974;2(872):81.

107. Toyama H, Takeshita G, Shibata K, et al. [Evaluation of the clinical usefulness of super dynamic 99mTc-HM-PAO SPECT in ischemic cerebrovascular disease: detection of hypoperfusion and hyperperfusion area.] *Kaku Igaku.* 1996;33(5):521. English abstract.

108. Tribl G, Howorka K, Heger G, et al. EEG topography during insulin-induced hypoglycemia in patients with insulin-dependent diabetes mellitus. *Eur Neurol.* 1996;36(5):303.

109. Tyler RH. Neurologic disorders in renal failure. *Am J Med.* 1968; 44:734.

110. Vas GA, Cracco JB. Diffuse encephalopathies. In: Daly DD, Pedley TA, eds. *Current Practice of Clinical Electroencephalography.* 2nd ed. New York: Raven Press; 1990:371.

111. Wengs WJ, Talwar D, Bernard J. Ifosfamide-induced nonconvulsive status epilepticus. *Arch Neurol.* 1993;50:1104.

112. Westmoreland BF, Klass DW, Sharbrough FW, Reagan TJ. Alpha coma: electroencephalographic, clinical, pathologic and etiologic correlations. *Arch Neurol.* 1975;32:713.

113. Wijdicks EFM. Determining brain death in adults. *Neurology.* 1995;45:1003. Special article.

114. Wijdicks EFM, Parisi JE, Sharbrough FW. The prognostic value of myoclonic status epilepticus in postanoxic coma. *Ann Neurol.* 1993;34: 298.

115. Windebank AJ, McEvoy. Diabetes and the nervous system. In: Aminoff MJ, ed. *Neurology and General Medicine.* 2nd ed. New York: Churchill Livingstone; 1995:349.

116. Yamada T, Young S, Kimura J. Significance of positive spike bursts in Reye's syndrome. *Arch Neurol.* 1977;34:376.

117. Young GB, Blume WT, Campbell VM, et al. Alpha, theta and alpha-theta coma: a clinical outcome study utilizing serial recordings. *Electroencephalogr Clin Neurophysiol.* 1994;91:93.

118. Zaret BS. Prognostic and neurophysiological implications of concurrent burst suppression and alpha patterns in the EEG of post-anoxic coma. *Electroencephalogr Clin Neurophysiol.* 1985;61(4):199.

119. Zwang HJ, Cohn D. Electroencephalographic changes in acute water intoxication. *Clin Electroencephalogr.* 1981;12:35.

# $9-1$

# Practice Parameters for Determining Brain Death in Adults

## (Summary Statement)

## OVERVIEW

Brain death is defined as the irreversible loss of function of the brain, including the brainstem. Brain death from primary neurologic disease usually is caused by severe head injury or aneurysmal subarachnoid hemorrhage. In medical and surgical intensive care units, however, hypoxic-ischemic brain insults and fulminant hepatic failure may result in irreversible loss of brain function. In large referral hospitals, neurologists make the diagnosis of brain death 25 to 30 times a year.

## JUSTIFICATION

Brain death was selected as a topic for practice parameters because of the need for standardization of the neurologic examination criteria for the diagnosis of brain death. Currently, there are differences in clinical practice in performing the apnea test and controversies over appropriate confirmatory laboratory tests. This document outlines the clinical criteria for brain death and the procedures of testing in patients older than 18 years.

## DESCRIPTION OF THE PROCESS

All literature pertaining to brain death identified by MEDLINE for the years 1976 to 1994 was reviewed. The key words "brain death" and "apnea test" (subheading, "adult") were used. Peer-reviewed articles with original work were selected. Current textbooks of neurology, medicine, pulmonology, intensive care, and anesthesia were reviewed for

This statement is provided as an educational service of the American Academy of Neurology. It is based on an assessment of current scientific and clinical information. It is not intended to include all possible proper methods of care for a particular neurologic problem or all legitimate criteria for choosing to use a specific procedure. Neither is it intended to exclude any reasonable alternative methods. The AAN recognizes that specific decisions on patient care are the prerogative of the patient and the physician caring for the patient and are based on all the circumstances involved. Regardless of the conclusions of this statement, the Quality Standards Subcommittee of the AAN recognizes the need to comply with the state law.

opinion. On the basis of this review and expert opinion, recommendations are presented as standards, guidelines, or options. *The recommendations in this document are guidelines unless otherwise specified (see boxed Definitions, p. 128).*

## I. DIAGNOSTIC CRITERIA FOR CLINICAL DIAGNOSIS OF BRAIN DEATH

A. Prerequisites. Brain death is the absence of clinical brain function when the proximate cause is known and demonstrably irreversible.

1. Clinical or neuroimaging evidence of an acute CNS catastrophe that is compatible with the clinical diagnosis of brain death
2. Exclusion of complicating medical conditions that may confound clinical assessment (no severe electrolyte, acid-base, or endocrine disturbance)
3. No drug intoxication or poisoning
4. Core temperature ≥32° C (90° F)

B. The three cardinal findings in brain death are coma or unresponsiveness, absence of brainstem reflexes, and apnea.

1. Coma or unresponsiveness—no cerebral motor response to pain in all extremities (nail-bed pressure and supraorbital pressure)
2. Absence of brainstem reflexes
   a. Pupils
      (i) No response to bright light
      (ii) Size: midposition (4 mm) to dilated (9 mm)
   b. Ocular movement
      (i) No oculocephalic reflex (testing only when no fracture or instability of the cervical spine is apparent)
      (ii) No deviation of the eyes to irrigation in each ear with 50 ml of cold water (allow 1 minute after injection and at least 5 minutes between testing on each side)
   c. Facial sensation and facial motor response
      (i) No corneal reflex to touch with a throat swab
      (ii) No jaw reflex
      (iii) No grimacing to deep pressure on nail bed, supraorbital ridge, or temporomandibular joint

127

## Definitions

**Classification of Evidence**
*Class I*
Evidence provided by one or more well-designed, randomized, controlled clinical trials.

*Class II*
Evidence provided by one or more well-designed clinical studies such as case-control and cohort studies.

*Class III*
Evidence provided by expert opinion, nonrandomized historical controls, or one or more case reports.

**Strength of Recommendations**
*Standards*
Generally accepted principles for patient management that reflect a high degree of clinical certainty (i.e., based on class I evidence or, when circumstances preclude randomized clinical trials, overwhelming evidence from class II studies that directly addresses the question at hand or from decision analysis that directly addresses all the issues).

*Guidelines*
Recommendations for patient management that may identify a particular strategy or range of management strategies and that reflect moderate clinical certainty (i.e., based on class II evidence that directly addresses the issue, decision analysis that directly addresses the issue, or strong consensus of class III evidence).

*Practice Options or Advisories*
Strategies for patient management for which clinical certainty is lacking (i.e., based on inconclusive or conflicting evidence or opinion).

*Practice Parameters*
Results, in the form of one or more specific recommendations, from a scientifically based analysis of a specific clinical problem.

---

d. Pharyngeal and tracheal reflexes
   (i) No response after stimulation of the posterior pharynx with tongue blade
   (ii) No cough response to bronchial suctioning
3. Apnea—testing performed as follows:
   a. Prerequisites
      (i) Core temperature ≥36.5° C or 97° F
      (ii) Systolic blood pressure 90 mm Hg
      (iii) Euvolemia. *Option:* positive fluid balance in the previous 6 hours
      (iv) Normal $P_{CO_2}$. *Option:* arterial $P_{CO_2}$ ≥40 mm Hg
      (v) Normal $P_{O_2}$. *Option:* preoxygenation to obtain arterial $P_{O_2}$ ≥200 mm Hg
   b. Connect a pulse oximeter and disconnect the ventilator.
   c. Deliver 100% $O_2$, 6 l/min, into the trachea. *Option:* place a cannula at the level of the carina.
   d. Look closely for respiratory movements (abdominal or chest excursions that produce adequate tidal volumes).
   e. Measure arterial $P_{O_2}$, $P_{CO_2}$, and pH after approximately 8 minutes and reconnect the ventilator.
   f. If respiratory movements are absent and arterial $P_{CO_2}$ is ≥60 mm Hg (*option:* 20 mm Hg increase in $P_{CO_2}$ over a baseline normal $P_{CO_2}$), the apnea test result is positive (i.e., it supports the diagnosis of brain death).

g. If respiratory movements are observed, the apnea test result is negative (i.e., it does not support the clinical diagnosis of brain death), and the test should be repeated.
h. Connect the ventilator if, during testing, the systolic blood pressure becomes ≥90 mm Hg or the pulse oximeter indicates significant oxygen desaturation and cardiac arrhythmias are present; immediately draw an arterial blood sample and analyze arterial blood gas. If $P_{CO_2}$ is ≥60 mm Hg or $P_{CO_2}$ increase is ≥20 mm Hg over baseline normal $P_{CO_2}$, the apnea test result is positive (it supports the clinical diagnosis of brain death); if $P_{CO_2}$ is <60 mm Hg or $P_{CO_2}$ increase is <20 mm Hg over baseline normal $P_{CO_2}$, the result is indeterminate, and an additional confirmatory test can be considered.

## II. PITFALLS IN THE DIAGNOSIS OF BRAIN DEATH

The following conditions may interfere with the clinical diagnosis of brain death, so that the diagnosis cannot be made with certainty on clinical grounds alone. Confirmatory tests are recommended.

A. Severe facial trauma
B. Preexisting pupillary abnormalities
C. Toxic levels of any sedative drugs, aminoglycosides, tricyclic antidepressants, anticholinergics, antiepileptic drugs, chemotherapeutic agents, or neuromuscular blocking agents
D. Sleep apnea or severe pulmonary disease resulting in chronic retention of $CO_2$

## III. CLINICAL OBSERVATIONS COMPATIBLE WITH THE DIAGNOSIS OF BRAIN DEATH

These manifestations are occasionally seen and should not be misinterpreted as evidence for brainstem function.

A. Spontaneous movements of limbs other than pathologic flexion or extension response
B. Respiratory-like movements (shoulder elevation and adduction, back arching, intercostal expansion without significant tidal volumes)
C. Sweating, blushing, tachycardia
D. Normal blood pressure without pharmacologic support or sudden increases in blood pressure
E. Absence of diabetes insipidus
F. Deep tendon reflexes; superficial abdominal reflexes; triple flexion response
G. Babinski reflex

## IV. CONFIRMATION LABORATORY TESTS (OPTIONS)

Brain death is a clinical diagnosis. A repeat clinical evaluation 6 hours later is recommended, but this interval is arbitrary. A confirmatory test is not mandatory but is desirable in patients in whom specific components of clinical testing cannot be reliably performed or evaluated. It should be emphasized that any of the suggested confirmatory tests may produce similar results in patients with catastrophic brain damage who do not (yet) fulfill the clinical criteria of brain death. The following confirmatory test findings are listed in the order of the most sensitive test first. Consensus criteria are identified by individual tests.

A. Conventional angiography. No intracerebral filling at the level of the carotid bifurcation or circle of Willis. The external carotid circulation is patent, and filling of the superior longitudinal sinus may be delayed.

B. Electroencephalography. No electrical activity during at least 30 minutes of recording that adheres to the minimal technical criteria for EEG recording in suspected brain death as adopted by the American Electroencephalographic Society, including 16-channel EEG instruments.

C. Transcranial Doppler ultrasonography
   1. Ten percent of patients may not have temporal insonation windows. Therefore, the initial absence of Doppler signals cannot be interpreted as consistent with brain death.
   2. Small systolic peaks in early systole without diastolic flow or reverberating flow, indicating very high vascular resistance associated with greatly increased intracranial pressure.

D. Technetium-99m hexamethylpropylene-amineoxime brain scan. No uptake of isotope in brain parenchyma ("hollow skull phenomenon").

E. Somatosensory evoked potentials. Bilateral absence of N20-P22 response with median nerve stimulation. The recordings should adhere to the minimal technical criteria for somatosensory evoked potential recording in suspected brain death as adopted by the American Electroencephalographic Society.

## V. MEDICAL RECORD DOCUMENTATION (STANDARD)

A. Etiology and irreversibility of condition
B. Absence of brainstem reflexes
C. Absence of motor response to pain
D. Absence of respiration with $P_{CO_2} \geq 60$ mm Hg
E. Justification for confirmatory test and result of confirmatory test
F. Repeat neurologic examination. *Option:* the interval is arbitrary, but a 6-hour period is reasonable.

## Acknowledgments

The Quality Standards Subcommittee wishes to express particular gratitude to Eelco F.M. Wijdicks, MD, for his work in preparing the background paper as well as this summary statement. Jasper R. Daube, MD, served as facilitator for this project. The Quality Standards Subcommittee thanks the Ethics and Humanities Subcommittee and the fifteen members of the AAN Member Reviewer Network who reviewed and returned comments on these practice parameters. The Subcommittee appreciates the reviews of several other critical care specialists.

*Quality Standards Subcommittee: Jay H. Rosenberg, MD (Chair); Milton Alter, MD, PhD; Thomas N. Byrne, MD; Jasper R. Daube, MD; Gary Franklin, MD, MPH; Benjamin Frishberg, MD; Michael L. Goldstein, MD; Michael K. Greenberg, MD; Douglas J. Lanska, MD; Shrikant Mishra, MD, MBA; Germaine L. Odenheimer, MD; George Paulson, MD; Richard A. Pearl, MD; and James Stevens, MD.*

Medical societies invited to comment on these practice parameters: the American Academy of Family Physicians (which provided comment), the American Association of Neurological Surgeons, and the American Academy of Pediatrics.

Approved by the Quality Standards Subcommittee July 20, 1994. Approved by the Practice Committee July 29, 1994. Approved by the Executive Board September 24, 1994.

From Report of the Quality Standards Subcommittee of the American Academy of Neurology. *Neurology.* 1995;45:1012-1014.

# 10

# Sleep Medicine

*Mark W. Mahowald*

Sleep medicine has become firmly established as a medical subspecialty. Sleep disorders are far more prevalent than initially suspected, and the socioeconomic consequences, at both personal and societal levels, are considerable. For instance, (1) obstructive sleep apnea is more prevalent than asthma; (2) in the United States, it is estimated that up to 200,000 motor vehicle accidents annually are due to the driver's falling asleep at the wheel; and (3) many major industrial catastrophes, including the Exxon Valdez, Three Mile Island, Chernobyl, and the Challenger disaster were officially attributed to sleepiness-related errors in judgment or performance in the workplace. Despite these impressive statistics, the average U.S. medical student is exposed to less than 2 hours of education related to sleep medicine during the entire 4-year medical school curriculum.[41]

This chapter reviews the major categories of sleep disorders, including symptoms, clinical findings, pathophysiology, and currently available laboratory techniques in the diagnosis of these disorders, with emphasis on the performance, indications, and interpretation of these studies.

## REVIEW OF NORMAL SLEEP

There are three states of mammalian being: wakefulness, non-rapid eye movement (NREM) sleep, and rapid eye movement (REM) sleep. Each of these states has its own distinct neuroanatomic, neurophysiologic, and neuropharmacologic correlates and behavioral features.[16,72,159,167]

It is now apparent that there are no single specific areas in the nervous system that control all the manifestations of the states of wakefulness, REM sleep and NREM sleep. Most of the state-determining mechanisms that result in the declaration of a given state depend on the brainstem (especially the pons) and basal forebrain regions. In general, the generators of wakefulness are diffusely located in the brainstem, particularly in the reticular activating system; those of NREM, in the medulla and basal forebrain; and those of REM, in the pons. There is recent evidence that the basal forebrain also plays a role in REM sleep. Although discrete regions of the pons have been identified as being responsible for the execution of elements of REM sleep—the perilocus ceruleus for the atonia and the vestibular nuclei for the gen-

eration of REMs—these areas are neither sufficient nor necessary for the occurrence of REM sleep.

For many years there was an ongoing search for specific "centers" of the brain that were thought to be responsible for the generation and declaration of the three states. It has become clear that the appearance of any of the states of being is extremely complex, involving multiple neural networks and many different levels of the nervous system. Factors involved in state generation are complex, and they include a wide variety of neural networks, neurotransmitters, neuromodulators, neurohormones, and a vast array of "sleep factors." Attesting to the complex nature of sleep are these two facts: (1) after suffering lesions of the brain, if an animal survives, it will eventually sleep, regardless of the area damaged; and (2) animals treated with antibodies directed against a number of sleep-inducing substances will sleep less than normal, but they will sleep. These facts lead to the conclusion that sleep is a fundamental property of neuronal groups, regulated by local factors, rather than a phenomenon that requires the whole brain.[77] It is clear that there are multiple state-determining variables that are recruited to occur in concert, resulting in the declaration of a given state. The fact that two-headed conjoined twins with a common circulatory system sleep independently speaks against a primary role of circulating sleep-inducing substances.[80,137]

Neurophysiologic and behavioral features of one state may intrude into another state, or states may oscillate rapidly, resulting in bizarre clinical phenomena.[89]

## DETERMINANTS OF SLEEPINESS/WAKEFULNESS

A number of different physiologic variables combine to determine the level of sleepiness/alertness at any given time. The homeostatic and chronobiologic (i.e., circadian) influences are the most important. The homeostatic factor is related to the duration of prior wakefulness: the longer the duration of wake, the greater the pressure to sleep. The chronobiologic factor is determined by the biologic clock, which has an inherent rhythm that is entrained by the environmental light-dark cycle.

In humans and other mammals the suprachiasmatic

nucleus (SCN) of the hypothalamus controls most circadian rhythms, such as rest-activity rhythm and drinking rhythm.[66] The biologic clock has an inherent rhythm that is entrained by the environmental light-dark cycle. Proof that the SCN is the "biologic clock" is compelling: (1) lesions of the SCN in humans and animals result in a random, irregular wake-sleep pattern; and (2) harvesting a lesion of the SCN in one strain of hamster with a given wake-sleep cycle and transplanting it with the SCN of another strain with a different cycle results in the recipient's developing the wake-sleep cycle of the donor.[121] There is good evidence that the SCN promotes wakefulness, not sleep, because animals whose SCN has been destroyed display an *increase* in total sleep time.[43]

The discovery of a retinohypothalamic tract in animals indicated that the biologic clock may be directly influenced by environmental light.[30,105,118,123] This finding has led to the application of bright light to reset rhythms of activity in animal studies and the wake/sleep cycle in humans.[38,82] The timing of exposure to bright light with respect to the intrinsic rhythm controls the nature of the resetting. Light at the beginning of the conventional sleep period will delay the sleep period, and light at the end of the conventional sleep period will advance it. Light administered in the middle of the day will have no effect. This variability of the effect of light on the wake-sleep cycle has led to the concept of the phase response curve (PRC), which indicates the various responses of advance, "dead zone," and delay of the cycle.[39,40,117] The PRC may differ substantially among individuals and will differ systematically with the intensity of the light.

The importance of the light-dark cycle on the human biologic clock is underscored by the fact that in totally blind humans, only one third will be entrained to the environment. One third will have a cycle that is 24-hours but is out of phase with the environment, and the remaining third will experience a free-running pattern longer than 24 hours.[135] The persistence of a retinohypothalamic tract that is independent of the tracts for vision is the proposed explanation for those blinded individuals who remain entrained to the external light-dark cycle. This fact should be taken into account prior to bilateral enucleation in entrained blind individuals. Treatment of totally blind people with a variety of pharmacologic agents may be useful in demonstrating the effect of these agents on biologic rhythms.[134]

# EVALUATION OF SLEEP-WAKE COMPLAINTS

The initial evaluation of sleep complaints begins with a thorough sleep history and physical examination. Particular attention should be paid to the cardiopulmonary, neurologic, and psychiatric examinations. A meticulous history of wake-sleep function must be detailed. Corroborating information from bed partners, other family members, coworkers, or caregivers is often required for a complete and accurate assessment of sleep behaviors.

## THE WAKE-SLEEP PATTERN

### Subjective Evaluation: Sleep-Wake Diaries

Prolonged sleep-wake diaries completed by the patient or observer may give an overview of wake-sleep patterns that are not obvious from the clinical history. Figure 10–1 shows a patient's self-perceived wake-sleep pattern.

### Objective Evaluation: Actigraphy

Analysis of sleep diaries may be insufficient to verify a tentative diagnosis in patients with reported insomnia or suspected wake-sleep cycle abnormalities. In such cases, definitive objective data may be obtained by actigraphy, a recently developed technique of recording activity during wake and sleep that supplements the subjective sleep log. An actigraph is a small wrist-mounted device that records the activity plotted against time—usually for 1 or 2 weeks.[165] When data collection has been completed, the results are transferred to a personal computer, where software displays activity vs. time. Figure 10–2 shows actigraphic reports and demonstrates how the rest/activity pattern is apparent at a glance. There is direct correlation between the rest/activity recorded by the actigraph and the wake-sleep pattern as determined by polysomnography (PSG).[27,28] Indications for the use of actigraphy include insomnia, wake-sleep schedule disorders, and monitoring of the treatment process.[10,138]

## SLEEP PHYSIOLOGY

### Polysomnography

The technology used for the physiologic diagnosis of sleep disorders employs standard electrophysiologic recording systems.[50] The basic PSG format has been standardized. It includes continuous monitoring of eye movements (EMs), at least one channel of electroencephalogram (EEG) (usually C3/A2 or C4/A1), respiratory parameters (at minimum, airflow), electrocardiography (ECG), submental electromyogram (EMG), and anterior tibialis EMG. Multiple respiratory parameters must be monitored to evaluate sleep-disordered breathing: (1) airflow (thermistors, thermocouples, or expired $CO_2$ sensors), (2) respiratory effort (strain gauges, inductance plethysmography, impedance pneumography, end esophageal pressure, intercostal EMG), and (3) gas exchange (oximetry). Other parameters may be monitored as clinically indicated, for example, extensive EEG for parasomnias, esophageal pH for gastroesophageal reflux, or penile tumescence for erectile function. The American Electroencephalographic Society has outlined specific polysomnographic recording techniques,[7] and sleep-stage scoring techniques have been standardized.[124]

By performance of an all-night PSG, sleep can be accurately quantified and sleep stages fully characterized. It is also possible to determine the presence of (1) sleep architecture disruption, (2) cardiopulmonary abnormalities, (3) sleep-related motor activity, and (4) other sleep-associated disorders. Visual scoring and interpretation of polysomnograms comprise the currently accepted standard. The reliability of computer-aided systems to evaluate sleep disorders awaits objective published verification.[62] The complex nature of normal and abnormal sleep, together with the complexities of the physiologic recording equipment (e.g., artifacts, maintenance of recording signals) are challenging.[87] It must be remembered that the EEG patterns of wakefulness and sleep in patients with underlying central nervous system (CNS) abnormalities may be highly abnormal, precluding the use of such "automated" scoring programs.

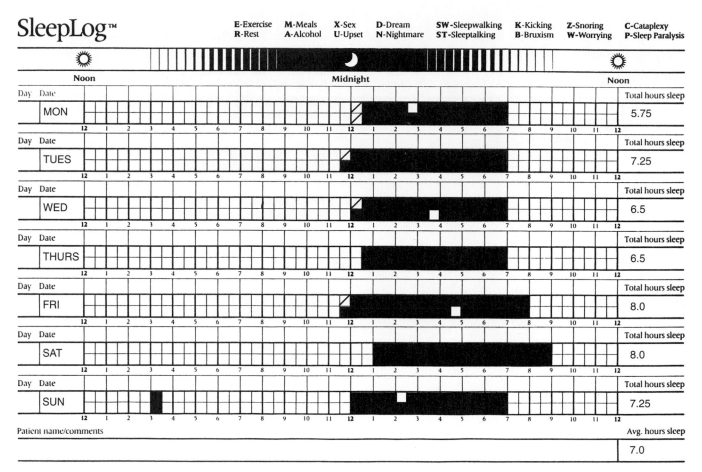

**FIGURE 10–1.** Normal sleep diary. Filled-in areas represent patient's perception of when sleep occurred. Sleep diaries provide "at a glance" overview of patient's impression of his or her wake-sleep pattern.

The following minimal information must be included in the sleep-disorder evaluation report[87]:

1. Parameters monitored
2. Duration and timing of day/night of study
3. Sleep staging (time and percent spent in each stage), total sleep time, sleep efficiency, number/duration of awakenings, and latency to both NREM and REM sleep
4. Respiratory patterns, including type (central, obstructive, or periodic), number, mean or range of duration, effect on oxygenation, sleep stage–body position relationship, and response to any diagnostic or therapeutic maneuvers
5. Cardiac rate or rhythm and any effect of sleep-disordered breathing on ECG
6. Medications taken during the preceding 24 hours

Detailed practice parameters for the indications for PSG have recently been developed.[11,36]

## DAYTIME ALERTNESS/SLEEPINESS

### Subjective Evaluation: Sleepiness Scales

Subjective introspective alertness-sleepiness scales, such as the Stanford Sleepiness Scale and the Epworth Sleepiness Scale (ESS), have been developed.[31,69] The ESS, frequently used as a screening tool for identifying excessive daytime sleepiness, generally correlates with other measures of sleep propensity.[70,71] It must be remembered that such instruments are limited by their lack of sensitivity: there may be a striking discrepancy between self-perceived sleepiness and the underlying true physiologic sleepiness in a given individual.[20,34] In one study neither patient nor partner ESS ratings were strong predictors of the degree of severity of sleep apnea.[75]

### Objective Evaluation

Numerous methods have been developed to measure physiologic sleepiness during the waking period.[101]

***Multiple Sleep Latency Test.*** The Multiple Sleep Latency Test (MSLT) is a standardized and well-validated measure of physiologic sleepiness. Parameters monitored are the same as for basic PSG: usually two eye movement and two EEG (central and occipital) channels, in addition to ECG, airflow, and submental EMG. The MSLT consists of four to five 20-minute nap opportunities offered at 2-hour intervals.[32] It is designed to (1) quantitate sleepiness by measuring how quickly an individual falls asleep on sequential naps during the day,[128] and (2) identify the abnormal occurrence of REM sleep during a nap. For each nap the latency between "lights out" and sleep onset is recorded. Pathologic ranges of sleep latency have been carefully defined. A mean latency of

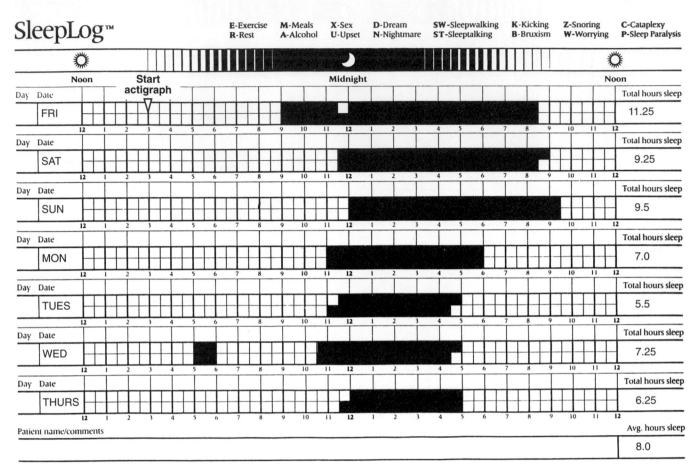

A

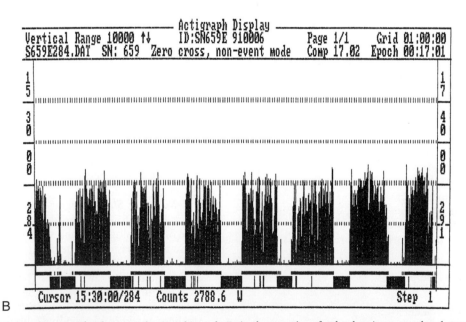

B

**FIGURE 10–2.** **A,** Normal sleep diary completed as part of actigraphic study. Patient's perception of wake-sleep is compared to that recorded objectively by actigraphy. **B,** Normal 1-week actigraphic study. Vertical bars represent activity levels plotted over seven consecutive 24-hour periods, allowing rapid assessment of rest-activity (sleep-wake) patterns.

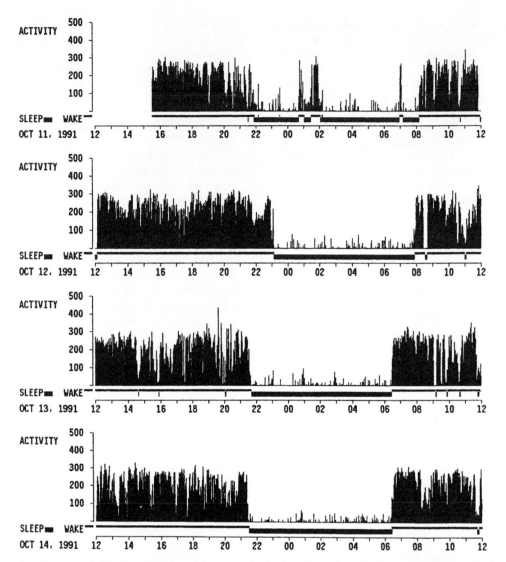

**FIGURE 10–2.** *Continued.* **C,** Expanded display of first four 24-hour periods of actigraphic study in *B* indicating clock time. Notice that brief awakening reported by patient about 2 hours after sleep onset on first night is reliably recorded by actigraph and is visible on full-week and expanded display.

5 minutes or less indicates severe excessive sleepiness. The number of naps during which REM sleep appears is also noted. Many factors can affect sleep latency during the daytime: prior sleep deprivation, sleep continuity, age, time of day, and medication use.[8,32,127] Proper interpretation requires a PSG done the preceding night to measure the quality and quantity of sleep obtained immediately prior to the MSLT. The MSLT is a most useful tool in quantifying daytime sleepiness and in differentiating the subjective complaints of "sleepiness," "tiredness," and "fatigue."

The final MSLT report must include the following minimal information:

1. Time of each nap
2. Individual subtest sleep latencies
3. Mean sleep latency
4. Number of REM occurrences

Other helpful information on the MSLT report includes data from the preceding night's PSG, such as time of lights out, wake-up time, total sleep time, sleep efficiency, and latencies to both NREM and REM sleep. All medications, including prescription drugs, over-the-counter drugs, and alcohol or recreational drugs, should be noted.

It must be remembered that false-negative MSLT results can and do occur and that there may be a discrepancy between the subjective complaint of sleepiness and the results of the MSLT.[35,131] REM sleep may also occur in subjects with no complaints of excessive daytime sleepiness.[22]

***Maintenance of Wakefulness Test.*** The Maintenance of Wakefulness Test (MWT) is a variation of the MSLT. Unlike the MSLT, in the MWT the subject is asked to resist sleep while sitting in a chair (rather than being asked to fall asleep lying in bed).[100] The MWT appears to offer no specific advantage over the MSLT.[132]

***Alpha Attenuation Test.*** This is a recently described technique to evaluate daytime sleepiness, based on the fact that EEG power in the alpha frequency range decreases when the eyes are closed. The ratio of mean eyes-closed to mean eyes-open alpha power during seated wakefulness is smaller in sleepy subjects.[6] Acceptance of this procedure will depend on more extensive validation studies.

***Pupillography.*** Static pupillography is based on the fact that the pupils constrict during sleep. The rate of pupillary constriction is determined and is considered to reflect the degree of underlying sleepiness.[150] Pupillography is used infrequently in the evaluation of excessive daytime sleepiness because it can be difficult to perform and interpret and gives no indication of the cause of the sleepiness. A variation of this test is dynamic pupillography, which measures the pupillary response to a sudden change in the amount of light entering the eye. Although once thought to measure underlying sleepiness, dynamic pupillography is not a valid indicator of sleepiness.[122]

Both subjective and objective measures of sleepiness have their limitations, and, as with many other tests in medicine, the results of both must be interpreted in light of the specific clinical situation.[4,71]

# SLEEP DISORDERS

## EXCESSIVE DAYTIME SLEEPINESS

The complaint of excessive daytime sleepiness (EDS) must be taken very seriously. True EDS is a manifestation of underlying physiologic sleepiness and, contrary to popular opinion, is rarely, if ever, due to psychologic or psychiatric conditions (e.g., depression, laziness, boredom). In the absence of sleep deprivation, daytime hypersomnia is almost inevitably due to an identifiable and treatable sleep disorder, such as sleep apnea, narcolepsy, or idiopathic CNS hypersomnia.

### Sleep Apnea

The prevalence of obstructive sleep apnea (OSA) in the general population is high: 2% of adult females and 4% of adult males.[177] It is most common in adults, males, snorers, postmenopausal women, elderly persons, and the overweight population. However, OSA is also seen in children, young women, and asthenic individuals. It must be emphasized that obesity is not present in approximately one third of individuals with OSA.[51] Conversely, the majority of obese males and the overwhelming majority of obese females do not have OSA.[156,168] The fact that sleep-disordered breathing is diagnosable and treatable in the vast majority of cases and can have devastating consequences prior to diagnosis and treatment mandates awareness of the availability of sleep-disorder centers staffed by experienced specialists.[163]

***Symptoms and Findings.*** The consequences of OSA fall into two major categories: (1) excessive daytime sleepiness due to the sleep fragmentation and (2) physiologic consequences of sleep-related desaturation, such as systemic and pulmonary hypertension, right-sided heart failure, and polycythemia. Morning headaches are a less reliable marker of OSA than previously thought.[3,120]

***Pathophysiology.*** The respiratory physiologic pattern is one of the most dramatic state-dependent phenomena: respiration may be profoundly altered by the transition from wakefulness to sleep, exaggerating wakeful pathologic conditions, with devastating consequences on the daytime alertness and physiologic state of the patient.[51] After sleep-disordered breathing (SDB) was first causally associated with the pickwickian syndrome in 1965,[48] it became apparent that SDB has a wide variety of presenting signs and symptoms.

***Clinical Diagnosis.*** The clinical diagnosis of OSA may be very difficult. Numerous studies have shown that there are often marked discrepancies between the clinically suspected and the laboratory-documented presence or severity of OSA. For this reason formal sleep studies are mandatory.[63,116,141,169]

Initially, SDB seemed straightforward and simple. Apnea was either obstructive or central. However, as monitoring techniques become more sophisticated and more diverse patient populations are studied, it has become increasingly apparent that pathologic conditions of respiratory physiology during sleep are complicated phenomena, requiring complex monitoring techniques with interpretation by experienced clinicians. For example, in some patients with OSA the underlying respiratory pattern is that of Cheyne-Stokes respiration (CSR), with a superimposed obstructive component. Elimination of the obstructive element is necessary before treatment of the residual CSR can be addressed. Therefore the patient may require two forms of treatment: nasal continuous positive airway pressure (CPAP) for the obstruction and supplemental oxygen for the CSR.

One important concept is the differentiation between OSA itself and the OSA syndrome (OSAS). Many individuals may be observed by a bed partner or parent to have periods of OSA. Formal evaluation is not indicated in the absence of symptoms or findings of the OSAS, such as hypersomnia, cor pulmonale, right-sided heart failure, or polycythemia.[115]

***Laboratory Diagnosis.*** The indications for formal sleep studies in suspected SDB are well accepted, and numerous clinical practice guidelines exist for adults[7,60,115,125] and children.[15]

*Polysomnography.* Continuous monitoring of sleep stages is mandatory. It is necessary to determine that adequate amounts of both NREM and REM sleep have occurred because it is well known that severe SDB can be exquisitely state-dependent. EEG monitoring is also important for the determination of arousals due to subtle SDB. A recently described condition called "upper airway resistance syndrome" may be associated with sleep fragmentation without significant hemoglobin oxygen desaturation or obvious abnormality of respiration.[42,56]

The determination of what constitutes an "arousal" remains controversial. Arousal scoring criteria have been developed[12]; however, there are no studies that have determined what degree of arousal or what frequency of arousals (per hour of sleep) actually impairs daytime alertness. There is growing evidence that "nonvisible sleep fragmentation," as determined by autonomic nervous system manifestations of arousal (increases in blood pressure or heart rate), in the absence of PSG evidence of arousal may be sufficient to result in impairment of daytime alertness and mood.[95,98]

The duration of the PSG is important because SDB may also be sleep-duration dependent.[170] Monitoring for extremity movements is also mandatory in cases of suspected SDB, since periodic movements of sleep (nocturnal myoclonus) may result in arousal-associated transitional hypopneas, which may mimic primary SDB.[54]

All studies performed to evaluate SDB must include assessment of both respiratory effort and effectiveness.[78] The presence of ventilatory effort is usually determined by chest and abdominal motion detectors (strain gauges, impedance, or inductance plethysmography). To detect paradoxical movement of the chest and diaphragm due to upper airway obstruction, sensitive recording of both chest and abdominal excursions must be performed. Quantitative estimates of effort require the more cumbersome measurement of pressure generated by the inspiratory muscles (esophageal pressure) or the sometimes elusive surface EMG activity of the inspiratory muscles (diaphragm, intercostal, or scalene muscles). These quantitative measurements are occasionally useful in detecting ventilatory effort when there is little mechanical movement. Arousal-dependent recruitment of accessory respiratory muscles, such as the sternocleidomastoid or the scalene muscle, can be documented by surface EMG in patients with neuromuscular disease.[64] The utility of monitoring accessory respiratory muscle activity is shown in Figure 10–3.

The effect of ventilatory effort on gas exchange may be estimated by measurement of hemoglobin oxygen saturation (oximetry) in appropriate situations. In patients not receiving oxygen, periodic oxygen desaturation with cycles of duration similar to those of apnea or hypopnea often reflects periods of inadequate ventilation. Transcutaneous or end-tidal $CO_2$ monitoring may be valuable in cases of suspected $CO_2$ retention. Continuous ECG monitoring is mandatory, both to determine any cardiac rate or rhythm consequences of SDB and for patient safety.

*Upper Airway Studies.* There is substantial evidence that, as a group, OSA patients have structural abnormalities of the upper airway; the airway is smaller than normal and narrowed laterally.[152] A number of techniques have been developed to evaluate the structure of the upper airway: cephalometric roentgenograms, somnofluoroscopy, acoustic reflection studies, flow-volume curves, and Müller or Valsalva maneuvers.[74,114,126] Such studies have been proposed as selective and predictive for the success of upper airway surgical procedures (particularly uvulopalatopharyngoplasty). Unfortunately, the predictive value, with few anecdotal exceptions, has been disappointing.[73,76,107]

*Daytime Nap Studies.* The use of daytime nap studies to evaluate the presence or severity of SDB is to be discouraged because the duration of the evaluation is usually inadequate to allow the presence of REM sleep. Furthermore, the sever-

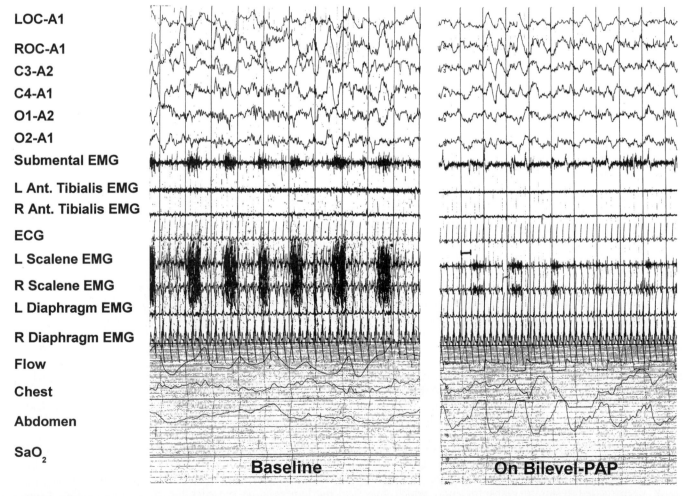

**FIGURE 10–3.** Polysomnogram demonstrating utility of accessory respiratory muscle EMG monitoring in a case of sleep-disordered breathing in patient with neuromuscular disease (48-year-old woman with amyotrophic lateral sclerosis who developed hypercapneic respiratory failure). Sleep was associated with hypercapnia, but no frank central or obstructive respiratory events and no hemoglobin oxygen desaturation were noted. Increased respiratory effort shown by EMG activity of scalenes on left panel is markedly reduced following administration of nasal bilevel positive airway pressure. Concomitantly, transcutaneous $CO_2$ fell substantially. *LOC/ROC,* Left/right outer canthus; *A1,* left mastoid; *C3/O1,* left central/occipital EEG; *EMG,* surface electromyogram.

ity of SDB tends to worsen as the night progresses[33,170]; therefore the short daytime study may not detect apnea, which is sleep-duration or circadian dependent. A negative nap study does *not* rule out significant SDB.[115]

*Nap, "Ambulatory (Screening)," and Automatic Titrating CPAP Studies.* There are ongoing efforts to develop "ambulatory" (home) or "screening" studies. These usually include ear oximetry and often do not include sleep monitoring. Although intended to be a less costly "screening" procedure, such studies more often become an "add on." They are prone to technical difficulties (i.e., keeping electrodes on) and may not indicate how much sleep was monitored or whether all stages of sleep occurred. These studies may not allow monitoring or observation of the patient's body position, which is most important in SDB. If the complaint is EDS and the study is negative, the patient needs formal sleep studies to rule out nonapneic causes of EDS. If the studies are positive for SDB, again, formal sleep studies are usually necessary to determine the exact nature of the apnea and any response to treatment.[24,81,83,154,160,176] Practice parameters for the use of portable recording in the assessment of OSA have recently been developed.[13,44] Before these techniques are widely adopted, each must be thoroughly evaluated.[45]

A number of automatically titrating CPAP devices are available, and they have been used with varying degrees of success.[46,153,162] Although promising, these devices cannot be used in all patients with OSA. In addition, it must be remembered that because a patient with EDS has snoring episodes and observed apneic episodes, it does not necessarily follow that that patient's EDS is due to OSA.

*"Computer-Aided Scoring".* Currently available computer-aided systems to evaluate sleep await objective published validation.[62] The difficulty in determining some forms of SDB with commonly used transducers, the masquerading of other sleep disorders as SDB, and the indeterminate nature of sleep stages in some patient populations (particularly those with CNS abnormalities) present a challenge.[87]

*Diagnostic and Therapeutic Maneuvers During Polysomnography.* The specific nature of SDB detected during PSG may not be obvious. Certain diagnostic and therapeutic maneuvers can be of diagnostic assistance. These include the administration of oxygen, $CO_2$, medications (benzodiazepines or acetazolamide); the application of CPAP, bilevel positive airway pressure (PAP), or a rocking bed; or the use of negative-pressure ventilators (i.e., iron lung, cuirass) alone or in combination: specifically, CPAP or bilevel PAP for OSA and CSA[17,58,67,139,164] and negative pressure ventilators for hypoventilation.[64] Experienced laboratories are equipped to perform such complex studies.

The use of "split-night" studies for CPAP titration remains controversial.[47,65,140] The likelihood of success undoubtedly depends on the experience of a given sleep laboratory.

*Interpretation of Data.* PSG interpretation requires experience and expertise because the spectrum of SDB is broad and encompasses OSA, central sleep apnea (CSA), CSR, and frank sleep-related respiratory insufficiency, which may occur in varying combinations. In addition, there are a number of conditions that may masquerade as SDB—even on formal PSG testing. These include periodic movements of sleep-induced oxygen saturation ($So_2$) oscillations associated with brief arousals[54] and nocturnal seizures resulting in apnea and desaturation.[102,171] It must also be remembered that some degree of SDB may be present in many individuals without clinical significance. The clinical relevance of any identified SDB must be determined in light of the patient's symptoms. For instance, the PSG finding of an apnea or hypopnea index of 20/h would hardly explain EDS severe enough to result in a fall-asleep motor vehicle accident or sleepiness in the workplace sufficient to jeopardize one's job.

Although there may be night-to-night variability in mild cases, a single PSG containing adequate amounts of both REM and NREM sleep will usually detect clinically significant SDB.[96,175]

## Narcolepsy

Narcolepsy is a relatively common disorder, with a prevalence of 0.09%, affecting at least 250,000 people in the United States. There is a clear genetic component, with more than 90% of individuals who have narcolepsy carrying the *HLA-DR2/DQ1* (under current nomenclature *HLA-DR15* and *HLA-DQ6*) gene (found in less than 30% of the general population).[1] It is currently thought that *DQ6*, which corresponds at the genomic level to the subregions *DQB1\*0602* and *DQA1\*0102* on chromosome 6, is one of the more reliable markers across ethnic groups.[18] This association is present in the different ethnic populations to varying degrees, and it represents the highest disease-HLA linkage known in medicine. Clearly, there is a genetic component; however, that component is neither necessary nor sufficient to cause narcolepsy.

The usual age of onset is adolescence or early adulthood, although the onset can range from early childhood to senescence (3 to 72 years). After a relatively brief period of progression as the disease declares itself, it tends to stabilize, but it rarely, if ever, completely remits.[53]

*Symptoms and Findings.* Excessive daytime sleepiness is the primary symptom. Unwanted or unanticipated sleep episodes, lasting seconds to minutes, may occur at inappropriate times, particularly during periods of reduced environmental stimulation, such as while reading, watching television, riding in or driving a motor vehicle, or attending classes or meetings. Such feelings of sleepiness are often dramatically, but briefly, reversed by a short nap. Aggressive treatment is needed because the psychosocial and socioeconomic consequences of narcolepsy are significant.[25,26]

Ancillary symptoms include cataplexy, hypnagogic hallucinations, and sleep paralysis. Cataplexy, which occurs in 65% to 70% of patients with narcolepsy, is a sudden loss of muscle tone, typically triggered by an emotion such as laughter, anger, excitement, delight, or surprise. Although the muscle weakness of cataplexy may be complete, resulting in falling down or being forced to sit, it is more often milder and more focal in nature, taking the form of facial sagging, slurred speech, localized weakness of an extremity, or the feeling that one's knees may "give way." Cataplexy may never occur in 30% of patients with narcolepsy. In many persons with narcolepsy the hypersomnia precedes the appearance of the ancillary symptoms, often by decades.[49,55] The absence of a history of cataplexy does not rule out the diagnosis of narcolepsy.

Sleep paralysis is experienced by up to 60% of patients with narcolepsy and consists of total body paralysis, with sparing of respiration and eye movements. It lasts from seconds to minutes and is very frightening to the patient.

Hypnagogic (at sleep onset) and hypnopompic (on awakening) hallucinations are seen in 12% to 50% of cases. These hallucinations are extremely vivid, often frightening dreams that occur during the transition between wakefulness and sleep. They may be associated with total body paralysis and the sensations of oppression and dread.

Notably, fewer than half (14% to 42%) of people with narcolepsy report all four symptoms of sleep attacks, cataplexy, hypnagogic hallucinations, and sleep paralysis.

Automatic behavior occurs in up to 80% of patients with narcolepsy. It is the simultaneous or rapidly oscillating occurrence of wake and sleep, during which the individual appears to be awake but is without full awareness. Such spells may result in extremely inappropriate behaviors and may lead to an erroneous diagnosis of partial complex seizures or psychogenic dissociative (fugue) states.

*Pathophysiology.* The pathophysiologic basis of narcolepsy results in impaired control of the boundaries that normally separate the states of wakefulness from REM and NREM sleep. The total sleep time per 24 hours in people with narcolepsy is similar to that in those without narcolepsy. However, the control of the onset-offset of both REM and non-REM sleep is impaired. This impairment explains in part both the nighttime sleep fragmentation and the intrusion of sleep into daytime wakefulness. Moreover, there is a clear dissociation of the various components of the individual wake and sleep states. Cataplexy and sleep paralysis simply represent the isolated and inappropriate intrusion or persistence of REM sleep–related atonia (paralysis) into wakefulness. The hypnagogic or hypnopompic hallucinations are (REM sleep–related) dreams occurring during wakefulness.[1]

No structural abnormalities of the brain have been consistently identified in humans with narcolepsy. Narcolepsy appears to be a neurotransmitter dysfunction.[110] The overwhelming percentage of cases are "idiopathic"; however, rare cases of "symptomatic" narcolepsy have been described in patients with associated abnormalities of the diencephalic, hypothalamic, or pontine regions of the brain.[5] Basal forebrain abnormalities have been reported in canine narcolepsy.[155]

*Clinical Diagnosis.* The diagnosis of narcolepsy may be suggested by the patient's history. Although it has been said that the report of cataplexy is pathognomonic of narcolepsy, that is not necessarily the case. A history of "classic" narcolepsy with cataplexy may be the manifestation of a somatoform disorder.[145] In view of the nature and duration of treatment with stimulant medications, objective sleep laboratory diagnosis is imperative.

### Laboratory Diagnosis

*Polysomnography and Multiple Sleep Latency Test.* An all-night PSG must be performed the night before the MSLT to determine the quality and quantity of the preceding night's sleep. On the MSLT patients with narcolepsy typically fall asleep in 5 minutes or less and usually display REM sleep on at least two of the daytime naps, an occurrence rarely seen in normals. The MSLT results must be interpreted in light of the patient's clinical symptoms and in view of the results of the preceding night's PSG. A "negative" MSLT does not absolutely rule out the possibility of narcolepsy. False-negative MSLTs do occur.[68] Stating that a "negative" MSLT absolutely rules out the diagnosis of narcolepsy in a hypersomnolent patient is analogous to saying that a normal ECG eliminates the diagnosis of cardiac disease in a patient with chest pain.

False-positive MSLT results may occur in the setting of prior severe sleep deprivation or withdrawal of REM sleep–suppressing agents, such as stimulants (methylphenidate, dextroamphetamine, or cocaine), alcohol, or tricyclic antidepressants. REM sleep may occur on MSLTs in the absence of narcolepsy in patients with myotonic dystrophy or the Prader-Willi syndrome.[61,113,166]

To date, there is no reliable objective measure of the compliance with or response to stimulant medication in patients with narcolepsy.[9] The response must be evaluated by the patient's subjective report.

*Human Leukocyte Antigen Typing.* Although the recent discovery of the association between narcolepsy and human leukocyte antigen (HLA) type is of intense scientific interest and research value, the variability of the presence of HLA associations in the general public and in patients with narcolepsy precludes its usefulness as a diagnostic test.[59,129] The associated HLA type is neither necessary nor sufficient for the appearance of narcolepsy.

*Neuroimaging Studies.* Narcolepsy is a clinical and sleep laboratory diagnosis. Symptomatic narcolepsy due to identifiable CNS abnormalities is rare. Further neurologic studies are indicated only in cases in which the history or neurologic examination strongly suggests a structural CNS pathologic condition.

## Idiopathic Central Nervous System Hypersomnia

Idiopathic CNS hypersomnia may represent a number of different conditions that present as unexplained excessive daytime sleepiness.

*Symptoms and Findings.* Idiopathic CNS hypersomnia is a condition characterized by excessive daytime sleepiness in the absence of sleep deprivation or other identifiable abnormality during sleep, such as obstructive sleep apnea.[52]

*Pathophysiology.* The pathophysiologic basis of idiopathic CNS hypersomnia is unknown.

*Clinical Diagnosis.* The diagnosis may be suspected by the history of unexplained excessive daytime sleepiness in the absence of symptoms suggestive of OSA, narcolepsy, or sleep deprivation. Formal studies are mandatory to confirm the absence of unsuspected sleep-related pathologic conditions and to confirm the subjective complaint of EDS. Chronic sleep deprivation must be aggressively ruled out as an explanation for EDS. As with narcolepsy, the treatment implications (stimulant medications indefinitely) require a formal objective diagnosis.

### Laboratory Diagnosis

*Polysomnography and Multiple Sleep Latency Test.* The all-night PSG is unremarkable, and the MSLT reveals objective hypersomnia, without the occurrence of REM sleep during the naps.[52]

*Human Leukocyte Antigen Studies.* These studies are not indicated.

*Neuroimaging Studies.* These studies are not indicated in the absence of clinical or neurologic examination findings suggestive of structural CNS abnormalities.

***Borderline Between Narcolepsy and Idiopathic Central Nervous System Hypersomnia.*** It is becoming clear that there is a great deal of overlap of symptoms and confusion in establishing a diagnosis between narcolepsy and idiopathic CNS hypersomnia.[19,29,108] A number of patients with narcolepsy and cataplexy may not demonstrate REM sleep on the MSLT, and, conversely, some with idiopathic CNS hypersomnia and without cataplexy may have REM sleep on the MSLT. One proposed classification is as follows[2]:

1. Narcolepsy with cataplexy (with or without REM sleep on the MSLT)
2. Hypersomnia without cataplexy
   a. With REM sleep on the MSLT
   b. Without REM sleep on the MSLT

## Recurrent Hypersomnia

This rare complaint may be the manifestation of a number of unusual but fascinating conditions including, Kleine-Levin syndrome, menstruation-related hypersomnia, and idiopathic recurring stupor.

***Kleine-Levin Syndrome.*** The Kleine-Levin syndrome is characterized by periodic hypersomnia, lasting days to weeks and occurring at intervals of days to years with intervening normal wake-sleep function and alertness. The classic form is idiopathic and seen in adolescent males, but the syndrome may affect both sexes and all age groups. The periodic hypersomnia may be associated with hyperphagia and hypersexuality and likely represents recurrent hypothalamic dysfunction. The often cited association with adolescent males and unusual behaviors (e.g., hypersexuality and megaphagia) have been overrated: the condition may occur in females, and it may not be associated with hyperphagia or hypersexuality.[157] This syndrome has been reported following mild head injury. No large-scale treatment studies are available. Stimulant medication has been proposed for the symptomatic period, and lithium has been apparently effective prophylactically.

***Menstruation-Related Hypersomnia.*** As the name implies, menstruation-related periodic hypersomnia is characterized by recurrent periods of hypersomnia related to menstruation. This condition may represent a variant of the Kleine-Levin syndrome.[21]

***Idiopathic Recurring Stupor.*** This strange condition was first reported in 1990 by Lugaresi's group. Idiopathic recurring stupor (IRS) is characterized by recurrent episodes of stupor, generally beginning in adulthood. The stupors occur at varying intervals, from multiple times weekly to only a few times a year. The duration of the stupor ranges from hours to a few days. There is a definite characteristic EEG pattern—a widely distributed, nonreactive 13 to 18 Hz EEG activity that has been present in all reported cases. The clinical and EEG manifestations are promptly, but briefly, reversed by the administration of flumazenil, a benzodiazepine antagonist.[84] Oral flumazenil, available in Europe, has been used to treat some patients with IRS.

IRS may be due to the action of "endozepines," which are endogenous ligands for the benzodiazepine recognition sites on gamma-aminobutyric acid (GABA) A receptors in the CNS. Endozepines are naturally occurring nonpeptide, nonbenzodiazepine substances that may play a role in CNS processes such as memory and learning and in pathologic processes such as panic disorders and hepatic encephalopathy. There is good evidence that a benzodiazepine-like substance plays a role in hepatic encephalopathy.[57,109,112] In IRS, CSF endozepine 4 levels were 300 times higher during an IRS spell than in control patients. The fact that elevated levels of endozepine 4 were present in both the CSF and blood indicate that this is a systemic disorder, not confined to the CNS.[133] The source of endozepine 4 and why it should be released intermittently are not known.

Although there are only about 15 cases reported in the literature, IRS is probably much more prevalent than currently thought, with many affected persons admitted to intensive care units for "stupor of unknown etiology," with the stupor being attributed to an overdose of a drug that was not identified by urine toxicology screen.

## INSOMNIA

Insomnia is the most common of all sleep-related complaints, affecting up to 30% of the adult population. It is a constitutional symptom, not a single diagnostic entity. Insomnia may be a manifestation of various underlying medical, psychiatric, or psychologic conditions. It may also be the presenting symptom of other primary sleep disorders. A clear understanding of the probable cause of insomnia in a given case is essential before rational and effective treatment can be determined.[178] The known socioeconomic consequences of this condition dictate thorough evaluation in all cases.[37,161]

## Symptoms and Findings

The primary symptom of insomnia is the complaint of the perception of an inability to sleep long enough to feel rested and restored on awakening. This effect may result from difficulty initiating or maintaining sleep.

## Clinical Diagnosis

A thorough history and physical examination are critical to the differential diagnosis of insomnia. Questioning should be directed at (1) duration and stability, (2) timing of night, and (3) daytime consequences. For practical purposes, insomnia may be arbitrarily categorized as transient (a few nights), short-term (less than 1 month), or chronic (longer than 1 month). With this information, the types of insomnia can be divided into transient, short-term, and chronic. Most cases of insomnia can be readily diagnosed and managed in the primary care setting.[172]

Interviewing the insomniac's bed partner can provide essential information regarding snoring and breathing patterns, unusual motor activity during sleep, or other signs of organic conditions that may disrupt sleep. The bed partner may know if there is a significant discrepancy between the amount of sleep and the number of awakenings the patient reports and the actual degree of sleep disruption.

Detailed sleep diaries may provide invaluable information as to the duration, continuity, and timing of sleep. Insomnia associated with circadian factors is readily identifiable by 2- to 3-week sleep diaries.

If a psychiatric condition is suspected, administration of a battery of standardized psychologic tests, such as the Minnesota Multiphasic Personality Inventory and the Beck Depression Inventory, may be helpful.

## Laboratory Diagnosis

*Actigraphy.* If the clinical interview, physical examination, and sleep diaries do not provide the desired clinical information regarding the overall wake-sleep pattern and do not suggest an underlying cause, actigraphy may be a valuable additional tool in the evaluation of insomnia. In some forms of insomnia, such as sleep-state misperception, the patient profoundly underestimates his or her total sleep time, reporting having only 1 to 2 hours of sleep per night, "documented" by sleep diaries. Actigraphy is the only practical means of confirming or refuting such reports. This is graphically displayed in Figures 10–4 and 10–5.

*Polysomnography.* In the absence of symptoms of severe daytime sleepiness, PSG is not indicated for the routine evaluation of insomnia. Consideration for polysomnographic assessment is appropriate when[14]:

1. SDB or periodic movements of sleep (see following section) are suspected

2. The initial diagnosis is uncertain, or behavioral or pharmacologic treatment has been unsuccessful
3. Precipitous arousals or violent behaviors during sleep are present, and the clinical diagnosis is uncertain
4. A persistent circadian rhythm disorder is suspected, and the clinical diagnosis is unclear
5. There are symptoms of severe excessive daytime sleepiness

Two special sleep-related conditions that may result in insomnia should be mentioned: (1) restless legs syndrome, and (2) periodic limb movement disorder of sleep. The difference between the two is that restless legs syndrome is a clinical complaint, whereas periodic limb movement disorder is a polygraphic finding.

## Restless Legs Syndrome

*Symptoms and Findings.* Restless legs syndrome (RLS) is a poorly understood, and occasionally incapacitating, disorder characterized primarily by a vague and difficult-to-describe sensation involving the lower extremities. This discomfort appears primarily during periods of inactivity, particularly during the transition from wake to sleep. These unpleasant sensations are typically relieved only by move-

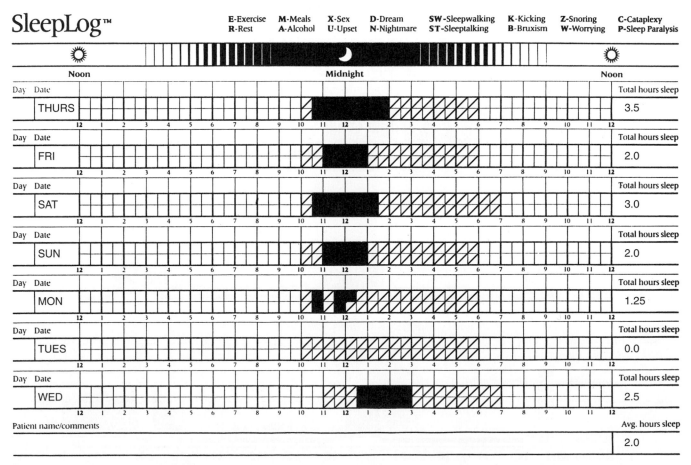

**FIGURE 10–4.** *A,* Sleep diary in case of sleep-state misperception insomnia. Patient is a 40-year-old businessman who had been treated with myriad medications for longstanding insomnia. Sleep diary indicates that he perceived obtaining 2 hours of sleep per night. Hatched portions are his self-perceived periods of wakefulness in bed.

*Figure continued on following page*

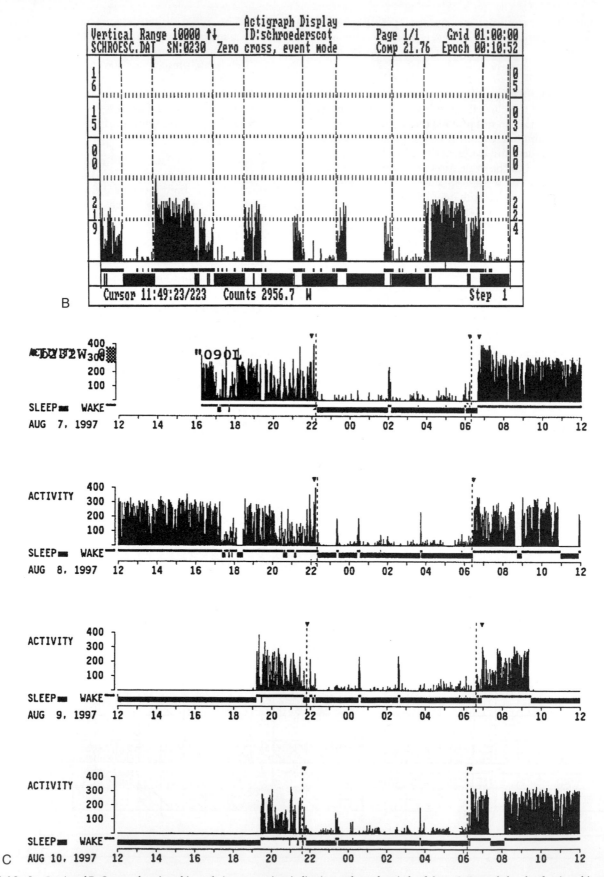

**FIGURE 10–4.** *Continued* **B,** One-week actigraphic study in same patient indicating prolonged periods of sleep. **C,** Expanded scale of actigraphic study in *B.* Sleep, between vertical dashed lines, actually averaged approximately 8 hours nightly. Periods of no activity during day indicated that patient usually only wore actigraph at night. This striking discrepancy between his perceived and actual sleep time was used to reassure patient and indicated that pharmacologic treatment was not appropriate because there was no true insomnia. This diagnosis would have been difficult, if not impossible, without actigraphic study.

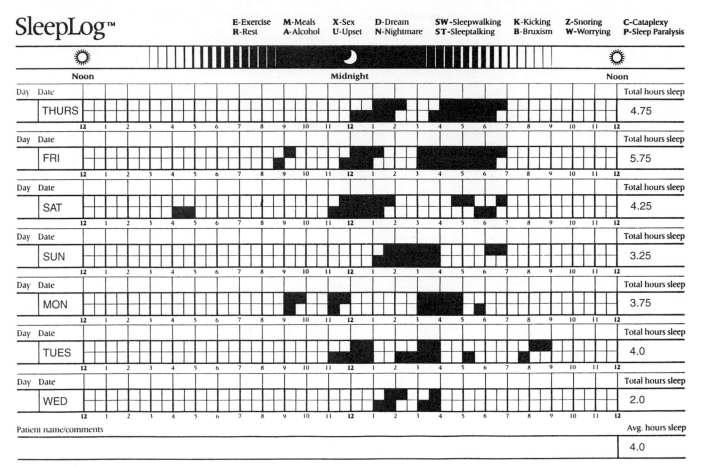

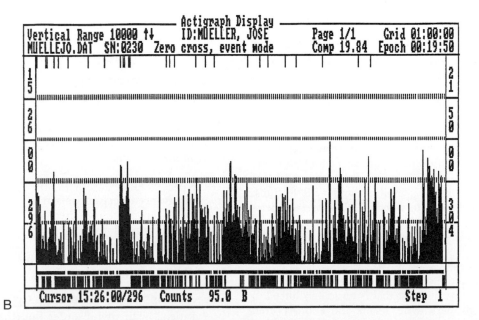

**FIGURE 10–5.** **A,** Sleep diary of a 32-year-old man who developed severe insomnia following spinal surgery for congenital malformation. Historically, his wake-sleep pattern was normal when he was receiving analgesics via epidural catheter, which had been removed. He was taking massive doses of oral analgesics and wearing fentanyl patch, which he stated did not help his insomnia. His physician (the author) was not convinced of the severity of insomnia and suspected drug-seeking behavior. **B,** Actigraphic study of this patient revealed profound insomnia. Although overall wake-sleep pattern can be seen, there were very few, and very brief, periods of consolidated sleep (actually worse than patient reported on his sleep diary). This information was presented to patient's neurosurgeon and anesthesiologist and led to reinsertion of the epidural catheter. Use of actigraphy in cases such as this—to confirm or refute an otherwise "unbelievable" wake-sleep complaint—provides invaluable information, often with very important therapeutic implications.

ment or stimulation of the legs. RLS is a major cause of insomnia and may also bother the patient's bed partner.[103]

*Pathophysiology.* RLS is very common, affecting 5% to 10% of the general population. The majority of cases are idiopathic or familial. A positive family history may be obtained in up to 50% of cases. Although RLS has been associated with a wide variety of other medical and neurologic conditions, such as iron deficiency anemia, renal failure, and various peripheral neuropathies, such cases are rare. Once believed to be psychiatric in nature, RLS has not been proven to be related to any psychologic or psychiatric problems.[103,104]

*Clinical Diagnosis.* RLS is a clinical diagnosis.

*Laboratory Diagnosis.* Formal sleep studies are not indicated in RLS. Likewise, extensive and expensive medical and neurologic evaluations are not warranted unless there are historical or physical examination suggestions of other underlying medical or neurologic disorders.

### Periodic Limb Movement Disorder

*Symptoms and Findings.* Periodic limb movement disorder (PLMD), formerly known as periodic movements of sleep or nocturnal myoclonus, is characterized by periodic (every 20 to 40 seconds) movements of the legs during sleep. These movements may be associated with arousals that are often too brief to be perceived by the individual. If these frequent arousals result in interruption of sleep, they may result in excessive daytime sleepiness. Almost all people with RLS have PLMD (80%), but the converse is not true. RLS is an unpleasant sensation perceived by the person during wakefulness, whereas in PLMD the movements occur during sleep and are most often not appreciated by the person (but may be bothersome to the bed partner).[103]

*Clinical Diagnosis.* PLMD may be suspected in difficult cases of insomnia or in otherwise unexplained EDS, but PSG confirmation is necessary.

*Laboratory Diagnosis.* PLMD is diagnosed by formal sleep studies. It must be remembered that periodic limb movements are common in the general population, increasing with advancing age, and may be completely asymptomatic.[103] Periodic limb movements are also common in individuals with narcolepsy.[23] The final diagnosis of PLMD must involve both clinical symptoms and PSG features. There is growing debate as to whether PSG-observed periodic limb movements in the absence of clinical symptoms of RLS are of any clinical significance.[97]

### CIRCADIAN RHYTHM DISTURBANCES

Most living creatures follow a relentless and pervasive daily rhythm of activity and rest that is ultimately linked to the geophysical light-dark cycle. Plants and animals, even unicellular organisms, show daily variations in metabolic activity, locomotion, feeding, and many other functions.[99,106,174] The importance of the light-dark cycle on the human biologic clock is underscored by the fact that in totally blind humans, only one third will be entrained to the environment. One third will have a cycle that is 24 hours long but is out of phase with the environment; the remaining third experience a free-running pattern longer than 24 hours.[135]

### Symptoms and Findings

The primary symptom of circadian rhythm disorders is the inability to sleep during the desired sleep time. Once the person falls asleep, there is no abnormality of the sleep per se. There is only an abnormality of the timing of sleep.

### Pathophysiology

The cause of all circadian rhythm disorders is an inability of the individual's biologic clock to adjust to the demands of the geophysical environment.

### Clinical Diagnosis

The wake-sleep schedule disorders fall into two categories: (1) primary (malfunction of the biologic clock per se) and (2) secondary (due to environmental effects on the underlying clock). The secondary disorders, such as jet-lag and shift work, are usually immediately apparent on simple questioning of the patient. The primary disorders may be much more difficult to diagnose because they typically masquerade as other sleep, medical, or psychiatric disorders, such as hypersomnia, insomnia, substance (sedative/hypnotic or stimulant) abuse, or psychiatric conditions.

Clinical evaluation must include a thorough medical and psychiatric history, physical examination, and a detailed analysis of the wake-sleep pattern. Careful attention must be paid to medication (prescription and other) use. One most important piece of historical information is whether once sleep has begun, it is uninterrupted and normal. It is not the sleep per se but the *timing* of sleep that is the abnormality. The patient's estimate of what his or her pattern would be (or has been) under "free-running" conditions may be invaluable. A subjective log reflecting at least 2 weeks of the patient's wake-sleep pattern should be available for the initial interview.[111] Some of the more common circadian rhythm disorders are summarized in the following sections.

### Delayed Sleep Syndrome

In delayed sleep phase syndrome (DSPS), the patient falls asleep late and rises late (Fig. 10–6). There is a striking inability to fall asleep at an earlier, more desirable time. This may present as either sleep-onset insomnia or EDS (particularly in the morning).

### Advanced Sleep Phase Syndrome

In advanced sleep phase syndrome (ASPS), the patient cannot stay up as late as desired and awakens far earlier than hoped. This condition may present as EDS (particularly in the evening) or sleep-maintenance insomnia. The undesirable early morning awakening in this condition often leads to the misdiagnosis of depression.

### Irregular or Non-24-Hour Sleep Cycles

Patients with this disorder find that their wake-sleep pattern gradually moves in and out of synchronization with their environment.

*Laboratory Diagnosis.* Actigraphy done for a period of 2 weeks or longer may be of great assistance in establishing the diagnosis of circadian rhythm disorders.

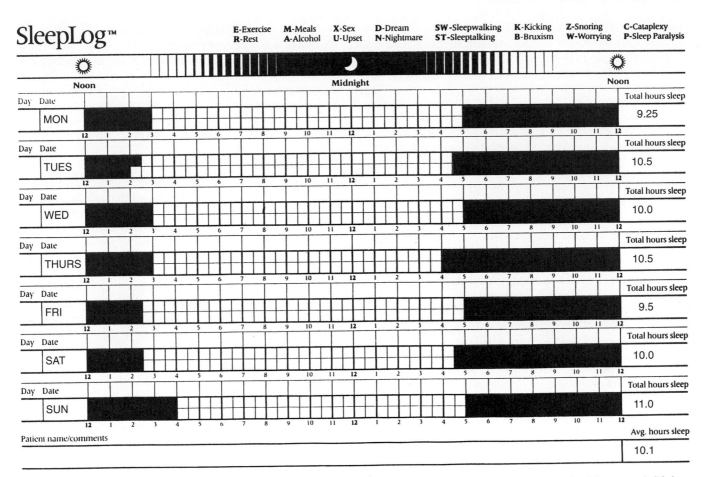

**SleepLog**™

| | E-Exercise | M-Meals | X-Sex | D-Dream | SW-Sleepwalking | K-Kicking | Z-Snoring | C-Cataplexy |
| | R-Rest | A-Alcohol | U-Upset | N-Nightmare | ST-Sleeptalking | B-Bruxism | W-Worrying | P-Sleep Paralysis |

**FIGURE 10–6.** Sleep diary in a "free-running" patient with delayed sleep-phase syndrome. This 38-year-old woman had suffered from a nearly life-long complete inability to fall asleep before approximately 4 AM and preferred to sleep until 3 PM. She was unable to retain employment, which required her to be at work in the morning. She had accommodated to her delayed biologic clock by obtaining employment that permitted her to work during her "wake" time. It is clear from this sleep diary that only abnormality is timing of her sleep period and that once she is asleep and permitted to sleep without interruption, there is nothing wrong with her sleep per se.

Identification of these often disabling disorders is important because there are effective therapeutic interventions to address them; these include chronotherapy, phototherapy, and pharmacologic agents.[111,136]

### Circadian Rhythms and Psychiatric Disorders

There is a striking relationship between circadian rhythms and certain psychiatric disorders—particularly seasonal affective disorder, primary depression, and bipolar affective disorder.[79,130,173] The clinical utility of formal sleep studies in individual cases remains to be determined.

### PARASOMNIAS

Parasomnias are defined as unpleasant or undesirable behavioral or experiential phenomena that occur predominately or exclusively during sleep. These were initially thought to represent a unitary event, often attributed to psychiatric disease. Recent clinical and polygraphic analysis has revealed that they are, in fact, the result of a large number of completely different conditions, most of which are diagnosable and treatable. Most are not the manifestation of psychiatric disorders and are far more prevalent than previously suspected.[93,146]

### Symptoms and Findings

Most parasomnias present with undesirable or unpleasant motor or vocal behaviors or unpleasant experiential phenomena during the sleep period. There are many different parasomnias, but most fall into one of the following categories[86]:

1. Disorders of arousal
2. REM sleep–behavior disorder
3. Nocturnal seizures
4. Miscellaneous (psychogenic dissociative states, nocturnal panic, posttraumatic stress disorder, rhythmic movement disorder)

### Disorders of Arousal

These disorders occur on a spectrum ranging from confusional arousals to sleepwalking to sleep terrors. They represent the simultaneous appearance or rapid oscillations of wake and NREM sleep—characterized by wakefulness that is sufficient for carrying out complex behaviors but insufficient for awareness of or responsibility for those actions. Such events are extremely common in children, and they are much more common in adults than previously suspected.

They may even begin in adulthood and are uncommonly associated with significant psychiatric disease. They tend to arise from the deepest stages of NREM sleep (slow-wave sleep) and therefore are most apt to occur during the first 2 hours of sleep. It is important to note that they may occur during *any* stage of NREM sleep and at any portion of the sleep period. They rarely occur during daytime naps. There is usually no remembered complex dream mentation. Full awakening following an episode is unusual, with the patient most often returning to sleep or being partially awake but extremely confused and disoriented.[86]

### REM Sleep Behavior Disorders

REM sleep behavior disorders (RBD) is a recently described condition that presents with the complaint of prominent motor behavior associated with vivid dreamlike mentation ("acting out of dreams"). Medical attention is sought when injury to the patient or the bed partner occurs or is feared. Unlike sleepwalking/sleep terrors, there is usually remembered vivid dreamlike mentation that correlates with the observed behavior, and the episode is followed by complete and immediate alertness. RBD is seen predominately in older men and is due to the absence of the generalized somatic paralysis that normally accompanies REM sleep. Approximately one third of cases will have an identifiable underlying neurologic disorder, but most are idiopathic. Extensive neurologic evaluation (evoked potentials, CT, MRI) is warranted only if the history or neurologic examination is suggestive of a structural CNS pathologic condition.[143] RBD is seen more often in patients with narcolepsy and may be exacerbated by medication prescribed for cataplexy.[144] There is a high correlation between RBD and degenerative neurologic disorders, such as Parkinson's disease and multiple system atrophy, and the RBD symptoms may antedate the appearance of the other features of the underlying disorder by many years.[119,142] A "parasomnia overlap" syndrome characterized by clinical and PSG features of both disorder of arousal and RBD has been recently described.[147] Figure 10–7 demonstrates the typical PSG finding of RBD.

The finding of REM sleep without atonia (RWA) on PSG does not necessarily mean that the patient has RBD. RWA without the clinical symptoms of dream-enacting behaviors may be seen in many other conditions, including neurodegenerative disorders such as Parkinson's disease and multiple system atrophy, or it may be a medication effect (selective serotonin-reuptake inhibitors, tricyclic antidepressants, or venlafaxine).[144,148,151]

### Nocturnal Seizures

Most nocturnal seizures present little diagnostic difficulty; however, it must be remembered that any behavior or experience, regardless of the clinical feature, that is recurrent, stereotyped, and inappropriate may be the manifestation of a seizure. Exclusively nocturnal seizures with extremely bizarre behaviors are not uncommon, but they are routinely misdiagnosed. Seizures emanating from the frontal lobe are a common culprit: their tendency for bizarre behaviors, exclusively nocturnal timing, and clustering in time all predispose to a psychiatric misdiagnosis. Interictal (and often ictal) EEGs may be unrevealing.[91,94]

### Miscellaneous Disorders

Psychogenic dissociative disorders are seen most frequently in women, and they may perfectly mimic complex sleepwalking or nocturnal seizures. A history (often difficult to obtain) of childhood physical or sexual abuse is almost always present. There may be few, if any, waking symptoms of dissociation.[149] Other unusual parasomnias include nocturnal panic and posttraumatic stress disorder.[91]

### Clinical Diagnosis

The history may lead to the suspicion of the actual diagnosis; however, experience has shown that in most cases the definitive diagnosis cannot be made by history alone; it must be confirmed by formal polygraphic study. Empiric medical treatment should be discouraged because the therapy for one disorder may actually worsen another. The vio-

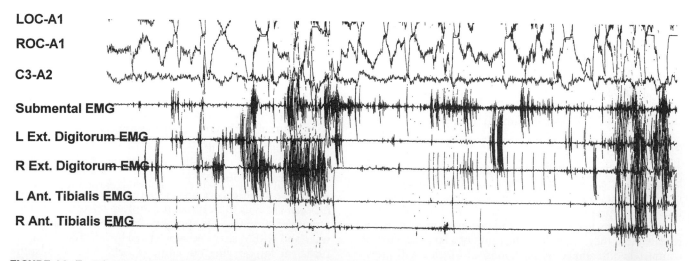

**FIGURE 10–7.** Polysomnogram of a patient with REM sleep-behavior disorder. This 65-year-old man complained of a 5-year history of progressively severe motor behaviors during sleep. He had kicked his wife and had fallen out of bed on a number of occasions during which he reported, "I was acting out my dreams." In contrast to anticipated muscle atonia during REM sleep, this polysomnogram reveals very prominent tonic and phasic muscle activity of submental and extremity muscles, associated with arm and leg flailing. If patient was awakened during these episodes, observed motor activity correlated with his recall of simultaneous dream mentation. *LOC/ROC*, Left/right outer canthus; *A1*, left mastoid; *C3/O1*, left central/occipital EEG; *EMG*, surface electromyogram.

lent behaviors exhibited during the various parasomnias may have forensic science implications.[85,92]

## Pathophysiology

Integral to the understanding of the parasomnias is the concept of state-dependent reorganization of the CNS. There is compelling evidence that extensive reorganization of the CNS activity occurs during sleep. Almost all portions of the nervous system are active across all three states of being, but active in a different mode. There are multiple state-determining variables that are recruited to occur in concert, resulting in the declaration of a given state. Parasomnias are clinical phenomena that, by and large, are related to the changes in brain organization across states of being; they are particularly apt to occur during the transition periods from one state to another.[158] Given the large number of neural networks, neurotransmitters, and other state-determining substances that must be recruited synchronously, and given the frequent transitions among the three states of being, it is surprising that parasomnias do not occur more frequently than they do. The concept of state dissociation in animals and humans has been extensively reviewed.[86,89,90]

## Laboratory Diagnosis

Isolated, often bizarre, sleep-related events may be experienced by perfectly healthy people, and most do not warrant further extensive or expensive evaluation. The initial approach to the complaint of unusual sleep-related behavior is to determine whether further evaluation is necessary. The patient should be queried regarding the exact nature of the events. Since many of these episodes may be associated with partial or complete amnesia, additional descriptive information from a bed-partner or other observer may prove helpful. Guidelines for the indications for further evaluation have been developed[88] and include behaviors that:

1. Are potentially violent or injurious
2. Are extremely disruptive to other household members
3. Result in the complaint of excessive daytime sleepiness
4. Are associated with medical, psychiatric, or neurologic symptoms or findings

Serious attention should be given to such parasomnia complaints under these circumstances. Formal PSG studies, appropriately performed, provide direct or indirect diagnostic information in the majority of cases. This information is of more than academic interest because most of these conditions are readily treatable. Emphasis must be placed on the types of studies required; routine PSGs performed for conventional sleep disorders are inadequate. In addition to the physiologic parameters monitored in the standard PSG, there must be an expanded EEG montage, the paper speed must be at least 15 mm/s, and there must be continuous audiovisual monitoring. Experienced technologist observation is invaluable. Multiple night studies may be required to capture an event. Unattended studies have no role in the evaluation of parasomnias.[91]

## SUMMARY

Sleep-wake complaints are ubiquitous. They may be associated with severe personal distress having personal and societal socioeconomic consequences. A thorough clinical evaluation coupled with judicious use of laboratory studies usually reveal a specific and treatable underlying condition.

## ACKNOWLEDGMENTS

Supported in part by a grant from Hennepin Faculty Associates, I am indebted to the physicians, nurses, polysomnographic technologists, and patients of the Minnesota Regional Sleep Disorders Center who offered their tireless support and to Ms. Traci Oletzke for her expert secretarial support.

## REFERENCES

1. Aldrich MS. The neurobiology of narcolepsy. *Prog Neurobiol.* 1992; 41:538-541.
2. Aldrich MS. The clinical spectrum of narcolepsy and idiopathic hypersomnia. *Neurology.* 1996;46:393-401.
3. Aldrich MS, Chauncey JB. Are morning headaches part of obstructive sleep apnea syndrome? *Arch Intern Med.* 1990;150:1265-1267.
4. Aldrich MS, Chervin RD, Malow BA. Value of the Multiple Sleep Latency Test (MSLT) for the diagnosis of narcolepsy. *Sleep.* 1997;20:620-629.
5. Aldrich MS, Naylor MW. Narcolepsy associated with lesions of the diencephalon. *Neurology.* 1989;39:1505-1508.
6. Alloway CED, Ogilvie RD, Shapiro CM. The alpha attenuation test: assessing excessive daytime sleepiness in narcolepsy-cataplexy. *Sleep.* 1997; 20:258-266.
7. American Electroencephalographic Society Ad Hoc Committee on Polysomnographic Guidelines. American Electroencephalographic Society guidelines for the polygraphic assessment of sleep-related disorders (polysomnography). *J Clin Neurophysiol.* 1991;9:88-96.
8. American Sleep Disorders Association. The clinical use of the Multiple Sleep Latency Test. *Sleep.* 1992;15:268-276.
9. American Sleep Disorders Association. Practice parameters for the use of stimulants in the treatment of narcolepsy. *Sleep.* 1994;17:348-351.
10. American Sleep Disorders Association. Practice parameters for the use of actigraphy in the clinical assessment of sleep disorders. *Sleep.* 1995; 18:285-287.
11. American Sleep Disorders Association. Practice parameters for the indications for polysomnography and related procedures. *Sleep.* 1997;20: 406-422.
12. American Sleep Disorders Association Atlas Task Force. EEG arousals: scoring rules and examples. *Sleep.* 1992;15:173-184.
13. American Sleep Disorders Association Standards of Practice Committee. Practice parameters for the use of portable recording in the assessment of obstructive sleep apnea. *Sleep.* 1994;17:372-377.
14. American Sleep Disorders Association Standards of Practice Committee. Practice parameters for the use of polysomnography in the evaluation of insomnia. *Sleep.* 1995;18:55-57.
15. American Thoracic Society. Standards and indications for cardiopulmonary sleep studies in children. *Am J Respir Crit Care Med.* 1996; 153:866-878.
16. Aserinsky A, Kleitman N. Regularly occurring periods of eye motility and concomitant phenomena during sleep. *Science.* 1953;118:273-274.
17. Badr MS, Grossman JE, Weber SA. Treatment of refractory sleep apnea with supplemental carbon dioxide. *Am J Respir Crit Care Med.* 1994; 150:561-564.
18. Basetti C, Aldrich MS. Narcolepsy. *Neurol Clin.* 1996;14:545-571.
19. Basetti C, Aldrich MS. Idiopathic hypersomnia: a series of 42 patients. *Brain.* 1997;120:1423-1435.
20. Benbadis SR, Perry MC, Mascha E, et al. Subjective vs. objective measures of sleepiness: correlation between Epworth Sleepiness Scale and MSLT. *Sleep Res.* 1997;26:641.
21. Billiard M, Guilleminault C, Dement WC. A menstruation-linked periodic hypersomnia. *Neurology.* 1975;255:436-443.
22. Bishop C, Rosenthal L, Helmus T, et al. The frequency of multiple sleep onset REM periods among subjects with no excessive daytime sleepiness. *Sleep.* 1996;19:727-730.
23. Boivin DB, Lorraine D, Montplaisir J. Effects of bromocriptine on periodic limb movements in human narcolepsy. *Neurology.* 1993;43: 2134-2136.
24. Broughton R, Fleming J, Fleetham J. Home assessment of sleep disorders by portable monitoring. *J Clin Neurophysiol.* 1996;13:272-284.
25. Broughton R, Ghanem Q, Hishikawa Y, et al. Life effects of narcolepsy: relationships to geographic origin (North American, Asian, or Euro-

pean) and to other patient and illness variables. *Can J Neurol Sci.* 1983; 10:100-104.

26. Broughton WA, Broughton RJ. Psychosocial impact of narcolepsy. *Sleep.* 1994;17:S45-S49.

27. Brown A, Smolensky M, D'Alonzo G, et al. Circadian rhythm in human activity objectively quantified by actigraphy. In: Hays DK, ed. *Chronobiology: Its Role in Clinical Medicine, General Biology, and Agriculture.* New York: John Wiley & Sons; 1990: pt A, 77-83.

28. Brown AC, Smolensky M, D'Alonzo GE, et al. Actigraphy: a means of assessing circadian patterns in human activity. *Chronobiol Int.* 1990; 7:125-133.

29. Bruck D, Parkes JD. A comparison of idiopathic hypersomnia and narcolepsy-cataplexy using self-report measures and sleep diary data. *J Neurol Neurosurg Psychiatry.* 1996;60:576-578.

30. Burchard JE. *Re-setting a biological clock.* Princeton, NJ: Princeton University; 1958. Thesis. Cited in Wever RA. *The Circadian System of Man: Results of Experiments Under Temporal Isolation.* New York: Springer-Verlag; 1979.

31. Carskadon MA, Dement WC. Normal human sleep: an overview. In: Kryger MH, Roth T, Dement WC, eds. *Principles and Practice of Sleep Medicine.* 2nd ed. Philadelphia: WB Saunders; 1994:16-25.

32. Carskadon MA, Dement WC, Mitler MM, et al. Guidelines for the Multiple Sleep Latency Test (MSLT): a standard measure of sleepiness. *Sleep.* 1986;9:519-524.

33. Charbonneau M, Marin JM, Olha A, et al. Changes in obstructive sleep apnea characteristics through the night. *Chest.* 1994;106:1695-1701.

34. Chervin RD, Aldrich MS, Pickett R, et al. Comparison of the results of the Epworth Sleepiness Scale and the Multiple Sleep Latency Test. *J Psychosom Res.* 1997;42:145-155.

35. Chervin RD, Kraemer HC, Guilleminault C. Correlates of sleep latency on the Multiple Sleep Latency Test in a clinical population. *EEG Clin Neurophysiol.* 1995;95:147-153.

36. Chesson Jr AL, Ferber RA, Fry JM, et al. The indications for polysomnography and related procedures. *Sleep.* 1997;20:423-487.

37. Chilcott LA, Shapiro CM. The socioeconomic impact of insomnia: an overview. *PharmacoEconomics.* 1996;10(suppl 1):1-14.

38. Czeisler CA, Kronauer RE, Allen JS, et al. Bright light induction of strong (type 0) resetting of the human pacemaker. *Science.* 1989;244: 1328-1333.

39. DeCorsey PJ. *Daily light sensitivity rhythm in the flying squirrel.* Madison, WI: University of Wisconsin; 1959. Thesis. Cited in Wever RA. *The Circadian System of Man: Results of Experiments Under Temporal Isolation.* New York: Springer-Verlag; 1979.

40. DeCorsey PJ. Daily light sensitivity rhythm in a rodent. *Science.* 1960; 131:33-35.

41. Department of Health and Human Services. *Report of the National Commission on Sleep Disorders Research.* Washington, DC: DHHS; 1992.

42. Downey III R, Perkin RM, MacQuarrie J. Upper airway resistance syndrome: sick, symptomatic but unrecognized. *Sleep.* 1993;16:620-623.

43. Edgar DM, Dement WC, Fuller CA. Effect of SCN lesions on sleep in squirrel monkeys: evidence for opponent process in sleep-wake regulation. *J Neurosci.* 1993;13:1065-1079.

44. Ferber R, Millman R, Coppola M, et al. Portable recording in the assessment of obstructive sleep apnea. *Sleep.* 1994;17:378-392.

45. Flemons WW, Remmers JE. Diagnosis of sleep apnea: questionnaires and home studies. *Sleep.* 1996;19:S243-S247.

46. Fleury B, Rakotonanahary D, Hausser-Hauw C, et al. A laboratory validation study of the diagnostic mode of the Autoset™ system for sleep-related respiratory disorders. *Sleep.* 1996;19:502-505.

47. Fleury B, Rakotonanahary D, Tehindrazanarivelo AD, et al. Long-term compliance to continuous positive airway pressure therapy (nCPAP) set up during a split-night polysomnography. *Sleep.* 1994;17:512-515.

48. Gastaut H, Tassinari C, Duron B. Etude polygraphique des manifestations épisodiques (hypniques et respiratoires) du syndrome de Pickwick. *Rev Neurol.* 1965;112:568-579.

49. Guilleminault C. Cataplexy. In: Guilleminault C, Dement WC, Passouant P, eds. *Narcolepsy.* New York: Spectrum; 1976:125-144.

50. Guilleminault C. *Sleeping and Waking Disorders: Indications and Techniques.* Menlo Park, CA: Addison-Wesley; 1982.

51. Guilleminault C. Clinical features and evaluation of obstructive sleep apnea. In: Kryger MH, Roth T, Dement WC, eds. *Principles and Practice of Sleep Medicine.* 2nd ed. Philadelphia: WB Saunders; 1994:667-677.

52. Guilleminault C. Idiopathic central nervous system hypersomnia. In: Kryger MH, Roth T, Dement WC, eds. *Principles and Practice of Sleep Medicine.* 2nd ed. Philadelphia: WB Saunders; 1994:562-566.

53. Guilleminault C. Narcolepsy syndrome. In: Kryger MH, Roth T, Dement WC, eds. *Principles and Practice of Sleep Medicine.* 2nd ed. Philadelphia: WB Saunders; 1994:549-561.

54. Guilleminault C, Crowe C, Quera-Salva MA, et al. Periodic leg movement, sleep fragmentation and central sleep apnea in two cases: reduction with clonazepam. *Eur Respir J.* 1988;1:762-765.

55. Guilleminault C, Dement WC, Passouant P. *Narcolepsy.* New York: Spectrum; 1976.

56. Guilleminault C, Stoohs R, Clerk A, et al. A cause of excessive daytime sleepiness: the upper airway resistance syndrome. *Chest.* 1993;104: 781-787.

57. Gyr K, Meier R. Flumazenil in the treatment of portal systemic encephalopathy: an overview. *Intensive Care Med.* 1991;17:S39-S42.

58. Hanly PJ, Millar TW, Steljes DG, et al. The effect of oxygen on respiration and sleep in patients with congestive heart failure. *Ann Intern Med.* 1989;111:777-782.

59. Hayduk R, Flodman P, Spence MA, et al. HLA haplotypes, polysomnography, and pedigrees in a case series of patients with narcolepsy. *Sleep.* 1997;20:850-857.

60. Health Technology Reports, US Department of Health and Human Services. *Polysomnography and Sleep Disorders Centers.* Washington, DC: Agency for Health Care Policy and Research; 1991. Publication No. 92-0027.

61. Hertz G, Cataletto M, Feinsilver SH, et al. Sleep and breathing patterns in patients with Prader-Willi syndrome (PWI): effects of age and gender. *Sleep.* 1993;16:366-371.

62. Hirshkowitz M, Moore CA. Issues in computerized polysomnography. *Sleep.* 1994;17:105-112.

63. Hoffstein V, Szalai JP. Predictive value of clinical features diagnosing obstructive sleep apnea. *Sleep.* 1993;16:118-122.

64. Iber C, Davies SF, Mahowald MW. Nocturnal rocking bed therapy: improvement in sleep fragmentation in patients with respiratory muscle weakness. *Sleep.* 1989;12:405-412.

65. Iber C, O'Brien C, Schluter J, et al. Single-night studies in obstructive sleep apnea. *Sleep.* 1991;14:383-385.

66. Ibuka N, Kawamura H. Loss of circadian rhythm in sleep-wakefulness cycle in the rat by suprachiasmatic nucleus lesions. *Brain Res.* 1975; 96:76-81.

67. Issa FG, Sullivan CE. Reversal of central sleep apnea using nasal CPAP. *Chest.* 1986;90:165-171.

68. Jahnke B, Aldrich MS. The Multiple Sleep Latency Test (MSLT) is not infallible. *Sleep Res.* 1990;19:240.

69. Johns MW. A new method for measuring daytime sleepiness. *Sleep.* 1991;14:540-545.

70. Johns MW. Daytime sleepiness, snoring, and obstructive sleep apnea. The Epworth Sleepiness Scale. *Chest.* 1993;103:30-36.

71. Johns MW. Sleepiness in different situations measured by the Epworth Sleepiness Scale. *Sleep.* 1994;17:703-710.

72. Jones B. Basic mechanisms of sleep-wake states. In: Kryger MH, Roth R, Dement WC, eds. *Principles and Practice of Sleep Medicine.* Philadelphia: WB Saunders; 1994:145-162.

73. Katsantonis GP, Maas CS, Walsh JK. The predictive efficacy of the Mueller maneuver in uvulopalatopharyngoplasty. *Laryngoscope.* 1989; 99:677-680.

74. Katsantonis G, Walsh JK. Somnofluoroscopy: its role in the selection of candidates for uvulopalatopharyngoplasty. *Otolaryngol Head Neck Surg.* 1986;94:56-60.

75. Kingshott RN, Sime PJ, Engleman HM, et al. Self-assessment of daytime sleepiness: patient versus partner. *Thorax.* 1995;50:994-995.

76. Koopman Jr CF, Moran Jr WB. Surgical management of obstructive sleep apnea. *Otolaryngol Clin North Am.* 1990;23:787-808.

77. Krueger JM, Obal Jr F, Kapas L, et al. Brain organization and sleep function. *Behav Brain Res.* 1995;69:177-185.

78. Kryger MH. Monitoring respiratory and cardiac function. In: Kryger MH, Roth T, Dement WC, eds. *Principles and Practice of Sleep Medicine.* 2nd ed. Philadelphia: WB Saunders; 1994:984-993.

79. Kupfer DJ, Monk TH, Barchas JD. *Biological Rhythms and Mental Disorders.* New York: Guilford Press; 1988:357.

80. Lahmeyer WH. Sleep in craniopagus twins. *Sleep.* 1988;11:301-306.

81. Levy P, Pepin JL, Deschaux-Blanc C, et al. Accuracy of oximetry for detection of respiratory disturbances in sleep apnea syndrome. *Chest.* 1996;109:395-399.

82. Lewy AJ, Wehr TA, Goodwin FK, et al. Light suppresses melatonin secretion in humans. *Science.* 1980;210:1267-1269.

83. Lloberes P, Montserrat JM, Ascaso A, et al. Comparison of partially attended night time respiratory recordings and full polysomnography in

patients with suspected sleep apnoea/hypopnoea syndrome. *Thorax.* 1996;51:1043-1047.

84. Lugaresi E, Montagna P, Tinuper P. Idiopathic recurring stupor. *Sleep Res.* 1993;22:229.

85. Mahowald MW, Bundlie SR, Hurwitz TD, et al. Sleep violence–forensic science implications: polygraphic and video documentation. *J Forensic Sci.* 1990;35:413-432.

86. Mahowald MW, Ettinger MG. Things that go bump in the night: the parasomnias revisited. *J Clin Neurophysiol.* 1990;7:119-143.

87. Mahowald MW, Iber C, Walsh JK. Evaluation of obstructive sleep apnea: considerations and caveats. Operative Techniques in *Otolaryngol Head Neck Surg.* 1991;2:73-80.

88. Mahowald MW, Rosen GM. Parasomnias in children. *Pediatrician.* 1990;17:21-31.

89. Mahowald MW, Schenck CH. Status dissociatus: a perspective on states of being. *Sleep.* 1991;14:69-79.

90. Mahowald MW, Schenck CH. Dissociated states of wakefulness and sleep. *Neurology.* 1992;42:44-52.

91. Mahowald MW, Schenck CH. Parasomnia purgatory: the epileptic/non-epileptic interface. In: Rowan AJ, Gates JR, eds. *Non-Epileptic Seizures.* Boston: Butterworth-Heinemann; 1993:123-139.

92. Mahowald MW, Schenck CH. Complex motor behavior arising during the sleep period: forensic science implications. *Sleep.* 1995;18:724-727.

93. Mahowald MW, Schenck CH. NREM parasomnias. *Neurol Clin.* 1996;14:675-696.

94. Mahowald MW, Schenck CH. Sleep disorders. In: Engel JJ, Pedley TA, eds. *Epilepsy: A Comprehensive Textbook.* Philadelphia: Lippincott-Raven; 1997:2705-2715.

95. Martin SE, Wraith PK, Deary IJ, et al. The effect of nonvisible sleep fragmentation on daytime function. *Am J Respir Crit Care Med.* 1997; 155:1596-1601.

96. Mendelson WB. Use of the sleep laboratory in suspected sleep apnea syndrome: is one night enough? *Cleve Clin J Med.* 1994;61:299-303.

97. Mendelson WB. Are periodic leg movements associated with clinical sleep disturbance? *Sleep.* 1996;19:219-223.

98. Mendelson WB. Sleep fragmentation and daytime wakefulness. *Am J Respir Crit Care Med.* 1997;155:1499-1500.

99. Minors DS. *Circadian Rhythms and the Human.* Bristol: Wright-PSG; 1981.

100. Mitler MM, Gujavarty KS, Browman CP. Maintenance of wakefulness test: a polysomnographic technique for evaluating treatment efficacy in patients with excessive somnolence. *EEG Clin Neurophysiol.* 1982; 53:568-661.

101. Mitler MM, Miller JC. Methods of testing for sleepiness. *Behav Med.* 1996;21:171-183.

102. Monod N, Peirano P, Plouin P, et al. Seizure-induced apnea. *Ann N Y Acad Sci.* 1988;533:411-420.

103. Montplaisir J, Godbout R, Pelletier G, et al. Restless legs syndrome and periodic limb movements during sleep. In: Kryger MH, Roth T, Dement WC, eds. *Principles and Practice of Sleep Medicine.* 2nd ed. Philadelphia: WB Saunders; 1994:589-597.

104. Montplaisir J, Lapierre O, Warnes H, et al. The treatment of the restless legs syndrome with or without periodic leg movements in sleep. *Sleep.* 1992;15:391-395.

105. Moore R. Retinohypothalamic projections in mammals: a comparative study. *Brain Res.* 1973;49:403-409.

106. Moore-Ede MC, Sulzman FM, Fuller CA. *The Clocks That Time Us: Physiology of the Circadian Timing System.* Cambridge, MA: Harvard University Press; 1982.

107. Moran Jr WB. Obstructive sleep apnea: diagnosis by history, physical exam, and special studies. In: Fairbanks DNF, Fujita S, Ikematsu T, et al, eds. *Snoring and Obstructive Sleep Apnea.* New York: Raven Press; 1987:19-38.

108. Moscovitch A, Partinen M, Guilleminault C. The positive diagnosis of narcolepsy and narcolepsy's borderland. *Neurology.* 1993;43:55-60.

109. Mullen KD, Mendelson WB, Martin JV, et al. Could an endogenous benzodiazepine ligand contribute to hepatic encephalopathy? *Lancet.* 1988;I:457-459.

110. Nishino S, Mignot E. Pharmacological aspects of human and canine narcolepsy. *Prog Neurobiol.* 1997;52:27-78.

111. Mahowald MW, Ettinger MG. Circadian rhythm disorders. In: Chokroverty S, ed. *Sleep Disorders Medicine: Basic Science, Technical Considerations, and Clinical Aspects.* 2nd ed. Boston: Butterworth-Heinemann; 1999:619-634.

112. Olasmaa M, Guidotti A, Costa E, et al. Endogenous benzodiazepines in hepatic encephalopathy. *Lancet.* 1989;I:491-492.

113. Park YD, Radtke R. Hypersomnolence in myotonic dystrophy: demonstration of sleep onset REM sleep. *J Neurol Neurosurg Psychiatry.* 1995; 58:512-513.

114. Partinen M, Guilleminault C, Quere-Salva MA, et al. Obstructive sleep apnea and cephalometric roentgenograms. *Chest.* 1988;93:1199-1205.

115. Phillipson EA, E. RJ, (Chairmen, American Thoracic Society Consensus Conference on Indications and Standards for Cardiopulmonary Sleep Studies). Indications and standards for cardiopulmonary sleep studies. *Am Rev Respir Dis.* 1989;139:559-568.

116. Pillar G, Peled N, Katz N, et al. Predictive value of specific risk factors, symptoms and signs in diagnosing obstructive sleep apnea and its severity. *J Sleep Res.* 1992;3:241-244.

117. Pittendrigh CS. Circadian rhythms and the circadian organization of living systems. *Cold Spring Harb Symp Quant Biol.* 1960;25:159-182.

118. Pittendrigh CS, Bruce VG. An oscillator model for biological clocks. In: Rudnick D, ed. *Rhythmic and Synthetic Processes in Growth.* Princeton, NJ: Princeton University Press; 1957:75-109.

119. Plazzi G, Corsini R, Provini F, et al. REM sleep behavior disorders in multiple system atrophy. *Neurology.* 1997;48:1094-1097.

120. Poceta JS, Dalessio DJ. Identification and treatment of sleep apnea in patients with chronic headache. *Headache.* 1995;35:586-589.

121. Ralph MR, Foster RG, Davis FC, et al. Transplanted suprachiasmatic nucleus determines circadian period. *Science.* 1990;247:925-978.

122. Ranzijn R, Lack L. The pupillary light reflex cannot be used to measure sleepiness. *Psychophysiology.* 1997;34:17-22.

123. Rawson KS. Homing behavior and endogenous activity rhythms. Cambridge, MA: Harvard University; 1956. Thesis. Cited in Wever RA. *The Circadian System of Man: Results of Experiments Under Temporal Isolation.* New York: Springer-Verlag; 1979.

124. Rechtschaffen A, Kales A. *A Manual of Standardized Terminology: Techniques and Scoring System for Sleep Stages of Human Subjects.* Los Angeles: UCLA Brain Information Service/Brain Research Institute; 1968.

125. Report of the Therapeutics and Technology Assessment Subcommittee of the American Academy of Neurology. Assessment: techniques associated with the diagnosis and management of sleep disorders. *Neurology.* 1992;42:269-275.

126. Rivlin J, Hoffstein V, Kalbfleisch J, et al. Upper airway morphology in patients with idiopathic obstructive sleep apnea. *Am Rev Respir Dis.* 1984;129:355-360.

127. Roehrs T, Roth T. Multiple Sleep Latency Test: technical aspects and normal values. *J Clin Neurophysiol.* 1992;9:63-67.

128. Roehrs T, Zorick F, Wittig R, et al. Predictors of objective level of daytime sleepiness in patients with sleep-related breathing disorders. *Chest.* 1989;95:1202-1206.

129. Rogers AE, Meehan J, Guilleminault C, et al. HLA DR 15 (DR2) and DQB1*0602 typing in 188 narcoleptic patients with cataplexy. *Neurology.* 1997;48:1550-1556.

130. Rosenthal NE, Blehar MC. *Seasonal Affective Disorders and Phototherapy.* New York: Guilford Press; 1989:386.

131. Rosenthal L, Folkerts M, Roehrs T, et al. Sleepiness and sleep onset REM periods in the absence of clinical symptomatology. *Biol Psychiatry.* 1994;36:341-343.

132. Roth T, Roehrs TA, Carskadon MA, et al. Daytime sleepiness and alertness. In: Kryger MH, Roth T, Dement WC, eds. *Principles and Practice of Sleep Medicine.* 2nd ed. Philadelphia: WB Saunders; 1994:40-49.

133. Rothstein JD, Guidotti A, Tinuper P, et al. Endogenous benzodiazepine receptor ligands in idiopathic recurring stupor. *Lancet.* 1992;340:1002-1004.

134. Sack RL, Lewy AJ, Blood ML, et al. Melatonin administration to blind people: phase advances and entrainment. *J Biol Rhythms.* 1991;6:249-261.

135. Sack RL, Lewy AJ, Blood ML, et al. Circadian rhythm abnormalities in totally blind people: incidence and clinical significance. *J Clin Endocrinol Metab.* 1992;75:127-134.

136. Sack RL, Lewy AJ, Hughes RJ. The use of melatonin for sleep and circadian rhythm disorders. *Ann Med.* 1998;30:115-121.

137. Sackett G, Korner A. Organization of sleep-waking states in conjoined twin neonates. *Sleep.* 1993;16:414-427.

138. Sadeh A, Hauri PJ, Kripke DF, et al. The role of actigraphy in the evaluation of sleep disorders. *Sleep.* 1995;18:288-302.

139. Sanders MH, Kern N. Obstructive sleep apnea treated by independently adjusted inspiratory and expiratory positive airway pressure via nasal mask: physiologic and clinical implications. *Chest.* 1990;98:317-324.

140. Sanders MH, Kern NB, Costantino JP, et al. Adequacy of prescribing positive airway pressure therapy by mask for sleep apnea on the basis of a partial-night trial. *Am Rev Respir Dis.* 1993;147:1169-1174.

141. Scharf SM, Garshick E, Brown R, et al. Screening for subclinical sleep-disordered breathing. *Sleep.* 1990;13:344-353.

142. Schenck CH, Bundlie SR, Mahowald MW. Delayed emergence of a parkinsonian disorder in 38% of 29 older men initially diagnosed with idiopathic rapid eye movement sleep behavior disorder. *Neurology.* 1996;46:388-393.

143. Schenck CH, Hurwitz TD, Mahowald MW. REM sleep behavior disorder: a report on a series of 96 consecutive cases and a review of the literature. *J Sleep Res.* 1993;2:224-231.

144. Schenck CH, Mahowald MW. Motor dyscontrol in narcolepsy: rapid eye movement sleep without atonia and REM sleep behavior disorder. *Ann Neurol.* 1992;32:3-10.

145. Schenck CH, Mahowald MW. Somatoform conversion disorder mimicking narcolepsy in 8 patients with nocturnal and diurnal dissociative disorders. *Sleep Res.* 1993;22:260.

146. Schenck CH, Mahowald MW. REM parasomnias. *Neurol Clin.* 1996; 14:697-720.

147. Schenck CH, Mahowald MW. A parasomnia overlap disorder involving sleepwalking, sleep terrors and REM sleep behavior disorder: report in 33 polysomnographically confirmed cases. *Sleep.* 1997;20:972-981.

148. Schenck CH, Mahowald MW, Kim SW, et al. Prominent eye movements during NREM sleep and REM sleep behavior disorder associated with fluoxetine treatment of depression and obsessive-compulsive disorder. *Sleep.* 1992;15:226-235.

149. Schenck CS, Milner DM, Hurwitz TD, et al. Dissociative disorders presenting as somnambulism: polysomnographic, video, and clinical documentation (8 cases). *Dissociation.* 1989;4:194-204.

150. Schmidt HS, Fortin LD. Electronic pupillography in disorders of arousal. In: Guilleminault C, ed. *Sleep and Waking Disorders: Indications and Techniques.* Menlo Park, CA: Addison-Wesley; 1981:127-141.

151. Schutte S, Doghramji K. REM behavior disorder seen with venlafaxine (Effexor). *Sleep Res.* 1996;25:364.

152. Schwab RJ, Gupta KB, Gefter WB, et al. Upper airway and soft tissue anatomy in normal subjects and patients with sleep-disordered breathing: significance of lateral pharyngeal walls. *Am J Respir Crit Care Med.* 1995;152:1673-1689.

153. Series F, Marc I. Efficacy of automatic continuous positive airway pressure therapy that uses an estimated required pressure in the treatment of the obstructive sleep apnea syndrome. *Ann Intern Med.* 1997;127: 588-595.

154. Series F, Marc I, Cormier Y, et al. Utility of nocturnal home oximetry for case finding in patients with suspected sleep apnea hypopnea syndrome. *Ann Intern Med.* 1993;119:449-453.

155. Siegel JM, Fahringer HM, Anderson L, et al. Evidence of localized neuronal degeneration in narcolepsy: studies in the narcoleptic dog. *Sleep Res.* 1995;24:354.

156. Sloan EP, Shapiro CM. Obstructive sleep apnea in a consecutive series of obese women. *Int J Eat Disord.* 1995;17:167-173.

157. Smolik P, Roth B. Kleine-Levin syndrome: etiopathogenesis and treatment. *Acta Univ Carol Med Monogr.* 1988;128:1-94.

158. Steriade M, Contreras D, Amzica F. Synchronized sleep oscillations and their paroxysmal developments. *Trends Neurosci.* 1994;17:199-210.

159. Steriade M, Hobson JA. Neuronal activity during the sleep-waking cycle. *Prog Neurobiol.* 1976;6:155-376.

160. Stiller RA, Strollo PJ, Sanders MH. Unattended recording in the diagnosis and treatment of sleep-disordered breathing: unproven accuracy, untested assumptions, and unready for routine use. *Chest.* 1994; 105:1306-1309.

161. Stoller MK. Economic effects of insomnia. *Clin Ther.* 1994;16:873-897.

162. Stradling JR, Barbour C, Pitson DJ, et al. Automatic nasal continuous positive airway pressure titration in the laboratory: patient outcomes. *Thorax.* 1997;52:72-75.

163. Strohl KP, Redline S. Recognition of obstructive sleep apnea. *Am J Respir Crit Care Med.* 1996;154:279-289.

164. Strumpf DA, Carlile CC, Millman RP, et al. An evaluation of the Respironics BiPAP bilevel CPAP device for delivery of assisted ventilation. *Respir Care.* 1990;35:415-422.

165. Tryon WK. *Activity Measurement in Psychology and Medicine.* New York: Plenum Press; 1991.

166. van der Meche FG, Bogaard JM, van der Sluys JC, et al. Daytime sleep in myotonic dystrophy is not caused by sleep apnea. *J Neurol Neurosurg Psychiatry.* 1994;57:626-628.

167. Vertes RP. Brainstem control of the events of REM sleep. *Prog Neurobiol.* 1984;22:241-288.

168. Vgontzas AN, Tan TL, Bixler EO, et al. Sleep apnea and sleep disruption in obese patients. *Arch Intern Med.* 1994;154:1705-1711.

169. Viner S, Szalai JP, Hoffstein V. Are history and physical examination a good screening test for sleep apnea? *Ann Intern Med.* 1991;115:356-359.

170. Walker JM, Farney RJ, Walker LE. Assessment of apnea/hypopnea across the night and between NREM and REM sleep. *Sleep Res.* 1986; 15:180.

171. Walls TJ, Newman PK, Cumming WJK. Recurrent apnoeic attacks as a manifestation of epilepsy. *Postgrad Med J.* 1981;57:575-576.

172. Walsh JK, Mahowald MW. Avoiding the blanket approach to insomnia. *Postgrad Med.* 1991;90:211-224.

173. Wehr TA. Effects of wakefulness and sleep on depression and mania. In: Montplaisir J, Godbout R, eds. *Sleep and Biological Rhythms: Basic Mechanisms and Applications to Psychiatry.* New York: Oxford University Press; 1990:42-86.

174. Wever RA. *The Circadian System of Man: Results of Experiments Under Temporal Isolation.* New York: Springer-Verlag; 1979.

175. Wittig RM, Romaker A, Zorick FJ, et al. Night-to-night consistency of apneas during sleep. *Am Rev Respir Dis.* 1984;129:244-246.

176. Yamashiro Y, Kryger MH. Nocturnal oximetry: is it a screening tool for sleep disorders? *Sleep.* 1995;18:167-171.

177. Young T, Palta M, Dempsey J, et al. The occurrence of sleep-disordered breathing among middle-age adults. *N Engl J Med.* 1993;328:1230-1235.

178. Zorick F. Overview of insomnia. In: Kryger MH, Roth T, Dement WC, eds. *Principles and Practice of Sleep Medicine.* 2nd ed. Philadelphia: WB Saunders; 1994:483-485.

# 11

# Neuropsychologic Testing

*Ola A. Selnes and Barry Gordon*

## SCOPE AND PURPOSE OF NEUROPSYCHOLOGIC ASSESSMENT

The purpose of the brain is behavior. Therefore assessment of behavior is the most direct measure of brain function and dysfunction. There are now many other methods of assessing brain mechanisms, including structural imaging with computed tomography (CT) and magnetic resonance imaging (MRI) and functional imaging of brain metabolism, blood flow, and electrical activity. However, none of these methods can be a substitute for direct measurement of the behavior that the brain is meant to do.

Neuropsychology has both scientific and clinical roots and purposes. The clinical face of neuropsychology concerns the assessment of behavior for medical purposes. This aspect is the focus of this chapter. The scientific side of neuropsychology deals with behavior-brain relationships. Although not the focus of this chapter, knowledge of behavior-brain relationships is important for choosing, using, and interpreting the results of clinical neuropsychologic testing, so these relationships are briefly reviewed. Since testing of behavior also raises issues of test reliability, validity, and testing procedures, these factors are also reviewed.

Neuropsychology clearly spans several disciplines but also can be considered a field in itself. There have been a number of debates as to where neuropsychology "belongs" professionally. Some have viewed neuropsychology as part of psychology; some, as part of neurology and behavioral neurology. However, this debate is ill-founded. Clinical neuropsychology draws not only on these disciplines but also on many others. It belongs to each and to all. Yet it should never be forgotten that clinical neuropsychology should serve the patient's medical purposes. Keeping this ultimate purpose in mind should help determine which discipline, and which perspective, is most important for each particular patient's purposes, at any particular time in its course.

In this general view, neuropsychology is any systematic assessment of function with the intent to quantify underlying brain function (or dysfunction) for those functions that are expressed through higher order abilities (e.g., language, memory, and reasoning) rather than elemental abilities (e.g., audition, tactile perception, and simple motor movements).

Depending on the specific question, the scope of neuropsychologic assessment can range from short, formalized mental status tests, such as the Mini Mental State Examination (MMSE) and the Neurobehavioral Cognitive Status Examination,[81] to a comprehensive assessment of all major cognitive domains. Although brief tests can have acceptable sensitivities and specificities in some clinical and epidemiologic situations,[139] they do require careful interpretation[99] and their sensitivity, specificity, and validity are too low for many clinical situations.[118] The neuropsychologic assessment referred to in this chapter is a more rigorous approach. As used here, the term refers to a combination of history and detailed examination. The degree of history taking may vary in both breadth and depth. The extent of the cognitive testing may also vary. However, the assessments discussed here typically take 2 to 5 hours or longer and rely on a number of standardized tests and subtests for each cognitive domain. The clinical motivations for such neuropsychologic assessment are varied, but in general they fall into several overlapping categories:

1. *Establish whether a patient's complaint is consistent with organic deficits.* A causal explanation may not be possible, but a correlation may be. Memory loss (whether reported by the patient or the family) is perhaps the most common such complaint. Another common one is word-finding difficulty. Memory loss and word-finding problems are common complaints of neurologically normal individuals. However, they can also be harbingers of Alzheimer's disease and other conditions. Establishing, by history or examination, the circumstances, specifics, and frequency of these problems is important for differentiating benign problems from pathologic ones.

2. *Establish whether there are impairments in functions for which a patient may or may not have complaints.* Lack of insight sometimes limits the usefulness of a history. A history may also not be revealing simply because some of the functions of the brain are not necessarily evident from behavior in everyday life or work. The patient may have a vague sense of something being wrong but may not be able to describe it. Also, there are functions that can be important clues to brain integrity but that cannot be directly tested by

everyday life. An example is the ability to repeat sentences, which is an important clue to the diagnosis of some types of aphasia.

3. *Establish bases for predicting functional recovery.* After a stroke, cardiac arrest, head injury or other known potential cause of cognitive dysfunction, neuropsychologic assessment can be useful for establishing whether deficits are present or not, predicting whether a patient might have difficulties with everyday functions, and predicting recovery.

4. *Establish baselines for purposes of diagnosis and prognosis.* Sometimes cognitive deficits are too subtle and individual variability is too great to permit any definitive conclusions as to whether clinically relevant deficits are actually present after only an initial evaluation. Under these circumstances, neuropsychologic assessment can be invaluable for objectively establishing a quantitative baseline for future comparison.

## APPROACHES TO NEUROPSYCHOLOGIC TESTING

When comprehensive neuropsychologic testing is to be done, two approaches may be contrasted: the fixed battery approach and the flexible battery approach. In the fixed approach the test battery is normally administered in its entirety, without regard for the specific referral question or complaints of the patient. Examples of the fixed battery approach are the Halstead-Reitan battery and the Luria-Nebraska Neuropsychological Battery (LNNB), which was developed by Golden, et al.[52] The fixed battery approach can be criticized on two grounds. One is self-evident. It does not allow any customization to answer the clinical question(s). The other concerns the specific tests chosen, which have often been of limited reliability and validity. Moreover, the summary scores and interpretations that have been derived from these fixed batteries have often been even less reliable or valid. Lezak[87] comments on these issues in more detail.

The flexible battery, or hypothesis-testing, approach allows selection of tests to be guided by the referral question, the patient's symptoms, the severity of these symptoms, the general physical health and stamina of the patient, and other factors such as occupational and educational background. The flexible battery approach has many virtues over the fixed battery approach apart from the merits or demerits of the specific test battery used.[13,75] A principal advantage of the flexible battery approach is that the assessment procedures can focus on the referral question. For example, if the question is whether the patient has early dementia, age-associated memory loss,[25,84] or depression, the examination focuses on various aspects of verbal and visual memory, measures of new learning, spontaneous recall, and recognition memory, as well as delayed recall. Since the diagnosis of dementia technically requires impairment in one or more cognitive domains in addition to the memory impairment, additional cognitive domains must be assessed. Rather than providing a yes/no answer to the question of brain damage, this approach can determine whether or not a cognitive impairment is present, and if so, whether the severity and specific pattern of impairment are consistent with a specific diagnosis. For assessing decline, a flexible battery typically includes measures with adequate dynamic range for detecting changes with progression of disease severity. A survey

among practicing neuropsychologists found that 82% preferred some type of flexible approach and only 18% preferred a standardized battery such as the Halstead-Reitan.[140]

The preferred approach in most cases is to have a core set of tests designed to sample the major cognitive domains, supplemented by additional tests dictated by the nature of the patient's problem and the specifics of the medical issues. This approach usually ensures the most efficient answer to the initial clinical questions and a basis for answering other clinical questions that may arise. An outline of the fixed-flexible testing schema that we use is given later.

## BASIC ASSUMPTIONS UNDERLYING NEUROPSYCHOLOGIC TESTING AND INTERPRETATION

Neuropsychologic testing is based on several postulates and empiric results. One postulate is that overt behavior is the product of internal functions, which are more or less hidden from the observer. A second postulate of neuropsychology is that the internal functions are modular; that is, they are to some extent functionally independent of one another. A third postulate of neuropsychology is that the number of internal functions is finite and that one internal function may participate in two or more overt behavioral functions. In other words, different overt behavioral abilities can and do make use of common internal functions. Understanding the meaning of a word that is heard uses the same internal mechanism as does understanding the meaning of a word that is seen, even though the routes required to reach that common stage differ because of the different input modalities.*

## TECHNICAL CONSIDERATIONS IN TEST INTERPRETATION

Technical issues such as reliability and validity have not received as much emphasis in neuropsychological testing as

---

*These postulates are not necessarily irreducible assumptions. It may be that internal-external differences and modularity arise in any sufficiently complex dynamic system, which is what the brain and mind are.[56] These theoretic postulates and empiric studies have suggested that the higher functions of the mind and brain are organized into broad functional components, such as attention, visual and auditory perception, tactile perception, language, construction (motor), planning and judgment, declarative memory, and motor and psychomotor speed. At the level of analysis being considered here, many of these functional units are strongly associated with anatomic divisions of the brain. The clearest example is the association between language and the dominant perisylvian area. For the abilities examined in clinical contexts, however, these relationships are far less direct. A function may be modular, but its brain implementation may involve multiple neurons and neural systems. Conversely, a single brain region, or even a single neuron or neural component, may participate in many different functions. Therefore the mapping from function to anatomy is not always one-to-one, and it cannot be expected to be. In clinical practice, these mappings are further complicated by the effects of preexisting individual differences (in basic abilities and in neuroanatomic organization), by the unique effects of that individual's disease (its location and time course), and by a host of responses to the deficit (ranging from functional work-arounds to neuronal reorganization and plasticity).

they have in other areas of psychology.[47] Nonetheless, most neuropsychologic tests in common use have acceptable reliability and validity. Of course, the actual reliability and validity of a given test depend on the specific patient population being evaluated. Thus the reliability and validity of a given test should ideally be evaluated separately for different disease states and different levels of severity of cognitive impairment.[16] A test that has proven validity for the assessment of moderate Alzheimer's disease may not prove useful for the assessment of cognitive symptoms in mild-to-moderate multiple sclerosis.

## TEST RELIABILITY

Test reliability can refer to one or all of several related concepts. It may mean test consistency or measurement precision, its stability over time (test-retest reliability), and comparability of results when the test is administered by different examiners (interrater reliability). Many medical professionals have the unwarranted impression that the reliability of neuropsychologic testing is much less than that of so-called objective tests. In reality, the reliability of standardized neuropsychometric tests can be as high as, if not higher than, that of many other medical tests. Published average internal consistency coefficients for subtests and composite scores of the Wechsler Memory Scale-Revised (WMS-R) range from 0.41 to 0.90 with a median of 0.74. Interscorer reliability for the two subtests requiring the most subjective judgment in scoring (logical memory and visual reproduction) were 0.99 and 0.97, respectively. By comparison, for example, the interrater reliability for determining regional brain atrophy by MRI has been reported to be in the 0.24 to 0.34 range.[122]

## TEST SENSITIVITY

Sensitivity refers to the ability of a test to detect a true difference or change. In the past, neuropsychologic tests were frequently evaluated in terms of their sensitivity to detect "brain dysfunction" or "organic brain injury." Today the emphasis has shifted to the ability of a test to detect decline or change in a given cognitive domain. Although the sensitivity of certain screening tests (e.g., MMSE) for detecting dementia is frequently reported, it often does not make much sense to evaluate the sensitivity of individual neuropsychologic tests for the detection of a specific disease. This is because the diagnostic usefulness is usually not in the individual test scores but in the profile or pattern of performance across different neuropsychologic tests.

## TEST VALIDITY

There are several types of validity. From a practical point of view, however, the most relevant validity aspect of neuropsychologic tests is construct validity, that is, whether the test actually provides a measure of what it purports to measure. Although many tests have acceptable "face validity," more formal assessment of construct validity is problematic. For example, although there is little doubt that the Rey Auditory Verbal Learning Test (RAVLT) provides a measure of verbal memory, the validity of its individual components (new learning, delayed recall, and recognition memory) is difficult to assess because of the lack of an accepted gold standard for these aspects of memory. Validity is of greater concern with more specialized tests, such as those measuring frontal lobe–type functions. For example, the validity of the Wisconsin Card Sorting Test (WCST) as a measure of frontal lobe impairment continues to generate controversy,[34,114] largely because its specificity has been called into question. Although there is no doubt that many patients with documented frontal lobe injury perform poorly on the WCST, this is also true of patients with lesions in other areas of the brain. Conversely, some patients with documented large frontal lobe lesions may actually show no abnormality on this test.[39] Thus, although the WCST probably does tap into aspects of frontal lobe–type functions, the interpretation of the results of performance on this test requires considerable caution. *Frontal lobe functions* is an umbrella term for a number of different functions, and it is not known which specific aspects of hypothetical frontal lobe–type functions (mental flexibility, abstraction, set shifting) are reflected in poor performance on the WCST.

Validity is often a major issue for brief screening tests for cognitive impairment. For example, Pierre Marie's Three Paper Test, which was formerly in common use as a measure of auditory comprehension in patients with aphasia, is not necessarily a valid test.[11] Educated patients pass the test even when their auditory comprehension is mildly impaired, and older, less well educated patients may fail the test because of reasons other than language impairment. Another example is the three-word memory test. It may come as a surprise to most neurologists that, depending on the specific choice of words, a substantial proportion of normal subjects will fail this test.[26] The Serial Sevens Test is another example of a test frequently failed by neurologically normal individuals, not because of attention deficits but because of low education level and poor mental arithmetic or calculation skills.[134]

# COMPONENTS OF A FLEXIBLE NEUROPSYCHOLOGIC BATTERY

Depending on background, training, and theoretic orientation, the choice of specific tests for a neuropsychologic evaluation may vary significantly among neuropsychologists. Typically, however, there is adequate overlap in terms of the actual cognitive domains assessed. The principal cognitive domains evaluated during a neuropsychologic examination are listed in Table 11–1, together with some representative tests for each domain. For a more complete discussion of other tests available for probing specific aspects of functioning within a specific cognitive domain, see Lezak.[87]

## ATTENTION

Mild, nonspecific deficits of attention are relatively common with most types of brain injury and can lead to impaired performance in a number of cognitive domains, including memory. Therefore it is important to include one or more measures of auditory or visual attention to control for possible confounding effects from attentional deficits. In some patients with mild closed head injury, deficits in attention may be the only measurable deficit in performance. The Digit Span subtest of the Wechsler Adult Intelligence Scale-revised (WAIS-R),[153] which requires the patient to repeat random sequences of digits of increasing length, is reliable and provides a rapid means for screening attentional abilities. Normal performance is $7 \pm 2$ for forward span and $5 \pm 2$ for backward span length, but clinically a significant dis-

## TABLE 11–1. Major Cognitive Domains and Relevant Tests

**General Intellectual Abilities**

| | |
|---|---|
| Wechsler Adult Intelligence Scale-Revised (WAIS-R) | Assessment of both verbal and nonverbal aspects of cognitive performance; provides separate verbal and performance IQ scores |
| Shipley Institute of Living Scale | Self-administered test of verbal and abstraction abilities; provides full-score IQ equivalent |
| Raven's Progressive Matrices | Nonverbal measure of IQ |
| National Adult Reading Test (NART) | Test of ability to read low-frequency, phonologically irregular words; provides full-scale IQ equivalent |

**Attention**

| | |
|---|---|
| Digit Span (Forward/Backward) | Measure of verbal attention span (subtest of WAIS-R) |
| Spatial Span (Forward/Backward) | Measure of visual attention span (subtest of WAIS-R) |
| Paced Auditory Serial Addition Test | Serial calculation measure of attention |
| Reaction Time (simple and choice) | Computerized measure of simple and choice reaction time |

**Language**

| | |
|---|---|
| Boston Diagnostic Aphasia Examination (BDAE) | Battery of language tests for aphasia assessment |
| Boston Naming Test | Visual confrontation naming, line drawings |
| Tactile Naming | Naming of everyday objects to touch (stereognosis) |
| Token Test | Test of auditory comprehension requiring patient to point to tokens of different size, shape, and color |
| Writing to Description | Subtest of BDAE; assesses ability to provide written description of a picture |
| Repetition | Subtest of BDAE; repetition of words and sentences |

**Memory**

| | |
|---|---|
| Wechsler Memory Scale-Revised (WMS-R) | Memory test battery with subtests that assess orientation, attention, verbal and visual memory |
| Rey Auditory Verbal Learning Test (RAVLT) | 15-word list learning test that evaluates verbal learning, delayed recall, and delayed recognition |
| California Verbal Learning Test | List-learning memory test similar to RAVLT; 16 words belong to four semantic categories[31] |
| Hopkins Verbal Learning Test | List-learning memory test; multiple alternate forms |
| Recognition Memory Test | Test of recognition memory for words and faces; forced-choice recognition testing |
| Benton Visual Retention Test | Paper-and-pencil test of visual memory for geometric designs |

**Visuoconstruction**

| | |
|---|---|
| Rey Osterreith Complex Figure Copy | Paper-and-pencil test of constructional skills requiring patient to copy a complex two-dimensional figure |
| Block Design (in WAIS-R) | Test requiring patient to assemble three-dimensional blocks to match a two-dimensional design |
| Clock Face Drawing | Brief test requiring patient to draw a circle with numbers representing clock-face and to set hands to indicate specified time |

**Visuoperception**

| | |
|---|---|
| Picture Completion (in WAIS-R) | Requires identification of missing details from line drawings |
| Line Discrimination Test | Evaluates ability of patient to match orientation of pair of lines to model |
| Clock Face Perception | Requires patient to tell time in photographs of clock faces |

**Abstraction/Problem Solving**

| | |
|---|---|
| Wisconsin Card Sorting Test (WCST) | Test of problem solving and abstraction requiring patient to infer decision making rules from feedback given during testing |
| Similarities (in WAIS-R) | Test of verbal abstraction requiring patient to state what two concepts have in common |
| Verbal Fluency | Verbal test requiring patient to generate as many words as possible that start with a certain letter in 60-second period |
| Stroop Interference Test | Test of resistance to interference and mental flexibility; requires patient to read out loud color of ink in which words are printed; words are names of colors printed in different color ink from name of color (e.g., word *red* is printed in blue ink) |

**Psychomotor Skills**

| | |
|---|---|
| Grooved Pegboard Test | Test of psychomotor speed that requires patient to insert grooved pegs into 5 × 5 array of slotted holes |
| Finger Tapping Test | Test of motor speed evaluating tapping speed in three 10-second trials |
| Trail Making Test | Test of psychomotor speed and mental flexibility; part A requires patient to connect numbered circles in sequence as quickly as possible; part B requires connecting alternating numbers and letters in sequence as quickly as possible |
| Digit Symbol (in WAIS-R) | Paper-and-pencil test of psychomotor speed, visual scanning, and new learning |

crepancy (± 3) between forward and backward span length is as informative as the absolute span length itself.[87] The Paced Auditory Serial Addition Test (PASAT) has been used frequently to evaluate patients with closed head injury and is considered sensitive to even mild residual attentional deficits.[59] The most sensitive evaluation of mild attentional deficits, however, can be accomplished through the use of computerized tests of simple and choice reaction time. Many different versions are now commercially available. Excellent normative data are available for the California Computerized Assessment Package (CALCAP),[102] which is a brief and

flexible program that is readily accepted by older patients or patients with no previous experience with computers. The complete version consists of seven subtests that can assess speed of processing, divided attention, sustained attention, and visual scanning. Instructions for each subtest are provided by the computer, along with practice trials to ensure that the patient understands the task. Scoring and display of the test results in graphic or numeric form is also included.

The most severe attention deficits are seen in patients with delirium, and patients with moderate to severe delirium are rarely able to focus their attention long enough to complete formal neuropsychologic testing. Consequently, bedside testing is often sufficient. Some of the bedside tests in common use, however, such as the Serial Sevens Test,[94] are confounded by mathematical and educational skills and typically result in a significant number of false-positive findings.[124,134]

## PSYCHOMOTOR SPEED

Assessment of psychomotor speed is particularly helpful for distinguishing between cortical and subcortical dementias, since psychomotor slowing is one of the early findings with subcortical disease. The CALCAP tests of reaction time referred to earlier are excellent tests of psychomotor speed with relatively little theoretic baggage. The Grooved Pegboard Test,[83] which requires the patient to place 25 slotted pegs into a 5 × 5 array of keyed holes, is one of the most sensitive tests of psychomotor speed. The patient must rotate the pegs to fit the keyed hole before they can be placed, thus relying on fine-motor control mediated by pyramidal tract systems. Both hands are tested, and subtle differences in motor speed between the two hands can be measured easily. The Grooved Pegboard Test is not only a measure of psychomotor speed but also of fine-motor control and agility. The Finger Tapping Test also provides a measure of motor speed, but without the element of agility. The Symbol Digit Test is another paper-and-pencil test of psychomotor speed.[135] It provides a measure of speed of visual scanning, memory, and writing speed, with additional elements of attentional and memory mechanisms. This test is sometimes confused with the Digit Symbol Test from the WAIS-R, another measure of psychomotor speed that requires conversion of numbers into symbols rather than symbols into numbers.

## LANGUAGE

In nonaphasic patients, assessment of language typically focuses on naming, reading, and writing. Evaluation of confrontation naming ability can be accomplished with the Boston Naming Test,[76] a carefully normed test that uses line drawings of objects with names ranging from high word frequency (easy to name) to very low frequency (more difficult to name). The short (30-item) version is usually adequate in most clinical situations.[92] Dysnomia is a ubiquitous finding in early dementia, and it may help to distinguish between cortical and subcortical dementias. It is also useful for discriminating a primary degenerative dementia from a dementia secondary to depression.[70] In patients with aphasia, language evaluation takes center stage and provides information on overall severity of impairment and prognostic information. The taxonomy or classification of aphasia type remains confusing to most nonexperts, and, depending on the duration of time after onset of symptoms, no more than 20% to 30% of patients will fit neatly into one of the major aphasia syndromes.[2] Detailed assessment of degree of intactness of comprehension, repetition, and speech fluency can provide a more reliable basis for prognosis than does the type of aphasia syndrome. In particular, assessment of single-word comprehension with tests such as the Word Discrimination subtest from the Boston Diagnostic Aphasia Examination (BDAE)[53] is useful because performance on this test has been shown to be highly predictive of degree of language recovery by 6 months after onset in patients with aphasia secondary to stroke.[130] Performance on tests of repetition is an indirect measure of degree of injury to the (dominant) postero-superior temporal lobe; it also carries prognostic information in that patients who present acutely with mild-to-moderate repetition disorders have an excellent prognosis for recovery.[129] Standard textbook accounts have emphasized the role of the arcuate fasciculus in repetition disorders.[1] Nevertheless, modern imaging studies have not supported a specific role for the arcuate fasciculus in repetition (only three cases with damage largely confined to the arcuate fasciculus have been reported to have conduction aphasia).[22,141] Recent MRI studies of patients with selective injury to the arcuate fasciculus as a result of demyelinating disease did not report repetition deficits in these patients.[111]

## MEMORY

Memory complaints are by far the most common reason for referral for neuropsychologic evaluation. Some of the dimensions of memory function for functional and neuroanatomic correlation have been recently reviewed.[55,57] The original version of the Wechsler Memory Scale (WMS) was among the most frequently administered tests of memory in clinical neuropsychologic practice, but the verdict is still out as to whether the revised version, the WMS-R,[154] will become equally popular.[29,37] Because of the time required to complete this memory battery, some neuropsychologists prefer a more focused evaluation of memory, such as the RAVLT[116] or the California Verbal Learning Test.[31] These are list-learning tasks that require the subject to learn as many words as possible from a 15- to 16-word list presented for five learning trials. The tests also allow for evaluating recall after interference, delayed recall (after 20 minutes or more), and recognition memory (patient selects the words from a list that also includes foils or distractor items). Delayed recall is particularly important for distinguishing impaired acquisition (new learning) from impaired retention of information, and it may be the only subtest that detects an abnormality in patients in the earliest stages of degenerative dementia such as Alzheimer's disease.

Assessment of recognition memory is helpful for distinguishing levels of severity of memory impairments. For example, recognition memory is typically better preserved in dementias with predominantly subcortical involvement, such as normal pressure hydrocephalus, human immunodeficiency virus (HIV)-dementia, and progressive supranuclear palsy, than in dementias with predominantly cortical involvement, even though performance on tests of free recall may be equally impaired in these two groups of patients. The Recognition Memory Test developed by Warrington[151] allows for assessment of both verbal and visual recognition memory. This test is particularly helpful for assessing patients with limited verbal output since the patient responds by pointing to one of two multiple choice answers for each test item. The test is limited by ceiling effects, however, and normative data are based on relatively small sample sizes.[77] Despite a resurgence of research interest in retrograde amnesia,[57] detailed formal assessment of remote or established memories is performed typically less often as part of a routine neuropsychologic examination. This is in part because remote memories tend to be relatively impervious to most types of brain injury and in part because they tend to be so individual in nature that standardized testing becomes a challenge. The Boston Famous Faces Test[3] may be used for this purpose, although its current version needs updating. The Rivermead Behavioural Memory Test[156] allows for quantitative assessment of remote autobiographic memories, but because of the time required for administration, its yield in routine clinical neuropsychologic examination may be relatively low.

## VISUOCONSTRUCTION

Tests of visuoconstructional abilities require the patient to assemble parts (lines in drawings, blocks, or pieces of a puzzle) into an integrated whole. Among neurologists, visuoconstructional assessment typically depends on information provided by the drawing subtest (interlocking pentagons) of the MMSE,[44] which may not be sensitive enough to detect either left parietal or right hemisphere abnormalities. Copying of complex two-dimensional drawings, such as the Rey Osterreith Complex Figure,[115] allows for relatively rapid assessment of constructional deficits. Performance on this test may also bring out evidence of subtle visual neglect. More detailed assessment of constructional abilities in mildly impaired or highly educated patients can be accomplished with the Block Design subtest from the WAIS-R, which requires manipulation of three-dimensional blocks to re-create designs of various levels of complexity. For patients with relatively severe impairment, the traditional clock-face drawing test can also provide useful information.[20,42] Asking the patient to draw the hands of the clock to show a specific time, such as 10 minutes past 11, increases the sensitivity of the test (since it requires integrating the concepts of number, time, and spatial information). In addition to testing the ability to construct a clock face, it is helpful in evaluating the patient's ability to tell time from photographs of clocks set at different times. Patients who fail both the constructional and the perceptual tasks typically have parietal lobe involvement, whereas patients who are impaired on the constructional test but have preserved ability to perceive time are more likely to have constructional deficits from subcortical or nondominant hemisphere involvement.

## VISUOPERCEPTION

Visuoperceptual deficits are encountered somewhat less frequently than are visuoconstructional deficits. Clues to the presence of perceptual difficulties may surface during tests that rely on pictures, such as the line drawings of the Boston Naming Test.[76] The Boston Diagnostic Aphasia Exam Cookie Theft Card is another quick screen to detect perceptual abnormalities and rare conditions such as simultanagnosia. More detailed assessment can be accomplished with the Picture Completion subtest of the WAIS-R, which requires the patient to point out "anomalies" or missing parts from line drawings. The Benton Line Orientation Test[14] also provides a measure of perceptual difficulties. More unusual perceptual impairments, such as prosopagnosia, are not routinely tested unless the history or examination suggests the presence of such a problem. A quick screen can be accomplished by showing the patient pictures of well-known individuals, such as past presidents of the United States, although it is important to distinguish naming difficulties from actual visual recognition difficulties. The Benton Face Recognition Test[14] provides a standardized measure of the ability to discriminate unfamiliar faces.

## ABSTRACTION/PROBLEM SOLVING

These are sometimes also termed "executive" or "frontal" type problems. Actually, a vast number of separable mental functions must be subsumed under these deceptively simple labels. Testing of these functions is thus constrained by our incomplete theoretic understanding. This disadvantage was recently underscored in a study by Duncan et al[36] showing that various tests of purported "executive function" showed almost no common variance when tested in a group of patients with putative "executive deficits," those with significant closed head injuries. As part of the clinical mental status examination, abstraction and problem-solving abilities are usually assessed by asking the patient to interpret well-known proverbs. However, this test is neither very sensitive nor very specific. Educated subjects typically pass this test regardless of an underlying cerebral pathologic condition, and less educated subjects may fail even in the absence of a true pathologic state. A standardized quantitative assessment of abstraction ability can be accomplished with the Similarities subtest of the WAIS-R. This test requires the subject to explain the common feature of two verbal concepts, such as a train and a car. A number of different tests are available to measure problem-solving abilities. Among the most time-efficient and sensitive is the Shipley Institute of Living Scale,[133] a self-administered paper-and-pencil test that incorporates both a vocabulary test and abstraction/problem-solving test, which together can be used to estimate full-scale IQ. The classic test of frontal-lobe type of abstraction/problem solving is the WCST. This test requires the patient to "sort" cards according to a principle that the patient must deduce from the feedback provided by the examiner as the test proceeds.[67] Another aspect of frontal- or executive-type functions that is useful to explore is mental flexibility and the ability to suppress habitual responses. The Stroop Interference Test[136] is a test of word/color reading that requires the patients to read color names that are printed in three different colors (red, green, or blue). The color of the ink is different from the color name; for example, the word *red* is printed in blue ink. The task is to read aloud, as quickly as possible, the color of the ink in which each word is printed rather than the word itself. This test requires that the patient inhibit or suppress the habitual response of reading the word itself.[105,145] A frequently used test to measure mental flexibility and resistance to interference is the Trail Making Test (parts A and B).[49,85] This paper-and-pencil test, which originally was developed for the U.S. Army, requires the patient to rapidly connect numbered circles in sequence for part A and alternating numbers and letters (1-A, 2-B, 3-C, etc.) for part B. It is the set-shifting aspect of part B, switching back and forth between numbers and letters of the alphabet, that assesses divided attention and cognitive flexibility. Wilson et al[157] have proposed a questionnaire and tests for "dysexecutive syndrome"; their utility and validity await wider testing.

## MOOD

Screening instruments such as the Beck Depression Inventory,[8] the Zung Self-Rating Depression Scale,[159] and the Center for Epidemiological Studies Depression Scale (CES-D)[112] are useful for obtaining a quick estimate of mood abnormalities, particularly if responses dealing directly with mood are considered apart from those that might index somatic problems. None of the screening tools for mood disorders is perfect; however, these tools should be able to detect the more severe impairments that could directly affect neuropsychologic test results and flag for the presence of milder problems that may be relevant to consider in an individual's case.

## SELECTION AND INTERPRETATION OF TESTS: BROAD ISSUES

The information that neuropsychology can provide relates to the status of the internal functions of the mind and brain. The ideal result of a neuropsychologic examination is to determine the maximal or near-maximal capabilities of each internal function. These in turn help establish how well the underlying neural substrates for these functions are capable of performing. The major barrier to straightforward interpretation of neuropsychologic test results is effort. If there is lack of effort, then overt performance will not reflect the true maximal capabilities on that task. Lack of effort is typically not a problem in the clinical setting. Fatigue and lapses in attention are often noted in a clinical setting but can usually be taken into account. Lack of effort is much more common, and more of a problem, in a forensic setting. Many subjects in such settings do not show the more florid hallmarks of lack of effort or subversion of test results. Nor can they be expected to be consistent in their lack of effort. Lack of effort in such settings may need to be inferred. Some of the findings may include the following: on any single test, easy items are failed and difficult items are passed; across tests, performance is worse on tests of the same or similar function that require effort, compared to that on tests that do not require as much effort; and the pattern of performance across tests may be incompatible with organic disease(s).

## STEPS IN THE INTERPRETATION OF NEUROPSYCHOLOGIC TEST SCORES

As with interpretation of other test results in medicine, the interpretation of neuropsychologic test results usually involves multiple steps. First, are there extraneous confounding issues, such as fatigue or peripheral sensory deficits? Second, are the test results normal or abnormal? Third, what is the degree of abnormality? Fourth, what is the potential clinical significance of any abnormal findings? Fifth, do the test results suggest a specific pattern of abnormality that may carry diagnostic implications? Sixth, what is the potential source or etiologic basis of any observed cognitive abnormalities? Seventh, do the results have any implications in terms of issues of localization or lateralization of the underlying disease? Each of these issues is considered in more detail in the following sections.

### CONFOUNDING ISSUES

Peripheral sensory deficits—most commonly visual problems, deafness, and peripheral neuropathies—may confound interpretation of neuropsychologic test results. Most of these should be obvious from the history or medical examinations.

### NORMAL VS. ABNORMAL TEST RESULTS

To determine whether any of the test results are abnormal, there must be a comparison of the test results with what is normal for the individual. The best such data come, of course, from premorbid testing; however, such data are rarely available. School records, particularly standardized tests, may be helpful for estimating verbal IQ, knowledge, and arithmetic capabilities. Knowledge of occupational history is also helpful. There are methods of estimating premorbid levels from current test performance, for example, using "hold" tests (e.g., vocabulary) that are relatively resistant to most brain injuries and diseases. However, these methods have limitations, such as their emphasis on verbal abilities.

Population-based estimates are therefore commonly used to estimate premorbid abilities. For most clinical situations it usually suffices to use available age- and education-based norms. However, these norms are typically limited at higher ranges of age and at lower ranges of education (below 10 years). Moreover, there are individuals and situations for whom these population-based norms may be misleading. Differences in neuropsychologic performance have been reported based on socioeconomic status, ethnicity,[93] native tongue and multilingualism, rural vs. nonrural background, literacy,[21] actual years of school attendance, whether grades were failed or not, and work history. Typically, such factors tend to cause false-positive test results (an interpretation of a test result as abnormal when it is actually normal for that individual).

Both individual- and population-based estimates of normative performance can be subject to a major interpretative error if performance on one set of neuropsychologic functions is used to infer what that individual's performance would have been like on another set of functions. This amounts to an assumption that individuals are homogeneous in their cognitive capacities. The assumption of homogeneity in the distribution of cognitive abilities on an individual level has never been proven, and everyday observation shows that it cannot be completely true. For example, it is entirely possible to find neurologically normal individuals with marked discrepancies between their verbal and nonverbal abilities. Full-scale IQ scores are often used as the "reference" for interpreting the level of other scores, with the expectancy that a full-scale IQ score in the superior range should imply a verbal memory score in the same range. This view amounts to the assumption that different aspects of human cognitive functions are normally highly intercorrelated, so that a high-average performance on tests of language and memory would imply that performance on visuospatial tests should also be in the high-average range. Although this correlation may be true in grouped data, it is much less reliable at the individual level. Some normal individuals have excellent verbal memories, whereas others rely more on their visual memories. Some individuals have an excellent sense of direction, whereas others do not. One example of how scores on one test do not necessarily predict scores on another is shown in Figure 11–1, which presents the relationship between memory test performance and IQ for individual subjects in a large multicenter study.

### DEGREE OF ABNORMALITY

Raw scores on test performance are typically transformed for interpretation and for comparison with other test scores. The most common such transformation is to reference the raw scores to those of a normative group, as dis-

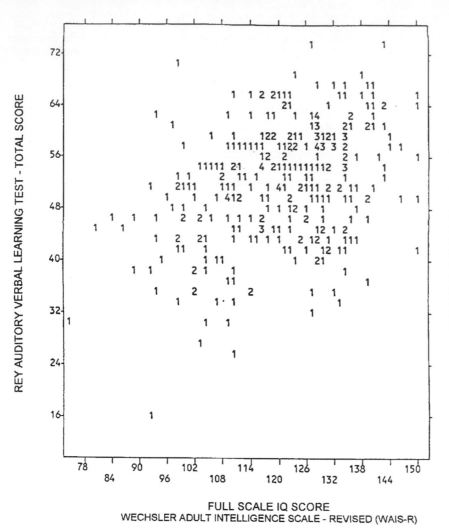

**FIGURE 11–1.** Scatterplot showing relationship between overall intelligence level (WAIS-R, full-scale IQ score) and memory performance (Rey Auditory Verbal Learning Test, total score). Although there is a trend suggesting that higher intelligence level is associated with higher scores on the memory test, note that the memory scores for subjects with very high intelligence levels (above 130 IQ) range from a low of 32 to a high of 75. 1, One observation; 2, two observations, etc. (From unpublished data, Multicenter AIDS Cohort Study.)

cussed earlier (usually based on age and education). Then a deviation score is calculated. The deviation score can be expressed quantitatively—as $z$ scores, $t$ scores, or percentiles—or it can be expressed qualitatively. A $z$ score is calculated by subtracting the observed patient score from the reference mean and then dividing by the standard deviation of the reference mean. The mean of a $z$ score is 0, and the standard deviation is 1. By convention, the "normal" group is ±1.96 SD on either side of the mean. A deviation of greater value is found in less than 5% of the normal group and is by common convention "abnormal." The $t$ scores are essentially $z$ scores, but they are transformed to have a mean of 50 and a SD of 10. One problem with $z$ scores and $t$ scores is that they may be inaccurate and misleading at the extremes of the group. Once a score is outside the normal range, there is typically relatively little normative data to use for comparison. Therefore, although a $z$ score of −5.7 can be computed, it can be relatively meaningless. For this reason some have suggested using percentiles. Table 11–2 shows how $t$ scores, percentiles, and the types of standard scores used on the WAIS-R are interrelated.

Such quantitative measures are generally preferred over categoric descriptions. However, for clinical use, it is sometimes helpful to provide such categories as *mildly impaired, moderately impaired,* and *markedly impaired.* There is no

uniform standard for these categories; they are typically established by reference to how much the observed patient score diverges from the population average or normal score. Frequently, but not always, the term *average performance* is used to describe a test score that falls within ±1 SD of the de-

**TABLE 11–2. Relationship of Standard Deviation (SD) Scores to Percentile Rankings, t Scores, and Wechsler Adult Intelligence Scale-Revised (WAIS-R) Full-Scale IQ Scores**

| SD | PERCENTILE | t SCORE | WAIS-R SCORE |
|---|---|---|---|
| 3.0 | 99+ | 80 | 145 |
| 2.5 | 99 | 75 | 137.5 |
| 2.0 | 98 | 70 | 130 |
| 1.5 | 93 | 65 | 122.5 |
| 1.0 | 84 | 69 | 115 |
| 0.5 | 69 | 55 | 107.5 |
| 0 | 50 | 50 | 100 |
| −0.5 | 31 | 45 | 92.5 |
| −1.0 | 16 | 40 | 85 |
| −1.5 | 7 | 35 | 77.5 |
| −2.0 | 2 | 30 | 70 |
| −2.5 | 1 | 25 | 62.5 |
| −3.0 | <1 | 20 | 55 |

mographically corrected mean score for that test. *Low average* is used to describe a test score that falls between 1 and 2 SD below the mean. Conversely, *above average* performance refers to a score between 1 and 2 SD above the mean. How the terms *mildly impaired, moderately impaired,* and *markedly impaired* are used is much less standardized. Their use is usually based on clinical experience with the range of possible cases, not necessarily with the degree of functional impairment that deficit represents for the individual.

## CLINICAL SIGNIFICANCE

If it is assumed that the neuropsychologic examination yielded some test scores in the impaired range, the next step is to determine whether any of these abnormal scores are clinically significant (i.e., signify that the observed score reflects an acquired abnormality in the brain's functioning) as opposed to representing a normal variability or a preexisting deficit. If the test abnormality is in the borderline to mild range, this decision can be difficult. In part because of the individual variability discussed earlier, considerable experience is required to translate a mild or borderline abnormal test finding into a conclusion regarding potential clinical significance. What is also necessary is the context in which the findings need to be put. Even a mild abnormality can be corroborative in the right context; conversely, in another context even a definite "abnormality" may be interpreted as normal for that individual.

If the patient's scores are all in the normal range, can it be concluded that from a cognitive point of view, nothing is "wrong" with the patient's brain functioning? This may depend (1) on the sensitivity of the individual neuropsychologic tests and (2) on whether the tests administered were the most appropriate for detecting a potential deficit. A mild deficit may not be picked up by the test. If, for example, the patient had a very high IQ before sustaining a brain injury, his or her score may have declined, but it may still be in the average or normal range of performance. The choice of specific tests is important, since some tests are clearly better than others for detecting particular problems. Despite these caveats, in general, neuropsychologic tests have adequate sensitivity for detecting abnormalities of cognitive functioning of sufficient magnitude to be of potential clinical significance.

## PATTERNS OF ABNORMALITY

Once a potentially clinically significant abnormality has been identified, examination of patterns of abnormalities may provide further clues to the clinical significance and possible etiologic basis of the cognitive abnormality. Is there evidence of convergent validity? If performance on two or more tests measuring the same cognitive domain is below average, this strengthens the case for an underlying abnormality, rather than an idiosyncrasy or artifact related to the testing. Pattern analysis can also help determine if the deficit is limited to a single cognitive domain (e.g., language) or more diffuse (involving multiple domains). Most important, the pattern analysis may provide clues as to whether the impaired cognitive domains are predominantly associated with cortical as opposed to subcortical functions. For example, impairment of naming and calculations typically results from cortical injury, whereas impairment of motor and psychomotor functions often signifies subcortical involvement.

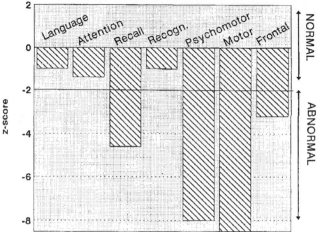

**FIGURE 11–2.** Example of neurocognitive profile consistent with possible subcortical disease. Performance on tests of cortical functions (e.g., language) is relatively preserved, whereas performance on tests of subcortical functions (e.g., psychomotor speed) is impaired. Memory performance is characterized by mild-to-moderate deficits of free recall but relatively preserved recognition memory.

A hypothetical cognitive profile is shown in Figure 11–2. The pattern indicates poor performance in areas of language, recall, and recognition memory but no abnormalities of motor speed. With no other history available, one may conclude (1) that there is a high likelihood of an actual acquired cognitive deficit and (2) that the pattern of the deficits is consistent with predominantly cortical involvement. However, these results by themselves do not point to a specific diagnosis. With additional data, principally the history from the patient, family members, and the referring physician, possible etiologic factors of the cognitive impairment can be determined.

## LESION LATERALIZATION AND LOCALIZATION

Neuropsychologic assessment (history and testing combined) assesses dysfunction. Any conclusions regarding anatomic localization made from the neuropsychologic examination are inferences about where the dysfunction is present in the brain. Different functions (and different tests) have varying degrees of lateralizing and localizing significance.

Language functions are reasonably well lateralized in most individuals, as are fine-motor functions. However, most other functions are not. The widespread use of discrepancies between verbal and performance IQ test scores on the WAIS-R to infer laterality of lesions is particularly problematic. The WAIS-R was not designed to provide such information, and the best available clinical evidence suggests that it does not.[152] Although handedness is generally correlated with the lateralization of language dominance, atypical patterns of lateralization occur with sufficient frequency to warrant the use of extra caution when making inferences about laterality of brain injury based on neuropsychologic test performance.[131,132]

Localization from neuropsychologic test performance is often even more problematic. Many functions are not "localized" in the traditional sense; other functions are precisely localizable but are not precisely delineated by standard clinical neuropsychologic testing. Some tests, such as measures of attention/concentration (e.g., the Digit Span subtest of the WAIS-R), have very little localizing value. Performance on other measures, for example, frontal lobe tests such as the Wisconsin Card Sorting Test, correlates with injury to the frontal lobes, but impaired performance on this test is not particularly specific to frontal lobe lesions.[114] Tests of constructional ability generally correlate with parietal lobe involvement, but subcortical lesions may also result in significant impairment on tests of constructional abilities.[82] There is also evidence that indistinguishable patterns of behavioral or cognitive deficit can be produced by different lesion locations. For example, discrete lesions involving the thalamus can produce behavioral changes that are for practical purposes indistinguishable from those produced by lesions of the frontal lobes.[137]

Once dysfunction has been established, determining whether the impairment is caused by a structural lesion requires further evidence and inference. Even localized impairments are not necessarily due to focal structural lesions; examples are postictal (Todd's) paralysis and migrainous scotomata. All dysfunctions do not have a macroscopic structural basis; vitamin $B_{12}$ deficiency is a classic example. Even localized structural lesions may not be readily discernible as such. Examples are the focal degenerations associated with posterior cortical degeneration or slowly progressive aphasia, which may not be apparent on standard MRI or CT. The opposite is also true. The presence of a lesion need not imply any cognitive symptoms or measurable deficits. Silent brain infarctions on MRI are increasingly recognized as a common finding.[48,90,109]

## ETIOLOGY

Once the degree and pattern of abnormality have been identified, the next step concerns the likely etiologic basis of the observed deficits. Etiologic inferences typically require information about such considerations as risk factors, time course, and possible pathophysiologic mechanisms. Is the patient in the early stages of Alzheimer's disease, or could the cognitive symptoms be secondary to more benign causes such as depression, side effects of medication, or normal aging? Alternatively, does the patient suffer from less common conditions such as posterior cortical degeneration or transient topographic amnesia? This step of the interpretation requires familiarity with a wide range of possible abnormalities or syndromes. The diagnostic significance of the neuropsychologic examination cannot be interpreted merely on the basis of individual test scores. The scores may establish whether the pattern and degree of cognitive impairment are consistent with a possible dementia syndrome, but they do not by themselves imply a specific etiologic basis for the dementia. Therefore the results must be integrated with the medical context of the patient's presentation.

## NEUROPSYCHOLOGIC EVALUATION OF SPECIFIC NEUROLOGIC CONDITIONS

### DEMENTIA

Neuropsychologic assessment is still the only procedure currently available to characterize the pattern and severity of cognitive impairment in patients with suspected dementia. It provides greater sensitivity and specificity for detecting de-

mentia than does any other individual diagnostic procedure.[9,50,148] Neuropsychologic assessment is particularly useful in patients with relatively early symptoms; it can also help to differentiate more benign conditions, such as age-associated memory loss or cognitive impairment secondary to depression, from early Alzheimer's disease. Certain diagnostic criteria, such as the National Institute of Neurological and Communicative Disorders and Stroke (NINCDS)–Alzheimer's Disease and Related Disorders Association (ADRDA), require neuropsychologic testing for establishing a diagnosis of Alzheimer's disease, whereas others, such as the *Diagnostic and Statistical Manual of Mental Disorders (DSM-IV)*, do not. Because the patterns of cognitive symptoms associated with different dementing illnesses may vary considerably, the results of neuropsychologic tests alone cannot establish a specific etiologic basis. Nevertheless, they can identify patterns of cognitive impairment that are consistent with a specific diagnosis, such as Alzheimer's disease. Converging evidence from both neuropathologic studies and functional imaging studies indicates that the earliest stages of neuronal degeneration in Alzheimer's disease involve the temporal lobes followed by parietal lobe involvement.[35,45,101] This translates into a pattern of early cognitive symptoms that includes memory impairment, dysnomia, and parietal lobe findings, such as constructional apraxia, dyscalculia, and dysgraphia. Several studies have demonstrated that the neuropsychologic tests most sensitive to the earliest cognitive manifestations of Alzheimer's disease include measures of delayed recall, confrontation naming, and visuoconstructional abilities.[73,88] If the results of the neuropsychologic testing do not uncover parietal lobe symptoms in a patient with suspected Alzheimer's disease, a diagnosis of Alzheimer's disease is less likely and a search for possible alternative etiologic factors should be pursued. As with all other diseases, the associated signs and symptoms, behavioral features (e.g., depression, urinary incontinence, gait changes), and other laboratory studies (CT, MRI, electroencephalography [EEG]) must be taken into account in weighing the probabilities of a particular diagnosis.

Although neuropsychologic testing may not be strictly necessary in all patients with suspected Alzheimer's disease, it is recommended whenever the patient presents with atypical features. This may include factors such as very early onset (before age 50), atypical features (e.g., preserved insight, personality, and self-care), or the presence of confounding conditions that by themselves may contribute to cognitive impairment (e.g., certain medications that affect the central nervous system, sleep apnea, metabolic abnormalities). With the advent of pharmacologic interventions, it may also be prudent to obtain baseline neuropsychologic testing before starting treatment. This approach allows for a more accurate and objective determination of any possible improvement in cognitive symptoms associated with the therapy.

Neuropsychologic testing is also helpful for evaluating dementias with atypical cognitive features, such as hippocampal sclerosis[24,143] and the more recently recognized syndromes of frontotemporal dementias,[43,104] posterior cortical degeneration,[12,147] and primary progressive aphasia.[100,121,128] Other more specialized focal progressive degenerative syndromes, such as progressive prosopagnosia[41] and progressive amusia and aprosody,[23] have also been described. Neuropsychologic and neurobehavioral evaluation early in the course

**TABLE 11–3. Patterns of Preserved and Impaired Functions in Focal Degenerative Syndromes**

| COGNITIVE DOMAIN | PRIMARY PROGRESSIVE APHASIA | POSTERIOR CORTICAL DEGENERATION | FRONTOTEMPORAL DEMENTIA |
|---|---|---|---|
| Attention | Normal | Normal | Impaired |
| New learning | Normal | Impaired | Impaired |
| Delayed recall | Normal | Impaired | Impaired |
| Naming | Impaired | Impaired | Impaired |
| Visuoconstruction | Normal | Impaired | Normal |
| Visuoperception | Normal | Impaired | Normal |
| Frontal | Normal | Normal | Impaired |
| Psychomotor | Normal | Normal | Normal |

of these focal degenerative syndromes (Table 11–3) can help to distinguish them from other degenerative syndromes (Alzheimer's disease, corticobasal degeneration, multisystem atrophy) for prospective clinical or investigational drug trials.[43] Although early identification of these syndromes at the present time may not necessarily offer any advantages in terms of therapeutic strategies, the time course and pattern of preserved cognitive and social skills differ sufficiently from typical Alzheimer's dementia to be potentially useful prognostic information for families and caregivers. Also, as pointed out by McKhann,[96] at the present stage of our knowledge, clinical trials with a small number of well-characterized patients may be preferable to larger studies with poorly characterized patients.

## CEREBROVASCULAR DEMENTIA

Interest in cerebrovascular disease as a potentially treatable or modifiable cause of dementia in late life has had a significant renaissance during the past two decades.[58] The term *multiinfarct dementia* was introduced by Hachinski et al,[61] but the concept of a single disease process characterized by stepwise cognitive decline and radiologic evidence of multiple brain infarcts has been replaced by a spectrum of conditions, ranging from diffuse periventricular microvascular ischemia to lacunar state and abnormalities involving hemodynamic mechanisms.[65,106] Consistent with this development, the *DSM-IV* has replaced the term *multiinfarct dementia* with *vascular dementia*.[7] Implicit in this redefinition of the concept of vascular dementia is the idea that the degree of cognitive impairment associated with cerebrovascular disease can range from subtle psychomotor slowing to full-blown dementia.[60] Although vascular dementia is believed to be the second most common cause of dementia after Alzheimer's disease,[68] there is still some controversy surrounding the clinical reality of this syndrome.[58,89] Several sets of diagnostic criteria for vascular dementia have been proposed.[117,155] Some studies have found relatively low sensitivity when these criteria were used,[51] but others have reported a high rate of diagnostic accuracy provided that a thorough workup, including neuropsychologic testing, is performed.[38]

The profile of neuropsychologic deficits is determined by multiple factors, such as degree and location of ischemic changes, atrophy, and ventricular enlargement. Nonetheless, in the early stages of the disease, the pattern of neuropsychologic deficits associated with cerebrovascular dementia is distinct from that associated with cortical dementias, such as Alzheimer's disease.[6,80] Because cerebrovascular dementias have disproportionate involvement of subcortical structures,

such as the basal ganglia and the thalamus, the neurocognitive profile is characterized principally by the presence of mild-to-moderate motor and psychomotor slowing relatively early in the disease process.[5,98,149] Psychomotor slowing, as measured by timed tests such as the Trail Making Test, Symbol Digit Test, and others, is the most critical neuropsychologic finding that helps to distinguish between subcortical and cortical dementias.[107] This is why screening tests such as the MMSE, which does not include measures of psychomotor speed, lacks sensitivity for the early detection of subcortical dementias. Psychomotor slowing does not occur until the very late stages of the illness in cortical dementias such as Alzheimer's disease or Pick's disease. Additionally, cortical features, such as dysnomia, dyscalculia, and agraphia, are less prominent in subcortical dementias.

Although new learning and memory may be disturbed to the same degree as in patients with Alzheimer's disease, patients with subcortical dementias typically show relative preservation of recognition memory. Severity of constructional deficits on tasks such as copying a cube or spontaneously drawing a clock face may not differentiate cortical from subcortical dementias, although the mechanisms underlying the deficits may be quite different.[82] The absence of parietal lobe type of perceptual deficits in vascular dementia, however, is very helpful in differentiating it from cortical dementias. Thus patients with subcortical vascular dementia are able to tell time from analog clocks, although this ability is typically impaired even in early Alzheimer's disease. Performance on tests traditionally thought of as relevant to frontal lobe functioning is typically impaired in vascular dementia.[80] This impairment is thought to be secondary to interruption of frontosubcortical connections rather than frontal lobe lesions.[72,137,158]

While the exact contribution of subcortical ischemic periventricular white matter lesions to the development of symptoms of cognitive impairment is still not understood, several studies now suggest that even nondemented patients with evidence of ischemic periventricular white matter disease show a characteristic pattern of psychomotor slowing on detailed cognitive testing.[19,74,123]

## EPILEPSY AND SURGICAL CONDITIONS

Neuropsychologic testing has played a prominent role in the evaluation and management of patients with epilepsy.[91] It has helped to characterize cognitive side effects associated with certain types and dosages of anticonvulsant medications[30,32,91] and to define patterns of cerebral language dominance in patients undergoing temporal lobectomy for medically intractable seizures.[33] The intracarotid amobarbital test introduced by Juhn Wada[150] continues to be the gold standard for establishing language laterality, but the specific cognitive tests used during this procedure have been refined substantially. Moreover, detailed cognitive testing in patients during direct cortical stimulation with indwelling subdural electrode arrays allows for a degree of refinement in presurgical mapping of language functions that was previously unobtainable.[64] As a result, unanticipated postoperative cognitive complications after temporal lobectomy have been greatly reduced.[15,142] Advances in many other areas of neurosurgical intervention have led to increased expectation for improved quality of the outcome following these procedures.[69] Thus preoperative and postoperative cognitive assessment in procedures such as aneurysm clipping, tumor resection, shunting for normal pressure hydrocephalus,[113] and other procedures[27] can help characterize the outcomes in terms of specific cognitive changes. With increasing competition for health care dollars, the importance of measuring cognitive outcomes is likely to become even more important for the future.

## HIV-DEMENTIA

Neuropsychologic testing played an important role in defining the natural history of cognitive impairment associated with HIV infection. Although some early cross-sectional studies concluded that cognitive impairment was prevalent at every stage of the infection, subsequent prospective cohort studies established that HIV-related cognitive impairment occurs only with late-stage disease, generally after the development of advanced immunosuppression or acquired immunodeficiency syndrome (AIDS).[126,127] The annual incidence of HIV-dementia is approximately 7% during the first 2 years after the diagnosis of AIDS.[95] Neuropsychologic testing remains an important part of the diagnostic workup for patients with suspected HIV-dementia.[63] The pattern of cognitive impairment in patients with HIV-dementia is characteristic of that seen with a frontosubcortical dementia. The principal abnormalities include psychomotor slowing, mild-to-moderate memory impairment (typically with relative preservation of recognition memory), visuoconstructional impairment, and poor performance on frontal lobe type of tests. Language and calculations typically remain relatively preserved until late stages of the disease. The cognitive profile of HIV-dementia resembles that of several other diseases with principally subcortical impairment, such as vascular dementia, normal pressure hydrocephalus, and progressive supranuclear palsy. Because most patients at risk for HIV-dementia tend to be much younger than patients at risk for vascular dementia, there is generally not much difficulty telling them apart. However, in a 65-year-old HIV-infected patient with a history of hypertension and diabetes, the finding of a subcortical pattern of cognitive impairment must be interpreted in light of additional laboratory findings such as CD4+ count and radiologic studies to differentiate among the most likely etiologic conditions.

A challenging aspect of diagnosing HIV-related cognitive impairment in younger patients is the need to rule out other possible confounding causes of mental status change. In this context the specific pattern of the observed cognitive impairment can be very helpful. Although there has been some confusion in the literature regarding variability in early cognitive features of HIV-dementia, in our experience the presentation of HIV-dementia is in fact stereotypical and usually fits a subcortical cognitive profile. Therefore, if a patient with HIV has memory or attentional deficits as principal presenting symptoms in the absence of significant psychomotor slowing, alternate etiologic factors for the cognitive changes should be explored. Some of the most common causes of non-HIV-related cognitive changes include side effects from medications, insomnia, fatigue, stress or mood changes, and polysubstance abuse. In addition, it is important to rule out common metabolic and nutritional causes of memory impairment, such as vitamin $B_{12}$ or folate deficiencies and thyroid abnormalities.

## NORMAL PRESSURE HYDROCEPHALUS

Neuropsychologic testing can be helpful in the workup of patients with suspected normal pressure hydrocephalus. Brief mental status tests, such as the MMSE, typically do not have the sensitivity to detect the cognitive abnormalities seen in early stages of this disorder.[146] The cognitive profile of patients with normal pressure hydrocephalus (NPH) is typical of subcortical dementia—with psychomotor slowing, memory impairment, and constructional deficits—but with relatively preserved naming and parietal lobe functions.[28] However, this profile is not specific for NPH and sometimes can be difficult to differentiate from cognitive impairment secondary to vascular dementia. Cognitive testing is also helpful to measure response to diagnostic procedures such as quantitative intracranial pressure monitoring and outcome following shunting.[79,113]

## CLOSED HEAD INJURY

Whether or not someone has suffered any symptoms or deficits as a result of a mild closed head injury is a question commonly posed to neuropsychologists. However, it is not always possible to answer this question definitively.

Although neural injury is a well recognized effect of severe head injuries, the pathologic substrate, if any, that might explain the effects of mild closed head injuries is still not established. Whether any structural impairments, and resulting cognitive impairments, can even occur with head injury that does not cause loss of consciousness remains controversial,[97] although our position has been that it is possible.[54]

The physiologic effects of a mild closed head injury can be approximately indexed by the presence and duration of any loss of consciousness or alteration of consciousness, by anterograde amnesia, and by retrograde amnesia. In general, the cognitive physiologic effects of closed head injury are maximal at the outset and then can be expected to lessen and, usually, disappear. Converging evidence from epidemiologic studies suggests that both symptoms and cognitive performance generally recover to within normal limits in approximately 3 months in most cases of initial mild-to-moderate closed head injury.[86] Milder cases of head injury seen in the general population can be expected to have a better prognosis.

Evaluation of symptoms after closed head injury is complicated by the fact that many of these symptoms, such as difficulty concentrating, difficulty remembering, and irritability and headache, are both fairly nonspecific and common in the normal population.[46] A study of a large group of patients involved in car accidents in Lithuania (where few subjects have personal injury insurance, thus removing the prospect of financial gain through symptom exaggeration) found no difference in the frequency of attention and memory complaints between cases and controls.[125] It is increasingly appreciated that many of the patients who report persistent problems after mild closed head injury have had preexisting psychologic and/or medical problems for which the closed head injury may be a convenient but inaccurate apparent origin.[4]

Evaluation of signs after mild closed head injury is complicated by the fact that little, if any, objective test evidence is expected in any individual case. The most common cognitive residuals that might occur from uncomplicated closed head injury are attentional deficits and deficits in new learning. However, although these effects are evident in group studies, in any individual case it may be impossible to detect them with current tests because of individual variability. Several factors need to be kept in mind in interpreting neuropsychologic test results in a case of suspected mild closed head injury. There should be some proportionality between the physiologic severity of the injury and the patient's symptoms and findings. The time course of symptoms and signs should be consistent. The deficits that occur after mild closed head injury theoretically can include all aspects of cognition, although in practice some are more susceptible than others, and some would not be expected to be affected at all. Deficits in attention, multitasking, and new learning are not unexpected. Deficits in vocabulary or prior semantic knowledge are generally incompatible with mild closed head injury.

### FORENSIC APPLICATIONS

Neuropsychology is frequently invoked in legal issues involving the question of central nervous system injury. In this context, many of the methodologic, procedural, and interpretative assumptions that underlie standard clinical use (the use assumed in this chapter) are not necessarily valid. We have earlier commented on the hazards of concluding that any outlier score reflects an acquired abnormality. Lack of effort on testing also deserves special mention.

### LEVEL OF EFFORT

Most neuropsychologic tests are effort dependent, and meaningful interpretation of the results of such tests assumes adequate effort on behalf of the patient. This is generally not a significant issue when patients are being evaluated for strictly clinical purposes. In the context of litigation, however, the patient's level of effort may become an issue.[40] The spectrum of lack of effort ranges from brief lapses of attention or effort, which even normal individuals may make from time to time, through pervasive lack of effort on testing and frank malingering. *Malingering* has been variously defined; what we mean here by frank malingering is a conscious attempt to deliberately subvert test results.

Several strategies can help to detect poor or uneven effort. Patterns of performance within tests, such as recency and primacy effects on memory testing, can provide important clues. Worse performance on "easier" tests of recognition memory compared to more demanding tests of free recall is also an indicator. Chance performance on tests, particularly when it is out of proportion to performance obtained on other tests or that expected from the individual's level of functioning (during the interview or in everyday life), also suggests a lack of effort.

Clues to the detection of possible malingering are similar to those discussed for level of effort. One may see inconsistencies in response to tests that measure similar functions and exaggeration of symptoms, which are believed to be characteristic features. For example, failing easy items but passing some of the more difficult ones is suggestive.[62,144] There have been several "tests" designed to detect malingering, typically by being so easy that poor performance is suspect.[17,78,110,120] The Rey 15-Item Visual Memorization Test is perhaps the simplest of these to administer and score.[18] However, this test is not necessarily sensitive.[103] The clearest evidence of all is performance that is significantly below chance on a test that allows such a measure, for example, the Warrington Recognition Memory tests.

In general, it must be remembered that lack of definite evidence of malingering is not proof that the subject was exerting full effort. Many patterns of abnormal test results can be generated by lack of effort, and by themselves these results may be difficult, if not impossible, to differentiate from abnormal results caused by pathologic brain dysfunction.

## SUGGESTIONS FOR BEDSIDE/OFFICE COGNITIVE SCREENING

Many neurologists will perform a detailed neurobehavioral assessment of cognition in patients before referring them for more formal neuropsychologic testing. The choice of specific screening tests is clearly a matter of personal preference, and the yield depends largely on the degree of experience with the test. Nonetheless, certain tests provide better sensitivity and specificity. Several excellent guides for office mental status examination are available, including the classic Strub and Black reference[138] and the very readable and up-to-date text by John Hodges.[71] The following are some suggestions for brief cognitive screening tests that are suitable for bedside or office administration.

### ORIENTATION

The standard questions concerning day, date, and place generally work well, although their specificity is poor, since many normal individuals will miss the date by 1 day. Asking the patient for the time of the day increases both the specificity and the sensitivity. Few normal individuals will be off by more than 1 hour, but patients with even mild dementia or delirium typically will make significant errors, often confusing morning with afternoon.

### ATTENTION

Despite its all too common use, the Serial Sevens Test is not a very good test of attentional functions because of its unacceptably high false-positive rate in patients with low education or poor calculation skills.[134] A standard forward and backward digit span test can be administered almost as quickly. Digit span backward adds considerably to the sensitivity of this test, and a discrepancy between forward and backward span of more than three digits is virtually diagnostic of an attentional impairment.[87]

### MEMORY

The three-word recall test (as in the MMSE) can detect gross memory impairments, but, depending on the patient's age and education, it is likely to miss mild-to-moderate memory problems.[66] As mentioned earlier, the choice of specific words has a significant effect on the sensitivity and specificity of this screening measure.[26] The memory subtest of the Neurobehavioral Cognitive Status Examination (NCSE),[81] which uses four words and incorporates a test of recognition memory, improves sensitivity without adding much time over the standard three-word recall test. Aspects of remote memory can be assessed easily through family and social history.

### LANGUAGE

Certain aspects of language, such as fluency in conversational speech and level of comprehension, can generally be evaluated from the clinical interview with the patient. Other features, such as naming, repetition, and writing, should be assessed through brief screening tests. The use of relatively difficult items for screening purposes, such as the phrase "no ifs, ands, or buts" for testing repetition, can be a time-saver. If the patient is able to do the task, repetition is clearly intact. If the patient fails the screening item, however, additional testing with easier items should be included to make sure that the deficit is real.

### SPATIAL ABILITIES

Visuoconstructional abilities can be assessed easily through quick screening tests such as having the patient draw a clock face or a three-dimensional cube. These tests are significantly more sensitive than the copying subtest of the MMSE (the interlocking pentagons). If spontaneous drawing is impaired, copying a model provided by the examiner should be attempted.

### PERCEPTUAL ABILITIES

Assessment of visuoperceptual abilities typically requires more specialized testing. Testing the patient's ability to tell time from pictures of standard analog clock faces can provide important clues to parietal lobe functioning. Patients with Alzheimer's disease typically have difficulty with time perception, even during the early stages of the illness.

### FRONTAL LOBE FUNCTIONS

The traditional approach to screening for frontal lobe–type symptoms by asking the patient to interpret proverbs may work for more educated patients, but it results in false-positive findings for less educated patients. Luria suggested several approaches for screening for frontal lobe impairment,[10] including the hand-position sequencing test (the Three-Hand Test).[119] Nonetheless, this is a challenging aspect of bedside higher cortical function assessment. Even detailed neuropsychologic tests of frontal lobe–type functions may not by themselves discriminate between the effects of frontocortical lesions and the remote effects of subcortical disease.

### PSYCHOMOTOR SPEED

By far the most neglected aspect of functioning in traditional mental status screening examinations is psychomotor and motor speed. The MMSE and other commonly used screening tests do not include any measures of motor speed, even though the finding of psychomotor slowing is one of the most important clues to subcortical involvement. A simple method for assessing psychomotor speed that does not require any instrumentation is to ask the patient to write the letters of the alphabet as quickly as possible. Neurologically normal individuals can generally perform this task in 20 seconds or less; a score of 30 seconds or more should be considered indicative of the presence of psychomotor slowing.[108]

When clinical suspicion is appreciable, or when the results of the mental status screening tests are equivocal, referral for more detailed neuropsychologic testing is appropriate.

## SUMMARY

Neuropsychologic testing can provide considerable diagnostic and prognostic input in patients with suspected or known cognitive symptoms. A specific referral question can help improve the yield of a neuropsychologic examination. A flexible battery approach that takes into account the nature and severity of the patient's problem is preferred by most neuropsychologists.

Neuropsychologic assessment is useful for detection and differentiation of dementia syndromes, particularly early in their course. This type of testing is increasingly used for measuring outcomes after surgical procedures, such as aneurysm clipping and shunting for NPH. With advances in pharmacologic treatments for the cognitive symptoms of Alzheimer's disease and other degenerative dementias, neuropsychologic testing will play an increasingly important role in measuring the degree and duration of improvement in response to these medications. With the extraordinary advances made over the past several decades in imaging the anatomy and physiology of the human brain, it seems only fitting that our measures of the cognitive and behavioral correlates of brain activity should become equally sophisticated and not be limited to crude 5-minute mental status screening examinations.

## ACKNOWLEDGMENT

The authors thank Dr. Pamela Talalay for her editorial assistance, and we also thank Dr. Sarah Reusing for her helpful comments on the manuscript.

## REFERENCES

1. Adams RA, Victor M, Ropper AH. *Principles of Neurology.* 6th ed. New York: McGraw-Hill; 1997.
2. Albert ML, Goodglass H, Helm NA, Rubens AB, Alexander MP. *Clinical Aspects of Dysphasia.* New York: Springer Verlag; 1991.
3. Albert MS, Butters N, Levin J. Temporal gradients in the retrograde amnesia of patients with alcoholic Korsakoff's disease. *Arch Neurol.* 1979;36:211-216.
4. Alexander MP. Mild traumatic brain injury: pathophysiology, natural history, and clinical management. *Neurology.* 1995;45:1253-1260.
5. Almkvist O. Neuropsychological deficits in vascular dementia in relation to Alzheimer's disease: reviewing evidence for functional similarity or divergence. *Dementia.* 1994;5:203-209.
6. Almkvist O, Backman L, Basun H, Wahlund LO. Patterns of neuropsychological performance in Alzheimer's disease and vascular dementia. *Cortex.* 1993;29:661-673.
7. American Psychiatric Association. *Diagnostic and Statistical Manual of Mental Disorders.* 4th ed. Washington, DC: APA; 1997.
8. Beck AT. *Beck Depression Inventory: manual.* San Antonio, Tex: Psychological Corporation; 1987.
9. Becker JT, Boller F, Lopez OL, Saxton J, McGonigle KL. The natural history of Alzheimer's disease: description of study cohort and accuracy of diagnosis. *Arch Neurol.* 1994;51:585-594.
10. Benson DF. My day with Luria. *J Geriatr Psychiatry Neurol.* 1996;9:120-122.

11. Benson DF, Ardila A. *Aphasia: A Clinical Perspective.* New York: Oxford University Press; 1996.
12. Benson DF, Davis JR, Snyder BD. Posterior cortical atrophy. *Arch Neurol.* 1988;45:789-793.
13. Benton A. Clinical neuropsychology: 1960–1990. *J Clin Exp Neuropsychol.* 1992;14:407-417.
14. Benton AL, Hamsher KS, Varney NR, Spreen O. *Contributions to Neuropsychological Assessment.* New York: Oxford University Press; 1983.
15. Bernstein JH, Prather PA, Rey-Casserly C. Neuropsychological assessment in preoperative and postoperative evaluation. *Neurosurg Clin North Am.* 1995;6:443-454.
16. Berry DTR, Allen RS, Schmitt FA. Rey-Osterreith Complex Figure: psychometric characteristics in a geriatric sample. *Clin Neuropsychologist.* 1991;5:143-153.
17. Binder LM. Assessment of malingering after mild head trauma with the Portland Digit Recognition Test. *J Clin Exp Neuropsychol.* 1993;15:170-182.
18. Boone KB, Savodnik I, Ghaffarian S, Lee A, Freeman D, Berman NG. Rey 15-Item Memorization and Dot Counting Scores in a "stress" claim worker's compensation population: relationship to personality (MCMI) scores. *J Clin Psychol.* 1995;51:457-463.
19. Breteler MM, van Amerongen NM, van Swieten JC, et al. Cognitive correlates of ventricular enlargement and cerebral white matter lesions on magnetic resonance imaging: The Rotterdam Study. *Stroke.* 1994;25:1109-1115.
20. Brodaty H, Moore CM. The Clock Drawing Test for dementia of the Alzheimer's type: a comparison of three scoring methods in a memory disorders clinic. *Int J Geriatr Psychiatry.* 1997;12:619-627.
21. Castro-Caldas R, Reis A, Guerriero M. Neuropsychological aspects of illiteracy. *Neuropsychol Rehabil.* 1997;7:327-338.
22. Chertkow H, Murtha S. PET activation and language. *Clin Neurosci.* 1997;4:78-86.
23. Confavreux C, Croisile B, Garassus P, Aimard G, Trillet M. Progressive amusia and aprosody. *Arch Neurol.* 1992;49:971-976.
24. Corey-Bloom J, Sabbagh MN, Bondi MW, et al. Hippocampal sclerosis contributes to dementia in the elderly. *Neurology.* 1997;48:154-160.
25. Coria F, Gomez de Caso JA, Minguez L, Rodriguez-Artalejo F, Claveria LE. Prevalence of age-associated memory impairment and dementia in a rural community. *J Neurol Neurosurg Psychiatry.* 1993;56:973-976.
26. Cullum CM, Thompson LL, Smernoff EN. Three-word recall as a measure of memory. *J Clin Exp Neuropsychol.* 1993;15:321-329.
27. Cumming S, Hay P, Lee T, Sachdev P. Neuropsychological outcome from psychosurgery for obsessive-compulsive disorder. *Aust N Z J Psychiatry.* 1995;29:293-298.
28. Cummings JL. *Subcortical Dementia.* New York: Oxford University Press; 1990.
29. D'Elia L, Satz P, Schretlen D. Wechsler Memory Scale: a critical appraisal of the normative studies. *J Clin Exp Neuropsychol.* 1989;11:551-568.
30. Deckers CL, Hekster YA, Keyser A, Meinardi H, Renier WO. Reappraisal of polytherapy in epilepsy: a critical review of drug load and adverse effects. *Epilepsia.* 1997;38:570-575.
31. Delis DC, Kramer JH, Kaplan E, Ober BA. *The California Verbal Learning Test (Research Edition).* New York: Psychological Corporation; 1987.
32. Devinsky O. Cognitive and behavioral effects of antiepileptic drugs. *Epilepsia.* 1995;36(suppl 2):S46-S65.
33. Dodrill CB. Preoperative criteria for identifying eloquent brain: intracarotid amytal for language and memory testing. *Neurosurg Clin North Am.* 1993;4:211-216.
34. Dodrill CB. Myths of neuropsychology. *Clin Neuropsychologist.* 1997;11:1-17.
35. Double KL, Halliday GM, Kril JJ, et al. Topography of brain atrophy during normal aging and Alzheimer's disease. *Neurobiol Aging.* 1996;17:513-521.
36. Duncan J, Johnson R, Swales M, Freer C. Frontal lobe deficits after head injury: unity and diversity of function. *Cogn Neuropsychol.* 1997;14:713-742.
37. Elwood RW. The Wechsler Memory Scale-Revised: psychometric characteristics and clinical application. *Neuropsychol Rev.* 1991;2:179-201.
38. Erkinjuntti T, Haltia M, Palo J, Sulkava R, Paetau A. Accuracy of the clinical diagnosis of vascular dementia: a prospective clinical and postmortem neuropathological study. *J Neurol Neurosurg Psychiatry.* 1988;51:1037-1044.
39. Eslinger PJ, Damasion AR. Severe disturbance of higher cognition after bilateral frontal ablation: patient EVR. *Neurology.* 1985;35:1731-1741.
40. Etcoff LM, Kampfer KM. Practical guidelines in the use of symptom validity and other psychological tests to measure malingering and symptom exaggeration in traumatic brain injury cases. *Neuropsychol Rev.* 1996;6:171-201.
41. Evans JJ, Heggs AJ, Antoun N, Hodges JR. Progressive prosopagnosia associated with selective right temporal lobe atrophy: a new syndrome? *Brain.* 1995;118:1-13.
42. Ferrucci L, Cecchi F, Guralnik JM, et al. Does the Clock Drawing Test predict cognitive decline in older persons independent of the Mini-Mental State Examination. *J Am Geriatr Soc.* 1996;44:1326-1331.
43. Filley CM, Kleinschmidt-De Masters BK, Gross KF. Non-Alzheimer fronto-temporal degenerative dementia: a neurobehavioral and pathologic study. *Clin Neuropathol* 1994;13:109-116.
44. Folstein MF, Folstein SE, McHugh PR. "Mini-Mental State": a practical method for grading the cognitive state of patients for the clinician. *J Psychiatr Res.* 1975;12:189-198.
45. Foundas AL, Leonard CM, Mahoney SM, Agee OF, Heilman KM. Atrophy of the hippocampus, parietal cortex, and insula in Alzheimer's disease: a volumetric magnetic resonance imaging study. *Neuropsychiatry Neuropsychol Behav Neurol.* 1997;10:81-89.
46. Fox D, Lees-Haley P, Earnest K, Dolezal-Wood S. Base rates of postconcussive symptoms in health maintenance organization patients and controls. *Neuropsychology.* 1995;9:606-611.
47. Franzen MD. *Reliability and Validity in Neuropsychology Assessment.* New York: Plenum; 1989.
48. Fukui T, Sugita K, Kawamura M, Takeuchi T, Hasegawa Y. Differences in factors associated with silent and symptomatic MRI T2 hyperintensity lesions. *J Neurol.* 1997;244:293-298.
49. Gaudino EA, Geisler MW, Squires NK. Construct validity in the Trail Making Test: what makes Part B harder? *J Clin Exp Neuropsychol.* 1995;17:529-535.
50. Geldmacher DS, Whitehouse PJ Jr. Differential diagnosis of Alzheimer's disease. *Neurology.* 1997;48:S2-S9.
51. Gold G, Giannakopoulos P, Montes-Paixao C, et al. Sensitivity and specificity of newly proposed clinical criteria for possible vascular dementia. *Neurology.* 1997;49:690-694.
52. Golden CJ, Purisch AD, Hammeke TA. *Luria-Nebraska Neuropsychological Battery: Forms I and II.* Los Angeles: Western Psychological Services; 1985.
53. Goodglass H, Kaplan E. *The Assessment of Aphasia and Related Disorders.* 2nd ed. Philadelphia: Lea & Febiger; 1983.
54. Gordon B. Postconcussion syndrome. In: Johnson RT, ed. *Current Therapy in Neurologic Disease.* 3rd ed. New York: BC Decker; 1990.
55. Gordon B. Memory systems and their disorders. In: McKhann GM, Asbury MA, McDonald WI, eds. *Diseases of the Nervous System.* Philadelphia: WB Saunders; 1992:703-717.
56. Gordon B. Models of naming. In: Goodglass H, Wingfield A, eds. *Anomia.* San Diego: Academic Press; 1997:31-64.
57. Gordon B. Neuropsychology and advances in memory function. *Curr Opin Neurol.* 1997;10:306-312.
58. Gorelick PB, Nyenhuis DL, Garron DC, Cochran E. Is vascular dementia really Alzheimer's disease or mixed dementia. *Neuroepidemiology.* 1996;15:286-290.
59. Gronwall DMA, Sampson H. *The Psychological Effects of Concussion.* Auckland, NZ: Auckland University Press; 1974.
60. Hachinski V. Vascular dementia: a radical redefinition. *Dementia.* 1994;5:130-132.
61. Hachinski VC, Lassen NA, Marshall J. Multi-infarct dementia: a cause of mental deterioration in the elderly. *Lancet.* 1974;2:207-210.
62. Haines ME, Norris MP. Detecting the malingering of cognitive deficits: an update. *Neuropsychol Rev.* 1995;5:125-148.
63. Harrison MJG, McArthur JC. *AIDS and Neurology.* Edinburgh: Churchill Livingstone; 1995.
64. Hart J, Lesser RP, Gordon B. Selective interference with the representation of size in the human by direct cortical electrical stimulation. *J Cogn Neurosci.* 1992;4:337-344.
65. Hatazawa J, Shimosegawa E, Satoh T, Toyoshima H, Okudera T. Subcortical hypoperfusion associated with asymptomatic white matter lesions on magnetic resonance imaging. *Stroke.* 1997;28:1944-1947.
66. Hawkins KA, Cooper ME. Limitations of cognitive status exams: a case-based discussion. *Psychiatry.* 1996;59:382-388.
67. Heaton RK. *Wisconsin Card Sorting Test Manual.* Odessa, Fla: Psychological Assessment Resources; 1981.

68. Hebert R, Brayne C. Epidemiology of vascular dementia. *Neuroepidemiology.* 1995;14:240-257.

69. Hermann BP. Developing a model of quality of life in epilepsy: the contribution of neuropsychology. *Epilepsia.* 1993;34(suppl 4):S14-S21.

70. Hill CD, Stoudemire A, Morris R, Martino-Salztman D, Markwalter HR, Lewison BJ. Dysnomia in the differential diagnosis of major depression, depression-related cognitive dysfunction and dementia. *J Neuropsychiatry Clin Neurosci.* 1992;4:64-69.

71. Hodges JR. *Cognitive Assessment for Clinicians.* Oxford: Oxford University Press; 1994.

72. Ishii N, Nishihara Y, Imamura T. Why do frontal lobe symptoms predominate in vascular dementia with lacunes. *Neurology.* 1986;36:340-345.

73. Jacobs DM, Sano M, Dooneief G, Marder K, Bell KL, Stern Y. Neuropsychological detection and characterization of preclinical Alzheimer's disease. *Neurology.* 1995;45:957-962.

74. Junque C, Pujol J, Vendrell P, et al. Leuko-araiosis on magnetic resonance imaging and speed of mental processing. *Arch Neurol.* 1990;47:151-156.

75. Kane RL. Standardized and flexible batteries in neuropsychology: an assessment update. *Neuropsychol Rev.* 1991;2:281-339.

76. Kaplan EF, Goodglass H, Weintraub S. *The Boston Naming Test.* 2nd ed. Philadelphia: Lea & Febiger; 1983.

77. Kapur N. Some comments on the technical acceptability of Warrington's Recognition Memory Test. *Br J Clin Psychol.* 1987;26:144-146.

78. Kapur N. The coin-in-the-hand test: a new "bed-side" test for the detection of malingering in patients with suspected memory disorder. *J Neurol Neurosurg Psychiatry.* 1994;57:385-386.

79. Kaye JA, Grady CL, Haxby JV, Moore A, Friedland RP. Plasticity in the aging brain: reversibility of anatomic, metabolic, and cognitive deficits in normal-pressure hydrocephalus following shunt surgery. *Arch Neurol.* 1990;47:1336-1341.

80. Kertesz A, Clydesdale S. Neuropsychological deficits in vascular dementia vs Alzheimer's disease: frontal lobe deficits prominent in vascular dementia. *Arch Neurol.* 1994;51:1226-1231.

81. Kiernan RJ, Mueller J, Langston JW, Dyke C. The neurobehavioral cognitive status examination: a brief but differentiated approach to cognitive assessment. *Ann Intern Med.* 1987;107:481-485.

82. Kirk A, Kertesz A. Subcortical contributions to drawing. *Brain Cogn.* 1993;21:57-70.

83. Klove H. Clinical neuropsychology. In: Forster FM, ed. *The Medical Clinics of North America.* Philadelphia: WB Saunders; 1963.

84. Koivisto K, Reinikainen KJ, Hanninen T, et al. Prevalence of age-associated memory impairment in a randomly selected population from eastern Finland. *Neurology.* 1995;45:741-747.

85. Larrabee GJ, Curtiss G. Construct validity of various verbal and visual memory tests. *J Clin Exp Neuropsychol.* 1995;17:536-547.

86. Levin HS, Mattis S, Ruff RM, et al. Neurobehavioral outcome following minor head injury: a three-center study. *J Neurosurg.* 1987;66:234-243.

87. Lezak M. *Neuropsychological Assessment.* 3rd ed. New York: Oxford University Press; 1995.

88. Locascio JJ, Growdon JH, Corkin S. Cognitive test performance in detecting, staging, and tracking Alzheimer's disease. *Arch Neurol.* 1995;52:1087-1099.

89. Loeb C, Meyer JS. Vascular dementia: still a debatable entity? *J Neurol Sci.* 1996;143:31-40.

90. Longstreth WT Jr, Manolio TA, Arnold A, et al. Clinical correlates of white matter findings on cranial magnetic resonance imaging of 3301 elderly people: The Cardiovascular Health Study. *Stroke.* 1996;27:1274-1282.

91. Loring DW. Neuropsychological evaluation in epilepsy surgery. *Epilepsia.* 1997;38(suppl 4):S18-S23.

92. Mack WJ, Freed DM, Williams BW, Henderson VW. Boston Naming Test: shortened versions for use in Alzheimer's disease. *J Gerontol.* 1992;47:154-158.

93. Manly JJ, Jacobs DM, Sano M, et al. Cognitive test performance among nondemented elderly African Americans and whites. *Neurology.* 1998;50:1238-1245.

94. Manning RT. The Serial Sevens Test. *Arch Intern Med.* 1982;142:1192.

95. McArthur JC, Hoover DR, Bacellar H, et al. Incidence, prevalence and risk factors of HIV associated dementia: a report from the Multicenter AIDS Cohort Study. *Neurology.* 1993;43:2245-2252.

96. McKhann GM. Clinical approaches to dementia. In: Svennerholm L, Asbury AK, Reisfeld RA, et al. *Progress in Brain Research.* New York: Elsevier Science; 1998:375-382.

97. McMillan TM. Minor head injury. *Curr Opin Neurol.* 1997;10:479-483.

98. McPherson SE, Cummings JL. Neuropsychological aspects of vascular dementia. *Brain Cogn.* 1996;31:269-282.

99. Meiran N, Stuss DT, Guzman DA, Lafleche G, Willmer J. Diagnosis of dementia: methods for interpretation of scores of 5 neuropsychological tests. *Arch Neurol.* 1996;53:1043-1054.

100. Mesulam M-M. Slowly progressive aphasia without generalised dementia. *Ann Neurol.* 1982;11:592-598.

101. Mielke R, Schroder R, Fink GR, Kessler J, Herholz K, Heiss WD. Regional cerebral glucose metabolism and postmortem pathology in Alzheimer's disease. *Acta Neuropathol (Berl).* 1996;91:174-179.

102. Miller EN, Satz P, Visscher BV. Computerized and conventional neuropsychological assessment of HIV-1 infected homosexual men. *Neurology.* 1991;41:1608-1616.

103. Millis SR, Kler S. Limitations of the Rey Fifteen-Item Test in the detection of malingering. *Clin Psychol.* 1995;9:241-244.

104. Neary D, Snowden JS, Mann DM, Northen B, Goulding PJ, Macdermott N. Frontal lobe dementia and motor neuron disease. *J Neurol Neurosurg Psychiatry.* 1990;53:23-32.

105. Osimani A, Alon A, Berger A, Abarbanel JM. Use of the Stroop phenomenon as a diagnostic tool for malingering. *J Neurol Neurosurg Psychiatry.* 1997;62:617-621.

106. Ott A, Breteler MM, de Bruyne MC, van Harskamp F, Grobbee DE, Hofman A. Atrial fibrillation and dementia in a population-based study: The Rotterdam Study. *Stroke.* 1997;28:316-321.

107. Padovani A, DiPiero V, Bragoni M, Iacoboni M, Gualdi GF, Lenzi GL. Patterns of neuropsychological impairment in mild dementia: a comparison between Alzheimer's disease and multi-infarct dementia. *Acta Neurol Scand.* 1995;92:433-442.

108. Power C, Selnes OA, Grim JA, McArthur JC. HIV Dementia Scale: a rapid screening test. *J Acquir Immune Defic Syndr Hum Retrovirol.* 1995;8:273-278.

109. Price TR, Manolio TA, Kronmal RA, et al. Silent brain infarction on magnetic resonance imaging and neurological abnormalities in community-dwelling older adults: The Cardiovascular Health Study. CHS Collaborative Research Group. *Stroke.* 1997;28:1158-1164.

110. Prigatano GP, Amin K. Digit Memory Test: unequivocal cerebral dysfunction and suspected malingering. *J Clin Exp Neuropsychol.* 1993;15:537-546.

111. Pujol P, Bello J, Deus J, Marti-Vilalta JL, Capdevila A. Lesions in the left arcuate fasciculus region and depressive symptoms in multiple sclerosis. *Neurology.* 1997;49:1105-1110.

112. Radloff LS. The CES-D scale: a self-report depression scale for research in the general population. *Appl Psychol Measurement.* 1977;1:385-401.

113. Raftopoulos C, Deleval J, Chaskis C, et al. Cognitive recovery in idiopathic normal pressure hydrocephalus: a prospective study. *Neurosurgery.* 1994;35:397-404.

114. Reitan RM, Wolfson D. A selective and critical review of neuropsychological deficits and the frontal lobes. *Neuropsychol Rev.* 1994;4:161-198.

115. Rey A. L'examen psychologique dans les cas d'encephalopathie traumatique. *Arch Psychol.* 1941;28:286-340.

116. Rey A. *L'Examen Clinique en Psychologie.* Paris: Presses Universitaires de France; 1964.

117. Rockwood K, Parhad I, Hachinski V, et al. Diagnosis of vascular dementia: Consortium of Canadian Centres for Clinical Cognitive Research consensus statement. *Can J Neurol Sci.* 1994;21:358-364.

118. Roper BL, Bielauskas LA, Peterson MR. Validity of the Mini-Mental-State Examination and the neurobehavioral cognitive status examination in cognitive screening. *Neuropsychiatry Neuropsychol Behav Neurol.* 1996;9:54-57.

119. Rothlind JC, Brandt J. A brief assessment of frontal and subcortical functions in dementia. *J Neuropsychiatry Clin Neurosci.* 1993;5:73-77.

120. Schagen S, Schmand B, de Sterke S, Lindeboom J. Amsterdam Short-Term Memory Test: a new procedure for the detection of feigned memory deficits. *J Clin Exp Neuropsychol.* 1997;19:43-51.

121. Scheltens P, Hazenberg GJ, Lindeboom J, Valk J, Wolters EC. A case of progressive aphasia without dementia: temporal? Pick's disease? *J Neurol Neurosurg Psychiatry.* 1990;53:79-80.

122. Scheltens P, Pasquier F, Weerts JG, Barkhof F, Leys D. Qualitative assessment of cerebral atrophy on MRI: inter- and intra-observer reproducibility in dementia and normal aging. *Eur Neurol* 1997;37:95-99.

123. Schmidt R, Fazekas F, Offenbacher H, et al. Neuropsychologic correlates of MRI white matter hyperintensities: a study of 150 normal volunteers. *Neurology.* 1993;43:2490-2494.

124. Schneider L. Serial Sevens Test. *Arch Intern Med.* 1983;143:612.

125. Schrader H, Obelieniene D, Bovim G, et al. Natural evolution of late whiplash syndrome outside the medicolegal context. *Lancet.* 1996;347:1207-1211.

126. Selnes OA, Galai N, Bacellar H, et al. Cognitive performance after progression to AIDS: a longitudinal study from the Multicenter AIDS Cohort Study. *Neurology.* 1995;45:267-275.

127. Selnes OA, Galai N, McArthur JC, et al. HIV infection and cognition in intravenous drug users: long-term follow-up. *Neurology.* 1997;48:223-230.

128. Selnes OA, Holcomb HH, Gordon B. Progressive dysarthria: structural and functional brain correlations. *Am J Psychiatry.* 1996;153:309-310.

129. Selnes OA, Knopman DS, Niccum N, Rubens AB. The critical role of Wernicke's area in sentence repetition. *Ann Neurol.* 1985;17:549-557.

130. Selnes OA, Niccum N, Knopman DS, Rubens AB. Recovery of single word comprehension: CT-scan correlates. *Brain Lang.* 1984;21:72-84.

131. Selnes OA, Pestronk A, Hart J, Gordon B. Limb apraxia without aphasia from a left-sided lesion in a right-handed patient. *J Neurol Neurosurg Psychiatry.* 1991;54:734-737.

132. Selnes OA, Rubens AB, Risse GL, Levy RS. Transient aphasia with persistent apraxia. *Arch Neurol.* 1982;39:122-126.

133. Shipley WC. *Institute of Living Scale.* Los Angeles: Western Psychological Services; 1946.

134. Smith A. The Serial Sevens Subtraction Test. *Arch Neurol.* 1967;17:78-80.

135. Smith A. *Symbol Digit Modalities Test.* Los Angeles: Western Psychological Services; 1982.

136. Stroop JR. Studies of interference in serial verbal reaction. *J Exp Psychol.* 1935;18:643-662.

137. Strub RL. Frontal lobe syndrome in a patient with bilateral globus pallidus lesions. *Arch Neurol.* 1989;46:1024-1027.

138. Strub RL, Black FW. *The Mental Status Examination in Neurology.* 2nd ed. Philadelphia: FA Davis; 1985.

139. Stuss DT, Meiran N, Guzman DA, Lafleche G, Willmer J. Do long tests yield a more accurate diagnosis of dementia than short tests? A comparison of 5 neuropsychological tests. *Arch Neurol.* 1996;53:1033-1039.

140. Sweet JJ, Moberg PJ. A survey of practices and beliefs among ABPP and non-ABPP clinical neuropsychologists. *Clin Neuropsychologist.* 1990;4:101-120.

141. Tanabe H, Sawada T, Inoue N, Ogawa M, Kuriyama Y, Shiraishi J. Conduction aphasia and arcuate fasciculus. *Acta Neurol Scand.* 1987;76:422-427.

142. Trenerry MR. Neuropsychologic assessment in surgical treatment of epilepsy. *Mayo Clin Proc.* 1996;71:1196-1200.

143. Troncoso JC, Kawas CH, Chang CK, Folstein MF, Hedreen JC. Lack of association of the apoE4 allele with hippocampal sclerosis dementia. *Neurosci Lett.* 1996;204:138-140.

144. Trueblood W, Schmidt M. Malingering and other validity considerations in the neuropsychological evaluation of mild head injury. *J Clin Exp Neuropsychol.* 1993;15:578-590.

145. Uttl B, Graf P. Color-Word Stroop Test performance across the adult life span. *J Clin Exp Neuropsychol.* 1997;19:405-420.

146. Vanneste JL. Three decades of normal pressure hydrocephalus: are we wiser now? *J Neurol Neurosurg Psychiatry.* 1994;57:1021-1025.

147. Victoroff J, Ross GW, Benson DF, Verity F, Vinters HV. Posterior cortical atrophy. *Arch Neurol.* 1994;51:269-274.

148. Villa G, Cappa A, Tavolozza M, et al. Neuropsychological tests and [99mTc]-HM PAO SPECT in the diagnosis of Alzheimer's dementia. *J Neurol.* 1995;242:359-366.

149. Villardita C. Alzheimer's disease compared with cerebrovascular dementia: neuropsychological similarities and differences. *Acta Neurol Scand.* 1993;87:299-308.

150. Wada J, Rasmussen T. Intracarotid injection of sodium amytal for the lateralization of cerebral speech dominance. *J Neurosurg.* 1960;17:266-282.

151. Warrington EK. *Recognition Memory Test.* Windsor: NFER-Nelson; 1984.

152. Warrington EK, James M, Maciejewsky C. The WAIS as a lateralizing and localizing diagnostic instrument: a study of 656 patients with unilateral cerebral excisions. *Neuropsychologia.* 1986;24:223-239.

153. Wechsler D. *Wechsler Adult Intelligence Scale-Revised.* New York: The Psychological Corporation; 1981.

154. Wechsler D. *Wechsler Memory Scale-Revised: Manual.* San Antonio: The Psychological Corporation; 1987.

155. Wetterling T, Kanitz RD, Borgis KJ. Comparison of different diagnostic criteria for vascular dementia (ADDTC, DSM-IV, ICD-10, NINDS-AIREN). *Stroke.* 1996;27:30-36.

156. Wilson B, Cockburn J, Baddeley AD. *The Rivermead Behavioural Memory Test.* Reading, England: Thames Valley Test Company; 1985.

157. Wilson BA, Evans JJ, Emslie H, Alderman N, Burgess P. The development of an ecologically valid test for assessing patients with a dysexecutive syndrome. *Neuropsychol Rehabil.* 1998;8:213-228.

158. Wolfe N, Linn R, Babikian VL, Knoefel JE, Albert ML. Frontal systems impairment following multiple lacunar infarcts. *Arch Neurol.* 1990;47:129-132.

159. Zung WWK. A self-rating depression scale. *Arch Gen Psychiatry.* 1965;12:63-70.

# 12

# Neuroimaging of Brain Tumors

*Norman E. Leeds, Ashok J. Kumar, and Edward F. Jackson*

The chapter is divided into four parts to address areas of interest in the imaging of a patient with a neurologic disorder who is suspected of having a brain tumor. First, the choice of imaging modality is discussed, specifically: What is the role of computed tomography vs. magnetic resonance imaging? Next, the importance of lesion location in understanding the type of tumor that may be present is considered. Then the potential pitfalls that may occur in the interpretation of the images of intracranial mass lesions and how to avoid them to reach the appropriate diagnosis are addressed. The brain may react in a limited number of ways because of tissue restrictions and the uniqueness of the blood-brain barrier (BBB). This explains the frequency of brain tumor mimics. These mimics are thus the focus of the discussion on pitfalls. Finally, new directions in magnetic resonance imaging that will improve diagnostic accuracy and surgical management are presented.

## COMPUTED TOMOGRAPHY VS. MAGNETIC RESONANCE IMAGING

Magnetic resonance imaging (MRI) is the choice in most patients with neurologic findings because of the excellent anatomic visualization it affords in multiple planes and because of the soft tissue discrimination made possible by variable pulse sequences. MRI signal changes highlight pathologic processes, not only leading to the early detection of lesions but also facilitating the more precise characterization of lesions. Other advantages of MRI include no ionizing radiation and absence of the beam-hardening artifact that may obscure subtle lesions and can be observed during a computed tomographic (CT) examination in the temporal region and posterior fossa. This artifact is caused by the bone–soft tissue interface (Hounsfield artifact).

In selected cases, CT is the examination of choice (Table 12–1). One example is a patient presenting with severe headache ("the worst headache of my life"), in whom CT is used to exclude a subarachnoid hemorrhage. Acute intracranial hemorrhages, including subarachnoid hemorrhage, are clearly delineated by CT. In these cases, contrast-enhanced helical CT (ultrafast CT) with reconstruction may be performed to identify the aneurysm.

CT may also be performed rapidly to exclude a treatable process in the acutely ill patient who is moving or has monitoring devices. It may also be used in the patient with a pacemaker, with other mechanical devices, or with metal objects (e.g., aneurysm clips) in whom MRI is contraindicated. CT can also optimally visualize calcification, which may be overlooked with MRI[35] (Fig. 12–1). In addition, CT is preferred for the follow-up of patients because it is less costly than MRI. In the immediate postoperative period, CT may also be used to exclude hemorrhage, an extradural collection, and/or hydrocephalus. CT with bone windows demonstrates osseous architecture to advantage. This can be of benefit in understanding patterns of bone production (Fig. 12–2A and B) and destruction and the associated soft tissue changes. Such a demonstration would be particularly advantageous in the evaluation of osseous components forming the base of the skull and the accompanying foramina, as well as in high-resolution examination of the petrous temporal bone. A preliminary CT of the orbits is also required in the patient to be examined by MRI who may have worked with metallic objects and could have a metal fragment in the eye that is potentially dangerous.

## MAGNETIC RESONANCE IMAGING EVALUATION OF MASS LESIONS

MRI is the imaging study of choice in the evaluation of the patient for an intracranial lesion. The most important

---

**TABLE 12–1. Indications for CT Examination**

A. Acute subarachnoid or intracranial hemorrhage
B. Three-dimensional reconstruction of aneurysm with helical scans
C. Acutely ill, agitated patient, to exclude intracranial process (e.g., hemorrhage, acute infarction, infection, or mass) because of rapid scan time
D. Patients in whom MRI is contraindicated: patients who have a pacemaker or metallic devices that may move during examination (i.e., aneurysm clips)
E. Calcified or ossified intracranial lesions, including skull base tumors and temporal bone lesions, to obtain more specific histologic diagnoses
F. Assessment for complications (e.g., hemorrhage or hydrocephalus) in the immediate postoperative interval
G. Visualization of metallic fragments within the orbit

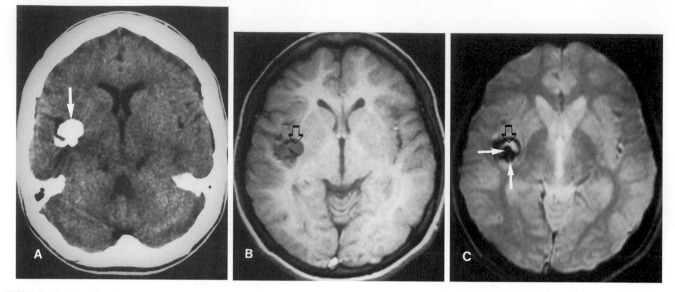

**FIGURE 12–1.** A heavily calcified mass: a cavernous angioma. **A,** Precontrast CT image. **B,** Precontrast axial T1-weighted MR image. **C,** Axial T2-weighted MR image. A heavily calcified mass in the right temporal lobe (*arrow* in **A**) is readily shown by CT. MR images (**B** and **C**) show that the mass is not completely calcified, but on the T1-weighted image it is seen to contain a central area of low signal intensity (*open black arrow* in **B**) that is bright on the T2-weighted image (*open black arrow* in **C**), which is evidence of old blood within the vascular malformation. Solid calcified mass is seen better by CT than by MRI, but MRI can show the intrinsic nature of the calcified mass for a precise diagnosis. Calcification (*white arrows* in **C**) is better seen on the T2-weighted sequence than on the T1-weighted sequence.

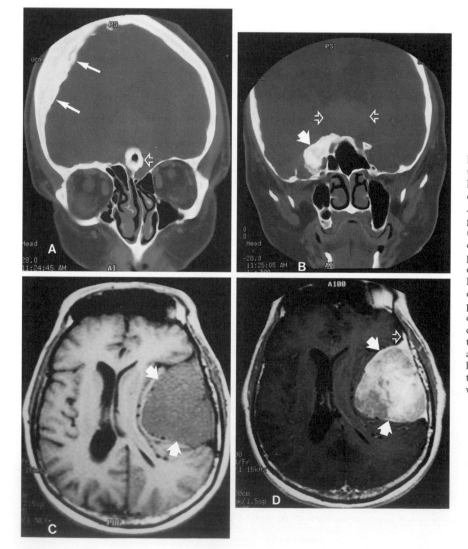

**FIGURE 12–2.** **A** and **B,** Coronal CT images of the calvarium in bone settings. **A,** Bone windows highlight bony architecture, revealing marked hyperostosis of the right side of the calvarium (*arrows* in **A**), produced by an underlying convexity meningioma obscured by bone settings. In brain settings (not shown), however, the striking enhancement characteristic of a meningioma was clearly seen. Hyperostosis of the crista galli (*arrowhead*) was produced by a meningioma in the anterior cranial fossa. **B,** Hyperostosis of the sphenoid bone (*arrow*) produced by a large suprasellar (*arrowheads*) and parasellar meningioma. (The enhancing tumors are out of focus in the bone settings.) **C** and **D,** A typical dural based meningioma with a dural tail. **C,** Precontrast axial T1-weighted MR image. **D,** Postcontrast axial T1-weighted MR image. A large dural based enhancing mass (*arrows* in **C** and **D**) with a broad base toward the inner table of the calvarium is associated with a dural tail (*open arrow* in **D**).

## TABLE 12–2. Lesion Locations as a Guide to Diagnosis

A. Dural based mass
  1. Meningioma
  2. Metastases
  3. Lymphoma
B. Cortical lesions
  1. Infarct
  2. Arteriovenous malformation
C. Subcortical lesion: glioma
D. Corticomedullary junction
  1. Metastases
  2. Abscess
  3. Watershed infarct
E. White-matter lesion
  1. Multiple sclerosis
  2. Disseminated necrotizing leuko-
     encephalopathy (DNL)
  3. Unidentified bright object (UBO)
  4. Encephalitis
  5. Acute disseminated encephalomyelitis
     (ADEM)
  6. Venous infarct
F. Paraventricular basal ganglia lesions
  1. Lymphoma
  2. Glioma

  3. Ependymoma
  4. Metastases
  5. Toxoplasmosis
G. Intraventricular lesion
  1. Glioma or ependymoma
  2. Neurocytoma
  3. Colloid cyst
  4. Subependymoma
  5. Metastases
  6. Meningioma
  7. Choroid plexus papilloma
  8. Pilocytic astrocytoma
H. Sellar mass
  1. Pituitary tumor
  2. Craniopharyngioma
  3. Arachnoid cyst
  4. Tumor arising from sphenoid sinus or
     nasopharynx
I. Suprasellar mass
  1. Craniopharyngioma
  2. Optic nerve glioma
  3. Hypothalamic glioma
  4. Meningioma

  5. Metastases
  6. Germinoma
  7. Epidermoid
  8. Sarcoidosis
  9. Langerhans histiocytosis
J. Pineal mass
  1. Germinoma
  2. Pineoblastoma
  3. Pineocytoma
  4. Meningioma
  5. Glioma
  6. Metastases
K. Posterior fossa lesion
  *Adult*
  1. Metastases
  2. Hemangioblastoma
  3. Primary glioma
  4. Infarct
  *Child*
  1. Medulloblastoma
  2. Pilocytic astrocytoma
  3. Fibrillary astrocytoma
  4. Ependymoma

observation shown by MRI is lesion location because this information often aids in determining the most likely type of pathologic process (Table 12–2). For example, dural-based lesions[29] should lead one to consider meningioma (Fig. 12–2*C* and *D*), metastases, and lymphoma. When the lesion is cortically oriented, a vascular lesion, such as an infarct or an arteriovenous malformation (AVM), should be considered. Subcortical lesions include primary brain tumors, which may be present with or without contrast enhancement (Figs. 12–3 and 12–4) or with enhancement (Fig. 12–5), or cerebral edema. The lack of enhancement favors either a low-grade neoplasm, such as oligodendroglioma[67] (see Fig. 12–3), or a fibrillary astrocytoma. Approximately 40% of nonenhancing astrocytomas are anaplastic (see Fig. 12–4), however, with the percentage increasing with age. Glioblastoma multiforme, which stereotypically presents as a thick-walled or complex ring with central necrosis, is the

most common neoplasm within the brain (see Fig. 12–5). Uncommonly, these neoplasms may show no enhancement (Fig. 12–6). Occasionally, primary brain tumors may cross cortical u-fibers and affect the adjacent gray matter (see Figs. 12–3 and 12–4).

Lesions in a corticomedullary location are hematogenous in origin and include metastases, abscesses (Fig. 12–7), and watershed infarcts (Fig. 12–8). White matter (medullary) lesions include multiple sclerosis (MS) plaques (Fig. 12–9*A*), allergic reactions, a variety of encephalitic processes, immune system–related lesions, and venous infarcts. Parasagittal lesions include meningiomas, metastases, lymphomas, and primary brain neoplasms (Fig. 12–10). Intraventricular masses include colloid cysts (Fig. 12–11), neurocytomas, subependymomas, metastases, meningiomas (Fig. 12–12), choroid plexus papillomas, and pilocytic astrocytomas. When a lesion is observed within the basal gan-

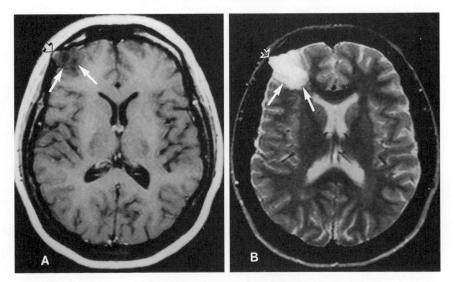

**FIGURE 12–3.** Oligodendroglioma of the right frontal lobe in a 15-year-old patient. **A,** Postcontrast axial T1-weighted MR image. **B,** Axial T2-weighted MR image. A superficial nonenhancing tumor (*white arrows* in **A**) is hyperintense on the T2-weighted image (*white arrows* in **B**). *Open arrows* in **A** and **B** demonstrate pressure erosion of the adjacent inner table of the calvarium by the slowly growing tumor.

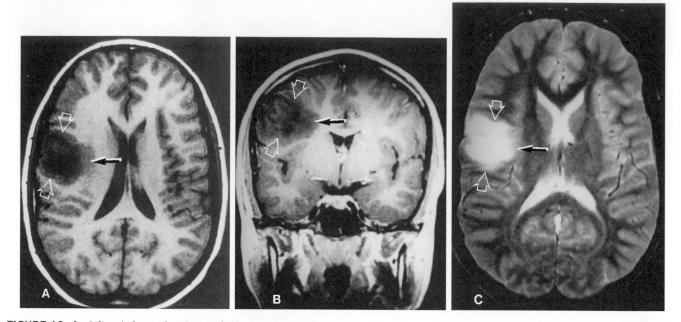

**FIGURE 12–4.** Subcortical nonenhancing anaplastic astrocytoma with invasion of the cortex in a 50-year-old patient. **A,** Precontrast axial T1-weighted MR image. **B,** Postcontrast coronal T1-weighted MR image. **C,** Axial T2-weighted MR image. A superficial nonenhancing anaplastic astrocytoma is seen involving the subcortical white matter (*arrows* in **A** through **C**) with cortical invasion (*open arrows* in **A** through **C**).

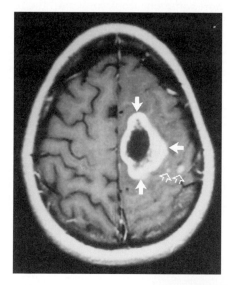

**FIGURE 12–5.** A stereotypical glioblastoma. Postcontrast axial T1-weighted MR image. An irregular, thick-walled enhancing ring lesion (*arrows*) with central necrosis is seen in the left frontal lobe. Small satellite nodules (*open arrows*) representing multifocal tumor spread. Note the obliteration of adjacent sulci secondary to surrounding edema.

**FIGURE 12–6.** An unusual nonenhancing glioblastoma. **A,** Postcontrast axial T1-weighted MR image. **B,** Axial T2-weighted MR image. A nonenhancing tumor (*arrows* in **A**) is seen in the right frontal lobe and has a small cystic component (*arrowhead* in **A**). On the T2-weighted image (**B**), the nonenhancing tumor (*arrows*) is better visualized with a larger area of involvement than that seen on the postcontrast T1-weighted image. This sequence also helps to distinguish edema (*E*) from tumor, with the edema appearing brighter than tumor.

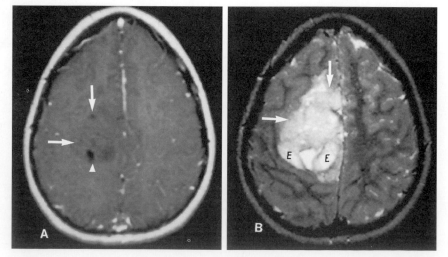

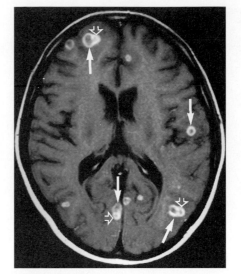

**FIGURE 12–7.** Multiple tuberculous abscesses. Postcontrast axial T1-weighted MR image. Multiple smooth-walled enhancing ring lesions are seen (*arrows*) scattered throughout both cerebral hemispheres. Some have daughter abscesses (*open arrows*), an important clue to the infectious etiologic basis. The lesions are seen in the corticomedullary junction and on the dural surface secondary to hematogenous spread.

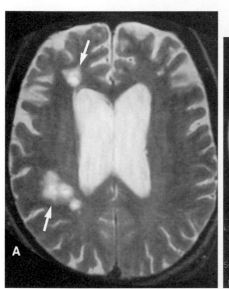

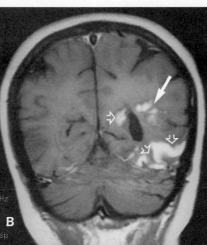

**FIGURE 12–8.** Acute cortical infarcts and watershed infarcts. **A,** Axial T2-weighted MR image. Watershed infarcts are seen in the corticomedullary junction (*arrows*). **B,** Postcontrast coronal T1-weighted MR image. Acute cortical infarcts are seen involving the left occipital lobe, with gyral enhancement (*open arrows*). Subcortical white-matter involvement (*large arrow*) is also seen.

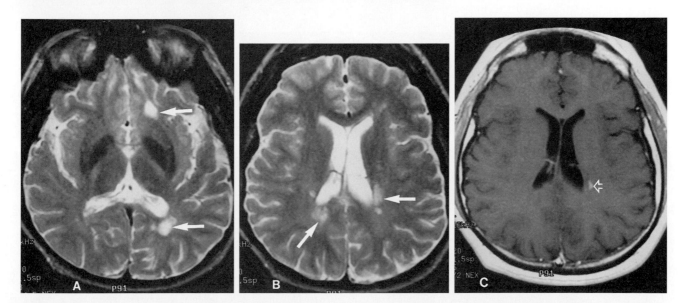

**FIGURE 12–9.** Multiple sclerosis. **A** and **B,** Axial T2-weighted MR images. **C,** Postcontrast axial T1-weighted MR image. Periventricular hyperintensities are seen on T2-weighted images (*arrows* in **A** and **B**), representing areas of demyelination resulting from multiple sclerosis. An acutely forming multiple sclerosis plaque may also enhance with contrast (*open arrow* in **C**).

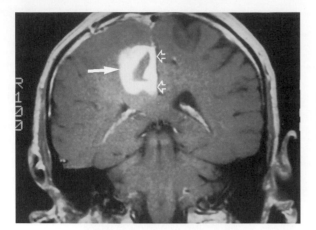

**FIGURE 12–10.** Glioblastoma simulating meningioma. Postcontrast coronal T1-weighted MR image. An enhancing and centrally necrotic glioblastoma (*large arrow*) invading the falx (*open white arrows*) is demonstrated.

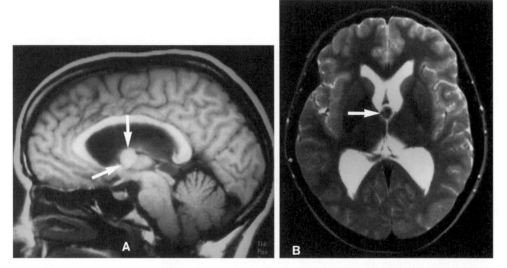

**FIGURE 12–11.** Anterior third ventricle/foramen Monro tumor: a colloid cyst. **A,** Precontrast sagittal T1-weighted MR image showing a colloid cyst in a typical anterior third ventricular location (*arrows*) with a bright signal. **B,** Axial T2-weighted MR image: the colloid cyst (*arrow*) is dark.

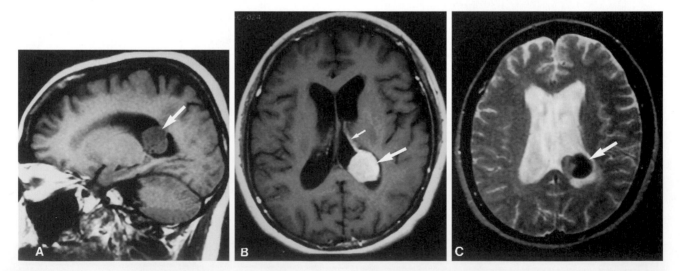

**FIGURE 12–12.** An intraventricular meningioma. **A,** Precontrast sagittal T1-weighted MR image. Arrow points to a tumor that is isointense with the gray matter and is situated within the atrium of the lateral ventricle. **B,** Postcontrast axial T1-weighted MR image. The tumor (*arrow*) shows the homogeneously intense enhancement typical of meningiomas. Small arrow points to prominent choroid plexus. **C,** Axial T2-weighted MR image. The tumor turns dark, indicating the presence of calcification.

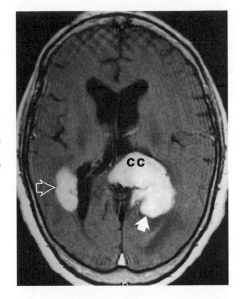

**FIGURE 12–13.** Lymphoma of the brain. Postcontrast axial T1-weighted MR image. An intensely enhancing mass is seen occupying the splenium of the corpus callosum (*cc*), left occipital lobe (*arrow*), and right paraventricular white matter (*open arrow*).

glion or paraventricular region, lymphoma (Fig. 12–13), glioma, metastasis, or toxoplasmosis (Fig. 12–14) should be considered. If the lesion affects the sella turcica,[39] the most likely diagnosis is a pituitary adenoma (Fig. 12–15). Rarely it is a tumor arising from the sphenoid sinus. If the mass is suprasellar in location,[39] the major possibilities include meningioma (Fig. 12–16), craniopharyngioma (Fig. 12–17), optic chiasm glioma, hypothalamic glioma, germ cell tumor, epidermoid tumor (Fig. 12–18), Langerhans histiocytosis, and sarcoidosis (Fig. 12–19).

If a lesion is seen in the pineal region, one must consider a tumor of pineal cell origin (Figs. 12–20 and 12–21), meningioma of the falx-tentorial junction, glioma arising in the thalamus or vermis, and metastasis. In the posterior fossa the possibilities depend on the age of the patient. In the adult patient, metastases, hemangioblastomas, primary gliomas, and infarcts must be considered. In the child the possibilities include medulloblastomas (Fig. 12–22), pilocytic astrocytomas (Fig. 12–23), fibrillary astrocytomas, astrocytomas of the brainstem (Fig. 12–24), and ependymomas (Fig. 12–25).

## BRAIN TUMOR MIMICS

This section discusses the potential pitfalls in the workup of the patient suspected of having a brain tumor. The patient who comes to the neurologist's office does not have a sign indicating that he or she has a brain tumor.

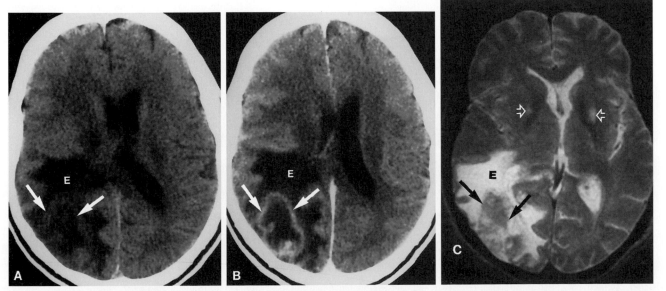

**FIGURE 12–14.** Toxoplasmosis. Axial precontrast (**A**) and postcontrast (**B**) CT scans of the brain. **C**, Axial T2-weighted MR image. An irregularly enhancing *Toxoplasma* abscess cavity (*arrows* in **B**) seen in the occipital lobe is associated with severe degree of edema (*E*), creating a mass effect. The abscess wall is vaguely outlined in the noncontrast scan (*arrows* in **A**). The axial T2-weighted MR image (**C**) demonstrates small lesions (*open arrows*) within the basal ganglia not seen by CT. *Black arrows* point to the abscess cavity that enhanced in the postcontrast MR study (not shown). (*E*, Edema.) The presence of multiple lesions and the basal ganglionic involvement in an immunocompromised patient strongly suggests a *Toxoplasma* infection.

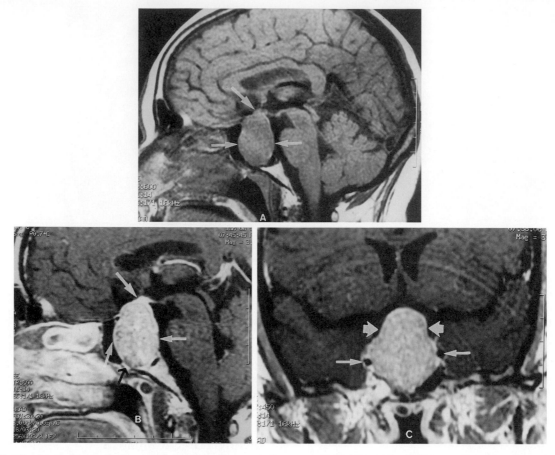

**FIGURE 12–15.** A typical intrasellar/suprasellar pituitary adenoma. **A,** Precontrast sagittal T1-weighted MR image. **B,** Postcontrast sagittal T1-weighted MR image. **C,** Postcontrast coronal T1-weighted MR image. A large intrasellar enhancing mass (*arrows* in **A** and **B**) has ballooned and eroded the floor of the sella turcica (*black arrow* in **B**). The suprasellar component of the tumor compresses the optic chiasm (*large arrow* in **A** and **B**). The coronal image demonstrates the typical hourglass appearance of a pituitary tumor (*large arrows* in **C**) as it emerges from the sella turcica into the suprasellar region through the diaphragma sella. *Small arrows* point to the carotid siphons displaced laterally by the intrasellar mass.

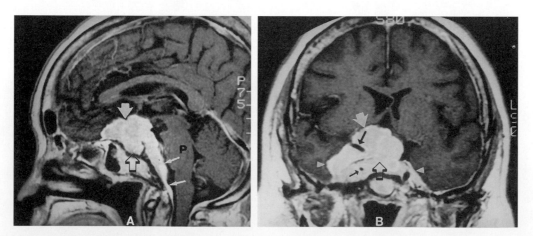

**FIGURE 12–16.** Suprasellar, intrasellar, retrosellar, and parasellar meningioma (not to be mistaken for pituitary adenoma). Postcontrast sagittal (**A**) and coronal (**B**) T1-weighted MR images. A large, brightly enhancing suprasellar meningioma (*large arrow* in **A** and **B**) with intrasellar extension (*open black arrow* in **A** and **B**) and retroclival extensions (*small arrows* in **A**) is noted. (*P,* Pons.) *White arrowheads* in **B** point to the parasellar tumor. *Small black arrow* in **B** points to cavernous sinus invasion resulting in encasement and narrowing of the cavernous portion of the right internal carotid artery. *Large black arrow* points to tumor encasing the supraclinoid portion of the right internal carotid artery.

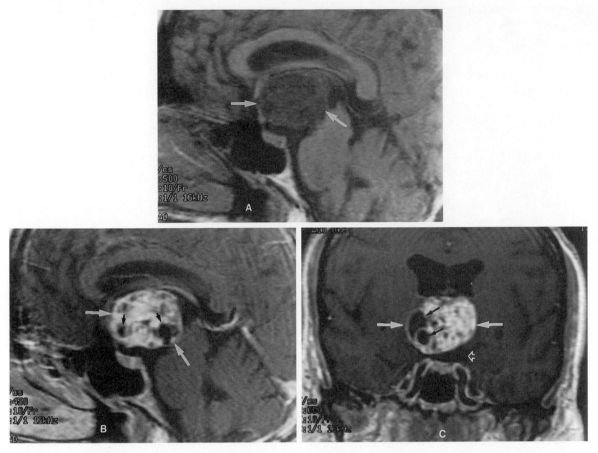

**FIGURE 12–17.**  Suprasellar craniopharyngioma. **A,** Precontrast sagittal T1-weighted MR image. **B,** Postcontrast sagittal T1-weighted MR image. **C,** Post-contrast coronal T1-weighted MR image. The suprasellar tumor is of low signal intensity on the T1-weighted image (*arrows* in **A**) and enhances with contrast (*arrows* in **B** and **C**). The tumor contains several small cystic areas (*black arrows* in **B** and **C**). *Open white arrow* in **C** points to suprasellar cistern.

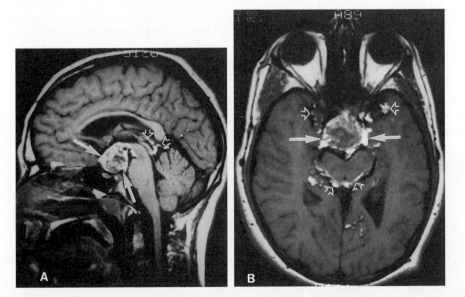

**FIGURE 12–18.**  Suprasellar epidermoid tumor. Precontrast sagittal (**A**) and axial (**B**) T1-weighted MR images. A large suprasellar epidermoid tumor (*large arrows* in **A** and **B**) with a heterogeneous bright and low signal intensity is observed. The fatty content of the epidermoid tumor has spilled into the subarachnoid space (*open white arrows* in **A** and **B**) outlining the adjacent cisterns.

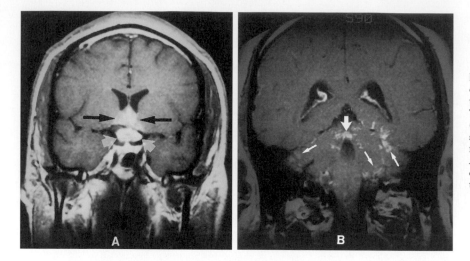

**FIGURE 12–19.** Suprasellar sarcoidosis with optic chiasm involvement and leptomeningeal infiltration of the cerebellar sulci. Postcontrast coronal T1-weighted MR images at the level of sella turcica (**A**) and the fourth ventricle (**B**). An enhancing suprasellar sarcoidosis (*black arrows* in **A**) with diffuse thickening of the optic chiasm (*white arrows* in **A**) is noted. **B** demonstrates leptomeningeal sarcoidosis infiltrating the vermian (*large arrow*) and the cerebellar sulci (*small arrows*).

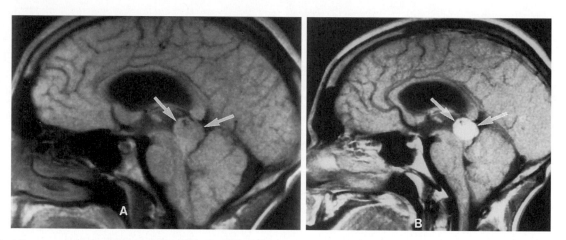

**FIGURE 12–20.** Posterior third ventricular and pineal tumor: germinoma. Precontrast (**A**) and postcontrast (**B**) sagittal T1-weighted MR images showing a germinoma (*arrows* in **A** and **B**), a common pineal region tumor in boys. The tumor intensely enhances with contrast agent (*arrows* in **B**).

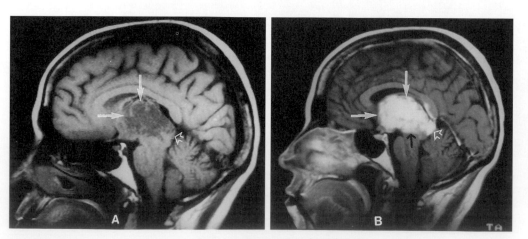

**FIGURE 12–21.** A highly malignant pineoblastoma infiltrating the third ventricle. Precontrast (**A**) and postcontrast (**B**) sagittal T1-weighted MR images. The pineoblastoma originated from the pineal region (*open arrow* in **A** and **B**) and grew anteriorly into the third ventricle (*arrows* in **A** and **B**), also infiltrating the midbrain (*black arrow* in **B**). The tumor intensely enhances with contrast agent (*arrows* in **B**).

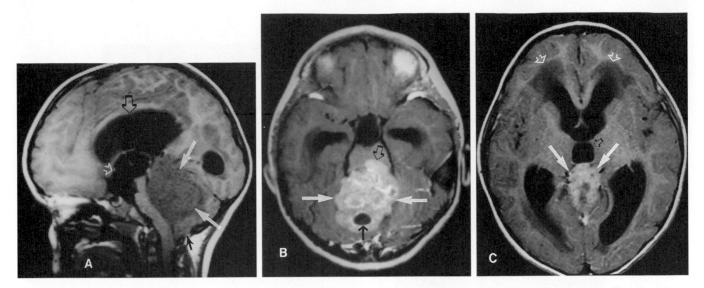

**FIGURE 12–22.** A midline vermian tumor in a child with medulloblastoma. **A,** Precontrast sagittal T1-weighted MR image. A tumor of low signal intensity (*arrows*) occupies the vermis, with resulting compression and forward displacement of the fourth ventricle, creating obstructive hydrocephalus with enlargement of the lateral ventricle (*open black arrow*) and third ventricle (*open white arrow*). The *black arrow* points to tonsillar herniation. **B,** Postcontrast axial T1-weighted MR image. A large enhancing vermian tumor (*arrows*) with a cyst posteriorly (*black arrow*) is seen infiltrating the pons anteriorly (*open black arrow*). **C,** Postcontrast axial T1-weighted image at the level of the third ventricle. A vermian tumor that is upwardly herniating through the tentorial hiatus (*arrows*) contributes to obstructive hydrocephalus with periventricular edema (*open white arrows*). The *open black arrow* points to an enlarged third ventricle.

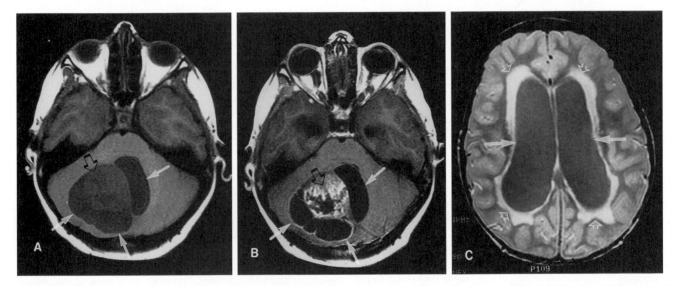

**FIGURE 12–23.** Pilocytic astrocytoma of the cerebellar hemisphere and vermis. Precontrast (**A**) and postcontrast (**B**) axial T1-weighted MR images. **C,** Axial proton density-weighted MR image. A pilocytic astrocytoma typically contains a cystic (*white arrows* in **A** and **B**) and a solid (*open black arrow* in **A** and **B**) enhancing tumor. **C** demonstrates obstructive hydrocephalus with enlargement of the lateral ventricles (*white arrows*) and periventricular edema (*open white arrows*) secondary to transependymal absorption.

**FIGURE 12–24.** Pontine glioma. **A,** Precontrast sagittal T1-weighted MR image. **B,** Postcontrast axial T1-weighted image. A nonenhancing pontine glioma (*large arrows* in **A** and **B**) is seen causing expansion of the pons and posterior displacement of the fourth ventricle (*arrowhead* in **A** and **B**). Pontine gliomas occasionally show exophytic components, as in this case (*open black arrow* in **A** and **B**), with tumor situated in front of the basilar artery (*open white arrow*).

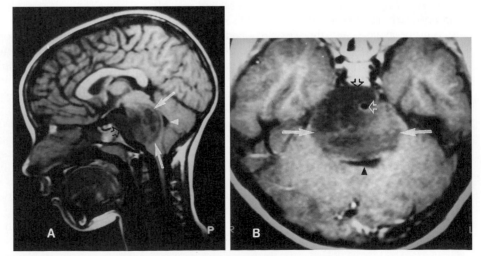

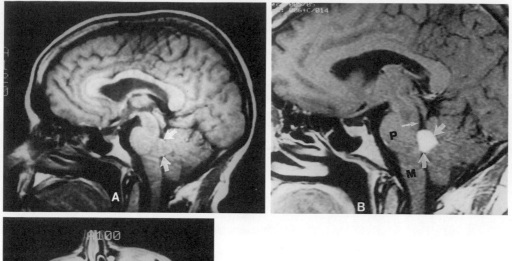

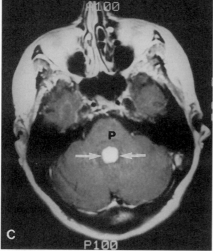

**FIGURE 12–25.** Fourth ventricular ependymoma. **A,** Precontrast sagittal T1-weighted MR image showing a tumor filling the fourth ventricle (*arrows*). **B,** Postcontrast sagittal T1-weighted image. The fourth ventricular tumor intensely enhances with contrast (*arrows*). The *small arrow* points to the superior aspect of the fourth ventricle. (*P,* Pons; *M,* medulla.) **C,** Postcontrast axial T1-weighted image. *Arrows* point to tumor within the fourth ventricle. (*P,* Pons.)

Rather, the patient presents with a series of complaints or physical findings that result in a workup and eventually necessitate imaging studies. MRI is the imaging study of choice in this setting, with the goal being to avoid being misled by mimics, which could result in incorrect management decisions. Therefore an optimized approach is required to increase diagnostic accuracy in patients with suspected brain tumors.

A retrospective study of patients presenting to The University of Texas M.D. Anderson Cancer Center with possible brain tumors was performed to reveal diagnostic dilemmas in various settings, appearances of the mimics, and possible misinterpretations. This approach was used so potential pitfalls could be avoided and the sensitivity and specificity of diagnosis could be improved. All MRI examinations were performed on superconductive systems operating at 1.5 T (General Electric Horizon, Milwaukee, Wis.). Our current method of examination of the brain includes the following sequences: axial T1-weighted spin-echo images (TR 500-550 ms, TE 8 ms) fast spin-echo T2-weighted images (TR 3500 ms, TE 98 ms), and fluid attenuation inversion recovery (FLAIR) images (TR 10,000 ms, TE 147 ms, IT 2200 ms) prior to the administration of contrast agent. Contrast study is then performed after intravenous injection of 0.1 ml/kg gadolinium-DTPA (Berlex Laboratories, Wayne, NJ). T1-weighted images of the brain are obtained in axial, coronal, and sagittal planes.

The examinations are performed with 5-mm-thick slices and an interslice gap of 1 to 2.5 mm. In addition, in some cases since 1994, dynamic studies have been performed to distinguish radiation effects from tumor. Currently, we are about to add diffusion and perfusion studies in the preoperative workup of some patients with brain tumors to examine the potential advantage of these new techniques. We are also investigating paradigms for performing functional studies to define better the relationship of neoplasm to active areas within the brain (motor function, receptive and expressive speech, memory and pain).

The potential pitfalls observed include distinguishing a cortical neoplasm from meningioma, a meningioma with a dural tail from a glioma or metastasis with a dural tail, a temporal lobe hamartoma or heterotopia from a neoplasm that may cause complex partial seizures, radiation effects from residual or recurrent tumor, intracerebral hematoma from hemorrhagic glioma, multiple sclerosis from a neoplasm, an infarct from a glioma, multifocal or multicentric glioma from metastasis and abscess, a cavernous angioma from metastasis, gliomatosis cerebri from encephalitis, and a giant aneurysm or vascular malformation from a neoplasm (Table 12–3). An additional difficulty is discerning the features that may aid in separating leptomeningeal disease in neoplasm from infection or meningeal fibrosis.

Cases that included these potential mimics were then carefully evaluated to identify characteristics that enabled

---

**TABLE 12–3. Potential Pitfalls in the Diagnosis of Intracranial Lesions**

A. Distinguishing cortical lesions from meningioma
B. Distinguishing dural tail in lesions other than meningioma
C. Distinguishing temporal lobe hamartoma or heterotopia from neoplasms that cause complex partial seizures
D. Distinguishing radiation effects from neoplasm
E. Distinguishing hemorrhagic gliomas and metastases from hematomas
F. Distinguishing multiple sclerosis from glioma
G. Distinguishing infarct from glioma
H. Appreciating a multifocal or multicentric glioma and distinguishing from metastases or abscess
I. Features that may aid in separating leptomeningeal disease in neoplasm from infection or meningeal fibrosis
J. Distinguishing cavernous angioma from metastases
K. Distinguishing gliomatosis cerebri from encephalitis
L. Distinguishing focal inflammatory process from glioma
M. Distinguishing giant aneurysm from neoplasm

---

the correct diagnosis to be made in the majority of cases. We envisioned that this information could be used to make the proper diagnosis either at the time of presentation or later, after the pathologic process had evolved. In either case, it was anticipated that the use of such information would lead to improved management and more successful therapy.

A superficial or cortical based lesion can often be difficult to separate from a meningioma. The most important feature that can lead to a correct diagnosis is expanded convolutions resulting from gyral involvement (Fig. 12–26). The superficial location of the mass often results in thinning or erosion of the overlying inner table of the calvarium. Other findings that may be common to both lesions include white-

matter buckling[58] and the occasional presence of border-forming vessels. The problem with the diagnosis in the patient whose MR study is shown in Figure 12–26 is that he had been treated with radiation to the brain for acute myelogenous leukemia. The superficial lesion seen could therefore be a chloroma or a radiation-induced meningioma. The identification of enlarged convolutions suggested the presence of an intracerebral lesion, which, in view of the acute myelogenous leukemia, was considered to be chloroma. This was confirmed by stereotactic biopsy findings.

A dural tail with meningeal enhancement has been observed in the setting of lesions other than meningioma.[68,78] It may occur in up to 60% of patients with meningioma.[30] A dural reaction and dural tail have also been observed in patients with metastatic lesions and glioblastoma multiforme.[78] In a metastatic lesion affecting the dura mater (Fig. 12–27), a dural reaction with layered thickening of the dura mater at the site of involvement can be observed together with a dural tail, as in the case illustrated. In another case of glioblastoma multiforme, a dural reaction with a dural tail was observed (Fig. 12–28). In this patient the imaging characteristics suggested the presence of an intraaxial mass because of expansion of the convolutions, the disproportionate edema, and the midline shift despite the dural reaction. The rapid onset and progression of symptoms in this patient supported a diagnosis of glioblastoma multiforme. The presence of necrosis within the lesion (not shown) supported this diagnosis. Pathologic evaluation confirmed the diagnosis of glioblastoma multiforme, with extension of the tumor via the Virchow-Robin spaces to the meninges and the development of dural infiltration, resulting in the formation of a dural tail. Leukemic infiltration may also mimic a meningioma by enveloping the falx (Fig. 12–29).

It is important to distinguish temporal lobe hamartoma or heterotopia[5] from temporal lobe tumors that cause complex partial seizures. The etiologic basis of complex partial seizures in most patients with temporal lobe lesions is a neoplasm[34] (Fig. 12–30). In such cases the tumor can often be

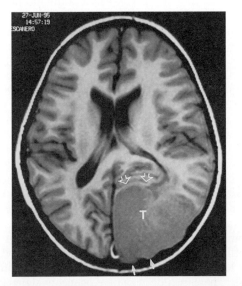

**FIGURE 12–26.** Axial T1-weighted MR image of a chloroma of the brain in an 18-year-old patient treated for acute myelogenous leukemia 10 years before and presenting acutely with seizure. A large superficial homogeneous lesion is isointense to gray matter and affects the superficial cortex and underlying white matter. Buckling of the white matter (*open arrows*) is seen. Question: Is this extraaxial? On postcontrast images (not shown), diffuse homogeneous enhancement of the lesion occurred. The critical finding is convolutional enlargement of the cortex with calvarial erosion (*arrows*). This lesion was called an intraaxial chloroma in view of the above findings and the history of acute myelogenous leukemia. This was confirmed pathologically. (*T*, tumor.)

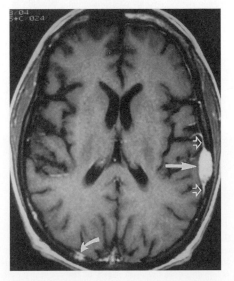

**FIGURE 12–27.** Metastasis with a dural tail. Postcontrast axial T1-weighted MR image reveals a dural based metastasis (*large arrow*) with a dural tail (*open arrows*) and a second calvarial metastases (*curved arrow*) in a 50-year-old patient with primary renal carcinoma.

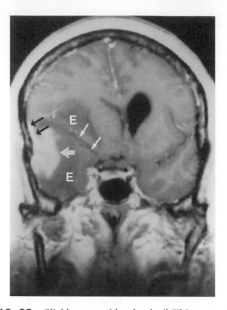

**FIGURE 12–28.** Glioblastoma with a dural tail. This postcontrast coronal T1-weighted MR image demonstrates a superficial intraaxial neoplasm (*large arrow*) with a dural tail (*black arrows*). There is extensive surrounding edema (*E*) with displacement of the sylvian fissure (*small white arrows*) and ventricular compression.

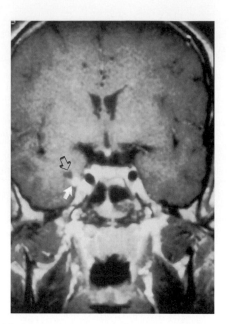

**FIGURE 12–30.** Pilocytic astrocytoma in a 13-year-old patient with complex partial seizures. This postcontrast coronal T1-weighted MR image reveals an enhancing nodule (*white arrow*) with a cystic component (*open arrow*) in the right medial temporal lobe.

recognized because of the presence of a localized intraaxial mass, which may be nodular or may have a cystic component (Fig. 12–30). The most common possibilities include juvenile pilocytic astrocytoma and ganglioglioma. Less common possibilities are benign lesions such as heterotopic gray matter (Fig. 12–31, see color plate) or hamartoma (Fig. 12–32).[5,10,11] In these cases, comparison of the two temporal lobes will reveal the loss of normal gray-white interface on the affected side and in some cases also an apparent discrete mass caused by clumping of the heterotopic tissue. The heterotopic mass has a signal intensity similar to that of normal gray matter.

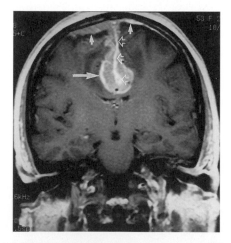

**FIGURE 12–29.** A leukemic infiltrate creating a tumorlike mass that envelopes the falx and mimics meningioma in a patient with acute lymphatic leukemia (ALL). This postcontrast coronal T1-weighted MR image reveals an inhomogeneous tumor (*large arrow*) coating the falx (*open arrows*) and extending over the dura mater of the convexity (*small arrows*). The lack of homogeneity of the tumor and the history of ALL enable the infiltrate to be differentiated from meningioma. The tumor completely regressed in response to radiotherapy.

Radiation effects may be difficult to differentiate from neoplasm. Patients with a glioma treated with radiation therapy may develop radiation effects alone or in combination with a glioma. Thus the ability to separate recurrent glioma from treatment effects is important. The more typical patterns of radiation effects after contrast enhancement include nodules, rings, a soap-bubble appearance, and flocculent lesions; these effects also have a predilection for the paraventricular regions (Fig. 12–33).[45,73] In addition, extensive edema is often present. Dynamic imaging, which measures contrast uptake over time, has been used to verify these cases. The uptake is slow and continuos in the setting of a radiation effect and more rapid in the presence of a tumor.[33] The temporal curves are therefore distinctively different (see Fig. 12–33) between tumor and radiation.

The ability to separate hemorrhagic glioma from an intracerebral hematoma is important from the standpoint of patient management (Fig. 12–34). In the CT era it was uncommon to recognize hemorrhage in a glioma (<1%); however, since the advent of MRI, hemorrhage is recognized more commonly (5% to 10%).[38] If the hemorrhage occupies a small portion of the glioma, differentiation from an intracerebral hematoma is not difficult since the character of the glioma is unchanged; however, differentiation may be more difficult when most of the tumor is affected.[3,20] Several features have been described[3,20,47] that allow for differential diagnosis. These include (1) a heterogeneous signal intensity or mass around or adjacent to hemorrhage; (2) an eccentric or central location of hemorrhage within the mass; (3) tumor opacification after the administration of intravenous contrast material; (4) hemorrhagic components of varying age; (5) delay in the temporal evolution of hemorrhage; (6) marked surrounding vasogenic edema; (7) a variable hemosiderin rim; and (8) appearance of tumor on imaging studies after the resolution of hemorrhage.

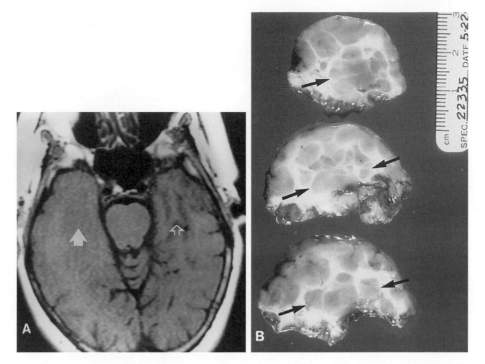

**FIGURE 12–31.** Heterotopic gray matter mimicking primary tumor. **A,** Precontrast axial T1-weighted MR image. **B,** Surgical specimen of the temporal lobe. Abnormal right temporal lobe white matter (*large arrow* in **A**), with loss of gray-white matter differentiation, is seen. The left temporal lobe white matter (*open arrow* in **A**) is normal. Temporal lobe resection revealed islands of heterotopic gray matter (*arrows* in **B**). (See Color Plate.)

In the majority of cases it is not difficult to distinguish MS from a glioma because MS is a white-matter lesion.[48] However, one must remember that white-matter tracts are present around the ventricles and within the corpus callosum. Solitary (Fig. 12–35) or multiple (Fig. 12–36) MS lesions in these locations can therefore simulate a glioma. An appropriate history and specific cerebrospinal fluid findings will often aid in establishing the correct diagnosis of MS.

Distinguishing an infarct from a glioma is not always easy. Infarcts affect the cortical structures or basal ganglia. The combined finding of a surface lesion and prominent gyri on T1-weighted, FLAIR, or T2-weighted images and the finding of gyral enhancement on postcontrast images should enable one to make the correct diagnosis (Fig. 12–37).[9,16,24,81] The history in most cases also aids in substantiating the diagnosis. In particular, the patient with a stroke usually presents with abrupt onset of symptoms. Gliomas also usually affect the subcortical region and spare gyri because they tend to be confined by subcortical u-fibers. In some cases, gliomas extend by satellitosis to the gray matter.[62] Incisural herniation with compression of the ipsilateral posterior cerebral artery may occur in some patients with neoplasms and result in an infarct that may be confused with a second focus of tumor (Fig. 12–38).

A multifocal glioma (Fig. 12–39) or multicentric glioma should be distinguished from metastases or abscesses. In a study of 100 patients with proven malignant gliomas performed at the University of Texas M.D. Anderson Cancer Center, multiple lesions were seen in 30%.[46] Multifocal lesions were seen in most of these patients; multicentric lesions were uncommon. Gliomas spread is via Scherer structures,[62] the subarachnoid space, and the subependymal or intraventricular spaces. At least one of the lesions should

have the pattern of a malignant glioma: a large, enhancing, complex ring lesion with necrosis or invasion of adjacent structures (see Fig. 12–5). The other lesions may have the appearance of nodules or rings of variable sizes and be present in multiple locations. Metastases and abscesses spread

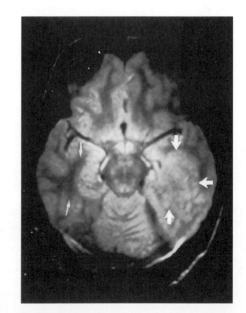

**FIGURE 12–32.** Hamartoma in a 20-year-old patient with a history of complex partial seizures. Axial proton-weighted MR image reveals loss of normal white matter in the left temporal lobe and distortion of the residual white matter (*white arrows*) compared with the normal white matter contralaterally (*small arrows*). The sharply defined lesion on the left was composed of gray and white matter and is featureless.

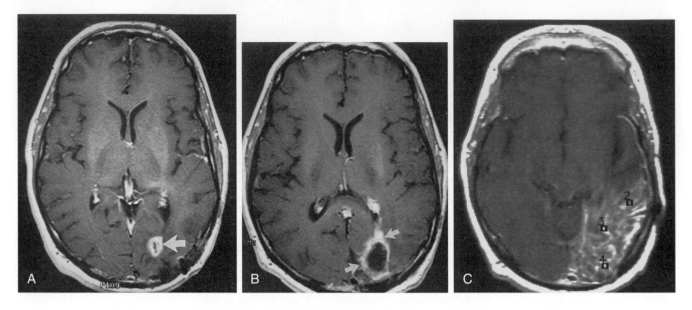

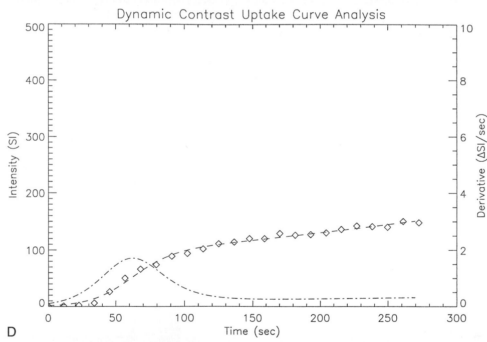

**FIGURE 12–33.** Left parietooccipital anaplastic astrocytoma in a 39-year-old patient. The tumor was resected in March 1995, and the patient was subsequently treated with accelerated radiotherapy and chemotherapy. **A through C,** Postcontrast axial T1-weighted MR images. **A,** This MR image obtained on June 26, 1996, revealed a thick-walled ring lesion (*large arrow*) with surrounding edema in the left posterior parietooccipital region without ventricular displacement of the occipital horn. Question: Is this tumor recurrence or a radiation effect? Surgery revealed predominant necrosis with scattered tumor cells of low activity. **B,** Five months later, despite complete resection, a larger enhancing ring lesion (*arrows*) affecting the surgical cavity was observed to extend to the ventricular wall. Dynamic scanning suggested a mixed radiation effect and islands of tumor. **C,** Follow-up examination 13 months later revealed an extensive gyral lesion with Swiss-cheese appearance encompassing the posterior half of the parietooccipital region without a mass effect. Dynamic scanning revealed a temporal slope consistent with a radiation effect. This illustrates the variable pattern and growth of radiation lesions and the value of dynamic scanning in such cases. Areas of interest for dynamic curves are noted as *2, 3,* and *4.* **D,** Typical curve from area of interest. The curve represented by dotted lines with a diamond represents a quantitative measure of the maximal rate of contrast agent uptake. This low curve represents the slow contrast uptake over time and indicates necrosis. The bell-shaped curve represents the derivatives of the fitted curve (see Fig. 12–50).

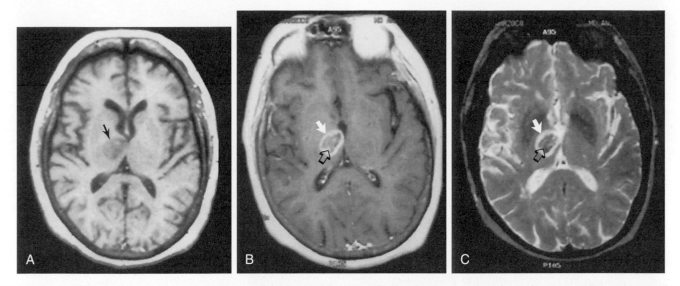

**FIGURE 12–34.** MR images in a 54-year-old patient with left hemiparesis suspected of having a brain tumor. Subacute hematoma mimics tumor. **A,** This precontrast axial T1-weighted MR image at the level of the thalamus reveals a hypointense lesion (*arrow*) with small foci of hyperintensity. **B,** This postcontrast axial T1-weighted MR image reveals that the rim enhances uniformly (*arrow*), with the central portion remaining hypointense (*open arrow*). **C,** This axial T2-weighted MR image demonstrates that the lesion has a bright rim (*arrow*), with the central portion showing mixed hypointensity and hyperintensity (*open arrow*). These findings are characteristic of a subacute hematoma. This is not a neoplasm.

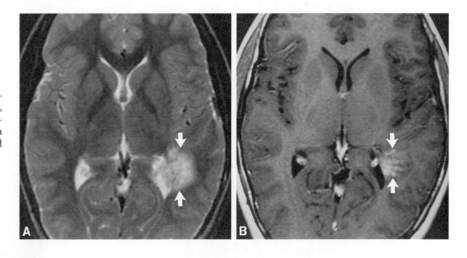

**FIGURE 12–35.** Multiple sclerosis in a 15-year-old patient. **A,** On this axial T2-weighted MR image, a flocculent white-matter lesion is observed extending to the ventricular wall (*arrows*), simulating a neoplasm. **B,** On this postcontrast axial T1-weighted image, the plaque is enhanced (*arrows*).

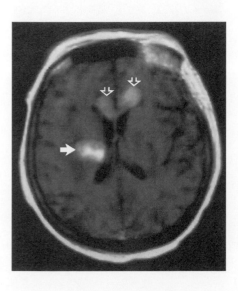

**FIGURE 12–36.** Multiple sclerosis in a 38-year-old patient. Postcontrast axial T1-weighted MR image in a 38-year-old patient who presented with left hemiparesis. Multiple enhancing lesions are seen in the paraventricular white matter affecting the ventricular wall (*large arrow*) and the corpus callosum (*open arrows*). This appearance could be confused with that of a lymphoma or glioma. Careful clinical and laboratory workup confirmed the diagnosis of tumefactive multiple sclerosis.

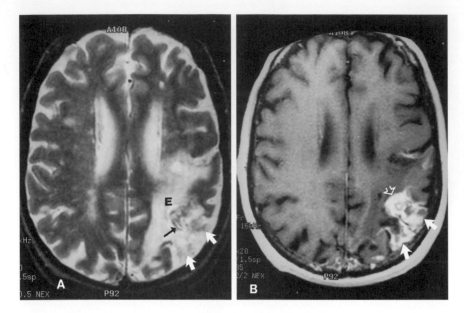

**FIGURE 12–37.** Subacute chronic infarct. MR images in a 62-year-old patient presenting with headaches and progressive right hemiparesis who was referred for evaluation for a brain tumor. **A,** This axial T2-weighted MR image reveals a lesion involving the cortex and adjacent white matter (*white arrows*) with laminar necrosis (*black arrow*) and surrounding diffuse edema (*E*). **B,** This postcontrast axial T1-weighted MR image demonstrates a superficial lesion conforming to the gyri (*white arrows*) and affecting the subcortical white matter (*open arrow*).

hematogenously and are seen either at the corticomedullary junction or on the surface of the brain (see Fig. 12–7).

The differentiation of leptomeningeal disease in the setting of infection from that in the setting of neoplasm and meningeal fibrosis[12,15,19,23,55,66] may be difficult (Fig. 12–40). The lesions are often similar because of the diffuse meningeal involvement that occurs in both settings, but variations may be observed in some patients. One rule of thumb is that the leptomeningeal disease in a patient seen at a general hospital is usually inflammatory, whereas it is more likely neoplastic in a patient seen at a cancer center. In addition, in leptomeningeal disease of infectious origin in the brain, thickening of the meninges is observed, and this area will

often have a smoother appearance than that seen in a patient with a neoplasm.[55] In the patient with neoplastic involvement, in addition to the thickening of the leptomeninges, the pial component of disease is also irregular and nodular (see Fig. 12–40) and can be localized.[44] The patient with meningeal fibrosis shows a smooth thickening of variable width without pial involvement (Fig. 12–41).

Cavernous angioma should be distinguished from metastases.[54] The cavernous angioma is seen as a round target lesion with a black rim and a bright center.[54] These lesions may be single or multiple; they may occur in white matter (Fig. 12–42); and edema or a mass effect is absent unless hemorrhage occurs. Metastatic lesions are more often associated with edema and are located at a corticomedullary junction, in a paraventricular location or on a dural surface. Black (hypointense) lesions may be observed on T2-weighted im-

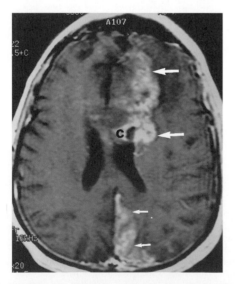

**FIGURE 12–38.** MR image in a 56-year-old patient with increasing somnolence and right hemiparesis. This postcontrast axial T1-weighted MR image reveals a large left frontal parasagittal glioblastoma multiforme (*large white arrows*) extending to the corpus callosum (*C*). Incisural herniation occurred prior to surgery as a result of the neoplasm, with a second lesion appearing in the left parietal parasagittal region and representing an enhancing infarct (*small arrows*) that affected cortical and subcortical tissue. This lesion should not be confused with a second neoplastic focus.

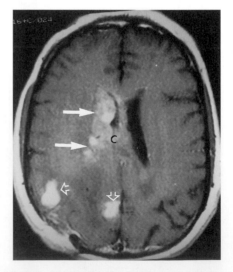

**FIGURE 12–39.** Multifocal malignant glioma in a 56-year-old patient. This postcontrast axial T1-weighted image reveals a paraventricular (*arrows*) and corpus callosal tumor (*C*) extending posteriorly along white matter tracts (Scherer structures) with other foci of tumor (*open white arrows*).

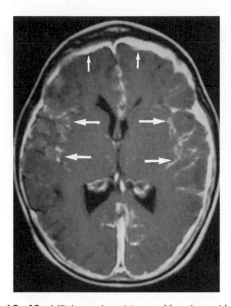

**FIGURE 12–40.** MR image in a 36-year-old patient with melanoma and leptomeningeal disease (carcinomatous meningitis). This postcontrast axial T1-weighted MR image reveals involvement of the arachnoid and pia mater of the sylvian fissure (*large arrows*) and the dura mater and leptomeninges (*small arrows*).

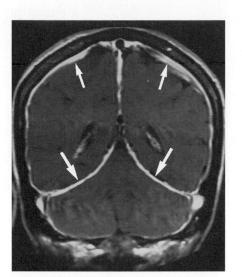

**FIGURE 12–41.** Aseptic dural fibrosis. This postcontrast coronal T1-weighted MR image reveals dural fibrosis (*small arrows*) and tentorial thickening (*large arrows*) resulting from multiple lumbar punctures.

ages in patients with melanoma, adenocarcinoma, hemosiderin deposits, or calcification.

It is important to distinguish gliomatosis cerebri from encephalitis. Gliomatosis cerebri may occur centrally or peripherally, and it affects more than one lobe of the brain.[64] The neoplasm is diffuse and does not respect subcortical u-fibers, so gray-white matter margins are breached (Fig. 12–43). Clinical symptoms progress slowly, and seizures may occur. In encephalitis the majority of lesions affect white matter (Fig. 12–44).[53] In addition, patients with encephalitis present acutely and are very ill.

It is important to separate a focal inflammatory lesion from a glioma. A patient presenting with a focal lesion and seizures may have either a localized infection (Figs. 12–45 and 12–46) or neoplasm, and it is important to distinguish between the two.[53] Both may be seen as a ring lesion on postcontrast studies. In most instances, however, the T2-weighted images will provide information that is critical in separating the two. Specifically, the boundary or rim of an inflammatory lesion will be black because of the presence of free radicals (see Fig. 12–45).[32] Also, as in other abscesses, the medial margin at the junction with the white matter may be thinner be-

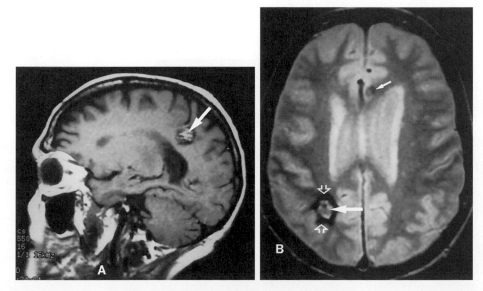

**FIGURE 12–42.** Cavernous angioma. **A,** Precontrast sagittal T1-weighted MR image. **B,** Axial T2-weighted MR image. A cavernous angioma typically demonstrates blood products at variable stages. Old blood is bright on a T1-weighted image (*arrow* in **A**) and on a T2-weighted image (*arrow* in **B**). Hemosiderin, an end product of hemorrhage, is seen as an area of dark signal intensity, blooming on a T2-weighted sequence (*open arrows* in **B**). A second small lesion is seen in the left cingulate gyrus (*small arrow*) in **B.** The stereotypical popcorn appearance of a cavernous angioma is well demonstrated.

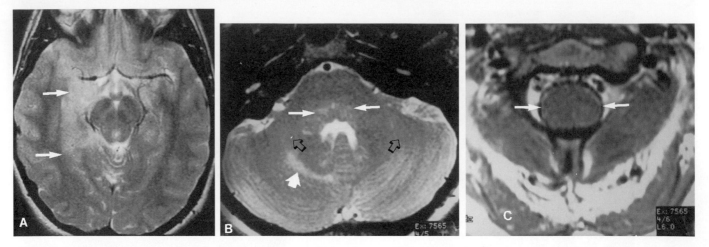

**FIGURE 12–43.** MR images in a 20-year-old patient with temporal lobe seizures and left-sided paresis: gliomatosis cerebri. **A,** This axial T2-weighted MR image through the temporal lobes reveals diffuse hyperintensity of the right medial temporal lobe crossing the gray-white matter junction (*arrows*). **B,** This axial T2-weighted image through the brainstem and fourth ventricle reveals hyperintensity within an enlarged pons (*arrows*) that extends to the middle cerebellar peduncles (*open black arrows*) and white matter of the cerebellar hemisphere (*large white arrow*). **C,** This postcontrast axial T1-weighted image through the upper cervical cord reveals enlargement of the cord without contrast enhancement (*arrows*). The presence of a diffuse lesion involving multiple lobes of the brain and crossing gray-white matter junctions is characteristic of gliomatosis cerebri. In this case, however, no contrast enhancement of the lesion occurred.

cause of the decreased vascularity of the white-matter surface compared with the vascularity of the gray matter.

A giant aneurysm may be confused with a neoplasm because of the mass effect that can occur in both settings. However, features are often present that may allow the correct diagnosis to be made.[54] Specifically, the giant aneurysm is usually related to the major arterial bifurcations (e.g., suprasellar in location), the middle cerebral artery trifurcation, and the basilar artery bifurcation. It may exhibit a target sign because of the whorls of clot that develop over time. A flow void is often recognized centrally or eccentrically, and this represents the remaining patent lumen (Fig. 12–47).[54]

## DISCUSSION

Superficial *intraaxial neoplasms* of the brain are often difficult to distinguish from *meningiomas* (Figs. 12–2C and D). For example, white-matter buckling,[58] a sign that is con-

sidered indicative of a dural-based or extraaxial lesion, is also infrequently seen in patients with intraaxial superficial tumors. It consists of a localized mass that lies adjacent to a dural surface (see Fig. 12–10), or a circumferential vessel (marginal vein) with occasional meningeal enhancement (see Fig. 12–28).[68,78] In the presence of an intraaxial neoplasm, however, there will be the unique finding of localized brain expansion and enlarged convolutions (see Fig. 12–26).

A dural tail was considered a characteristic sign of a meningioma (see Fig. 12–2D).[30,77] In fact, however, in a study of a large series of patients with meningiomas, Goldsher et al[30] observed dural enhancement with a dural tail in only 60% of patients. A further important point made by Tokumaru et al[69] was that the dural tail may reveal a meningioma, but it may also conceivably signify only a dural reaction. In line with this finding, Wilms et al[78] demonstrated that a dural reaction or a dural tail could be recognized in the MR studies of dural-based nonmeningioma neoplasms

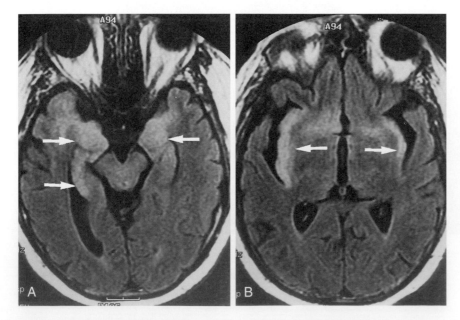

**FIGURE 12–44.** Axial FLAIR images in a patient with herpes simplex encephalitis. A nonenhancing high signal intensity lesion is seen involving the regions of the limbic system, namely, the medial temporal lobes (*arrows* in **A**) and insular cortex (*arrows* in **B**) bilaterally. This finding in an acutely ill patient is highly suggestive of herpes simplex encephalitis.

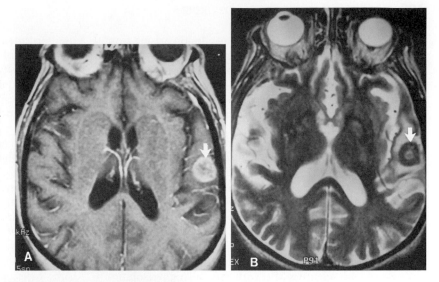

**FIGURE 12–45.** MR images in a 45-year-old patient with a history of seizures. **A,** Postcontrast axial T1-weighted image reveals a left temporal lobe lesion with rim enhancement (*arrow*) and a central component of mixed intensity. **B,** Axial T2-weighted image at the same level. The wall of the lesion is seen as a thick black rim (*arrow*) with a central hyperintense component. A rim that turns dark on the sequence is a characteristic of a lesion with an infectious etiologic basis. This lesion was determined to be a histoplasmoma.

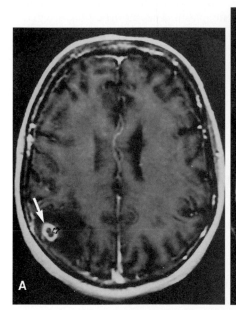

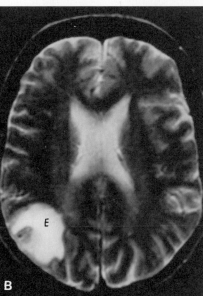

**FIGURE 12–46.** Cysticercosis mimicking metastasis. **A,** Postcontrast axial T1-weighted image. **B,** Axial T2-weighted image. Cysticercosis is seen within the right parietal lobe and appears as an enhancing ring lesion (*large arrow* in **A**) with a central scolex (*open arrow* in **A**) that is creating significant edema (*E* in **B**).

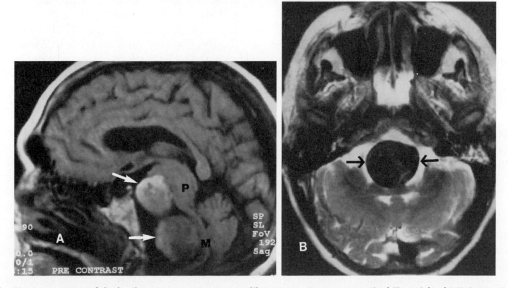

**FIGURE 12–47.** Giant aneurysms of the basilar artery creating a tumorlike mass. **A,** Precontrast sagittal T1-weighted MR image. **B,** Axial T2-weighted image. A giant bilobed, partially thrombosed basilar artery aneurysm (*arrows* in **A**) is seen compressing the pons (*P*) and medulla (*M*). The thrombosed component of the aneurysm is seen as a bright signal intensity (*arrows*) on this T1-weighted image. Flowing blood within the aneurysm creates a signal loss, producing a dark signal intensity on the T2-weighted image (*arrows* in **B**), a characteristic appearance of a giant aneurysm on MR images, which should not be mistaken for tumor. (Courtesy of Lisa Hinckley, M.D., Baylor College of Medicine, Houston, Tex.)

(see Figs. 12–27 and 12–28). Therefore a lesion arising from the dura mater or within the brain in proximity to the dura mater may affect the dura mater directly by invasion or indirectly by irritating the adjacent dura mater (see Fig. 12–10). Thus dural involvement may be observed in non-meningiomas, and critical evaluation is necessary to exclude other possibilities.

In the patient presenting with *complex partial seizures,* an organic lesion intrinsic to the brain is usually the cause.[34] Affected patients stereotypically have a neoplasm such as an astrocytoma (see Fig. 12–30), oligodendroglioma, or gangli-oglioma. Infrequently, developmental lesions may occur, such as hamartomas (see Fig. 12–32) or gray-matter hetero-topias (Fig. 12–31; see color plate).[5,11] In all instances, surgical resection is required to correct the problem. The examination of choice to precisely define the relevant anatomy in the patient with seizure is MRI with coronal, high-resolution T1-weighted and T2-weighted images with 3 mm sections with a reverse angle to the temporal lobe.[14,37] Microscopically, *hamartomas* consist of mature ganglion cells scattered haphazardly in a normal neuropil. Grossly, the affected portion of the brain may appear normal or disorganized.[11] *Heterotopic gray matter* is normal gray matter in an unusual location and is related to a migrational anomaly.[5]

*Radiation therapy or chemotherapy effects on the brain* are well known. Radiologic changes in particular are being recognized with greater frequency as the result of more aggressive therapy and the improved imaging capabilities of MRI.[7,10,43,71,72,79] Often, however, it is not possible to discriminate posttreatment changes from residual or recurrent tumor (see Fig. 12–33).[33,80] In fact, this is a serious problem at our institution. Thus we have started to use dynamic scanning with MRI to discriminate between the two and have found it to be a highly reliable method.[33] In particular, the variation in appearance of the temporal curves of contrast seen over time has helped significantly in distinguishing between the two entities (see Figs. 12–33 and 12–50). The pathophysiologic changes that are due to radiation therapy include vascular damage with thickening of the blood vessel walls and also hyalinization.[7] Another change is damage to oligodendrocytes affecting the myelin sheath, with direct effects on microglia and axons.[7,10] In addition, Sawaya et al[61] have demonstrated that the fibrinolytic enzyme system in brain tumors is affected, leading to increased vascularity and an increased likelihood of hemorrhage, necrosis, or infarction.[60,70] A tumor-host interaction also may contribute to the pathophysiologic changes that occur. The patterns associated with radiation effects should therefore be carefully sought to differentiate the two lesions. Perfusion imaging may be of value in distinguishing tumor from necrosis.[1,57] It is also important to understand that necrosis provokes the development of cerebral edema.[17] In fact, in some cases only necrosis has been observed at autopsy with no residual neoplasm.[45]

In a patient with a *nontumoral intracerebral hematoma,* it is important to distinguish this lesion from a hemorrhagic neoplasm since many hematomas may not require surgical intervention if they are not large enough or not in a critical location. In the case illustrated in Figure 12–34, variable opinions were expressed about the nature of the lesion, but if one examines the imaging characteristics, an appropriate diagnosis can be made. An intracerebral hematoma follows a well-accepted temporal pattern.[31] In the acute phase, images are usually of mixed intensity, with foci of hypointensity and hyperintensity intermixed in a well-defined mass with minimal surrounding edema. By 24 hours to 7 days after the ictus, the lesions are isointense to slightly hypointense on T1-weighted images and hypointense on T2-weighted images. After a week a hyperintense rim is seen on the T1-weighted image, with the interior slowly becoming hyperintense over the following weeks. T2-weighted images remain hypointense slightly longer but then also gradually become hyperintense. After approximately 2 weeks, both sequences reveal bright lesions that may persist over months. Therefore an intracranial hematoma assumes a relatively consistent pattern over time[31] and should be distinguishable from a hemorrhagic glioma.[3,20,47]

*In patients with MS, the mass may become tumefactive.* In such cases, solitary (see Fig. 12–35) or multiple (see Fig. 12–36) large masses that are paraventricular in location may be confused with a neoplasm. The important feature that is characteristic of an MS lesion is that it originates from deep white matter; gray matter is rarely involved and necrosis is uncommon in MS. The clinical presentation in a patient with MS should also be quite different from that in a patient with a neoplasm. For example, in the patient with MS the lesion does not usually explain the patient's symptoms. In addition, the symptoms and physical findings vary, and patients often have remissions and exacerbations of variable duration.

*Infarcts should be separated from tumors by imaging.* Patients, however, may be sent in for evaluation for a tumor because of positive MRI findings and a clinical history that does not suggest a stroke. Specifically, the symptoms of stroke may be slowly progressive as the stroke evolves, rather than presenting acutely. In addition, in the acute stage of stroke, prominent gyri are observed, with gyral enhancement seen following the intravenous administration of contrast material by MRI.[9,24] In the subacute stage the subcortical tissues may also be affected, resulting in a larger lesion (see Fig. 12–37). The involvement of subcortical tissue may cause confusion, but the characteristic changes within the gyri should enable one to make the appropriate diagnosis and avoid this pitfall (see Fig. 12–38). In strokes the earliest changes observed on MRI are seen 24 to 72 hours after the ictus and include gyral enlargement on T2-weighted images and vascular opacification on postcontrast images.[24] The gyral enhancement on postcontrast studies is related to BBB breakdown and luxury perfusion.[41] On the other hand, linear bands observed acutely in the ischemic area represent slow flow or occlusion of the regional arteries.[24,81] These changes may occur earlier than the gyral enhancement, although in some cases they may occur simultaneously. Complex metabolic changes develop as a consequence of the reduction in arterial blood flow locally and regionally, and these are accompanied by local vasodilatation and anoxia. The breakdown in the sodium-potassium pump contributes to the development of vasogenic and cytotoxic edema. The combination of pathophysiologic changes affecting the gyri, subcortical structures, adjacent white matter, and regional vasculature is responsible for the appearance seen on MRI (see Fig. 12–38). The changes observed over time reflect the brain damage that may result from these pathophysiologic alterations.

*Multicentric gliomas* (multiple histologically separate foci of glioma) and *multifocal gliomas* (tumors that are histologically interconnected) (see Figs. 12–5 and 12–39) may mimic metastases or abscesses.[74] In a review of 500 patients with gliomas, Kyritsis et al[40] noted a 10% incidence of multifocal and multicentric gliomas. However, in a recent review by Leeds et al,[46] a 30% incidence was noted in 100 patients with pathologically proven glioblastoma multiforme who had MRI examinations and underwent surgery. Although one can usually separate multifocal or multicentric glioma from metastases, there are occasions when the lesions look similar, and in these instances the correct diagnosis can be made only at surgery. The reason why it is sometimes difficult to distinguish between the two is that gliomas spread via the subarachnoid space, extend via the Virchow-Robin spaces adjacent to the dura mater, and then reach other portions of the brain. However, although metastatic tumors and abscesses typically spread either by hematogenous extension into the brain at corticomedullary junctions or on the dural surface, these lesions, particularly with metastases, may also then spread to other locations via the subarachnoid space. This explains the occasional similar appearance of metastases and gliomas. Glioblastoma multiforme usually presents as a complex ring, whereas metastases or abscesses present as noncomplex rings.[8] An abscess is observed to have a black rim on T2-weighted images[32] with budding or new offshoots occurring with the formation of new lesions, whereas the medial wall adjacent to the white matter is thinner because of decreased vascularity. Metastases usually assume the appearance of solid nodules or simple rings. Multicentric gliomas rarely have an appearance inseparable from that of metastases on the basis of imaging findings.[40] In these cases only biopsy may separate the two processes.

To determine whether the dura mater or leptomeninges are involved in a patient suspected of having *dural disease or leptomeningeal disease,* an understanding of these structures is important. The dura mater consists of two layers. The superficial, or outer, layer lies on the surface and is closely applied and fused to the periosteum in the adult; the inner layer, though closely applied to the outer layer, separates to form the falx and tentorium. The leptomeninges consists of the arachnoid mater, which covers the brain and forms the outer layer of the subarachnoid space, and the pia mater, which is closely applied to the brain surface and actually covers the gyri and dips into the sulci. The pia mater forms the inner surface of the subarachnoid space. The subdural space lies between the dura mater (outer surface) and the arachnoid mater (inner surface). Lesions that involve the leptomeninges are often attributed to meningitis, which may be inflammatory or neoplastic (see Fig. 12–40); the two processes can be indistinguishable.[15,44,55] The lesions may be localized, multifocal or diffuse.[44,55,66] However, confusion may occur despite the apparent anatomic variances. As a result, it can still be difficult to distinguish dural from leptomeningeal involvement.[66] In patients suspected of harboring leptomeningeal disease, findings from lumbar puncture may help to distinguish the two lesions. Various authors[28,44,52,76] have reported that lumbar puncture is positive in only 56% to 64% of patients with carcinomatous meningitis, even after two to three lumbar punctures were performed in patients with pleocytosis and an elevated protein level. On the other hand, lumbar puncture is often positive

in patients with bacterial meningitis, and this difference in the frequency of positive findings may be used to distinguish carcinomatosis from bacterial meningitis. A further problem is posed by the bone marrow depression that occurs in cancer patients undergoing radiation therapy and chemotherapy. These immunocompromised patients are susceptible to a variety of inflammatory processes. Thus the two meningitic processes often have a similar appearance on imaging studies and may be difficult to separate.[15,55,66] A possible distinguishing feature in the patient with inflammatory meningitis is that vasogenic and cytotoxic edema may develop secondary to the formation of a brain abscess or arterial and venous ischemia, resulting in infarction. In a patient with a neoplasm, carcinomatous meningitis may develop when tumor cells from metastases within the brain are shed into the subarachnoid spaces or spread when the neoplasm extends to meningeal vessels. Dural involvement may represent either a reaction to calvarial lesions or may result from direct extension from meningeal vessels or from the calvarial disease. However, a dural reaction that may not be related to an infectious or neoplastic process and one that must also be considered when localized or diffuse dural thickening is recognized may also stem from surgery, trauma, shunt placement, lumbar puncture (see Fig. 12–41), subdural hematomas, subacute infarcts, and postural hypotension.[12,19,23]

In differentiating *cavernous angioma from metastases,* knowledge of the typical appearance of angioma aids in making the correct diagnosis (see Fig. 12–42).[2] In particular, cavernous angiomas can be multiple and not associated with a mass effect or edema (unless bleeding occurs).

In *encephalitis,* the lesions tend to be localized or diffuse within white matter and do not usually affect the gray-white matter interface (see Fig. 12–44). The patient becomes acutely ill, and early recognition is important so that treatment can be started immediately. *Herpes encephalitis* usually is observed to affect both temporal lobes, the limbic system, and then the insular cortex; for this reason it can simulate gliomatosis cerebri. The difference is that the encephalitis is acute in onset and the anatomic involvement is predictable. In addition, in *gliomatosis cerebri* the lesions are distinctly different in that they are diffuse and may affect the cortical surface and adjacent white matter and do not respect gray-white matter boundaries.[64] They may also be central in location. Gliomatosis cerebri can also spread along white matter tracts from the cerebral hemisphere into the brainstem and spinal cord (see Fig. 12–43).

*Abscesses can mimic metastases or glioblastoma.* However, a well-formed abscess will have an enhancing rim produced by a capsule, and it will have a central area of necrotic debris (see Fig. 12–45). In addition, the inner margin of the abscess cavity has a smooth margin, whereas the margin of metastatic tumors and glioblastoma tends to be irregular, nodular, and shaggy. A larger ring surrounded by daughter rings is a classic finding in a patient with an abscess (see Fig. 12–7). An abscess in immunocompromised patients with unusual opportunistic organisms, however, may have a thick and irregular wall mimicking metastasis or glioblastoma multiforme.[53] *Toxoplasma* infections are the most common opportunistic infections in patients with acquired immunodeficiency syndrome (AIDS). When single or multiple enhancing ring lesions in the region of basal ganglia and corticomedullary junctions are recognized in immunocompromised patients, a diagnosis of toxoplasmosis should be considered (see Fig. 12–14). Fungal infections of the brain are rare, but they occur with greater frequency in immunocompromised patients. Fungal abscesses are seen as an enhancing ring lesion on postcontrast T1-weighted images, similar to the appearance of a pyogenic abscess, but the capsule tends to show dark signals on T2-weighted images as a result of paramagnetic contents (see Fig. 12–45). Cysticercosis is the most common parasitic infection, and 60% to 90% of affected patients have central nervous system lesions.[53] The imaging findings vary with the stages of infection, from a nonenhancing cyst to a ring-enhancing target lesion to a calcified nodule (see Fig. 12–46).

It is necessary to distinguish an *aneurysm from a tumor* because of the significant difference in the management of the two entities. It is extremely important to consider a giant aneurysm, particularly in a patient with a large enhancing mass centered along the course of a major intracranial bifurcation, such as in the suprasellar or anterior sellar region, in the region of middle cerebral artery bifurcation, or at the tip of the basilar artery. Giant aneurysms may assume the appearance of a large space-occupying mass that mimics tumor.[54] If an aneurysm is mistakenly diagnosed as tumor when a surgical biopsy is attempted, the consequences can be catastrophic. However, because of flowing blood, the presence or absence of thrombus, and wall calcification within the aneurysm, there are magnetic resonance (MR) signals characteristic of a giant aneurysm[54] that allow it to be distinguished from a neoplasm. Specifically, an aneurysm with flowing blood will typically show a high-velocity signal loss (flow void) on T1-weighted and T2-weighted images and thus will appear dark. Signal heterogeneity may be observed if turbulent flow is present within the aneurysm (see Fig. 12–47). The aneurysm wall may also show circular peripheral wall enhancement as a result of vasa vasorum. Partially thrombosed aneurysms will have concentric layers of multilaminated clot of variable signal intensity on T1-weighted and T2-weighted images (see Fig. 12–47). Completely thrombosed aneurysms will be hyperintense on T1-weighted and T2-weighted images. Multilayered clots can be seen in thrombosed aneurysms, and these result from repeated episodes of hemorrhage.[54]

*Large unruptured AVMs can rarely mimic vascular tumor.* The differentiation is easy on the basis of MR findings because AVMs demonstrate large, serpiginous feeding arteries and draining veins around a nidus. In addition, unlike tumors, AVMs usually are not associated with edema. On standard spin-echo images (T1-weighted and T2-weighted), AVMs appear as a tightly paired "honeycomb" of "flow voids" caused by high-velocity signal loss.[54] A diagnosis of AVM should be entertained when a hemorrhagic mass is found to be associated with large serpentine arteries that feed the mass and also with large veins that drain into adjacent sinuses. Cerebral angiography is recommended to confirm the diagnosis and to understand the vascular anatomy so that the most appropriate treatment (e.g., embolotherapy, surgery, or both) can be determined.

# NEW DIRECTIONS IN NEUROIMAGING USING MAGNETIC RESONANCE IMAGING

Proton density–weighted (PDW), T1-weighted (T1W), T2-weighted (T2W), and T1W postcontrast images have been the standard means of evaluating intracranial lesions with MRI since the mid-1980s. With the recent advent of magnetization transfer and FLAIR techniques, the capabilities of conventional imaging sequences have been extended and the conspicuity of lesions has been significantly improved. However these techniques are not radical departures from the standard imaging sequences. In contrast, recent improvements in MR scanner hardware, particularly the magnetic gradient field subsystems, have opened up entirely new neuroimaging options. This section discusses some of these options, all of which involve very high speed imaging techniques.

## PERFUSION IMAGING PULSE SEQUENCES IN MAGNETIC RESONANCE IMAGING

Two MR-based techniques have been proposed for the direct mapping of relative cerebral blood volume (rCBV) and relative cerebral blood flow (rCBF). The first technique, sometimes referred to as dynamic susceptibility change (DSC) mapping, takes advantage of the transient susceptibility change that occurs when a bolus of paramagnetic contrast agent passes through the microvasculature. Since susceptibility changes are effectively local magnetic field inhomogeneities, such changes cause enhanced dephasing of nearby nuclear spins by decreasing the "apparent" T2 relaxation time (T2*). This results in a transient decrease in the signal intensity on T2W or T2*W images as the bolus passes through the microvasculature (Fig. 12–48). The higher the local perfusion, the greater the magnitude of the signal loss. Therefore areas of increased perfusion will appear hypointense relative to regions of decreased perfusion on T2W or T2*W images. Operating under the assumption that the contrast agent remains intravascular (i.e., that there is no breakdown of the BBB), such images can be used to construct maps of rCBV (Fig. 12–49) or rCBF.[57,63] If, however, the BBB is significantly fenestrated and contrast agent "leaks" from the vascular space into the interstitial space, bolus-infusion perfusion mapping will underestimate the value of rCBV. An advantage of this technique, as opposed to other nonbolus techniques, in terms of mapping rCBV, is the favorable signal-to-noise ratio of the perfusion images, particularly if double-dose or triple-dose bolus injections of contrast agent are used.

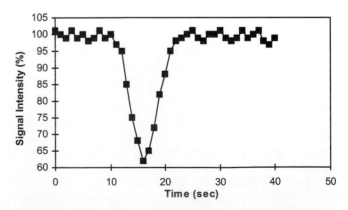

**FIGURE 12–48.** Time-vs.–signal intensity curve from a well-perfused region of interest in a bolus-infusion (dynamic susceptibility contrast) study. The area under the curve is proportional to the relative cerebral blood volume.

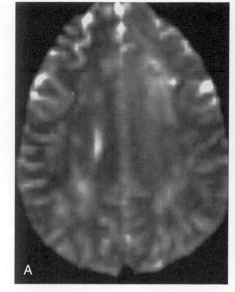 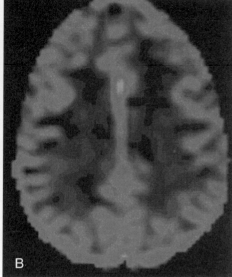

**FIGURE 12–49.** Spin-echo EPI T2-weighted image (**A**) and a dynamic susceptibility charge perfusion map (**B**). A 0.2 mmol/kg dose of gadolinium-DTPA was used for the bolus. Note the expected contrast between the gray matter and white matter in the perfusion map.

It is commonly accepted that tumors frequently induce angiogenesis and that highly vascular tumors are often more malignant than tumors that are not associated with increased local vascularity. Treatment-related changes and benign lesions, on the other hand, do not typically exhibit the same level of angiogenesis. Therefore the ability to assess vascularity using perfusion mapping should improve the characterization of lesions. Bolus-infusion perfusion mapping has been proposed as a tool for improving our ability to differentiate tumor from treatment-related changes and to assess tumor grade.[1] Such methods of quantitating rCBV should also improve our ability to assess the efficacy of antiangiogenesis drug therapy.

A further advance has been the development of gadolinium-based contrast agents with chelates that have larger molecular weights than does DTPA. These chelates make the agent a predominantly blood-pool agent, which can be used in whole-body imaging or in the imaging of intracranial lesions with compromised BBBs. Several such agents are being developed, and preliminary reports of their ability to estimate perfusion and vascularity in animal models have been published.[65,75]

The second MRI technique for evaluating perfusion relies on time-of-flight techniques. This technique, called EPISTAR (*echo-planar MRI imaging and signal targeting with alternating radiofrequency*), uses a variation of the inversion recovery technique and requires no injection of contrast agent.[22] However, the signal-to-noise ratio, compared with that produced by the bolus-injection technique, is inferior, imaging multiple slices is more difficult, and care must be taken to minimize unwanted magnetization transfer effects. On the other hand, the EPISTAR technique does not require a bolus infusion of contrast medium and can be used to assess rCBV in a totally noninvasive manner.

It should be noted that both the DSC mapping and EPISTAR techniques require very rapid imaging. Typically, this is best performed with systems capable of single-shot echo-planar imaging (EPI) techniques, which allow images to be acquired at a rate as high as 100 to 500 ms per image.

## DYNAMIC CONTRAST MAGNETIC RESONANCE IMAGING

Although the use of precontrast and postcontrast T1-weighted images is routine in neuroimaging studies, the kinetics of the contrast agent uptake are not typically considered. The rapid acquisition of T1-weighted images before, during, and after the infusion of a bolus of contrast agent, however, allows the rates of contrast agent uptake and washout from a lesion to be assessed. In theory, such data provide a means of quantitating the relative vascularity and permeability with two- or three-compartment rate kinetic models. Such noninvasively obtained information on vascularity and permeability can be extremely valuable in the practice of oncology. In addition, methods to quantitatively assess BBB permeability can be highly useful in determining the potential success of chemotherapeutic agents and in assessing the efficacy of novel therapeutic agents, such as receptor-mediated permeabilizers, that locally and temporarily increase the BBB permeability and thereby allow a larger concentration of drug to cross into the interstitial space.

Qualitative or semiquantitative applications of dynamic contrast MRI to the imaging of the brain in patients with suspected tumors have been reported.[33,80] Figure 12–50 shows typical gadolinium-DTPA uptake curves from regions of interest (ROIs) in pathologically proven cases of anaplastic astrocytoma, small cell lung cancer metastasis, meningioma, and radiation necrosis. The utility of dynamic contrast MR data in differentiating these types of intracranial lesions was recently reported by Hazle et al,[33] and correlations of patient outcome and dynamic contrast MRI indexes have been reported by Wong et al.[80] In addition to such qualitative or empiric model dynamic MRI studies, several quantitative pharmacokinetic techniques have been described that estimate the local permeability or vascularity in human brain neoplasms. In addition to extracting pharmacokinetic data from single user– or multiple user–defined ROIs, several groups have generated parametric maps that overlay color-coded maps of the pharmacokinetic parameters of interest on a standard high-resolution anatomic image. This method decreases the sampling error inherent in ROI tech-

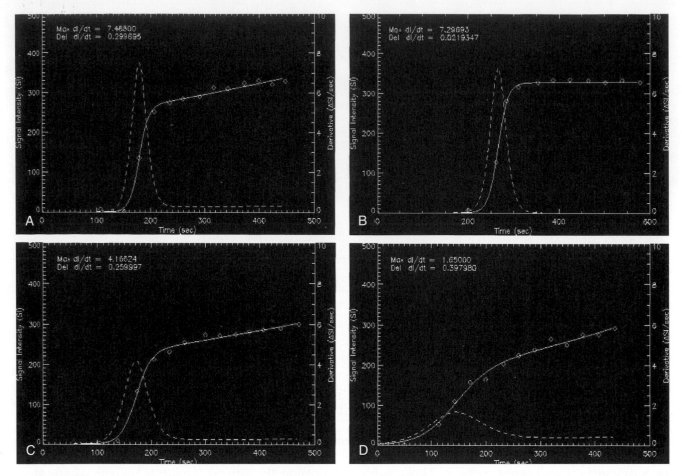

**FIGURE 12–50.** Dynamic MRI contrast agent uptake curves obtained from histopathologically proven cases of anaplastic astrocytoma (**A**), meningioma (**B**), metastatic lesion (**C**), and radiation necrosis (**D**). The solid lines are sigmoidal-exponential fits to the data, and the dashed lines are the first derivatives of the fitted curves. The peak of the derivative provides a quantitative measure of the maximal rate of contrast agent uptake. In general, faster uptake rates are observed in most high-grade lesions, and slower rates are observed in the setting of treatment-related changes.

niques and greatly enhances the assessment of lesion heterogeneity (Fig. 12–51; see color plate).

However, as with perfusion mapping studies, dynamic contrast MRI requires good temporal resolution, particularly when vascularity must be quantitated. Although some groups have used EPI for such studies, others have optimized the acquisition time of gradient-echo or fast spin-echo sequences.

### DIFFUSION-WEIGHTED PULSE SEQUENCES

If appropriate gradient pulses are added within the echo time of an EPI spin-echo sequence, image contrast is generated that depends heavily on the rate of diffusion of the nuclear spins.[57,63] In general, T2-weighted images are acquired with and without such diffusion-sensitizing gradient pulses. In the diffusion-sensitized images, tissues with freely diffusing spins are *hypo*intense relative to tissues with spins that have restricted motion. The contrast between the freely diffusing and restricted spins increases as the area of the diffusion-sensitizing gradient pulses increases, and this area is directly related to the often quoted "*b*-factor" value.[42,59,63] More specifically, the attenuation of the signal from a given tissue in diffusion-weighted images is proportional to $e^{-bD}$ where $b$ is the $b$-factor and $D$ is the diffusion coefficient. Therefore, for a given $b$-factor, the larger the diffusion coef-

ficient, the greater the signal loss that results from the application of the diffusion-sensitizing gradients. Similarly, for a given diffusion coefficient value, the signal attenuation resulting from the application of the diffusion-sensitizing gradients increases with the $b$-factor. Appropriate postprocessing of the images also allows the calculation of an "apparent diffusion coefficient" (ADC) image in which the pixel intensity is proportional to the diffusion coefficient.[42,59,63] In such ADC images, regions of freely diffusing spins are *hyper*intense relative to regions where diffusion is restricted. Furthermore, if the diffusion-sensitizing gradients are applied appropriately along the three orthogonal directions, anisotropic diffusion images can be generated in addition to an isotropic diffusion image that is obtained from the trace of the diffusion tensor.[49] There are advantages and disadvantages to both the isotropic and anisotropic diffusion images. For example, because water diffuses more freely along white-matter tracts than it does transverse to the tracts, the intensity of normal white matter in anisotropic ADC images depends on the direction of the applied diffusion-sensitizing gradients (Fig. 12–52). This could cause confusion in the characterization of a lesion if the directionality of the white-matter tracts is not fully appreciated. Therefore it is frequently useful to examine the isotropic diffusion-weighted or ADC images, in which the directional information is removed, rather than the anisotropic images. On the other hand, the anisotropic images may be useful for evaluating disease processes that disrupt the normal white-matter tracts, and subtle changes in the tracts may occur before a frank lesion is recognized.

Several clinical applications of diffusion-weighted imaging have been reported. Most often, diffusion-weighted imaging is used for detecting acute stroke and delineating the extent of tissue damage.[57,63] It has also been used for distinguishing tumor core from other components (e.g., cysts, necrosis, and edema) and for evaluating cysts containing high levels of paramagnetic proteins that would otherwise disguise their fluidlike nature and make them more difficult to distinguish from tumors.[57,63] In addition, diffusion-weighted imaging has been used for mapping temperature during hyperthermia induced by radiofrequency or laser applicators and for three-dimensional mapping of large white-matter tracts in the brain.[57,63]

Practically, high-quality diffusion-weighted images are difficult to obtain with many current MRI scanners because the motion caused by diffusion is quite small compared with gross motion and perfusion. Therefore diffusion-weighted images are highly susceptible to motion artifacts and typically require very stable gradient subsystems with EPI capabilities that allow the acquisition of diffusion data in times that "freeze" most other sources of physiologic motion. As more snapshot EPI-capable scanners are being installed in clinical sites, and with the recent approval by the U.S. Food and Drug Administration of several commercial diffusion imaging packages, applications of diffusion imaging should certainly expand.

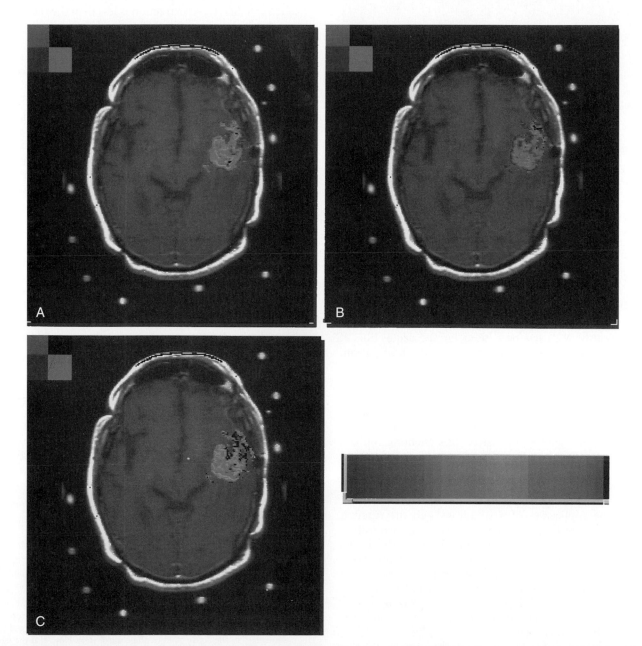

**FIGURE 12–51.** Parametric pharmacokinetic maps in which the pixel color is proportional to the relative degree of vascularity (**A**), permeability (**B**), and washout rate (**C**). Such studies have been useful in guiding stereotactic biopsies of patients who have multiple possible targets, particularly those who have undergone prior therapy. (See Color Plate.)

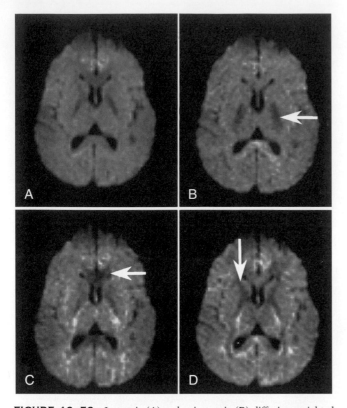

**FIGURE 12–52.** Isotropic (**A**) and anisotropic (**B**) diffusion-weighted images of normal human brain, with diffusion-sensitizing gradients applied in the superior-inferior (**B**), right-left (**C**), and anterior-posterior (**D**) directions. For all images, the *b*-value was 600 s/mm². The *arrows* indicate areas showing the expected directional dependence of the diffusion of water protons; that is, white matter tracts along the diffusion-sensitizing gradient become hypointense since diffusion along the tracts is less restricted than diffusion across the tracts.

## FUNCTIONAL MAGNETIC RESONANCE IMAGING PULSE SEQUENCES

Previously, MRI has been used for the acquisition of high-resolution anatomic, not functional, information. However, two techniques exist for acquiring functional MRI (fMRI) data. The underlying physiologic principle for both techniques is that the neural activation that occurs in response to a stimulus, such as a motor task, results in local vasodilation and a concomitant local increase in rCBV. The first fMRI technique to capitalize on this phenomenon was based on the infusion DSC mapping technique involving use of bolus contrast agent, as described earlier.[6] In this technique two bolus infusions are performed. The first bolus is infused during image acquisition in a control state, (i.e., without the application of a stimulus), and the rCBV is mapped in the resting condition. Following the acquisition of this control state data, a second bolus is infused while images are acquired during the application of a stimulus. Since the stimulus-induced neuronal activation produces a local vasodilation and a subsequent increase in rCBV, the DSC near the activated areas is increased relative to that occurring in the control state as a result of the increased local concentration of the contrast agent.

The advantage of bolus infusion techniques for fMRI is that they produce a significant change in the signal intensity between the control and activated states (typically approxi-

mately 30% at 1.5 T). The disadvantage, however, is that they require the infusion of a contrast agent, which limits the number of times fMRI maps can be acquired during a single session and how soon sessions can be repeated.

Contrast agent does not need to be infused in the second technique of performing fMRI studies, which is currently the most commonly used technique. This technique is known as *blood oxygen level dependent* (BOLD) contrast. It takes advantage of the fact that deoxyhemoglobin is a paramagnetic substance that causes increased local dephasing of the spins resulting from T2* (susceptibility) effects, whereas oxyhemoglobin is a diamagnetic substance that has minimal T2* effects. When neuronal activation occurs, local vasodilation leads to a local increase in the concentration of oxyhemoglobin compared with that in the control (resting) state. Positron emission tomography (PET) studies have shown that the rate of oxygen extraction is less than the rate of oxyhemoglobin delivery.[26] Therefore the deoxyhemoglobin-to-oxyhemoglobin ratio is decreased locally. This results in less T2* dephasing in areas near neuronal activation, and the areas of activation on T2*-weighted images are therefore hyperintense relative to their condition in the control state. Unfortunately, this change in signal intensity is relatively small (approximately 1% to 5% at 1.5 T and approximately 20% at 4 T).[59,63] However, the BOLD contrast phenomenon does provide a completely noninvasive means of indirectly mapping areas of activation by measuring the hemodynamic response changes secondary to the neuronal activation. With the BOLD technique, multiple stimulation paradigms can be applied in a single imaging session, and this method generally compensates for the lower percentage in the signal change than that yielded by the bolus infusion technique. Since reports of the first BOLD studies were published in 1992, there have been many reports of BOLD studies for widely varying applications, including studies of visual stimulation,[21,59,63] auditory stimulation,[13,21,25,59] memory,[18,27,51] language,[4,25,36] sensory and motor stimulation,[1,13,21,50,59,63] psychiatric disorders, and pain.[56] Typical signal intensity curves obtained during the control and activated states in a motor task are shown in Figure 12–53. Examples of BOLD

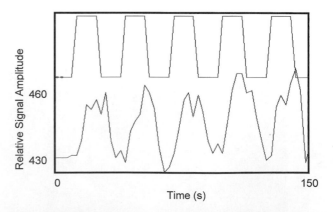

**FIGURE 12–53.** BOLD functional MRI signal intensity curve obtained from a region of interest in the motor strip (bottom tracing). The top tracing is the known stimulus timing. Note the small percentage change in the signal intensity in the active state vs. the control state. Note also the latent period between the applied stimulus and the signal change resulting from the fact that BOLD mapping techniques measure the hemodynamic response as opposed to the actual neuronal activation.

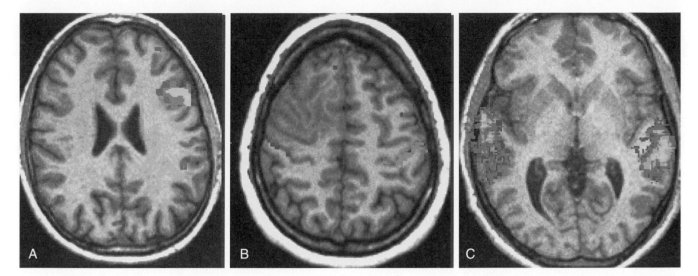

**FIGURE 12–54.** BOLD fMRI activation maps obtained by cross-correlation of the known stimulus pattern with the signal intensity curve on a pixel-by-pixel basis. **A,** Expressive speech task. **B,** Bilateral hand mapping, with *blue* corresponding to a left-hand task and *yellow* corresponding to a right-hand task. **C,** Auditory stimulation. (See Color Plate.)

fMRI activation maps for language, motor, and auditory tasks are shown in Figure 12–54 (see color plate).

Regardless of the technique used to acquire the fMRI data, the demands on the MRI scanner are extreme in terms of the required acquisition rates, with the studies typically performed with single-shot EPI sequences.

## SUMMARY

In the workup of the patient with a suspected intracranial mass, the neurologist must choose the appropriate imaging examination to visualize any intracranial abnormality. In most cases, MRI is the study of choice. However, CT has advantages in certain circumstances.

It is important to know the lesion location because this information improves the accuracy of the diagnosis. However, since the brain can react to an intracranial lesion in only a limited number of ways, many lesions have a similar appearance. To avoid potential pitfalls in diagnosis, cases have been selected to show the variances in appearance and presentation.

New imaging techniques that have led to improvements in diagnostic accuracy and surgical management have also been described. These include dynamic scanning, perfusion and diffusion imaging, and functional imaging, which demonstrates the neuronal activation that occurs in response to an external stimulus, such as motor tasks, visual stimulation, auditory stimulation, memory, language, pain, and psychologic disorders.

## ACKNOWLEDGMENTS

The authors wish to thank Danisha L. Branch, Senior Secretary, Division of Diagnostic Radiology, M.D. Anderson Cancer Center, for her tireless and adept proficiency in the support, preparation, and coordination of this manuscript.

## REFERENCES

1. Aronen HJ, Gazit IE, Louis DN, et al. Cerebral blood volume maps of gliomas: comparison with tumor grade and histologic findings. *Radiology.* 1994;191:41-51.
2. Atlas SW. Intraaxial brain tumors. In: Atlas SW, ed. *Magnetic Resonance Imaging of the Brain and Spine.* New York: Raven Press; 1991:223-326.
3. Atlas S, Grossman RI, Gomori JM, et al. Hemorrhagic intracranial malignant neoplasms: spin echo MRI imaging. *Radiology.* 1987;164:71-77.
4. Atlas SW, Howard RSI, Maldjian J, et al. Functional magnetic resonance imaging of regional brain activity in patients with intracerebral gliomas: findings and implications for clinical management. *Neurosurgery.* 1996;38:329-338.
5. Barkovich AJ, Kjos BO. Grey matter heterotopias: MRI characteristics and correlation with developmental and neurologic manifestations. *Radiology.* 1992;182:493-499.
6. Belliveau JW, Kennedy DN, McKinstry RC, et al. Functional mapping of the human cortex by magnetic resonance imaging. *Science.* 1991;254:716-719.
7. Boyko OB. Neuroimaging of radiation injury to the central nervous system. *Neuroimaging Clin North Am.* 1993;3:803-815.
8. Braun IF, Chambers B, Leeds NE, et al. The value of unenhanced scans in differentiating lesions producing ring enhancement. *AJNR.* 1982;3:643-647.
9. Bryan RN, Levy LM, Whitlow WD. Diagnosis of acute cerebral infarction: comparison of CT and MRI imaging. *AJNR.* 1991;12:611-620.
10. Burger PC, Boyko OB. The pathology of central nervous system radiation injury. In: Gutin PH, Liebel SA, Sheline GF, eds. *Radiation Injury to the Nervous System.* New York: Raven Press; 1991:191-208.
11. Burger PC, Scheithauer VB, Vogel FS, eds. *Surgical Pathology of the Nervous System and Its Covering.* New York: Churchill Livingstone; 1991:336-338.
12. Burke JW, Podrasky AE, Bradley WG Jr. Meninges: benign post-operative enhancement on MRI images. *Radiology.* 1990;174:99-102.
13. Calvert GA, Bullmore ET, Brammer MJ, et al. Activation of auditory cortex during silent lipreading. *Science.* 1997;276:593-596.
14. Chan S, Erickson JK, Yoon SS. Limbic system abnormalities associated with mesial/temporal sclerosis: model of chronic cerebral changes due to seizures. *Radiographics.* 1997;17:1095-1110.
15. Chang KH, Han MH, Roh JK, et al. Gd-DTPA–enhanced MRI imaging of the brain in patients with meningitis comparison with CT. *AJNR.* 1990;11:69-76.
16. Crain MR, Yuh WTC, Greene GM. Cerebral ischemia: evaluation with contrast-enhanced MRI imaging. *AJNR.* 1991;12:631-639.
17. Curnes JT, Laster DN, Ball MR, et al. MRI of radiation injury to the brain. *AJNR.* 1986;7:389-394.
18. D'Esposito M, Detre JA, Alsop DC, et al. The neural basis of the central executive system of working memory. *Nature.* 1995;378:279-281.
19. Destian S, Heier LA, Zimmerman RA, et al. Differentiation between meningeal fibrosis and chronic subdural hematoma after ventricular shunting: value of enhanced CT and MRI scans. *AJNR.* 1989;10:1021-1026.
20. Destian S, Sze G, Krol G, et al. MRI imaging of hemorrhagic intracranial neoplasms. *AJNR.* 1988;9:1115-1122.

21. DeYoe EA, Bandettini P, Neitz J, et al. Functional magnetic resonance imaging (FMRI) of the human brain. *J Neurosci Methods.* 1994;54:171-187.

22. Edelman RR, Siewert B, Darby DG, et al. Qualitative mapping of cerebral blood flow and functional localization with echo-planar MRI imaging and signal targeting with alternating radio frequency. *Radiology.* 1994;192:513-520.

23. Elster AD, DiPiersio DA. Cranial post-operative site: assessment with contrast-enhanced MRI imaging. *Radiology.* 1990;174:93-98.

24. Elster AD, Moody DM. Early cerebral infarction: gadopentetate dimeglumine enhancement. *Radiology.* 1990;177:627-632.

25. FitzGerald DB, Cosgrove GR, Ronner S, et al. Location of language in the cortex: a comparison between functional MRI imaging and electrocortical stimulation. *AJNR.* 1997;18:1529-1539.

26. Fox P, Raichle M. Focal physiological uncoupling of cerebral blood flow and oxidative metabolism during somatosensory stimulation in human subjects. *Proc Natl Acad Sci U S A.* 1986;83:1140-1144.

27. Gabrieli JDE, Brewer JB, Desmond JE, Glover GH. Separate neural bases of two fundamental memory processes in the human medial temporal lobe. *Science.* 1998;276:264-266.

28. Glass JP, Melameed M, Chernik NL, Posner JB. Malignant cells in cerebrospinal fluid (CSF): the meaning of a positive cytology. *Neurology.* 1979;29:1369-1375.

29. Goldberg, HI. Extraaxial brain tumors. In: Atlas, SW. *Magnetic Resonance Imaging of the Brain and Spine.* New York: Raven Press; 1991:327-378.

30. Goldsher D, Litt AW, Pinto RS, et al. Dural "tail" associated with meningiomas on Gd-DTPA–enhanced MRI images: characteristics, differential diagnostic value, and possible implications for treatment. *Radiology.* 1990;176:447-450.

31. Gomori JM, Grossman RI. Mechanisms responsible for the MRI appearance and evolution of intracranial hemorrhage. *Radiographics.* 1988;8:427-440.

32. Haimes AB, Zimmerman RD, Morgello S, et al. MRI images of brain abscesses. *AJNR.* 1989;10:279-291.

33. Hazle JD, Jackson EF, Schomer DF, Leeds NE. Dynamic imaging of intracranial lesions using fast spin-echo imaging: differentiation of brain tumors and treatment effects. *J Magn Reson Imaging.* 1997;7:1084-1093.

34. Heinz ER, Crain BJ, Radtke RA, et al. MRI imaging in patients with temporal lobe seizures: correlation of results with pathologic findings. *AJNR.* 1990;11:827-832.

35. Henkelman RW, Watts JF, Kurcharczyk W. High-signal intensity in MRI images of calcified brain tissue. *Radiology.* 1991;179:199-200.

36. Hertz-Pannier L, Gaillard WD, Mott SH, et al. Noninvasive assessment of language dominance in children and adolescents with functional MRI: a preliminary study. *Neurology.* 1997;48:1003-1012.

37. Jack CR Jr, Rydberg CH, Krecke KN, et al. Mesial temporal sclerosis: diagnosis with fluid-attenuated inversion-recovery versus spin-echo MR imaging. *Radiology.* 1996;367-373.

38. Kondziolka D, Bernstein M, Resch L, et al. Significance of hemorrhage into brain tumors: clinicopathological study. *J Neurosurg.* 1987;67:852-857.

39. Kucharczyk W, Montanera WJ. The sella and parasellar region. In: Atlas, SW. *Magnetic Resonance Imaging of the Brain and Spine.* New York: Raven Press; 1991:625-667.

40. Kyritisis AP, Levin VA, Yung WKA, Leeds NE. Imaging patterns of multifocal gliomas. *Eur J Radiol.* 1993;16:163-170.

41. Lassen NA. The luxury perfusion syndrome and its possible relation to acute metabolic acidosis localized within the brain. *Lancet.* 1966;2:1113-1115.

42. Le Bihan D, Turner R, Douek P, Patronas N. Diffusion MRI imaging: clinical applications. *AJR.* 1992;159:591-599.

43. Lee AWM, Cheng OC, Ng SH, et al. Magnetic resonance imaging in the clinical diagnosis of late temporal lobe necrosis following radiotherapy for nasopharyngeal cancer. *Clin Radiol.* 1990;42:24-31.

44. Lee YY, Tien RD, Bruner JW. Loculated intracranial leptomeningeal metastases: CT and MRI characteristics. *AJNR.* 1989;10:1171-1179.

45. Leeds NE, Kumar AJ, Fuller FN, Jackson EF. MR findings of radiation damage to the brain with histopathologic correlation. Scientific exhibit presented at the American Society of Neuroradiology Meeting; April 23-27, 1995; Chicago.

46. Leeds NE, Kumar AJ, Fuller GN, et al. Spread of malignant gliomas. Scientific exhibit presented at the 83rd Radiological Society of North America Scientific Meeting; Nov. 30-Dec. 5, 1997; Chicago.

47. Leeds NE, Sawaya R, Van Tassel P, Hayman LA. Intracranial hemorrhage in the oncologic patient. *Neuroimaging Clin North Am.* 1992;2:119-136.

48. Loevner LA, Grossman RI, McGowan JC, et al. Characterization of multiple sclerosis plaques with T1-wtd, MR and quantitative magnetization transfer. *AJNR.* 1995;16:1473–1479.

49. Moseley ME, Cohen Y, Kucharczyk J, et al. Diffusion-weighted MR imaging of anisotropic water diffusion in cat central nervous system. *Radiology.* 1990;176:439-445.

50. Mueller WM, Yetkin FZ, Hammeke TA, et al. Functional magnetic resonance imaging mapping of the motor cortex in patients with cerebral tumors. *Neurosurgery.* 1996;39:515-521.

51. Ojemann JG, Buckner RL, Corbetta M, Raichle ME. Imaging studies of memory and attention. *Neurosurg Clin North Am.* 1997;8:307-319.

52. Olson ME, Chernik NL, Posner JB. Infiltration of the leptomeninges by systemic cancer: a clinical and pathologic study. *Arch Neurol.* 1974;30:122-137.

53. Osborn AG. Infections of the brain and its linings. In: Osborn AG, ed. *Diagnostic Neuroradiology: A Text/Atlas.* St. Louis: Mosby; 1994:673-715.

54. Osborn AG. Intracranial aneurysm/intracranial vascular malformations. In: Osborn AG, ed. *Diagnostic Neuroradiology: A Text/Atlas.* St. Louis: Mosby; 1994:248-329.

55. Phillips ME, Ryals TJ, Kambhu SA, Yuh WTC. Neoplastic vs. inflammatory meningeal enhancement with Gd-DTPA. *J Comput Assist Tomogr.* 1990;14:536-541.

56. Rainville P, Duncan GH, Price DD, et al. Pain affect encoded in human anterior cingulate but not somatosensory cortex. *Science.* 1997;277:968-971.

57. Rosen BR, Aronen HJ, Cohen MS, et al. Diffusion and perfusion fast scanning in brain tumors. *Neuroimaging Clin North Am.* 1993;3:631-648.

58. Russell EJ, George A, Kricheff E II. Atypical computed tomographic features of intracranial meningioma. *Radiology.* 1980;136:673-682.

59. Sanders JA, Orrison WWJ. Functional magnetic resonance imaging. In: Orrison WWJ, Lewine JD, Sanders JA, Hartshorne MF, eds. *Functional Brain Imaging.* St. Louis: Mosby; 1995:239-326.

60. Sawaya R. The fibrinolytic enzymes in the biology of brain tumors. In: Sawaya R, ed. *Fibrinolysis and the Central Nervous System.* Philadelphia: Hanley & Belfus; 1990:106-126.

61. Sawaya R, Ramo J, Glas-Greenwalt P, Wu FZ. Plasma fibrinolytic profile in patients with brain tumors. *Thromb Haemost.* 1991;65:15-19.

62. Scherer HJ. Structural development in gliomas. *Am J Cancer.* 1938;34:333-351.

63. Sorenson AG, Rosen BR. Functional MRI of the brain. In: Atlas SW, ed. *Magnetic Resonance Imaging of the Brain and Spine.* Philadelphia: Lippincott-Raven; 1996:1501-1545.

64. Spagnoli MV, Grossman RI, Packer RJ, et al. Magnetic resonance imaging determination of gliomatosis cerebri. *Neuroradiology.* 1987;29:15-18.

65. Su M-Y, Najafi AA, Nalcioglu O. Regional comparison of tumor vascularity and permeability parameters measured by albumin-Gd-DTPA and Gd-DTPA. *Magn Reson Med.* 1995;34:402-411.

66. Sze G, Soletsky S, Bronen R, Krol G. MRI imaging of the cranial meninges with emphasis on contrast enhancement and meningeal carcinomatosis. *AJNR.* 1989;10:965-975.

67. Tice H, Barnes PD, Goumnerova L, Scott RM, Tarbell NJ. Pediatric and adolescent oligodendrogliomas. *AJNR.* 1993;14:1293-1300.

68. Tien RD, Yang PJ, Chu PK. "Dural tail sign": a specific MRI sign for meningioma? *J Comput Assist Tomogr.* 1991;15:64-66.

69. Tokumaru A, Toshihiro O, Tsuneyoshi E, et al. Prominent meningeal enhancement adjacent to meningioma on Gd-DPTA–enhanced MRI images: histopathologic correlation. *Radiology.* 1990;175:431-433.

70. Ts'ao C, Ward WF. Acute radiation effects on the content and release of plasminogen activator activity in cultured aortic endothelial cells. *Radiat Res.* 1985;101:394-401.

71. Tsuruda JS, Kortman KE, Bradley WG Jr, et al. Radiation effects on cerebral white matter, MRI evaluation. *AJR.* 1987;149:165-171.

72. Valk PE, Dillon WP. Radiation injury of the brain. *AJNR.* 1991;12:45-62.

73. VanTassel P, Bruner JM, Maor MH, Leeds NE, et al. MRI of toxic effects of accelerated fractionation radiation therapy and carboplatin chemotherapy for malignant gliomas. *AJNR.* 1995;16:715-726.

74. VanTassel P, Lee YY, Bruner JM. Synchronous and metachronous malignant gliomas: CT findings. *AJNR.* 1988;9:725-732.

75. Vexler V, Clement O, Schmitt-Willich H, Brasch R. Effect of varying the molecular weight of the MRI contrast agent Gd-DTPA-polysine on blood pharmacokinetics and enhancement patterns. *J Magn Reson Imaging.* 1994;4:381-388.

76. Wasserstrom WR, Glass JP, Posner JB. Diagnosis and treatment of leptomeningeal metastases from solid tumors. experience with 90 patients. *Cancer.* 1982;49:759-772.

77. Wilms G, Lammens M, Marchal G, et al. Thickening of dura surrounding meningiomas: MRI features. *J Comput Assist Tomogr.* 1989;13:763-769.

78. Wilms G, Lammens M, Marchal G, et al. Prominent dural enhancement adjacent to non-meningiomatous malignant lesion on contrast-enhanced MRI images. *AJNR.* 1991;12:761-764.

79. Wilson DA, Nitschke R, Bowman ME, et al. Transient white matter changes on MRI images in children undergoing chemotherapy for acute lymphocytic leukemia: correlation with neuropsychologic deficiencies. *Radiology.* 1991;180:205-209.

80. Wong ET, Jackson EF, Hess K, et al. Correlations between dynamic MRI and outcome in patients with malignant glioma. *Neurology.* 1998;50: 777-781.

81. Yuh WTC, Crain MR, Loes DJ, et al. MRI imaging of cerebral ischemia findings in the first 24 hours. *AJNR.* 1991;12:621-629.

# 13

# Gait Disorders

*Joseph C. Masdeu*

There exists a large group of cases where the gait in old people becomes considerably disordered, although the motor power of the legs is comparatively well preserved. A paradoxical state of affairs is the result: testing of the individual movements of the legs while the patient reclines upon the couch shows little, if any, reduction in the strength. The tonus may not be grossly altered and the reflexes may betray only minor deviations. Sensory tests show no unusual features. But when the patient is instructed to get out of bed and to walk, remarkable defects may be witnessed. The patient, first of all, appears most reluctant to make the attempt. His stance is bowed and uncertain. He props himself against the end of the bed and seeks the aid of the bystanders. Encouraged to take a few steps, he advances warily and hesitatingly. Clutching the arms of two supporters, he takes short, shuffling steps. The legs tend to crumble by giving way suddenly at the knee joints. Progression, as far as it is possible, is slow and tottery. The patient veers to one side or the other. Frequently the legs cross, so that one foot gets in the way of the other.

*McDonald Critchley*[29]

Diagnostic testing for gait disorders presupposes an understanding of the clinical presentation. Tools should be used that can clarify the diagnosis, not confuse the diagnostician. Because gait disorders abound in old age, age-related changes in diagnostic tests can be mistakenly taken to explain the disorder. A frequent clinical picture, described masterfully in the quote by Critchley that introduces this chapter, presents to many physicians "a paradoxical state of affairs." Thus this chapter contains an introduction on the classification and clinical diagnosis of gait disorders, which should be read before the review of diagnostic methods.

*Stance, equilibrium,* and *balance* are terms that refer to the ability or act of maintaining an erect posture. Gait, or ambulation, presupposes the ability to stand, although the neural mechanisms underlying these two motor functions are far from identical. Surprisingly, some patients experience more difficulty standing than walking, for instance, those with orthostatic tremor.[24] The emphasis of this chapter is not on the diagnosis of neurologic disorders that secondarily result in ambulation difficulties (e.g., stroke causing hemiplegia) but on disorders that primarily affect the ability to stand or walk, often without overt weakness. Disorders of stance and gait can be the presenting syndrome of many different pathologic conditions along the neuraxis. Clinical localization prior to the use of ancillary diagnostic testing is essential if ancillary procedures are to be applied in a focused and economical manner that will minimize the likelihood of false-positive findings.[96]

During the diagnosis of gait disorders, it is useful to think about the neurologic systems underlying the control of gait and balance.[105,108] At the simplest level, gait requires sensory information and a motor output. Sensory information includes proprioception, vision, and vestibular input. On the motor side, the corticospinal, vestibulospinal, and reticulospinal tracts convey to the cord output from higher centers. In turn, the anterior horn cells, through their axons, stimulate muscles, which transform that output into specific movements.

Sensory systems can be tested by exploring the performance of the patient while one or two varieties of sensory input are removed and the functions of gait or balance depend on the remaining sensory information. For instance, Romberg's test explores the patient's ability to maintain a steady, upright posture when vision is removed and the base of support is reduced (i.e., patient must keep feet together). Proprioceptive or vestibular loss will result in difficulty maintaining balance. To test the intactness of the corticospinal tract, spinal cord, peripheral nerves, and muscles, the examiner asks the patient to wiggle the toes, draw a circle on the floor with each foot, and extend the big toe against resistance. Proximal muscle strength in the legs can be tested by asking the patient to rise from a low chair without using the arms for support. Despite the patient's ability to perform all these tasks well, he or she may still have difficulty walking and have a propensity to falling. This apparent discrepancy highlights the importance of neural systems that are critical for gait but are distinct from the system mediating volitional leg and foot movements.[105] In addition to vestibular and cerebellar input, the basal ganglia and several brainstem nuclei, including the pedunculopontine nucleus, play an important role in the control of postural and locomotor activity. Normally, this activity is unconscious, carried out, for instance, while the person concentrates his or her attention on getting something from the refrigerator rather than on the activity of walking itself.

## PEDIATRIC GAIT DISORDERS

Developmental gait delay and gait disorders of childhood represent an important part of the diagnostic work of pediatricians and pediatric neurologists. The vast differential diagnosis of these disorders is outside the scope of this chapter, which focuses on gait disorders of the adult, particularly of the older adult.

## GAIT DISORDERS IN THE YOUNGER ADULT

In the younger adult, gait disorders are commonly related to specific neurologic or neuromuscular disorders. Some of these disorders primarily affect a functional system, for example, motor strength impaired by myasthenia gravis. Others involve multiple motor and sensory systems, such as Guillain-Barré syndrome, which affects motor pathways and fibers conveying proprioceptive information. The patient with multiple sclerosis can have an assortment of proprioceptive loss, cerebellovestibular dysfunction, visual impairment, faulty basal-ganglionic feedback, and corticospinal tract damage. Thus a gait disorder in the young adult is likely to be related to a single disease process. Therefore a review of diagnostic testing of gait disorders in the young adult closely follows a review of diagnostic testing in neurologic diseases. The examiner confronted with a young adult who has a gait disorder is likely to see someone with hemiparesis, paraparesis, limb weakness, a sensory disorder, or cerebellar incoordination syndrome. Many of these disorders are reviewed in other chapters of this book. The reader is referred to the chapters on cerebrovascular disorders (Chapter 5), multiple sclerosis (Chapter 6), hydrocephalus (Chapter 7), neuroimaging of brain tumors (Chapter 12), neurotoxicology (Chapter 17), infectious disorders (Chapter 18), peripheral nerve disease (Chapter 19), neuromuscular disorders (Chapter 21) and rheumatologic disorders (Chapter 27).

## GAIT DISORDERS IN THE OLDER ADULT

### EPIDEMIOLOGY

Stance and gait disorders are particularly common in the elderly population. The Duke Study of Normal Aging estimated that gait disturbances affect 15% of the elderly, being the most common neurologic impairment in this age group.[112] Among the elderly, falls are the leading source of injury-related deaths.[11] In the United States, approximately 9500 deaths among persons age 65 years or older annually are attributed to a falling episode. Falling is also a major cause of morbidity among older individuals. Eighty-four percent of the approximately 200,000 hip fractures that occur yearly affect people older than 65. Most of these cases are related to a fall. Hip fracture is the most common injury leading to hospitalization in this age group.[60]

### Falls

Gait and balance impairment result in falls. Falls are very common in the older population.[110] Cross-sectional surveys of communities in Western societies find that from one quarter to one third of persons aged 65 and older report a fall in the previous year. From one third to one half of elderly persons who report falling in the previous year have fallen two or more times. The rate of falls is higher in women than in men and increases with age, rising from about 30 to 50 falls per 100 person-years at ages 65 to 74 to about 60 to 90 falls per 100 person-years in those 75 and older.[110]

### Consequences of Falls

Falls frequently cause physical injuries and are usually followed by a restriction of activities, which may precipitate another fall. Thus a vicious circle is created in which the curtailment of mobility results in further deconditioning, so that the individual becomes more prone to falling.

*Injuries Caused by Falls.* Between 10% and 15% of falls in the elderly result in a serious injury.[110] Approximately 5% to 10% of falls in the elderly result in a fracture (involving the hip in 1% to 2% of total falls), and about 5% of falls cause other serious injuries, requiring medical care or causing disability. In a Florida study, the fall injury rate in women age 75 and older was approximately 120 per 1000 per year; and in men of that age, about 85 per 1000 per year.[139] More than 40% of these subjects were hospitalized, with an average length of stay of 12 days. Other serious injuries resulting from falls include hematoma, head injury with loss of consciousness, dislocation and other severe joint injury, severe laceration, sprain, and disabling soft tissue injury. Injuries to the head comprise a substantial proportion of serious nonfracture injuries.[110] Most falls, however, do not cause sufficient injury to require medical attention.

*Disability Resulting From Falls.* The psychologic and functional consequences of falls can be substantial, whether or not an injury occurs.[110] The inability to get up and a "long lie" after a fall may lead to serious physical complications, including pneumonia and hypothermia. Even in the absence of physical morbidity, a long lie may result in reduced self-confidence, feelings of helplessness, and loss of function. About one quarter of falls in the community result in an immediate activity limitation related to injury or fear of falling.[110] Falls are responsible for 1 in 5 of all days of restricted activity in the elderly, a higher proportion than for any other health condition.[80] In 1986 most of the 58.9 million days of restricted activity and the 18.8 million bed days among the elderly related to all forms of injury were due to falls.[109] The functional consequences of hip fracture are devastating: 20% to 30% of previously community-dwelling patients with hip fracture remain in long-term care 1 year after the injury.[121] Of elderly living at home who are hospitalized for a fall injury other than a hip fracture, nearly 40% die or are discharged to a nursing facility.[110]

### ETIOLOGY

Unlike in younger adults, gait impairment in older individuals seldom results from a single etiologic basis. Most often, partial impairment of multiple systems is responsible for the impaired balance and gait witnessed by the clinician. In about one fourth of the cases, however, one of the factors contributing to gait impairment can be corrected enough to reverse the disability. The task of the clinician is to identify the causes contributing to gait impairment and identify the correctable ones. Still, a large number of elderly patients have idiopathic gait impairment: the identifiable causes do not satisfactorily explain why an individual patient has a tendency to fall.

The multifactorial genesis of gait and balance impairment in the older adult cannot be overemphasized. Studies of falls have illustrated that individuals who fall typically have more than one risk factor for falling.[130] Robbins et al[127] found that the predicted 1-year risk of falling ranged from 12% for persons with none of three risk factors (i.e., hip weakness assessed manually, unstable balance, and taking four or more prescribed medications) to 100% for persons with all three risk factors. It is also likely that older persons with vestibular dysfunction alone will not experience gait difficulties, but the rule is that proprioception and vision will also be impaired to some extent. As a result, the vestibular dysfunction becomes symptomatic. Impairment of central processing is added to sensory deficits in many older adults. Cortical-basal-ganglionic-thalamic-cortical mechanisms can be affected by a loss of dopaminergic neurons or neurons belonging to other systems, by fiber damage caused by chronic ischemia in the white-matter watershed, lateral to the ventricular angles, or by other mechanisms still poorly understood.

Emphasis on one or another etiologic factor as being mainly responsible for gait impairment has changed throughout the history of neurology in parallel with a growing understanding of brain disorders. For instance, in a monograph on "senile paraplegia" published in 1907, Lhermitte attributed to lacunar disease the kind of gait impairment described by Critchley in the introductory quotation to this chapter. Extensive autopsy experience had given the neurologists of the time a sense that vascular disease was often present in patients with gait impairment. When Adams et al[2] described "normopressure hydrocephalus" in 1965, the attention of neurologists turned to this etiologic factor, which is eminently treatable but much rarer than thought in the late 1960s. In the 1960s and 1970s the characterization of Parkinson's disease turned the attention of neurologists to dopaminergic dysfunction as an explanation of gait disorders of the elderly. In the mid 1980s, the term *lower-body parkinsonism* was coined to highlight the slowness and clumsiness of lower extremity function that many elderly patients have while walking, although their isometric strength is normal.[41,151] Unlike patients with parkinsonism, however, they generally move their feet accurately when performing a volitional activity, such as drawing a circle on the floor, and they do not improve by taking dopaminergic agents.[99] Some of these patients have vascular disease of the brain.[41,151] This brief historical account illustrates a common phenomenon in medicine. It highlights the fact that many gait disorders remain poorly understood and therefore the current diagnostic algorithm is both incomplete and tentative.

In some published series the majority of patients were assigned a primary cause for their gait disorder.[145,146] Other authors failed to find a cause in the majority of patients.[1] This discrepancy may reflect (1) different patient populations: a single diagnosis may be more readily identifiable in a general medical or neurologic practice, whereas in gait-disorders clinics the proportion of idiopathic gait disorders is larger, possibly because patients with Parkinson's disease and other readily identifiable disorders are not referred to specialized centers for evaluation; (2) a different diagnostic approach: sensory deficits, for instance, are very prevalent in the elderly with or without gait disorders; when some clinicians discover a sensory deficit, they may consider it responsible for the gait disorder, whereas others may decide that a different etiologic complex must be at work to explain the clinical picture. Whether a given etiologic factor is the main source of the patient's gait difficulties is often not the key question. Instead, whether a correctable cause can be found and addressed is the real issue. Even a modest functional improvement can forestall the dismal consequences of repeated falls.

In a series of 120 older adults referred to a neurologist for an undiagnosed gait disorder, Sudarsky[145] reported the frequency of each etiologic factor (Fig. 13–1). Sensory deficits represented the largest single neurologic cause of gait instability. As etiologic factors, myelopathy and multiple infarcts accounted for half of the cases. In 14% of the cases the etiologic factor remained undetermined. The rest fell under the categories of parkinsonism, cerebellar degeneration, hydrocephalus, an assortment of other causes (including neoplasms and subdural hematoma), psychogenic gait disorders, and toxic or metabolic causes (see Fig. 13–1). In 50 consecutive patients older than 50 who were admitted to a neurologic service because of walking difficulty, Fuh et al[43] identified the following causes: multiple cerebral infarcts, 24%; myelopathy, 22%; parkinsonism, 12%; cerebellar degeneration, 8%; brain tumor, 6%; Binswanger's disease, 4%; Alzheimer's disease, 4%; other diseases, 10%; and unknown etiology, 10%. The miscellaneous category included a patient with chronic inflammatory demyelinating polyneuropathy. Patients with undetermined gait disorder were older than 60 and had "senile gait." Potentially treatable causes of gait impairment were found in nearly one third of patients.

The following section lists anatomically the major etiologic categories responsible for gait impairment. The causes are listed from the more peripheral ones, including muscle weakness, to the primary ones, affecting the control centers of the brain.

## Muscle Weakness

Many older adults with gait difficulties blame their problem on muscle weakness. With age, both muscle mass and strength decrease, even in normal individuals. Muscle mass is lost at a rate of 0.5% to 1% annually in women and men over 60 years; muscle strength loss ranges from 20% to 40% from the third to the eighth decades and may be even higher in the eighth decade.[74] Weakness is due to loss of muscle mass and contractility (force/cm$^2$ of muscle cross section). The good news is that vigorous physical activity is associated with maintaining muscle strength, mass, and contractility.[74]

Diseases of muscle or the neuromuscular junction are rarely responsible for gait impairment in the older adult. Polymyalgia rheumatica may cause muscle claudication but more often causes pain, affects the jaw muscles, and gives rise to the headaches characteristic of temporal arteritis. Palpation of poorly pulsatile, swollen temporal arteries helps to determine the diagnosis. An elevated erythrocyte sedimentation rate is present in the majority of the cases, and a biopsy of the temporal artery may show giant cell infiltration of the media of the vessel, with destruction of the elastic membrane. Polymyositis can give rise to proximal weakness. In such a case isometric weakness would be more pronounced than the gait impairment, alerting the clinician to the possi-

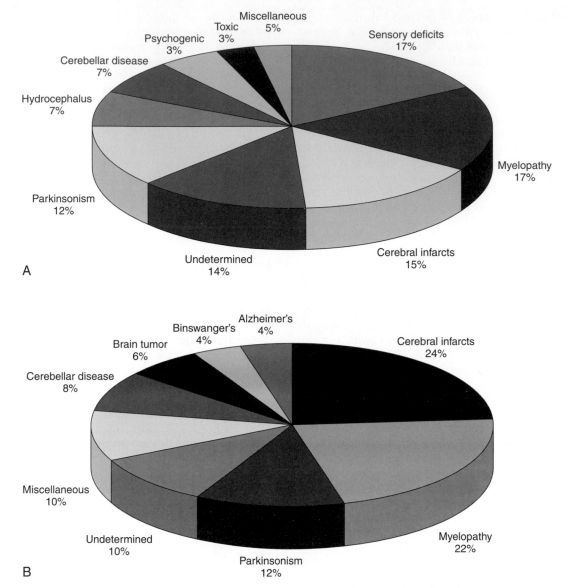

**FIGURE 13–1.** Distribution of main etiologic categories in two groups of patients referred to a neurologist for undiagnosed gait disorder. **A,** N = 120 patients.[145] **B,** N = 50 patients.[43] Note similarity and discrepancies of the two series. Diagnostic criteria, particularly for patients who do not have stroke, myelopathy, or cerebellar degeneration, is responsible for some of the differences. Series **A** more often contains diagnosis of sensory deficits. Of miscellaneous diagnoses in series **B,** only two patients with polyneuropathy (4%) would fit under *sensory deficits* category.

bility of muscle disease. Diagnostic testing for this disorder, and for myasthenia gravis and the Lambert-Eaton syndrome, is discussed in Chapters 21 and 27.

## Sensory Deficits

Sensory deficits ranked first as the etiologic factor in some series of unselected patients referred for gait impairment.[145] Although proprioception, vestibular function, and vision are all often affected, there are specific disorders that involve one modality more than the other two. To clarify testing for sensory function crucial for gait, it is important to review briefly the physiologic basis of sensory postural control. Proprioception, vestibular function, and vision are all required because no single sense can directly measure the center of gravity of the body to place it within the base of support, a condition of stability in bipedal stance and gait.[108] The somatosensory input provides information on the ori-

entation of body parts relative to one another and to the support surface. Vision measures the orientation of the eyes and head in relation to surrounding objects. The vestibular system measures gravitational, linear, and angular accelerations of the head in relation to inertial space. As the person stands or walks, the brain must quickly select the appropriate sensory inputs to provide accurate information. Often, one or more of the three sensory systems may provide information that is misleading for the purpose of balance control. For instance, when a person stands beside a large bus that begins to move slowly, the visual system conveys the false impression that the person is moving in the opposite direction. Nashner[108] has called *sensory organization* the process of selecting and combining sensory information appropriate for balance control. Faulty sensory organization, or one that relies primarily on an impaired sensory system, may lead to unsteadiness in walking. Although some simple clinical maneuvers, such as Romberg's test, can help to identify gross deficiencies in one sensory modality, specialized testing with posturography may be needed to evidence subtler changes.

***Proprioception.*** Somatosensory input dominates the control of balance when the support surface is steady. Even with vision removed, a patient with bilateral vestibular loss but good proprioception can stand normally.[108] Several disorders that can affect primarily proprioception will be reviewed in turn. Many other disorders can affect proprioception in the older adult, including toxic neuropathies induced by cisplatin or nitrous oxide. A more extensive treatment of peripheral nerve diseases is presented in Chapter 19.

### Vitamin-Induced Neuronopathies

VITAMIN B$_{12}$ DEFICIENCY. Pernicious anemia, involving deficient production of intrinsic factor, is the most common cause of vitamin B$_{12}$ deficiency, with many cases occurring in older people.[134] Vitamin B$_{12}$ deficiency is also observed as a result of chronic intestinal malabsorption and, rarely, dietary deficiency. The daily requirement for vitamin B$_{12}$ is only 5 µg/d. Neuropathy and myelopathy (subacute combined systems degeneration) can occur without hematologic manifestations.

The onset of vitamin B$_{12}$ deficiency is insidious, beginning with distal paresthesias, weakness, and unsteadiness of gait (particularly difficulty walking in the dark). Proprioceptive loss in the legs and sensory ataxia can become severe. Lhermitte's sign is often present, reflecting damage of the dorsal columns. Tendon reflexes are typically depressed to absent. An extensor plantar response is characteristically observed, and, with time, a spastic-ataxic gait is also noted.

Vitamin B$_{12}$ assay is used for screening. A Schilling test is done for confirmation of true addisonian pernicious anemia. This disorder is important to recognize because it is occasionally encountered in the elderly and is a treatable cause of imbalance and gait disorder. Gait improves fully in a majority of patients when neurologic signs last less than 3 months.[134]

MEGADOSE PYRIDOXINE NEUROPATHY. Chronic ingestion of megadoses of pyridoxine (2 to 6 g/d) has also been associated with an ataxic peripheral neuropathy.[134] Both proximal and distal parts of the body are simultaneously affected by sensory loss of the large fiber modalities. The other major clinical features are ataxia and pseudoathetosis without severe weakness. Sensory loss may be heralded by Lhermitte's sign, severe paresthesias, or dysesthesias.[3] Pyridoxine intoxication kills dorsal root ganglia cells at high doses and impairs their metabolism at lower toxic doses, so that the peripherally and centrally directed axons both degenerate. Axonal regeneration can occur when excessive pyridoxine is eliminated.[134] Diagnostic testing for this disorder relies on the history and the improvement subsequent to elimination of excessive pyridoxine intake.

### Chronic Immune-Mediated Disorders

PARANEOPLASTIC SENSORY NEURONOPATHY (ANTI-HU). This disorder primarily affects the dorsal-root ganglia cells. Paresthesias or dysesthesias generally move from a distal to a proximal direction, but some cases have shown early sensory changes in proximal areas, including the face.[134] Position and vibration sense are most severely affected, with consequent severe sensory ataxia and pseudoathetosis in the out-

stretched limbs.[5] There is early widespread absence of reflexes. The associated neoplasm is most often a small cell cancer of the lung. The neuropathy may precede the clinical appearance of the carcinoma for longer than 3 years but more often by only a few months. The neuropathy often progresses in a subacute fashion but may then level off to a plateau. Although treatment of the underlying neoplasm usually has no effect on the neuropathy, there are some dramatic individual cases associated with reversal after effective treatment of the primary neoplasm.

Pathologic observations show a lymphocytic infiltration of dorsal root ganglia with a marked depopulation of dorsal root ganglion cells and Nageotte nodules. The peripheral sensory axons degenerate, but there is also degeneration in the centrally directed axon since the dorsal columns, particularly the gracile sectors, are severely affected.

This type of carcinomatous neuropathy is often associated with cerebrospinal fluid and serum antibodies, which react with dorsal root ganglia (IgG anti-Hu antibodies). These antibodies also react with a brain nuclear protein and an identical antigen that is highly specific for small cell lung cancer.[5] The spinal fluid of these patients often contains a few mononuclear cells (5 to 50/mm$^3$) with elevations of protein as high as several grams.

SENSORY NEURONOPATHY OF SJÖGREN'S SYNDROME. Sjögren's syndrome, characterized by keratoconjunctivitis sicca, xerostomia, and rheumatoid arthritis, is often accompanied by a sensory polyneuropathy or polyganglionopathy.[54,148] More common in women, this disorder can present with gait disorder caused by deafferentation.[138,148] Minor salivary gland biopsy is frequently positive.[54] Vasculitic neuropathy or nonspecific epineurial inflammation may be found on nerve biopsy. Antibodies to extractable nuclear antigens are the most specific serologic marker of Sjögren's syndrome, but they were present in only 10% of patients with the sicca complex and neuropathy but no arthritis.[54]

CHRONIC IDIOPATHIC ATAXIC NEUROPATHY. Chronic ataxic sensory neuropathy is a slowly progressive illness with distal paresthesias and sensory ataxia, areflexia, normal strength, and a profound loss of proprioceptive and kinesthetic sensation extending upward to the most proximal joints.[30] Many affected patients have uncomfortable paresthesias with a severe loss of balance in the dark. The ataxia may be accompanied by pseudoathetosis. Sabin[134] has studied several patients with sensory ganglionopathies who complained bitterly of very uncomfortable "pulling" and "stretching" sensations when they tried to move about and as a result confined themselves to a bed and chair existence. Response to immunosuppressant strategies has been poor.[30]

Electrophysiologic studies show normal motor conduction velocities and electromyography (EMG) but no sensory potentials. Biopsy of the sural nerve shows loss of large heavily myelinated fibers. Many patients have a serum monoclonal (mostly immunoglobulin M [IgM]) or polyclonal gammopathy, and some have elevated cerebrospinal fluid gamma globulin levels in spite of low normal total cerebrospinal fluid (CSF) protein levels.[30]

GALOP SYNDROME. Some of the milder cases of chronic ataxic neuropathy may actually be GALOP (*g*ait disorder, *a*utoantibody, *l*ate-age *o*nset, *p*olyneuropathy), a milder syndrome that is often responsive to treatment.[116,117] GALOP is characterized by the presence of IgM antibodies, which are reactive with central myelin antigen (CMA). Pestronk et al[117] described nine patients, with an average age of 70 years, with anti-CMA antibodies, eight of whom had disabling difficulty with ambulation, "out of proportion to that expected for age." The gait disorder developed over a period of 2 to 15 years and presented as slow ambulation and frequent falling, particularly backward. Patients walked with small steps and had difficulty turning. Some of them had moderate distal weakness in the legs, but a sensory loss in a stocking distribution was common, although not as pronounced as that seen in ataxic sensory neuronopathies. Romberg's sign was strikingly positive. The five patients who were treated with intravenous immunoglobulin or cyclophosphamide experienced improvement.[117]

Most helpful for diagnostic testing is an enzyme-linked immunosorbent assay (ELISA) detecting very high titers (>1:10,000) of serum IgM binding to a CNS myelin antigen (CMA) preparation that copurifies with myelin-associated glycoprotein (MAG).[116] Electrophysiologic studies can be heterogeneous. Features suggesting demyelination are common, such as prolonged distal latencies and slow nerve conduction velocities, but conduction block is absent.

CHRONIC INFLAMMATORY DEMYELINATING POLYNEUROPATHY. Although not typically the main presentation, gait impairment can occur in the demyelinating polyneuropathies.[134] Hyperacute Guillain-Barré syndrome (GBS) is misdiagnosed in the emergency department when a healthy-appearing patient is observed to stagger about with a bizarre ataxia and complain of only tingling paresthesias. Examination reveals good strength (which may be sustained only in irregular bursts), dampened reflexes, and normal sensation as tested routinely. The patient is often released from the emergency department with a diagnosis of hysteria, but hours later the individual may require emergency care for evolving widespread flaccid paralysis. This early ataxic phase of GBS might also be due to a physiologic effect of large-fiber demyelination, which is concentrated in the posterior roots. Some patients recovering from GBS go through a phase of ataxia that is out of proportion to the loss of strength or position sense. Likewise, chronic inflammatory demyelinating polyneuropathy (CIDP) may present as an ataxic syndrome. The degree of gait impairment corresponds to the degree of motor-sensory loss.[36] Diagnostic testing for these disorders is discussed in Chapter 19.

Occasionally, CIDP may cause a vestibular syndrome. Frohman et al[42] described a 45-year-old woman with CIDP manifested by foot numbness, limb weakness, gait and postural instability, and oscillopsia. Bilateral vestibulopathy was documented by clinical examination, bithermal calorics, rotary chair testing, brainstem auditory evoked responses (BAERs), and dynamic posturography. MRI with gadolinium demonstrated enhancement of cranial nerve VIII bilaterally. Over the next 6 years, there was a striking synchronization between the activity of this patient's CIDP and vestibulopathy with respect to clinical course, including relapses and responses to immune therapy.

***Vestibular Disorders.*** Older people who complain of unsteadiness when walking often have a normal standard neurologic examination. Fife and Baloh[38] studied 26 patients older than 75 who complained of disequilibrium and in whom no cause was evident after clinical evaluation.

Each patient and each of 26 age-matched controls underwent a comprehensive evaluation that included a history and physical examination, a questionnaire, functional scales, a gait and balance scale, Mini-Mental State testing, audiometry, visual acuity, visual tracking, rotational vestibular testing, and quantitative posturography. Although none had Romberg's sign, the patients tended to sway more and do poorer on semiquantitative gait and balance testing than did controls. Their base of support was slightly widened, their turns were unsteady, and they tended to stagger when pushed and to veer when walking. Patients showed few differences from controls for most other measurements. However, 7 patients had profoundly reduced vestibular function, as determined by rotational vestibular testing and quantitative posturography. In the remaining 19 patients, the average vestibular function was still significantly lower than that of controls. Fife and Baloh[38] concluded that quantitative measurement of vestibular function should be considered in older people complaining of disequilibrium, particularly if the cause is not apparent after the initial evaluation.

Lesions of the vestibular region may present with unilateral or bilateral findings. Unilateral findings are not uncommon in vascular disorders, such as Wallenberg's syndrome (Fig. 13–2), with multiple sclerosis, and with neoplasms of the cerebellopontine angle. With infarction, patients tend to fall to the side of the infarct. Their gait is broad based and lurching. Removal of vision by environmental darkness or impaired eyesight impacts negatively their ability to ambulate and predisposes them to falls. Initially, most of these patients have a prominent headache and are nauseous. In addition to the impairment of balance and ataxia ipsilateral to the lesion, they have a crossed sensory loss (on the ipsilateral face and contralateral body), an ipsilateral Horner's syndrome, and ipsilateral palatal weakness, with hoarseness and dysphagia. Atherosclerotic vascular dis-

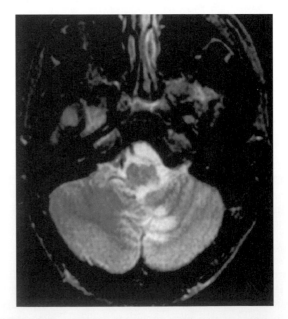

**FIGURE 13–2.** Wallenberg's syndrome. MRI of 31-year-old man with left lateral medullary infarction after spontaneous dissection of left vertebral artery. Cerebellar tonsil is also affected.

ease of the vertebral or posterior-inferior cerebellar arteries may occlude these vessels, and it is responsible for this syndrome in about half of the cases.[75] Most of the rest are due to cardiogenic emboli. Spontaneous dissection of the arterial wall is a frequent cause in younger patients[103] but not in older ones, in whom temporal arteritis should be suspected, particularly in very old individuals with a high sedimentation rate.[123] In a small autopsy series of patients with temporal or giant cell arteritis, the vertebral arteries were found to be affected in all cases.[159] Polymyalgia rheumatica may be present but is not a universal finding. The superficial temporal arteries are often tender and swollen, with a faint pulse.

Bilateral findings are present in Wernicke's encephalopathy of vitamin $B_1$ deficiency. On magnetic resonance imaging (MRI), changes have been documented in the periventricular gray matter, consisting of reversible high intensity on T2-weighted images and transient gadolinium enhancement.[45,141]

MRI is the procedure of choice for the diagnosis of demyelinating, ischemic, and neoplastic disease affecting the vestibular nuclei (Fig. 13–2). Recent plaques of multiple sclerosis in this region present as areas of increased T2 signal and may rarely enhance after the infusion of gadolinium. They are apparent on both heavily T2-weighted and proton-density spin-echo sequences, with the second sequence becoming more sensitive as gliosis develops. A new MRI sequence, fluid attenuated inversion recovery (FLAIR), suppresses the high signal from the cerebrospinal fluid (CSF) and therefore allows for better visualization of lesions causing T2-weighted hyperintensity in the area of filled spaces. However, several studies have shown that this sequence is less sensitive than conventional spin echo in detecting demyelinating lesions of the brainstem and spinal cord.[15,77,143] Unlike in the hemispheres, chronic plaques seldom become hypointense on T1-weighted images. Demyelinating disease most often affects other areas of the brain; the subtle findings in the lateral medulla are often accompanied by periventricular ovoids, which are hyperintense on T2-weighted images, facilitating the diagnosis. FLAIR MRI is sensitive for supratentorial multiple sclerosis and ischemic lesions.[4,15,21,113,129,163] Tumors are easily visualized on MRI and are discussed in Chapter 12. The diagnostic workup for peripheral vestibular disorders is discussed more fully in Chapter 16.

*Vision.* Visual loss and, particularly, distorted visual input can have a major effect in the gait of an older person who already has some sensory loss in the other two modalities essential for maintaining balance—proprioception and vestibular function. Before lens implants became commonplace, older adults having cataract surgery often went through a period of time when they found it difficult to walk normally and were afraid of falling. Eventually their brain learned to integrate the new visual information for the purpose of maintaining balance. To a lesser degree, some of the same difficulty can result from a change in prescription glasses in persons who have proprioceptive or vestibular impairment. On the other hand, these patients find it helpful to walk in areas that are well lighted, optimizing the use of visual clues and thus facilitating steadiness. The diagnostic workup for visual disorders is discussed in Chapter 15.

## Spinal Claudication

The term *spinal claudication* comprises several disorders that cause the patient to experience radicular pain or leg weakness after having walked or stood still for a while. It differs from vascular claudication in the localization and nature of the pain, but more so in that the peripheral pulses are not markedly depressed. Spinal claudication generally results from compression of the cauda equina and the lumbosacral roots by a narrow spinal canal, with tight lateral recesses leaving little room for the exiting roots. In some patients compression of the radicular arteries, particularly the artery of Adamkiewicz, feeding the conus and epiconus, may cause cord ischemia and leg weakness. Three factors are involved in this anatomic situation: (1) the patient was born with a narrow canal; (2) degenerative disease of the spine, with facet joint and ligament hypertrophy, contributes to crowding even further the space available to the cauda equina, roots, and radicular vessels; and (3) exaggeration of the lumbar lordosis in the upright position worsens the compression of these structures.

Although this syndrome is real, it is rare. Unfortunately, some older adults who complain of gait difficulties have a lumbosacral MRI performed "just in case." When this test shows marked degenerative changes in their spine, with a narrow canal, the tendency is to diagnose the disease based on the imaging findings. Particularly in such cases, it is extremely important to correlate the imaging findings carefully with the clinical presentation. Severe degenerative changes are the rule in MRI of the lumbosacral spine in persons older than 70 years, but they may be found in asymptomatic subjects of all ages.[17,71,140] The clinical history is more important than the imaging findings in making the diagnosis. The history needs to be scrutinized. Other causes of gait impairment cause "gait claudication" because patients tire from having to attend to their gait and being fearful of a fall. For instance, many patients with parkinsonism need to sit after having stood for a short while because their "legs get heavy." Anxiety over a fall can cause "weak legs." Onset or worsening of characteristic radicular pain, on the other hand, favors spinal claudication. MRI findings are helpful to plan the surgery, but some surgeons prefer to rely on CT, which shows bone changes better than MRI does. EMG may show denervation changes in a radicular distribution or, rarely, may be normal in the resting state. By themselves, EMG changes are not diagnostic.

## Cervical Myelopathy

Although lumbosacral stenosis is seldom the cause of gait difficulties in the older adult, cervical myelopathy from cervical spondylosis was the second most common cause in a series by Sudarsky[145] and one by Fuh et al.[43] Because it is potentially treatable, cervical myelopathy should be considered in any older adult presenting with gait impairment. Some patients have the characteristic clinical picture of cervical radicular pain and spastic paraparesis, but most do not have radicular pain. Initially, at the time when surgery is most likely to be successful and prevent further deterioration, the gait impairment may be very subtle, noticeable only to the patient and yielding minimal findings on neurologic examination.[135] The paucity of findings may delay the diagnosis. In the Yale series,[135] the investigators estimated that the diagnosis had been delayed by 6.3 years on average. The earliest consistent symptom in all their 22 patients was a gait abnormality. These patients may become unsteady when they close their eyes and stand with their feet together. They are unable to walk in tandem. The brachioradialis reflex may be depressed; instead, a brisk finger flexor response is elicited when the brachioradialis tendon is percussed (inverted radial reflex). Careful testing of vibratory sense may reveal a sensory level in the cervical region. Sometimes the patient perceives the stimulus better in the thumb than in the small finger. Early diagnosis is important because the myelopathy of cervical spondylosis is often progressive if untreated.[135] Occasionally, thoracic myelopathy can produce similar gait impairment.

In terms of diagnostic testing, all the precautions discussed in the previous section on spinal stenosis also apply here. MRI of the cervical spine is helpful, but, in the absence of clinical findings, the presence of spondylitic changes by themselves does not confirm the diagnosis. Rather severe changes can be seen in asymptomatic older adults.[62,65,125,158] Plain x-ray films are helpful in determining the shape of the cervical spine, the alignment of the vertebrae, the status of the bone, the vertical extent of the disease process, the degree of anterior and posterior osteophytes, and the nature of the disk spaces (Fig. 13–3A). Baseline plain x-ray films are also

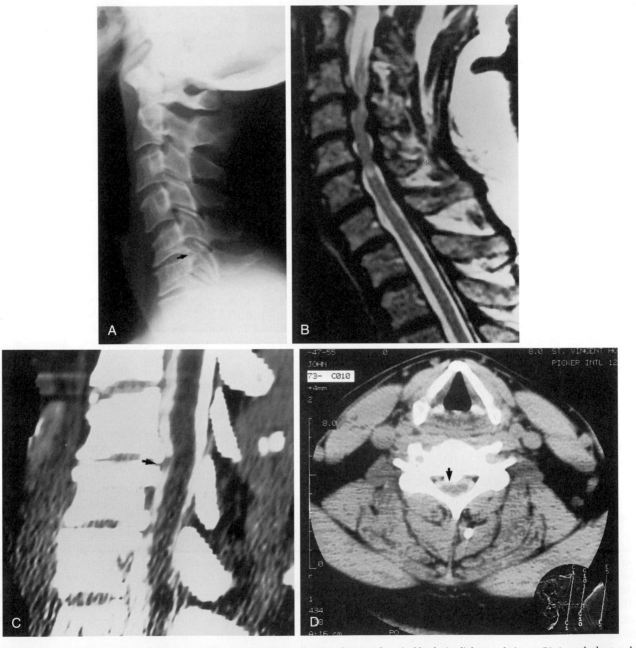

**FIGURE 13–3.** Cervical spondylosis. **A,** Plain x-ray film of cervical spine showing absence of cervical lordosis, slight angulation at C5-6, marked osteophyte formation at C5-6 (*arrow*), narrow disk spaces at C5-6 and C6-7 levels and canal stenosis. **B,** Cervical spondylosis with cervical myelopathy. MRI of 67-year-old woman with progressive quadriparesis and spastic gait. Spinal cord is compressed at C3-4-5 levels. Increased signal intensity in substance of cord indicates presence of myelopathy. **C,** CT myelogram with sagittal reconstruction of same patient as in **A** showing distortion and displacement of spinal canal by osteophyte formation and narrow canal at C5-6 (*arrow*) and C6-7 levels. **D,** CT myelogram in axial projection showing ossification of posterior longitudinal ligament in midline (*arrow*), indenting thecal sac. (*A, C,* and *D* from Murali R, Masdeu J. Cervical spondylotic myelopathy. In: Masdeu J, Sudarsky L, Wolfson L, eds. *Gait Disorders of Aging: Falls and Therapeutic Strategies.* Philadelphia: Lippincott-Raven; 1997:197-208.)

useful when surgery is being considered for later comparison with postoperative x-ray films or when the patient cannot undergo MRI, for instance, if he or she has a pacemaker. Several recent studies agree that MRI is the screening test of choice in most instances.[135,142] Bony osteophytes can be seen as black ridges compressing the canal and, if the compression is severe, causing high-intensity changes in the spinal cord on T2-weighted images (Fig. 13–3B). The patient whose MRI is shown in Figure 13–3 had quadriparesis with a spastic-ataxic gait.

In addition to narrowing of the spinal canal by spondylitic hypertrophy of bones and ligaments, two changes are frequently observed in the cord itself: decreased diameter and a hyperintense signal on T2-weighted images. How often a hyperintense area is observed depends on the stage of progression, with gliosis and microcavitation of the gray matter, and other poorly understood factors. In some series as many as 40% of the patients have this finding.[162] Although some investigators have determined that the presence of this finding and its irreversibility after surgery predicts a poor outcome, others have not.[102,162] MRI may show other changes within the spinal cord itself caused by chronic compression, such as syrinx formation. MRI is also of great value in the differential diagnosis of myelopathy because conditions such as tumor and infection can be ruled out easily. In multiple sclerosis an abnormal signal may be found in the spinal cord and elsewhere in the brain because of the presence of plaques.

However, MRI scan is not as good as CT in showing osteophytes or ossification of the posterior longitudinal ligament. If surgical treatment is contemplated, thin-slice CT of the cervical spine after intrathecal introduction of a nonionic water-soluble contrast material is of great help (Fig. 13–3C). MRI scan, CT scan, and CT myelography are all complementary tests; they are not mutually exclusive. CT myelography is most valuable for deciding on the surgical approach, either anterior or posterior. CT myelography also allows for accurate measurement of the spinal canal in the axial, sagittal, and coronal planes. A canal diameter of <12 mm in the anteroposterior plane is considered stenotic. Ossification of the posterior longitudinal ligament (OPLL) is sometimes found in patients with cervical spondylotic myelopathy. OPLL may be segmental or continuous in the cervical spine. CT myelography is particularly useful for diagnosing this entity, which has significant bearing on the type of surgical procedure to be performed (Fig. 13–3D).

Statham et al[142] assessed the need for additional testing after MRI in patients with suspected cervical spondylotic myelopathy. A total of 102 patients were prospectively investigated, with MRI used as the initial imaging technique. The aim was to discover if clinicians could manage patients with MRI alone or if they would find a second investigation necessary. Management of 82 patients involved the use of MRI alone; 34 of this group were treated surgically. A second investigation was done for 20 patients: a myelogram was used in 18 patients and a CT myelogram in 2. Only 5 of these 20 patients had surgical treatment. The diagnosis changed after the second investigation in 4 patients, but management was not influenced in any of these cases. The authors concluded that MRI is a satisfactory alternative to myelography for most patients with suspected cervical spondylotic myelopathy.

Somatosensory evoked responses (SERs) can be normal in half of the patients with symptomatic cervical myelopathy.[149] Motor responses from magnetic stimulation and spinal cord evoked potentials (EPs) are more sensitive.[9,10,90] Occasionally, these electrophysiologic tests may be useful when the clinical picture is less than conclusive.[124] More often, in mild cases they are also inconclusive. Postdecompression improvement of SERs predicted faster recovery but did not match the 1-year outcome of surgical patients.[18] Most neurosurgeons do not require SERs as part of the presurgical battery.

## Cerebellar Disorders

Cerebellar lesions may affect gait by causing disequilibrium and by altering limb and trunk kinematics and interlimb coordination.[31] The cerebellum does not appear to actually generate postural and gait synergies because these automatic responses, although very dysmetric, are present in dogs with total cerebellectomies.[119]

Disturbances of gait and balance are primarily caused by lesions of the vestibulocerebellum and spinocerebellum or their connections. Lesions of the cerebellar hemispheres cause irregular timing, force, and cadence of leg movements, leading to inaccurate and variable stepping.[59] Lesions of the *vestibulocerebellum*, or floccular-nodular lobe, can produce balance and gait disturbances that resemble those caused by vestibular lesions.[31] Tremor of the head and trunk, truncal imbalance, and swaying and falling in all directions are characteristic of vestibulocerebellar lesions. Vestibular nystagmus may be present. The clinical syndrome caused by lesions of the *spinocerebellum* is best characterized by alcoholic cerebellar degeneration, which primarily affects the anterior lobe of the cerebellum but also involves the olivary complex and the vestibular nuclei.[156] Patients with alcoholic cerebellar degeneration have a widened base, instability of the trunk, and slow and halting gait with irregular steps and superimposed lurching. The gait abnormalities are accentuated at the initiation of gait, on turning, and with changes in gait speed. Affected patients may have severe gait ataxia without nystagmus, dysarthria, or arm dysmetria. Even the heel-to-shin test may give little indication of the severity of the gait disturbance. Interestingly, if patients stop drinking alcohol and have adequate nutrition, the gait improves so that the steps are no longer irregular and tandem walking or sudden movements are necessary to demonstrate the gait ataxia.[156] Although most often patients with cerebellar lesions tend to fall to the side of the lesion, some patients with lesions in the tonsillar area develop increased tone (and increased reflexes) in the ipsilateral side and fall to the contralateral side. This was the case with the 69-year-old whose CT is shown in Figure 13–4.

Ischemic and hemorrhagic strokes are the most frequent causes of cerebellar dysfunction in the older adult.[31] The clinical presentation of infarction in the territory of the posterior inferior cerebellar artery was described earlier, in the section on vestibular dysfunction (see Fig. 13–2). Gait impairment is the most common presentation of infarcts in the territory of the superior cerebellar artery.[75] In the older age group infarction in the territory of the posterior-inferior cerebellar artery is caused by atheromatous vascular disease as often as by embolic disease. Presumed cerebral embolism was the predominant stroke mechanism in patients with superior cerebellar artery distribution infarcts.[75]

The clinical presentation of cerebellar hemorrhage may be acute, subacute, or chronic.[22,93] Variations in location, size, and development of the hematoma; brainstem compression; fourth ventricular penetration; and development of hydrocephalus result in variations in the mode of presentation of cerebellar hemorrhage. The hemorrhages most frequently occur in the region of the dentate nucleus. Patients present with occipital or frontal headache, dizziness, vertigo, nausea, repeated vomiting, and inability to stand or walk. They often have truncal or limb ataxia, ipsilateral gaze palsy, and small reactive pupils. Horizontal gaze paresis, paretic nystagmus, and facial weakness are also common. Frank hemiparesis is absent. Ocular bobbing and skew deviation may be present. Not all patients present such a dramatic picture. Those with small (usually <3 cm in diameter) cerebellar hematomas may present only with vomiting and without headache, gait instability, or limb ataxia.

Degenerative diseases of the cerebellum include disease restricted to the cerebellum and diseases with extracerebellar involvement, such as olivo-ponto-cerebellar ataxia (OPCA) or multisystem atrophies.[31] Spinocerebellar degenerations typically begin at a younger age.

Paraneoplastic cerebellar syndromes can be seen with bronchial, breast, and ovarian cancer.[31] The symptoms include ataxia of gait and stance, limb ataxia, terminal tremor, gaze-evoked nystagmus, and disturbed smooth-pursuit eye movements.

Toxic cerebellar syndromes in older people are frequently due to slower drug metabolism and reduced tolerance.[31] All centrally acting drugs may lead to cerebellar disturbances of stance and gait. The drugs most frequently responsible for toxic disturbances include alcohol, antiepileptic drugs, lithium, and tranquilizers.

### Vascular Disease of the Brain

Vascular disease of the brain ranks among the top three causes of gait impairment in the older adult.[43,145] Affected patients are referred for progressive gait impairment; they are not stroke patients with secondary hemiparesis and gait difficulty. Vascular disease causing this syndrome most often affects the supratentorial compartment in the form of lacunar disease or ischemic disease of the white matter. Less

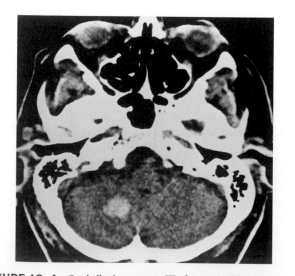

**FIGURE 13–4.** Cerebellar hematoma. CT of 64-year-old man with sudden onset of inability to walk and tendency to fall to left side. Hemorrhage involves right supratonsillar region.

often, it involves the posterior circulation, involving vestibular or cerebellar structures, and, very rarely, other brainstem structures important for gait, such as the mesencephalic locomotor center. Lacunar disease will be discussed first, followed by white-matter disease, and finally the syndrome of the mesencephalic locomotor center. CT and MRI are the diagnostic tests most useful for the study of these syndromes.

*Lacunar Disease.* Ischemic brain disease tends to follow one of three patterns, discernible by clinical evaluation and through neuroimaging procedures: (1) cortical infarcts, most often related to embolic disease; (2) subcortical disease, often in the form of widespread lacunes and white-matter changes, most often related to arteriolar disease; and (3) a mixture of the two patterns, often related to atheromatous disease of the major vessels.[96] The second and third types of cerebrovascular disease tend to cause gait and balance impairment early in the course of the disease. Subcortical infarcts strategically located may impair equilibrium and gait with little or no limb weakness demonstrated on isometric testing. These lesions tend to affect structures with a critical role in gait and balance mechanisms, including the cortical-basal-ganglionic/thalamic/cortical loop (Fig. 13–5A). Although acute stroke tends to be associated with overt neurologic findings, gait impairment may be neglected as a neurologic finding but may be the result of small "silent" lacunar strokes.[16] In a cohort of clinically asymptomatic patients studied during the Asymptomatic Carotid Atherosclerosis Study, Brott et al[25] documented lacunar strokes with CT in 11% of the patients. These patients were more likely to have gait impairment.

*Thalamic Astasia.* The inability to stand or walk despite minimal weakness has been recorded with thalamic infarction[26,83,98] and hemorrhage, particularly when the superior portion of the ventrolateral nucleus or suprathalamic white matter was involved (Fig. 13–5B).[98,155] It has also been reported in patients with lesions in the internal capsule or corona radiata who had the syndrome of unilateral ataxia and crural paresis (ataxic hemiparesis).[40,66,68,136] Alert, with normal or near-normal strength on isometric muscle testing and a variable degree of sensory loss, these patients could not stand, and some with acute lesions could not sit up unassisted. They fell backward or toward the side contralateral to the lesion. These patients appeared to have a deficit of overlearned motor activity of an axial and postural nature. In the vascular cases the deficit improved in a few days or weeks. However, these patients had a tendency to sustain falls during the rehabilitation period.

*Capsular and Basal Ganglia Lesions.* A tendency to fall despite good strength was recorded by Groothuis et al[56] in a patient with a small medial capsular hemorrhage involving the most lateral portion of the ventrolateral nucleus of the thalamus and by Labadie et al[82] in patients with acute lesions in the basal ganglia. Multiple bilateral lacunes involving the basal ganglia can be attended by gait impairment (see Fig. 13–5A).

*White-Matter Disease.* Disorders of gait were pronounced among 41 well-documented cases of progressive arteriopathic white-matter disease described with histologic evidence since 1978 (males, 23; females, 18; mean age of onset, 60 ± 9.7 years; mean length of illness, 5.8 ± 4.2 years).[27,32,34,51,55,67,69,128] Impairment of ambulation preceded

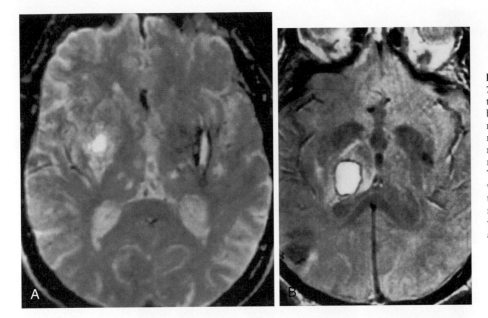

**FIGURE 13–5.** **A,** Lacunar disease. MRI of 73-year-old man, a chronic hypertensive, with transient episode of mild left-sided weakness but progressive gait impairment. In addition to multiple thalamic lacunes and larger infarct in right lenticular nucleus, there is organizing hematoma in left external capsular region, surrounded by dark-appearing hemosiderin. **B,** Thalamic hematoma. MRI of 86-year-old man with transient mild left hemiparesis but inability to walk for 8 weeks, despite recovery of isometric strength. Right thalamic hematoma involves ventrolateral and ventral posterior nuclei, as well as pulvinar nucleus.

cognitive impairment in 43% of the cases, whereas in only 17% dementia developed before gait impairment; in 20% the two conditions evolved simultaneously, and in 20% insufficient data precluded the timing of gait abnormality vs. dementia. Comparing demented elderly subjects with controls for dementia, several authors failed to find a significant correlation between white-matter disease and dementia, but white-matter disease correlated with gait impairment.[47,63] Periventricular white-matter changes were present in cases of "lower body parkinsonism."[41,151] In controlled studies of elderly who were prone to falling, impaired gait and balance correlated with the presence of white-matter disease on CT or MRI.[14,64,100,150]

White-matter changes on CT or MR are very common in older people (Fig. 13–6). On MR, some degree of white-matter changes is present in about 30% of subjects over the age of 65.[35] Areas of the periventricular white matter that show hypodensity on CT appear markedly hyperintense on T2-weighted images and hypointense on T1-weighted images[78] (see Fig. 13–6A). However, high-intensity areas on T2-weighted MR are often undetected on CT. On T2-weighted MR images, it may be difficult to differentiate areas of increased water content because of dilation of perivascular spaces with normal aging or transependymal CSF absorption from areas of tissue damage since both have increased intensity values.[7,79,164] For this reason it seems preferable to make the diagnosis of significant white-matter changes only when the abnormalities are visible on T1-weighted images. However, there are no data available exploring the functional significance of white-matter changes on only T2-weighted images vs. changes on both T2- and T1-weighted images.

Because the histology underlying these changes remains elusive in some cases, Hachinski et al[58] coined the descriptive term *leuko-araiosis* for the CT findings. Several authors have reported normal histologic findings, but ischemic changes similar to the findings in subcortical arteriosclerotic encephalopathy (SAE) have been present in cases with pronounced changes on T1-weighted MRI or CT.[20,72,78,89,94,126,128,161] Cerebrovascular disease and hypertension are frequent correlates of subcortical arteriosclerotic encephalopathy.[8,154] Amyloid angiopathy has been incriminated in the genesis of white-matter disease in some elderly individuals.[32,55] In addition to white-matter changes, amyloid angiopathy results in subcortical hemorrhages (Fig. 13–6B).

Some ischemic leukoencephalopathies, such as CADASIL, are familial.[133] CADASIL stands for *c*erebral *a*utosomal *d*ominant *a*rteriopathy with *s*ubcortical *i*nfarcts and *l*eukoencephalopathy.[28] CT and MRI show an abnormal white matter—hypodense on CT, hyperintense on T2-weighted MR images, and hypointense on T1-weighted MR images (Fig. 13–6C to F). Imaging changes are often present in presymptomatic individuals.[28] CADASIL has been mapped to a mutation of the notch 3 gene, on chromosome 19.[33,73] A PAS-positive granular material is deposited in the media of the arterioles of the brain and other organs, including skin.[132] When the result is positive, a skin biopsy is helpful, but there are genetically proven cases with a negative skin biopsy result.[131] Other vascular familial leukoencephalopathies include familial amyloid angiopathy and disorders that are less well characterized.[55,57,70,118]

***Pontomesencephalic Gait Failure.*** The laterodorsal region of the midbrain contains the mesencephalic locomotor region, which plays an important role in locomotion in animals.[46] Stimulation of this region in the cat induces rapid walking, followed by running. This area contains the cuneiform nucleus and the cholinergic pedunculopontine nucleus. In humans, loss of neurons in the pedunculopontine nucleus has been found in progressive supranuclear palsy and Parkinson's disease but not in patients with Alzheimer's disease, implying a possible role of this nucleus in ambulatory mechanisms. The patient whose MRI is shown in Figure 13–7 had acute onset of inability to walk without hemiparesis or sensory loss.[97] She was able to draw a circle with either leg when sitting down but could not generate regular stepping movements with her feet. Holding onto a walker and stooped forward, she could walk with short, shuffling, irregular steps. Her base of ambulation was only minimally wide. This patient was unable to initiate reg-

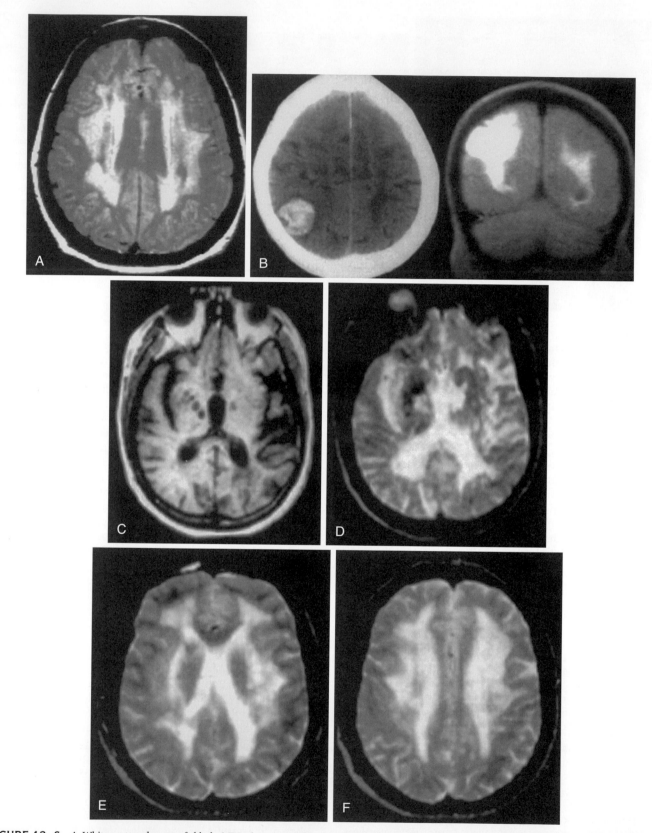

**FIGURE 13—6. A,** White-matter changes of elderly. MRI of normotensive 75-year-old woman with normal mentation but slow, hesitating gait and propensity to falling. Ventricular fluid is dark in proton-density MRI. Periventricular white matter is hyperintense, suggesting presence of extensive gliosis. **B,** Amyloid angiopathy. CT scan of 79-year-old woman showing recent hemorrhage in right supramarginal gyrus (*left*). On T2-weighted MRI, lesion appears bright because of high methemoglobin content and abnormal white matter is hyperintense in both hemispheres (*right*). **C** to **F,** Cerebral autosomal dominant arteriopathy with subcortical infarcts and leukoencephalopathy (CADASIL). **C, D,** T1-weighted and T2-weighted MR images of 40-year-old who had sustained several strokes, leaving him with quadriparesis. CADASIL was confirmed by brain biopsy and genetic typing. **E, F,** T2-weighted MR images of asymptomatic 40-year-old relative of previous patient at 50% genetic risk of having CADASIL, showing abnormally hyperintense periventricular white matter. (*C* to *F* from Sabbadini G, Francia A, Calandriello L, et al. Cerebral autosomal dominant arteriopathy with subcortical infarcts and leukoencephalopathy (CADASIL). Clinical, neuroimaging, pathological and genetic study of a large Italian family. *Brain.* 1995;118:207-215. By permission of Oxford University Press.)

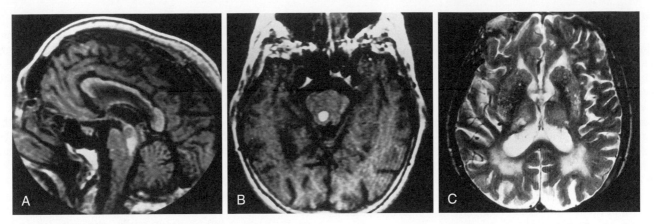

**FIGURE 13–7.** Pedunculopontine gait failure. MRI of 83-year-old woman with gait failure after hemorrhage in locomotor mesencephalic region. Lesion is shown in sagittal (**A**) and coronal (**B**) planes. In addition, periventricular white-matter changes and small thalamic lacunes were present in this chronic hypertensive individual (**C**).

ular stepping either in attempted walking or in response to loss of balance. There was no cadence or rhythmicity to this patient's gait. The deficit of gait observed in this case bears a striking resemblance to the idiopathic gait failure experienced by many elderly individuals, which usually does not have a clear anatomic correlate.[114] These persons lack the ability to generate spontaneous, rhythmic stepping movements. In acute pontomesencephalic gait failure, imaging studies may show hemorrhagic or ischemic lesions.[37,137]

### Toxic or Metabolic Encephalopathies

Because these disorders are often treatable causes of gait impairment, it is important to recognize metabolic or toxic agents, most often in the form of medications. Psychotropic, diuretic, antihypertensive, and antiparkinsonian medications, especially if used in improper doses, may contribute to falls in the elderly by decreasing alertness, depressing psychomotor function, or causing weakness, fatigue, dizziness, or postural hypotension.[110,120,122] These adverse physiologic effects may be exacerbated by altered drug metabolism in elderly individuals.

Although not confirmed by all studies, there is good evidence that the use of hypnotic-anxiolytic drugs, particularly benzodiazepines, increases the risk of falls.[88,111,127,144] The role of diuretic, antihypertensive, and other medications linked to orthostatic hypotension in increasing the risk of falls is uncertain and needs further investigation.[120] Several studies have found an association between falls and the number of medications being taken. This situation could reflect the synergistic effects among drugs, but it could also be due to the poorer health of individuals taking multiple medications.

Patients with metabolic encephalopathy often display an insecure gait and may fall over backward if displaced. This phenomenon is particularly dramatic with uremia and hepatic failure, in which asterixis may impair stance.[145]

### Parkinsonian Syndromes

Gait abnormalities are the presenting complaint in 12% to 18% of patients with Parkinson's disease.[115] Early in the disease, when one side is affected, the patient appears to drag a leg during ambulation. When the opposite leg is also involved, the steps are short and the feet appear to barely clear the floor, giving the impression of a shuffling gait (marche à petits pas). The patient turns with small steps and moves the trunk in a rigid manner (en bloc turning) because associated body movements, including arm swing, are decreased. The difficulty that patients with Parkinson's disease have with taking the first step has been termed *start hesitation*. As the disease progresses, the center of gravity is shifted forward. During ambulation, the flexed trunk precedes the lower limbs, leading the patient to take increasingly frequent short steps, which often end with the patient's fall. This phenomenon is known as festination, which is one of the characteristics of advanced Parkinson's disease. Instead of the propulsive gait, the patient might develop retropulsion, which is a tendency to fall backward or to take rapid, short backward steps. Resting tremor is often exacerbated while walking.[115]

"Freezing" may be seen in Parkinson's disease.[115] It refers to the patient's feet getting stuck to the ground while walking and the patient being unable to initiate movements of the lower limbs. This phenomenon is noted especially in doorways, on elevators, and in turns. After a few seconds to minutes, the patient may be able to walk again, first taking multiple small steps and then resuming normal stride. As a general term, freezing episodes and related phenomena are called *motor blocks*. Giladi et al[50] reported that 32% of their 990 patients with Parkinson's disease had motor blocks. Start hesitation occurred in 86% of the patients; blocking on turning, in 45%; and blocking in narrow spaces, in 25%. When the initial symptoms of Parkinson's disease occur in the upper body, the likelihood of motor blocks is lesser. Giladi et al also reported that a longer duration of the disease, a higher Hoehn and Yahr stage, and a longer duration of levodopa therapy were significantly associated with the presence of motor blocks.

Falling is another major disability in Parkinson's disease. Although there are multiple causes of this falling, the most important ones are postural instability, gait abnormalities, cognitive impairment, difficulties in sitting and rising, orthostatic hypotension, dyskinesias, and age-related deconditioning.[115] Gait abnormalities, such as start-hesitation, festination, retropulsion, and freezing, frequently lead to falls. At times the patient may trip or stumble over rough surfaces because each step is too small to clear the obstacle. In the later stages of the disease, frequent falling is often caused by postural instability.[115]

## Late-Life Hydrocephalus

Although not a frequent cause of gait disorders in older adults, symptomatic hydrocephalus presents initially with gait impairment; it is important to recognize this potentially treatable disorder.[157] Particularly after CT became available, several authors found enlarged ventricles to be present frequently in patients with gait disorders.[39] From this finding they concluded that symptomatic hydrocephalus was common, and the use of shunting procedures increased. However, even in series with carefully selected patients, some patients failed to improve after shunting, which suggests that hydrocephalus was not the cause of their gait disorder.[52] For this reason it is important to apply more sensitive diagnostic criteria in the workup of affected patients.[53] CSF manometrics are not predictive of which patients will improve after shunting.[92] MRI and single photon emission computed tomography (SPECT) are more helpful.[53] Chapter 7 describes diagnostic testing for symptomatic hydrocephalus in greater detail.

## Psychogenic Conditions

Gait disorders caused by psychogenic factors are rare and generally do not present a diagnostic dilemma. It is important, however, not to mislabel an organic gait disorder as a psychogenic one. Therefore some of the characteristics of these disorders will be reviewed briefly here. On the other hand, psychogenic factors often play a role in aggravating the functional consequences of an organic gait disorder, and sometimes they are amenable to specific treatment.[147]

During panic attacks, patients may feel that their legs are weak and they become unsteady. To protect themselves from a perceived risk of falling, they may adopt a gait pattern described as "walking on ice."[85] They crouch forward, abduct their arms and shorten their stride. Sometimes these patients cling to walls or furniture and may not venture away from the house.[147] A similar gait pattern, described as cautious gait, is very common in patients with organic gait disorders. A major difference is that the cautious gait in patients with

anxiety tends to occur episodically, in the context of a panic attack, whereas organic gait disorders are generally more persistent. Other features that differentiate psychogenic from organic gait disorder include dramatic moment-to-moment fluctuations in performance, excessive hesitation (e.g., slow motion or walking as through a viscous fluid), and buckling of the knees without falling.[85] A psychogenic Romberg test is characterized by buildup of sway, with a consistent tendency to fall toward the observer. This effect can often be overcome by distraction, for instance, by examining the pupils while the patient quietly stands.[147]

Of the 60 patients with "hysterical gait disorders" described by Keane,[76] some manifested a hemiparesis or paraparesis, but the largest group had an assortment of ataxic gaits, characterized by dramatically exaggerated sway with avoidance of falls. Some patients exhibited "tightrope balancing": walking on a narrow base while keeping their arms abducted. Others were described as "tremblers," who are not to be confused with patients having orthostatic tremor, an organic disorder.[24] Overall, a neurologic examination can easily pinpoint the nature of the problem in about 75% of patients with psychogenic gait disorders.[85]

## Rare Etiologies—Neoplasms and Subdural Hematoma

Occasionally, an older person with a worsening gait disorder may harbor a frontal tumor (Fig. 13–8A and B) or a subdural hematoma (Fig. 13–8C). Meningiomas carry a better prognosis, but they are not as common as glioblastomas or metastases in the older age group. By the time the patient becomes symptomatic, these lesions can be easily identified by MRI scanning. CT is less sensitive than MRI, particularly for glioblastoma. Also, poor definition of cortical boundaries may make it difficult to differentiate a glioma from a meningioma on CT or a noncontrast study. On a contrast study, the more homogeneous pattern of a meningioma and the presence of a dural tail are characteristics that help differentiate this lesion from a glioblastoma. However, some meningiomas may have cystic areas that enhance poorly.

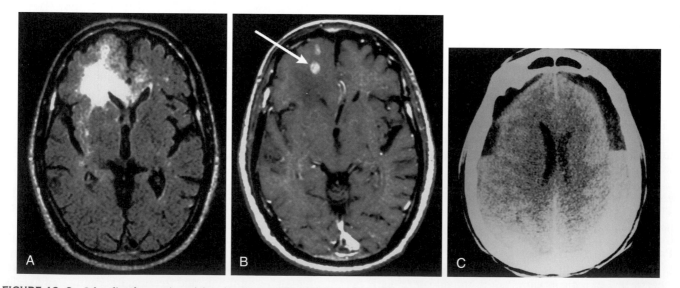

**FIGURE 13–8.** Other disorders causing gait impairment. **A** and **B,** Frontal lobe tumor. This 80-year-old experienced progressive deterioration of gait over 3-week period. T2-weighted MRI showed hyperintense lesion with edema in centrum semiovale of right frontal lobe, causing thickening of corpus callosum (**A**). Lesion had contrast-enhancing nodule (**B,** *arrow*) suggestive of malignancy. It proved to be glioblastoma multiforme. **C,** Bilateral subdural hematomas in older person with increasing difficulty ambulating. Note more dense blood elements sedimenting in deponent portion of hematomas, with bilateral fluid levels.

Calcification in a meningioma and changes in the cortical bone are better appreciated on CT, but these characteristics are seldom critical for the diagnosis. Also, in the case of glioblastomas, the extent of the tumor is better visualized by MRI than by CT. Neither technique, however, accurately shows the extent of brain infiltrated by malignant glial cells. MRI is also more sensitive than CT for the detection of metastatic brain disease. More details of diagnostic testing for brain tumors are found in Chapter 12

In patients who are prone to falls, a subacute deterioration should raise the suspicion of a subdural hematoma, particularly when a worsening in gait is accompanied by changes in mental status (Fig. 13–8C). Although MRI depicts these lesions with more accuracy than CT does, symptomatic subdural hematomas are visualized well with CT and can be adequately managed neurosurgically without the need for MRI.

### Idiopathic Gait Disorders

A large proportion of older patients with gait disorders have none of the disease processes discussed previously. Although in Sudarsky's series[145] this group comprises only 14% of the patients referred to a neurologist for gait disorders, and the experience of Fuh et al[43] was similar, other researchers looking for the cause of progressive gait impairment in selected populations have failed to find a cause in a larger proportion of patients.[6,114] Because the progression of the disorder is slow, over the course of months or years, poorly understood "degenerative" disorders involving the neural centers or pathways for gait control are likely to be responsible.

#### APPROACH TO DIAGNOSTIC TESTING

From the foregoing sections, it is clear that before selecting ancillary tests, the clinician needs to have an idea of the location of the pathologic process, by means of the neurologic examination, and of the likely etiologic basis, by means of the history.

### History

In older patients with gait disorders, it is often difficult to ascertain the precise timing of the disorder. The witness of someone else close to the patient should be sought. Most central and peripheral disorders described earlier develop insidiously over the course of months or years. Initially, many patients feel that their balance is "off." This complaint is elicited not only from patients whose loss of proprioception or vestibular function renders them unsteady but also from patients with disorders of central motor control, as those with Parkinson's disease or thalamic lacunes. Patients should be questioned about falls. Falls are often considered by patients misjudgments or accidents and not a result of the disorder that brings them to consult the physician. The circumstances of the most recent fall should be analyzed in detail. Did it happen at night, with poor ambient lighting? Did it come out of the blue, when the patient was trying to turn?

### Physical Examination

The neurologic examination is most helpful in defining the likely localization of the pathologic condition responsible for the gait disorder. Peripheral neuropathies that are severe enough to cause gait impairment are accompanied by a

positive Romberg sign. In this context the Romberg sign is defined as increased unsteadiness with eye closure while the patient stands with the feet together. Muscle stretch reflexes are reduced or absent. However, an absent ankle jerk is a common finding in older individuals.[29] Distal paresthesias or sensory loss to pinprick may be present. Vibratory sense is uniformly decreased, out of proportion to the distal loss in the feet characteristic of old age.[29] Conspicuously absent are findings characteristic of central processing impairment, such as difficulty initiating a step.

Patients with cervical spondylosis have a mixture of sensory and motor findings. Romberg's sign is often positive. Gait may be spastic, rigid, or even apractic. An inverted radial reflex or a cervical cord level for vibratory sense are very helpful in uncovering cervical myelopathy. The Romberg sign is also positive in patients with vestibular disorders. The deficit is often bilateral, and a clear lateralization is uncommon. Nystagmus may be present.

Patients with a disorder of central processing caused by parkinsonism or vascular disease are unsteady, particularly when walking without paying attention to their gait. They often do better in a physician's office than at home, when they are concentrating on preparing the next meal rather than walking carefully across a carpeted room. Cortical mechanisms take over when the patients attend to their gait. It is the "automatic pilot," mediated by the cortical-basal-ganglionic-thalamic-cortical loop and other pathways, that is impaired in these patients. The Romberg sign is often absent. Many of these patients also have difficulty shifting in bed. When lying prone on the examining table, they may be unable to slide horizontally. Typically, when asked to do this, they grab the sides of the examining table with their hands and push themselves up. One would think that their axial muscles are paralyzed, except that the isometric strength of these muscles on purposeful movements is normal.

### Evaluation of Gait and Balance

Quantification of the degree of balance and gait impairment is useful to assess the effect of therapeutic interventions or to detect individuals at risk for falling. Several semiquantitative scales have been described with this purpose. In the "Get Up and Go" test, subjects stand up from a chair, walk 3 meters, turn around, and return. Performance is judged subjectively and graded with the following scale: 1 = normal; 2 = very slightly abnormal; 3 = mildly abnormal; 4 = moderately abnormal; 5 = severely abnormal. It has been shown that older adults who scored 3 or higher on this test had an increased risk for falls.[101] When timed, this test correlates well with other functional scales, such as the Barthel Index.[91] Neurologically normal adults who are independent in balance and movement skills can finish the test in less than 10 seconds while patients who are independent in basic transfers can finish the test in less than 20 seconds. Patients who required more than 30 seconds to finish the test were dependent in most activities of daily living.[160] A similar, but more elaborate, test is the Tinetti Balance and Mobility Scale.[152] In clinical practice it is difficult to monitor mild changes in the gait and balance performance of a single individual by the use of these scales, which are more attuned to screening populations for gait and balance problems.

A simple, more sensitive method is to videotape a sequence of the patient's performance on a given date and

| TABLE 13–1. **Videotaped Motor Sequence** |
| --- |

- Supine to side-lying to supine
- Move up toward head of bed while supine
- Supine to sitting over side of bed
- Short-distance ambulation
- Sit in chair
- Balance sitting on chair
- Drawing circle and cross
- Alternating heel-toe tapping
- Sit to stand from chair
- Standing with eyes closed for 30 seconds, feet together, no support; arms stretched, supinated, in front
- Finger-to-nose coordination test
- Standing and rising to toes, heels
- Unilateral stance for 10 seconds on each foot
- Walking on heels, toes, 5 meters
- Tandem gait, 5 meters

compare it with similar videotaped sequences obtained at other times. The sequence of performance should be standardized. We use the sequence outlined in Table 13–1.

### Ancillary Tests: Indications

Once the physical examination and the history have suggested the most likely localization, targeted testing should be done. The appropriate tests for each condition were enumerated in the preceding sections. Here they will be reviewed briefly, starting from the test to the conditions in which it is indicated.

#### Chemistries

*Thyroid Function Tests.* Thyroid function tests should be performed in patients with a peripheral neuropathy, particularly when it is accompanied by vestibular and cognitive impairment. They should also be done in patients with vestibular impairment unexplained by other causes.

*Vitamin $B_{12}$ Levels.* Vitamin $B_{12}$ levels should be obtained in patients with an insidious thick-fiber peripheral neuropathy, particularly if posterolateral cord findings are also present. Hematologic abnormalities need not be present.[61] If cobalamin levels are normal but the condition is strongly suspected, levels of serum methylmalonic acid and homocysteine should be obtained because these metabolites rise when intracellular cobalamin is deficient.[86]

*Toxicology.* Heavy metal levels, particularly mercury levels, should be obtained in patients with a possible toxicologic exposure who have a proprioceptive loss.

#### Immunochemistry

*GALOP IgM Serum Antibody.* This antibody binds to a CNS myelin antigen that copurifies with myelin-associated glycoprotein.[116] Because the GALOP disorder is probably rare and its manifestations mimic common etiologic factors for gait impairment, the role of this test in the workup of patients with gait disorders needs further evaluation.[117] It should probably be reserved for patients with a slowly progressive ataxic neuropathy for which other causes have not been found.

*Anti-Hu Antibodies.* Anti-Hu antibodies should be obtained in patients with a subacute sensory neuronopathy. Many of these patients have paresthesias or dysesthesias, which are not as common in other peripheral neuropathies

with ataxia. Finding a positive titer of these antibodies encourages a search for the primary malignancy.

*Neurophysiology.* Although important for a thorough understanding of gait disorders, neurophysiologic testing has a limited value in clinical practice.

*Nerve Conduction Velocities.* Nerve conduction velocity testing may be helpful in documenting a thick-fiber peripheral neuropathy. Many of the disorders of peripheral nerves have common findings, with prolonged distal latencies and slow nerve conduction velocities. Normal motor nerve conduction velocities but absent sensory responses are noted in sensory neuronopathies.

*Somatosensory Evoked Responses and Motor Magnetic Stimulation.* Disorders with impaired proprioception typically delay the SERs. This test is generally not needed for the workup of a patient with gait disorders, but it may be helpful for assessing the degree of proprioception impairment in some patients. SERs have also been used to assess patients with cervical myelopathy. However, even in symptomatic patients, the sensitivity of SERs averages only about 75%.[9,124] A normal study does not rule out the disorder. In some hands motor evoked responses have been more sensitive.[90] Many neurosurgeons do not use evoked responses in the diagnosis or management of cervical spondylitic myelopathy, although the technique may help predict which patients are likely to have a faster recovery.[18]

*Visual Evoked Responses.* Abnormal visual evoked responses in a patient with a myelopathy increase the likelihood of demyelinating disease. This test may be helpful in patients with findings attributable to the cervical cord who have a stenotic lesion when the MRI appearance is atypical, for instance, showing a thickened, rather than thinned, cord.

*Posturography.* Posturography records the body sway of the person standing on a static platform (static posturography) or the movements of a person while the platform moves horizontally or vertically (dynamic posturography). Additionally, the sensory inputs to the person undergoing posturography can be modified to select balance strategies that rely primarily on visual, somatosensory, or vestibular information. Static posturography uses a static platform, or "force plate," to record vertical, and in some cases horizontal (shear), force exerted by the feet on the ground during upright stance. A computer records the forces for brief periods and stores the data. Subjects may stand with their eyes open or closed, and their feet may be together, apart, or in tandem or single-foot stance.

Dynamic posturography uses a similar force plate to record forces exerted by the feet, but the plate can move in the horizontal plane and rotate about an axis colinear with the ankles, thus pitching forward or backward. The rotational movement of the platform may be matched to the rotational movement of the subject, so that the angle between the foot and the lower leg remains constant, thereby removing proprioceptive clues. In addition, the platform is surrounded by a visual environment that can present disorienting visual clues. For instance, as the subject tilts forward, the visual environment may move forward at the same speed as the subject's body, giving the subject the impression that he or she is not tilting forward. When both proprioception and visual information are misleading, the subject needs to rely on vestibular information, unaltered by the testing equipment. Therefore dynamic posturography has been extensively used to assess vestibular function in patients with balance problems.

Dynamic posturography also allows for the measurement of the latency of responses the subject makes to destabilizing stimuli. For instance, in response to a toes-up movement of the platform, the subject will contract the anterior tibial muscle to effect a corrective forward movement of the leg and body that will keep him or her from falling backward. The latency of such a movement can be measured by (1) recording the onset of forward displacement of the center of force on the force plate; (2) recording EMG from the anterior tibial or other muscles, or (3) using motion sensors attached to the knees, hips, shoulders, or head.

In 1992 the American Academy of Neurology published a technical assessment on the clinical usefulness of posturography.[48] It concluded that posturography does not help localize lesions in the nervous system and does not help make a specific diagnosis. Although it was considered doubtful that static posturography would become an efficacious diagnostic test, dynamic posturography was considered promising for use in specialized environments dedicated to the analysis and management of vestibular dysfunction. Different conclusions were reached by an evaluation of the same technology that was approved by the American Academy of Otolaryngology–Head and Neck Surgery Foundation and published in 1997.[104] This assessment considers posturography an established test of postural stability, useful in a number of conditions:

1. Balance rehabilitation
2. Patients with disequilibrium for whom conventional tests are negative
3. Balance impairment after trauma
4. Return-to-work assessment for patients with vestibular or neurologic disorders
5. Individuals exposed to vestibulotoxic medications or substances
6. Patients with a history of falls and aging patients with disequilibrium
7. Patients who have a nonorganic sensation of imbalance

Regarding gait impairment in older adults, Baloh et al[12] concluded that posturography provided little information about the cause of the imbalance and did not correlate with the frequency of reported falls.

Dynamic posturography may help distinguish patients with psychogenic gait disorders or malingering from patients with imbalance resulting from vestibular disorders.[87] However, trained observers have done just as well in separating these two groups.[153] In summary, posturography may be helpful in further defining the sensory or motor components of a complex balance disorder. However, it will not define the specific location of the lesion in the neuraxis nor its etiologic basis.

***Magnetic Resonance Imaging and Computed Tomography.*** MRI has replaced CT as the test of choice for imaging many of the disorders causing gait disorders. For detailed discussions on the role of MRI in the workup of the different disorders for which it is helpful, the reader is referred to the corresponding section in this chapter. For instance, the applicability of MRI for the study of cervical myelopathy secondary to cervical spondylosis is discussed under cervical myelopathy.

### Spine

LUMBOSACRAL SPINE. For the workup of spinal claudication, MRI is not needed in most instances. CT will depict a narrow canal with crowding of the lateral recesses caused by facet hypertrophy. CT will also show the thickened ligamentum flavum and, possibly, calcification of the posterior longitudinal ligament. However, if CT is negative, MRI may be needed to rule out other lesions in the region of the cauda equina, such as a terminal filament ependymoma or a neurilemoma.

CERVICAL SPINE. MRI is the diagnostic tool of choice for the workup of patients with a clinical picture suggestive of cervical spondylosis[135,142] (Fig. 13–3*B*). Spin-echo sequences should be obtained, including T2-weighted images depicting any possible edema or microcavitation in the cord itself. At first glance, the recently popularized FLAIR sequence appears ideal for the study of changes within the cord because it combines the sensitivity for local water increase of a T2-weighted image with a background free of the bright signal of CSF. Although the FLAIR sequence has not been studied in this process, its lack of sensitivity for other lesions of the spinal cord may be a harbinger of poor results here also.[77,143,163]

### Brain

CEREBELLAR AND VESTIBULAR DISEASE. Cerebellar atrophy can be visualized with CT, but it is depicted with greater accuracy by MRI. In patients with symptoms of disorders such as olivo-ponto-cerebellar degeneration, the changes are so prominent that they can be easily visualized with CT. On the other hand, ischemic lesions in the cerebellum or vestibular nuclei are reliably seen only with MRI (see Fig. 13–2). Even MRI may be negative in the first few hours or even days after the event. T2-weighted images are most sensitive for the intraparenchymal changes. The FLAIR sequence is more sensitive than spin-echo T2-weighted sequences for supratentorial, but not infratentorial, ischemic lesions.[21] Because the location of an infarct can often be deduced from the clinical examination, MRI helps more by depicting the vascular changes than by showing the exact localization of the infarct. The most characteristic pattern in MRI of the posterior circulation is dissection of the vertebral artery. On T1-weighted images, a bright semilunar ring can be seen encircling the narrowed lumen of the vessel. Vessels occluded by local atheromatous changes or by emboli can be seen, as well as perforator occlusion by atheromatous plaques in the wall of the basilar artery. Changes in the vessel wall are best visualized by MRI, but MR angiography allows for three-dimensional visualization of the lumen of large to middle-sized vessels.

MRI is also the procedure of choice to image other potentially treatable lesions of the posterior fossa causing gait impairment, such as tumors (Fig. 13–9) or arteriovenous malformations.

LACUNAR DISEASE. Acutely, ischemic lacunar disease is poorly visualized by either CT or MRI. MRI is eventually more sensitive than CT for the detection of lacunes (Fig. 13–5*A*). Because lacunes can cause unexplained gait and balance impairment in an older adult, MRI of the brain should

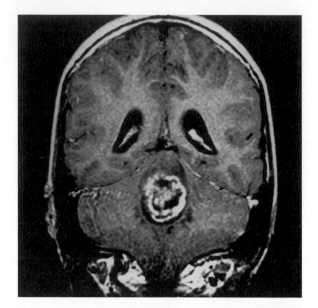

**FIGURE 13–9.** Cerebellar astrocytoma. Gadolinium-enhanced MRI of 14-year-old boy with progressive difficulty running.

be obtained a few days after an acute onset of balance or gait impairment. Depending on the location and extent of the lesion, it will be more likely related to either small vessel disease (lipohyalinosis, arteriosclerosis, CADASIL) or embolic. Giant lacunes are often embolic, but they seldom present with pure gait impairment, a frank hemiparesis being more common. The management of these lesions differs, and therefore a precise etiologic diagnosis is important. For ischemic lesions of the supratentorial compartment, FLAIR sequences are more sensitive than conventional spin-echo sequences.[21,113]

WHITE-MATTER DISEASE. White-matter disease of aging can be visualized either with CT or MRI[14,23] (Fig. 13–6A and B). Actually, MRI may be too sensitive for white-matter disease. High-intensity areas on T2-weighted MR are often undetected on CT. On T2-weighted MR images, it may be difficult to differentiate areas of increased water content caused by dilation of perivascular spaces with normal aging or transependymal CSF absorption from areas of tissue damage because both have increased intensity values.[7,164] For this reason it seems preferable to make the diagnosis of significant white-matter changes only when the abnormalities are visible

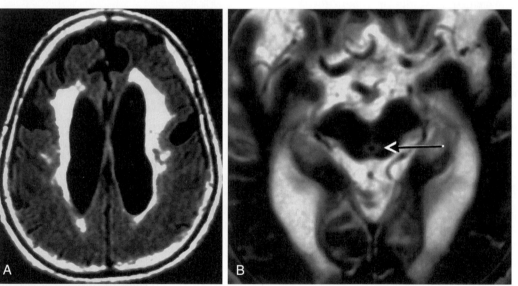

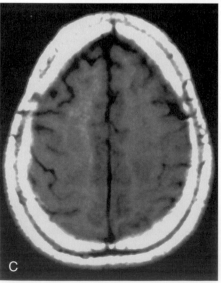

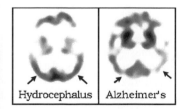

**FIGURE 13–10.** Hydrocephalus. MRI and SPECT of 71-year-old woman with gait impairment and incontinence that had progressed over 2-year period and worsened to point of patient being wheelchair bound for 3 months before neuroimaging studies were obtained. Cognition was preserved, except for mild impairment of executive functions and memory. **A,** FLAIR axial image at level of lateral ventricles. Note ventricular dilation, abnormal periventricular high signal, and dilation of interhemispheric fissure and central sulci. **B,** T2-weighted axial MRI at level of midbrain showing increased flow-void in sylvian aqueduct (*arrow*). Note enlargement of temporal horns and basal cisterns. **C,** T1-weighted axial MRI of same patient at high supraventricular level, showing compression of sulci at high frontoparietal region, near vertex. **D,** Patient's SPECT (*left*) is compared to SPECT of patient with Alzheimer's disease and large ventricles. Note preserved activity in parietotemporal association cortex (*arrows*) in patient with hydrocephalus but decreased perfusion in patient with Alzheimer's disease.

on T1-weighted images. However, there are no data available for exploring the functional significance of white-matter changes on only T2-weighted images vs. changes on both T2- and T1-weighted images. Proton-density images are also helpful. High-intensity changes on this sequence seem to correlate with the presence of gliosis, a pathologic finding in some patients with white-matter disease and gait disorder.[13]

HYDROCEPHALUS. Although hydrocephalus can be visualized with CT as well as with MRI, MRI shows CSF flow-related findings that may help separate hydrocephalus from communicating hydrocephalus (Fig. 13–10). The flow void in the sylvian aqueduct is prominent in patients with communicating hydrocephalus and decreases after shunting.[49,95] Bradley et al[19] studied CSF stroke volume and aqueductal CSF-flow void score before and after shunting. All 12 patients with CSF stroke volumes >42 μL responded favorably to CSF shunting. They and others failed to find a relationship between aqueductal CSF flow void score and responsiveness to shunting.[81] Because older subjects often have atrophy, the sulci at the base may be dilated, sometimes markedly, in communicating hydrocephalus (Fig. 13–10A and B). In some cases compression of the cortical sulci in the high convexity helps to define symptomatic hydrocephalus (Fig. 13–10C).

***Single Photon Emission Computed Tomography and Positron Emission Tomography.*** SPECT can be used to evaluate cerebral perfusion in patients with brain disorders. With PET, regional cerebral blood flow and metabolism can be measured. Both techniques can also be used to depict the regional density of a number of neurotransmitters. The role of these two procedures in the workup of patients with gait disorders is still in an investigational stage, except that the lower frontal to posterior perfusion ratio on SPECT was found to predict which patients with hydrocephalus will improve after shunting (Fig. 13–10D).[52] Patients with decreased perfusion in the parietotemporal association cortex are more likely to have Alzheimer's disease and enlarged ventricles caused by atrophy (Fig. 13–10D). This information is important because shunting at any age, and particularly in the elderly, is not without risk.[157]

After the standard workup of patients with gait disorders has been completed, about one fifth of them, or more, may be undiagnosed.[6,145] Because most of these patients have gait patterns suggestive of dysfunction of the control centers in the brain, it is logical to investigate for changes in these brain structures with techniques that are potentially more sensitive than MRI.[44] For this reason PET or SPECT may be used to image the medial frontal region, putamen, and lateral thalami to assess hypoperfusion changes or decreased metabolism that still has not resulted in structural changes. Multiple examples exist of the greater sensitivity of functional neuroimaging in degenerative disorders of the brain, including Huntington's chorea and Alzheimer's disease.[84] Nakamura et al[107] studied a group of 45 patients with Alzheimer disease at different clinical stages and 15 controls with *N*-isopropyl-p-[[123]I]iodoamphetamine SPECT. At a moderate stage, reduced mean values of cortical perfusion, particularly in the frontal lobe, were associated with increased postural sway, stride length variability, and decreased stride length. At a severe stage reduced perfusion in the basal ganglia and the frontal lobe also were associated with increased postural sway, double support time, stride length variability, and decreased walking speed and stride length.

## REFERENCES

1. Achiron A, Ziv I, Goren M, et al. Primary progressive freezing gait. *Mov Disord.* 1993;8:293-297.
2. Adams R, Fisher C, Hakim S, Ojemann R, Sweet W. Symptomatic occult hydrocephalus with "normal" cerebrospinal fluid pressure. *N Engl J Med.* 1965;273:117-126.
3. Albin R, Albers J, Greenberg H, et al. Acute sensory neuropathy-neuronopathy from pyridoxine overdose. *Neurology.* 1987;37:1729-1732.
4. Alexander JA, Sheppard S, Davis PC, Salverda P. Adult cerebrovascular disease: role of modified rapid fluid-attenuated inversion-recovery sequences. *AJNR.* 1996;17:1507-1513.
5. Anderson NE, Rosenblum MK, Graus F, Wiley RG, Posner JB. Autoantibodies in paraneoplastic syndromes associated with small-cell lung cancer. *Neurology.* 1988;38:1391-1398.
6. Atchison PR, Thompson PD, Frackowiak RS, Marsden CD. The syndrome of gait ignition failure: a report of six cases. *Mov Disord.* 1993; 8:285-292.
7. Awad I, Johnson P, Spetzler R, Hodak J. Incidental subcortical lesions identified on magnetic resonance imaging in the elderly. II. Postmortem pathological correlations. *Stroke.* 1986;17:1090-1097.
8. Awad I, Spetzler R, Hodak J, Awad C, Carey R. Incidental subcortical lesions identified on magnetic resonance imaging in the elderly. I. Correlation with age and cerebrovascular risk factors. *Stroke.* 1986;17: 1084-1089.
9. Baba H, Kawahara N, Tomita K, Imura S. Spinal cord evoked potentials in cervical and thoracic myelopathy. *Int Orthop.* 1993;17:82-86.
10. Baba H, Maezawa Y, Imura S, Kawahara N, Tomita K. Spinal cord evoked potential monitoring for cervical and thoracic compressive myelopathy. *Paraplegia.* 1996;34:100-106.
11. Baker S, Harvey A. Fall injuries in the elderly. In: Radebaugh T, Hadley E, Suzman R, ed. *Falls in the Elderly: Biologic and Behavioral Aspects.* Philadelphia: WB Saunders; 1985;1:501-512.
12. Baloh RW, Spain S, Socotch TM, Jacobson KM, Bell T. Posturography and balance problems in older people. *J Am Geriatr Soc.* 1995;43:638-644.
13. Baloh RW, Vinters HV. White matter lesions and disequilibrium in older people. II. Clinicopathologic correlation. *Arch Neurol.* 1995;52: 975-981.
14. Baloh RW, Yue Q, Socotch TM, Jacobson KM. White matter lesions and disequilibrium in older people. I. Case-control comparison. *Arch Neurol.* 1995;52:970-974.
15. Bastianello S, Bozzao A, Paolillo A, et al. Fast spin-echo and fast fluid-attenuated inversion-recovery versus conventional spin-echo sequences for MR quantification of multiple sclerosis lesions. *AJNR.* 1997;18:699-704.
16. Boon A, Lodder J, Heuts-van-Raak L, Kessels F. Silent brain infarcts in 755 consecutive patients with a first-ever supratentorial ischemic stroke: relationship with index-stroke subtype, vascular risk factors, and mortality. *Stroke.* 1994;25:2384-2390.
17. Boos N, Rieder R, Schade V, Spratt KF, Semmer N, Aebi M. 1995 Volvo Award in clinical sciences. The diagnostic accuracy of magnetic resonance imaging, work perception, and psychosocial factors in identifying symptomatic disc herniations. *Spine.* 1995;20:2613-2625.
18. Bouchard JA, Bohlman HH, Biro C. Intraoperative improvements of somatosensory evoked potentials: correlation to clinical outcome in surgery for cervical spondylitic myelopathy. *Spine.* 1996;21:589-594.
19. Bradley W Jr, Scalzo D, Queralt J, Nitz WN, Atkinson DJ, Wong P. Normal-pressure hydrocephalus: evaluation with cerebrospinal fluid flow measurements at MR imaging. *Radiology.* 1996;198:523-529.
20. Braffman B, Zimmerman R, Trojanowski J, et al. Pathologic correlation with gross and histopathology. 2. Hyperintense white-matter foci in the elderly. *AJNR.* 1988;9:629-636.
21. Brant-Zawadzki M, Atkinson D, Detrick M, Bradley WG, Scidmore G. Fluid-attenuated inversion recovery (FLAIR) for assessment of cerebral infarction: initial clinical experience in 50 patients. *Stroke.* 1996; 27:1187-1191.
22. Brennan RW, Bergland RM. Acute cerebellar hemorrhage: analysis of clinical findings and outcome in 12 cases. *Neurology.* 1977;27:527.
23. Briley DP, Wasay M, Sergent S, Thomas S. Cerebral white matter changes (leukoaraiosis), stroke, and gait disturbance. *J Am Geriatr Soc.* 1997;45:1434-1438.

24. Britton TC, Thompson PD, van der Kamp W, et al. Primary orthostatic tremor: further observations in six cases. *J Neurol.* 1992;239:209-217.

25. Brott T, Tomsick T, Feinberg W, et al. Baseline silent cerebral infarction in the Asymptomatic Carotid Atherosclerosis Study. *Stroke.* 1994;25:1122-1129.

26. Cambier J, Elghozi D, Strube E. Lésions du thalamus droit avec syndrome de l'hémisphère mineur: discussion du concept de négligence thalamique. *Rev Neurol (Paris).* 1980;136:105-116.

27. Caplan L, Schoene W. Clinical features of subcortical arteriosclerotic encephalopathy (Binswanger disease). *Neurology.* 1978;28:1206-1215.

28. Chabriat H, Vahedi K, Iba-Zizen MT, et al. Clinical spectrum of CADASIL: a study of 7 families—cerebral autosomal dominant arteriopathy with subcortical infarcts and leukoencephalopathy. *Lancet.* 1995;346:934-939.

29. Critchley M. On senile disorders of gait, including the so-called "senile paraplegia." *Geriatrics.* 1948;3:364-370.

30. Dalakas MC. Chronic idiopathic ataxic neuropathy. *Ann Neurol.* 1986;19:545-554.

31. Diener H, Nutt J. Vestibular and cerebellar disorders of equilibrium and gait. In: Masdeu J, Sudarsky L, Wolfson L, eds. *Gait Disorders of Aging: Falls and Therapeutic Strategies.* Philadelphia: Lippincott-Raven; 1997:261-272.

32. Dubas F, Gray F, Roullet E, Escourolle R. Leucoencéphalopathies artériopathiques (17 cas anatomo-cliniques). *Rev Neurol (Paris).* 1985;141:93-108.

33. Ducros A, Nagy T, Alamowitch S, et al. Cerebral autosomal dominant arteriopathy with subcortical infarcts and leukoencephalopathy, genetic homogeneity, and mapping of the locus within a 2-cM interval. *Am J Hum Genet.* 1996;58:171-181.

34. Dupuis M, Brucher J, Gonsette R. Observation anatomo-clinique d'une encéphalopathie sous-corticale artérioscléreuse ("maladie de Binswanger") avec hypodensité de la substance blanche au scanner cérébral. *Acta Neurol Belg.* 1984;84:131-140.

35. Fazekas F, Niederkorn K, Schmidt R, et al. White matter signal abnormalities in normal individuals: correlation with carotid ultrasonography, cerebral blood flow measurements, and cerebrovascular risk factors. *Stroke.* 1988;19:1285-1288.

36. Feasby T. Inflammatory-demyelinating polyneuropathies: a review of GBS and CIDP with analysis of clinical, laboratory and pathologic findings in these conditions. *Neurol Clin.* 1992;10:651-670.

37. Felice K, Keilson G, Schwartz W. 'Rubral' gait ataxia. *Neurology.* 1990;40:1004-1005.

38. Fife TD, Baloh RW. Disequilibrium of unknown cause in older people. *Ann Neurol.* 1993;34:694-702.

39. Fisher C. Hydrocephalus as a cause of disturbances of gait in the elderly. *Neurology.* 1982;32:1358-1363.

40. Fisher C, Cole M. Homolateral ataxia and crural paresis; a vascular syndrome. *J Neurol Neurosurg Psychiatry.* 1965;28:48-55.

41. FitzGerald P, Jankovic J. Lower body parkinsonism: evidence for vascular etiology. *Mov Disord.* 1987;4:249-260.

42. Frohman EM, Tusa R, Mark AS, Cornblath DR. Vestibular dysfunction in chronic inflammatory demyelinating polyneuropathy. *Ann Neurol.* 1996;39:529-535.

43. Fuh JL, Lin KN, Wang SJ, Ju TH, Chang R, Liu HC. Neurologic diseases presenting with gait impairment in the elderly. *J Geriatr Psychiatry Neurol.* 1994;7:89-92.

44. Fukuyama H, Ouchi Y, Matsuzaki S, et al. Brain functional activity during gait in normal subjects: a SPECT study. *Neurosci Lett.* 1997;228:183-186.

45. Gallucci M, Bozzao A, Splendiani A, Masciocchi C, Passariello R. Wernicke encephalopathy: MR findings in five patients. *AJNR.* 1990;11:887-892.

46. Garcia-Rill E. The pedunculopontine nucleus. *Prog Neurobiol.* 1991;36:363-389.

47. George A, de Leon M, Gentes C, et al. Leukoencephalopathy in normal and pathologic aging: CT of brain lucencies. *AJNR.* 1986;7:561-566.

48. George B, Zerah M, Lot G, Hurth M. Oblique transcorporeal approach to anteriorly located lesions in the cervical spinal canal. *Acta Neurochir (Wien).* 1993;121:187-190.

49. Gideon P, Stahlberg F, Thomsen C, Gjerris F, Sorensen PS, Henriksen O. Cerebrospinal fluid flow and production in patients with normal pressure hydrocephalus studied by MRI. *Neuroradiology.* 1994;36:210-215.

50. Giladi N, McMahon D, Przedborski S, et al. Motor blocks in Parkinson's disease. *Neurology.* 1992;42:333-339.

51. Goto K, Ishii N, Fukasawa H. Diffuse white-matter disease in the geriatric population: a clinical, neuropathological, and CT study. *Radiology.* 1981;141:687-695.

52. Graff-Radford N, Godersky J, Jones M. Variables predicting outcome in symptomatic hydrocephalus in the elderly. *Neurology.* 1989;39:1601-1604.

53. Graff-Radford N, Godersky J. A clinical approach to symptomatic hydrocephalus in the elderly. In: Masdeu J, Sudarsky L, Wolfson L, eds. *Gait Disorders of Aging: Falls and Therapeutic Strategies.* Philadelphia: Lippincott-Raven; 1997:245-259.

54. Grant IA, Hunder GG, Homburger HA, Dyck PJ. Peripheral neuropathy associated with sicca complex. *Neurology.* 1997;48:855-862.

55. Gray F, Dubas F, Roullet E, Escourolle R. Leukoencephalopathy in diffuse hemorrhagic cerebral amyloid angiopathy. *Ann Neurol.* 1985;18:54-59.

56. Groothuis D, Duncan G, Fisher C. The human thalamocortical sensory path in the internal capsule: evidence from a small capsular hemorrhage causing a pure sensory stroke. *Ann Neurol.* 1977;2:328-333.

57. Gutierrez-Molina M, Caminero Rodriguez A, Martinez Garcia C, Arpa Gutierrez J, Morales Bastos C, Amer G. Small arterial granular degeneration in familial Binswanger's syndrome. *Acta Neuropathol.* 1994;87:98-105.

58. Hachinski V, Potter P, Merskey H. Leuko-araiosis. *Arch Neurol.* 1987;44:21-23.

59. Hallett M, Stanhope S, Thomas S, Massaquoi S. Pathophysiology of posture and gait in cerebellar ataxia. In: Shimamura M, Grillner S, Edgerton V, eds. *Neurobiological Basis of Human Locomotion.* Tokyo: Japan Scientific Societies Press; 1991:275-283.

60. Haupt B, Graves E. Detailed diagnoses and surgical procedures for patients discharged from short-stay hospitals (1979). In: DHHS Pub. No. (PHS) 82-1274-1. Washington, DC: Department of Health and Human Services; 1982.

61. Healton EB, Savage DG, Brust JC, Garrett TJ, Lindenbaum J. Neurologic aspects of cobalamin deficiency. *Medicine.* 1991;70:229-245.

62. Healy JF, Healy BB, Wong WH, Olson EM. Cervical and lumbar MRI in asymptomatic older male lifelong athletes: frequency of degenerative findings. *J Comput Assist Tomogr* 1996;20:107-112.

63. Hendrie H, Farlow M, Austrom M, Edwards M, Williams M. Foci of increased T2 signal intensity on brain MR scans of healthy elderly subjects. *AJNR.* 1989;10:703-707.

64. Hennerici MG, Oster M, Cohen S, Schwartz A, Motsch L, Daffertshofer M. Are gait disturbances and white matter degeneration early indicators of vascular dementia? *Dementia.* 1994;5:197-202.

65. Herzog RJ, Wiens JJ, Dillingham MF, Sontag MJ. Normal cervical spine morphometry and cervical spinal stenosis in asymptomatic professional football players: plain film radiography, multiplanar computed tomography, and magnetic resonance imaging. *Spine.* 1991;16:S178-S186.

66. Huang C, Lui F. Ataxic-hemiparesis, localization and clinical features. *Stroke.* 1984;15:363-366.

67. Huang K, Wu L, Luo Y. Binswanger's disease: progressive subcortical encephalopathy or multi-infarct dementia? *Can J Neurol Sci.* 1985;12:88-94.

68. Iragui V, McCutchen C. Capsular ataxic hemiparesis. *Arch Neurol.* 1982;39:528-529.

69. Janota I. Dementia, deep white matter damage and hypertension: 'Binswanger's disease.' *Psychol Med.* 1981;11:39-48.

70. Jen J, Cohen AH, Yue Q, et al. Hereditary endotheliopathy with retinopathy, nephropathy, and stroke (HERNS). *Neurology.* 1997;49:1322-1330.

71. Jensen MC, Brant-Zawadzki MN, Obuchowski N, Modic MT, Malkasian D, Ross JS. Magnetic resonance imaging of the lumbar spine in people without back pain. *N Engl J Med.* 1994;331:69-73.

72. Johnson K, Davis K, Buonanno F, Brady T, Rosen T, Growdon J. Comparison of magnetic resonance and roentgen ray computed tomography in dementia. *Arch Neurol.* 1987;44:1075-1080.

73. Joutel A, Vahedi K, Corpechot C, et al. Strong clustering and stereotyped nature of Notch 3 mutations in CADASIL patients. *Lancet.* 1997;350:1511-1515.

74. Judge J. Resistance training. In: Masdeu J, Sudarsky L, Wolfson L, eds. *Gait Disorders of Aging: Falls and Therapeutic Strategies.* Philadelphia: Lippincott-Raven; 1997:381-393.

75. Kase CS, Norrving B, Levine SR, et al. Cerebellar infarction: clinical and anatomic observations in 66 cases. *Stroke.* 1993;24:76-83.

76. Keane J. Hysterical gait disorders. *Neurology.* 1989;39:586-589.

77. Keiper MD, Grossman RI, Brunson JC, Schnall MD. The low sensitivity of fluid-attenuated inversion-recovery MR in the detection of multiple sclerosis of the spinal cord. *AJNR.* 1997;18:1035-1039.

78. Kinkel W, Jacobs L, Polachini I, Bates V, Heffner RJ. Subcortical arteriosclerotic encephalopathy (Binswanger's disease): computed tomographic, nuclear magnetic resonance, and clinical correlations. *Arch Neurol.* 1985;42:951-959.

79. Kirkpatrick J, Hayman L. White-matter lesions on MR imaging of clinically healthy brains of elderly subjects: possible pathologic basis. *Radiology.* 1987;162:509-511.

80. Kosorok M, Omenn G, Diehr P, Koepsell T, Patrick D. Restricted activity days among older adults. *Am J Public Health.* 1992;82:1263-1267.

81. Krauss JK, Regel JP, Vach W, Jungling FD, Droste DW, Wakhloo AK. Flow void of cerebrospinal fluid in idiopathic normal pressure hydrocephalus of the elderly: can it predict outcome after shunting? *Neurosurgery.* 1997;40:67-73; discussion 73-74.

82. Labadie E, Awerbuch G, Hamilton R, Rapcsak S. Falling and postural deficits due to acute unilateral basal ganglia lesions. *Arch Neurol.* 1989; 261:492-496.

83. Laplane D, Escourolle R, Degos J, Sauron B, Massiou H. La négligence motrice d'origine thalamique: à propos de deux cas. *Rev Neurol (Paris).* 1982;138:201-211.

84. Leblhuber F, Brucker B, Reisecker F, et al. Single photon emission computed tomography in subjects at risk for Huntington's chorea. *J Neurol.* 1990;237:496-498.

85. Lempert T, Brandt T, Dieterich M, Huppert D. How to identify psychogenic disorders of stance and gait. *J Neurol.* 1991;238:140-146.

86. Lindenbaum J, Healton EB, Savage DG, et al. Neuropsychiatric disorders caused by cobalamin deficiency in the absence of anemia or macrocytosis. *N Engl J Med.* 1988;318:1720-1728.

87. Lipp M, Longridge NS. Computerised dynamic posturography: its place in the evaluation of patients with dizziness and imbalance. *J Otolaryngol.* 1994;23:177-183.

88. Lipsitz L, Jonsson P, Kelley M, Koestner J. Causes and correlates of recurrent falls in ambulatory frail elderly. *J Gerontol Med Sci.* 1991;46: M114-M122.

89. Lotz P, Ballinger W, Quisling R. Subcortical arteriosclerotic encephalopathy: CT spectrum and pathologic correlation. *AJR.* 1986;147: 1209-1214.

90. Maertens de Noordhout A, Remacle JM, Pepin JL, Born JD, Delwaide PJ. Magnetic stimulation of the motor cortex in cervical spondylosis. *Neurology.* 1991;41:75-80.

91. Mahoney R, Barthel D. Functional evaluation: the Barthel Index. *Maryland Med J.* 1965;14:61-65.

92. Malm J, Kristensen B, Karlsson T, Fagerlund M, Elfverson J, Ekstedt J. The predictive value of cerebrospinal fluid dynamic tests in patients with idiopathic adult hydrocephalus syndrome. *Arch Neurol.* 1995;52:783-789.

93. Marshall J. Cerebellar vascular syndromes. In: Toole J, ed. *Vascular Diseases.* Part III. New York: Elsevier; 1989:89-94.

94. Marshall V, Bradley W, Marshall C, Bhoopat T, Rhodes R. Deep white matter infarction: correlation of MR imaging and histopathologic findings. *Radiology.* 1988;167:517-522.

95. Mascalchi M, Arnetoli G, Inzitari D, et al. Cine-MR imaging of aqueductal CSF flow in normal pressure hydrocephalus syndrome before and after CSF shunt. *Acta Radiol.* 1993;34:586-592.

96. Masdeu J. Disorders of stance and gait. In: Greenberg J, ed. *Neuroimaging: A Companion to Adam's and Victor's Principles of Neurology.* New York: McGraw-Hill; 1995:25-40.

97. Masdeu J, Alampur U, Cavaliere R, Tavoulareas G. Astasia and gait failure with damage of the pontomesencephalic locomotor region. *Ann Neurol.* 1994;35:619-621.

98. Masdeu J, Gorelick P. Thalamic astasia: inability to stand after unilateral thalamic lesions. *Ann Neurol.* 1988;23:596-603.

99. Masdeu J, Wolfson L. Lower body (vascular) parkinsonism. *Arch Neurol.* 1990;47:748.

100. Masdeu J, Wolfson L, Lantos G, et al. White matter disease in the elderly prone to falling. *Arch Neurol.* 1989;46:1292-1296.

101. Mathias S, Nayak US, Isaacs B. Balance in elderly patients: the "get-up and go" test. *Arch Phys Med Rehabil.* 1986;67:387-389.

102. Matsuda Y, Miyazaki K, Tada K, et al. Increased MR signal intensity due to cervical myelopathy: analysis of 29 surgical cases. *J Neurosurg.* 1991;74:887-892.

103. Mokri B, Houser OW, Sandok BA, Piepgras DG. Spontaneous dissections of the vertebral arteries. *Neurology.* 1988;38:880.

104. Monsell EM, Furman JM, Herdman SJ, Konrad HR, Shepard NT. Computerized dynamic platform posturography. *Otolaryngol Head Neck Surg.* 1997;117:394-398.

105. Mori S. Neurophysiology of locomotion: recent advances in the study of locomotion. In: Masdeu J, Sudarsky L, Wolfson L, eds. *Gait Disorders of Aging: Falls and Therapeutic Strategies.* Philadelphia: Lippincott-Raven; 1997:55-78.

106. Murali R, Masdeu J. Cervical spondylotic myelopathy. In: Masdeu J, Sudarsky L, Wolfson L, eds. *Gait Disorders of Aging: Falls and Therapeutic Strategies.* Philadelphia: Lippincott-Raven; 1997:197-208.

107. Nakamura T, Meguro K, Yamazaki H, et al. Postural and gait disturbance correlated with decreased frontal cerebral blood flow in Alzheimer disease. *Alzheimer Dis Assoc Disord.* 1997;11:132-139.

108. Nashner L. Physiology of balance, with special reference to the healthy elderly. In: Masdeu J, Sudarsky L, Wolfson L, eds. *Gait Disorders of Aging: Falls and Therapeutic Strategies.* Philadelphia: Lippincott-Raven; 1997:37-53.

109. National Center for Health Statistics. *Current Estimates From the National Health Interview Survey, United States, 1986.* In: Vital and Health Statistics Series. Washington, DC: US Government Printing Office; 1987;10(164):16-52.

110. Nevitt M. Falls in the elderly: risk factors and prevention. In: Masdeu J, Sudarsky L, Wolfson L, eds. *Gait Disorders of Aging: Falls and Therapeutic Strategies.* Philadelphia: Lippincott-Raven; 1997:13-36.

111. Nevitt M, Cummings S, Kidd S, Black D. Risk factors for recurrent nonsyncopal falls: a prospective study. *JAMA.* 1989;261:2663-2668.

112. Newman G, Dovenmuehle R, Busse E. Alterations in neurologic status with age. *J Am Geriatr Soc.* 1960;8:915-917.

113. Noguchi K, Ogawa T, Inugami A, et al. MRI of acute cerebral infarction: a comparison of FLAIR and T2-weighted fast spin-echo imaging. *Neuroradiology.* 1997;39:406-410.

114. Nutt J, Marsden C, Thompson P. Human walking and higher-level gait disorders, particularly in the elderly. *Neurology.* 1993;43:268-279.

115. Pahwa R, Koller W. Gait disorders in parkinsonism and other movement disorders. In: Masdeu J, Sudarsky L, Wolfson L, eds. *Gait Disorders of Aging: Falls and Therapeutic Strategies.* Philadelphia: Lippincott-Raven; 1997:209-220.

116. Pestronk A. Chronic immune polyneuropathies and serum autoantibodies. In: Rolak L, Harati Y, eds. *Neuroimmunology for the Clinician.* Boston: Butterworth-Heinemann; 1997:237-251.

117. Pestronk A, Choksi R, Bieser K, et al. Treatable gait disorder and polyneuropathy associated with high titer serum IgM binding to antigens that copurify with myelin-associated glycoprotein. *Muscle Nerve.* 1994;17:1293-1300.

118. Quattrocolo G, Leombruni S, Vaula G, et al. Autosomal dominant late-onset leukoencephalopathy: clinical report of a new Italian family. *Eur Neurol.* 1997;37:53-61.

119. Rademaker G. The physiology of standing. In: Denny-Brown D, ed. Minneapolis: University of Minnesota Press; 1980.

120. Ray W, Griffin M. Prescribed medications, falling, and fall-related injuries. In: Weindruch R, Ory M, eds. *Frailty Reconsidered: Reducing Frailty and Fall-Related Injuries in the Elderly.* Springfield, Ill: Charles C Thomas; 1991:76-89.

121. Ray W, Griffin M, Baugh D. Mortality following hip fracture before and after implementation of the prospective payment system. *Arch Intern Med.* 1990;150:2109-2114.

122. Ray W, Griffin M, Schaffner W, et al. Psychotropic drug use and the risk of hip fracture. *N Engl J Med.* 1987;316:363-369.

123. Reich KA, Giansiracusa DF, Strongwater SL. Neurologic manifestations of giant cell arteritis. *Am J Med.* 1990;89:67-72.

124. Restuccia D, Valeriani M, Di Lazzaro V, Tonali P, Mauguiere F. Somatosensory evoked potentials after multisegmental upper limb stimulation in diagnosis of cervical spondylotic myelopathy. *J Neurol Neurosurg Psychiatry.* 1994;57:301-308.

125. Reul J, Gievers B, Weis J, Thron A. Assessment of the narrow cervical spinal canal: a prospective comparison of MRI, myelography and CT-myelography. *Neuroradiology.* 1995;37:187-191.

126. Rezek D, Morris J, Fulling K, Gado M. Periventricular white matter lucencies in senile dementia of the Alzheimer type and in normal aging. *Neurology.* 1987;37:1365-1368.

127. Robbins A, Rubenstein L, Josephson K, et al. Predictors of falls among elderly people: results of two population-based studies. *Arch Intern Med.* 1989;149:1628-1633.

128. Rosenberg G, Kornfeld M, Stovring J, Bicknell J. Subcortical arteriosclerotic encephalopathy (Binswanger): computerized tomography. *Neurology.* 1979;29:1102-1106.

129. Rovaris M, Yousry T, Calori G, Fesl G, Voltz R, Filippi M. Sensitivity and reproducibility of fast-FLAIR, FSE, and TGSE sequences for the MRI assessment of brain lesion load in multiple sclerosis: a preliminary study. *J Neuroimaging*. 1997;7:98-102.

130. Rubenstein L, Josephson K. Interventions to reduce the multifactorial risks for falling. In: Masdeu J, Sudarsky L, Wolfson L, eds. *Gait Disorders of Aging: Falls and Therapeutic Strategies*. Philadelphia: Lippincott-Raven; 1997:309-326.

131. Rubio A, Rifkin D, Powers JM, et al. Phenotypic variability of CADASIL and novel morphologic findings. *Acta Neuropathol*. 1997; 94:247-254.

132. Ruchoux MM, Maurage CA. CADASIL: cerebral autosomal dominant arteriopathy with subcortical infarcts and leukoencephalopathy. *J Neuropathol Exp Neurol*. 1997;56:947-964.

133. Sabbadini G, Francia A, Calandriello L, et al. Cerebral autosomal dominant arteriopathy with subcortical infarcts and leucoencephalopathy (CADASIL): clinical, neuroimaging, pathological and genetic study of a large Italian family. *Brain*. 1995;118:207-215.

134. Sabin T. Peripheral neuropathy: disorders of proprioception. In: Masdeu J, Sudarsky L, Wolfson L, eds. *Gait Disorders of Aging: Falls and Therapeutic Strategies*. Philadelphia: Lippincott-Raven; 1997:273-282.

135. Sadasivan KK, Reddy RP, Albright JA. The natural history of cervical spondylotic myelopathy. *Yale J Biol Med*. 1993;66:235-242.

136. Sage J, Lepore F. Ataxic hemiparesis from lesions of the corona radiata. *Arch Neurol*. 1983;40:449-450.

137. Sand J, Biller J, Corbett J, Adams H, Dunn V. Partial dorsal mesencephalic hemorrhages: report of three cases. *Neurology*. 1986;36:529-533.

138. Satake M, Yoshimura T, Iwaki T, Yamada T, Kobayashi T. Anti-dorsal root ganglion neuron antibody in a case of dorsal root ganglionitis associated with Sjögren's syndrome. *J Neurol Sci*. 1995;132:122-125.

139. Sattin R, Huber D, DeVito C, et al. The incidence of fall injury events among the elderly in a defined population. *Am J Epidemiol*. 1990;131: 1028-1037.

140. Savage RA, Whitehouse GH, Roberts N. The relationship between the magnetic resonance imaging appearance of the lumbar spine and low back pain, age and occupation in males. *Eur Spine J*. 1997;6:106-114.

141. Schroth G, Wichmann W, Valavanis A. Blood-brain-barrier disruption in acute Wernicke encephalopathy: MR findings. *J Comput Assist Tomogr*. 1991;15:1059-1061.

142. Statham PF, Hadley DM, Macpherson P, Johnston RA, Bone I, Teasdale GM. MRI in the management of suspected cervical spondylotic myelopathy. *J Neurol Neurosurg Psychiatry*. 1991;54:484-489.

143. Stevenson VL, Gawne-Cain ML, Barker GJ, Thompson AJ, Miller DH. Imaging of the spinal cord and brain in multiple sclerosis: a comparative study between fast FLAIR and fast spin echo. *J Neurol*. 1997;244: 119-124.

144. Studenski S, Duncan P, Chandler J, et al. Predicting falls: the role of mobility and nonphysical factors. *J Am Geriatr Soc*. 1994;42:297-302.

145. Sudarsky L. Clinical approach to gait disorders of aging: an overview. In: Masdeu J, Sudarsky L, Wolfson L, eds. *Gait Disorders of Aging: Falls and Therapeutic Strategies*. Philadelphia: Lippincott-Raven; 1997:147-157.

146. Sudarsky L, Ronthal M. Gait disorders among elderly patients. *Arch Neurol*. 1983;40:740-743.

147. Sudarsky L, Tideiksaar R. The cautious gait, fear of falling, and psychogenic gait disorders. In: Masdeu J, Sudarsky L, Wolfson L, eds. *Gait Disorders of Aging: Falls and Therapeutic Strategies*. Philadelphia: Lippincott-Raven; 1997:283-295.

148. Tajima Y, Mito Y, Owada Y, Tsukishima E, Moriwaka F, Tashiro K. Neurological manifestations of primary Sjögren's syndrome in Japanese patients. *Intern Med*. 1997;36:690-693.

149. Tang XF, Ren ZY. Magnetic transcranial motor and somatosensory evoked potentials in cervical spondylitic myelopathy. *Chin Med J (Engl)*. 1991;104:409-415.

150. Tell GS, Lefkowitz DS, Diehr P, Elster AD. Relationship between balance and abnormalities in cerebral magnetic resonance imaging in older adults. *Arch Neurol*. 1998;55:73-79.

151. Thompson P, Marsden C. Gait disorder of subcortical arteriosclerotic encephalopathy: Binswanger's disease. *Mov Disord*. 1987;2:1-8.

152. Tinetti ME. Performance-oriented assessment of mobility problems in elderly patients. *J Am Geriatr Soc*. 1986;34:119-126.

153. Uimonen S, Laitakari K, Kiukaanniemi H, Sorri M. Does posturography differentiate malingerers from vertiginous patients? *J Vestib Res*. 1995;5:117-124.

154. van Swieten JC, Geyskes GG, Derix MM, et al. Hypertension in the elderly is associated with white matter lesions and cognitive decline. *Ann Neurol*. 1991;30:825-830.

155. Verma A, Maheshwari M. Hypoesthetic-ataxic-hemiparesis in thalamic hemorrhage. *Stroke*. 1986;17:49-51.

156. Victor M, Adams R, Mancall E. A restricted form of cerebellar cortical degenerative occurring in alcoholic patients. *Arch Neurol*. 1959;1:577-588.

157. Weiner HL, Constantini S, Cohen H, Wisoff JH. Current treatment of normal-pressure hydrocephalus: comparison of flow-regulated and differential-pressure shunt valves. *Neurosurgery*. 1995;37:877-884.

158. Weis E Jr. Abnormal magnetic-resonance scans of the cervical spine in asymptomatic subjects. *J Bone Joint Surg Am*. 1991;73:1113.

159. Wilkinson I, Russell R. Arteries of the head and neck in giant cell arteritis. *Arch Neurol*. 1972;27:378-391.

160. Woollacott M, Shumway-Cook A. Clinical and research methodology for the study of posture and balance. In: Masdeu J, Sudarsky L, Wolfson L, eds. *Gait Disorders of Aging: Falls and Therapeutic Strategies*. Philadelphia: Lippincott-Raven; 1997:107-121.

161. Yamanouchi H. Loss of white matter oligodendrocytes and astrocytes in progressive subcortical vascular encephalopathy of Binswanger type. *Acta Neurol Scand*. 1991;83:301-305.

162. Yone K, Sakou T, Yanase M, Ijiri K. Preoperative and postoperative magnetic resonance image evaluations of the spinal cord in cervical myelopathy. *Spine*. 1992;17:S388-S392.

163. Yousry TA, Filippi M, Becker C, Horsfield MA, Voltz R. Comparison of MR pulse sequences in the detection of multiple sclerosis lesions. *AJNR*. 1997;18:959-963.

164. Zimmerman R, Fleming C, Lee B, Saint-Louis L, Deck M. Periventricular hyperintensity as seen by magnetic resonance: prevalence and significance. *AJR*. 1986;146:443-450.

# 14

# Neurolaryngology

*David B. Rosenfield and Nagalapura S. Viswanath*

This chapter discusses the differential diagnosis and testing of patients with abnormal speech. Speech, a priori, is motor output. It reflects the motor execution of verbal communication, and in that regard it is (clinically) independent of language (e.g., word choice, syntax, selection of appropriate sounds) compromise, which is the hallmark of aphasia. Patients with dysarthria, dysphonia, or dysfluency may have disturbance of speech without any compromise of language.

Speech is produced by a complex interaction of neuromuscular systems, including respiration, laryngeal activity, and articulation. These systems are controlled by the brain and therefore are subject to perturbations and disruptions resulting from neurologic disease. Weakness of the articulators, respiratory system, or laryngeal system can disrupt speech production, as can movement disorders. The result may be difficulty in formulating correct sounds or disturbance in their fluent production.

Before proceeding with a discussion of speech disorders, we will briefly review the basic mechanisms of speech production. These mechanisms have clinical relevance in understanding how neuraxis compromise can cause abnormalities in the sounds we produce.

## NORMAL SPEECH MOTOR PRODUCTION

In order to be effective in communication, speech requires high-fidelity transfer of a message from the speaker's brain to the listener's brain. The execution of the motor output program involves intricate movements of respiratory, laryngeal, and articulative structures that produce sound waves, which vary in time (i.e., time-varying acoustic patterns). The output is not a linear concatenation of a motor pattern underlying segments of phonation (phonemes) produced in isolation. Rather, there is a smooth blending of movements across different segments of output, such that movements at the end of one segment blend into those of another, providing the necessary ingredients for intonation and linguistic stress (i.e., suprasegmental features).[5,9]

This complex process is controlled by the brain. The larynx provides the sound source, but the manipulation underlying laryngeal function and the subsequent changes of the sound waves it produces, are all under cerebral control.[5,9,14]

Speech normally occurs during expiration, beginning with relaxation of diaphragm muscles and contraction of internal intercostal muscles. The external intercostal muscles counteract the internal intercostals, prolonging the expiratory phase. When the expiratory phase begins, the vocal folds move toward the midline, decreasing the size of the glottis (the opening between the vocal folds, also known as the "glottal chink"). Vocal fold movement to the midline primarily results from contraction of the interarytenoid muscles, located in the posterior aspect of the vocal folds. When these muscles contract, the vocal folds are approximated.[5]

As air pressure below the glottis (subglottal pressure) increases, it exceeds the pressure above the vocal folds (supraglottic pressure) and the impedance of the approximated folds, causing the vocal folds to separate (abduct). Rapid flow of air through the now-separated folds causes a "negative" pressure in the glottis, producing the Bernoulli effect. This aerodynamic effect, coupled with the natural elasticity of the muscles comprising the vocal folds, causes them to readduct toward the midline. This process then occurs again, resulting in a to-and-fro vocal fold motion that produces sound output. The number of times that the folds cycle to and fro per second is described in cycles per second (hertz), which defines the fundamental frequency of the acoustic wave produced. The degree of vocal movement of the folds from the center, before reabducting forces prevail, corresponds to the amplitude or intensity of the signal produced. An adult male vibrates the vocal folds during speech between 100 and 150 Hz; the adult female, 200 and 250 Hz.[1,5]

The preceding description is known as the neuro-muscular-aerodynamic theory of phonation. The resulting "fundamental frequency" reflects the subglottal pressure (an increase of which usually causes increased fundamental frequency and intensity) and the length and tension of the vocal folds. Pitch is the clinical correlate of fundamental frequency.[5]

The larynx consists of several muscles, all but one of which are adductors. Contraction of each muscle has a

This work was supported by the Lowin Medical Research Foundation and the M.R. Bauer Foundation.

unique effect on the distribution of mass within the vocal fold; it also alters the position and shape of the edge of the vocal fold. Thus each of the several laryngeal muscles has a different effect on phonation. These muscles are all striated, and each receives neural input from the central and peripheral nervous systems.[7,16]

The production of sound (phonation) requires appropriate stiffness/slackness of laryngeal vocal folds, a finite dimension of the laryngeal opening, and a specific volume and velocity of air moving through that opening. A narrow range of values exists for these three variables to initiate and maintain phonation.[8,22] Compromise of any of these variables (e.g., dystonia, tremor, weakness, slowed movements) can alter sound output. This is a very sensitive system, and clinically it is subject to minimal perturbations. Mild laryngeal tremor can produce major symptoms, as can minimal disruption of the mucosa or weakness of the respiratory or laryngeal muscles.

The source-filter theory of speech production purports that a "spectrum" of sound waves is produced at the source of the sound production (i.e., the glottis) and subsequently it is modified (filtered) as the waves traverse the space (resonant cavities) that lies above the glottis. This filtering alters the relative distribution of energy within the component frequencies (Fourier's theorem permits a complex wave being analyzed into component frequencies), creating unique sound entities called vowels. Each vowel has a particular set of spectral (e.g., energy) peaks and is dependent on the shape of the cavity above the glottis. The relationship between the first two spectral peaks, referred to as the first and second formant frequencies, is sufficient to determine the identity of each vowel.[1,5]

One can easily demonstrate the relationship between these cavities and the vowels on oneself. Make a long "ah" sound, then lower the jaw, and then raise it. Simultaneously, move the tongue into various positions and move the lips. Note that the sounds change, covering a large expanse of vowel sounds, without changing the vibrations within the larynx.

Vowel production also requires the shutting off of the nasal cavity from the oral cavity and the alteration of the shape of the oral cavity by moving the tongue, lips, and jaw. Elevating the soft palate, thus separating the nasal cavity from the oral cavity, is performed through contraction of the levator palatini and superior cricopharyngeal muscles. Weakness of these muscles produces hypernasality of the vowel sounds. Obstruction of the nasal cavity (e.g., rhinitis) produces hyponasality.[5]

The source-filter theory also explains the production of consonants. Some consonants are turbulent noise sounds, shaped by constricting air passage in the oral cavity (e.g., /s/ and /ch/ sounds), whereas others employ two separate sources of sound (e.g., the "quasi-periodic" sounds from the glottis and the constriction noise in the oral cavity, such as the /z/ and /th/ sounds).[5]

The spectral differences (the location of the different energies in their respective parts of the sound waves) among the different significant sounds (referred to as phonemes) of any human language can be described in terms of the source of the sound and the changing configuration of the cavities through which those sound waves must travel. However, there are other differences among sounds that result from differences in the timing of brief movements ("gestures")

within the laryngeal and oromotor subsystems of the speech motor control system. This principle is best illustrated by describing the six "stop consonants" (/p/, /b/, /t/, /d/, /k/, /g/).[5]

The stop consonants are so named because of their shared manner of production. They are achieved by elevating the soft palate, shutting off the nasal cavity from the oral cavity. Further, the breath stream is stopped for a brief interval (approximately 250 milliseconds), resulting in increased supraglottal pressure, and then suddenly released.[5]

Two features of this production denote the differences among the six stop consonants. The first feature is the place of articulation, which is the point at which the vocal tract is closed to stop the breath stream. For /p/ and /b/, the lips are closed (therefore the sounds are referred to as "bilabials"). For /t/ and /d/, contact is made between the tip of the tongue and the alveolus (referred to as "alveolars"). For /k/ and /g/, contact is between the back of the tongue and the soft palate, known as the velum (hence "velars"). The acoustic consequence of different places of articulation is reflected in differences in the intensities of component frequencies of the sounds at the instant of the air release, which is when the sound is produced.[5]

The importance of timing in engendering segmental or phonemic differences is illustrated by a feature that distinguishes how pairs of stop consonants with the same place of articulation are realized (e.g., pairs /p/ and /b/, /t/ and /d/, and /k/ and /g/). The first of each pair is traditionally referred to as "voiceless," and the second as "voiced." An important acoustic difference between these voiced and voiceless stops occurs when they appear at the beginning of a word (e.g., contrast "pin" vs. "bin"); there is a difference between the timing and sequential arrangement of the upper articulatory "release" and the onset of vocal fold vibrations. If the vocal folds vibrate before release, are coincidental with release, or follow release within a brief interval, voiced stops are produced. On the other hand, if vocal fold vibrations begin after release but are delayed beyond a brief interval, voiceless stops are produced.[1,5]

Thus, if voicing begins within 15 to 20 milliseconds after release, /b/ is heard. However, if voicing begins after 20 ms, /p/ is heard. Thus precise timing is essential for the distinction between the stop pairs.[1,5]

Because of their clinical importance, the three nasal consonants (/m/, /n/, and /ng/) also require discussion. The important element in the manner of production of these nasals is that the air stream is simultaneously directed through the nasal and oral cavities. The consonant /m/ is similar to /b/ as well as /p/ in that they are all bilabial; /n/ is similar to /t/ and /d/ because they are alveolar; /ng/ (the last sound in "going") is velar, as are /k/ and /g/. All nasals are voiced sounds, that is, there is continuous vocal fold activity during their production. The differences and similarities between nasals and stops is important for knowing how to evaluate patients with a weak velum.[1,5]

The preceding discussion provides a brief overview of the speech production process. Throughout the production of these sounds, there is a rich tapestry of feedback within the speech motor control system, involving input from the auditory, tactile, and kinesthetic systems. All these systems are controlled by the brain and its neural output and input. Disturbance of these systems can produce dysarthria, dysphonia, or dysfluency.

Most clinicians view dysarthria as resulting from neurologic compromise of the articulators and dysphonia as being caused by focal disruption of the laryngeal sound source. Although dysphonia can reflect neurologic or mechanical compromise to the sound production system, dysphonia actually is a dysarthria.

## SYMPTOMS

Complete a full neurologic history (including family history for movement disorders, motor neuron disease, neuropathy, myopathy, myasthenia) regarding nonspeech but neurologic abnormalities. If there is suspicion of other symptoms that indicate compromise of the neuraxis, suspect a similar problem for the patient's speech complaints.

Assess whether the patient has a problem in language or speech, or both. If the patient uses incorrect words or has problems with syntax or comprehension, suspect language compromise. This necessitates that the patient be evaluated for brain disease (usually cortical left hemisphere). Even if there is associated speech compromise, the presence of language disturbance mandates an evaluation for aphasia, including consideration of stroke, infection, and tumor. If there is a complaint of altered speech but not language compromise, the focus is on identifying what level of the neuraxis is disrupted and what diseases are suspect.

Ask about the specific problem that the patient has with his or her voice. In particular, ask whether it "gets stuck," shakes, or improves with alcohol. (All these suggest tremor.) Is the speech weak, hypernasal, lacking appropriate stresses in the sentence, associated with short rushes, or slurred? (All these imply neurologic dysfunction.) Improvement after resting a few minutes suggests neuromuscular junction dysfunction. Has the patient seen an otolaryngologist, and, if so, does the patient have a videotape of his or her larynx during ongoing speech?[14]

Inquire whether the patient has had any recent trauma (including trauma to the neck) or undergone intubation. Trauma can cause dislocation or distortion of the posterior portion of the vocal folds (dislocated arytenoid cartilage). Intubation can also cause focal laryngeal mucosa damage and focal nerve compromise.[2]

If the patient's voice is hoarse or raspy without a sensation of strain, suspect vocal abuse (e.g., screaming at a rock concert) or voice misuse (e.g., lecturing to a class). Inquire whether the patient has problems with swallowing (e.g., nasal regurgitation, aspiration, frequent pneumonia, choking on food), which can suggest neurologic compromise.[14]

Ask about the onset of the speech disturbance. Organically induced speech motor disturbances usually have a gradual onset, unless they result from stroke. Psychogenic disturbances frequently present with an abrupt onset. Is the speech abnormality always present? Neurologic causes of abnormal speech production are rarely associated with episodes of true normality. Although the patient may state that at times his or her speech is normal, careful questioning usually reveals that the speech is more normal at some times than at others (e.g., less abnormal) but is never truly normal. A patient who does have intermittent periods of true normality is more likely to have a psychogenic disturbance.[14]

Augmentation of speech disturbance when the patient is under stress is not a helpful sign for differentiating organic from nonorganic disease. Speech motor output is a finely controlled motor system that is very sensitive to one's emotional milieu.[14]

Is there laryngeal pain or discomfort when the patient is not talking? Most speech motor disruptions are not associated with laryngeal pain during silence. When pain is present, suspect a focal laryngeal pathologic condition or acid reflux involving the vocal folds.

Patients with gastroesophageal reflux may present with voice symptoms. These patients need not have obvious signs of reflux and may only occasionally have reflux. When an acidic agent makes contact with the vocal folds, even only intermittently, it can cause laryngeal discomfort and damage the mucosa, producing dysphonia or strained, hoarse speech. Suspect acid reflux if the patient complains of heartburn or an intermittent sour taste in the mouth.

When patients complain of a strained sensation or any type of pain while talking, consider spasmodic dysphonia and its accompanying differential diagnoses, including tremor and dystonia. Remember that a sensation of tightness and strain may reflect the patient's coping strategies in dealing with the underlying sound production deficit. Encourage the patient to speak without these maneuvers, which might then cause production of glottal stops (staccato-like catches) and phonation tremor.[13,15]

The inability to produce anything but a whispered voice can be seen in bilateral vagal compromise, vocal fold lesions, abductor spasmodic dysphonia, or psychogenic aphonia. If an aphonic patient has normal cough or laughter, this does not mandate a psychogenic cause. To make a definitive diagnosis of functional aphonia, one should have bona fide evidence of a conversion reaction. One can have a functional disorder and not meet these criteria, but it is then difficult to be certain about the diagnosis.[13–15]

## SIGNS

There is an expanding literature on the acoustic structure of human speech, which can be parsed into signs for examination. Further, there are descriptions of how dysfunction of each cranial nerve impacts speech output. Too often, these analyses are nonpractical, and the neurologist's auditory perceptual acumen is nonsophisticated in their detection. The following discussion is based on a practical and focused examination, directed at ascertaining disease processes.

Perform a full neurologic examination, in addition to examining the patient's speech. If there is evidence of neurologic compromise in the nonspeech domain (e.g., tremor, dystonia, neuropathy, myopathy, brain disease), suspect similar abnormality in the domain of speech. During the examination of speech, presumably done in part during the patient's account of the history of complaints, listen for evidence of strain, tremor, weakness, slurring, harshness, and hypernasality.

Ask the patient to produce an /a/ sound in a slow, easy mode and to increase slowly, and then decrease slowly, the pitch. This should be done effortlessly, without signs of tremor or "voice arrest," which can imply vocal fold nonoscillation resulting from underlying tremor. Encourage the patient not to use any coping strategies when doing this maneuver. Often, patients bear down and strain when they have underlying phonatory tremor, which masks the tremor and produces a nontremor speech pattern in sound output.

When the patient attempts to sustain the /a/ sound, flaccid laryngeal muscles will produce a breathy sound and decreased volume. Unilateral vocal fold weakness produces a voice that is less breathy but more hoarse than does bilateral vocal fold paralysis. Diplophonia, the simultaneous production/perception of two separate pitches, is common in unilateral vocal cord paralysis, but its phonatory basis is poorly understood. Patients with bilateral vocal cord paralysis can have inspiratory stridor.[13–15]

Strained/strangled hoarseness with vowel prolongation can indicate hyperadduction of the vocal cords. This can result from spasmodic dysphonia or increased tone (upper motor neuron lesions), or it may reflect the patient's coping strategy for trying to overcome the speech deficit produced by underlying tremor or mild weakness. The coexistence of pseudobulbar crying or laughing suggests bilateral upper motor neuron damage.[13,15]

Ask the patient to cough. If the cough is a weak, explosive sound, the patient may have vocal adductor weakness. The sound of the cough is usually minimally compromised in unilateral vocal cord paralysis (results in abduction) from recurring laryngeal nerve damage; it is very compromised (reduced) with higher unilateral vagal lesions above the take-off of the superior laryngeal nerve. Bilateral vagal lesions at this level cause a defective or absent cough and are often associated with aspiration.[14,18]

Ask the patient to say, "Ambling along rainy island avenue." This is an all-voiced phrase that usually increases sound abnormalities associated with tremor and dysphonia. Also, ask the patient to say, "He saw half a seashell." This sentence requires several abductor/adductor movements of the vocal folds and increases the speech disturbance associated with abductor spasmodic dysphonia.[14]

Is the volume normal? Does it vary? Is there a hypernasal component? Evaluate the latter by asking the patient to repeat "Coca-cola" several times. Listen carefully for hypernasality. Disturbances in these domains all reflect neurologic disease.[13–15]

Since speech is viewed as a motor output, assess it just as you would the other motor functions, such as tapping one's finger. The neurologist is interested in power, rapidity, and dexterity of movements, as well as other functions. The repetitive assessment of the /pa/, /ta/, /ka/ sounds offers good assessment of articulatory dynamics. Just as rapid finger tapping can produce stigmata of cerebellar dysfunction (e.g., irregular tapping) as well as upper motor neuron compromise (slow but regular rate), so do the repetitive utterances of these sounds.[8,13,18]

The clarity of the /pa/ sound, in addition to reflecting adequate respiratory and phonatory power, depends on good orbicularis oris power (cranial nerve [CN] VII). The crispness of /ta/ depends on distal genioglossus strength (CN XII), and, likewise, the /ka/ reflects posterior tongue strength, as well as palate strength (CN IX, X, XII). These sounds all depend on appropriate laryngeal (phonatory) support, inclusive of adequate respiratory flow, as well as appropriate mandibular movement. Air wastage through the nares (which will cause a mirror held under the nostrils to fog) suggests palate weakness.[8,13,18]

The sounds should be crisp and clear, with normal volume, and the rate should be regular and fast. A slow but rhythmic rate implies bilateral upper motor neuron com-

promise. An irregularly irregular rhythm applies cerebellar disease. It is important to test these sounds with both a fast rate and a slow rate. Rapid rate can fatigue the muscles; slow rate may not. Patients with weak palate muscles may substitute /ba/ for /pa/, proceeding to /ma/. Similarly, weak palate muscles can change /ta/ into /da/ and then /na/, and /ka/ can become /ga/ and then /nga/. These changes reflect acoustic consequences of aerodynamic changes.[8,13,18]

The patient should be able to elevate the palate normally and symmetrically, without tremor or myoclonus. The patient should also be able to apply good pressure from the tongue against the interior of the cheek. Fasciculations, atrophy, and anteroposterior furrows of the tongue suggest lower motor neuron compromise. Unilateral CN XII damage causes deviation to the afflicted side on attempted protrusion but rarely causes major speech compromise. Bilateral involvement of CN XII produces severe dysarthria, distorting virtually all lingual consonants (e.g., /l/, /r/).[8]

The patient should be able to pucker the lips (CN VII) well and have enough power in the cheeks (CN VII) to permit applying significant air pressure against pursed lips without leakage. Unilateral lower motor neuron facial weakness can cause the mouth to droop and the cheek to bulge when this procedure is attempted, as well as during the production of "plosive" sounds (e.g., /p/, /b/). Usually, the intact opposite side provides sufficient compensation during compression of the lips, resulting in a mild deficit. However, bilateral facial nerve damage causes the lips to bulge markedly during plosive sound production, resulting in severe speech deficit. Weakness of the lower lip can result in compromise of labiodental fricatives (e.g., /f/, /v/).[14]

Damage to the motor division of CN V produces mandible weakness, compromising tongue and lower lip approximation to the upper lip, teeth, and hard palate. Unilateral lesions seldom disrupt normal speech, but bilateral lesions severely affect all speech sounds. Be certain to test the jaw jerk. If this is exaggerated, suspect bilateral upper motor neuron damage above the pons.[14]

Spasticity resulting from bilateral corticobulbar tract lesions can cause slow rate and a harsh, strained output. The consonants and vowels are imprecise, and pitch can be low (some patients strain, producing high pitch) and monotonous. Phrases are short, stresses within the sentence are inappropriate, and volume is poorly controlled and often loud. Frequently, the speech is hypernasal. Also, the patient may demonstrate inappropriate crying and laughter (pseudobulbar palsy).[14]

Cerebellar lesions can also cause abnormalities in contextual speech, producing irregular random breaks in articulation, vowel distortions, excesses in stress, prolongation of sounds, increased intervals between words, varying degrees of harshness, and decreased rate. Cerebellar speech is different among cerebellum-afflicted patients, and therefore it is often difficult to ascertain. When cerebellar abnormalities are suspected, check the arms, midline, and legs of the patient carefully for other signs of cerebellar disturbance.[14]

Hypokinetic dysarthria, typically noted in Parkinson's disease, can produce short rushes of speech, increased rate, monopitch, decreased volume, monoloudness, altered stress, breathiness, imprecise consonants, harshness, low pitch, and palilalia. It is rare for a patient to have speech disruption from bradykinesia without stigmata of neurologic dysfunction elsewhere being noted on examination (e.g., cogwheeling, rigidity, masked facies, festinating gait, resting tremor).[14]

Dysarthria can also be associated with hyperkinetic movement disturbances. The type of speech abnormality depends on the etiologic basis. The most prominent findings are variable rate, inappropriate silences, and irregular distortion of consonants, vowels, and volume. Usually, the patient has obvious evidence of the hyperkinesis on examination.

Test for oral apraxia. This condition is associated with lesions that are located anteriorly, approximating Broca's area. It can also be associated with cortical-basal-ganglionic degeneration, one of the Parkinson-plus syndromes. Affected patients often cannot follow commands requiring them to pretend to kiss, suck, stick out their tongue, or lick crumbs off their lips. Often, especially early in the disease course, their language deficits are nonexistent or very subtle, and they have difficulty in producing their intended speech targets. They complain of difficulty with speech production and are very frustrated.[19,23]

The preceding maneuvers are used to screen the neurologic axis for deficits in speech production. However, the perceptual-acoustic-physiologic relationships are far more complex. Despite a certain homogeneity of perceptual dimensions for any particular type of dysarthria, a wide variety of movement in motor control problems can exist for any member of that group. The etiologic relationships have not yet been established between perceptual-acoustic dimensions or neurologic signs (e. g., flaccidity, rigidity, spasticity) and associated motor control problems.[5,7–9,14]

## CLINICAL SYNDROMES

### DYSARTHRIA

If a patient has symptoms or signs suggesting phonation compromise, whether the cause is related to the upper or lower motor neuron, unless the condition is clearly essential tremor, the patient should be examined by a qualified otorhinolaryngologist to exclude a focal laryngeal pathologic condition (e.g., tumor, polyp).

The best method for observing laryngeal movements, normal or otherwise, is with a nasopharyngeal fiberoptiscope, which permits examination of the vocal folds at rest and during ongoing speech. Ask for a video recording. Otorhinolaryngologists frequently do not focus on whether movement disorders of the larynx (or tongue or pharynx) are present at rest or during phonation. Their focus is usually on ascertaining the presence of a tumor or polyp or vocal fold weakness. Often, the neurologist detects tremor or another movement abnormality that would otherwise be undetected. Be certain that the evaluation includes fiberoptic visualization of the vocal folds, not just evaluation with a laryngeal mirror. The mechanics of the mirror examination render evaluation of the larynx during running speech impossible. Further, after the neurologist has seen video recordings of a few larynxes during speech, his or her expertise in evaluating laryngeal function will increase dramatically.

The fiberoptic evaluation should cost less than a few hundred dollars. The procedure is simple and safe and can be done in an office without anesthesia. It should always be accompanied by a video recording for the referring physician's review. Usually, accompanying detailed acoustic evaluations performed on special equipment are expensive and unnecessary, providing data that have minimal additional clinical relevance.[21]

Visual stroboscopy is a technique for evaluating the vocal folds that is very helpful in excluding lesions of the mucosa, which can disrupt phonation. This technique requires an expertise not achieved by many otorhinolaryngologists, but one that is helpful in elucidating mucosa abnormalities causing disturbance in oscillation.[21]

As noted earlier, acid reflux can damage the vocal folds. Usually there is evidence of esophageal erosion, and the vocal cords appear irritated and inflamed. However, the latter is not necessarily true, especially if the acid reflux is intermittent. Strings that are sensitive to pH changes can be inserted into the esophagus, by a gastroenterologist or an otorhinolaryngologist, to elucidate this possibility further.[6]

The most frequent cause of compromise of speech due to myopathy is hypothyroidism and polymyositis. If a patient is suspected of having myopathy (stigmata of myopathy noted elsewhere on examination, speech characterized by hoarseness/breathiness/hypernasality/weak speech-related muscles), the evaluation is the same as for any other myopathy. If these symptoms and findings improve with rest, evaluate the patient for neuromuscular junction dysfunction.[14]

When peripheral nerve lesions to the larynx are suspected, consider the full differential diagnosis for neuropathy. In particular, attention should focus on tumor compressing the nerve, viral disturbance (most common), diabetes, and alcohol-related illness. Affected patients may have stigmata of peripheral neuropathy elsewhere on examination; their speech is usually breathy, hoarse, low in volume, and diplophonic and may be hypernasal. In addition to the evaluation for neuropathy, obtain a chest x-ray film and computed tomographic (CT) scan from the base of the skull through the lower portions of the thyroid gland, extending to the carina of the bronchus. This approach will exclude thyroid tumors, which account for over one half of patients with bilateral vocal fold paralysis, and other neoplasms (e.g., pulmonary, metastatic, esophageal, glomus jugulare, lymphoma). If signs of central nervous system (CNS) compromise, including other cranial nerves, are present, MRI of the brain and lumbar puncture may be required to exclude collagen disease, tumor, and infection. All patients with such signs should be examined by a qualified otorhinolaryngologist.[14]

If these studies are normal and the patient has pain when swallowing as well as when talking, consider rheumatoid arthritis of the joints within the larynx. A sedimentation rate and rheumatoid factor tests are helpful, as may be x-ray film and CT scan of the larynx. Similarly, CT scans of the larynx are excellent for excluding arytenoid dislocation (many otorhinolaryngologists miss this diagnosis on indirect laryngoscopy). Strongly consider this diagnosis when a patient has voice complaints following intubation.[2]

If disease of the bulbar nuclei (CN IX, X, XII) is suspected, consider a lower motor neuron pathologic condition, especially amyotrophic lateral sclerosis (ALS). Many patients with ALS can have only bulbar compromise; all should undergo a detailed evaluation, including electromyography of the peripheral, thoracic paraspinous, and genioglossus muscles. Many of these patients present with slow, strained, gravelly, hypernasal speech. On examination, be certain to have them repeat /pa/, /ta/, and /ka/ several times, both rapidly and slowly. Substitution of voiced cognates (/pa/ > /ba/ > /ma/; /ta/ > /da/ > /na/; /ka/ > /ga/ > /nga/) strongly suggests palate weakness, thereby extending involvement beyond what may be only laryngeal weakness. This finding, coupled with slow output (e.g., spasticity) of these sounds, strongly suggests motor neuron disease.[18]

If the patient has a weak, hoarse voice with unchanging pitch and imprecise consonants and vowels, suspect hypokinetic dysarthria, usually Parkinson's disease. Almost all such patients will demonstrate stigmata of their movement disorder elsewhere on examination. They may also have an accelerated rate of speech while talking and repetitive dysfluencies (palilalia). Patients with cortical-basilar-ganglionic degeneration, one of the Parkinson-plus syndromes, can present only with speech complaints (e.g., substitution of incorrect sounds) early in their disease course, but most will have oral apraxia on examination and signs of abnormalities in their nonspeech domain.[14]

Similarly, patients with speech disruption due to hyperkinesia (e.g., sudden alterations in pitch, volume, consonant/vowel precision) usually have movement abnormality on visual inspection. Further, patients with cerebellar disease (e.g., phonatory tremor, irregular variations of articulatory abnormalities and imprecise consonants, excessive or equal stress on all syllables) usually have stigmata of cerebellar disease elsewhere on examination.[14]

Some patients with movement disorders, especially tremor and focal laryngeal dystonia, present with only phonation compromise. These patients, as well as others, may have spasmodic dysphonia. This disturbance is becoming increasingly recognized, in part because of the sometimes effective (and expensive) treatment with botulinum toxin injections. The evaluation of these patients is discussed in the following section.[14]

## SPASMODIC DYSPHONIA

Spasmodic dysphonia (SD) is a speech disturbance characterized by strained phonation with staccato-like catches in sound output. There are two types of SD: one type is due to vocal fold hyperadduction, and the other is due to intermittent abduction. Either type may be associated with reduced volume and may have a tremor component to the sound. The first type is characterized by uncomfortable, effortful, choppy breaks in phonation, staccato-like catches, and straining of the sound output. The abductor type of SD is characterized by breathy, effortful voice quality with sudden cessation of phonation, resulting in speech segments that are whispered. Both types of dysphonia can exist in a single patient.[13–15]

The diagnosis of adductor spasmodic dysphonia is clearer when the patient complains of strain and strangle during speech production. If these symptoms are absent, the physician should suspect voice misuse or abuse and disturbances that relate to poor voice habits and vocal hygiene.[13–15]

In a recent series of 100 patients being evaluated for SD, 71 patients had tremor, 25 had oromandibular dystonia, 12 had hypothyroidism, and 27 had either a functional disturbance or focal dystonia (6 had the abductor type). The evaluation for SD is similar to that for the underlying movement disorder, if one is suspected. Otherwise, the patient should also have indirect laryngoscopy, especially if he or she has

not responded to the usual therapies for movement disorders. If a positive response to therapy still is not noted and the laryngeal fiberoptic examination is normal, evaluation for acid reflux by a qualified gastroenterologist is indicated.[15]

## DYSFLUENCY

Stuttering is a disturbance of human speech production characterized by repetition and lengthening of sounds and syllables and by inappropriate pauses. In the past, stuttering was differentiated from stammering. Stutterers repeated the sound until they achieved their target (e.g., c-c-c-car), whereas stammerers held onto the sound until they achieved their target (e.g., c...ar). This distinction is no longer valid because it is now known that these different outputs can readily change because they represent the stutterer's coping mechanism for achieving a fluent target rather than a separate disease process.[3]

The grimacing, closing of eyes, and other accessory muscle activities frequently associated with stuttering are "secondary symptoms" that the stutterer probably has "learned" to employ as he or she attempts to "get the word out." These can be self-controlled readily and are not true dystonias.[3,14]

Stuttering is a pancultural global disturbance that has been recognized since the earliest times. It is mentioned on Mesopotamian clay tablets and in Egyptian hieroglyphics and is referred to in the Old Testament and the Holy Koran. Stuttering afflicts at least 1% of the world adult population and at least 4% of children. The condition is much more common among males then females. Affected individuals do not stutter in all of their speech; the majority of their output is fluent. The location of their dysfluencies is not random; most occur at the beginning of words, sentences, and phrases. There is a significantly higher concordance of stuttering among identical twins than fraternal twins, which suggests a genetic component.[12]

There are several fluency-evoking maneuvers, the most potent of which is singing (no stutterer stutters when he or she sings). Other such maneuvers include repetitive reading of the same passage (known as adaptation) and loud playing of "white noise" in the person's ear to prevent the hearing of his or her own speech.[3,12]

No psychiatry-oriented therapy has cured stuttering, although such therapy can decrease some of the associated anxiety and stress. A 10-year old stutterer may be terrified to present a book report in front of his class because of his stuttering; he may be just as nervous about singing yet can sing without any dysfluencies. Stutterers are more dysfluent when under stress, just as all symptoms of motor control disturbance are more pronounced when the patient is under stress.[3,12]

Nudelman et al[10] model stuttering as an instability in a feedback system, but they do not know the anatomic locations of the brain responsible for dysfluency. In 1972 Rosenfield[11] reported on a previously fluent adult who became dysfluent, without aphasia, following brain compromise. Later expanded literature pertaining to previously fluent patients who were rendered dysfluent from brain injury has included multiple locations of brain lesions: posterior or anterior, right or left, cortical or subcortical, and usually very small.[17]

These "acquired stutterers," as opposed to "developmental stutterers," demonstrate dysfluencies throughout a sentence; they do not improve with fluency-evoking maneuvers and are seldom personally distraught over their speech. Most developmental stutterers began stuttering as young children, whereas most of the acquired stutterers became afflicted as adults.[17]

Since developmental stutterers usually have a normal neurologic examination, their evaluation need not include neurologic studies. However, the acquired stutterer, who may have an abnormal examination (depending on the cause), should be evaluated for acquired brain disease (through MRI, electroencephalography, vascular and tumor workup) and, possibly, psychogenic disturbance.

Another type of dysfluency is cluttering, which is characterized by rapid speed, repetitions, omissions, interjections, and disturbed prosody. Affected persons may omit sounds, syllables, and whole words and invert the order of the sounds. Clutterers often repeat initial sounds and may prolong several sounds within a word. A listener usually has the sensation that the clutterer's speech is extremely rapid, although speech analysis often shows otherwise. Unlike developmental stutterers, who are usually very concerned about their speech deficit, clutterers commonly are not and may become perturbed when others point out their speech abnormality. Evaluation for cluttering seldom involves formal neurologic studies, unless disturbance in learning or attention is found.[17,20]

Palilalia, another type of dysfluency, is characterized by compulsive repetition of words or phrases at increasing speed with a decrescendo phonatory volume. This condition is usually associated with Parkinson's disease, but it can also occur in pseudobulbar palsy. With palilalia, speech improves considerably when the patient speaks with a metronome, pronouncing each syllable (not each word) in a stable cadence. The evaluation is the same as for Parkinson's disease.[4,17]

## SUMMARY

There is an expanding body of knowledge of the neurologic causes of speech abnormalities. Similarly, the differential diagnosis that the neurologist needs to be familiar with is also expanding, as is the range of diagnostic studies. This chapter provides an armamentarium of information to help neurologists in their clinical assessment of individuals with speech abnormalities and indicates which investigations are appropriate.

## REFERENCES

1. Baken RJ. *Clinical Measurement of Speech and Voice.* Boston: College Hill Press; 1987.
2. Benjamin B. Laryngeal trauma from intubation: endoscopic evaluation and classification. In: Cummings CC, Fredrickson JM, Harker LA, Krause CJ, Schuller DE, eds. *Otolaryngology—Head and Neck Surgery.* 3rd ed. St. Louis: Mosby; 1998:2013.
3. Bloodstein O. *A Handbook on Stuttering.* 5th ed. San Diego: Singular Publishing Group; 1995.
4. Boller F, Albert M, Denes F. Palilalia. *Br J Disord Comm.* 1975;10:92-97.
5. Borden GJ, Harris KS, Raphael KJ. *Speech Science Primer: Physiology, Acoustics, and Perception of Speech.* 3rd ed. Baltimore: Williams & Wilkins; 1994.
6. Fraser AG. Review article: gastroesophageal reflux and laryngeal symptoms. *Aliment Pharmacol Ther.* 1994;8:265-272.
7. Hirano M. *Clinical Examination of Voice.* New York: Springer-Verlag; 1981:7.
8. Hirano M. Objective evaluation of the human voice: clinical aspects. *Folia Phoniatr.* 1989;41:89-144.
9. Kent RD, Read C. *The Acoustic Analysis of Speech.* San Diego: Singular Publishing Group; 1992.
10. Nudelman HB, Herbrich KE, Hoyt BD, Rosenfield DB. A neuroscience model of stuttering. *J Fluency Dis.* 1989;14:399-427.
11. Rosenfield DB. Stuttering and cerebral ischemia. *N Engl J Med.* 1972; 287:991.
12. Rosenfield DB. Stuttering. *CRC Crit Rev Clin Neurobiol.* 1984;1:117-139.
13. Rosenfield DB. Clinical aspects of speech motor compromise. In: Jankovic J, Hallett M, eds. *Therapy With Botulinum Toxin.* New York: Marcel Dekker; 1994:397.
14. Rosenfield DB, Barroso AO. Difficulties with speech and swallowing. In: Bradley WG, Darroff RB, Fenichel GM, Marsden CD, eds. *Neurology in Clinical Practice: Principles of Diagnosis and Management.* 2nd ed. Boston: Butterworth-Heinemann, 1996;1:155.
15. Rosenfield DB, Donovan DT, Sulek M, Viswanath NS, Inbody GP, Nudelman HS. Neurologic aspects of spasmodic dysphonia. *J Otolaryngol.* 1990;19:231-236.
16. Rosenfield DB, Miller RH, Sessions RB, Patten BM. Morphologic and histochemical characteristics of laryngeal muscle. *Arch Otolaryngol.* 1982;108:662-666.
17. Rosenfield DB, Viswanath NS, Callis-Landrum L, DiDanato R, Nudelman HB. Patients with acquired dysfluencies: what they tell us about developmental stuttering. In: Peters HFM, Halstijn W, Starkweather CW, eds. *Speech Motor Control in Stuttering.* Amsterdam: Excerpta Medica; 1991:277.
18. Rosenfield DB, Viswanath NS, Herbrich KE, Nudelman HB. Evaluation of the speech motor control system in amyotrophic lateral sclerosis. *J Voice.* 1991;5:224-230.
19. Schneider JA, Watts RL, Gearing M, Brewer RP, Mirra SS. Corticobasal degeneration: neuropathologic and clinical heterogeneity. *Neurology.* 1997;48:959-969.
20. St. Louis KO, Hinzman AR, Hull FM. Studies of cluttering: disfluency and language measures in young possible clutterers and stutterers. *J Fluency Dis.* 1985;10:151-172.
21. Stasney CR. *Atlas of Dynamic Laryngeal Pathology.* San Diego: Singular Publishing Group; 1996.
22. Stevens KN, Klatt DH. Current models of sound sources for speech. In: Wyke B, ed. *Ventilatory and Phonatory Control Systems: An International Symposium.* Oxford: Oxford University Press; 1974:279.
23. Strand EA, McNeil MR. Effects of length and linguistic complexity on temporal acoustic measures in apraxia of speech. *J Speech Hear Res.* 1996;39:1018-1033.

Section III

# NEURO-OPHTHALMOLOGY, NEURO-OTOLOGY, AND NEUROTOXICOLOGY

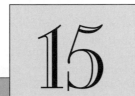

# Neuro-ophthalmology

*Steven L. Galetta, Grant T. Liu, and Nicholas J. Volpe*

This chapter reviews the diagnostic tests used in the evaluation of several common neuro-ophthalmologic entities, including optic nerve disease, pseudotumor cerebri, anisocoria, ptosis, and ocular motor palsies. Emphasis is placed on those bedside tests that help establish the diagnosis of these common clinical problems. The utility of the cocaine test and the Tensilon (edrophonium chloride) test and the role of neuroimaging in these conditions is analyzed.

## OPTIC NERVE DISEASE

### APPROACH TO THE PATIENT WITH VISION LOSS AND POSSIBLE OPTIC NEUROPATHY

There are several aspects of the neuro-ophthalmic examination that help localize visual loss to the optic nerve. Patients with optic neuropathies usually have reduced acuity, dyschromatopsia, an afferent pupil defect, nerve fiber–type defects on visual field testing, and an abnormal optic nerve appearance (pallor or swelling). The final cause of an optic neuropathy relies heavily on the historical details of the visual loss and the result of diagnostic testing.

### Visual Field Testing

A visual field evaluation is vital to establish the nature of the visual loss. On visual field examination, patients with optic neuropathies may have central, centrocecal, arcuate, altitudinal, or nasal step defects. Visual fields should be as-

sessed one eye at a time. Static perimetry tested on an automated perimeter (i.e., Humphrey perimeter) allows for threshold testing of the central 30 degrees and is very sensitive in detecting visual field defects common in optic neuropathies. The kinetic technique (Goldmann perimeter) may be more appropriate for some patients because it can be performed more quickly and allows for interaction with the examiner. Similar information can be obtained from a tangent screen examination. The least sensitive method of field testing relies on confrontation techniques with finger counting or comparison of red test objects. The examiner should concentrate on the central 30 degrees of the field and the relative differences in temporal vs. nasal and upper vs. lower aspects of the visual field.

### OPTIC NEURITIS

Optic neuritis is an acute, sporadic inflammatory optic neuropathy. It is the most common cause of acute vision loss from optic neuropathy in young adults. Peak incidence is in the third and fourth decade, and it is more common in women.[84] Patients usually present with acute vision loss with pain exacerbated by eye movements.[64] Young age and the presence of pain are strong predictors that inflammation is the cause of the optic neuropathy. In middle-aged patients without pain, distinction from ischemic optic neuropathy can be difficult.[92]

Diagnostic evaluation of suspected optic neuritis is undertaken for two reasons. The first is to rule out an underly-

231

ing, potentially treatable systemic illness that is causing the inflammatory optic neuropathy. The second is to help predict whether the patient is at risk for developing multiple sclerosis (MS) and therefore might benefit from intravenous steroids, as recommended by the Optic Neuritis Treatment Trial (ONTT).

## Laboratory Testing

Inflammatory optic neuropathy may occur in a variety of clinical settings. Underlying systemic illnesses that are recognized as causes of inflammatory optic neuropathy include syphilis, systemic lupus erythematosus, sarcoidosis, and opportunistic infections in immunocompromised hosts. Since optic neuritis secondary to demyelination is a clinical diagnosis based on the history and physical examination, many would argue that no testing is indicated in an otherwise typical case. In idiopathic optic neuritis some improvement almost always occurs within 30 days.[6] Therefore from a diagnostic standpoint it is not unreasonable to defer diagnostic testing until the patient fails to improve 1 month after onset.

Patients enrolled in the ONTT had antinuclear antibody (ANA), fluorescent treponemal antibody absorption test (FTA-ABS), chest x-ray examination, lumbar puncture, and magnetic resonance imaging (MRI) of the brain performed. These studies were of limited value in excluding other causes of optic neuritis.[5,6,84] Several patients had positive ANA, but these patients did not differ in their clinical course or treatment response. Criteria that favor aggressive workup include age younger than 20, progression beyond 14 days, failure to begin recovery within 30 days, bilateral involvement, and systemic symptoms or signs. If there is any doubt, a serologic evaluation, including erythrocyte sedimentation rate, rapid plasma reagin (RPR), FTA-ABS, angiotensin-converting enzyme (ACE), and ANA, should be performed.

Cerebrospinal fluid (CSF) analysis also has a limited role in the diagnosis of optic neuritis. In a 2-year follow-up study, the presence of oligoclonal bands was associated with increased risk of developing clinically definite MS.[93] However, the finding of oligoclonal bands added little to the risk assessment of MS since most of the patients also had abnormal MRI scans. Thus we do not perform lumbar punctures in patients with the typical profile of optic neuritis.

## Neuroimaging

Previous data have shown that both computed tomography (CT) scanning and MRI scanning may document abnormalities in the optic nerves of patients with optic neuritis.[42,73,75] About two thirds of patients with optic neuritis will have enhancing optic nerve lesions on MRI scan.[73,75] This enhancement may also be seen in other inflammatory optic neuropathies, such as sarcoidosis, meningeal processes, and radiation optic neuropathy. Demyelinating lesions in other parts of the brain may also be evident on MRI.[4] The ONTT found that the MRI scan was a powerful predictor of the 5-year risk of developing MS.[85] It has been well established that the majority of patients who have optic neuritis will ultimately develop MS, and the white-matter burden on MRI may correlate with the risk of this development.[10,30,91] In the ONTT, 51% of patients with three or more white-matter lesions that were >3 mm developed MS within 5 years. In contrast, only 16% of patients with normal MRI scans developed MS in the first five years.[85] In this 5-year follow-up period,

MS did not develop in any patient with a normal MRI who had (1) painless visual loss, (2) severe optic disc edema, (3) disc or peripapillary hemorrhage, or (4) macular exudate.[85] The ONTT also showed the 2-year risk of MS in patients with abnormal MRI scan to be significantly reduced by treatment with intravenous methylprednisolone when compared to those treated orally or with placebo.[7] However, the 4-year data suggest that this protective effect is short-lived, with no difference between treated and untreated groups.[62]

To conclude, magnetic resonance (MR) scanning of the optic nerves and brain should be ordered in all cases of acute optic neuritis to help establish the diagnosis, rule out alternative causes of acute optic neuropathy, and help determine the patient prognosis. When white-matter lesions are detected on MRI scan, intravenous steroid therapy seems to reduce the short-term risk of developing MS.

## Other Tests

Visual evoked potentials will often demonstrate prolonged latencies in both acute and resolved optic neuritis. The test is probably of little use at the time of the acute presentation. Reduced acuity, impaired color vision, an abnormal visual field, and an afferent pupil defect will generally establish the presence of an optic neuropathy. Therefore the visual evoked response will only be confirmatory and probably will not alter the acute management.

Currently, it has not been proven that evoked responses can reliably distinguish different causes of optic neuropathy. The evoked response may have a role in cases of unexplained vision loss or incidental recognition of optic nerve head pallor. In the former situation a normal visual evoked response suggests nonorganic vision loss. An abnormal response does not necessarily confirm damage to the anterior visual pathway since this test can be voluntarily altered by the patient.[15] With a pale optic nerve, a prolonged latency may suggest a previous episode of optic nerve demyelination.

Whether the physician chooses to obtain other evoked potentials (i.e., somatosensory, brainstem auditory) and spinal fluid analysis for oligoclonal banding in patients with optic neuritis is a matter of approach. These tests have little direct role in establishing the etiologic basis of acute vision loss. They may give prognostic information regarding the risk of subsequent development of multiple sclerosis. However, they do not alter the initial management, and currently there is insufficient information to warrant treatment with intravenous steroids based on these tests. Therefore we do not recommend obtaining evoked potentials or performing oligoclonal banding in typical cases.

## Pediatric Optic Neuritis

The causes of optic neuritis in children are different from those of adults. Idiopathic demyelination is a less common cause. Unlike adults, most affected children have swollen optic nerves, bilateral involvement is common, and there is often a prodrome of a viral illness.[55,61,86] Pediatric optic neuritis frequently occurs in conjunction with, or during the recovery phase of, a viral illness such as mumps, chickenpox, or influenza. It also is well recognized as occurring in association with vaccinations such as mumps, measles, and rubella. The visual outcome is almost always favorable, and the risk of subsequent MS is probably low.[86] In a life-table analysis of 79 patients, Lucchinetti et al[68] found that 13% would develop clinical or laboratory-supported MS in 10 years. By 20 years, this risk rose to 19%. By comparison, the 5-year risk in adults is approximately 30%.

Despite these differences, as with adults, the diagnosis is a clinical one. Depending on the examiner's comfort with the presentation, no tests may be ordered or an extensive battery of tests, including MR scanning, blood tests, and lumbar puncture, may be pursued. Since the history is often unclear, a workup is usually performed. In addition to the previously mentioned serologic workup, a Lyme disease titer should be considered in endemic areas or in patients with a clear history of exposure. The presence of the characteristic erythema chronicum migrans skin lesion will establish the diagnosis even before serologic studies show a positive result.

## ISCHEMIC OPTIC NEUROPATHY

The most common optic neuropathy in middle-age and older adults is anterior ischemic optic neuropathy (AION). By definition, patients with AION have optic disc swelling. Visual field defects are typically altitudinal, nasal, or arcuate. Patients with posterior ischemic optic neuropathy (PION) may have a normal-appearing fundus. PION is much rarer than AION and is frequently associated with an underlying systemic vasculitis. AION is believed to result from a non-embolic occlusion of one of the posterior ciliary arteries.

Evaluation of patients with ischemic optic neuropathy is directed first to excluding inflammatory, compressive, or infiltrative causes and then to distinguishing arteritic (associated with temporal arteritis) from nonarteritic forms. Finally, the examiner must consider a diagnostic evaluation for underlying systemic illnesses known to predispose to this condition. As previously mentioned, distinction from optic neuritis or an infectious optic neuropathy can be difficult since considerable overlap exists. The vast majority of patients are diagnosed on clinical grounds based on age and the presence of sudden unilateral vision loss with optic disc edema. Although not completely reliable signs, the presence of disc hemorrhages and altitudinal disc swelling favor the presence of ischemic optic neuropathy over optic neuritis.[119] If there are no atypical features on review of symptoms and examination, the diagnostic algorithm should be focused on excluding temporal arteritis. If there is a question of progressive vision loss, investigation for possible compressive lesions and inflammation and infection should be performed. Because idiopathic, bilateral nonarteritic AION is very rare, older patients with sudden simultaneous bilateral optic neuropathy should be assumed as having temporal arteritis until proven otherwise. Consideration should also be given to a meningeal process (infectious or carcinomatous), and the threshold for lumbar puncture should be low.

### Arteritic vs. Nonarteritic Ischemic Optic Neuropathy

This distinction is the most important diagnostic issue. Its importance lies in the fact that arteritic cases will often become bilateral within days and that aggressive treatment with intravenous steroids may salvage vision and protect better against further vision loss.[66,72] Patients with giant cell arteritis are typically older, have premonitory systemic and visual symptoms, and have more severe (often bilateral) vision loss. The first value to be obtained in all patients with AION is the Westergren sedimentation rate. Any result >40 mm/h is reported as abnormal, although the sedimentation rate is usually proportionally higher in older patients.[74] Although most patients with giant cell arteritis will have markedly elevated sedimentation rates (>90 mm/h), approximately one fifth of patients will have normal values.[46,66] Therefore, if the clinical suspicion is high, the patient should be treated with corticosteroids, regardless of the sedimentation rate, while awaiting temporal artery biopsy. We have added a C-reactive protein to our list of initial diagnostic tests for the patient with suspected giant cell arteritis. In a recent study,[40] an elevated C-reactive protein level (>2.45 mg/dl) was more sensitive (100%) than the erythrocyte sedimentation rate (>47 mm/h) for the diagnosis of giant cell arteritis. The combination of an elevated sedimentation rate and C-reactive protein yielded a specificity of 97% for the diagnosis of giant cell arteritis.

Fluorescein angiography can help to distinguish arteritic and nonarteritic ischemic optic neuropathy (ION). Delayed and patchy choroidal filling (Fig. 15–1) is characteristic of arteritic ION.[70,89]

All patients with suspected temporal arteritis should undergo temporal artery biopsy. Because of the possibility of skip areas,[2] biopsies of at least 2 cm each should be obtained.[18] The issue of whether to obtain a bilateral or unilateral temporal artery biopsy remains controversial. In many instances a unilateral biopsy will suffice. We obtain a bilateral biopsy only when the initial biopsy is negative or equivocal and the clinical suspicion for giant cell arteritis (GCA) remains high. In a series of 182 patients who had bilateral biopsies, only six (3.3%) had a different pathologic condition between the two sides.[9] In three cases the findings were consistent with healed arteritis, and in the other three cases early arteritis was suggested. Thus the added value of a second contralateral temporal biopsy is relatively low. It is presently well established that a biopsy will still reflect diagnostic pathologic evidence several weeks, and possibly even years, after steroid therapy has begun.[1,66,107] Therefore therapy should never be delayed until the biopsy report is received.[9] With PION (no disc swelling), the diagnosis is temporal arteritis until proven otherwise. PION has also been reported with atherosclerotic disease, herpes zoster, lupus erythematosus, and polyarteritis nodosa. In addition, consideration should be given to carcinomatous or infectious meningitis, and a lumbar puncture is recommended.

When the examiner is confident with the diagnosis of ischemic optic neuropathy and has excluded temporal arteritis, the remaining diagnostic testing is geared toward eliminating systemic predilections to this condition. Diabetes mellitus and hypertension should be excluded. In the appropriate clinical setting profound anemia and uremia should be excluded because these are potential causes of AION.

AION rarely occurs in conjunction with carotid artery disease or embolic cardiac disease. Noninvasive carotid artery studies, transcranial Doppler ultrasonography, and cardiac echocardiography have limited diagnostic value in the evaluation of patients with AION. Patients with AION associated with severe carotid artery occlusive disease usually have hemispheric signs or other signs of ocular ischemia.

## COMPRESSIVE OPTIC NEUROPATHIES

Both unilateral and bilateral vision loss can result from compressive lesions affecting the anterior visual pathways. Any patient who has experienced progressive vision loss over

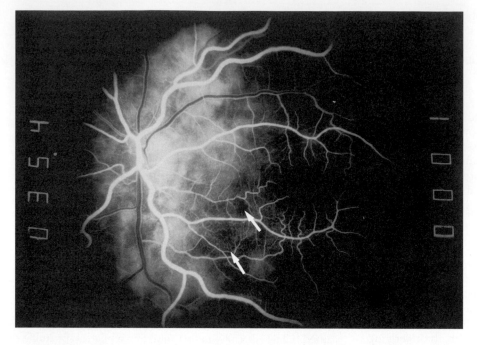

**FIGURE 15–1.** Fluorescein angiogram demonstrating delayed and patchy choroidal filling (*arrows*) in a patient with biopsy-proven giant cell arteritis.

a period of weeks or longer should be assumed to have a compressive lesion until proven otherwise. Some compressive lesions are associated with abrupt vision loss, as with pituitary apoplexy, mucocele enlargement, and aneurysm expansion. Common causes of compressive optic neuropathy and chiasmal syndromes include pituitary tumor, meningioma (suprasellar or optic nerve sheath), craniopharyngioma, glioma (nerve or chiasm), aneurysm, sinus tumor, and thyroid ophthalmopathy.

When the diagnosis of a compressive lesion is suspected, neuroimaging is mandatory. Both CT scan and MR scan have their advantages, and they are often complementary. Gadolinium-enhanced MR imaging with surface coil and fat suppression techniques usually provides images superior to CT scanning. CT continues to be superior for evaluation of bone (destruction or hyperostosis) and for detecting tumor calcification (meningioma). CT is also more widely available and less expensive, making it an acceptable screening tool for most compressive lesions. CT should include axial and coronal views. MR images are far superior for evaluation of the optic chiasm and tract. The lack of ionizing irradiation and improved orbital images make MR the better initial diagnostic testing in most instances. The study should focus particular attention on the orbits, and gadolinium enhancement will increase the sensitivity.

### OTHER OPTIC NEUROPATHIES

In addition to inflammatory, infectious, ischemic, and compressive optic neuropathies, visual loss can result from toxic, nutritional, and hereditary insults. The diagnosis of toxic optic neuropathies is usually established by clinical history and suspicion. Testing has little role except to identify known toxins in the blood (i.e., methanol). When nutritional or deficiency optic neuropathies are suspected, vitamin $B_{12}$ and folate levels should be checked.

Finally, precipitous, sequential vision loss from an optic neuropathy (particularly in young men) may be the result of Leber's hereditary optic neuropathy (LHON). This condition is inherited through the maternal lineage and has been found to result from a mitochondrial mutation. Initially, a nucleotide substitution at position 11778 was identified.[98,117] This mutation is a guanine-to-adenine base substitution and results in an amino acid change from arginine to histidine. This switch results in an abnormal subunit 4 of NADH dehydrogenase, which is the first enzyme in the pathway of oxidative phosphorylation. Since the time of that identification, as many as 10 other mutations have been identified in patients with LHON. In addition to the 11778 mutation, the other commonly identified mutations include substitutions at position 3460, 4160, 5244, 4917, 13708, 14484, 15257, and 15812 in the mitochondrial DNA.[14,43,47–50,67,81] None of these other mutations occur in the same gene as the 11778 mutation. However, they do affect other subunits of the same respiratory chain complex. Any patient with an unexplained optic neuropathy should have blood testing (commercially available through Athena Diagnostics, Worcester, Mass.) for one of the several LHON mutations that have been identified. A positive result for one of these mutations will occur in most, but not all, patients, and therefore in certain patients the diagnosis remains a clinical one. Genetic testing can also be used in asymptomatic family members so that recommendations for lifestyle changes can be made (e.g., cessation of smoking and alcohol intake) and to aid in genetic counseling. Although all patients with LHON probably have a genetic predisposition that is ultimately responsible for the vision loss, it is not yet understood why some patients with the mutation remain unaffected or what determines the time at which vision loss occurs in affected individuals.

## PSEUDOTUMOR CEREBRI

Pseudotumor cerebri (idiopathic intracranial hypertension) typically affects young obese women; the common symptoms include headache, transient visual obscurations (seconds), pulsatile intracranial noises, or double vision.[114,116] Almost uniformly, individuals with this disorder have papilledema (optic disc swelling in association with elevated intracranial pressure). Patients should satisfy the following (modified Dandy) diagnostic criteria: (1) signs and symptoms due to elevated intracranial pressure, (2) a normal neurologic examination, except for an abducens palsy, (3) neuroimaging excluding a cause of the elevated intracranial pressure, and (4) normal CSF parameters, except for an elevated opening pressure.[100] The only permanent sequela is visual loss related to optic nerve dysfunction, and sometimes the deficits are severe.[22] The exact cause is uncertain.

## PSEUDOPAPILLEDEMA

Optic disc abnormalities that may mimic papilledema ophthalmoscopically (pseudopapilledema) include congenital anomalies, tilting, hypoplasia, and drusen. Often the distinction is difficult, and the diagnosis may be aided by serial dilated fundus examinations and review of stereo disc photographs. Discs with true papilledema will leak during fluorescein angiography, in contrast to those with pseudopapilledema, which tend not to leak.[20] CT scanning of the orbits and B-scan ultrasonography can be used to identify calcified drusen at the globe-nerve junction.[31]

## NEUROIMAGING

Although either method is acceptable, MRI of the brain without gadolinium is preferred over CT scanning with contrast material to exclude hydrocephalus or another cause of elevated intracranial pressure (e.g., a mass lesion, venous sinus thrombosis, or dural arteriovenous malformation). Common radiographic findings in pseudotumor cerebri include an empty sella, dilation of the optic nerve sheaths, and elevation of the optic disc.[35] Many patients will have "slit-like" ventricles,[120] but in at least two recent studies[35,45] age-matched controls had similar ventricular sizes.

## CEREBROSPINAL FLUID

Following normal neuroimaging, lumbar puncture is necessary to rule out meningitis, for example, and to document the CSF opening pressure. The lumbar puncture should be performed with the patient relaxed in a lateral decubitus position, with the head and spine at the same level and the neck and knees slightly flexed. To establish the diagnosis of pseudotumor cerebri, the CSF opening pressure should exceed 250 mm $H_2O$, the upper limit of normal for most obese and nonobese individuals.[21] Approximately 20 to 30 ml of CSF can be removed, although the optimal amount has not been studied. In suspected cases with a normal CSF opening pressure, monitoring for 1 hour with an epidural transducer or subarachnoid bolt may be considered,[38,90] but this is rarely done in clinical practice. The cell count and glucose should be normal, and the protein normal or low. One study[19] found an inverse relationship between CSF opening pressure and CSF protein, whereas another[51] refuted this finding and documented CSF protein <20 mg/dl in only 26% of patients. Many patients will experience headache relief after the first lumbar puncture. Serial lumbar punctures, done either to withdraw more fluid or to monitor the CSF pressures, probably have no role in the management of this disorder.[88]

## VISUAL FUNCTION

Visual function guides management of the patient. Severe or progressive visual loss at presentation, or despite optimum medical management with acetazolamide or furosemide, is an indication for optic nerve sheath decompression surgery.[23] Thus neurologists need to enlist ophthalmologists or neuro-ophthalmologists to help monitor the vision of their patients with pseudotumor cerebri.

Visual field testing is the most sensitive method for detecting visual loss in these patients, and precise documentation requires kinetic or threshold perimetry with each eye (Fig. 15–2). The most common abnormalities are blind-spot enlargement, generalized constriction of isopters, and inferior nasal field loss,[114] which are all due to compression of ganglion cell axons by the swollen optic disc. As discussed earlier, Goldmann perimetry is a kinetic technique (moving stimuli)[115] that is shorter in duration than visual field testing. It allows interaction with the examiner and may be more appropriate for patients with significant visual loss. Computerized threshold perimetry of the central 30 degrees of vision (stationary targets, Humphrey 30-2 program), although lengthy and tedious, in most instances is a better objective and more reproducible test for patients with pseudotumor cerebri. Each field can be quantified by using the average of all the threshold values (in decibels) for each measured area, allowing for an objective numeric comparison of serial fields. In a prospective study by Wall and George,[116] 96% of patients had some abnormality detected through Goldmann perimetry, whereas 92% had deficits noted by computerized testing. However, automated perimeters are more widely available, and because of their advantages, most patients with pseudotumor cerebri should be followed up with serial threshold field examinations. Finger confrontation methods and tangent screen visual field examinations are too insensitive to detect subtle visual loss.[113]

It is important to note that some patients are unable to perform reliably on computer visual fields for one reason or another, and their suspected field loss should be confirmed by Goldmann perimetry, especially before optic nerve surgery is considered. In addition, we have encountered many patients with pseudotumor cerebri who have a component of functional visual loss. In such persons, tangent screen examination may be necessary to document nonphysiologic field constriction.

In contrast to the high incidence of visual field deficits, visual acuity, color vision, and pupillary reactivity are typically normal in affected patients, and about one half have abnormal contrast sensitivity.[116] Therefore these parameters are considered to be insensitive measures of alteration in visual function when compared to visual field testing.[114] The latency of visual evoked potentials (VEPs) was found to be correlated with CSF opening pressure by one group of investigators,[101] but others[110] found most VEPs to be normal despite the presence of visual field deficits and abnormal contrast sensitivity. Most experts therefore discourage the use of VEPs to monitor patients with pseudotumor cerebri.[114]

Patients should have weekly or biweekly follow-up initially. Then, if their vision stabilizes or improves, the interval between examinations can be lengthened. Each examination should consist of documentation of visual acuity, color vision, visual fields, pupillary reactivity, and fundus appearance.

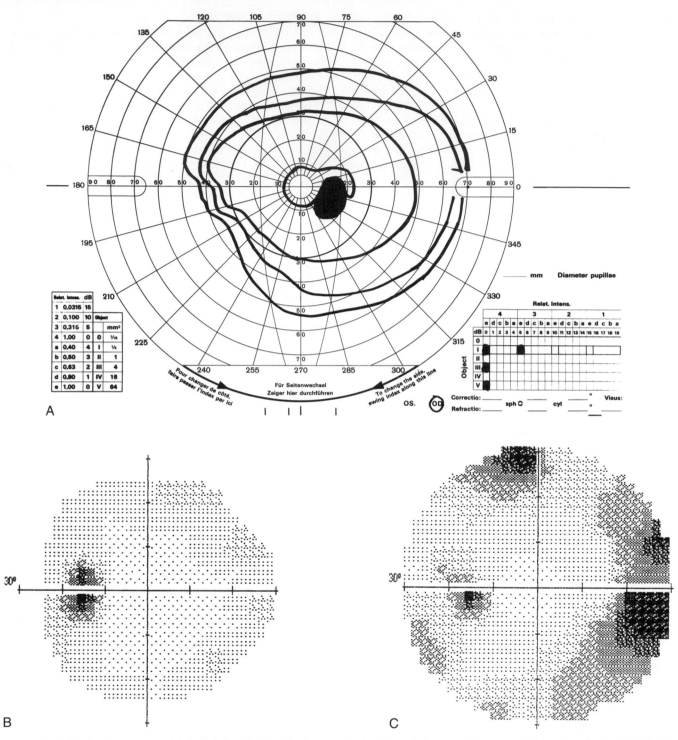

**FIGURE 15–2. A,** Goldmann (kinetic) visual field typical of visual loss associated with pseudotumor cerebri. Enlarged blind spot and infranasal constriction are present. **B** and **C,** Examples of Humphrey (threshold) 30-2 computerized perimetry demonstrating typical enlarged blind spot (**B**) and infranasal constriction associated with pseudotumor cerebri (**C**). The gray scale plots the central 30 degrees of vision.

## UNEQUAL PUPILS (ANISOCORIA)

### THE DILATED PUPIL

The first issue to resolve when evaluating a patient with asymmetric pupils is to determine which pupil is the abnormal one. The process begins by examining the pupillary light reflex (Fig. 15–3).[106] If one pupil is sluggish to light stimulation, the abnormal pupil has been identified. A sluggish pupil implies parasympathetic pathway dysfunction since sympathetic denervation does not alter pupillary reactivity to light. Parasympathetic impairment is confirmed by demonstrating that the pupil inequality is greatest in bright illumination, whereas sympathetic dysfunction is established by pupil asymmetry, which is greatest in the dark. Patients with physiologic anisocoria have normoreactive pupils without much change in the net amount of anisocoria under light and dark conditions.[99] Naturally, the presence of ptosis on one side can also help identify the affected pupil.

If a pupil is poorly reactive to light but the near response is intact or shows a slow constriction to a near stimulus, a tonic pupil is the most likely diagnosis. Further confirmation of a tonic pupil may be established by demonstrating segmental constriction of the pupil to light stimulation on slit-lamp examination.[104] The combination of an idiopathic tonic pupil and absent deep tendon reflexes is referred to as Adie's syndrome. Patients with tonic pupils may demonstrate pupillary constriction to dilute pilocarpine (1/8%), indicating denervation supersensitivity.[8] Most normal pupils typically do not respond to dilute pilocarpine. Corneal reflex testing and applanation tonometry should not be performed before the administration of pilocarpine because these tests may alter corneal permeability. Some caution is also necessary in interpreting the dilute pilocarpine test since Jacobson has shown that some patients with preganglionic parasympathetic dysfunction will also respond to dilute pilocarpine.[44] Since tonic pupils may be a manifestation of neurosyphilis, FTA-ABS or microhemagglutination assay–*Treponema pallidum* (MHA-TP) testing should be done in those patients without a defined cause for their dilated pupil.[29]

Slit-lamp examination is also necessary in the patient with pupillary mydriasis to look carefully for iris tears, uveitis, or evidence of angle-closure glaucoma. If an isolated

dilated pupil does not respond to light or near stimulation and the slit-lamp examination is normal, pharmacologic blockade should be suspected. One percent pilocarpine constricts both the normal pupil and the dilated pupil from preganglionic and postganglionic parasympathetic dysfunction.[105] However, it typically does not constrict the pharmacologically blocked pupil. The 1% pilocarpine test should be interpreted with caution if it is performed near the termination of pharmacologic blockage, because the affected pupil may constrict.[16]

If the patient has isolated pupillary dilation along with other signs of a third nerve palsy, an aneurysm of the posterior communicating artery should be considered until proven otherwise. In this situation it is often useful to obtain an emergent CT or MRI scan before proceeding with angiography since other compressive lesions may be found, eliminating the need for an invasive procedure. However, if the scan cannot be obtained immediately, we recommend proceeding directly to angiography. If the scan is negative, even if it includes MR angiography, conventional angiography is still necessary to exclude an aneurysm. Keane and Ahmadi[53] have documented two patients with third nerve palsy and posterior communicating artery aneurysms measuring 5 to 6 mm missed by MRI angiography. A study evaluating the accuracy of three-dimensional MR angiography in the detection of intracranial aneurysms found a mean sensitivity of 63% among five observers who used conventional an-

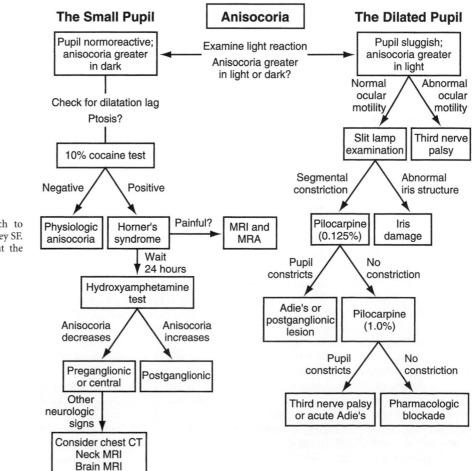

**FIGURE 15–3.** The diagnostic approach to anisocoria. (Adapted from Thompson HS, Pilley SF. Unequal pupils: a flow chart for sorting out the anisocorias. *Surv Ophthalmol.* 1976;21:45.)

giography as the gold standard.[60] Furthermore, higher diagnostic sensitivity was found for anterior communicating and middle cerebral aneurysms compared to internal carotid artery aneurysms.

### THE SMALL PUPIL

The sympathetically denervated pupil is small and is often associated with partial ptosis. Horner's syndrome is strongly suggested when the anisocoria increases in the dark or a dilation lag of the affected pupil is observed. Dilation lag may be demonstrated at the bedside by quickly turning off the room lights and observing the rate of pupillary dilation. The sympathetically denervated pupil will be delayed in reaching its final resting state in the dark.[87] Typically, measurements of pupil size are made at 5 and 15 seconds to document this dilation disparity in darkness.

Since many individuals have physiologic anisocoria and an unrelated ptosis, a pseudo-Horner's syndrome is a relatively common clinical occurrence.[103] In this situation, or to confirm a Horner's syndrome, cocaine testing is necessary. Again, no applanation tonometry or corneal testing should be performed before administration of cocaine. We suggest using a 10% solution since cocaine is a relatively weak pupillary dilator. The pupil should be assessed at baseline and again 40 to 60 minutes after the cocaine eyedrops have been administered. Sometimes neither pupil has responded, requiring a second instillation of drops and observation for another 30 minutes. In a positive test, the cocaine fails to dilate the sympathetically impaired pupil or does so very poorly. Kardon and colleagues[52] have determined that a postcocaine anisocoria of 0.8 mm or greater has a mean odds ratio of 1054:1 that a Horner's syndrome is present.

Once Horner's syndrome is established, it is useful to perform 1% hydroxyamphetamine (Paredrine) testing to distinguish between postganglionic and preganglionic sympathetic interruption. It is important that at least 24 hours separate the cocaine test and the hydroxyamphetamine test. Hydroxyamphetamine produces the release of norepinephrine from the postganglionic neurons. If both pupils dilate, a preganglionic process is likely, whereas failure to dilate after administration of 1% hydroxyamphetamine supports a postganglionic localization. In a study of normal individuals, hydroxyamphetamine produced a symmetric 2 mm mean increase in the size of the pupils.[25]

The pupil should be assessed at baseline and 45 minutes after administration of hydroxyamphetamine. Cremer et al[24] studied the amount of hydroxyamphetamine induced mydriasis necessary to establish the presence of a postganglionic sympathetic defect. The difference in pupillary dilatation to hydroxyamphetamine between the two eyes was used to determine the amount of drug-induced mydriasis. A logistic regression analysis was created to predict the probability of a postganglionic defect. For instance, a 1 mm increase in the amount of anisocoria provides an 85.5% probability that the lesion is postganglionic. A 2 mm increase is associated with a 99% probability of a postganglionic defect. The hydroxyamphetamine test is not perfect, however; Maloney et al[71] found that the diagnostic specificity for postganglionic Horner's syndrome was only 84%. In other words, 16% of patients who failed to have pupillary dilation had a preganglionic lesion. However, when both pupils dilated, the diagnostic specificity was 97% for a preganglionic lesion. In a more recent study, Cremer et al[24] found an increase in the anisocoria in 93% of postganglionic cases. The anisocoria decreased or did not change in 90% of preganglionic patients.

If the lesion can be localized to the postganglionic neuron, we recommend evaluation only if Horner's syndrome is painful because most postganglionic Horner's syndromes have a benign etiologic basis (e.g., vasculopathic). In the case of a painful Horner's syndrome, we suggest that MRI and MR angiography of the neck be performed to exclude a carotid dissection.[26,58,59] It is not unreasonable to obtain chest radiographs of a patient with suspected postganglionic Horner's syndrome since hydroxyamphetamine testing is not perfect in localization. If the process is found to be preganglionic, the other neurologic signs should be used to guide the investigation. For instance, accompanying hemianesthesia or ataxia mandate a brain MRI to exclude a brainstem lesion. On the other hand, a sensory level lesion accompanying a Horner's syndrome should be evaluated with a spine MRI. If the preganglionic Horner's syndrome is isolated or is associated with brachial plexopathy, a chest CT or MRI with attention to the lung apex is indicated. A congenital Horner's syndrome is usually associated with a lighter colored iris on the affected side (iris heterochromia). In children without birth trauma, including those with iris heterochromia, diagnostic testing should be performed to exclude neuroblastoma.[80] MRI of the head, neck, and chest and urinary catecholamine screening is one recommended protocol.

## PTOSIS

The evaluation of the patient with ptosis includes a careful history and ophthalmologic examination. In fact, most patients require no further diagnostic testing after a complete examination. In normal individuals the upper lid covers the superior margin (1 to 2 mm) of the cornea (limbus), and the lower lid borders its inferior aspect. The palpebral fissure is the opening between the upper and lower lids. In most normal individuals it measures between 9 and 12 mm. However, since lower lid position may vary greatly, it is best to measure the distance between the pupillary light reflex and the upper lid margin to assess the amount of ptosis. This measurement is referred to as the margin reflex distance, and it typically measures 4 to 5 mm.[82]

Measurement of levator palpebrae superioris muscle function helps to narrow the differential diagnosis of ptosis. Levator function is assessed by fixing the brow manually and asking the patient to look downward.[95] A ruler is then placed at the lid margin, and the number of millimeters of lid elevation is measured as the patient looks upward (Fig. 15–4). Normal levator function is >12 mm.[82] Ptosis produced by levator dehiscence and Horner's syndrome is usually associated with normal levator function. In contrast, levator function is reduced in ptosis associated with myasthenia gravis, congenital ptosis, third nerve palsies, and myopathic conditions such as chronic progressive ophthalmoparesis and myotonic dystrophy. The following section reviews the common causes of ptosis that may require further diagnostic evaluation, even after a complete history and examination.

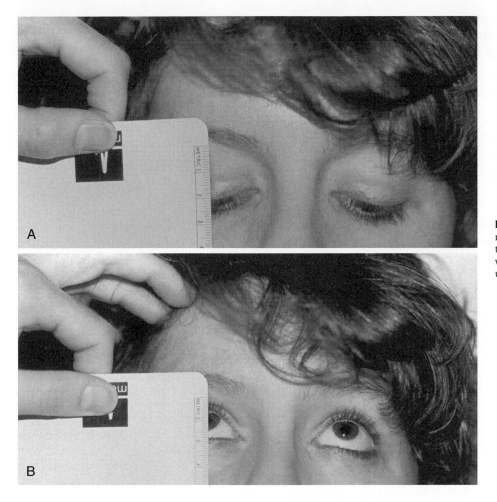

**FIGURE 15–4.** **A,** To measure levator muscle function, a ruler is placed over the center of the eyelid as the patient gazes downward. **B,** The distance the lid travels to reach upgaze is recorded.

## SPECIFIC DISORDERS

### Myasthenia Gravis

Levator function in myasthenia gravis is related to the amount of ptosis; patients with prominent ptosis will have the most impaired levator function. Normal levator function in the setting of marked ptosis argues against the diagnosis of myasthenia.[82] Documentation of a change in levator function is one objective method for assessing improvement of ptosis.

A Tensilon test can verify the diagnosis of myasthenia.[36,97] This test is positive in 80% to 90% of patients.[54,78] Tensilon may be drawn up in a 1 ml tuberculin syringe and administered intravenously in 2 mg increments, separated by 30 to 60 seconds, up to a total of 10 mg. The advantage of this incremental method of administration is that the full 10 mg dose may not be required to produce a positive response. If a tuberculin syringe is used, flushing of an intravenous line is not necessary. Alternatively, a 2 mg test dose is injected, and 1 minute later the remaining 8 mg of Tensilon is administered. If an intravenous line is used instead of a tuberculin syringe, flushing the line with normal saline is necessary to ensure that the Tensilon has been delivered to the bloodstream. The response to Tensilon is often dramatic and occurs within minutes of injection. Paradoxical worsening of ptosis should not be considered a positive test.[76] Atropine 0.4 mg should be ready in a separate syringe and administered intravenously if symptomatic bradycardia occurs. Optimally, a Tensilon test requires a team effort, with one individual administering the drug, another documenting the clinical findings, and a third monitoring the blood pressure and pulse. Cardiac monitoring or avoiding the test is suggested in patients with a history of heart disease or arrhythmia. One may not require the full dose of Tensilon to achieve a response, and eyelid twitching, tearing, and abdominal cramping are signs that the Tensilon has taken effect.[36]

Intramuscular neostigmine (Prostigmin) may be used instead of Tensilon in children who may not cooperate for an intravenous infusion, children who are too agitated to monitor over a short period, or adults whose signs are subtle and require a longer period of observation.[36,77] For adults, 1.5 mg of neostigmine and 0.6 mg of atropine sulfate are drawn up into a syringe and injected intramuscularly. The pediatric dose of neostigmine is .04 mg/kg, not to exceed a total of 1.5 mg.[76] The effect of intramuscular neostigmine usually begins by 15 minutes and is maximal by 30 minutes.[76]

If the patient has a history of cardiac disease, a noninvasive ice pack test or a sleep test can be used.[83,96] In the ice pack test, a bag of ice is placed over the affected lid for 1 minute, and then the response of the lid is assessed. In one study 8 of 10 patients with myasthenia gravis displayed unequivocal improvement of levator strength.[96] Furthermore, one myasthenic patient with a negative Tensilon test result had a positive ice pack test result, demonstrating this added diagnostic benefit.[96] The precise mechanism by which cooling improves myasthenic weakness is unclear. Enhanced transmitter release, reduced acetylcholinesterase activity, and increased receptor sensitization are possible mechanisms.[96] In the sleep test the patient is allowed to sleep for approximately 30 minutes to see if rest improves the ptosis.[83]

Anti-acetylcholine receptor antibodies are positive in 50% to 75% of patients with ocular myasthenia and in 80% to 90% of those with generalized disease.[65,102,111] Antibody tests that measure the accelerated degradation or blockage of acetylcholine receptors may occasionally be positive in seronegative individuals.[28]

Single-fiber electromyography (EMG) studies may be helpful if the Tensilon test and antibody studies are nondiagnostic or cannot be performed. A recent study of single-fiber EMG verified its benefit in the diagnosis of ocular myasthenia.[109] Extraocular muscle single-fiber EMG was positive in all 24 myasthenic patients tested. In this series the Tensilon test was positive in 16 of 22 (72.7%) tested patients. Another study of single-fiber EMG compared its diagnostic utility in distinguishing ocular myasthenia from chronic progressive external ophthalmoparesis (CPEO).[78] By testing the orbicularis oculi muscle, the investigators noted abnormal findings in 13 of 14 (93%) myasthenic patients. None of the patients with CPEO had an abnormal study. These two studies support the use of single-fiber EMG as the most sensitive diagnostic test for ocular myasthenia.[78,109] In patients with mild myasthenia, the combination of single-fiber EMG, anti-acetylcholine receptor antibody studies, and the Tensilon test should provide laboratory confirmation of myasthenia gravis in at least 95% of patients.[54]

### Myopathic Ptosis

Patients with myopathic ptosis often give a long history of droopy lids. Occasionally, the ptosis will be the only manifestation of a myopathic condition. However, many patients have other neurologic signs. These patients often have levator function between 5 and 11 mm.[82] In the Kearns-Sayre syndrome, patients have ophthalmoparesis, pigmentary retinopathy, and ataxia. The CSF protein is usually elevated (>100 mg/dl) in this condition. Since affected patients often have cardiac conduction abnormalities, they require electrocardiographic (ECG) assessment or Holter monitoring. Other useful diagnostic tests in patients with Kearns-Sayre syndrome and those with progressive external ophthalmoparesis include a muscle biopsy to detect ragged red fibers and mitochondrial DNA deletions.[79]

In myotonic dystrophy, findings other than ptosis include orbicularis oculi weakness, frontal balding, testicular atrophy, cataracts, and cardiac conduction abnormalities. The hallmark of the disorder is myotonia confirmed by examination or EMG.

### Nuclear and Supranuclear Ptosis

Ptosis may also be caused by injury to ill-defined supranuclear pathways. A predominance of right hemispheric lesions has been observed.[63] Brain MRI provides the most useful diagnostic test for evaluating the patient with suspected supranuclear ptosis. Rare cases of bilateral ptosis caused by injury to the central caudal nucleus of CN III are also best assessed with MRI.

### Ptosis and Pupil Inequality

Mild ptosis associated with miosis and pupillary dilation lag in the dark strongly suggests a Horner's syndrome.

On the other hand, pupillary dilation in combination with impaired adduction, elevation, and depression implies a third nerve palsy. Tests used in the diagnosis and management of these two conditions are discussed under anisocoria. There has been a single case report of a posterior communicating aneurysm manifesting as unilateral ptosis in isolation.[37]

## OCULAR MOTOR (CN III, IV, AND VI) PALSIES

A complete, isolated infranuclear oculomotor (CN III) nerve palsy causes ipsilateral elevation, adduction, and depression weakness accompanied by pupillary mydriasis and ptosis.[11] The trochlear (CN IV) nerve supplies the superior oblique muscle, which internally rotates the eye and depresses it in adduction.[12] Patients with CN IV nerve paresis may have vertical diplopia, an ipsilateral hypertropia that worsens on contraversive (contralateral conjugate) horizontal gaze, and ipsilateral head tilt (Parks three-step test). The abducens (CN VI) nerve innervates the lateral rectus muscle, which abducts the eye. Patients with a lateral rectus palsy complain of binocular horizontal double vision that worsens on ipsiversive gaze and at distance. The ocular motor nerves arise from the brainstem and course through the subarachnoid space before reaching the cavernous sinus and the orbit to innervate the muscles of the eye.

Although many patients with acquired ocular motor palsies require neuroimaging or laboratory evaluation, some subgroups can be managed without further testing. General guidelines are given in the following discussion, and some are based on the age of the patient. The "rules" regarding isolated (i.e., no other neurologic or ophthalmic signs) CN III palsies are summarized in Table 15-1.[108]

In patients older than 10 years with acquired, isolated pupil-involving complete or partial CN III palsies, a posterior communicating aneurysm should be excluded emergently (see discussion of pupils). We still recommend emergent brain MRI or CT prior to angiography because some individuals may have a mesencephalic infarction,[56] mesencephalic hemorrhage,[34] cavernous sinus mass, or pituitary apoplexy. Aneurysms causing acquired CN III palsies are rare in young children. More common causes in this age group include trauma, meningitis, and neoplasms.

In middle-aged and older adults, the most common identifiable cause of isolated, acquired complete pupil-sparing CN III palsies is vascular insufficiency associated with advanced age, diabetes, hypertension, or atherosclerosis.[94] Pre-

**TABLE 15-1. Recommendations for Neuroimaging in Adult Patients with Acquired Isolated CN III Palsies**

| OPHTHALMOPARESIS | PUPIL | RECOMMENDATIONS |
|---|---|---|
| Complete | Involved | CT or MRI, then angiography |
| Partial | Involved | CT or MRI, then angiography |
| Complete | Spared | Observation |
| | | MRI if no improvement within 8 wk |
| Partial | Spared | Serial observation of the pupil for 1 wk |
| | | MRI if no improvement within 8 wk |
| | | MRI for superior division paresis |

sumably, these nerves develop ischemia within the subarachnoid space or cavernous sinus.[11] CN IV and CN VI may be similarly affected. The prognosis for spontaneous improvement within 3 months is excellent. Currently, in patients over 50 with vascular risk factors and isolated complete pupil-sparing CN III, IV, or VI palsies, we recommend observation and MRI only in those who worsen or fail to improve within 8 weeks.[17] Those without identified vascular risk factors should have their blood pressure and fasting glucose, lipids, and cholesterol levels measured. Exceptional cases of isolated, complete pupil-sparing CN III palsies have been reported with small infarcts in the mesencephalon[13,41] and a basilar artery aneurysm.[69] Isolated spontaneously remitting CN VI palsies have been observed with small pontine infarcts[27,32] and intracranial masses.[112] We have also encountered a patient with an isolated CN IV palsy from a small midbrain hemorrhage. The recent recognition of isolated palsies resulting from brainstem lesions has been largely due to advances in MRI. We now have a low threshold for scanning patients with isolated ocular motor palsies early in their course.

Individuals with acquired isolated, pupil-sparing partial CN III palsies should be observed serially for 1 week for evidence of pupillary involvement. In one study[57] 14% of patients with CN III palsies due to posterior communicating aneurysms presented with normal pupils and partial motility deficits, but pupillary mydriasis developed within days in most of these cases. Thus, if the pupil remains uninvolved after 1 week, an aneurysm should be considered less likely, and a vasculopathic cause can be assumed if the patient has appropriate risk factors. Patients with superior division partial CN III paresis (levator and superior rectus weakness only), which is frequently associated with compressive lesions,[39] are the exception and should undergo neuroimaging.

Processes that may mimic isolated pupil-sparing CN III, IV, and VI palsies in adults include myasthenia gravis, thyroid eye disease, and giant cell arteritis (caused by muscle ischemia[3]). When these disorders are considered, an edrophonium test, thyroid function tests, orbital neuroimaging, and erythrocyte sedimentation rate may be helpful.

Virtually all patients younger than 50 (especially those without vasculopathic risk factors) with an isolated, acquired ocular motor palsy should undergo neuroimaging to exclude the presence of a mass lesion. One exception is an individual with an acquired superior oblique paresis, large vertical fusional amplitude, and longstanding head tilt consistent with a decompensated congenital CN IV palsy.

Any combination of CN III, IV, or VI palsy with an ipsilateral Horner's syndrome or sensory abnormality in the $V_1$ or $V_2$ distribution is an indication for an MRI of the brain with gadolinium, coronal views, and special attention to the cavernous sinus.[33] The usual etiologic factors are mass lesions, aneurysms, inflammatory conditions, and infectious processes. In cases with sparing of $V_2$ but involvement of the optic nerve, scanning should be directed toward the orbital apex.

Any individual with an ocular motor palsy accompanied by ataxia or long tract sign (usually crossed) should obtain an MRI of the brain, with special attention to the brainstem. Infarction, mass lesions, and vascular malformations are the usual culprits in such a setting.

We have a low threshold for neuroimaging in patients with traumatic ocular motor palsies, even when they are isolated. Such individuals may have a pseudoaneurysm or a posteriorly draining cavernous sinus fistula. Some ocular motor palsies from minor trauma are harbingers of an underlying aneurysm or a mass lesion.[118] Extraocular muscle entrapment resulting from orbital wall fracture may mimic an ocular motor palsy.

Meningeal processes also should be considered in patients with ocular motor palsies, especially when they occur bilaterally or in combination, and when other cranial nerves or nerve roots are involved. MRI with gadolinium may disclose meningeal enhancement. CSF examination, including cultures and cytologic studies, should be performed to exclude acute bacterial and chronic fungal meningitis, tuberculosis, syphilis, Lyme disease, sarcoidosis, and carcinomatous or lymphomatous meningitis. In ocular motor palsies due to Guillain-Barré syndrome, the Fisher variant, or chronic inflammatory demyelinating polyneuropathy, the CSF protein level should be elevated.

## REFERENCES

1. Achkar AA, Lie JT, Hunder GG, et al. How does previous corticosteroid therapy affect the biopsy findings in giant cell (temporal) arteritis? *Ann Intern Med.* 1994;120:987-992.
2. Albert DM, Ruchman ML, Keltner JL. Skip areas in temporal arteritis. *Arch Ophthalmol.* 1976;94:2072-2077.
3. Barricks ME, Traviesa DB, Glaser JS, et al. Ophthalmoplegia in cranial arteritis. *Brain.* 1977;100:209-221.
4. Beck RW, Arrington J, Murtagh FR. Brain MRI in acute optic neuritis: experience of the Optic Neuritis Study Group. *Arch Neurol.* 1993;8: 841-846.
5. Beck RW, Cleary PA, Anderson MM, et al. A randomized, controlled trial of corticosteroids in the treatment of acute optic neuritis. *N Engl J Med.* 1992;326:581-588.
6. Beck RW, Cleary PA, Backlund JC, et al. The course of visual recovery after optic neuritis: experience of the optic neuritis treatment trial. *Ophthalmology.* 1994;101:1771-1778.
7. Beck RW, Cleary PA, Trobe JD, et al. The effect of corticosteroids for acute optic neuritis on the subsequent development of multiple sclerosis. *N Engl J Med.* 1993;329:1764-1769.
8. Bourgon P, Pilley SF, Thompson HS. Cholinergic supersensitivity of the iris sphincter in Adie's tonic pupil. *Am J Ophthalmol.* 1978;85:373-377.
9. Boyev LR, Harris LL, Miller NR, et al. Efficacy of unilateral versus bilateral temporal artery biopsies in detecting temporal arteritis. *Invest Ophthalmol Vis Sci.* 1997;38:S382.
10. Bradley WG, Whitty CWM. Acute optic neuritis and the prognosis for multiple sclerosis. *J Neurol Neurosurg Psychiatry.* 1976;39:283-289.
11. Brazis PW. Localization of lesions of the oculomotor nerve: recent concepts. *Mayo Clin Proc.* 1991;66:1029-1035.
12. Brazis PW. Localization of lesions of the trochlear nerve: diagnosis and localization—recent concepts. *Mayo Clin Proc.* 1993;68:501-509.
13. Breen LA, Hopf HC, Farris BK, et al. Pupil-sparing oculomotor nerve palsy due to midbrain infarction. *Arch Neurol.* 1991;48:105-106.
14. Brown MD, Voljavec AS, Lott MT, et al. Mitochondrial DNA complex I and III mutations associated with Leber's hereditary optic neuropathy. *Genetics.* 1992;130:163-173.
15. Bumgartner J, Epstein CM. Voluntary alteration of visual evoked response. *Ann Neurol.* 1982;12:475.
16. Burde RM, Savino PJ, Trobe JD. *Clinical Decisions in Neuroophthalmology.* St. Louis: Mosby; 1992:338.
17. Capo H, Warren F, Kupersmith MJ. Evolution of oculomotor nerve palsies. *J Clin Neuroophthalmol.* 1992;12:21-25.
18. Chambers WA, Bernadino VB. Specimen length in temporal artery biopsies. *J Clin Neuroophthalmol.* 1988;8:121-125.
19. Chandra V, Bellur SN, Anderson RJ. Low CSF protein concentration in idiopathic pseudotumor cerebri. *Ann Neurol.* 1986;19:80-82.
20. Corbett JJ. Problems in the diagnosis and treatment of pseudotumor cerebri. *Can J Neurol Sci.* 1983;10:221-229.
21. Corbett JJ, Mehta MP. Cerebrospinal fluid pressure in normal obese subjects and patients with pseudotumor cerebri. *Neurology.* 1983;33: 1386-1388.

22. Corbett JJ, Savino PJ, Thompson HS, et al. Visual loss in pseudotumor cerebri: follow-up of 57 patients from five to 41 years and a profile of 14 patients with permanent severe visual loss. *Arch Neurol.* 1982;39:461-474.

23. Corbett JJ, Thompson HS. The rational management of idiopathic intracranial hypertension. *Arch Neurol.* 1989;46:1049-1051.

24. Cremer SA, Thompson HS, Digre KB, et al. Hydroxyamphetamine mydriasis in Horner's syndrome. *Am J Ophthalmol.* 1990;110:71-76.

25. Cremer SA, Thompson HS, Digre KB, et al. Hydroxyamphetamine mydriasis in normal subjects. *Am J Ophthalmol.* 1990;110:66-70.

26. Digre KB, Smoker WR, Johnston P, et al. Selective MR imaging approach for evaluation of patients with Horner's syndrome. *Am J Neuroradiol.* 1992;13:223-227.

27. Donaldson D, Rosenberg NL. Infarction of abducens nerve fascicle as cause of isolated sixth nerve palsy related to hypertension. *Neurology.* 1988;38:1654.

28. Drachman DB. Medical progress: myasthenia gravis. *N Engl J Med.* 1994;330:1797-1810.

29. Fletcher WA, Sharpe JA. Tonic pupils in neurosyphilis. *Neurology.* 1986;36:188-192.

30. Francis DA, Compston DAS, Batchelor JR, et al. A reassessment of the risk of multiple sclerosis developing in patients with optic neuritis after extended follow-up. *J Neurol Neurosurg Psychiatry.* 1987;50:758-765.

31. Froula PD, Bartley GB, Garrity JA, et al. The differential diagnosis of orbital calcification as detected on computed tomography scans. *Mayo Clin Proc.* 1993;68:256-261.

32. Fukutake T, Hirayama K. Isolated abducens nerve palsy from pontine infarction in a diabetic patient. *Neurology.* 1992;42:2226.

33. Galetta SL. Cavernous sinus syndromes. In: Margo CE, Hamed LM, Mames RN, eds. *Diagnostic Problems in Clinical Ophthalmology.* Philadelphia: WB Saunders; 1994:609-615.

34. Getenet J-C, Vighetto A, Nighoghossian N, et al. Isolated bilateral third nerve palsy caused by a mesencephalic hematoma. *Neurology.* 1994;44:981-982.

35. Gibby WA, Cohen M, Goldberg HI, et al. Pseudotumor cerebri: CT findings and correlation with vision loss. *Am J Radiol.* 1993;160:143-146.

36. Glaser JS, Bachynski B. Infranuclear disorders of eye movement. In: Glaser JS, ed. *Neuroophthalmology.* Philadelphia: JB Lippincott; 1990:396-397.

37. Good EF. Ptosis as the sole manifestation of compression of the oculomotor nerve by an aneurysm of the posterior communicating artery. *J Clin Neuroophthalmol.* 1990;10:59-61.

38. Green JP, Newman NJ, Stowe ZN, et al. "Normal pressure" pseudotumor cerebri. *J Neuroophthalmol.* 1996;16:241-246.

39. Guy JR, Day AL. Intracranial aneurysms with superior division paresis of the oculomotor nerve. *Ophthalmology.* 1989;96:1071-1076.

40. Hayreh SS, Podhajsky PA, Ramvan R, et al. Giant cell arteritis: validity and reliability of various diagnostic criteria. *Am J Ophthalmol.* 1997;123:285-296.

41. Hopf HC, Gutmann L. Diabetic third nerve palsy: evidence for a mesencephalic lesion. *Neurology.* 1990;40:1041-1045.

42. Howard CW, Osher RW, Tomsak RL. Computed tomographic features in optic neuritis. *Am J Ophthalmol.* 1980;89:699-702.

43. Howell N, Kubacka I, Xu M, et al. Leber hereditary optic neuropathy: involvement of the mitochondrial NDI gene and evidence for an intragenic suppressor mutation. *Am J Hum Genet.* 1991;48:935-942.

44. Jacobson DM. A prospective evaluation of cholinergic supersensitivity of the iris sphincter in patients with oculomotor nerve palsies. *Am J Ophthalmol.* 1994;118:377-383.

45. Jacobson DM, Karanjia PN, Olson KA, et al. Computerized tomography ventricular size has no predictive value in diagnosing pseudotumor cerebri. *Neurology.* 1990;40:1454-1455.

46. Jacobson DM, Slamovitz TL. Erythrocyte sedimentation rate and its relationship to hematocrit in giant cell arteritis. *Arch Ophthalmol.* 1987;105:965-967.

47. Johns DR, Heher KL, Miller NR, et al. Leber's hereditary optic neuropathy: clinical characteristics of the 14484 mutation. *Arch Ophthalmol.* 1993;111:495-498.

48. Johns DR, Neufeld MJ. Cytochrome b mutations in Leber hereditary optic neuropathy. *Biochem Biophys Res Commun.* 1991;181:1358-1364.

49. Johns DR, Smith KH, Miller NR. Leber's hereditary optic neuropathy: clinical characteristics of the 3460 mutation. *Arch Ophthalmol.* 1992;110:1577-1581.

50. Johns DR, Smith KH, Savino PJ, et al. Leber's hereditary optic neuropathy: clinical characteristics of the 15257 mutation. *Ophthalmology.* 1993;100:981-986.

51. Johnston PK, Corbett JJ, Maxner CE. Cerebrospinal fluid protein and opening pressure in idiopathic intracranial hypertension (pseudotumor cerebri). *Neurology.* 1991;41:1040-1042.

52. Kardon RH, Denison CE, Brown CK, et al. Critical evaluation of the cocaine test in the diagnosis of Horner's syndrome. *Arch Ophthalmol.* 1990;108:384-387.

53. Keane JR, Ahmadi J. Third nerve palsies and angiography. *Arch Neurol.* 1991;48:470.

54. Kelly JJ, Daube J, Lennon VA. The laboratory diagnosis of mild myasthenia gravis. *Ann Neurol.* 1982;12:238-242.

55. Kennedy C, Carroll FD. Optic neuritis in children. *Arch Ophthalmol.* 1960;63:747-755.

56. Kim JS, Kang JK, Lee SA, et al. Isolated or predominant ocular motor nerve palsy as a manifestation of brain stem stroke. *Stroke.* 1993;24:581-586.

57. Kissel JT, Burde RM, Klingele TG, et al. Pupil-sparing oculomotor palsies with internal carotid-posterior communicating artery aneurysms. *Ann Neurol.* 1983;13:149-154.

58. Kline LB. The neuroophthalmologic manifestations of spontaneous dissection of the internal carotid artery. *Semin Ophthalmol.* 1992;7:30-37.

59. Kline LB, Vitek JJ, Raymon BC. Painful Horner's syndrome due to spontaneous carotid artery dissection. *Ophthalmology.* 1987;94:226-230.

60. Korogi Y, Takahashi M, Mabuchi M, et al. Intracranial aneurysms: diagnostic accuracy of three dimensional time of flight MR angiography. *Radiology.* 1994;193:181-186.

61. Kriss A, Francis DA, Cuendet B. Recovery of optic neuritis in childhood. *J Neurol Neurosurg Psychiatry.* 1988;51:1253-1258.

62. Kupersmith M, Kaufman D, Paty DW, et al. Megadose corticosteroids in multiple sclerosis. *Neurology.* 1994;44:1-4.

63. Lepore FE. Bilateral cerebral ptosis. *Neurology.* 1987;37:1043-1046.

64. Lepore FE. The origin of pain in optic neuritis. *Arch Neurol.* 1991;48:748-749.

65. Lindstrom JM, Seybold M, Lennon V, et al. Antibody to acetylcholine receptor in myasthenia: prevalence, clinical correlates, and diagnostic value. *Neurology.* 1976;26:1054-1059.

66. Liu GT, Glaser JS, Schatz NJ, et al. Visual morbidity in giant cell arteritis: clinical characteristics and prognosis for vision. *Ophthalmology.* 1994;101:1779-1785.

67. Lott MT, Voljavec AS, Wallace DC. Variable genotype of Leber's hereditary optic neuropathy patients. *Am J Ophthalmol.* 1990;109:625-631.

68. Lucchinetti CF, Kiers L, O'Duffy A, et al. Risk factors for developing multiple sclerosis after childhood optic neuritis. *Neurology.* 1997;49:1413-1418.

69. Lustbader JM, Miller NR. Painless, pupil-sparing but otherwise complete oculomotor nerve paresis caused by basilar artery aneurysm. *Arch Ophthalmol.* 1988;106:583-584.

70. Mack HG, O'Day J, Currie JN. Delayed choroidal perfusion in giant cell arteritis. *J Clin Neuroophthalmol.* 1991;11:221-227.

71. Maloney WF, Younge BR, Moyer NJ. Evaluation of the causes and accuracy of pharmacologic localization in Horner's syndrome. *Am J Ophthalmol.* 1980;90:394-402.

72. Matzkin DC, Slamovits TL, Sachs R, et al. Visual recovery in two patients after intravenous methylprednisolone treatment of central retinal artery occlusion secondary to giant-cell arteritis. *Ophthalmology.* 1992;99:68-71.

73. Merandi SF, Kudryk BT, Murtagh FR, et al. Contrast enhanced MR imaging of optic nerve lesions in patients with acute optic neuritis. *AJNR.* 1991;12:923-926.

74. Miller A, Green M, Robinson D. Simple rule for calculating normal erythrocyte sedimentation rate. *Br Med J Clin Res Ed.* 1983;286:266.

75. Miller DH, Newton MR, van der Pool JC. Magnetic resonance imaging of the optic nerve in optic neuritis. *Neurology.* 1988;38:175-179.

76. Miller NR. *Walsh & Hoyt's Clinical Neuro-ophthalmology.* 4th ed. Baltimore: Williams & Wilkins; 1985;2:851-854.

77. Miller NR, Morris JE, Maguire M. Combined use of neostigmine and ocular motility measurements in the diagnosis of myasthenia. *Arch Ophthalmol.* 1982;100:761-763.

78. Milone M, Monarco ML, Evoli A, et al. Ocular myasthenia: diagnostic value of single fiber EMG in the orbicularis oculi muscle. *J Neurol Neurosurg Psychiatry.* 1993;56:720-721.

79. Moraes CT, Dimauro S, Zeviani M, et al. Mitochondrial DNA deletions in progressive external ophthalmoplegia and Kearns-Sayre syndrome. *N Engl J Med.* 1989;30:1293-1299.

80. Musarella M, Chan HS, DeBoer G, et al. Ocular involvement in neuroblastoma: prognostic implications. *Ophthalmology.* 1984;91:936-940.

81. Newman NJ. Leber's hereditary optic neuropathy: new genetic considerations. *Arch Neurol.* 1993;50:540-548.

82. Nunery WR, Cepela M. Levator function in the evaluation and management of blepharoptosis. *Ophthalmol Clin.* 1991;4:1-16.

83. Odel JG, Winterkorn JMS, Behrens MM. The sleep test for myasthenia gravis: a safe alternative to tensilon. *J Clin Neuroophthalmol.* 1991;11:228-292.

84. Optic Neuritis Study Group. The clinical profile of optic neuritis: experience of the Optic Neuritis Treatment Trial. *Arch Ophthalmol.* 1991;109:1673-1678.

85. Optic Neuritis Study Group. The 5-year risk of MS after optic neuritis: experience of the Optic Neuritis Treatment Trial. *Neurology.* 1997;49:1404-1413.

86. Parkin PJ, Hierons R, McDonald WI. Bilateral optic neuritis: a long term follow-up. *Brain.* 1984;107:951-964.

87. Pilley SF, Thompson HS. Pupillary "dilatation lag" in Horner's syndrome. *Br J Ophthalmol.* 1975;59:731-735.

88. Practice parameters: lumbar puncture (summary statement). *Neurology.* 1993;43:625-627.

89. Quillen DA, Cantore WA, Schwartz SR, et al. Choroidal nonperfusion in giant cell arteritis. *Am J Ophthalmol.* 1993;116:171-175.

90. Radhakrishnan K, Ahlskog JE, Garrity JA, et al. Idiopathic intracranial hypertension. *Mayo Clin Proc.* 1994;69:169-180.

91. Rizzo JF, Lessell S. Risk of developing multiple sclerosis after uncomplicated optic neuritis. *Neurology.* 1988;38:185-190.

92. Rizzo JF, Lessell S. Optic neuritis and ischemic optic neuropathy: overlapping clinical profiles. *Arch Ophthalmol.* 1991;100:1668-1672.

93. Rolak LA, Beck RW, Paty DW, et al. Cerebrospinal fluid in acute optic neuritis: experience of the optic neuritis treatment trial. *Neurology.* 1996;46:368-372.

94. Rush JA, Younge BR. Paralysis of cranial nerves III, IV, and VI. *Arch Ophthalmol.* 1981;99:76-79.

95. Sedwick LA. Ptosis. In: Margo C, Hamed L, Mames R, eds. *Diagnostic Problems in Clinical Ophthalmology.* Philadelphia: WB Saunders; 1994:38-42.

96. Sethi K, Rivner MH, Swift TR. Ice pack test for myasthenia gravis. *Neurology.* 1987;37:1383-1385.

97. Seybold ME, Daroff RB. The office tensilon test for ocular myasthenia. *Arch Neurol.* 1986;43:842.

98. Singh G, Lott MT, Wallace DC. A mitochondrial DNA mutation as a cause of Leber's hereditary optic neuropathy. *N Engl J Med.* 1989;320:1300-1305.

99. Slamovits TL, Glaser JS. The pupils and accommodation. In: Glaser JS, ed. *Neuroophthalmology.* Philadelphia: JB Lippincott; 1990:459-486.

100. Smith JL. Whence pseudotumor cerebri? (editorial). *J Clin Neuroophthalmol.* 1985;5:55-56.

101. Soelberg Sørensen P, Trojaborg W, Gjerris F, et al. Visual evoked potentials in pseudotumor cerebri. *Arch Neurol.* 1985;42:150-153.

102. Soliven BC, Lange DT, Penn AS. Seronegative myasthenia gravis. *Neurology.* 1988;38:514.

103. Thompson BM, Corbett JJ, Kline LB, et al. Pseudo-Horner's syndrome. *Arch Neurol.* 1982;39:108-111.

104. Thompson HS. Segmental palsy of the iris sphincter in Adie's syndrome. *Arch Ophthalmol.* 1978;96:1615-1620.

105. Thompson HS, Newsome DA, Loewenfield ID. The fixed dilated pupil. *Arch Ophthalmol.* 1971;86:21-27.

106. Thompson HS, Pilley SF. Unequal pupils: a flow chart for sorting out the anisocorias. *Surv Ophthalmol.* 1976;21:45-48.

107. To KW, Enzer YR, Tsiaras WG. Temporal artery biopsy after one month of corticosteroid therapy. *Am J Ophthalmol.* 1994;117:265-267.

108. Trobe JD. Third nerve palsy and the pupil: footnotes to the rule. *Arch Ophthalmol.* 1988;106:601-602.

109. Uyama J, Mimura O, Ikeda N, et al. Single fiber electromyography of extraocular muscles in myasthenia gravis. *Neuroophthalmology.* 1993;13:253-261.

110. Verplanck M, Kaufman DI, Parsons T, et al. Electrophysiology versus psychophysics in the detection of visual loss in pseudotumor cerebri. *Neurology.* 1988;38:1789-1792.

111. Vincent A, Newsom DJ. Anti-acetylcholine receptor antibodies. *J Neurol Neurosurg Psychiatry.* 1980;43:590-600.

112. Volpe NJ, Lessell S. Remitting sixth nerve palsy in skull base tumors. *Arch Ophthalmol.* 1993;111:1391-1395.

113. Wall M. Sensory visual testing in idiopathic intracranial hypertension: measures sensitive to change. *Neurology.* 1990;40:1859-1864.

114. Wall M. Idiopathic intracranial hypertension. *Neurol Clin.* 1991;9:73-95.

115. Wall M, George D. Visual loss in pseudotumor cerebri: incidence and defects related to visual field strategy. *Arch Neurol.* 1987;44:170-175.

116. Wall M, George D. Idiopathic intracranial hypertension: a prospective study of 50 patients. *Brain.* 1991;114:155-180.

117. Wallace DC, Singh G, Lott MT, et al. Mitochondrial DNA mutation associated with Leber's hereditary optic neuropathy. *Science.* 1988;242:1427-1430.

118. Walter KA, Newman NJ, Lessell S. Oculomotor palsy from minor head trauma: initial sign of intracranial aneurysm. *Neurology.* 1994;44:148-150.

119. Warner JEA, Lessell S, Rizzo JF, et al. Does optic disc appearance distinguish ischemic optic neuropathy from optic neuritis? *Arch Ophthalmol.* 1997;115:1408-1410.

120. Weisberg LA. Computerized tomography in benign intracranial hypertension. *Neurology.* 1985;35:1075-1078.

# 16

# Neuro-otology

*Robert W. Baloh and Kathleen M. Jacobson*

The neural pathways of the auditory and vestibular systems are anatomically proximate in much of their course from their end organs in the inner ear to their termination in the cortex. Because of the close anatomic linkage, disorders that affect hearing often affect balance and equilibrium and vice versa. For this reason they are considered together in the field of neuro-otology. Despite their anatomic closeness, however, substantial pathophysiologic differences make clinical examination of the two systems quite different. The auditory system is physiologically relatively isolated, so that its function and dysfunction can be tested independently of other neural systems. The vestibular system, in contrast, has many close physiologic links with other sensorimotor systems and can be tested only indirectly by noting secondary effects on oculomotor and balance functions. Abnormalities in the auditory system lead to only a few well-defined and unique symptoms (i.e., hearing loss or tinnitus). Abnormalities of the vestibular system can cause symptoms that mimic disorders of many other neural structures. Such symptoms result from impaired spatial orientation (dizziness), oculomotor dysfunction (oscillopsia), motor abnormalities (including disequilibrium and falls), and autonomic dysfunction (including nausea, vomiting, and syncope).

Since dizziness can represent several different overlapping sensations and can be caused by many different pathophysiologic mechanisms, it is critical that the examining physician take a careful history to determine the type of dizziness before proceeding with diagnostic studies.[2] The history provides direction for both the examination and diagnostic workup (Table 16–1). For example, the focus in a patient presenting with presyncopal light-headedness should be on the cardiovascular system, not the vestibular system. Although such a distinction seems obvious, we still have many referrals to our laboratory for vestibular function testing in patients complaining of presyncopal light-headedness.

Vertigo, defined as an illusion of movement (usually rotation), always indicates an imbalance within the vestibular system, although the symptom itself does not indicate where in the system the imbalance originates. The same sensation can result from lesions in such diverse locations as the inner ear, the deep paravertebral stretch receptors of the neck, the visual-vestibular interaction centers in the brainstem and cerebellum, or the subjective sensation pathways of the thalamus or cortex.[1] Distinction between peripheral and central causes of vertigo can usually be made based on certain features obtained in the history. In general, peripheral vertigo is more severe than central vertigo, is more likely to be associated with hearing loss and tinnitus, and often leads to nausea and vomiting. Vertigo of central origin is typically associated with neurologic symptoms, such as diplopia, dysarthria, incoordination, numbness, and weakness. Lesions within the internal auditory canal produce a combination of vertigo, hearing loss, and facial weakness because of damage to cranial nerves (CN) VII and VIII.

Hearing loss is typically divided into conductive, sensorineural, or central—based on the anatomic site of the lesion. Conductive hearing loss results from lesions involving the external or middle ear. It is typically characterized by an approximately equal loss of hearing at all frequencies and by well-preserved speech discrimination once the threshold for hearing is exceeded. Sensorineural hearing loss results from lesions of the cochlea and/or auditory division of CN VIII. With sensorineural hearing loss, the hearing levels for different frequencies are usually unequal, typically resulting in better hearing for lower than for higher frequency tones. Patients with sensorineural hearing loss often have difficulty hearing speech that is mixed with background noise and may be annoyed by loud speech. Central hearing disorders result from lesions of the central auditory pathways. As a rule, patients with central lesions do not have impaired hearing for pure tones, and they can understand speech as long as it is clearly spoken in a quiet environment.

Tinnitus refers to noises that arise spontaneously in one or both ears. With objective tinnitus, the patient hears a sound arising external to the auditory system, a sound that can usually be heard by the examiner with a stethoscope. Subjective tinnitus can arise from sites anywhere in the auditory system. Sounds most frequently noted are metallic ringing, buzzing, blowing, and roaring; less often mentioned are clanging, popping, or nonrhythmic beating. Tinnitus

Supported by NIH Grants NIDCD DC 01404 and NIA AG 09693.

245

**TABLE 16–1.  Diagnostic Workup for Several Common Types of Dizziness**

| TYPE OF DIZZINESS | MECHANISM | FOCUS OF WORKUP |
|---|---|---|
| Vertigo | Imbalance in tonic vestibular signals | Auditory and vestibular function |
| Presyncopal light-headedness | Cerebral hypoperfusion | Cardiovascular function |
| Psychophysiologic dizziness | Impaired central integration of sensory signals | Psychiatric assessment |
| Disequilibrium | Loss of vestibulospinal, proprioceptive, or cerebellar function | Vestibular, peripheral nerve, and cerebellar function |

without observable hearing loss appears sporadically and for variable lengths of time in many individuals without any evidence of an ongoing pathologic process.

The focus of this review is the diagnostic workup of patients presenting with vertigo, hearing loss, and tinnitus. We will first briefly review the bedside and laboratory tests of auditory and vestibular function and then address the diagnostic workup in common clinical situations.

## BEDSIDE TESTING

### VESTIBULAR TESTS

Bedside tests of vestibular function can be subdivided into those of vestibulo-ocular and vestibulospinal function. As a general rule, tests of vestibulospinal function are insensitive because most patients can use vision and proprioceptive signals to compensate for any vestibular loss. Patients with an acute unilateral peripheral vestibular lesion may past point or fall toward the side of the lesion, but within a few days balance returns to normal. Patients with bilateral peripheral vestibular loss have more difficulty compensating and usually show some imbalance on the Romberg test and tandem walking tests, particularly when the eyes are closed.

It can be difficult to separate vestibulo-ocular control from the other ocular control systems, but since the vestibulo-ocular system is the only ocular control system that works at high frequencies and high velocities, one can usually obtain a rough assessment of vestibular function at the bedside. If the patient is instructed to focus on the examiner's nose and the patient's head is rapidly moved to the side, normally there will be a smooth compensatory eye movement that is roughly equal and opposite to the head movement. In patients with vestibular lesions, the compensatory eye movement is inadequate and the patient requires catch-up saccades to maintain fixation on the examiner's nose. This "head-thrust test" can be used to identify both unilateral and bilateral deficits in the vestibulo-ocular reflex, based on whether the catch-up saccades occur in only one direction or in both directions.[16] Another qualitative bedside test of the vestibulo-ocular reflex is to have the patient shake the head back and forth at frequencies above one cycle per second while reading a standard visual acuity chart.[10] A decrease in visual acuity of more than one line compared to testing with the head held still indicates an abnormal vestibulo-ocular reflex.

Spontaneous nystagmus secondary to peripheral vestibular lesions is inhibited with fixation and may only be seen with recordings in the dark (one of the major uses of electronystagmography). One can partially inhibit fixation by using Frenzel glasses (+30 lenses) or by covering one eye and looking into the other eye with an ophthalmoscope.[20] As a general rule, nystagmus that is noted only when fixation is inhibited indicates a peripheral vestibular lesion. By contrast, spontaneous nystagmus that is noted on routine examination while the patient is fixating is nearly always due to a central lesion.

Two different types of positional testing are routinely used: (1) a rapid change from the erect sitting position to the supine head-hanging position (Dix-Hallpike test, Fig. 16–1), and (2) a quick head turn to the side while the patient is lying supine. Paroxysmal positional nystagmus occurs transiently after the position is reached, whereas static positional nystagmus persists as long as the position is held. The most common type of paroxysmal positional nystagmus (benign

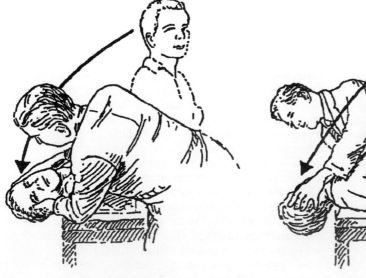
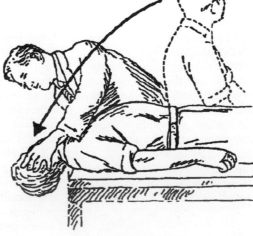

**FIGURE 16–1.** Dix-Hallpike positional test for benign positional vertigo.

Head-hanging right                    Head-hanging left

positional nystagmus) is induced by the Dix-Hallpike test. It usually has a 3- to 10-second latency before onset and rarely lasts longer than 30 seconds. The nystagmus has combined torsional and vertical components consistent with its originating from the posterior semicircular canal. A key feature is that the patient has severe vertigo with the initial positioning, but with repeated positioning, the vertigo and nystagmus fatigue. As discussed later, when this characteristic paroxysmal positional nystagmus is identified, the diagnosis of benign positional vertigo is made and one can proceed with a simple curative maneuver.

## AUDITORY FUNCTION TESTING

A quick test for hearing loss in the speech range is to observe the patient's response to spoken commands at different intensities (whisper, conversation, shouting). Tuning fork tests permit a rough assessment of hearing for pure tones of known frequency, and the clinician can use his or her own hearing as a reference standard. In the Rinne test nerve conduction is compared to bone conduction by holding a tuning fork against the mastoid process until the sound can no longer be heard. It is then placed 1 inch from the ear and in normal subjects can be heard twice as long by air conduction as by bone conduction. If bone conduction is better than air conduction, the hearing loss is conductive, but care must be taken to ensure that the bone conduction sound is not heard in the normal ear. In the Weber test, the tuning fork is placed on the patient's forehead or upper teeth. Normally this sound is referred to the center of the head. If it is referred to the side of a unilateral hearing loss, the hearing loss is conductive; if it is referred away from the side of a unilateral hearing loss, the loss is sensorineural.

# LABORATORY TESTS

## ELECTRONYSTAGMOGRAPHY

Electrooculography (EOG) is the simplest and most readily available method for recording eye movements.[4] With this technique, a voltage surrounding the orbit is measured whose magnitude is proportional to the amplitude of eye movement. When used for evaluating vestibular function, the technique has been termed electronystagmography (ENG). However, often the terms *EOG* and *ENG* are used interchangeably. With ENG, the velocity, frequency, and amplitude of spontaneous or induced nystagmus and the changes in these measurements brought about by loss of fixation (either with the eyes closed or with the eyes open in darkness) can be quantified. Also, visually guided eye movements can be quantitatively assessed.

ENG can be used to evaluate many types of eye movement disorders by adapting the testing procedure for specific abnormalities. It is useful, however, to have a standard test battery that screens all important areas. A typical battery includes tests for spontaneous and positional nystagmus, the bithermal caloric test of horizontal vestibulo-ocular reflex function, and tests of visual ocular control (saccades, smooth pursuit, and optokinetic nystagmus). With the bithermal caloric test, each ear is irrigated with cool (30° C) and warm (44° C) water for 30 to 40 seconds, and the peak slow-phase velocity of induced nystagmus is measured. The four responses are compared with two standard formulas:

Caloric asymmetry =
$$\frac{(\text{Right } 30° + \text{Right } 44°) - (\text{Left } 30° + \text{Left } 44°)}{\text{Right } 30° + \text{Right } 44° + \text{Left } 30° + \text{Left } 44°} \times 100$$

Directional preponderance =
$$\frac{(\text{Right } 30° + \text{Left } 44°) - (\text{Right } 44° + \text{Left } 30°)}{\text{Right } 30° + \text{Left } 44° + \text{Right } 44° + \text{Left } 30°} \times 100$$

### Interpretation

Like testing for spontaneous nystagmus at the bedside, nystagmus present only in the dark (inhibited with fixation) suggests a peripheral vestibular lesion. By contrast, if the spontaneous nystagmus changes direction with gaze and if it is present with fixation, this suggests a central vestibular lesion. A caloric asymmetry >25% indicates a unilateral peripheral vestibular lesion, which includes the root entry zone of the vestibular nerve at the brainstem.[5] A directional preponderance >30% is a nonspecific finding indicating a vestibular lesion anywhere within the vestibular system.[5] Abnormalities of saccades, smooth pursuit, and optokinetic nystagmus usually indicate a lesion of the central nervous system (if it is assumed that the patient is alert, cooperative, and not taking sedating medications)[4] (Table 16–2).

## ROTATIONAL TESTING

Rotational testing of the vestibulo-ocular reflex is becoming more widely used because modern motor-driven platforms can be precisely controlled and multiple graded stimuli can be delivered in a relatively short time.[4] Also, the head can be moved voluntarily in the frequency range of natural head movements so that it is possible to make quantitative measurements of the vestibulo-ocular reflex at the bedside. Most attention has been focused on the horizontal vestibulo-ocular reflex since it is the easiest to stimulate and record. Unlike caloric testing, rotational testing depends only on the inner ear and is unrelated to the physical features of the external ear or temporal bone. Thus rotational testing is a more reliable vestibular stimulus. A major disadvantage of rotational testing is that both ears are stimulated simultaneously; therefore it is less useful than caloric testing for identifying unilateral peripheral vestibular lesions.

### Interpretation

Results of rotational testing of the horizontal vestibulo-ocular reflex are typically reported in terms of gain (peak slow-phase eye velocity divided by peak stimulus velocity) and timing measurements (phase or time constant) (Table 16–2).[6] Although patients with complete unilateral peripheral vestibular deficits show an asymmetry in rotation-induced nystagmus, particularly at high velocities and high frequencies, such testing is insensitive for identifying partial unilateral loss of vestibular function. Patients with bilateral vestibular loss typically show a decrease in gain (beginning in the low-frequency range and involving the higher frequencies in later stages), an increase in the low-frequency phase lead, and a shortening of the time constant. Because of its greater sensitivity in comparison to caloric testing, rotational testing is ideal for the follow-up of patients receiving potentially ototoxic drugs. Patients with cerebellar lesions usually have normal rotational responses in the dark, but

**TABLE 16–2. Main Indications for Different Diagnostic Tests and Meaning of Abnormal Findings**

| TEST | INDICATIONS | ABNORMAL FINDINGS | LIKELY MEANING |
|---|---|---|---|
| Electronystagmography | To document a unilateral vestibular lesion or peripheral vs. central vestibular lesion | Unidirectional spontaneous or positional nystagmus in dark | Peripheral vestibular lesion |
| | | Direction-changing spontaneous or positional nystagmus with fixation | Central vestibular lesion |
| | | Caloric asymmetry >25% | Unilateral peripheral vestibular lesion |
| | | Caloric directional preponderance >30% | Vestibular lesion (nonspecific) |
| | | Saccade overshoots | Cerebellar lesion |
| | | Impaired pursuit, optokinetic nystagmus | Central lesion (nonspecific) |
| Rotational testing | To document bilateral peripheral vestibular lesion | Decreased gain, increased phase lead, and shortening of time constant in dark | Bilateral peripheral vestibular lesion |
| | To document peripheral vs. central vestibular lesion | Impaired fixation-suppression | Cerebellar lesion |
| Posturography | Not a diagnostic test | | |
| Audiometry | To screen all cases of vertigo, tinnitus, or hearing loss of unknown cause | Progressive unilateral high frequency | Acoustic neuroma or other CN VIII lesion |
| | | Fluctuating unilateral low frequency | Meniere's syndrome |
| | | Bilateral 4000 Hz notch | Noise-induced |
| | | Bilateral symmetric sloping | Presbycusis |
| Brainstem auditory evoked responses | To separate nerve vs. cochlear | All waves absent | Not helpful |
| | | All waves delayed | Conductive or cochlear loss |
| | | Delayed I-V interval | CN VIII or brainstem lesion |

they are unable to inhibit the vestibulo-ocular reflex when they are rotated with a fixation target.[6]

## POSTUROGRAPHY

The neural pathways that underlie the vestibular contributions to the control of the head, body, and limbs are collectively called the vestibulospinal system. To date, vestibular tests have concentrated on the vestibulo-ocular system, mainly because it is difficult to accurately assess the role of the vestibular system in isolation from other sensory systems, namely, vision and somatosensation. Motor-driven force platforms have been designed to control the relative contributions of the visual, somatosensory, and vestibular inputs that are normally used to maintain an upright posture.[12] With such a device, the platform on which a patient stands can be moved simultaneously with the visual surround. By coupling the platform to the sway of the subject (sway referencing), it is possible to maintain a constant angle between the foot and lower leg, thereby reducing a major source of somatosensory input to the postural control system. If the subject closes the eyes or if the movement of the visual enclosure is coupled to body sway, the patient is deprived of visual information about postural sway. In this way the influence of the labyrinth on the upright posture through the vestibulospinal system can be studied in relative isolation.

### Interpretation

There is little evidence to suggest that specific patterns of abnormality on posturography are associated with specific neuro-otologic disorders. Patients with acute peripheral vestibular lesions show a transient increase in sway, particularly when the vestibular system is partially isolated with sway referencing and eye closure, but these abnormalities are transient, lasting only a few weeks, even if the unilateral vestibular lesion is permanent.[13] Similarly, patients with bilateral reduction in peripheral vestibular function have abnormal postural sway with sway referencing and eye closure,

but these findings are also seen with central lesions such as cerebellar atrophy.[7] Thus posturography, in its current state, is not a diagnostic test. However, it may be useful for follow-up of balance function as patients compensate for or are treated for vestibular disorders.

## AUDIOMETRY

An audiogram is one of the most informative and cost-effective screening tests available to neurologists. We order a screening audiogram in nearly all patients who present with vertigo, tinnitus, or hearing loss if there is no obvious cause identified through the history and physical examination. Most audiograms include pure tone, speech, and acoustic impedance testing.[9] Pure tone testing is the nucleus of the examination. Pure tones at selected frequencies are presented by either earphones (air conduction) or a vibrator pressed against the mastoid portion of the temporal bone (bone conduction), and the minimal level that the subject can hear is determined for each frequency. Hearing levels are recorded in decibels (dB) with reference to normal hearing ears. Two speech tests are routinely used. The speech reception threshold (SRT) is the intensity at which the patient can correctly repeat 50% of the words presented. The SRT is a test for hearing sensitivity for speech and should reflect the hearing level for pure tones in the speech range. The speech discrimination test is a measure of the patient's ability to understand speech when it is presented at a level that is easily heard. Acoustic impedance measurements are useful for assessing the mobility of the tympanic membrane and ossicular chain as well as for measuring stapedius muscle contraction.

### Interpretation

The pattern of pure-tone hearing loss often suggests the likely cause of the hearing loss (Table 16–2). In patients with CN VIII lesions, speech discrimination can be severely reduced, even when pure tone thresholds are normal or nearly normal, whereas in patients with cochlear lesions, discrimination tends to be proportional to the magnitude of the hearing loss. If a normal tympanic membrane and ossicular chain are assumed, an abnormal stapedius reflex indicates a lesion of CN VII or VIII or the interconnecting pathways in the brainstem.

### BRAINSTEM AUDITORY-EVOKED RESPONSES

Brainstem auditory-evoked responses (BAERs) can be recorded from scalp electrodes at 0 to 10 ms (early), 10 to 50 ms (middle), and 50 to 500 ms (late) following a click stimulus.[19] The early potential reflects electrical activity at the cochlea, CN VIII, and brainstem; the later potentials reflect cortical activity. Computer averaging of the responses to 1000 to 2000 clicks separates the evoked potential from background noise. We will consider only the early evoked responses, which are used to estimate the magnitude of hearing loss and to differentiate among cochlear, CN VIII, and brainstem lesions.

### Interpretation

The most common BAER abnormality is an absence of all waves associated with a profound unilateral sensorineural hearing loss (see Table 16–2). This finding is of little localizing value since it can be associated with any lesion that severely impairs hearing. It also points out the importance of obtaining a standard pure-tone audiogram before ordering a BAER. Another common finding is a delay in all waves, typically associated with either a conductive or a cochlear hearing loss, also of relatively little localizing value. A more specific finding is a delay in the I-V or I-III-V interval, which indicates involvement of the auditory division of CN VIII and the central auditory pathways.

## DIAGNOSTIC WORKUP FOR COMMON CLINICAL PRESENTATIONS

### ACUTE VERTIGO

Acute spontaneous vertigo (Fig. 16–2) results from a sudden unilateral impairment of vestibular function. It can result from sudden loss of peripheral input due to damage to the labyrinth or vestibular nerve, or it can be due to a sudden unilateral impairment of vestibular nuclear or vestibulocerebellar activity. The patient experiences an intense sense of rotation that is aggravated by head motion and often by lying down but relieved by sitting upright and keeping the head still or by lying with the intact side undermost. There also may be a sense of self-tilting toward the affected side. The patient usually notices that the visual world is moving slowly in one direction and quickly back in the other direction because of the spontaneous nystagmus. Standing and

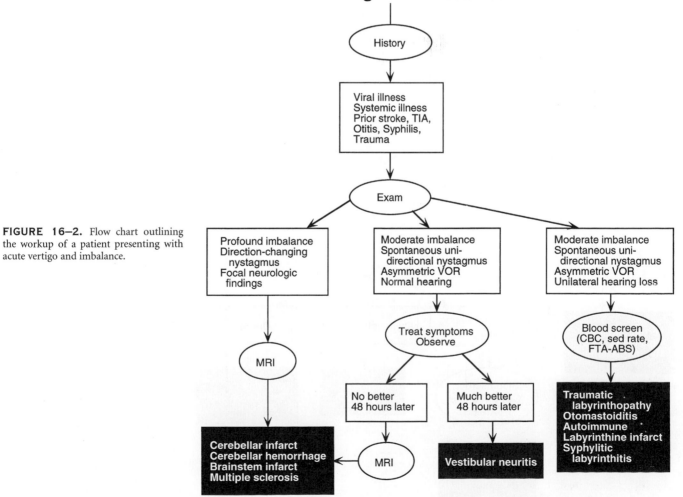

**FIGURE 16–2.** Flow chart outlining the workup of a patient presenting with acute vertigo and imbalance.

walking is difficult, and falls may occur toward the affected side. There are nearly always associated autonomic symptoms, including malaise, pallor, sweating, nausea, vomiting, and sometimes diarrhea. The first task of the examining physician is to determine whether the vertigo is of central or peripheral origin because some central causes of acute vertigo can be life-threatening and may require immediate intervention.

As noted earlier, the history often provides critical information on deciding whether the vertigo is of peripheral or central origin. The age of the patient and a history of hypertension, atherosclerotic vascular disease, or stroke suggest whether brain infarction or hemorrhage is a possible consideration. Associated unilateral hearing loss or prior trauma or infection involving the ear points toward a peripheral source. On physical examination, patients with peripheral vestibular lesions have impaired balance, but they are able to walk even during the acute phase. By contrast, patients with

central vestibular lesions are often unable to stand or take even a single step without falling. Because this distinction is so critical, patients should try to stand and walk even though they are extremely uncomfortable and prefer to lie still in bed. Spontaneous nystagmus of peripheral origin does not involve a change of direction with gaze to either side, although it increases in amplitude with gaze in the direction of the fast phase and decreases in amplitude with gaze away from the fast phase. By contrast, spontaneous nystagmus of central origin typically involves a change of direction when the patient looks away from the direction of the fast phase. Peripheral spontaneous nystagmus is inhibited with fixation; therefore the nystagmus is usually prominent only for the first 12 to 24 hours and may be completely inhibited, even with gaze in the direction of the fast phase, within a few days. By contrast, spontaneous nystagmus of central origin often persists for weeks to months. Because of these features, if there is a question regarding the peripheral or central ori-

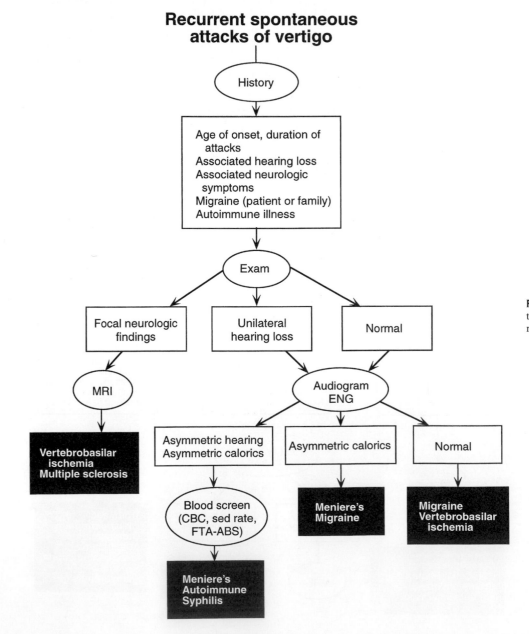

**FIGURE 16–3.** Flow chart outlining the workup of a patient presenting with recurrent spontaneous attacks of vertigo.

gin of vertigo on presentation, the patient should simply be observed for 24 to 48 hours to see if the course is typical of a peripheral or central vestibular lesion.

There are a few occasions in neuro-otology when magnetic resonance imaging (MRI) is indicated immediately:

- Vertigo and profound imbalance (patient cannot stand)
- Vertigo and focal neurologic findings
- Vertigo and new-onset severe headaches
- Horizontal spontaneous nystagmus that changes direction with gaze
- Vertical spontaneous or positional nystagmus

Note that one instance is when a patient presents with acute vertigo that likely is due to cerebellar infarct or hemorrhage. Such central lesions must be identified as soon as possible since both can lead to a mass effect with compression of the brainstem. If the indications are not clear after the physical examination, the patient should be observed. If the patient's condition is no better within 24 to 48 hours, an MRI scan should be performed. Cerebellar infarct is probably the only central lesion that could masquerade as a peripheral vestibular lesion, particularly during the first few hours, when it may be difficult to assess gait and balance and the spontaneous nystagmus.[17]

### RECURRENT SPONTANEOUS ATTACKS OF VERTIGO

Recurrent attacks of vertigo (Fig. 16–3) occur when there is a sudden temporary and largely reversible impairment of resting neural activity of one labyrinth or its central connections with subsequent recovery to normal or near-normal function. Such attacks typically last minutes to hours, rather than days, and terminate not through compensation, as with prolonged attacks, but through restoration of normal neural activity. The history provides one additional key piece of information in such patients—the duration of attacks. Vertigo of vascular origin (transient ischemic attacks [TIAs]) typically last minutes,[15] whereas peripheral inner ear causes of recurrent vertigo typically last hours. Migraine is a common cause of recurrent attacks of vertigo often beginning in childhood.[3] Vertigo is the initial symptom of multiple sclerosis in about 5% of cases. If there are focal neurologic findings on examination, it is routine to proceed directly to an MRI scan. However, it is important to keep in mind that patients with vertebrobasilar TIAs often have a completely normal neurologic examination between attacks. A screening audiogram and an electronystagmogram (ENG) examination are indicated in any patient who is having recurrent attacks of vertigo that likely are of peripheral origin (no neurologic symptoms and signs, with or without hearing loss). The diagnosis of Meniere's disease rests on finding the characteristic fluctuating low-frequency hearing loss. However, early in the disease process, hearing and vestibular function can be normal with Meniere's disease. Asymmetric caloric responses are occasionally seen with migraine, but hearing loss is infrequent with this disorder.

### RECURRENT EPISODES OF POSITIONAL VERTIGO

The history can usually separate positional vertigo (Fig. 16–4) from spontaneous attacks of vertigo, although sometimes patients will report having vertigo for several days when what they mean is that they were susceptible to episodes of positional vertigo during that time. Also, they

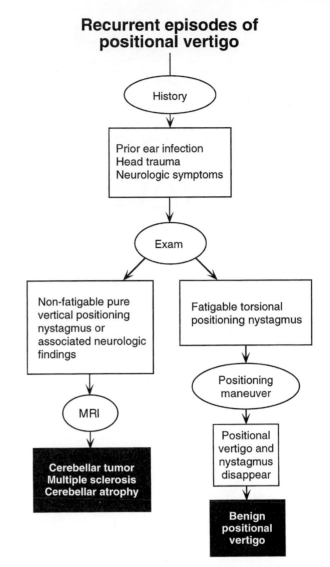

**FIGURE 16–4.** Flow chart outlining the workup of a patient presenting with recurrent episodes of positional vertigo.

may complain of a nonspecific motion-sickness type of dizziness between attacks of positional vertigo. Positional vertigo is nearly always a benign condition that can be easily cured at the bedside, but rarely it can be a symptom of a central lesion, particularly a lesion near the fourth ventricle. The diagnosis is usually clear after the standard positional testing has been performed (see Fig. 16–1). If the patient exhibits the characteristic fatigable torsional-positioning nystagmus that lasts <30 seconds, the diagnosis of benign positional vertigo is made.[1] Any deviation from this characteristic nystagmus profile should raise suspicion of a central lesion. Typically, central positional nystagmus is nonfatiguing and purely vertical (either upbeating or downbeating). Most cases of central positional nystagmus also have other associated neurologic findings. Since there are horizontal canal variants of benign positional vertigo, transient direction-changing horizontal nystagmus induced by turning the head to the side is also usually of benign peripheral origin.[1]

The cause of benign positional vertigo has convincingly been shown to result from debris (calcium carbonate crystals) moving freely within the semicircular canals (usually the

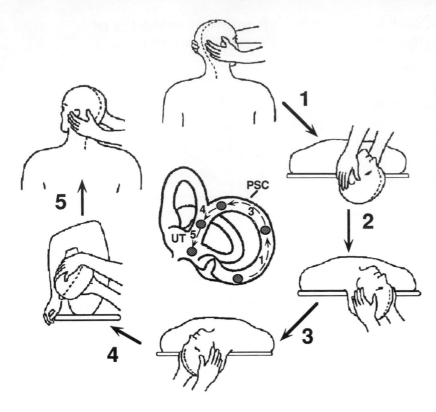

**FIGURE 16–5.** Treatment maneuver for benign positional vertigo affecting the right ear. The procedure can be reversed for treating the left ear. *1,* The patient is seated upright, with the head facing the examiner, who is standing on the right. The patient should grasp the forearm of the examiner with both hands for stability. The patient is then moved into the supine position, with the head allowed to extend just beyond the end of the examining table and the right ear downward. This position is maintained until the nystagmus ceases. *2,* The examiner moves to the head of the table, repositioning the hands as shown. *3,* The patient's head is rotated toward the left, stopping with the right ear upward. This position is maintained for 30 seconds. *4,* The patient rolls onto the left side while the examiner rotates the patient's head leftward until the nose is directed toward the floor. This position is held for 30 seconds. *5,* The patient is lifted into the sitting position, facing left. The entire sequence should be repeated until no nystagmus can be elicited. Labyrinth in the center shows the position of the debris (*shaded oval*) before and after each position change as it moves around and out of the posterior semicircular canal (*PSC*) and into the utricle (*UT*). (Adapted from Foster CA, Baloh RW. Episodic vertigo. In: Rakel RE, ed. *Conn's Current Therapy.* Philadelphia: WB Saunders; 1995;837-841.)

**FIGURE 16–6.** Flow chart outlining the workup of a patient presenting with disequilibrium without vertigo.

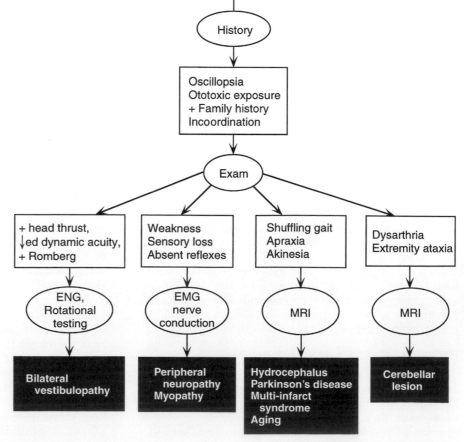

posterior semicircular canal).[1] This condition can be cured at the bedside with a simple positioning maneuver[11] designed to remove the debris from the semicircular canal (Fig. 16–5). If the characteristic fatigable positioning nystagmus is identified after the Dix-Hallpike test and the nystagmus disappears after the maneuver is performed, the diagnosis of benign positional vertigo is confirmed. Unfortunately, a small percentage of patients with benign positional vertigo (<5%) are not cured by this maneuver, possibly because the debris is lodged in the canal and not easily moved out. Lack of success after the positional maneuver, therefore, does not rule out a benign peripheral origin if the other features of the nystagmus are characteristic.

### DISEQUILIBRIUM WITHOUT VERTIGO

Patients who present with disequilibrium but without vertigo (Fig. 16–6) present a diagnostic challenge since the cause can be a lesion at such varied locations as the inner ear, the peripheral nerves and muscles, and multiple sites within the CNS. Patients who lose vestibular function symmetrically (e.g., after exposure to ototoxic drugs) have no vertigo but complain of oscillopsia due to loss of the vestibuloocular reflexes and imbalance due to loss of the vestibulospinal reflexes. Bilateral vestibular loss in young patients leads to only modest imbalance, but in older patients the vestibular loss can be disabling.[14] There are several bedside tests that indicate a bilateral vestibular loss (see bedside testing), but a definitive diagnosis requires vestibular function testing, preferably with quantitative rotational testing. Balance and gait disorders in older patients are often multifactorial. So-called multisensory dizziness occurs when there is partial loss of multiple sensory inputs (e.g., diabetic peripheral neuropathy and retinopathy). The normal deterioration in gait and balance that occurs with aging can mimic potentially

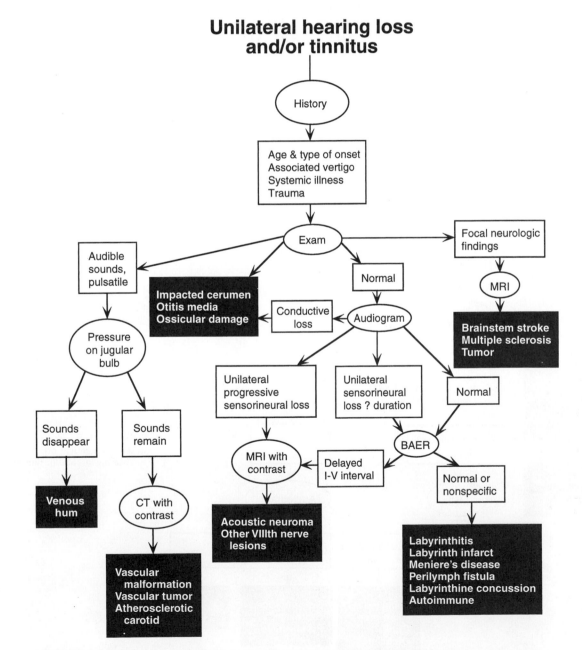

**FIGURE 16–7.** Flow chart outlining the workup of a patient presenting with unilateral hearing loss and/or tinnitus.

treatable disorders, such as occult hydrocephalus, Parkinson's disease, and multiinfarct syndrome. An MRI of the brain helps to distinguish between these different entities.

## UNILATERAL HEARING LOSS AND TINNITUS

As a general rule, a patient presenting with unilateral hearing loss or tinnitus or both (Fig. 16–7) will have an identifiable cause if a careful diagnostic workup is undertaken.[2] As with vertigo, the patient's age, the type of onset, the duration of symptoms, and whether there are associated vestibular or neurologic symptoms should be noted in the history. A prior history of trauma, infection, or systemic illness may be critical for determining the diagnosis. The examination should include a careful search for audible sounds in the ear and over the mastoid, the neck, and the external auditory canal. Carotid bruits are often transmitted to the ear. A venous hum is typically caused by turbulent flow in an enlarged jugular bulb. If the examiner can hear the same localized pulsatile sound that the patient reports, and if the sound does not disappear after gentle pressure over the jugular bulb, one should consider obtaining a computed tomography (CT) scan with contrast to rule out a vascular malformation or vascular tumor. The external auditory canal should be carefully examined to rule out impacted cerumen, infection, or obvious results of trauma.

The key laboratory test in every patient who complains of unilateral hearing loss or tinnitus is the audiogram since the pattern of hearing loss provides important diagnostic information (Table 16–2). Any patient with documented progressive unilateral sensorineural hearing loss should have an MRI with contrast performed to rule out an acoustic neuroma or other CN VIII tumor.[14] Although more than 95% of patients with acoustic neuroma present with unilateral hearing loss, occasionally a patient will present with unilateral tinnitus without hearing loss.[18] In the latter case, an abnormal BAER indicating CN VIII involvement leads to an MRI with contrast. Since acoustic neuromas are invariably slow growing and rarely present with normal hearing, it is reasonable to simply follow up patients who present with unilateral hearing loss of unknown duration or with unilateral tinnitus and normal hearing by repeating audiograms every 3 to 6 months. If evidence of a progressive hearing loss develops, an MRI with contrast is indicated.

## BILATERAL HEARING LOSS AND TINNITUS

Unlike a case with unilateral hearing loss or tinnitus or both, a treatable cause is rarely found in patients presenting with bilateral hearing loss or tinnitus or both (Fig. 16–8).[2] One exception is the identification and discontinuation of a drug known to produce bilateral tinnitus. As in patients with unilateral auditory symptoms, the key laboratory test in assessing patients with bilateral symptoms is the audiogram. By far the most common abnormalities identified are a bilateral notched (at 4000 Hz) sensorineural hearing loss due to noise exposure and a bilateral symmetric sloping sensorineural hearing loss typical of presbycusis. Patients with both of these disorders often complain of bilateral tinnitus. Sometimes amplification not only improves hearing in such patients but also improves tinnitus, probably because it introduces background sounds that help mask the tinnitus. Neurologic causes of bilateral hearing loss and/or tinnitus are rare. Finally it is rare to find a cause for bilateral tinnitus in a patient with normal hearing.

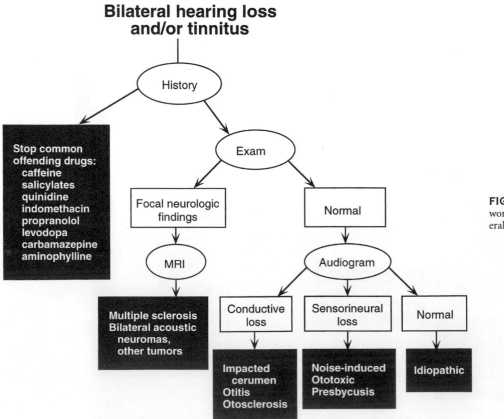

**FIGURE 16–8.** Flow chart outlining the workup of a patient presenting with bilateral hearing loss and/or tinnitus.

# SUMMARY

As in most areas of clinical medicine, the history is often the key to the diagnosis in patients presenting with neuro-otologic symptoms. The most common type of vertigo, benign positional vertigo, can be diagnosed at the bedside based on the characteristic history and the finding of fatigable positional nystagmus on the Dix-Hallpike positional test. Furthermore, this condition can be cured with a simple positioning maneuver. Quantitative auditory and vestibular function testing are important for documenting the site and the severity of deficit in patients with chronic neuro-otologic symptoms. Only a few presentations (see discussion of acute vertigo) require neuroimaging.

Dizziness, tinnitus, and hearing loss are common symptoms caused by many different diseases. Laboratory studies can help localize the lesion (peripheral, central, inner ear, CN VIII), but the diagnosis usually rests on finding the characteristic combination of symptoms and signs. The logic used to diagnose the common clinical presentations in neuro-otology are presented through flow diagrams.

# REFERENCES

1. Baloh RW. Benign positional vertigo. In: Baloh RW, Halmagyi GM, eds. *Disorders of the Vestibular System.* New York: Oxford University Press; 1996:238.
2. Baloh RW. *Dizziness, Hearing Loss and Tinnitus.* New York: Oxford University Press; 1998.
3. Baloh RW. Neurotology of migraine. *Headache.* 1997;37:615.
4. Balow RW, Furman JMR. Modern vestibular function testing. *West J Med.* 1989;150:59.
5. Baloh RW, Honrubia V. *Clinical Neurophysiology of the Vestibular System.* 2nd ed. Philadelphia: FA Davis; 1990.
6. Baloh RW, Honrubia V, Yee RD, et al. Changes in the human vestibulo-ocular reflex after loss of peripheral sensitivity. *Ann Neurol.* 1984;16:222.
7. Baloh RW, Jacobson KM, Beykirch K, Honrubia V. Static and dynamic posturography in patients with vestibular and cerebellar lesions. *Arch Neurol.* 1998;55:649.
8. Baloh RW, Yee RD, Honrubia V. Late cortical cerebellar atrophy: clinical and oculographic features. *Brain.* 1986;109:159.
9. Beagley HA, ed. *Audiology and Audiologic Medicine.* New York: Oxford University Press; 1981.
10. Demer JL, Honrubia V, Baloh RW. Dynamic visual acuity: a test for oscillopsia and vestibulo-ocular reflex function. *Am J Otol.* 1994;15:340.
11. Epley JM. The canalith repositioning procedure: for treatment for benign positional vertigo. *Otolaryngol Head Neck Surg.* 1992;107:399.
12. Fetter M, Dichgans J. Vestibular tests in evolution. II. Posturography. In: Baloh RW, Halmagyi GM, eds. *Disorders of the Vestibular System.* New York: Oxford University Press; 1996:256.
13. Fetter M, Diener HC, Dichgans J. Recovery of postural control after an acute unilateral vestibular lesion in humans. *J Vestib Res.* 1991;1:373.
14. Fife TD, Baloh RW. Disequilibrium of unknown cause in older people. *Ann Neurol.* 1993;34:694.
15. Grad A, Baloh RW. Vertigo of vascular origin: clinical and ENG features in 84 cases. *Arch Neurol.* 1989;46:281.
16. Halmagyi GM, Curthoys IS. A clinical sign of canal paresis. *Arch Neurol.* 1988;45:737.
17. Huang CY, Yu YL. Small cerebellar strokes may mimic labyrinthine lesions. *J Neurol Neurosurg Psychiatry.* 1985;48:263.
18. Kim HN, Jenkins HA. Vestibular schwannomas and other cerebellopontine angle tumors. In: Balow RW, Halmagyi GM, eds. *Disorders of the Vestibular System.* New York: Oxford University Press; 1996;461.
19. Stockard JJ, Stockard JE, Sharbough FW. Brain stem auditory evoked potentials in neurology: methodology, interpretation, and clinical application. In: Aminoff MJJ, ed. *Electrodiagnosis in Clinical Neurology.* New York: Churchill Livingstone; 1986:467.
20. Zee DS, Fletcher WA. Bedside examination. In: Baloh RW, Halmagyi GM, eds. *Disorders of the Vestibular System.* New York: Oxford University Press; 1996;178.

# 17

# Neurotoxicology

*James W. Albers and Stanley Berent*

The evaluation of a patient with a suspected neurotoxic disorder is no different from the evaluation of any patient with symptoms or signs referable to the nervous system. The patient's complaints (symptoms) and findings on clinical examination (signs) are used to localize the problem to broad regions of the nervous system and to generate a differential diagnosis. At that point any number of tests are sometimes selected to refine the differential diagnosis.[2] In the process, some items may be eliminated from the differential diagnosis and others may be added. This iterative process of formulating a clinical hypothesis and then performing additional studies, when indicated, to refine the diagnosis forms the basis of clinical medicine. Available tests include quantitative neuropsychologic measures of cognition and affect, imaging studies of anatomy and structure, metabolic studies of neuroanatomic function, electrophysiologic studies of the central and peripheral nervous systems, and a variety of ancillary laboratory studies directed toward evaluation of other organ systems or measurement of the body burden of a specific toxin.

Occasionally the results of a laboratory test will suggest the cause of a neurotoxic problem. Only rarely, however, are clinical findings so characteristic as to suggest a specific disorder. More commonly, the cause (etiologic basis) of a problem is inferred by addressing a series of questions referred to as the Hill criteria.[43] This process probably has its most direct application to infectious diseases, but it is an exercise that clinicians use daily in identifying any number of vascular, metabolic, infectious, neoplastic, or toxic etiologic complexes. Of the criteria, the most directly relevant to establishing a neurotoxic cause include appropriate exposure, biologic plausibility, and elimination of competing causes. Of these, the most difficult criterion to satisfy is that related to eliminating competing explanations. It is this role that is often deferred to the expertise of the experienced clinician. For the most part, few of the tests available are of sufficient specificity to establish a specific neurotoxic disorder in isolation.

In addition to their use in evaluation of individual patients, neurologic tests frequently are employed to compare groups of individuals in an attempt to identify group differences. The most familiar use involves neurologic testing in pharmacologic trials. This testing includes attempts to identify the efficacy of a drug that purports to improve neurologic function and to discover an unsuspected neurotoxicity. Most pharmaceutical trials are cohort studies in which patients are followed up over time in a controlled manner. In these studies the groups differ only by the presence of the pharmaceutical agent. This chapter focuses on the use of neurologic testing to identify differences among individuals who presumably differ only by their exposure to a certain neurotoxic agent. In the occupational setting, such a test most commonly is a cross-sectional study in which control subjects are matched to workers exposed to some substance, with the groups presumably differing only by exposure. Occasionally, specific neurologic tests are developed to measure a particular attribute by making them particularly sensitive to the neurotoxic agent being studied. It is well known that evaluations of this type are vulnerable to unidentified confounders, limiting the power of cross-sectional studies. In general, these studies are considered *hypothesis generating* rather than *hypothesis testing*. This terminology acknowledges that cross-sectional studies identifying differences between groups cannot necessarily assume that the differences are related to the variable in question (e.g., a suspected neurotoxin). Once a difference is identified, a cohort study, in which individuals can be examined before and after exposure, remains one of the best methods of evaluating the hypothesis that the suspected neurotoxin is producing the adverse effect.

A variety of tests are important in the evaluation of neurotoxic disorders. The objective of any test is to sample aspects of function or structure that are relevant to clinical questions and to provide support for diagnostic conclusions. They also are used to ensure the organic nature of a suspected neurotoxic disorder and to screen groups of subjects with suspected neurotoxic disorders, particularly toxic neu-

Supported in part by a DOW Chemical Company Foundation SPHERE (Supporting Public Health and Environmental Research Efforts) Award, and funding from CSX Transportation, Inc., and the National Institutes of Health (NS 15655, AG 08671 and AG 07378). The authors wish also to thank Christine Swartz, Ph.D., and Bruno Giordani, Ph.D., for their assistance in preparing the sections on neuropsychology.

ropathy. The role of neurologic testing is limited until the tests themselves have been evaluated. At minimum, the sensitivity and specificity of any measure must be known before it can be effectively used in any neurologic evaluation. The application and limitations of conventional studies are best established for individual patient evaluations. All tests have limitations, and indiscriminate use in suspected occupational or environmental disorders is inconsistent with their intended application. For most disorders, abnormalities are nonspecific and of limited use in establishing the cause of neurologic impairment. This is because few neurotoxic problems have cardinal electrophysiologic features that are sufficiently characteristic to be considered diagnostic. Further, measures purporting to identify subclinical group differences in suspected neurotoxic disorders must be interpreted cautiously because of numerous confounders that influence such data.

Neurotoxins exist that damage the nervous system at different levels. A selection of tests frequently used by the neurologist during the evaluation of an individual patient are listed in Table 17–1. The most important role of neuropsychologic, electrophysiologic, and imaging studies relates to the sensitivity in identifying an abnormality, sometimes in the absence of clinical symptoms or signs. Some tests, such as electromyographic (EMG) studies, localize the abnormality to a degree not clinically possible, and most clinicians consider these tests extensions of the clinical neurologic examination. The material that follows reviews neurologic tests used in studies of neurotoxic disorders. Following a brief discussion of toxic encephalopathy, the chapter is divided into two sections. The first relates to conventional neuropsychologic measures of various aspects of behavior. The second reviews those studies that are more familiar to the neurologist, including EMG, evoked potential studies, and imaging studies. Other than laboratory tests, which may be useful in establishing an elevated body burden of a specific potential neurotoxin, the remaining tests are general studies used in the evaluation of any patient with suspected neurologic disease that are not restricted to the evaluation of neurotoxic disorders.

---

### TABLE 17–1. Tests Frequently Used by the Neurologist

**Selected Neuropsychologic Tests**
*Mental Status*
Mini-Mental State Examination (MMSE)

*Intellect*
Wechsler Adult Intelligence Scales-Revised (WAIS-R)
    Verbal (information, comprehension, arithmetic, similarities,
        vocabulary, digit span)
    Performance (picture completion, picture arrangement, block
        design, object assembly, digit symbol)
Peabody Picture Vocabulary Test-Revised (PPVT-R)

*Language*
The Boston Naming Test
Verbal Fluency

*Scholastic Achievement*
Wide Range Achievement Test-Third Edition (WRAT-3)
    (reading, spelling, arithmetic)

*Memory*
Buschke Selective Reminding Test (SRT)
Wechsler Memory Scale-Russell Modification (WMS)
    Personal and current information
    Orientation
    Mental control
    Logical memory
    Memory span (digit span)
    Visual reproduction
    Associate learning

*Attention*
Test of Variables of Attention (TOVA)

*Executive Function/Complex Problem Solving*
Halstead-Reitan Category Test

*Motor and Psychomotor Areas*
Strength of Grip
Finger Tapping Speed
Reaction Time
Grooved Pegboard
Trail Making Test

*Affect*
SCL-90-R
Minnesota Multiphasic Personality Inventory (MMPI)
Hamilton Rating Scale for Depression (HRSD)

**Evaluating the Central Nervous System**
*Electrophysiology*
Electroencephalogram (EEG)
Quantitative EEG (QEEG) and EEG brain mapping
Evoked potential studies
    Visual evoked responses (VER)
    Brainstem auditory evoked responses (BAER)
    Somatosensory evoked potentials (SSEP)
Event-related potentials (e.g., P-300)
Blink reflexes

*Imaging*
Computerized tomography (CT)
Magnetic resonance imaging (MRI)
Single photon emission computed tomography (SPECT)
Positron emission tomography (PET)

**Evaluating the Autonomic and Peripheral Nervous Systems**
*Autonomic Nervous System*
Q-SART
Sympathetic skin response (SPR)
R-R interval

*Peripheral Nervous System*
*Quantitative Measures*
Quantitative sensory testing (QST)
Posturography

*Electrophysiology*
Electromyography
    Nerve conduction studies (sensory and motor)
    Repetitive motor nerve stimulation
Needle electromyography
    Conventional
    Single-fiber
Blink reflexes

*Neuropathology*
Nerve and muscle biopsy

# CENTRAL NERVOUS SYSTEM EVALUATIONS

The most common neurotoxic syndromes involving the central nervous system (CNS) are those producing acute or chronic encephalopathy. Patients with acute mild encephalopathy may complain of headache and light-headedness but demonstrate few neurologic signs. Symptoms rapidly resolve after removal from exposure. More severe forms of acute encephalopathy produce confusion, increased irritability, and altered levels of consciousness. Examination may demonstrate altered judgment and disorientation, nystagmus, and ataxia prior to more severe alteration of consciousness. In the absence of hypoxia, resolution typically is rapid after removal from exposure. A nonspecific psychoorganic syndrome or solvent encephalopathy has been attributed by some to chronic low-level or repeated high-level exposure to common organic solvents. Substantial controversy exists as to whether exposure to these substances, in the absence of hypoxia, produces permanent CNS damage in the form of a chronic toxic encephalopathy. Of note, the psychoorganic syndrome typically does not progress to the level of impairment at which neurologic or electrophysiologic signs are evident. At this mild or equivocal level of abnormality, conventional neuropsychologic (not neurophysiologic) testing is important.[63] Other toxins, however, produce CNS abnormalities when present in sufficient quantities for sufficient periods of time. In several the early nonspecific behavioral abnormalities (irritability, confusion, and anxiety) associated with mild toxic encephalopathy are followed by more apparent personality change, inappropriate behavior, impaired cognition, and disorientation. At this level of impairment the neurologic examination demonstrates postural tremor, slowed coordination, and restlessness, typically in association with asterixis, dysarthria, akathisia, gross ataxia, and the appearance of primitive reflexes (snout, suck, and grasp). As delirium develops, reflexes become hyperactive and pathologic Babinski and Chaddock reflexes become evident, sometimes in association with myoclonus. With progressive deterioration of consciousness, decerebrate posturing develops. Regardless of the nature of the resultant CNS syndrome, few would dispute the limited impact of electrophysiologic evaluations in this setting other than to indicate the magnitude of abnormality.

## Neuropsychometric Evaluation*

The neuropsychometric evaluation is guided by the patient's expressed complaints (symptoms). These symptoms, together with symptoms of other potential problems associated with encephalopathy, are translated into questions that can be answered by behavioral measurement. The procedure used to quantify behavioral aspects of human function employs psychologic tests. To quote from Anastasi, "A psychological test is essentially an objective and standardized measure of a sample of behavior."[15, p. 23] The demands for test standardization and objectivity have been formalized as "standards."[14] Each test carries a unique set of desired attributes and capabilities, as well as limitations and sources of error. There are literally thousands of neuropsychologic tests,

each designed for measuring some aspect of behavior that is relevant to a specified clinical inquiry. Most often, it is necessary to measure several aspects of behavior in order to arrive at a definitive conclusion regarding an individual's functioning. The various measures are clustered in a battery of tests, which are then administered to the person. To understand how decisions are made with regard to which behaviors to measure in a given case and how individual tests are chosen requires some discussion. The following paragraphs address some of the critical issues that underlie this decision process.

Table 17–1 lists a number of tests with established validity and reliability and presents their corresponding behavioral domains. This table is intended to be only illustrative of tests employed in a neuropsychologic test battery. The tests are typical of those used in clinical evaluations. These tests listed have been chosen based on their established validity and reliability and their frequent use. They also have been selected as representative measures of intellect, language, cognition (e.g., learning, memory, problem solving), attention, sensation, perception, motor and psychomotor behavior, affect (e.g., anxiety, depression), and personality (e.g., coping style and effectiveness, presence and type of psychopathology).

The Mini-Mental State Examination (MMSE) is a brief, easily scored test of several cognitive functions. The scale assesses a subject's orientation to time and place, instantaneous recall, short-term memory, and ability to perform serial subtractions or reverse spelling. The MMSE also measures constructional capacities (the ability to copy a design) and the use of language. The examination consists of 30 questions that relate to major cognitive domains such as orientation, attention, memory, language, and visual-spatial abilities. The MMSE score is produced by adding the points assigned to each successfully completed task, for a total score of 0 to 30. As a formal mental status examination, the MMSE is probably the most widely employed brief screening measure for dementia that is used alone or as a component of a larger battery. On the Buschke Selective Reminding Test (SRT), subjects are asked to recall as many words as they can, in any order, from a list of 10 words just read to them. After each trial the examiner repeats all the words that the patient omitted in that trial. Scores for verbal retention, storage, and retrieval can be obtained over each trial, as well as scores for delayed recall and recognition. The Test of Variables of Attention (TOVA) is a standardized continuous performance test that assesses sustained attention. The TOVA is administered with the use of a personal computer. It involves a 23-minute vigilance task, during which an individual must observe a screen on which one of two visual stimuli is randomly presented on the computer screen for 100 ms every 2 seconds. The person is instructed to press a microswitch every time he or she sees the target stimulus. Scores include the number of omissions, commissions, mean response time for correct responses, and standard deviation of response time for correct responses. Norms are supplied with the test manual. The TOVA's use of standard geometric shapes (i.e., squares) as stimuli has been shown to preclude strong practice effects, as well as performance effects related to learning disabilities. The primary measure of interest for this study will be the TOVA commission (impulsivity) measure, although other scores will also be examined in secondary analyses. The TOVA is linked to recent neuropsychologic theories of memory that posit multiple dimensions, including encoding and sustaining, mediated by many brain structures.

---

*Material in this discussion relies heavily on Berent's previous publications, most notably, Berent, S., and Swartz, CL. Essential psychometrics. In: Sweet, J., ed. Forensic Neuropsychology: Fundamentals and Practice. Berwyn, PA: Swets & Zeitlinger; 1999:1-24.

Psychometry-based assessment is a dynamic and interactive process between the examiner and the examinee; the neuropsychologist is responsible for selecting a test, overseeing administration and scoring of the test, and interpreting scores.[16] The application of psychometrics aims to achieve a scientifically based, objective, and systematic approach to establish signs that substantiate and elucidate the patient's clinical status. A series of clinically relevant questions can be addressed by the psychometric examination, including those listed in Table 7–2. The first question formally addressed by the neuropsychometric examination is the presence or absence of abnormality. Answering it requires a knowledge of normal and abnormal behavior and how each is reflected in psychologic test results. In answering the question of normality, the problem of individual differences is addressed because people vary one from another, sometimes substantially, along a continuum for any given behavior. This variability of human behavior is one of the great challenges for psychometric examination.

A systematic and objective approach based on sound principles of science is critical to the clinical enterprise because of the inferential nature of the information and the lack of precision at every level of involvement. For example, the patient may mistakenly complain of a memory deficit when, in fact, he or she is experiencing a problem with attention or some other aspect of cognition. On the other hand, problems may exist that are not obvious to the patient. There are relatively few specific nervous system responses to trauma or disease, and the etiologic basis usually cannot be established by association alone without violating basic clinical and scientific principles.

The psychometric approach is also complicated by the fact that behavioral measures are not usually specific to a given kind of neurologic disorder. For example, decreased memory may result from a toxic encephalopathy, although an identical complaint may be associated with a progressive disorder such as Alzheimer's disease or clinical depression. A complaint of memory impairment alone, whether made by self-report or by someone close to the patient, is insufficient to establish a diagnosis. Information obtained directly from the patient or indirectly from family members or others can be important, but the clinical evaluation of patients with suspected neurologic disease requires a balance of established clinical and laboratory measures that ultimately produce a differential diagnosis.

The clinician also is responsible for identifying disorders whose symptoms mimic neurotoxic damage but are unrelated to an environmental toxic etiologic factor. In establishing a diagnosis of neurotoxic disease, interpretation of abnormal neuropsychologic test findings must account for findings that are unrelated to toxic exposure (e.g., a preexisting pathologic condition such as previous head injury) or represent a normal physiologic or psychologic variation (e.g., low intelligence level or depressed mood). The goal is to arrive at an objective reality concerning the patient's problem and to identify the cause (or etiologic complex), the anticipated course, and the treatment.

### Essential Psychometric Test Criterion

Four essential psychometric test requirements—validity, reliability, procedural standardization, and availability of normative data—are important for any neuropsychologic test.

*Validity.* A test must reflect, through published research, the established validity of the instrument to measure what it purports to measure. Validity is a technical aspect of test development. As stated in the standards, validity is the most important consideration in test evaluation because it refers to the ". . . appropriateness, meaningfulness, and usefulness of the specific inferences made from test scores."[14] Validity can be examined in a number of different forms. One of the most straightforward is *face validity*. Face validity refers to the overt meaningfulness or relatedness of an instrument. For example, an individual question, such as "Are you depressed?" would reflect a high degree of face validity for the assessment of depression because the apparent purpose of the question is directly related to the desired inference. Face validity can be deceptive in its simplicity, however, and is not sufficient to qualify an instrument as a formal psychologic test. Although the face validity of a test item may make it a good candidate for inclusion in the final instrument, other, (higher) forms of validity must derive from formal statistical inquiry. Through a formal statistics-based study, an item that first appears to relate to an underlying theoretic construct may be found to have very little relationship to that behavior. On the other hand, some seemingly unrelated items may be found to vary strongly with the construct of interest. The face validity of an instrument can affect the respondent's motivation and interact with the patient's response set. For persons with a "malingering" and "naive" response set, particularly high inflation in symptoms and areas of deficits may be most apparent on tasks with high face validity but less evident on tasks with low face validity. Thus correlation methods are important to the establishment of a test's actual validity. Although beyond the scope of the present chapter, more complex aspects of validity are often discussed with regard to issues of content, criteria, or construct validity.

*Sources of Bias.* Even though a neuropsychologic test can exhibit adequate validity, individual performances on a test can be affected by multiple factors that may compromise the accuracy or meaningfulness of a particular set of test scores. These factors may include the characteristics of the test, such as clarity of directions, degree of novelty, and degree of cultural bias. Sources of test bias, such as cultural factors, can be particularly important issues to consider. These factors may also interact with characteristics of the individual test taker, such as skill level, anxiety, motivation, physical

---

### TABLE 17–2. Questions Potentially Addressed by the Psychometric Examination

Is the person functioning normally or abnormally?
What is the specific nature of the abnormality?
What is the magnitude of severity?
Does the abnormality represent a change from historical baseline?
Is the abnormality acute, subacute, or chronic?
Is the problem worsening, static, or resolving?
Is there focal or generalized neurologic involvement?
To what extent are motivation, depression, and other nonneurologic factors involved?
What is the functional significance for other aspects of the individual's life?
Are there implications for diagnosis, treatment, prognosis, or etiology?

limitations, degree of bilingualism, deficiencies in educational opportunities, or unfamiliarity with testing situations.[32] Motivational factors of the test taker may be particularly salient in forensic settings. Persons involved in litigation may reflect a unique subpopulation with differing characteristics, including base rates of reported symptoms.[37] In addition, issues related to inappropriate standardization samples, examiner language bias, or inequitable social consequences may have an impact on the validity of an instrument for a given person.[64] Interpersonal variables, such as differences in age, socioeconomic status, or cultural background, may affect motivation for testing, response set, or test-taking approach. For example, some research has suggested that the "tempo of life" traditionally associated with a cultural group may affect the "speed" of response to test items.[44] Members of minority cultural groups may not have experienced certain task demands in testing situations, and this differential motivation for a task may confound the results of their performance.[24,50] These moderating variables may result in a different validity coefficient for a particular subgroup and should be reported in validation studies and taken into account in the interpretation of test results.

*Reliability.* Reliability refers to the degree to which test scores are free from errors of measurement.[14] It is an indication of the test's consistency, either between items in a given administration or between two or more administrations of the same test. The reliability of a test establishes the upper limit for the validity of the test. Although the user of a test is not generally required to establish a test's reliability independently, the user does need to know to what extent differences between forms or administrations of a particular test reflect errors of measurement vs. the effects of disease progression (e.g., metastasis of a malignant tumor) or other clinical event.

Every test score includes some error. This error is expressed as the error of measurement and should be specified by the test publisher in the published manual. The error of measurement is used to construct intervals for a particular score. It is the test user's responsibility to consider this error in reaching conclusions regarding a given score. For instance, the published error of measurement on a commonly used intelligence test is ±5 points. Thus a score ($s$) derived on any given occasion would actually be $s \pm 5$. If $s = 100$, it is likely that the actual score is 95 or 105. If the test is administered in a given case on two separate occasions, yielding scores of 95 and 102, respectively, in practice these results would be considered to be the same. All conclusions that are based on psychologic test findings, as in all scientific enterprise, are probability statements, which include an error of measurement. This error score will vary depending on the exactness required in a given instance.

The reliability of an instrument is often reported in terms of test-retest, alternate form, split-half, and other measures of internal consistency. As in the case of validity, reliability is established through formal scientific inquiry and is represented by correlation analysis. Measurements of reliability can be influenced by extraneous factors. Reliability can also be influenced by the variability in scores or a restriction in range of scores. When the distribution of scores is restricted in range, the reliability coefficient is lower. Studies of test-retest reliability are affected by the length of the interval between administration of the tests, which may be influenced by practice effects, real learning, and maturation. External factors, such as an individual's attempts at "guessing," "malingering," or other variations in the test situations, may act as confounding factors in assessment of a test's reliability.

## Other Issues in Test Construction and Utilization

*Standardization.* To be formally termed a "test," a measurement device must be "standardized"; that is, a standard procedure for administering the test needs to be specified and adhered to in all instances of test administration. The concept of standardization is important in psychology, as in science in general, and its importance in the measurement of behavior can not be overestimated. Standardization applies to all aspects of the test, including such seemingly extra-test considerations as instructions and examples given, timing of stimulus presentations, how to respond to the subject's questions, the testing environment, and other details of the test situation. If the standardized procedure of administration is altered, the reliability and validity of the instrument is compromised. As already mentioned, standardization refers to uniformity in the administration of the test, but it also extends to test scoring. Some tests are relatively simple instruments that require very little on the part of the examiner to ensure uniform administration and scoring. In other instances the test procedure or scoring may be complex and may require substantial training for professionally acceptable use. In all cases there are basic considerations of test administration that require formal training to be qualified as a tester. This area of practice is another that is sometimes abused, and the consumer of test information must determine that proper procedure has been followed in any given instance. Published guidelines and texts address these issues.[1,34]

*Normative Data.* Finally, a test is "normed"; that is, there is some prescribed method for relating the test scores to a representative population sample. It should be mentioned that norms do not remove the paramount importance placed on validity and reliability issues. They simply aid in understanding what a particular score on a test means. A relatively low score on a verbal learning task might be expected of someone with a life-long record of low intellect and academic achievement, for instance, whereas in another person it might reflect a cognitive impairment. Normative data are usually derived through formal research, in which the test being developed is administered to a large group of subjects. Important factors to consider in evaluating the adequacy of a particular normative group include representativeness, size, and relevance. Results from tests often generate standardized scores or a percentile rank, based on the normative sample, which allow comparison of an individual's performance across different tests. These standardized scores and percentile ranks are usually based on the assumption that the population's performance on this measure eventuates in a characteristic numeric distribution, usually approximating a normal distribution, the normal or bell-shaped curve.

The performance of the "normative" group determines the average performance anticipated for a given individual on the specified test and provides an indication of "normally" expected variability in performance. It is through such normative testing that "raw" test scores that are earned by a given individual take on clinically relevant meaning. By scaling the raw score, the psychologist is able to compare that individual performance against a meaningful referent group and determine the score's significance in the individual case. For example, most commonly used tests of intelligence have been "normed" against a sample that reflects an average scaled score of 100, with a standard deviation of ±15. The psychologist who gives this test to a person who obtains a scaled score of 85 knows that this individual falls one standard deviation below the average and is functioning at the 15th percentile in comparison to the referent population (i.e., better than only 15% of the referent population). As can be seen from this description, the adequacy of the test is often determined by the adequacy of the sample against which the test has been normed. Some measurements may also generate age-equivalent or grade-equivalent scores, and not all measured variables are normally distributed (e.g., relative handedness is not normally distributed in the general population). The reference group(s) will determine the shape of the distribution, as well as its average performance level and variability.

## Test Selection

There are many published psychologic tests to choose from and a variety of nontest procedures (i.e., tasks). The designation "task" is designed to distinguish these procedures from "psychological tests," which are bona fide in the technical sense. Simple and choice reaction-time procedures, for example, lend themselves to computerization and have become important in studies of neuropharmacology and behavior. In the use of such instruments, standardization of procedure becomes as important as the task itself in determining the instrument's usefulness and appropriateness in a given instance.

On what basis is a given test selected to be used in a particular case? There are several factors to consider in answering such a question. A test provides a sample of behavior, usually expressed as a collection of numeric data, and the neuropsychologist must consider how the test's results will relate to the patient's complaints and symptoms as well as to the referral question(s). The technical merits of the test must also be evaluated, and the methodology required for test administration must be considered. Finally, there are factors such as customary practice, training background, and professional competencies and other practical considerations. The capacity of a given instrument to generate data that will address the person's complaints or symptoms must be considered. The question posed might be as follows: Are there observable behaviors whose measurement will help answer the referral question(s)? Relevant variables become "operationally defined" as performance on a given task. In many instances, more than one kind of data may be required to answer a given question. For example, a question about a student's readiness to return to a regular classroom setting following a period of hospitalization may require test data that reflect, among other things, past school performance (e.g., reading level), general level of ability (e.g., intellect), presence or absence of cognitive dysfunction (e.g., impairment of memory), and factors that may interfere with optimal performance (e.g., depression). Particular instruments may be selected on the basis of their ability to assess multiple areas of functioning vs. a more narrow-band instrument, which would assess a single skill. Other factors to be considered may be the age of the patient and the appropriateness of a measure across the age span.

The technical merits of a given test instrument, from a psychometric point of view, will be evaluated. Are the available norms suitable for comparison to the present sample? Does the test measure the theoretic construct as needed to answer the referral question? (For example, is it valid?) Will the chosen test allow for a repeat examination at a future date, or are practice effects too great to allow for such retesting when it is needed? Other considerations might include the availability of qualitative analysis of performances, and the use of objective scoring criteria. Given particular referral questions, the propensity of the instrument to minimize false-positives or false-negatives may also be particularly important.[22] A number of tests have used a technique based on the forced-choice psychophysical procedure known as "symptom validity testing" to assess for signs and to make quantitative estimates of the probability of malingering or "faking bad."[19,39,45,46,57]

Another area to consider in choosing a test can be termed "convention." There are certain instruments that have been used so extensively that they have become standard components in most neuropsychologic test batteries. A prime example of such a "standard" is the Wechsler Adult Intelligence Scale-Revised (WAIS-R) and its recent revision (WAIS-III), or its counterpart, the Wechsler Intelligence Scale for Children-Third Edition (WISC-III).[79] The Wechsler intelligence scales, in fact, have been translated into many languages and have been "normed" to many cultures. These scales are almost universally used by neuropsychologists everywhere.

## ASSESSMENT DOMAINS

Behavior can be divided into a number of areas, and tests have been devised to measure these various domains. These behavioral categories are not entirely arbitrary since arguments can be made about the relative exclusiveness of each domain in addition to the interactive quality of the domains. In addition to an objective appraisal of the patient's history, some of the most important areas to measure include intellect, language, cognition (e.g., learning, memory, problem solving), attention, sensation, perception, motor and psychomotor behavior, affect (e.g., anxiety, depression), and personality (e.g., coping style and effectiveness as well as presence and type of psychopathology). Advances in neuroscience in the past few decades have taught us that the question of neurologic dysfunction is a complex one that requires a comprehensive examination to address; this is because of psychometric reasons but also because of the myriad functions of the brain. When a different kind of question is posed, the nature of the behavioral data needed for its answer will also be different, as will the construction of the test battery. This allows the neuropsychologist to also examine the pattern of an individual's performance in order to assess convergent (or supporting) findings and discriminative (or differentiating) evidence that contributes to a differential diagnosis.

## ELECTROPHYSIOLOGY

### Electroencephalogram

The electroencephalogram (EEG) consists of electrical signals recorded from the scalp that are generated by neural tissue within the brain. The resultant waveforms are inspected visually and interpreted subjectively. Interpretation includes evaluation of the waveform amplitude, frequency, coherence, symmetry, and responsiveness. Criteria for abnormality are somewhat arbitrary, and minor interobserver differences exist in the determination of normal and abnormal. In addition, the EEG is influenced by numerous factors that may be difficult to control, including the level of arousal.

The EEG plays an important role in the evaluation of encephalopathy by providing an objective measure of severity. There is a relatively good relationship between the EEG abnormality and the level of encephalopathy in acute encephalopathy.[52] Sensitivity for detection of encephalopathy is modest, but most patients with clinically evident encephalopathy have an abnormal EEG. The characteristic finding in encephalopathy is diffuse intermittent or continuous slowing of the background rhythm. The earliest slowing appears in the posterior rhythm, with progressive reduction into the low alpha- or high theta-frequency range. With progressive deterioration, a dominant theta frequency becomes widespread and the EEG demonstrates poor reactivity, especially to visual stimuli. As the level of encephalopathy deteriorates, intermittent delta frequency appears, maximal over anterior regions. In patients with severe encephalopathy, large-amplitude irregular delta activity predominates, followed by progressive loss of amplitude and reactivity. Burst-suppression patterns precede loss of all electrical activity, coinciding to loss of cerebral function.

A major limitation relates to the poor specificity of slowing of the EEG background rhythm. Slowing is a nonspecific finding that does not distinguish between the many forms of encephalopathy.[52] Triphasic waves are recorded in hepatic encephalopathy, but they also occur with other forms of encephalopathy, including those associated with water intoxication, hypercalcemia, thyroid disease, renal failure, and hypoxia. The presence of triphasic waves best correlates with the level of consciousness, and these waves are prominent in obtunded patients.[52] The EEG is more likely to be abnormal in acute (vs. chronic) encephalopathy. In the latter any objective evidence of cerebral dysfunction is an important contribution. For example, in chronic renal failure, the EEG often becomes abnormal only when deterioration of mental status is clinically evident. The best examples of toxic encephalopathy occur with barbiturate intoxication. EEG abnormalities are as described earlier, and the degree of abnormality correlates well with the degree of mental alteration and the level of intoxication. An additional finding is symmetrical beta activity in the frontal head regions. Degenerative disorders producing encephalopathy also demonstrate reduced frequency and abnormal background rhythm regulation. Disorders that produce cortical gray-matter dysfunction primarily cause irregular slowing and reduced amplitude. Those associated with subcortical gray-matter involvement demonstrate bilateral synchronous, semirhythmic slow activity or spike-wave complexes.[52]

## Quantitative EEG and EEG Brain Mapping

Quantitative EEG (QEEG) is the result of mathematical manipulation or processing of the conventional EEG signal to highlight particular components of interest, such as epileptiform discharges, or to transform the signal to emphasize some particular information, such as slow-frequency activity. Because of excessive slow activity in toxic encephalopathy, one potential application might be a frequency domain analysis to quantify the power of signal. Quantification of this type permits statistical comparisons between individual patients and normative data, between groups of patients, and between successive measurements of the same individual. Brain mapping is the result of a topographic display of the QEEG data. This method includes amplitude and frequency representations. QEEG and brain mapping have theoretic potential advantages over conventional EEG studies, but they remain research tools that have had limited application in the evaluation of encephalopathy or dementia. As such, they have unknown sensitivity and specificity.

QEEG has had limited application in identifying differences between groups of subjects. A primary difficulty encountered in such comparisons involves the possibility that any identified differences may simply reflect different levels of arousal that are too subtle to be detected in the conventional EEG. Assessments by committees of the American Academy of Neurology (AAN) and the American Clinical Neurophysiology Society (ACNS) concluded that QEEG and brain mapping are predisposed to false-positive results, which limit their clinical potential.[56] QEEG techniques vary substantially between laboratories, and demonstrating the clinical usefulness of one technique cannot be generalized to other techniques. EEG artifacts that are easily identified by an experienced electroencephalographer on conventional EEG sometimes appear in unusual ways in QEEG analyses. In addition, data-processing algorithms generate new artifacts that are difficult to identify, and analyses sometimes include hundreds of comparisons, producing multiple "abnormalities" by chance alone. In the evaluation of a patient with suspected dementia or encephalopathy, the finding of focal or generalized background slowing supports an organic disorder as opposed to an affective disorder (e.g., depression). For such evaluations, QEEG likely parallels the role of conventional EEG.

The American Psychiatric Association (APA) Task Force on Electrophysiological Assessment reported that QEEG can assist in detecting excessive slow activity in organic disorders.[13] However, retrospective evaluations of QEEG techniques comparing disparate groups are usually uncontrolled because they are neither random nor masked, making it difficult to evaluate their clinical utility. Further, evaluations of individual techniques frequently are conducted by investigators involved in the commercialization of the instrument, making it difficult to assess bias.[56] There is little information on how EEG brain mapping can impact the diagnosis of individual patients, and the information on sensitivity and specificity fails to substantiate a role for these tests in the clinical diagnosis of individual patients. Abnormalities identified by these techniques are nonspecific for the cause and type of pathologic condition and do not necessarily correspond to any symptoms.[10] The AAN and the ACNS assessed medicolegal abuse in relationship to brain mapping and QEEG.[56] Difficulties identified were "false-positive" and "false-negative" results at odds with other clinical measures. Both reports expressed concern that results can be influenced dramatically during the relatively subjective process of selecting portions of the EEG signal for evaluation and quantitative analyses. Test-retest reproducibility is poor, and there are few objective safeguards to limit statistical or selection-bias errors.[56] The major concern in application of studies of unproved sensitivity, specificity, and reproducibility is the resultant confusion caused by their introduction. Prospective controlled studies have not yet satisfactorily evaluated test specificity or sensitivity of QEEG techniques. At present, QEEG and brain mapping should be used only by physicians who are highly skilled in conventional EEG, and then only as an adjunct to interpretation of the traditional EEG. Use in any other context has been classified as class III quality (evidence provided by expert opinion, nonrandomized historical controls, or case reports).[56]

### Evoked Potential Studies

Evoked potential (EP) studies refer to recordings of electrical signals generated within the nervous system in response to a specific peripheral stimulus (tactile, electrical, visual, or auditory). Surface recordings are made of electrical activity resulting from peripheral nerve, plexus, spine, or brain, reflecting the functional integrity of the afferent pathways.

Visual evoked potentials (VEPs) are recorded from the scalp in response to visual stimuli, usually a shifting checkerboard pattern. They are sensitive to optic nerve and anterior chiasm disorders. Brainstem auditory evoked potentials (BAEPs) evaluate the integrity of the auditory portion of cranial nerve (CN) VIII or the auditory pathways in the brainstem. Somatosensory evoked potentials (SSEPs) are analogous to sensory nerve conduction studies. As such, they reflect activity in large myelinated peripheral axons and posterior and lateral afferent spinal cord pathways. The SSEP amplitude is lower than sensory nerve recordings and varies considerably in response to averaging technique, electrode montage, muscle activity, and stimulation paradigm, limiting the usefulness of SSEP amplitude measures. The most reliable abnormalities are those related to afferent pathway conduction slowing. Most neurotoxins produce neuronal death and axonal loss. This results in loss of response but little in the way of conduction slowing, limiting the sensitivity of SSEP measures to detect neurotoxic injury. In addition, selective loss of small myelinated fibers typically does not produce SSEP abnormalities, although SSEPs recorded in response to thermal stimuli provide a possible mechanism to evaluate small-fiber neuropathy.

EP studies are frequently used to identify clinically silent lesions in demyelinating disease, such as multiple sclerosis, and they have had application in neurotoxicology studies.[17] MRI imaging is particularly sensitive to myelin abnormalities, resulting in a decrease in the demand for EP studies because of their relative insensitivity and lack of specificity. Nevertheless, EP studies are occasionally abnormal when other clinical and laboratory studies are normal. There are few reports related to detection of neurotoxic disease. BAER abnormalities were reported in some toluene abusers at a time when no other clinical or electrophysiologic abnormalities were identified, suggesting a potential screening role for this test.[68] Nevertheless, at present, this proposed application has yet to be evaluated in a controlled environment.

### Event-Related Potentials

Event-related potentials are specialized EEG techniques used to explore specific cortical processes, including those purportedly related to cognition and attention.[54] In these recordings a specific event is time-locked to the EEG in order to explore temporally associated activity. One such event-related potential is the P-300, a potential generated in response to a random auditory signal that the patient is instructed to count, thereby encouraging attention to the stimuli. The P-300 is sometimes referred to as a cognitive EP, attributing some cognitive significance to its presence. Nevertheless, the role of this signal in relation to cognition is controversial, and the P-300 may be an electrophysiologic correlate of selected attention.[40,54,59] At present, application of this technique is limited and the sensitivity and specificity of the test is undefined.

### Blink Reflexes

Blink reflex studies are evoked responses recorded from the orbicularis oculi muscles in response to percutaneous electrical stimulation of the supraorbital nerve. They reflect neural activity along peripheral and central pathways, including a polysynaptic pathway component that crosses the midline.[72] The afferent limb of the blink reflex is mediated by the trigeminal nerve, and the efferent component is mediated by the facial nerve. Blink reflex measures include ipsilateral and contralateral response latencies. Like other evoked response measures, their utility has not been established in neurotoxic disorders. This complex polysynaptic reflex is sensitive to cueing, indicating that attention influences test results.[70] It is likely that numerous other intervening factors also influence results. Like many other electrophysiologic measures, the sensitivity and specificity of these measures are unknown.

## IMAGING

The most important role of imaging studies in suspected intoxication is to provide objective evidence of neuronal loss and to identify disorders other than neurotoxic exposure to account for the neurologic findings. Computed tomography (CT) and magnetic resonance imaging (MRI) are capable of identifying structural abnormalities. Both are sensitive to disorders that result in cerebral atrophy. Any neurotoxin that produces neuronal death has the potential to produce atrophy identifiable by imaging studies, depending upon the location and extent of involvement. In patients with acute encephalopathy, imaging studies are unremarkable unless a preexisting condition is involved. In chronic encephalopathy of sufficient magnitude, imaging abnormalities reflect the magnitude of neuronal loss. A useful model of neurotoxicity and the sensitivity of imaging studies is hypoxia. Depending on the magnitude and duration of hypoxia or anoxia, a spectrum of identifiable imaging abnormalities exist. Like any disorder that produces neuronal death, the abnormalities are not necessarily immediately apparent but develop subsequent to the injuries.

The administration of imaging studies indiscriminately, rather than in response to a clinical suspicion, is never justified. Some functional neuroimaging studies, such as single photon emission computed tomography (SPECT) and positron emission tomography (PET), are specialized tests of uncertain sensitivity or specificity that have little general application or acceptance for establishing specific diagnoses. SPECT measures regional blood flow, and, in general, findings reflect regional cerebral metabolism.[8] PET uses positron-emitting radiopharmaceuticals to provide images of the distribution of these biologic compounds that reflects the metabolic, biochemical, or pharmacologic processes.[7] Both studies demonstrate abnormality in response to neurotoxic injury, and even those neurotoxins that are highly selective for one specific cell type (e.g., MPTP and neuronal damage in the zona compacta of the substantia nigra) produce identifiable PET abnormalities.[26,27] PET is complimentary to structural imaging studies, and it has proven clinical efficacy in the differential diagnosis of dementia and movement disorders and in the localization of brain tumors and seizure foci.[7] At present, however, there are few controlled experimental studies of SPECT or PET and no available sensitivity and specificity rates.[73] Most current information is derived from non-replicated, unpublished, or anecdotal observations. This situation makes the application of such information, particularly in forensic situations, inappropriate. The Society of Nuclear Brain Imaging Council[73] has cautioned that use of these studies to provide "objective evidence" of impairment potentially leads to insupportable conclusions when the studies are used to link a neurophysiologic parameter (e.g., blood flow or metabolism) to clinical dysfunction. It is equally inappropriate to interpret SPECT or PET information to infer evidence that any neurologic condition is caused by a specific substance-induced illness or injury.

# PERIPHERAL NERVOUS SYSTEM MEASURES

## TOXIC NEUROPATHY

There are numerous neurotoxins that produce toxic neuropathy.[4,30,41,42,69] Nevertheless, the diagnosis of "toxic neuropathy" is probably overused in terms of attributing idiopathic neuropathies not otherwise classified to toxic-metabolic causes in the absence of a defined association. The importance of toxic neuropathies exceeds their number because of the expected improvement after identification and reduction or removal from further exposure. In general, toxic neuropathies are associated with distal paresthesias, sensory loss, and weakness, although pure sensory or motor neuropathies exist. The type, rate of onset, and severity reflect the specific toxin and exposure history. Distal weakness, stocking-glove sensory loss, and reflex loss are easily recognized. With the exception of the sensory examination, the findings are relatively objective and are not influenced by extrinsic factors such as motivation, education, or fatigue.

A variety of electrophysiologic tests are available to confirm the presence of neuropathy and refine the differential diagnosis. Of these tests, the most important is the electrodiagnostic examination.[2] Nerve conduction studies and needle EMG are sensitive and specific for disorders of the lower motor neuron and the dorsal root ganglion and its peripheral axon. Most neurologists consider these evaluations extensions of the clinical examination, and most of the resultant information is clinically relevant, with measures such as compound muscle action potential amplitude directly reflecting clinical examination findings. Other measures, such as quantitative sensory testing, are less specific for peripheral dysfunction, but occasionally they are important in the assessment of toxic neuropathy, particularly as screening instruments.

## QUANTITATIVE MEASURES

### Quantitative Sensory Testing

Quantitative sensory testing (QST) is used by many investigators in the assessment of toxic neuropathy, and these psychomotor tests have application in clinical, pharmacologic, and neurotoxicologic studies.[20,21] The validity of QST is established, and interexaminer comparisons are favorable, including comparison of paramedical personnel. Different sensory modalities, such as vibration and thermal sensations, can be evaluated, corresponding to different nerve fiber populations. The testing is noninvasive and well tolerated, and the quantitative results allow parametric statistical analyses and detection of subtle group differences when used under controlled conditions. QST also is useful in monitoring longitudinal change over time. In some comparisons, such as the prospective study of pyridoxine neurotoxicity, thermal changes detected by QST occurred earlier and were more severe than changes in vibration sensation or in sural nerve action potential amplitude.[18] In contrast, others have compared QST and nerve conduction study (NCS) results in the evaluation of diabetic polyneuropathy and found QST complimentary but ancillary to nerve conduction studies, with the sural recording being the best single predictor of mild neuropathy.[61] Disadvantages of QST include the time required to perform such studies; the need for patient cooperation; sensitivity to subtle motivational factors, learning, and age effects; and the inability to distinguish central from peripheral disorders.

### Posturography

Static posturography records minute swaying of the body during quiet stance, providing a quantitative measure of postural movement. The static platform senses vertical and shear forces exerted by the feet. These measures allow calculation of the amplitude and rate of sway. Dynamic posturography uses the same techniques to record sway in response to perturbation of the platform, often combined with visual stimuli. The most common application is in the evaluation of patients with suspected vestibular disorders. The AAN Therapeutics and Technology Assessment Subcommittee has reviewed the clinical utility of posturography.[9] This report indicated that specificity is poor and that the patterns of abnormality reported for vestibular disorders do not exclude central or peripheral dysfunction. An additional limitation is that the implied stimulus-response measure actually requires volitional cooperation of the subject in maintaining a stable upright posture. For example, small volitional shifts in posture dramatically influence the test results. In a cooperative, motivated subject, test results are repeatable. However, posturography is not useful in localizing lesions in the nervous system, nor does it help make a specific diagnosis.[35,37] The subcommittee concluded that it is doubtful that this functional measure will become an efficacious diagnostic test. Information regarding test sensitivity is limited.

## ELECTROPHYSIOLOGY

### Electromyography

*Electromyography* is the term used to describe NCSs and the needle electromyography examination (NEE). The evaluation for neuropathy includes sensory and motor NCSs, evaluation of late responses, the NEE, and, occasionally, other studies such as sympathetic responses and measures used to confirm clinical findings and localize specific abnormalities to a degree not clinically possible. The electrodiagnostic evaluation is an extension of the clinical examination, with established reference values, reproducibility, limitations, and guidelines for appropriate utilization.[11,12,28,29,38] The evaluation allows classification of the neuropathies into broad categories that focus the differential diagnosis, direct the subsequent evaluation, and often suggest a specific diagnosis based on findings that suggest the underlying pathophysiologic complex. Factors such as age, temperature, and body size influence normal values, and recognition of this influence increases the sensitivity and accuracy of these tests.[31,67,75–77] Electrodiagnostic studies also play an increasingly important role in clinical trials, including evaluation of therapeutic agents and identification of potential neurotoxicity.

Sensory and motor NCSs and the NEE are important in the evaluation of neuropathy because they evaluate slightly different components of the nervous system.[3] NCSs are noninvasive and provide the most useful information in the evaluation of neuropathy. These tests technically are "evoked response" studies, in that an electrical signal generated by peripheral nerve or muscle is recorded in response to a percutaneous stimulus. The NEE has a less prominent role in the evaluation of neuropathy. It is used primarily to document the distribution of axonal lesions and identify disorders such as polyradiculopathy, which may be clinically indistinguishable from neuropathy.

The electrodiagnostic examination identifies potential causes of neuropathy, including those associated with peripheral neurotoxins, but it cannot diagnose toxic neuropathy in isolation. One conventionally used classification scheme separates peripheral disorders into broad categories based on electrodiagnostic evidence of sensory or motor involvement combined with uniform or multifocal demyelination or pure axonal loss.[35] Table 17–3 classifies several types of toxic neuropathies by using electrophysiological test results. This classification scheme reduces the number of disorders that must be considered in the differential diagnosis of any possible neuropathy. The definition of decreased motor nerve conduction velocity is important in this classification system. There are criteria useful in identifying conduction slowing that results from segmental demyelination. Nevertheless, other abnormalities, including axonal degeneration, axonal stenosis, channelopathies, and selective loss of large myelinated motor fibers, occasionally produce substantial slowing. Conduction slowing is used in this classification scheme to include any slowing that cannot be attributed to axonal loss lesions alone. For the most part, conduction velocities <80% of the lower limit of normal or distal latencies and F wave latencies >125% of the upper limit of normal usually fulfill this requirement.[25,62] The results of the electrodiagnostic examination also distinguish acquired neuropathies, including those associated with neurotoxic disorders, from hereditary disorders associated with conduction slowing.[49] Partial conduction block along motor axons and increased temporal dispersion are important features associated with some acquired neuropathies. Their absence suggests uniform involvement of all fibers and supports a hereditary rather than an acquired etiologic basis.

### TABLE 17–3. Toxic Neuropathy Classified by Electrodiagnostic Findings

**Motor or Motor > Sensory, Conduction Slowing**
Arsenic (shortly after acute exposure)
Amiodarone
Carbon disulfide
Cytosine arabinoside (ara-C)
Methyl n-butyl ketone
n-Hexane
Saxitoxin (sodium channel blocker)
Suramin
Swine flu vaccine

**Motor or Motor > Sensory, No Conduction Slowing**
Cimetidine
Dapsone
Disulfiram (carbon disulfide?)
Doxorubicin
Hyperinsulin/hypoglycemia
Nitrofurantoin
Organophosphorus esters (OPIDN)
Vincristine

**Sensory Only (Neuropathy or Neuronopathy)**
Cisplatin
Ethyl alcohol
Metronidazole
Pyridoxine
Styrene
Thalidomide
Thallium (small fiber)

**Sensorimotor, No Conduction Slowing**
Acrylamide
Amitriptyline
Arsenic (chronic)
Carbon monoxide
Colchicine (neuromyopathy)
Ethambutol
Ethyl alcohol
Ethylene oxide
Elemental mercury
Gold
Hydralazine
Isoniazid
Lithium
Metronidazole
Nitrofurantoin
Nitrous oxide (myeloneuropathy)
Paclitaxel
Perhexiline
Phenytoin
Thallium
Vincristine

The NEE is a sensitive indicator of partial denervation of any cause, and even mild axonal loss of motor fibers produces easily identified fibrillation potentials.

### Repetitive Motor Nerve Stimulation

The most frequently used technique available to evaluate neuromuscular transmission is repetitive motor nerve stimulation. This technique identifies impaired neuromuscular transmission as a decline (decrement) in the motor response recorded with repeated depolarization (e.g., 3 Hz) of the nerve.[6,53] Ordinarily, acetylcholine released from the nerve terminal in response to depolarization produces an endplate potential larger than necessary to generate a muscle action potential, and the normal neuromuscular junction shows no variation in amplitude or configuration with repetitive stimulation. The normal response depends on the availability of acetylcholine, inactivation of acetylcholine in the synaptic cleft, and functioning acetylcholine receptors. Abnormality of any of these may result in impairment of neuromuscular transmission. Application of this technique in neurotoxic disease is limited to demonstrating abnormal neuromuscular transmission in acute organophosphorus intoxication.[48,55]

## TESTS OF AUTONOMIC NERVOUS SYSTEM FUNCTION

The sympathetic skin potential (SSP) is an easily assessed measure of autonomic function.[71] Whereas standard conduction studies primarily evaluate large myelinated nerve fibers, SSPs evaluate small nerve fiber function. The SSP is differentially recorded from skin between areas of high and low sweat gland density. SSPs normally appear spontaneously or in response to a variety of stimuli, such as electrical stimulation, loud noise, or an emotionally charged question. The purpose of the stimulus is to illicit an autonomic response to startle, not to directly depolarize the nerve. SSPs are used to document autonomic impairment in disorders such as inflammatory or diabetic neuropathy, but they have limited application in neurotoxic disorders. In general, neither their sensitivity nor their specificity is known. Other tests of autonomic nervous system function exist (e.g., R-R interval, Q-SART) but are beyond the scope of this review. At present, none of these has had extensive application or evaluation in neurotoxic disorders.

## OTHER LABORATORY TESTING

The role of traditional laboratory measures in the evaluation of suspected neurotoxic disorders is related to identifying systemic disorders associated with neurologic dysfunction. For example, arsenic-induced toxic neuropathy is associated with anemia, pancytopenia, and abnormal liver function tests, and L-tryptophan intoxication is associated with an increased total eosinophil count.[36,47,78,81] In addition, the excretion of arsenic and certain heavy metals can be measured in the urine and other tissues (e.g., hair).[58,80] Nevertheless, the metabolism of most other chemicals is sufficiently rapid that detection in body tissues is difficult. In select situations, such as acute organophosphate intoxication, plasma butyryl (pseudo) cholinesterase (BuChE) and red blood cell acetylcholinesterase (AChE) are reduced when measured soon after poisoning.[51,65] Although evaluation of individual laboratory tests of blood and urine is beyond the scope of this chapter, it is important to recognize that the role of random screening is limited and finding an abnormal value does not ensure that the cause has been established because competing explanations commonly exist (e.g., in relationship to increased arsenic excretion associated with ingestion of some seafoods). In patients with solvent-induced neuropathy, such as in association with n-hexane, biopsy of the peripheral nerve shows focal axonal swellings consisting of neurofilament aggregates. Biopsy of skin, fascia, muscle, and nerve from patients with eosinophilia-myalgia syndrome associated with L-tryptophan intoxication typically demonstrates perivascular inflammation with lymphocytes and rare eosinophils in connective tissue. In other situations tissue biopsy is rarely indicated, other than to document the presence of disorders unrelated to toxic exposure. None of these measures is useful for screening purposes, other than in association with a specific chemical in an industrial setting.

## ESTABLISHING ETIOLOGY

For the most part, it is difficult to establish the etiologic basis of a neurotoxic disorder because there is no single specific presentation. There are, however, several characteristic presentations that suggest the possibility of a toxic cause for the neurologic presentation. Like any clinical diagnosis, the initial clue in suspecting a toxic etiologic basis may be recognition of a cardinal systemic feature that suggests exposure to a specific toxin. This recognition usually stems from a high level of suspicion after other competing causes have been eliminated. Occasionally, a toxic cause is proposed because no immediate etiologic factor is apparent (as in probable "toxic-metabolic" neuropathy). Unfortunately, competing causes frequently are only superficially evaluated or addressed in reports of diagnostic conclusions. Patients with a neurologic disorder of uncertain cause understandably search for any possible explanation for their problem. Exposure to potential neurotoxins occurs frequently, and a neurotoxic explanation for a given problem subsequently becomes self-evident. Nevertheless, association is only one of several criteria used to identify a cause-effect relationship between a potential toxin and a neurologic disorder. For example, any patient with a history of excessive alcohol use who is found to have a pure sensory neuropathy, with stocking-glove sensory loss, areflexia, and absent sensory nerve action potentials, may have an alcohol-associated sensory neuropathy. Nevertheless, a clinically indistinguishable neuropathy occurs in association with Sjögren's syndrome, neoplasm (paraneoplastic syndrome), hereditary sensory neuropathy, (e.g., Friedreich's ataxia), cisplatin, metronidazole, pyridoxine, styrene, thalidomide, thallium, human immunodeficiency virus, idiopathic sensory ganglionitis, nutritional disorders (e.g., vitamin E deficiency), and the Fisher variant of Guillain Barré syndrome.[3,35]

Although it is difficult to establish the cause of some neurotoxic disorders, there are criteria useful in establishing the etiology. The cause of a problem is commonly inferred by addressing a series of questions sometimes referred to as the Bradford Hill criteria.[43] This process probably has its most direct application to infectious diseases, but it is an exercise that clinicians use daily in identifying any number of vascular, metabolic, infectious, neoplastic, or toxic etiologic complexes. Table 17–4 lists several of the questions that are important in determining whether a specific toxin is capable of causing toxic neuropathy, as modified from those first

---

**TABLE 17–4. Questions Useful in Establishing a Toxic Etiology**

Appropriate timing of exposure and signs?
High relative risk based on epidemiologic studies or case reports?
Biologically plausible?
Dose-response relationship?
Removal from exposure modifies effect?
Existence of animal model?
Consistency among studies conducted at different times and in different settings?
Relative specificity of cause-effect?
Evidence of analogous problems caused by similar agents?
Other causes eliminated?

Data from Hill AB. The environment and disease: association or causation? *Proc R Soc Med.* 1965;58:295-300.

outlined by Sir Austin Bradford Hill.[43] These questions are used to distinguish causation from association. Of the criteria, the most directly relevant to establishing a neurotoxic cause include appropriate exposure, biologic plausibility, and elimination of competing causes. In the appropriate clinical setting, several laboratory tests are useful in establishing an increased body burden of a potential neurotoxin or identifying the characteristic pathologic features of toxic exposure. Unfortunately, the most difficult diagnostic step usually is recognizing the potential relationship of a toxic exposure and the neurologic disorder.

## NEUROLOGIC TESTING IN GROUP COMPARISONS

The selected tests described in the preceding section have the greatest utility in individual patient evaluations, and many are used conventionally in the evaluation of patients with suspected neurologic disorders. Unfortunately, for the most part, few abnormalities are indicative of a neurotoxic impairment, as opposed to an abnormality of any other cause. In most clinical situations the most difficult diagnostic step in patient evaluation is recognizing the potential relationship of a toxic exposure to the neuropathology. Neurologic tests occasionally are applied to groups of individuals. This application may be less familiar to the clinical neurologist, and in this setting, understanding the numerous forms of unintentional bias become important in interpreting group differences.

### PHARMACEUTICAL INVESTIGATIONS

Quantitative neurologic tests, including electrophysiologic measures such as NCSs, play an important role in clinical pharmacologic trials.[2,60] Electrophysiologic measures are frequently used to fulfill entry criteria and identify appropriate candidates for inclusion in the trial. In addition, the quantitative nature of many of the tests makes them appropriate end-point measures. In their most common application, electrophysiologic measures are used to evaluate the efficacy of a specific treatment in prospective controlled studies. One example is the Diabetic Care and Complication Trial (DCCT), which compared intensive diabetic therapy to conventional diabetic care.[33] In this study, significant nerve conduction differences were observed between the treatment groups (cohorts), all favoring better performance (faster conduction velocities, shorter F wave latencies) in the intensive therapy group. Nonparametric multivariate tests of the NCS measures established a strong effect in favor of intensive treatment, establishing that the electrophysiologic abnormalities associated with diabetic neuropathy are delayed or prevented by intensive treatment. NCSs were among the best measures demonstrating the beneficial effect, indicating their excellent sensitivity relative to other measures. Electrophysiologic measures are frequently monitored in pharmaceutical trials to identify suspected or unsuspected neurotoxicity of the study medication. Prospective studies have the advantage of using the patient as his or her own control, thereby minimizing the extraneous effects.

Electrophysiologic measures also have been used to evaluate individuals exposed to occupational or environmental neurotoxins. Typically, cross-sectional comparisons are made between the group of interest and unexposed or historical controls. A major limitation of cross-sectional studies is selection bias because of the many unsuspected factors that potentially influence the test results. It is for this reason that cross-sectional studies are considered hypothesis generating and incapable of establishing the cause of any identified group differences. This contrasts with the hypothesis-testing capability of cohort or case-control studies. One example of inadvertent selection bias in a cross-sectional study follows.

An evaluation of 138 chlor-alkali workers with occupational exposure to elemental mercury was conducted in the 1980s by using electrodiagnostic and clinical evaluations to document neurologic impairment.[5] This cross-sectional study was designed so that examiners were masked to mercury exposure levels and workers were unaware of the specific study question. In an effort to minimize selection bias, workers were randomly selected from those eligible to participate. The evaluation identified abnormalities suggestive of a mild asymptomatic neuropathy among exposed workers, including electrodiagnostic evidence of a mild sensorimotor polyneuropathy. Of the 138 workers, 18 were found to have mild clinically evident neuropathy, and when they were compared to the remaining 120 workers, they demonstrated significantly elevated urine mercury indexes, prolonged distal latencies, and reduced sensory amplitudes. Further comparison of NCS results for all workers to historical control data matched by sex and age demonstrated many significant differences, all favoring poorer performance in the mercury-exposed workers. Important findings included lower median and ulnar sensory amplitudes and prolonged distal latencies in the worker population compared to the historical control group. Sural amplitudes were lower only for those workers with clinically evident neuropathy. This finding was surprising because sural NCSs are generally considered to be the most sensitive indicator of sensory neuropathy.

Multiple linear regression analyses of the clinical and electrodiagnostic measures vs. urine mercury indexes demonstrated several significant correlations of the clinical grading of sensory loss and the ulnar and median sensory latencies with mercury indexes. These differences persisted even when age, height, and weight were accounted for in the analyses. The findings were thought to identify a toxic neuropathy associated with mercury exposure. Alternatively, the reduced sensory amplitudes could have been explained by hand size because the manual laborers studied probably had larger hands than did the controls. This argument does not explain the longer latencies, however. Although the relationship between mercury and weight was not explained, it was hypothesized that larger individuals were more likely to work as manual laborers in the exposed areas. It was even hypothesized that larger workers might accumulate greater amounts of mercury, producing increased toxicity.

It now is established that many anthropometric factors, including height, weight, body mass index, and finger circumference account for substantial variability in electrodiagnostic measures.[67,74,75] The relationship with finger size is clear, with increasing finger diameter producing a decreased sensory amplitude because the recording electrode is separated farther from the digital nerves than with smaller finger size.[23,75] However, the relationships between other variables, such as body mass index (BMI) and sensory latencies, are not intuitively obvious. Nevertheless, given this new information, at least some of the electrodiagnostic results obtained for the chlor-alkali workers likely reflected BMI, not mercury exposure. In retrospect, "normal" values for unexposed workers matched for age and BMI are comparable to those reported in the original manuscript, indicating that mercury exposure probably did not explain the findings.[66,76] The inadvertent relationship between mercury exposure and BMI was unsuspected and unappreciated as important. Unfortunately, it produced an unexpected selection bias that no statistical manipulation is capable of correcting.

## CONCLUSION

The neurologic and neuropsychologic examinations are the most fundamental form of standardized clinical testing capable of detecting subtle abnormalities that are potentially associated with neurotoxic exposure. The neurologist routinely interprets symptoms and signs in establishing the extent and clinical significance of neurologic dysfunction. The neurologist also is responsible for defining the etiologic basis of a specific problem prior to recommending treatment. The process of establishing a diagnosis includes interpreting results from appropriate laboratory, electrodiagnostic, and imaging studies. During the evaluation, systemic illnesses with neurologic manifestations are often detected, as are normal patterns of physiologic or psychologic variation that mimic neurologic disease.

When cognitive dysfunction is suspected, the neurologist uses the results of standardized clinical neuropsychologic evaluations performed in consultation with a clinical neuropsychologist. The formal neuropsychologic test measures are important in quantifying cognitive impairments and in evaluating nonspecific complaints, such as decreased memory or concentration. In addition, the neuropsychologic evaluation may be important in identifying altered mood, abnormal anxiety states, motivational factors, and psychopathologic conditions. Occasionally, selected psychomotor or psychosensory tests supplement the neurologic and neuropsychologic examinations. Such tests are most often used in identifying subtle differences between exposed and unexposed populations, particularly when a specific abnormality (e.g., diminished sensation, impaired coordination, or abnormal tremor) is suspected. In this context, results are subject to selection bias. Few of these specialized measures have had widespread application in standardized form, and their sensitivity and specificity have undergone limited evaluation.

Several electrophysiologic tests are well standardized, with widespread application being part of the clinical neurologic evaluation. The peripheral nervous system is a common target of neurotoxic substances, and the conventional EMG examination is used to evaluate patients with suspected peripheral neuropathy. The sensitivity and specificity of NCSs are established, and they are objective measures that are independent of patient cooperation or motivation. Other electrodiagnostic studies, such as conventional EEG and evoked responses, have extensive clinical application, although their application in potential neurotoxic evaluations is less well established.

Standard imaging techniques are most useful in identifying anatomic or structural CNS abnormalities. In clinical neurotoxicologic evaluations, imaging studies typically are used to exclude other disorders. They are not screening examinations, and their use usually is not justified unless there is a demonstrable neurologic impairment or strong suspicion of a structural defect. SPECT and PET are specialized tests of uncertain sensitivity or specificity that presently have little general application or acceptance for establishing specific diagnoses.

Identification of individual patient abnormalities differs from identification of exposed group vs. control group differences. The evaluation of the individual patient uses standard neurologic and neuropsychologic examinations to develop a differential diagnosis that is useful in determining what additional testing may be helpful in establishing the final diagnosis and cause of the patient's problem. In addition, these conventional examinations are important in establishing the clinical significance of a specific effect. Group evaluations often include additional quantitative measures that are important in determining whether any effect can be demonstrated. Group comparisons may be important in establishing dose-response relationships, but cross-sectional studies of this type are sensitive to selection bias and are considered hypothesis generating rather than hypothesis-testing studies. The neurologist's experience in evaluating adverse neurologic effects from pharmaceutical agents is directly applicable to the evaluation of symptomatic or asymptomatic individuals with occupational or environmental exposure to potential neurotoxins. Clinical neurotoxicology is a multidisciplinary effort; the standardized neurologic and neuropsychologic evaluations are the most important and tests useful for defining clinical abnormalities and establishing cause-effect relationships.

## REFERENCES

1. Adams KM, Rourke BP. *The TCN Guide to Professional Practice in Clinical Neuropsychology.* Berwyn, PA: Swets & Zeitlinger; 1992.
2. Albers JW. Standardized neurological testing in neurotoxicology studies. In: Johnson BL, ed. *Advances in Neurobehavioral Toxicology: Applications in Environmental and Occupational Health.* Chelsea, England: Lewis Publishers; 1990:151-164.
3. Albers JW. Clinical neurophysiology of generalized polyneuropathy. *J Clin Neurophysiol.* 1993;10:149-166.
4. Albers JW, Bromberg MB. Chemically induced toxic neuropathy. In: Rosenberg NL, ed. *Occupational and Environmental Neurology.* Boston: Butterworth-Heinemann; 1996:175-233.
5. Albers JW, Cavender GF, Levine SP, et al. Asymptomatic sensorimotor polyneuropathy in workers exposed to elemental mercury. *Neurology.* 1982;32:1168-1174.
6. Albers JW, Leonard JA, Jr. Nerve conduction and electromyography. In: Crockard A, Hayward R, Hoff JT, eds. *Neurosurgery: The Scientific Basis of Clinical Practice.* Oxford, England: Blackwell Scientific Publications Ltd; 1992:735-757.
7. American Academy of Neurology. Assessment: positron emission tomography. *Neurology.* 1991;41:163-167.
8. American Academy of Neurology. SPECT and neurosonology qualifications approved. *Neurology.* 1991;41:13A.
9. American Academy of Neurology. Assessment: posturography. Report of the Therapeutics and Technology Assessment Subcommittee. Minneapolis: American Academy of Neurology; 1992.
10. American Academy of Neurology. Assessment: EEG brain mapping. Report of the Therapeutics and Technology Assessment Committee (unpublished, 1994).
11. American Association of Electrodiagnostic Medicine. Guidelines in electrodiagnostic medicine. *Muscle Nerve.* 1992;15:229-253.
12. American Association of Electrodiagnostic Medicine. *Proposed Policy for Electrodiagnostic Medicine.* Rochester, Minn: AAEM; 1997:1-16.
13. American Psychiatry Association. Quantitative electroencephalography: a report on the present state of computerized EEG technology—American Psychiatry Association Task Force on Quantitative Electrophysiological Assessment. *Am J Psychiatry.* 1991;148:961-964.

14. American Psychological Association. *Standards for Educational and Psychological Testing.* Washington, DC: APA; 1985.

15. Anastasi A. *Psychological Testing.* 4th ed. New York: Macmillan Publishing; 1976.

16. Anastasi A. What counselors should know about the use and interpretation of psychological tests. *J Counsel Devel.* 1992;70:610-615.

17. Arezzo JC, Simson R, Brennan NE. Evoked potentials in the assessment of neurotoxicity in humans. *Neurobehav Toxicol Teratol.* 1985;7:299-304.

18. Berger AR, Schaumburg HH, Schroeder C, et al. Dose response, coasting, and differential fiber vulnerability in human toxic neuropathy: a prospective study of pyridoxine neurotoxicity. *Neurology.* 1992;42:1367-1370.

19. Binder LM, Pankratz L. Neuropsychological evidence of a factitious memory complaint. *J Clin Exp Neuropsychol.* 1987;9:167-171.

20. Bleecker ML. Quantifying sensory loss in peripheral neuropathies. *Neurobehav Toxicol Teratol.* 1985;7:305-308.

21. Bleecker ML. Vibration perception thresholds in entrapment and toxic neuropathies. *J Occup Med.* 1986;28:991-994.

22. Boll TJ, La Marche JA. Neuropsychological assessment of the child: myths, current status, and future prospects. In: Walker CE, Roberts MC, eds. *Handbook of Clinical Child Psychology.* 2nd ed. New York: John Wiley & Sons; 1992:133-148.

23. Bolton CF, Carter KM. Human sensory nerve compound action potential amplitudes: variation with sex and finger circumference. *J Neurol Neurosurg Psychiatry.* 1980;43:925-928.

24. Brescia W, Fortune JC. Standardized testing of American Indian students. *Coll Student J.* 1989;23:94-104.

25. Bromberg MB. Comparison of electrodiagnostic criteria for primary demyelination in chronic polyneuropathy. *Muscle Nerve.* 1991;14:968-976.

26. Calne DB, Eisen A, McGeer E. Alzheimer's disease, Parkinson's disease, and motoneuron disease: abiotrophic interaction between aging and environment? *Lancet.* 1986;2:1067-1070.

27. Calne DB, Snow BJ. PET imaging in Parkinsonism. *Adv Neurol.* 1993;60:484-487.

28. Campbell WW, Robinson LR. Deriving reference values in electrodiagnostic medicine. *Muscle Nerve.* 1993;16:424-428.

29. Chaudhry V, Cornblath DR, Mellits ED. Inter- and intra-examiner reliability of nerve conduction measurements in normal subjects. *Ann Neurol.* 1991;30:841-843.

30. Critchley EMR. Neuropathies due to drugs. In: Vinkin PJ, Bruyn GW, Klawans HL, eds. *Handbook of Clinical Neurology.* Amsterdam: Elsevier; 1987:301-302.

31. Denys EH. The influence of temperature in clinical electrophysiology. *Muscle Nerve.* 1991;14:795-811.

32. Deutsch M, Fishman JA, Kogan L, et al. Guidelines for testing minority group children. *J Soc Iss.* 1964;20:129-145.

33. Diabetes Control and Complications Trial (DCCT) Research Group. Effect of intensive diabetes treatment on nerve conduction in the Diabetes Control and Complications Trial. *Ann Neurol.* 1995;38:869-880.

34. Division 40 Task Force on Education Accreditation and Credentialing. Guidelines regarding the use of nondoctoral personnel in clinical neuropsychological assessment. *Clin Neuropsychol.* 1989;3:23-24.

35. Donofrio PD, Albers JW. Polyneuropathy: classification by nerve conduction studies and electromyography. *Muscle Nerve.* 1990;13:889-903.

36. Donofrio PD, Wilbourn AJ, Albers JW, et al. Acute arsenic intoxication presenting as Guillain-Barré-like syndrome. *Muscle Nerve.* 1987;10:114-120.

37. Dunn JT, Lees-Haley PR, Brown RS, et al. Neurotoxic complaint base rates of personal injury claimants: implications for neuropsychological assessment. *J Clin Psychol.* 1995;51:577-584.

38. Dyck PJ. Invited review: limitations in predicting pathologic abnormality of nerves from the EMG examination. *Muscle Nerve.* 1990;13:371-375.

39. Faust D, Hart K, Guilmette TJ. Pediatric malingering: the capacity of children to fake believable deficits on neuropsychological testing. *J Consult Clin Psychol.* 1988;56:578-582.

40. Geisler MW, Polich J. P300 and individual differences: morning/evening activity preference, food, and time-of-day. *Psychophysiology.* 1992;29:86-94.

41. Gilliatt RW, Schaumburg HH, Asbury AK, et al. Environmental and toxic hazards. In: Persson A, ed. *Symposium 5: Neurophysiological Methods for the Early Detection of Neuromyopathies.* Stockholm: Sixth International Congress for Electromyography; 1979.

42. He F. Occupational toxic neuropathies: an update. *Scand J Work Environ Health.* 1985;11:321-330.

43. Hill AB. The environment and disease: association or causation? *Proc R Soc Med.* 1965;58:295-300.

44. Hinkle JS. Practitioners and cross-cultural assessment: a practical guide to information and training. *Measure Eval Counsel Devel.* 1994;27:103-115.

45. Hiscock CK, Branham JD, Hiscock M. Detection of feigned cognitive impairment: the two-alternative forced-choice method compared with selected conventional tests. *J Psychopath Behav Assess.* 1994;16:95-110.

46. Hiscock M, Hiscock CK. Refining the forced-choice method for the detection of malingering. *J Clin Exp Neuropsychol.* 1989;11:967-974.

47. Kamb ML, Murphy JJ, Jones JL, et al. Eosinophilia-myalgia syndrome in L-tryptophan-exposed patients. *JAMA.* 1992;267:77-82.

48. Kinnby B, Konsberg R, Larsson A. Immunogenic potential of some mercury compounds in experimental contact allergy of the rat oral mucosa. *Scand J Dent Res.* 1988;96:60-68.

49. Lewis RA, Sumner AJ. Electrodiagnostic distinctions between chronic familial and acquired demyelinative neuropathies. *Neurology.* 1982;32:592-596.

50. Loewenstein DA, Arguelles T, Arguelles S, et al. Potential cultural bias in the neuropsychological assessment of the older adult. *J Clin Exp Neuropsychol.* 1994;16:623-629.

51. Lotti M. The pathogenesis of organophosphate polyneuropathy. *Crit Rev Toxicol.* 1991;21:465-487.

52. Markand ON. Electroencephalography in diffuse encephalopathies. *J Clin Neurophysiol.* 1984;1:357-407.

53. Massey JM. Electromyography in disorders of neuromuscular transmission. *Semin Neurol.* 1990;10:6-11.

54. Matsumoto JY. Movement-related potentials and event-related potentials. In: Daube JR, ed. *Clinical Neurophysiology.* Philadelphia: FA Davis; 1996:141-144.

55. Namba T, Nolte CT, Jackrel J, et al. Poisoning due to organophosphate insecticides: acute and chronic manifestations. *Am J Med.* 1971;50:475-492.

56. Nuwer M. Assessment of digital EEG, quantitative EEG, and EEG brain mapping: report of the American Academy of Neurology and the American Clinical Neurophysiology Society. *Neurology.* 1997;49:277-292.

57. Pankratz L. A new technique for the assessment and modification of feigned memory deficit. *Percept Mot Skills.* 1983;57:367-372.

58. Poklis A, Saady JJ. Arsenic poisoning: acute or chronic? suicide or murder? *Am J Forensic Med Pathol.* 1990;11:226-232.

59. Polich J, Moore AP, Wiederhold MD. P300 assessment of chronic fatigue syndrome. *J Clin Neurophysiol.* 1995;12:186-191.

60. Potvin AR, Tourtellotte WW, Potvin JH, et al. *Quantitative Examination of Neurologic Functions.* Vol. I. *Scientific Basis and Design of Instrumented Tests.* Vol. II. *Methodology for Test and Patient Assessments and Design of a Computer-Automated System.* Boca Raton, Fla: CRC Press; 1985.

61. Redmond JMT, McKenna MJ, Feingold M, et al. Sensory testing versus nerve conduction velocity in diabetes polyneuropathy. *Muscle Nerve.* 1992;15:1334-1339.

62. Report from an Ad Hoc Subcommittee of the American Academy of Neurology AIDS Task Force: research criteria for diagnosis of chronic inflammatory demyelinating polyneuropathy (CIDP). *Neurology.* 1991;41:617-618.

63. Report of the Therapeutics and Technology Subcommittee of the American Academy of Neurology: assessment: neuropsychological testing in adults—considerations for neurologists. *Neurology.* 1996;47:592-599.

64. Reynolds CR, Brown RT. *Perspectives on Bias in Mental Testing.* New York: Plenum; 1984.

65. Richardson RJ. Assessment of the neurotoxic potential of chlorpyrifos relative to other organophosphorus compounds: a critical review of the literature. *J Toxicol Environ Health.* 1995;44:135-165.

66. Rivner MH, Swift TR, Crout BO, et al. Toward more rational nerve conduction interpretations: the effect of height. *Muscle Nerve.* 1990;13:232-239.

67. Robinson LR, Rubner DE, Wahl PW, et al. Influences of height and gender on normal nerve conduction studies. *Arch Phys Med Rehabil.* 1993;74:1134-1138.

68. Rosenberg NL, Spitz MC, Filley CM, et al. Central nervous system effects of chronic toluene abuse: clinical, brainstem evoked response and magnetic resonance imaging studies. *Neurotoxicol Teratol.* 1988;10:489-495.

69. Sanek Z. Toxic neuropathies. *Semin Neurol.* 1987;7:9-17.

70. Sanin LC, Kronenberg MF, Stetkarova I. Potentiation of the R component of blink reflex by anticipation. *Neurology.* 1993;43:A289-A290.

71. Shahani BT, Halperin JJ, Bolu P, et al. Sympathetic skin responses: a method of assessing unmyelinated axon dysfunction in peripheral neuropathies. *J Neurol Neurosurg Psychiatry.* 1984;47:536-542.

72. Small GW, Borus JF. Outbreak of illness in a school chorus: toxic poisoning or mass hysteria? *N Engl J Med.* 1983;308:632-635.

73. Society of Nuclear Brain Imaging Council. Ethical clinical practice of functional brain imaging. *J Nucl Med.* 1996;37:1256-1259.

74. Stetson DS. *Median and Ulnar Conduction Measures in Control and Industrial Populations: Associations with Ergonomic Risk Factors.* Ann Arbor: University of Michigan, 1991. Thesis.

75. Stetson DS, Albers JW, Silverstein BA, et al. Effects of age, sex, and anthropometric factors on nerve conduction measures. *Muscle Nerve.* 1992;15:1095-1104.

76. Stetson DS, Silverstein BA, Keyserling WM, et al. Median sensory distal amplitude and latency: comparisons between nonexposed managerial/professional employees and industrial workers. *Am J Ind Med.* 1993; 24:175-189.

77. Swift TR, Ward LC, Soudmand R. Height determines nerve conduction velocity in the legs. *Neurology.* 1981;31(pt 2):66.

78. Troy JL. Eosinophilia-myalgia syndrome. *Mayo Clin Proc.* 1991;66:535-538.

79. Wechsler D. *Manual for the Wechsler Intelligence Scale of Children.* 3rd ed. New York: Psychological Corp; 1991.

80. Windebank AJ. Metal neuropathy. In: Dyck PJ, Thomas PK, Griffin JW, Low PA, Poduslo JF, eds. *Peripheral Neuropathy.* 3rd ed. Philadelphia: WB Saunders; 1993:1549-1570.

81. Winkelmann RK, Connolly SM, Quimby SR, et al. Histopathologic features of the L-tryptophan-related eosinophilia-myalgia (fasciitis) syndrome. *Mayo Clin Proc.* 1991;66:457-463.

# NEUROMUSCULAR DISORDERS

## 18

# Peripheral Nerve Disease

*John W. Griffin, Justin C. McArthur, and D.R. Cornblath*

Peripheral neuropathies result from a large number of possible causes, and the range of phenotypic expression is often frustratingly limited. The most successful peripheral nerve diagnosticians use a sequence of differential diagnosis that first classifies the patient's neuropathy clinically, then uses electrodiagnostic testing to evaluate the nature of the underlying pathophysiology, and finally selects the appropriate laboratory tests. Such a strategy minimizes the use of laboratory testing. For example, in a patient with a large-fiber predominantly motor neuropathy, genetic screening for heritable amyloidosis is not indicated, but a lumbar puncture to determine cerebrospinal fluid (CSF) protein may be necessary. Conversely, in a patient presenting with neuropathic pain and impotence there are fewer indications for lumbar puncture, but amyloid is a major feature of the differential diagnosis. The economic implications of unfocused laboratory testing deserve emphasis. For example, it is possible to spend as much as $1000 on serologic testing for antiglycolipid antibodies alone. Similarly, genetic testing for Charcot-Marie-Tooth disease, heritable amyloidosis, and other heritable neuropathies can each cost more than magnetic resonance imaging (MRI) scans. Following reviews of the use of each of the major testing modalities, this chapter outlines the approach to some common clinical presentations

## ELECTRODIAGNOSTIC TESTING

Electrodiagnostic studies—nerve conduction studies and electromyography (EMG)—are integral to the evaluation of patients with peripheral neuropathy. These studies are an extension of the clinical examination and an indicator of the underlying pathophysiology of the specific neuropathy. Close coordination between the peripheral nerve diagnostician and the neuromuscular electrodiagnostician ensures that the electrodiagnostic studies will have maximal value in differential diagnosis.

The clinician should frame a series of questions that can be specifically answered by the electrodiagnostician. The simplest question is whether or not a peripheral nerve disorder is present. Although this may sound self-evident, many patients with numbness in the feet do not have a disturbance of the peripheral nerves as the basis of their symptoms. With a few exceptions, described below, patients with peripheral nerve diseases have abnormal electrodiagnostic studies.

The next question deals with the anatomic distribution of the peripheral nerve disease present: Is it a mononeuropathy, multiple mononeuropathy, or a symmetrical polyneuropathy? This question is best answered after consultation with the referring physician and a brief neuromuscular examination by the electrodiagnostician. Although it would seem that this question could be answered solely on clinical grounds, on occasion electrodiagnostic studies reveal answers that alter the approach to the patient. For example, an individual who comes with what appears clinically as a simple compressive mononeuropathy may be found to have other mononeuropathies or a systemic polyneuropathy. In such an individual the diagnosis of the underlying systemic neuropathy may be suggested. Another example is the patient who is referred with the clinical presumption of a symmetrical polyneuropathy but who proves to have a widespread multiple mononeuropathy on the basis of detailed electrodiagnostic studies. In such an individual the diagnosis of vasculitis would be suspected.

This work was supported in part by NIH NS 26643, RR00722, and a grant from Genentech, Inc.

**TABLE 18–1. Clinical Features Useful in Categorizing Neuropathies for Differential Diagnosis***

Time course
  Acute
  Subacute
  Chronic
  Lifelong
Functional modalities affected
  Motor
  Sensory
    Large fiber
    Small fiber
    Global
  Autonomic
Distribution
  Distally predominant
  Proximal involvement
  Patchy
Age of onset
Family history
Other medical conditions

*The diagnoses associated with these features are reviewed in reference 20.

The next question posed for the electrodiagnostician is whether the neuropathy is primarily due to axonal degeneration, demyelination, or a combination of both. This question is usually the most important for electrodiagnosticians and the one most clinically relevant. Much has been written on the electrodiagnostic distinction between axonal and demyelinating neuropathies, and the reader is referred to those volumes.[4,34,55]

Normal function of a nerve fiber depends on the integrity of both the axon and the surrounding myelin. In general, neuropathies characterized by predominantly distal axonal degeneration have reduced motor and sensory evoked amplitudes with preservation of distal and F-wave latencies and motor and sensory conduction velocities. Conversely, patients whose neuropathies are characterized predominantly by demyelination have alterations in conduction parameters, such as distal and F-wave latency and conduction velocity, with relative preservation of distal evoked amplitudes. Marked reductions in conduction velocity are often the first clues to the presence of a predominantly demyelinating neuropathy. An example is hereditary motor sensory neuropathy type I (Charcot-Marie-Tooth disease type I), a disorder in which the patient is often unaware of the family history. Similarly, a more patchy pattern of peripheral nerve demyelination with variable prolongations of terminal and F-wave latencies and reductions in conduction velocities may first raise the possibility of chronic inflammatory demyelinating polyneuropathy (CIDP). The determination and detection of partial motor conduction block (PMCB) requires special comment.[9] PMCB describes the finding of lower amplitudes and areas of compound muscle action potentials (CMAPs) with proximal, rather than with distal, stimulation of individual nerves in the absence of nerve anastomoses or other explanations. PMCB suggests an acquired demyelinating neuropathy and can be seen in CIDP. PMCB, with preserved sensory conduction across the same nerve segments, is the major electrodiagnostic feature in multifocal motor neuropathy (MMN).[7]

Much has also been written on the potential pitfalls of electrodiagnostic studies.[33] The main caveat to bear in mind when interpreting electrodiagnostic studies is that they concentrate on the large myelinated fiber population, virtually ignoring the unmyelinated fiber population. Thus, in patients with pure small-fiber sensory neuropathies, electrodiagnostic studies are typically normal. Similarly, the rare patient with true dorsal radiculopathies, such as tabes dorsalis and the dorsal root degeneration occasionally seen in association with human immunodeficiency virus (HIV) infection, may have normal or nearly normal electrodiagnostic studies. Electrodiagnostic testing may identify irrelevant findings in some settings and thereby divert attention from the clinically important issues. An example is the elderly patient with cervical spondylosis and myelopathy whose electrodiagnostic studies detect a mild neuropathy. Although this may suggest vitamin $B_{12}$ deficiency, for example, compressive myelopathy is considerably more likely. Similarly, in patients with diabetic polyneuropathy, electrodiagnostic testing can identify trivial nerve compressions of no symptomatic significance and thereby potentially lead to unnecessary surgery. Last, electrodiagnostic studies may not be needed when the cause and extent of the neuropathy are evident. For example, the very large number of patients with diabetic polyneuropathy or with alcohol-related polyneuropathy do not require electrodiagnostic testing.

## QUANTITATIVE SENSORY TESTING

In recent years, quantitative sensory testing (QST) equipment has become available. QST studies should also be looked upon as an extension of the neurologic examination. Depending on the specific piece of equipment used, vibration, thermal, and pain thresholds can be tested reliably. A variety of methodologies are in use, as are different testing algorithms.[12] In any case the psychophysical measurement of a patient's sensory perception is valuable; in particular, this methodology provides one of the few quantitative ways to look at small-fiber sensory function. There are a number of critical questions to be answered in evaluating the commercially available equipment,[12] and one must be assured of the validity of the normative data. With these caveats in mind, QST in our hands has proved to be a useful measure in the evaluation of patients with peripheral neuropathy, especially those with small-fiber neuropathy.

## ANTIBODY ASSAYS

The availability of serologic tests whose results correlate with specific neuropathies has increased dramatically within the past few years. In a few instances, detection of an antibody is virtually diagnostic of a specific disorder, and in even fewer examples the antibody has been proved to cause the nerve injury. In other instances the association of specific antibodies with specific patterns of neuropathy is much weaker, and their general application is premature. Antibody assays will be a rapidly changing area, but for the clinician at the moment the challenge is to sort judiciously among the various serologic tests available. This is particularly important because of the cost of some of these assays. In general, the clinician is well advised to avoid the predetermined "packages" offered by various laboratories because in most instances they provide a mix of useful tests and irrelevant tests. For example, it is possible to purchase a "package" for CIDP in which one component is molecular genetic testing for Charcot-Marie-Tooth disease type I, a differential possibility that is relevant in only a small proportion of patients with CIDP.

### ANTIGLYCOLIPID ANTIBODIES

Antiglycolipid antibodies can cause peripheral nerve disease. A firmly established example is the role of "anti-MAG" antibodies in causation of peripheral neuropathy. In other instances, such as anti-GM$_1$ antibodies in multifocal motor neuropathy, the association between specific antiglycolipid antibody patterns and specific neuropathies is sufficiently clear-cut to warrant their use in cases of neuropathy with compatible clinical pictures, but their role in pathogenesis remains uncertain.

### "ANTI-MAG" ANTIBODIES

Latov et al[37] first described a patient with peripheral neuropathy and a monoclonal immunoglobulin M (IgM) paraprotein that bound to myelin. The monoclonal antibody was shown to bind to a specific glycoprotein on electrophoretic gels, the myelin-associated glycoprotein (MAG).[3,19,28,42] Of all patients with IgM paraproteins and peripheral neuropathy, as many as 50% appear to have these "anti-MAG" antibodies. The clinical manifestations usually correlated with this antibody include a slowly progressive sensory neuropathy that is dominated by large-fiber sensory dysfunction and often gait ataxia, with lesser degrees of weakness and small-fiber sensory dysfunction. Electrodiagnostically, there are clear features of demyelination, with a variable degree of axonal loss. The pathologic picture, at least until secondary axonal loss supervenes, is dominated by evidence of demyelination and remyelination, often with scattered "onion bulbs," the whorls of supernumerary Schwann cells that reflect the Schwann cell proliferation that accompanies demyelination. A distinctive feature of the pathology is the presence of "myelin wide spacing," in which neighboring myelin lamellae approximately double their intraperiod distances[42] (Fig. 18–1). The myelin

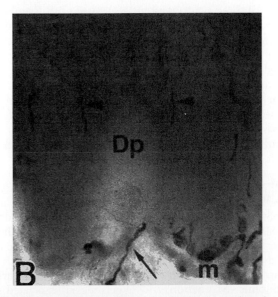

**FIGURE 18–1.** Plastic embedded section of skin with the dermal papilla (*Dp*) and the darker epidermis above. Note the numerous intraepidermal nerve fibers. The sample has been immunostained with the panaxonal marker PGP9.5. (From Crawford TO, Hsieh S-T, Schryer BL, et al. Prolonged survival in transected nerves of C57BL/Ola mice is independent of age. *J Neurocytol.* 1995;24:333-340.)

wide spacing reflects the deposition of IgM within the myelin sheath. In addition, the monoclonal IgM has been used to transfer the neuropathy,[24,54,63] most convincingly by systemic administration to chicks.[56]

The antigen toward which this antiglycoconjugate antibody is directed has been a complex issue. The myelin-associated glycoprotein, identified by Quarles et al[48] more than 20 years ago, is a component of peripheral nerve Schwann cells. It is heavily glycosylated and contains sulfated oligosaccharides. However, myelin also contains glycolipids reactive with antibodies against the same epitope. Among these is sulfate-3-glucuronylneolactotetraosyl-seramide (SGNLC), often termed sulfate-3-glucuronyl paragloboside (SGPG).[8,49] Because MAG itself is not a constituent of compact myelin,[57–59] it is likely that the binding responsible for the myelin wide spacing is directed toward these intrinsic sulfated glycolipids of myelin. In any event, in older patients with predominantly sensory neuropathies and demyelinating electrophysiology, consideration of anti-MAG neuropathy begins by obtaining immunofixation to detect the presence of monoclonal proteins. If a monoclonal IgM spike is present, assessment for anti-MAG antibodies is worthwhile; in nearly half of such patients the antibodies will be detectable. A small number of patients with anti-MAG reactivity are said not to have demonstrable IgM paraproteins, but the significance of such a pattern is uncertain.

The treatment of IgM paraproteinemia with anti-MAG reactivity is currently uncertain. Although some patients respond to intensive plasmapheresis or the use of plasmapheresis combined with cytotoxic drugs,[43] the advisability of treatment is usually doubtful. In general, these are very slowly changing neuropathies occurring in older patients, and the clinician must weigh the limited evidence for efficacy with the expense and potential danger of aggressive treatment in this patient population.

### ANTI-GM$_1$ AND ANTI-GQ$_{1b}$ ANTIBODIES

Antibodies against ganglioside epitopes, including GM$_1$, GD$_{1a}$, asialoGD$_{1a}$, GQ$_{1b}$, and LM$_1$, have been described in peripheral neuropathies. At present the clinical relevance is greatest for GM$_1$ and GQ$_{1b}$, and they will be the focus of the following discussion.

### GM$_1$

GM$_1$ is a major ganglioside of peripheral nerve, present in both the myelin and the axon In the axon, it is concentrated in the axolemma of the nodes of Ranvier of myelinated fibers, and recent data have confirmed that anti-GM$_1$ antibodies can alter impulse conduction. Anti-GM$_1$ antibodies have been identified in two major settings, multifocal motor neuropathy and Guillain-Barré syndrome (GBS). Initially the possibility that these antibodies were useful in the diagnosis of amyotrophic lateral sclerosis (ALS) was considered,[45] but the levels are in general low and inconsistent, and they have no role in either the diagnosis or treatment decisions in ALS at present.

***Multifocal Motor Neuropathy.*** High titers of IgM antibodies against the ganglioside GM$_1$ are found in approximately 70% of patients with the clinical and electrodiagnostic picture of MMN.[2,7,44,46] When electrodiagnosis and clinical evaluation are inconclusive, a high IgM anti-GM$_1$ antibody level is useful as supporting evidence for the diagnosis of MMN. Security of diagnosis in this disorder is an important issue because the condition is usually responsive to intravenous gammaglobulin, and treatment can sometimes dramatically improve the level of function of patients with MMN.[6,22] However, the presence of anti-GM$_1$ antibodies, particularly in lower titers, is in no way specific for the diagnosis of MMN; nor is their presence necessary for the diagnosis.

***Guillain-Barré Syndromes.*** There is increasing interest in the role of antiglycoconjugate antibodies in the pathogenesis of the various forms of GBS, but at present they are diagnostically useful primarily in Fisher syndrome, as discussed later. Antibodies to GM$_1$ or other gangliosides have been reported in several series of GBS, but the patterns remain controversial. The clearest association is between anti-GM$_1$ antibodies and the predominantly axonal forms of GBS.[25,64,65] At least two forms of "axonal" GBS can be distinguished: the syndrome of acute motor and sensory axonal neuropathy (AMSAN) described by Feasby et al,[14,15,23] and the purely motor disorder, acute motor axonal neuropathy (AMAN), described by Griffin et al[22] and McKhann et al.[41] Both of these disorders can follow *Campylobacter jejuni* infection. In AMAN there is increasing evidence to suggest that IgG anti-GM$_1$ antibodies may be pathogenically important. This epitope is expressed in a lipopolysaccharide of the *Campylobacter* strains isolated from patients with acute motor axonal neuropathy.[65,66] Pathologic studies have demonstrated that in autopsies of patients with AMAN there is deposition of IgG in the nodes of Ranvier and in the internodal periaxonal space of myelinated motor fibers. Markers of complement activation appear in the same sites and are followed by the appearance of macrophages. This disorder has very little evidence of lymphocytic inflammation.[22,41] Taken together, these findings strongly suggest that IgG anti-GM$_1$ antibodies may be binding to epitopes in the nodes of motor fibers and producing the disorder.

Kornberg et al[35] have pointed out the high correlation between IgG anti-GM$_1$ antibodies and acute motor axonal syndromes in clinical samples. A difficulty at this time appears to lie in the sensitivity of IgG anti-GM$_1$ testing. The sensitivity of the assay in patients with AMAN is currently <50%.[25] At present, antiganglioside antibody testing is not an important aspect of diagnosis of GBS.

## GQ$_{1b}$

In contrast, a very specific and apparently relatively sensitive assay is testing for anti-GQ$_{1b}$ antibodies in Fisher syndrome.[16] The Fisher syndrome of ataxia, ophthalmoparesis, and areflexia has long been linked to GBS, and recent data have clarified the pathogenetic similarities. The GQ$_{1b}$ glycoconjugate is expressed in the lipopolysaccharide of *Campylobacter jejuni* in those patients with *Campylobacter* infection preceding development of Fisher syndrome, suggesting that an immune response to the organism is targeting shared epitopes with motor nerves and other sites in the peripheral nervous system and probably the central nervous system. This antibody is present in up to 90% of patients with Fisher syndrome and has also been identified in patients with more typical GBS associated with ophthalmoparesis. Anti-GQ$_{1b}$ antibodies are clinically useful in confirmation of this uncommon disorder.

## Antiglycoconjugate Antibodies Accompanying Sensory Syndromes

Pestronk et al[47] identified eight patients with axonal predominantly sensory neuropathies and antibodies reactive with sulfatides. Some but not all of these patients also had monoclonal proteins. The data remain insufficient to determine the value of antisulfatide antibodies in patients with painful sensory neuropathies, but it is noteworthy that antisulfatide antibodies bind to dorsal root ganglion neurons of the rat. Establishing the clinical usefulness of these assays requires larger prospective studies.

## ANTI-HU (ANNA-1) ANTIBODIES IN CARCINOMATOUS SENSORY NEURONOPATHY

The idea that neuropathy could be a remote effect of carcinoma was first suggested by Denny-Brown[11] in 1948 in his description of patients with a subacute ataxic sensory neuropathy. The concept was expanded by the London Hospital Group in the 1960s, and for a certain period, screening for occult carcinoma was an accepted aspect of evaluation for almost any neuropathy. In retrospect, many of the distally predominant sensory motor neuropathies occurred in the late stages of cancer, and neuropathy is a very uncommon presenting manifestation of underlying carcinoma. At present, in our opinion extensive cancer screening (beyond a chest x-ray examination and stool guaiac) is not indicated in patients with bland distally predominant sensory motor neuropathies.

In contrast, extensive investigation is mandatory for the group of patients with subacute ataxic neuropathies that were originally described by Denny-Brown.[11] Typically, over a few weeks these individuals develop widespread paresthesias or pain and progressive loss of kinesthetic sensation, resulting in gait ataxia, pseudoathetosis of the outstretched arms, rombergism, and difficulty with coordination of the hands. A similar picture can occur in association with Sjögren's syndrome, as indicated earlier, or on an idiopathic basis. All three syndromes are associated with lymphocytic infiltration into the dorsal root ganglia. In distinguishing among these forms of sensory ganglionitis, a particularly valuable assay is the anti-Hu antibody.[18] This antibody is directed against a 37 kD nuclear antigen that is shared between neurons and cells of the underlying tumor, which is most often oat cell carcinoma of the lung. Both the specificity and the sensitivity are high.[5] Although this assay is not of value in patients with, for example, predominantly motor neuropathies, it is an invaluable test in patients with subacute ataxic neuropathies.

## ANTI–CALCIUM CHANNEL ANTIBODIES IN LAMBERT-EATON SYNDROME

Strictly speaking, Lambert-Eaton myasthenic syndrome (LEMS) should be considered a peripheral neuropathy because the disorder is produced by antibodies against voltage-gated calcium channels of the motor nerve terminals.[62] The clinical picture of easy fatigability, muscle weakness, variable autonomic dysfunction, and hyperreflexia associated with increased strength and reflexes after exercise suggests the diagnosis. The most useful confirmatory test is the response to high-rate (50 Hz) repetitive nerve stimulation. The initial compound muscle action potential amplitudes are reduced, usually with amplitudes <15% of normal. With high rates of nerve stimulation, there is a two- to forty-fold increment in amplitude. This facilitation is classic in a presynaptic disorder of neuromuscular transmission and in the appropriate clinical setting is diagnostic of LEMS.

## CUTANEOUS NERVE BIOPSIES

The value of nerve biopsies in differential diagnosis is limited. A fundamental distinction should be made between settings in which a nerve biopsy can be interpreted in routine clinical pathology laboratories and conditions in which evaluation by specialized units is essential. Two disorders fall into the former category: vasculitis and amyloid infiltration of nerve. Even in these settings, experience in the special features of peripheral nerve pathology is useful, and usually other diagnoses that may require more specialized evaluation are under consideration. In most other neuropathies, for the nerve biopsy to be useful, its assessment should include embedding in plastic and inspection of 1 μm plastic sections, as well as standard paraffin-embedded sections. Teased nerve fibers, although not essential in every case, are the most sensitive means of detecting demyelination and remyelination and should be available in a laboratory. Last, electron microscopy can be useful in certain special situations, and its availability is desirable. For these reasons, in selecting laboratories to evaluate nerve biopsies, it is necessary for the referring physician to check both the methods by which nerve biopsies are processed and the number of nerve biopsies assessed annually.

Nerve biopsy is rarely indicated to establish the diagnosis of peripheral neuropathy; in general, the recognition of neuropathy is accomplished by clinical evaluation and electrodiagnostic testing. Pure "small-fiber" neuropathies, which may be "invisible" by standard electrodiagnostic testing, may be an occasional exception. Even in this example the clinical features, quantitative sensory testing, autonomic testing, or skin biopsy to examine intracutaneous innervation may be sufficient.

Some of the specific indications for nerve biopsy are outlined in the following discussion.

### VASCULITIS

Nerve biopsy is an important part of the evaluation of patients with suspected vasculitic neuropathies. The neuropathic picture suggesting underlying vasculitis usually includes the presence of multiple mononeuropathy, often painful. Biopsy of tissues other than nerve may be diagnostic in systemic vasculitis, and the general evaluation may suggest appropriate sites. An uncommon but important group of patients have been characterized as having "vasculitis restricted to the peripheral nervous system." Such patients have normal sedimentation rates and lack any other cutaneous, ocular, renal, or other identifiable target-organ involvement. However, even in such patients, necrotizing arteritis can be seen in muscle biopsy as well as in nerve biopsy, and combined nerve, and muscle biopsy is indicated.[52]

For many pathologists a diagnosis of vasculitis will not be made unless there is definite evidence of necrotizing changes in blood vessel walls; inflammation of the vessel wall or of the perivascular region is insufficient. Because of sampling variability, the absence of arteritis cannot exclude the diagnosis of vasculitis. Other suggestive but nondiagnostic

features of angiopathic nerve involvement include marked fascicle-to-fascicle variation in nerve fiber affectation, crescentic infarcts of the perineurium, and proliferation of new vessels around epineurial or, occasionally, around endoneurial vessels (reflecting occlusion of those vessels near the site of the biopsy) (see Fig. 18–1). Immunocytochemistry, demonstrating deposition of immunoglobulins and terminal complement complexes in the vessel wall in association with CD8 cytotoxic T cells and T4 cells, is a helpful adjunctive approach.

### AMYLOIDOSIS

Nerve biopsy is often the only practical means of identifying amyloid infiltration of nerve. In our institution the clinical picture of small-fiber neuropathy with pain, loss of pain sensibility (often associated with spontaneous neuropathic pain), and autonomic involvement represents one of the most common indications for cutaneous nerve biopsy. Amyloid is deposited as nonbranching fibrils measuring 10 to 20 nm in diameter. A variety of different proteins can be deposited in the nerve as amyloid. The most frequently encountered in peripheral nerve clinics is deposition of immunoglobulin light chains in association with monoclonal gammopathies. Although the monoclonal gammopathy is usually detected by immunofixation electrophoresis of serum, light-chain deposition can occur with only small levels of a paraprotein. The familial amyloidoses represent deposition of mutant transthyretin, gelsolin, or apolipoprotein A-I. Molecular genetic tests are available for the specific point mutations in these disorders, but their expense and relative unavailability mean that a pathologic diagnosis of amyloidosis is usually required before proceeding to molecular genetic analysis.

Amyloid is demonstrated in tissue sections by Congo red staining, which produces the characteristic birefringent pattern under polarized light. Immunocytochemistry can detect the protein composition of the amyloid deposits. In primary amyloidosis, antibodies to immunoglobulin light chains identify the nature of the deposits, whereas in familial amyloidoses antibodies to transthyretin, gelsolin, or apolipoprotein A-I can be diagnostic.

As noted in the following section, simply to document the presence of a small-fiber neuropathy, skin biopsy to examine intracutaneous innervation may prove to be a simple and powerful technique.

## SKIN BIOPSIES TO EXAMINE INTRACUTANEOUS INNERVATION

Skin biopsy has become a useful means of assessing small-caliber sensory and autonomic fibers. These fibers are "invisible" to standard electrodiagnostic testing. Quantitative thermal testing is a useful adjunct to assessing warm and cool sensors, and measures of cardiovascular autonomic function and of sweating are available in some centers. Such testing is extensively available and represents an attractive method of assessing, in particular, small-nerve fibers. First, skin biopsy is simple and only minimally invasive; cutaneous nerve biopsies are more elaborate and expensive undertakings with some morbidity involved. Second, skin biopsies allow assessment of whether the fiber populations of interest actually reach their targets. With a cutaneous nerve biopsy, in contrast, the investigation is restricted to a single spatial "window" on the nerve, and fiber terminals may be missing more peripherally yet appear relatively normal at the level of the sural nerve biopsy. Third, skin biopsy allows multiple sampling in time and space, providing an indication of the temporal progression or the response to treatment. Fourth, skin biopsies allow selective assessment of specific fiber populations of interest. For example, the C-fiber terminals are easily assessed by examination of the intraepidermal axon terminals.[30,40] The sympathetic innervation of sweat glands can be judged relatively easily,[30] and by means of special stains other specific nerve populations can be evaluated. For example, staining for tyrosine hydroxylase and blood vessel markers in combination can identify the extent of innervation of intracutaneous blood vessels.

Since the first descriptions of intraepidermal fibers by Langerhans and by Retzius, several groups have attempted to develop this biopsy as a diagnostic technique.[1,30,40,50,51] The technical breakthroughs that have allowed easy assessment of these small fibers came from the development of antibod-ies for immunocytochemistry that could intensely label even the finest axons and from the use of preparations that allow examination of relatively thick (50 to 100 µm) sections (Fig. 18–2). In addition, sufficient normative data have been developed to understand the degree of site-to-site variation within specific target areas (e.g., the distal leg or the thigh), the degree of interindividual variation, and the extent of age-related change.[31,32,39]

The major indication for skin biopsies currently is assessment of epidermal innervation by small-caliber sensory fibers. The epidermis, thought for a long period to be virtually devoid of nerve fibers, has proved to have a rich innervation. The axons of the epidermis, as illustrated in Figure 18–3, are truly "free nerve endings" that pass between the adjacent keratinocytes without a Schwann cell ensheathment.[60] They reach the stratum corneum, occasionally branching within the epidermis. These axons are exclusively sensory, as demonstrated by the complete elimination of epidermal innervation by dorsal root ganglionectomy.[38] They arise from C fibers and probably A delta fibers. All are stained with the

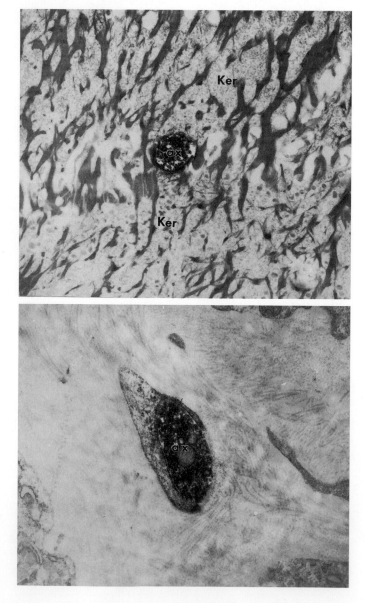

**FIGURE 18–2.** Electron micrograph from a plastic-embedded section, cut tangentially to the surface of the skin, so that the nerve fibers are cut in cross-section. The immunostained nerve fibers have a black reaction product and are labeled *ax.* In the epidermis (*upper panel*) the axons run without Schwann cell investment between neighboring keratinocytes (*Ker*), distinguished by their prominent keratohyaline, forming dark bands running through the cells. The lower panel shows an axon within the dermis. Note that it has a surrounding Schwann cell investment. (From Crawford TO, Hsieh S-T, Schryer BL, et al. Prolonged axonal survival in transected nerves of C57BL/Ola mice is independent of age. *J Neurocytol.* 1995;24:333-340.)

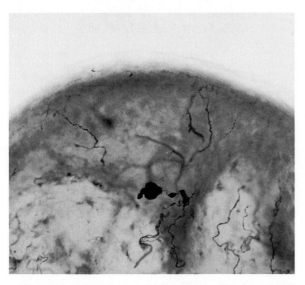

**FIGURE 18–3.** There are prominent axonal swellings in this biopsy from the proximal thigh of a patient with a painful small-fiber neuropathy. (From Holland NR, Crawford TO, Hauer P, et al. Small-fiber sensory neuropathies: clinical course and neuropathology of idiopathic cases. *Ann Neurol.* 1998;44:47.)

polyaxonal marker PGP 9.5 directed against a ubiquitin carboxyterminal hydrolase, and a portion of them are stained intensely with antibodies against the calcitonin and gene-related peptide and substance P.[27]

The best-established clinical indication for skin biopsy at present is assessment of painful neuropathies in patients without evidence of large-fiber involvement (i.e., normal tendon reflexes and electrodiagnostic studies). Among the small-fiber neuropathies studied to date, the large idiopathic group predominantly involves older patients[26] and patients with diabetes,[30,32] painful sensory neuropathy associated with HIV infection,[40] Fabry's disease,[53] or leprosy.[29]

In a recent study of idiopathic painful sensory neuropathy, biopsies were taken from at least three sites—the distal leg above the ankle, the distal thigh above the knee, and the proximal thigh. The typical pattern consisted of depletion of epidermal nerve fibers distally (Fig. 18–4), with more normal densities, but often with predegenerative changes in the axons at more proximal levels. These predegenerative changes included axonal swellings and increased varicosity[53] and an increased tendency toward intraepidermal branching. Although this population has not yet been rigorously tested, it appears that patients with intraspinal disease producing radiculopathies do not have changes in epidermal innervation.

## BLOOD TESTS

The specific blood tests valuable in the individual patient are defined by the clinical picture, but several general comments apply to most patients. Screening for diabetes is almost universally done, but there is an important caveat: *Although diabetic neuropathy is the most prevalent peripheral nerve disease in developed countries, it is also the most overdiagnosed.* Most cases of diabetic polyneuropathy develop in individuals with established diabetes of many years' duration.[13] If there is no previous history of diabetes and if the fasting blood sugar level is normal, glucose tolerance testing

is usually not necessary and may produce results that divert attention from other potential causes. For example, mild-to-moderate hyperglycemia at 1 or 2 hours is irrelevant to the patient with new onset of a predominantly motor neuropathy and is of doubtful relevance even in patients with a picture otherwise compatible with the predominantly sensory neuropathy usually associated with diabetes. Determination of glycated hemoglobin is a valuable means of assessing diabetic populations and following individual patients with diabetes, but it is not a primary means of diagnosing diabetes in individual patients.

Routine laboratory tests and thyroid function studies can help identify those patients in whom unsuspected metabolic disease is present. Abnormal liver function tests may suggest the possibility of occult alcoholism. Vitamin $B_{12}$ testing may identify the rare patient with pernicious anemia who develops primary peripheral nerve disease rather than myelopathy.

Special comment should be made about the group of patients with purely sensory neuropathies and gait ataxia who have markedly elevated antinuclear antibody (ANA) titers but few other laboratory abnormalities. These patients often prove to have sensory ganglionitis associated with features of Sjögren's syndrome.[21] They constitute a discrete patient population and are noteworthy in part because they present initially to neurologists rather than to rheumatologists. In most of these patients there is little evidence of other extraglandular effects of Sjögren's syndrome.[21] A lip biopsy, showing the typical inflammation of minor salivary glands, can be a useful and confirmatory test.

Detection of monoclonal gammopathies has become increasingly important as the spectrum of paraproteinemic

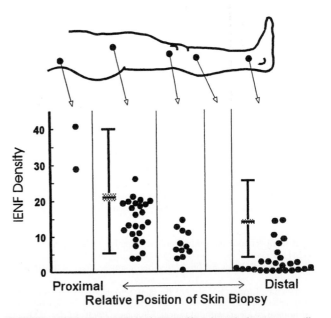

**FIGURE 18–4.** Intraepidermal nerve fiber (*IENF*) densities are illustrated in skin biopsies from various levels in the leg in patients with idiopathic painful small-fiber sensory neuropathy. In the proximal thigh and the distal leg, the bars represent the 5% to 93% range for normal controls. Note that even in proximal regions the intraepidermal nerve fiber density is on the average lower than in controls but is within the normal range. In contrast, only a few individuals have fiber densities within the normal range at the level of the distal leg, and most have no intraepidermal fibers. (From Holland NR, Crawford TO, Hauer P, et al. Small-fiber sensory neuropathies: clinical course and neuropathology of idiopathic cases. *Ann Neurol.* 1998;44:47.)

neuropathies has broadened. Monoclonal proteins that cause neuropathy can be missed by serum protein electrophoresis because they usually do not increase the total amount of gammaglobulin. Immunofixation electrophoresis is the most sensitive assay, and monoclonal spikes may be detectable only by this method. However, immunofixation is sufficiently sensitive that irrelevant paraproteins can be detected in a significant proportion of elderly patients. Therefore the role of monoclonal gammopathies in causation of nerve disease must always be interpreted cautiously. Detection of a monoclonal immunoglobulin mandates a skeletal survey (to exclude solitary plasmacytoma or multiple myeloma[17,36,61]) and urine immunofixation (to search for excessive light-chain excretion, a finding that may raise the suspicion of associated amyloidosis). A bone marrow aspirate and biopsy are usually advised as part of evaluation for possible myeloma, although the yield in patients with chronic peripheral neuropathies and paraproteins is low. In any event such patients require continued monitoring for the possible evolution of a more aggressive plasma cell disorder.

## SUMMARY

Selecting appropriate laboratory testing in diagnosing peripheral neuropathies is important because it increases the yield of correct diagnoses and is cost-effective. A large number of tests are available. This chapter provides a guide to selecting appropriate tests and reviews the clinical situations that suggest specific tests. Electrodiagnostic testing is valuable in almost all patients with peripheral neuropathy. Quantitative sensory testing adds additional information and is especially useful in patients with small-fiber neuropathy. On occasion, routine blood tests may detect metabolic disorders causing a patient's disorder. A number of antibody assays for neuropathies are commercially available, with the most useful being anti-MAG, anti-GM$_1$, anti-GQ$_{1b}$, anti-Hu, and anti–calcium channel antibodies, but these tests should be used only in very select situations and not as "screening studies." The role of cutaneous nerve and skin biopsies in selected disorders is also discussed.

## REFERENCES

1. Bolton CF, Winkleman RK, Dyck PJ. A quantitative study of Meissner's corpuscles in man. *Neurology.* 1966;16:1-9.
2. Bouche P, Moulonguet A, Ben Younes-Chennoufi A, et al. Multifocal motor neuropathy with conduction block: a study of 24 patients. *J Neurol Neurosurg Psychiatry.* 1995;59:38-44.
3. Braun PE, Frail DE, Latov N. Myelin-associated glycoprotein is the antigen for a monoclonal IgM in polyneuropathy. *J Neurochem.* 1982;39:1261-1265.
4. Brown WF, Bolton CF. *Clinical Electromyography.* Boston: Butterworth; 1987.
5. Chalk CH, Lennon VA, Stevens JC, et al. Seronegativity for type 1 antineuronal nuclear antibodies ("anti-Hu") in subacute sensory neuronopathy patients without cancer. *Neurology.* 1993;43:2209-2211.
6. Chaudhry V, Corse AM, Cornblath DR, et al. Multifocal motor neuropathy: response to human immune globulin. *Ann Neurol.* 1993;33:237-242.
7. Chaudhry V, Corse AM, Cornblath DR, et al. Multifocal motor neuropathy: electrodiagnostic features. *Muscle Nerve.* 1994;17:198-205.
8. Chou KH, Ilyas AA, Evans JE, et al. Structure of a glycolipid reacting with monoclonal IgM in neuropathy and with HNK-1. *Biochem Biophys Res Commun.* 1985;128:383-388.
9. Cornblath DR, Sumner AJ, Daube J, et al. Issues and opinions: conduction block in clinical practice. *Muscle Nerve.* 1991;14:869-871.
10. Crawford TO, Hsieh S-T, Schryer BL, et al. Prolonged axonal survival in transected nerves of C57BL/Ola mice is independent of age. *J Neurocytol.* 1995;24:333-340
11. Denny-Brown D. Primary sensory neuropathy with muscular changes associated with carcinoma. *J Neurol Neurosurg Psychiatry.* 1948;11:73-87.
12. Dyck PJ, Arezzo JC, Bolton CF, et al. Quantitative sensory testing: a consensus report from the Peripheral Neuropathy Association. *Neurology.* 1993;43:1050-1052.
13. Dyck PK, Dratz KM, Karnes JL, et al. The prevalence by staged severity of various types of diabetic neuropathy, retinopathy, and nephropathy in a population-based cohort: the Rochester Diabetic Neuropathy Study [published erratum appears in *Neurology* 1993;43:2345]. *Neurology.* 1993;43:817-824.
14. Feasby TE, Gilbert JJ, Brown WF, et al. An acute axonal form of Guillain-Barré polyneuropathy. *Brain.* 1986;109:1115-1126.
15. Feasby TE, Hahn AF, Brown WF, et al. Severe axonal degeneration in acute Guillain-Barré syndrome: evidence of two different mechanisms? *J Neurol Sci.* 1993;116:185-192.
16. Fisher M. An unusual variant of acute idiopathic polyneuritis (syndrome of ophthalmoplegia ataxia and areflexia). *N Engl J Med.* 1956;255:57-65.
17. Gosselin S, Kyle RA, Dyck PJ. Neuropathy associated with monoclonal gammopathies of undetermined significance. *Ann Neurol.* 1991;30:54-61.
18. Graus F, Elkon KB, Cordon-Cardo C, et al. Sensory neuronopathy and small cell lung cancer: an antineuronal antibody that also reacts with the tumor. *Am J Med.* 1986;80:45-52.
19. Gregson NA, Leibowitz S. IgM paraproteinaemia, polyneuropathy and myelin-associated glycoprotein (MAG). *Neuropathol Appl Neurobiol.* 1985;11:329-347.
20. Griffin JW, Cornblath DR. Diseases of the peripheral nervous system. In: Rosenberg RN, ed. *Comprehensive Neurology.* New York: Raven Press; 1991;421-450.
21. Griffin JW, Cornblath DR, Alexander E, et al. Ataxic sensory neuropathy and dorsal root ganglionitis associated with Sjögren's syndrome. *Ann Neurol.* 1990;27:304-315.
22. Griffin JW, Li CY, Ho TW, et al. Guillain-Barré syndrome in northern China: the spectrum of neuropathologic changes in clinically defined cases. *Brain.* 1995;118:577-595.
23. Griffin JW, Li CY, Ho TW, et al. Pathology of the motor-sensory axonal Guillain-Barré syndrome. *Ann Neurol.* 1996;39:17-28.
24. Hays AP, Latov N, Takatsu M, et al. Experimental demyelination of nerve induced by serum of patients with neuropathy and an anti-MAG IgM M-protein. *Neurology.* 1987;37:242-256.
25. Ho TW, Mishu B, Li CY, et al. Guillain-Barré syndrome in northern China: relationship to *Campylobacter jejuni* infection and anti-glycolipid antibodies. *Brain.* 1995;118:597-605.
26. Holland NR, Crawford TO, Hauer P, et al. Small-fiber sensory neuropathies: clinical course and neuropathology of idiopathic cases. *Ann Neurol.* 1998;44:47.
27. Hsieh S-T, Choi S, Lin W-M, et al. Epidermal denervation and its effects on keratinocytes and Langerhans cells. *J Neurocytol.* 1996;25:513-524.
28. Ilyas AA, Quarles RH, MacIntosh TD, et al. IgM in a human neuropathy related to paraproteinemia binds to a carbohydrate determinant in the myelin-associated glycoprotein and to a ganglioside. *Proc Natl Acad Sci U S A.* 1984;81:1225-1229.
29. Karanth SS, Springall DR, Lucas S, et al. Changes in nerves and neuropeptides in skin from 100 leprosy patients investigated by immunocytochemistry. *J Pathol.* 1989;157:15-26.
30. Kennedy WR, Wendelschafer-Crabb G. The innervation of human epidermis. *J Neurol Sci.* 1993;115:184-190.
31. Kennedy WR, Wendelschafer-Crabb G. Quantification of nerve in skin biopsies from control and diabetic subjects. *Neurology.* 1994;44(suppl 2):A275. Abstract.
32. Kennedy WR, Wendelschafer-Crabb G, Johnson T. Quantification of epidermal nerves in diabetic neuropathy. *Neurology.* 1996;47:1042-1048.
33. Kimura J. Principles and pitfalls of nerve conduction studies. *Ann Neurol.* 1984;16:415-429.
34. Kimura J. *Electrodiagnosis in Diseases of Nerve and Muscle: Principles and Practice.* Philadelphia: FA Davis; 1989.
35. Kornberg AJ, Pestronk A, Bieser K, et al. The clinical correlates of high-titer IgG anti-GM$_1$ antibodies. *Ann Neurol.* 1994;35:234-237.
36. Kyle RA, Dyck PJ. Osteosclerotic myeloma (POEMS syndrome). In: Dyck PJ, Thomas PK, Griffin JW, et al, eds. *Peripheral Neuropathy.* Philadelphia: WB Saunders; 1993:1288-1293.
37. Latov N, Sherman WH, Nemni R, et al. Plasma-cell dyscrasia and pe-

ripheral neuropathy with a monoclonal antibody to peripheral-nerve myelin. *N Engl J Med.* 1980;303:618-621.

38. Li Y, Hsieh S-T, Chien H-F, et al. Sensory and motor denervation influence epidermal thickness in rat foot glabrous skin. *Exp Neurol.* 1997; 147:452-462.

39. McArthur JC, Stocks A, Hauer P, et al. Epidermal nerve fiber density: normative reference range and diagnostic efficiency. *Arch Neurol.* 1998; 55:1513-1520.

40. McCarthy BG, Hsieh S-T, Stocks EA, et al. Cutaneous innervation in sensory neuropathies: evaluation by skin biopsy. *Neurology.* 1995;45: 1848-1855.

41. McKhann GM, Cornblath DR, Griffin JW, et al. Acute motor axonal neuropathy: a frequent cause of acute flaccid paralysis in China. *Ann Neurol.* 1993;33:333-342.

42. Mendell JR, Sahenk Z, Whitaker JN, et al. Polyneuropathy and IgM monoclonal gammopathy: studies on the pathogenetic role of anti-myelin–associated glycoprotein antibody. *Ann Neurol.* 1985;17:243-254.

43. Nobile-Orazio E, Baldini L, Barbieri S, et al. Treatment of patients with neuropathy and anti-MAG IgM M-proteins. *Ann Neurol.* 1988;24:93-97.

44. Parry GJ, Clarke S. Multifocal acquired neuropathy masquerading as motor neuron disease. *Muscle Nerve.* 1988;11:103-107.

45. Pestronk A, Adams RN, Clawson L, et al. Serum antibodies to GM$_1$ ganglioside in amyotrophic lateral sclerosis. *Neurology.* 1988;38:1457-1461.

46. Pestronk A, Cornblath DR, Ilyas AA, et al. A treatable multifocal motor neuropathy with antibodies to GM$_1$ ganglioside. *Ann Neurol.* 1988;24: 73-78.

47. Pestronk A, Li F, Griffin JW, et al. Antibodies to myelin-associated glycoprotein and sulfatide in predominantly sensory polyneuropathies. *Ann Neurol.* 1990;28:239. Abstract.

48. Quarles RH, Everly JL, Brady RO. Evidence for the close association of a glycoprotein with myelin. *J Neurochem.* 1973;21:1177-1191.

49. Quarles RH, Ilyas AA, Willison HJ. Antibodies to glycolipids in demyelinating diseases of the human peripheral nervous system. *Chem Phys Lipids.* 1986;42:235-248.

50. Ridley A. Silver staining of nerve endings in human digital glabrous skin. *J Anat.* 1969;104:41-48.

51. Ridley A. Silver staining of the innervation of Meissner corpuscles in peripheral neuropathy. *Brain.* 1991;196:539-552.

52. Said G, Lacroix-Ciaudo C, Fujimura H, et al. The peripheral neuropathy of necrotizing arteritis: a clinicopathological study. *Ann Neurol.* 1988;23:461-465.

53. Scott LJC, Griffin JW, Barton NW, et al. Quantitative analysis of epidermal innervation in Fabry's disease and comparison with sural nerve morphometry. *Neurology.* 1998.

54. Steck AJ, Murray N, Justafre JC, et al. Passive transfer studies in demyelinating neuropathy with IgM monoclonal antibodies to myelin-associated glycoprotein. *J Neurol Neurosurg Psychiatry.* 1985;48:927-929.

55. Sumner AJ. *The Physiology of Peripheral Nerve Disease.* Philadelphia: WB Saunders; 1980.

56. Tatum AH. Experimental paraprotein neuropathy, demyelination by passive transfer of human IgM anti-myelin–associated glycoprotein. *Ann Neurol.* 1993;33:502-506.

57. Trapp BD, Andrews SB, Wong A, et al. Co-localization of the myelin-associated glycoprotein and the microfilament components F-actin and spectrin in Schwann cells of myelinated fibers. *J Neurocytol.* 1989; 18:47-60.

58. Trapp BD, Quarles RH. Immunocytochemical localization of the myelin-associated glycoprotein: fact or artifact? *J Neuroimmunol.* 1984; 6:231-249.

59. Trapp BD, Quarles RH, Griffin JW. Myelin-associated glycoprotein and myelinating Schwann cell–axon interaction in chronic B-B′ iminodipropionitrile neuropathy. *J Cell Biol.* 1984;98:1272-1278.

60. Uldry P-A, Steck A-J. Plasma exchange in neurology. *Curr Stud Hematol Blood Transfus.* 1990;57:167-183.

61. Victor M, Banker BQ, Adams RD. The neuropathy of multiple myelomas. *J Neurol Neurosurg Psychiatry.* 1958;21:73-88.

62. Vincent A, Lang B, Newsom-Davis J. Autoimmunity to the voltage-gated calcium channel underlies the Lambert-Eaton myasthenic syndrome, a paraneoplastic disorder. *Trends Neurosci.* 1989;12:496-502.

63. Willison HJ, Trapp BD, Bacher JD, et al. Demyelination induced by intraneural injection of human anti-myelin–associated glycoprotein antibodies. *Muscle Nerve.* 1988;11:1169-1176.

64. Yuki N, Handa S, Taki T, et al. Cross-reactive antigen between nervous tissue and a bacterium elicits Guillain-Barré syndrome: molecular mimicry between ganglicide GM$_1$ and lipopolysaccharide from Penner's serotype 19 of *Campylobacter jejuni. Biomed Res.* 1992;13:451-453.

65. Yuki N, Yoshino H, Sato S, et al. Acute axonal polyneuropathy associated with anti-GM$_1$ antibodies following *Campylobacter jejuni* enteritis. *Neurology.* 1990;40:1900-1902.

66. Yuki N, Yoshino H, Sato S, et al. Severe acute axonal form of Guillain-Barré syndrome associated with IgG anti-GD$_{1a}$ antibodies. *Muscle Nerve.* 1992;15:899-903.

# 19

# Mononeuropathies

*Daniel M. Feinberg and David C. Preston*

Patients with disorders of the peripheral nervous system are common in the practice of neurology and internal medicine. Among disorders of the peripheral nervous system, isolated mononeuropathies of individual peripheral nerves occur most frequently. Each peripheral nerve has its own unique motor and sensory innervation leading to well-recognized patterns of the mononeuropathies. Some are extremely familiar, such as in median neuropathy at the wrist (i.e., carpal tunnel syndrome), whereas others are distinctly unusual, such as suprascapular neuropathy under the suprascapular notch. The mononeuropathies, especially when mild or early in their course, are often mistaken for more proximal lesions in the brachial and lumbosacral plexus or for lesions at the level of the nerve roots. Most are readily diagnosable on the basis of clinical and electrodiagnostic findings and in selected cases with appropriate imaging studies.

## MONONEUROPATHIES OF THE UPPER EXTREMITY

### MEDIAN NEUROPATHY (Fig. 19–1)

#### Median Neuropathy at the Wrist: Carpal Tunnel Syndrome

Carpal tunnel syndrome (CTS) is the most common entrapment neuropathy affecting the upper extremity.[1] It results from compression of the median nerve as it passes under the flexor retinaculum (i.e., transverse carpal ligament) at the wrist. In most cases, a pathologic condition of the transverse carpal ligament shows edema, vascular sclerosis, and fibrosis—findings consistent with repeated stress to connective tissue. Demyelination follows compression and ischemia of the median nerve, and, if severe enough, wallerian degeneration and axonal loss follow. Occupations or activities that involve repetitive hand use clearly increase the risk of CTS. Other predisposing causes and associations of CTS include the presence of a ganglionic cyst or tumor in the canal, degenerative arthritis (especially rheumatoid arthritis), amyloidosis, circulatory disturbances (e.g., compression via a persistent median artery), pregnancy, hemodialysis, and metabolic abnormalities (including hypothyroidism and diabetes mellitus).

The clinical syndrome is often heralded by nocturnal awakening, usually a few hours after falling asleep, because of a sensation of pressure and paresthesias in the hand. The fingers may be perceived as stiff or swollen, but often no objective correlates to these symptoms are found, especially early in the course. Commonly, pain and pressure extend into the forearm, arm, or, less often, the shoulder. Patients may also report exacerbation of symptoms during routine activities, such as driving, holding the phone, or reading a book or paper. In some patients these symptoms may persist for years before any objective sensory loss or motor deterioration is apparent. Women are more commonly affected than men, and the syndrome is rare in children.

On physical examination, several provocative maneuvers are often employed. Tapping of the median nerve over the carpal tunnel may cause paresthesias in the first 3½ digits (Tinel's sign). Passively flexing the wrist for only 30 seconds may also provoke median paresthesias (Phalen's sign). Flexing the wrist increases pressure within the carpal tunnel, resulting in ischemia and paresthesias. A wide range of sensitivities and specificities for Tinel's sign and Phalen's maneuver have been reported in the literature. Tinel's sign is present in more than half of CTS cases; however, false-positive Tinel's signs are common in the general population. A Phalen's maneuver is more sensitive than Tinel's sign and has fewer false-positives.

Weakness and atrophy of the thenar muscles may be present if there is significant axonal loss. Objective sensory loss, hyperesthesia, or allodynia on the first 3½ digits may be found. Of importance, sensation over the thenar area is spared in CTS; this territory is supplied from the palmar cutaneous sensory branch of the median nerve that arises proximal to the carpal tunnel.

The main differential diagnosis of CTS includes a more proximal median neuropathy in the region of the elbow, brachial plexopathy, and cervical radiculopathy. A proximal lesion should be suspected if any of the upper extremity reflexes are abnormal, if sensory loss extends beyond the median nerve territory, or if strength of arm pronation, wrist flexion, elbow flexion, or extension are impaired. In early or mild cases, however, the symptoms and signs of CTS may overlap with lesions of the proximal median nerve, brachial

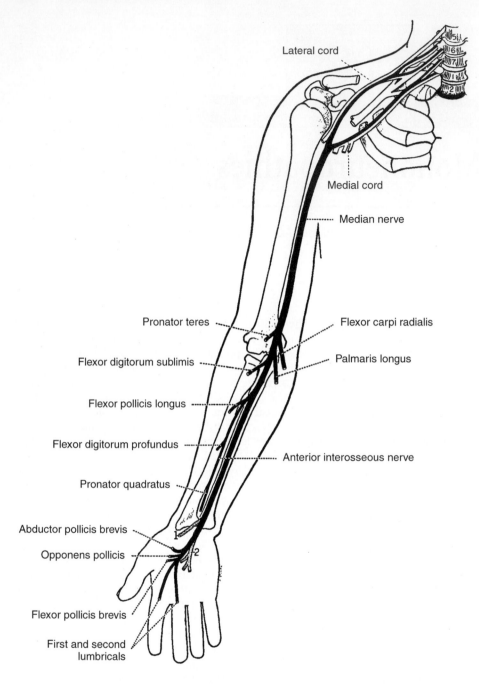

Lateral cord

Medial cord

Median nerve

Pronator teres

Flexor carpi radialis

Flexor digitorum sublimis

Palmaris longus

Flexor pollicis longus

Flexor digitorum profundus

Anterior interosseous nerve

Pronator quadratus

Abductor pollicis brevis

Opponens pollicis

Flexor pollicis brevis

First and second lumbricals

**FIGURE 19–1.** Anatomy of the median nerve. The median nerve is derived from a combination of the lateral and medial cords of the brachial plexus. Motor innervation is supplied to forearm muscles and muscles of the thenar eminence. Sensation is supplied to the thenar eminence by the palmar cutaneous sensory branch (*1*) and to the first three and one half digits by several digital sensory branches (*2*). (Adapted from Haymaker W, Woodhal B. *Peripheral Nerve Injuries.* Philadelphia: WB Saunders; 1953.)

plexus, and most often the cervical roots. In these cases laboratory diagnostic confirmation is essential, especially when the clinical syndrome is not obvious.

The principal diagnostic tests in suspected median neuropathy are nerve conduction studies (Protocol 19–1) and needle electromyography (EMC). Imaging of the carpal tunnel is only useful in selected cases when a tumor or cyst is suspected. In CTS the primary underlying pathophysiologic condition is demyelination of the median nerve. Nerve conduction studies are extremely sensitive in their ability to demonstrate demyelination. Routine electrodiagnostic testing should include median motor and sensory nerve conduction studies. The motor latency is usually prolonged across the wrist in CTS but is normal distal to the transverse carpal ligament. In the Rochester study of more than 829 hands with a clinical diagnosis of CTS, 37.5% had prolonged

median motor distal latency (>4.6 ms). The median nerve motor distal latency can also be compared with the ulnar nerve motor distal latency. A difference of >1.8 ms is considered abnormal.[26] Comparisons to the contralateral median motor distal latency are generally not as useful since CTS is bilateral in 55% of patients. The compound muscle action potential (CMAP) amplitude of the abductor pollicis brevis was abnormal in 15.4% of hands studied in the Rochester study. A reduced CMAP amplitude may indicate either axonal loss or conduction block. To distinguish these, palmar stimulation may be used to assess the CMAP amplitude with stimulation distal to the carpal tunnel (Fig. 19–2).[13] Reduced amplitudes with stimulation both distal and proximal to the carpal tunnel indicate axonal loss, whereas reduced amplitudes proximal to the carpal tunnel with normal or improved amplitudes on palmar stimulation denote conduction block. Often, a combination of axonal loss and conduction block is present. Forearm median motor conduction velocity may be reduced in some cases of CTS (11% of the limbs in the Rochester series). The explanation for this is loss of large, rapidly conducting myelinated fibers in the carpal tunnel compression.[24]

Median sensory nerve conduction studies are more sensitive than motor studies in the evaluation for CTS. Orthodromic sensory nerve conduction studies were first described, but antidromic stimulation produces larger sensory nerve action potential (SNAP) amplitudes with no difference in distal latency. The median sensory nerve distal latencies were abnormal in 64% of the Rochester series patients. The antidromic median SNAP amplitudes were reduced in 88% of those patients. In contrast, only 39% of orthodromic median SNAP amplitudes were reduced. Similar to motor studies, reduced SNAP ampiitudes may result from either axonal loss or conduction block across the wrist. Palmar stimulation also can be employed for sensory fibers to make this differentiation.[13]

In patients with typical CTS, the median distal motor and sensory latencies are moderately to markedly prolonged. However, a group of patients remains with clinical symptoms and signs of CTS in whom these routine studies are normal (approximately 10% to 25% of CTS patients). In these patients the electrodiagnosis of CTS will be missed unless further testing is performed with more sensitive nerve conduction studies (Fig. 19–3). These studies usually involve a comparison of the median nerve to another nerve of similar length and size in the same hand. The ulnar nerve is the nerve most commonly used for comparison, and less often the radial nerve is used. In each of these comparison studies, identical distances are used between the stimulator and recording electrodes for the median and ulnar nerve studies. These techniques create an ideal internal control in which several variables known to affect conduction time are held constant, including distance, temperature, age, and nerve and/or muscle size. Ideally, the only factor that varies in these paired comparison studies is that although the median nerve traverses the carpal tunnel, the other nerve does not.

The median and ulnar palm-to-wrist mixed latency is more sensitive than antidromic or orthodromic SNAP measurements in the diagnosis of CTS. The amplitudes of the responses are larger since this technique stimulates and records mixed nerve potentials, which includes the group Ia afferents from muscle spindles. Hence it is less likely that

---

**PROTOCOL 19–1. Recommended NCS Protocol for Carpal Tunnel Syndrome (CTS)**

**Routine Studies**
1. Median motor study recording abductor pollicis brevis, stimulating wrist and elbow
2. Ulnar motor study recording abductor digiti minimi, stimulating wrist, below groove, and above groove
3. Median and ulnar F responses
4. Median sensory response, recording second or third digit, stimulating wrist
5. Ulnar sensory response, recording fifth digit, stimulating wrist

*The study is highly suggestive of isolated CTS if*
1. The median studies are abnormal, showing marked slowing across the wrist (prolonged distal motor and sensory latencies) and prolonged minimum F wave latencies. The median CMAP and SNAP amplitudes may be diminished if there is secondary axonal loss or if demyelination has led to conduction block at the wrist.
   and
2. The ulnar motor, sensory, and F wave studies are normal (making a polyneuropathy unlikely).

*If the median motor, sensory, and F response studies are normal or equivocal,* proceed with the median vs. ulnar comparison tests or inching across the wrist.

*Median vs. Ulnar Comparisons*
1. Comparison of the median vs. ulnar mixed palm-to-wrist peak latencies, stimulating the median and ulnar palm one at a time, 8 cm from the recording electrodes placed over the median and ulnar wrist, respectively
2. Comparison of the median lumbrical and ulnar interosseous distal motor latencies, stimulating the median and ulnar wrist at identical distances (8 to 10 cm), recording with the same electrode over the second lumbrical/interosseous
3. Comparison of the median and ulnar digit 4 sensory peak latencies, stimulating over the median and ulnar wrist one at a time, at identical distances (11 to 13 cm), and recording digit 4

*Median Inching Across the Wrist*
1. Motor inching across the wrist into the palm at 1 cm intervals looking for an abrupt change in latency (>0.3 ms) or significant increase in CMAP amplitude (distal/proximal ratio >1.2)

2. Sensory inching across the wrist into the palm at 1 cm intervals looking for an abrupt change in latency (>0.3 ms) or significant increase in SNAP amplitude (distal/proximal ratio >1.6).

If two or three of the median vs. ulnar comparison tests or the inching studies are abnormal, there is a high likelihood of mild CTS. Proceed to the EMG.

*If the ulnar motor or sensory studies are also abnormal,* the case is more complex. There are now two fundamental issues that must be addressed at this point:
1. If the median abnormalities localize to the wrist, then what is the significance of the ulnar abnormalities? The patient may have
   a. CTS and a coexistent ulnar neuropathy at the elbow (a common situation)
   b. CTS and a coexistent polyneuropathy resulting in ulnar abnormalities
   c. CTS and a brachial plexopathy
2. If the median nerve abnormalities do not localize to the wrist, then what is the significance of the ulnar abnormalities? The patient may have a
   a. Brachial plexopathy
   b. Polyneuropathy

Performing the median vs. ulnar comparison studies or median inching studies across the wrist will often answer whether or not the median nerve abnormalities localize to the wrist, even if there are ulnar abnormalities. Whether the ulnar nerve abnormalities represent ulnar neuropathy at elbow, brachial plexopathy, or polyneuropathy will depend on further nerve conduction studies. If the ulnar motor studies show clear-cut slowing or conduction block across the elbow, then the ulnar abnormalities are undoubtedly due to ulnar neuropathy at the elbow. If this is not the case, then lower extremity motor and sensory studies (tibial and peroneal motor, sural sensory, tibial F responses) should be performed to exclude a polyneuropathy. Further upper extremity sensory studies (radial, lateral antebrachial, and medial antebrachial) as well as more extensive EMG may be necessary to exclude a brachial plexopathy if lower extremity studies are normal.

---

From Preston DC, Shapiro BE. *Electromyography and Neuromuscular Disorders.* Boston: Butterworth-Heinemann; 1998. Reprinted with permission.

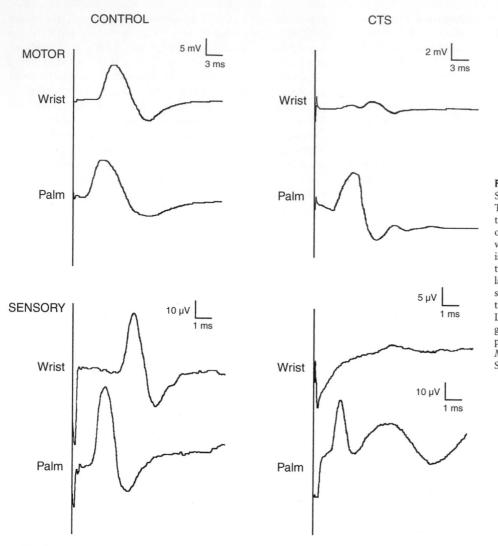

**FIGURE 19–2.** Change in CMAP and SNAP amplitude across the carpal tunnel. To assess possible conduction block across the carpal tunnel, either the median CMAP or SNAP can be recorded, stimulating the wrist and palm. Note that in controls, there is only a slight increase in amplitude between palm and wrist stimulation sites. A large difference between palm and wrist sites in carpal tunnel syndrome (CTS) patients signifies conduction block. (From Lesser EA, Venkatesh S, Preston DC, Logigian EL. Stimulation distal to the lesion in patients with carpal tunnel syndrome. *Muscle Nerve.* 18:503, © 1995; John Wiley & Sons, Inc.)

median mixed responses will be absent in contradistinction to the routine SNAP in severe CTS. A difference of 0.4 ms between median and ulnar mixed palm-to-wrist latencies is considered significant. The overall rate of abnormality in this test in the Rochester study was 91%. Kimura[10] found that the latency from palm to wrist was abnormal in 21% of hands with normal SNAP latencies.

The second commonly employed median-to-ulnar comparison study is the Digit 4 Sensory study. In most patients the lateral half of the fourth digit is supplied by the median nerve; the medial half, by the ulnar nerve. An antidromic sensory study recording over digit 4 and stimulating median and ulnar sensory fibers at the wrist can be performed to compare the latencies. A difference of 0.5 ms is considered significant. Uncini et al[27] found that the digit 4 comparison studies were the most sensitive method for the electrodiagnosis of CTS. Martinez Cruz[15] found that digit 4 recordings were abnormal in 85% of patients with mild CTS but noted that the palm-to-wrist study was abnormal in 92.5% of patients.

The third commonly employed median-ulnar study involves comparing motor latencies from the second lumbrical (median) and interosseous (ulnar) muscles.[19] With an active recording electrode placed slightly lateral to the third metacarpal in the palm, stimulation of the median nerve re-

sults in the recording of a CMAP from the second lumbrical, whereas stimulation of the ulnar nerve at the wrist with the same recording electrodes results in a CMAP from the deeper ulnar innervated interossei muscles. A latency difference of 0.5 ms is considered significant.

Using the median-ulnar comparisons increases the diagnostic yield to approximately 95%. However, these sensitive median vs. ulnar comparison studies rely on very small differences between the median and ulnar latencies (0.4 to 0.5 ms) as a measure of median nerve dysfunction. Thus each of these studies requires meticulous attention to distance measurements, electrode placement, stimulus and recording artifact, and supramaximal stimulation. The other main use of these comparative studies is identifying CTS in the presence of superimposed polyneuropathy. In polyneuropathy, all latencies may be prolonged. The key question is whether the median latencies are prolonged out of proportion to what would be expected for the polyneuropathy.

Enthusiasm over the highly sensitive median-to-ulnar comparisons and other electrodiagnostic tests must be weighed against their lack of specificity and the possibility of false-positive results if these methods are not used in the proper clinical content. The probability of any diagnostic test demonstrating a true positive depends not only on the sensitivity of the test but also on the prevalence of the disease in the population (Bayes' theorem). The chance of a false-positive result increases dramatically when the prevalence of the disease in a population being studied is low, even when the test is highly sensitive and specific (Table 19–1). Thus, if these highly sensitive electrodiagnostic tests were used as a screening tool in a population with a low incidence of CTS, most "positive" tests would actually be false-positives. However, this is generally not a problem if patients are referred for diagnostic testing with a high clinical suspicion of the disorder (e.g., patients with wrist and arm pain, median paresthesias, and Phalen's sign have a high prevalence of CTS). In these patients a positive result on one of the median-ulnar comparison tests is likely to be a true positive.

**TABLE 19–1. Predictive Value of a Positive Test With 95% Sensitivity and 95% Specificity Based on Prevalence of the Disease in the Population Being Studied**

| PREVALENCE (%) | PREDICTIVE VALUE OF POSITIVE TEST (%) |
|---|---|
| 75 | 98 |
| 50 | 95 |
| 20 | 83 |
| 10 | 68 |
| 5 | 50 |
| 1 | 16 |
| 0.1 | 2 |

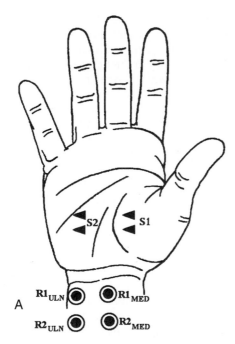

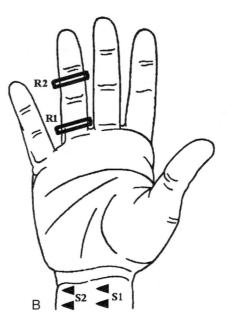

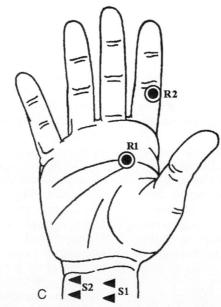

**FIGURE 19–3.** Median vs. ulnar comparison studies. **A,** Palmar mixed, **B,** digit 4 sensory, and **C,** lumbrical-interossei studies. *S1,* Median stimulation point; *S2,* ulnar stimulation point; *R1,* active recording electrode; *R2,* reference recording electrode. In each study identical distances between stimulation and recording sites are used for the median and ulnar nerves. (From Preston DC, Ross MH, Kothari MJ, Plotkin GM, Venkatesh S, Logigian EL. The median-ulnar latency difference studies are comparable in mild carpal tunnel syndrome. *Muscle Nerve.* © 1994; John Wiley & Sons, Inc.)

In median neuropathy at the wrist, needle EMG is used to confirm localization and to assess the chronicity and severity of axonal loss. On routine needle EMG in patients with CTS, only the distal median muscles are abnormal (i.e., abductor pollicis brevis, opponens pollicis). However, in every patient it is useful to study additional proximal muscles to distinguish CTS from proximal median neuropathy, brachial plexopathy, peripheral neuropathy, and cervical radiculopathy (especially C6-C7). Needle EMG examination of the flexor carpi radialis, pronator teres, triceps, biceps, and cervical paraspinal muscles can usually be used to make that differentiation.

## Median Neuropathy in the Forearm: Anterior Interosseous Nerve Syndrome

Anterior interosseous nerve (AIN) syndrome was first described in 1952 by Kiloh and Nevin.[9] The clinical features of the syndrome include weakness of the flexor pollicis longus, flexor digitorum profundus (to digits 3 and 4), and pronator quadratus. The AIN has no cutaneous sensory supply, but it does supply proprioception and pain sensation to deep tissues, including the wrist joint. Thus deep, aching forearm and wrist pain are common symptoms of the AIN syndrome.

AIN arises from the median nerve after the nerve passes through the two heads of the pronator teres. The syndrome is often thought to be idiopathic; however, numerous etiologic complexes have been described (Table 19–2). The differential diagnosis includes tendon rupture and a forme fruste of brachial neuritis. All patients with AIN syndrome should have electrophysiologic evaluation that includes proximal and shoulder girdle muscles. The patients may only complain of thumb pain or weakness but may have less bothersome proximal signs and symptoms.

The electrophysiologic evaluation in a patient with suspected AIN syndrome is primarily guided by needle EMG of muscles supplied by the AIN. In addition, a fundamental understanding of Martin-Gruber types of anastomoses is critical since 50% of these anastomoses arise from the AIN. Therefore a patient with AIN syndrome may present with ulnar intrinsic hand weakness in addition to weakness of AIN muscles.

## Median Nerve Compression by Ligament of Struthers

The median nerve may be compressed by a ligament of Struthers that runs from the medial epicondyle to a bone spur on the anteromedial surface of the humerus about 4 to 6 cm proximal to the medial epicondyle. Approximately 2% of the population have this bone spur, but only a fraction develop median nerve compression at that site. Patients report tenderness above the elbow, but otherwise the signs and symptoms are often vague. Exploration of the median nerve above the elbow may allow release of the ligament. Needle EMG is most useful for localizing this type of compression, although proximal median nerve motor conduction studies may also be of value if conduction block or focal slowing is present.

## Pronator Syndrome

The median nerve can become compressed when it passes between the superficial and deep heads of the pronator teres if the muscle is hypertrophied or if there is a fibrous

**TABLE 19–2. Most Common Causes of Anterior Interosseous Nerve Syndrome**

| REFERENCE NO. | NO. OF CASES | REPORTED CAUSE |
|---|---|---|
| 10 | 10 | Tendinous origin of deep head of the pronator teres |
| | | Strap from shoulder bag |
| | | Trauma (radial fracture) |
| 11 | 13 | Trauma |
| | | Fibrous band |
| | | Arterial thrombosis |
| 12 | 33 | Fibrous bands from pronator teres or flexor digitorum superficialis |
| | | Compression by pronator teres |

band within its substance. The symptoms of this compression are aching pain in the proximal forearm that is exacerbated by repetitive elbow motions. Sensory symptoms may be present, but they are not characteristically worst at night or worsened by wrist movements, as in CTS. The most important sign in pronator syndrome is tenderness over the proximal forearm. Weakness of forearm and hand intrinsic muscles may be present; however, a large series[7] showed no measurable weakness in median-innervated muscles. Based on anatomy, one would expect that sensory abnormalities would include the median palmar cutaneous branch to the thenar eminence, but in practice the sensory examination is not sensitive for this entrapment. The differential diagnosis includes median neuropathy at the wrist, brachial plexopathy, C6 or C7 radiculopathy, and chronic compartmental syndrome.

Electrophysiologic evaluation for pronator syndrome relies on careful needle EMG examination. EMG will show abnormalities in distal and proximal median muscles.[5] It is also important to recognize that the amplitude of the action potential of the median nerve sensory nerve may be affected in compression of the proximal median nerve and that this finding should not be confused with a lesion at the wrist.

## ULNAR NEUROPATHY (Fig. 19–4)

### Ulnar Neuropathy at the Elbow

Ulnar neuropathy at the elbow is the second most common entrapment neuropathy in the upper extremity. In most cases paresthesias and hypesthesias are initial symptoms. These symptoms are especially bothersome with either persistent flexion or repetitive movements of the elbow, as well as leaning on the elbow (e.g., at a desk or on an armchair). The symptoms may be intermittent or, in more severe cases, persistent. Patients may note waking from sleep with elbow pain and paresthesias into the fourth and fifth digits. There may be cramping or aching in the forearm and hand. Motor signs are the most significant and important. Since the majority of intrinsic hand function is ulnar innervated, unrecognized ulnar neuropathy may lead to significant dysfunction of the hand and loss of dexterity.

On physical examination, there may be tenderness at and around the elbow. There may be a thickened nerve in the cubital tunnel, which may be exquisitely tender. Tinel's sign may be present at this site, with paresthesias radiating into the fourth and fifth digits. Motor examination may reveal at-

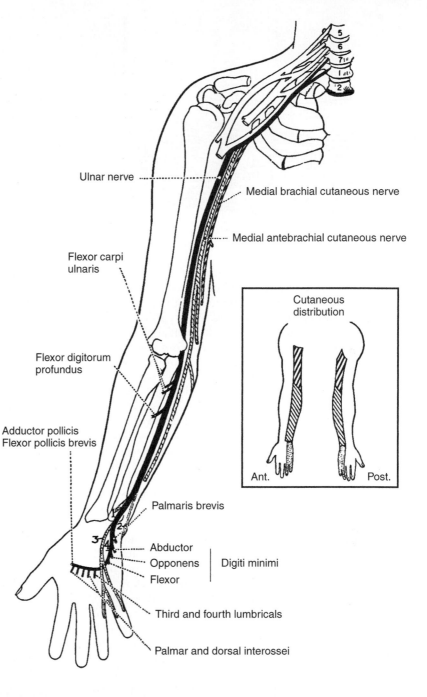

**FIGURE 19–4.** Ulnar nerve anatomy. The ulnar nerve, along with the medial brachial and medial antebrachial cutaneous nerves, is derived from the medial cord of the brachial plexus. *Inset:* Cutaneous distributions of the ulnar, medial brachial cutaneous, and medial antebrachial nerves. (From Haymaker W, Woodhal B. *Peripheral Nerve Injuries.* Philadelphia: WB Saunders; 1953.)

rophy of the interossei, hypothenar, and thenar muscles. The major motor disability results from diminished (1) strength of pinch between the thumb and other digits, (2) coordination between the thumb and digits in precise tasks, (3) synchrony of digital flexion during grasp, and (4) strength of grasp.[4] A positive Froment's sign (attempts to adduct the thumb are accompanied by flexion of the distal interphalangeal joint) indicates weakness of the adductor pollicis, flexor pollicis brevis, and the first dorsal interosseous (FDI) muscle. The flexor carpi ulnaris (FCU) and flexor digitorum profundus to the fourth and fifth digits (FDP4/5) are often relatively spared. Although not clinically weak, these muscles are frequently abnormal on needle EMG.

Sensory examination often reveals loss of sensation in the medial fourth digit and the entire fifth digit. The territory of the dorsal cutaneous branch may also be abnormal,

and this is an important finding in excluding ulnar neuropathy at the wrist. The dorsal cutaneous branch of the ulnar nerve arises 6 to 8 cm above the wrist and supplies the skin on the medial side of the dorsum of the hand and proximal portions of the dorsum of the fifth finger and medial half of the dorsum of the fourth finger.

The differential diagnosis of ulnar neuropathy at the elbow includes lower trunk brachial plexopathy, C8-T1 radiculopathy, and ulnar neuropathy at the wrist. The causes of ulnar neuropathy at the elbow include acute or chronic external pressure, bony or scar-tissue impingement, cubital tunnel syndrome, and chronic subluxation of the nerve. Cubital tunnel syndrome refers specifically to constriction of the ulnar nerve as it passes under the aponeurosis of the FCU (Fig. 19–5).[4] From 30% to 50% of surgical cases reveal no specific etiologic basis.

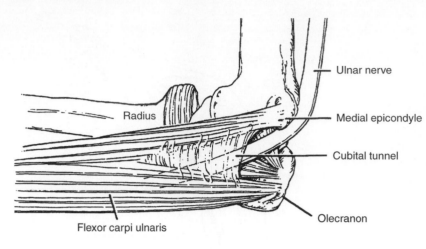

Radius

Ulnar nerve

Medial epicondyle

Cubital tunnel

Olecranon

Flexor carpi ulnaris

**FIGURE 19–5.** Ulnar nerve anatomy at the elbow. Entrapment of the ulnar nerve can occur either at the ulnar groove between the medial epicondyle and the olecranon or distally at the cubital tunnel. (Adapted from Kincaid JC. AAEE Minimonograph #31. The electrodiagnosis of ulnar neuropathy at the elbow. *Muscle Nerve.* 11:1005, © 1988; John Wiley & Sons, Inc.)

The electrodiagnostic evaluation of ulnar neuropathy at the elbow is not as clearly agreed upon as for median neuropathy at the wrist. Nerve conduction studies should include ulnar and median motor and sensory studies (Protocol 19–2). In addition, if lower trunk brachial plexopathy is suspected, the medial antebrachial cutaneous nerve sensory study should be obtained to assess the sensory nerve supplying the medial, ventral forearm. Ulnar nerve motor conduction studies include recording over the abductor digiti quinti or the first dorsal interosseous and stimulating at the wrist and below and above the cubital tunnel. A flexed elbow is the preferred patient position when ulnar motor studies are being performed because the surface-measured nerve length is more accurate than when the study is performed with the straight-elbow position.[12] When this technique is used, a drop in conduction velocity of >11 m/s between the forearm and the across-the-elbow segments indicates focal demyelination. A distance of at least 10 to 12 cm should be used between the below- and above-elbow sites of stimulation.

In addition to slowed conduction velocities across the elbow in ulnar neuropathy, the other reliable electrophysiologic marker of demyelination is conduction block. A >20% reduction in CMAP amplitude between the below- and the above-elbow stimulation sites is generally suggestive of conduction block of ulnar neuropathy across the elbow. To localize the site of demyelination exactly, one can "inch" across the elbow in 1 cm increments, looking for either an abrupt fall in amplitude or an increase in latency (>0.5 ms). This technique can then be useful in planning subsequent surgery. Ulnar neuropathy at the cubital tunnel (typically 1 to 2 cm distal to the medial epicondyle) may be treated by simple decompression, whereas ulnar neuropathy at the retrocondylar groove may require ulnar transposition surgery.

Ulnar sensory nerve conduction studies are helpful in identifying an ulnar neuropathy and differentiating it from a cervical radiculopathy. They can be performed either orthodromically (stimulating digit 5 and recording over the ulnar nerve at the wrist) or antidromically (stimulating the ulnar nerve at the wrist and recording over digit 5). Since orthodromic surface-recorded sensory responses are lower in amplitude, antidromic responses are generally preferred. Sensory studies are more sensitive than motor studies in detecting ulnar neuropathy but cannot localize the lesion to the elbow. In some patients, especially those with early or

---

**PROTOCOL 19–2. Recommended Nerve Conduction Protocol for Ulnar Neuropathy at the Elbow (UNE)**

**Routine Studies**
1. Ulnar motor study recording abductor digiti minimi, stimulating wrist, below-elbow, and above-elbow in the flexed elbow position
2. Median motor study recording abductor pollicis brevis, stimulating wrist and elbow
3. Median and ulnar F responses
4. Ulnar sensory response, recording fifth digit, stimulating wrist
5. Median sensory response, recording second or third digit, stimulating wrist

**Patterns That May Result**
*UNE With Demyelinating and Axonal Features*
- Normal or low-amplitude CMAP with normal or slightly prolonged distal latency
- Unequivocal evidence of demyelination at the groove (conduction block or slowing of >10 to 11 m/s across the groove compared to the forearm segment, in the flexed elbow position)
- Low ulnar SNAP

*UNE With Pure Demyelinating Features*
- Normal distal ulnar CMAP and SNAP amplitudes and latencies
- Unequivocal evidence of demyelination at the groove (conduction block or slowing of >10 to 11 m/s across the groove compared to the forearm segment)

*Nonlocalizable Ulnar Neuropathy (Axonal Features Alone)*
- Normal or low-amplitude CMAP with normal or slightly prolonged distal latency
- Low ulnar SNAP

If the ulnar neuropathy is nonlocalizable, the following should be considered:
- Repeat motor studies recording the first dorsal interosseous, stimulating wrist, below-elbow, and above-elbow in the flexed elbow position
- Motor inching across the elbow
- Sensory or mixed studies across the elbow
- Recording the dorsal ulnar cutaneous SNAP (bilateral studies) (Remember that the dorsal ulnar cutaneous SNAP can be normal in some patients with UNE.)
- Recording the medial antebrachial cutaneous SNAP (bilateral studies) if sensory loss extends above the wrist on clinical exam or if there is a suggestion of lower brachial plexus lesion by history

From Preston DC, Shapiro BE. *Electromyography and Neuromuscular Disorders.* Boston: Butterworth-Heinemann; 1998. Reprinted with permission.

mild ulnar neuropathy at the elbow, a mixed nerve study across the elbow can be performed to compare conduction velocity in the forearm to across the elbow. This study is performed by stimulating the ulnar nerve at the wrist and co-recording with surface electrodes over the ulnar nerve below and above the elbow. Any drop in conduction velocity of 22 m/s in the straight-elbow position is significant and is suggestive of demyelinative slowing across the elbow.[20]

Needle examination is critical in determining the localization of the lesion and the pathophysiologic process (Protocol 19–3). Most studies have documented fibrillations in 47% to 64% of ulnar hand intrinsics.[2,18] Proximal ulnar innervated muscles (i.e., FCU, FDP4/5) may also have active or chronic denervation; however, they may be normal in spite of a lesion at the elbow, especially in early or mild cases. Active denervation was less common in proximal muscles but correlated with more severe lesions. To exclude a lower brachial plexopathy and cervical radiculopathy, it is essential to sample nonulnar C8-T1 innervated muscles (e.g., abductor pollicis brevis, extensor indicis, flexor pollicis longus), which should all be normal in isolated ulnar neuropathy.[11]

### Ulnar Neuropathy at the Wrist (Fig. 19–6)

At the wrist the ulnar nerve enters Guyon's canal and divides into deep and superficial branches. The superficial branch is a sensory, and the deep branch is predominantly motor. The deep branch then divides into a hypothenar branch and a palmar branch to the interossei and lumbricals. The neurologic sign most important to recognize when assessing for ulnar neuropathy at the wrist is sparing of the sensory territory supplied by the dorsal ulnar cutaneous branch. This territory is always normal in ulnar neuropathy at the wrist. There are various lesions that affect either the hypothenar branch, the deep branch distal to the hypothenar branch, the superficial branch alone, or a combination of these. The etiologic complex of ulnar neuropathy at the wrist includes mass lesions (especially ganglion cysts) and repetitive trauma (common in bicyclists, mechanics, etc.).

Imaging studies (i.e., MRI scan) are quite sensitive in identifying a ganglionic cyst or other mass lesion. Otherwise, diagnosis is usually confirmed by electrophysiologic testing. The electrophysiologic findings depend on which branches are affected—sensory branch, hypothenar muscle branches, deep palmar motor branch, or all three. If there is a distal lesion affecting only the deep palmar motor branch, then routine ulnar sensory and motor conductions recording the fifth digit and the abductor digiti minimi (ADM), will be normal. In all cases of suspected ulnar neuropathy at the wrist, however, it is important to perform motor studies recording the FDI. In lesions of the deep palmar motor branch, the latency to the FDI may be prolonged with a decreased CMAP amplitude, whereas the ADM latency and amplitude remain normal. Comparison with the contralateral asymptomatic side is often helpful. If the lesion is more proximal, affecting the hypothenar branches, the distal motor latency to the ADM may also be prolonged. However, even in such proximal lesions, the deep palmar motor branch is often affected out of proportion to the hypothenar branch, and the latency to the FDI will still be relatively longer than to the ADM.

The other potentially helpful nerve conduction study to perform is the lumbrical-interossei distal latency comparison.

---

**PROTOCOL 19–3. Recommended EMG Protocol for Ulnar Neuropathy at the Elbow**

1. Ulnar muscle distal to the wrist (first dorsal interosseous or abductor digiti minimi)
2. Ulnar muscles in the forearm (flexor digitorum profundus–digit 5 and flexor carpi ulnaris)

If any of the ulnar muscles are abnormal, the following additional muscles should be studied:
- At least two nonulnar lower trunk/C8-T1 muscles (e.g., abductor pollicis brevis, flexor pollicis longus, extensor indicis proprius) to exclude a lower brachial plexopathy, polyneuropathy, or C8-T1 radiculopathy
- C8 and T1 paraspinals

**Special Considerations**
- If the ulnar neuropathy is superimposed on another condition (e.g., polyneuropathy, plexopathy, radiculopathy), a more detailed EMG examination will be required.
- The abductor digiti minimi is frequently painful and difficult for some patients to tolerate.
- In ulnar neuropathy at the elbow, the flexor carpi ulnaris may be spared even when the flexor digitorum profundus–digit 5 is abnormal.
- If no evidence of ulnar neuropathy is found on nerve conduction studies, EMG should focus on evaluation for lower brachial plexopathy or C8-T1 radiculopathy if clinically indicated.

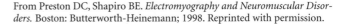

From Preston DC, Shapiro BE. *Electromyography and Neuromuscular Disorders.* Boston: Butterworth-Heinemann; 1998. Reprinted with permission.

---

This test is usually performed in patients with suspected CTS to identify relative slowing of the median nerve across the wrist, but it is equally useful in identifying subtle slowing of the distal ulnar nerve. Since the ulnar interossei are innervated by the deep palmar motor branch, this test can be very useful in identifying differential ulnar slowing at the wrist in lesions that involve the deep palmar motor branch. A distal motor latency difference >0.4 ms comparing the ulnar interossei to the second lumbrical suggests focal slowing across the wrist.

If the lesion involves the distal sensory branch, the routine ulnar SNAP recording over the fifth digit will be abnormal. In contrast, the dorsal ulnar cutaneous SNAP will be normal in all lesions at the wrist. This combination of an abnormal ulnar SNAP and a normal dorsal ulnar cutaneous SNAP is highly suggestive of a lesion at the wrist.

The needle EMG examination of suspected ulnar neuropathy at the wrist is straightforward. The FDI and ADM must be sampled to detect involvement of the deep palmar motor and hypothenar branches, respectively. The FDP (ulnar slip) and FCU must be sampled to exclude an ulnar neuropathy proximal to the wrist. Finally, median and radial C8-T1 muscles (e.g., abductor pollicis brevis, flexor pollicis brevis, extensor indicis) and the lower cervical paraspinal muscles must be sampled to exclude a cervical root or motor neuron lesion.

As is often the case with ulnar neuropathy at the elbow, the lesion in ulnar neuropathy at the wrist may be purely axonal (low CMAP amplitude recording ADM and FDI, with a normal or only mildly prolonged distal latency). This situation makes it difficult to differentiate a pure motor lesion at the wrist from a lesion proximal to the dorsal root ganglion (cervical root or motor neuron). In such cases the clinical presentation and serial follow-up remain important.

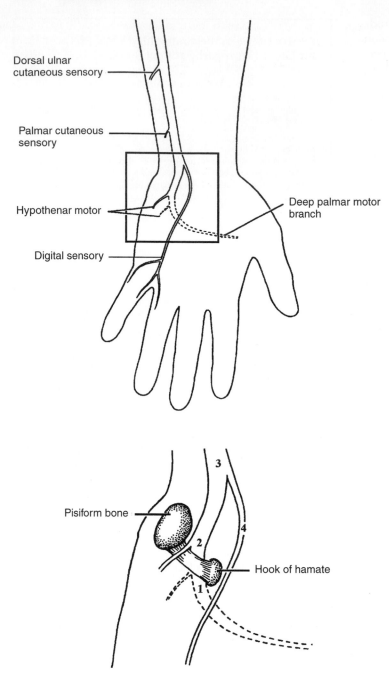

Dorsal ulnar
cutaneous sensory

Palmar cutaneous
sensory

Hypothenar motor

Digital sensory

Deep palmar motor
branch

Pisiform bone

Hook of hamate

**FIGURE 19–6.** Ulnar nerve at the wrist anatomy. Entrapment of the ulnar nerve at the wrist can have several patterns: (1) pure motor lesion affecting only the deep palmar motor branch; (2) pure motor lesion affecting the deep palmar and hypothenar motor branches; (3) motor and sensory lesion (proximal canal lesion) affecting the hypothenar and deep palmar motor and digital sensory branches; and, rarely, (4) pure sensory involving only the digital sensory fibers to the volar fourth and medial fifth fingers. (Adapted from Olney RK, Hanson M. AAEE Case report #15. Ulnar neuropathy at or distal to the wrist. *Muscle Nerve.* © 1988; John Wiley & Sons.)

## RADIAL NEUROPATHY (Fig. 19–7)

The radial nerve is derived from the posterior cord of the brachial plexus and the C5-T1 nerve roots. Just distal to its origin, several sensory branches leave the radial nerve, including the posterior cutaneous nerve of the arm, the lower lateral cutaneous nerve of the arm, and the posterior cutaneous nerve of the forearm. The radial nerve then runs alongside the axillary artery into the upper arm. Between the long and medial heads of the triceps, it winds around the humerus in a spiral. An important point for electromyographers is that the branch to the triceps and anconeus muscles leaves the radial nerve proximal to the spiral groove. Distal to the spiral groove, the radial nerve sends motor branches to the brachioradialis and the extensor carpi radialis longus. Just distal to the elbow, the radial nerve then divides into the superficial and deep branches (Fig. 19–8). The superficial branch supplies cutaneous sensation to the lateral aspect of the dorsum of the hand, the lateral thenar eminence, the proximal portions of the dorsum of the second and third fingers, and the lateral portion of the fourth finger. The deep branch continues as the posterior interosseous nerve. The posterior interosseous nerve innervates the extensor carpi radialis brevis and the supinator. It then enters the arcade of Frohse of the supinator muscle to innervate the extensor digitorum, extensor digiti minimi, extensor carpi ulnaris, abductor pollicis longus, extensor pollicis longus, extensor pollicis brevis, and the extensor indicis proprius muscles.

### Radial Neuropathy Above the Spiral Groove

Radial neuropathy above the spiral groove may occur secondary to trauma or compression by soft tissues or in the axilla by use of a crutch. A nerve lesion at this site will cause weakness of all radial innervated muscles, including the triceps brachii. The triceps reflex will be diminished or absent, and there will be sensory loss in the arm, forearm, and radial-innervated hand. Electromyographically, all radial muscles, including the triceps brachii, will be abnormal. Importantly, the deltoid and the latissimus dorsi, both supplied by nerves derived from the posterior cord, will be normal.

### Radial Neuropathy at the Spiral Groove

This entrapment neuropathy, also known as Saturday night palsy, is the most common type of radial neuropathy, characteristically occurring when a person has fallen asleep with the arm draped over a chair or bench, especially during a deep sleep or following intoxication. The resultant prolonged immobilization leads to compression and demyelination of the radial nerve. Other lesions at this location may occur following fracture of the humerus, infarction from vasculitis or intravenous drug injection, or strenuous muscular effort.[3]

Clinically, patients present with a marked wrist and finger drop, along with mild weakness of supination (due to weakness of the supinator muscle) and elbow flexion (due to weakness of the brachioradialis). Notably, elbow extension (triceps brachii) is spared. The triceps reflex is usually normal, and the brachioradialis reflex is reduced or absent. Sensation is disturbed over the lateral dorsal hand and the dor-

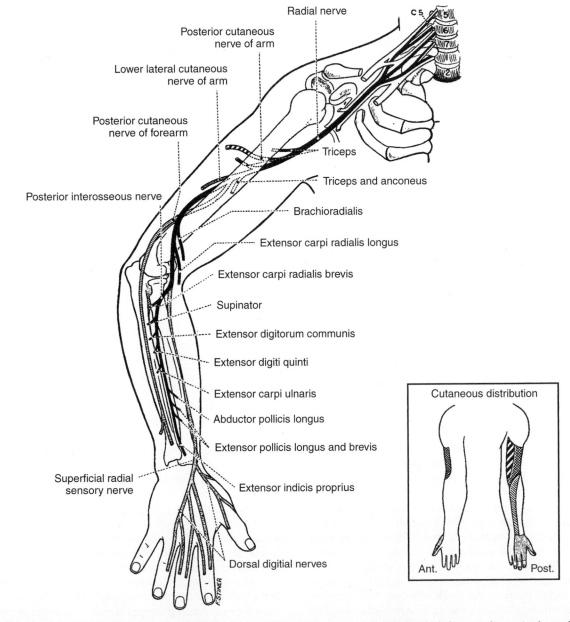

**FIGURE 19–7.** Anatomy of the radial nerve. The radial nerve is derived from the posterior cord of the brachial plexus. In the proximal arm, the radial nerve first gives off the posterior cutaneous nerve of the arm, lower lateral cutaneous nerve of the arm, and the posterior cutaneous nerve of the forearm, followed by muscular branches to the triceps brachii and anconeus. The nerve then wraps around the humerus, descending into the region of the elbow, where muscular branches are given off to the brachioradialis, extensor carpi radialis (long head), and supinator. More distally, the nerve bifurcates into the superficial radial sensory and posterior interosseous nerves. The posterior interosseous nerve supplies the remainder of the wrist and finger extensors and the supinator and abductor pollicis longus. *Inset:* Sensory territories supplied by the radial nerve. (Adapted from Haymaker W, Woodhal B. *Peripheral Nerve Injuries.* Philadelphia: WB Saunders; 1953.)

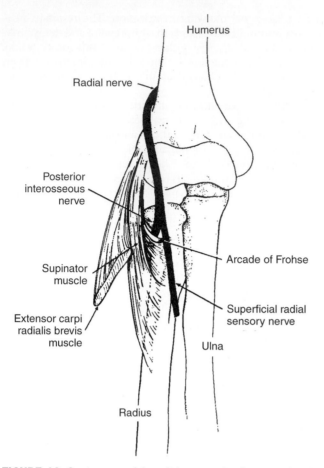

Humerus

Radial nerve

Posterior
interosseous
nerve

Supinator
muscle

Extensor carpi
radialis brevis
muscle

Arcade of Frohse

Superficial radial
sensory nerve

Ulna

Radius

**FIGURE 19–8.** Anatomy of the radial nerve at the elbow. Distal to the elbow, the radial nerve bifurcates into the superficial radial sensory and posterior interosseous nerves. The posterior interosseous nerve enters the supinator muscle under the arcade of Frohse to supply most of the extensors of the wrist and the thumb and finger extensors. (Adapted from Wilbourn AJ. Electrodiagnosis with entrapment neuropathies. In 1992 AAEM Plenary Session I. Entrapment Neuropathies. Rochester, Minn: American Association of Electrodiagnostic Medicine, 1992, p 29. Copyright © 1992 American Association of Electrodiagnostic Medicine. Used by permission.)

sal aspects of digits 1 through 4 in the distribution of the superficial radial sensory nerve.

## Posterior Interosseous Neuropathy

Superficially, PIN may resemble entrapment of the radial nerve at the spiral groove. In both, the patient presents with wrist and finger drop but sparing of elbow extension.[4] However, several important features easily separate the two. In PIN, radial innervated muscles above the takeoff to the posterior interosseous nerve (i.e., brachioradialis, extensor carpi radialis [long head], triceps) are spared. When a patient with PIN attempts to extend the wrist, he or she may do so weakly, with a radial deviation. The wrist deviates radially in extension because of the relative preservation of the extensor carpi radialis, in comparison to the weak extensor carpi ulnaris, which comes off distally to the lesion. The second major difference involves the sensory findings. In PIN there is no cutaneous sensory loss. There may be pain in the forearm from dysfunction of the deep sensory fibers supplying the interosseous membrane and the joint capsules. In contrast, radial neuropathy at the spiral groove results in cutaneous sensory loss in the dorsal hand and digits 1 through 4.

PIN usually results from entrapment of the nerve under the tendinous arcade of Frohse. Rarely, other mass lesions (e.g., ganglionic cysts, tumors) also may result in PIN.

### Superficial Radial Sensory Neuropathy

The superficial radial sensory nerve is derived from the main radial nerve in the region of the elbow. It runs subcutaneously adjacent to the radius in the distal third of the forearm. This superficial location next to bone makes it extremely susceptible to compression. Tight-fitting bands, such as watches or bracelets, may result in compression. Wearing handcuffs, especially when excessively tight, characteristically result in a superficial radial sensory neuropathy. Because the superficial radial sensory nerve is purely sensory, there is no associated weakness. A characteristic patch of altered sensation develops over the lateral dorsum of the hand, part of the dorsal thumb, and the dorsal proximal phalanges of the index, middle, and ring fingers.

### Differential Diagnosis and Diagnostic Evaluation of Radial Neuropathy

The differential diagnosis of a wrist drop—other than a radial neuropathy at the spiral groove, axilla, and PIN—includes typical presentations of C7-C8 radiculopathy, brachial plexus lesions, and central causes. Since most muscles that extend the wrist and fingers are innervated by the C7 nerve root, radiculopathy may rarely present solely with a wrist and finger drop, with relative sparing of nonradial C7 innervated muscles. However, several key features differentiate these conditions clinically. Radial neuropathy at the spiral groove or axilla should result in weakness of the brachioradialis, a C5-C6 muscle, which should not be weak in a lesion of the C7 nerve root. On the other hand, radial neuropathy at the spiral groove should spare the triceps, which would be expected to be weak in a C7 radiculopathy. If a C7 radiculopathy is severe enough to cause muscle weakness, other nonradially innervated C7 muscles should also be weak (e.g., pronator teres, flexor carpi radialis), leading to weakness of arm pronation and wrist flexion. However, in rare situations nonradial C7 muscles may be relatively spared, and the clinical differentiation is quite difficult.

Although lesions of the posterior cord of the brachial plexus result in weakness of radial innervated muscles, the deltoid (axillary nerve) and latissimus dorsi (thoracodorsal nerve) should also be weak. Central lesions may also result in a wrist and finger drop. The typical upper motor neuron posture results in flexion of the wrist and fingers, which in the acute phase, or when the lesion is mild, may superficially resemble a radial neuropathy. Central lesions are identified by increased muscle tone and deep tendon reflexes (unless acute), slowness of movement, associated findings in the lower face and leg, and the absence of altered sensation in the superficial radial distribution.

The most important nerve conduction study to perform is the radial motor test. A radial CMAP can be recorded over the extensor indicis proprius muscle. The radial nerve can be stimulated in the forearm, at the elbow (in the groove between the biceps and brachioradialis muscles), and below and above the spiral groove. It is always important to compare the radial CMAP amplitude with the contralateral asymptomatic side. Any axonal loss will result in a decreased distal CMAP amplitude. In fact, the best way to assess the degree of axonal loss is to compare the CMAP amplitude of the involved side with that of the contralateral side. Notable exceptions include hyperacute lesions (before wallerian degeneration has taken place) and chronic lesions (if complete reinnervation has occurred).

The value of performing radial motor studies usually lies in looking for a focal conduction block between the proximal and distal sites and in determining the relative CMAP amplitude (to assess axonal loss). In radial neuropathy at the spiral groove, CMAPs recorded with stimulation at the forearm, elbow, and below the spiral groove may be completely normal if the lesion is purely demyelinative. However, stimulation proximal to the spiral groove will result in marked temporal dispersion or a decrease in the CMAP amplitude or area (i.e., electrophysiologic evidence of a conduction block). The relative drop in proximal to distal CMAP amplitude will give some indication of the proportion of fibers blocked.

In contrast to radial motor studies, the superficial radial sensory nerve is easy to stimulate and record. If there has been secondary axonal loss, the response will be diminished in amplitude. As with motor studies, it is often useful to compare the response with the contralateral asymptomatic side. If the pathologic condition is one of pure or predominant demyelination, an interesting phenomenon occurs: while the patient reports marked numbness in the distribution of the superficial radial sensory nerve, the SNAP will be normal, even when compared side to side. A normal superficial radial sensory response is also seen in PIN, as expected, because the nerve carries no cutaneous sensory fibers.

The EMG approach in radial neuropathy is directed at differentiating among PIN, radial neuropathy at the spiral groove, radial neuropathy in the axilla, a lesion of the posterior cord of the brachial plexus, a C7 radiculopathy, and a central lesion. In PIN, abnormalities are limited to those muscles innervated by the posterior interosseous nerve. As one moves more proximally to radial neuropathy at the spiral groove, the brachioradialis, the extensor carpi radialis (long head), and the supinator will also be affected. If the lesion is even more proximal at the axilla, the triceps and the anconeus will be involved. As one moves more proximally to a lesion of the posterior cord of the plexus, additional abnormalities are seen in the deltoid (axillary nerve) and latissimus dorsi (thoracodorsal nerve). A C7 radiculopathy includes abnormalities in the cervical paraspinal muscles and nonradial-innervated C7 muscles (e.g., pronator teres, flexor carpi radialis). Finally, in central lesions, motor unit action potentials (MUAPs) and the recruitment pattern are normal in weak muscles, although there may be decreased activation of normal MUAPs.

## SUPRASCAPULAR NEUROPATHY (Fig. 19–9)

The suprascapular nerve arises from the upper trunk of the brachial plexus (C5-6). It then travels under the upper

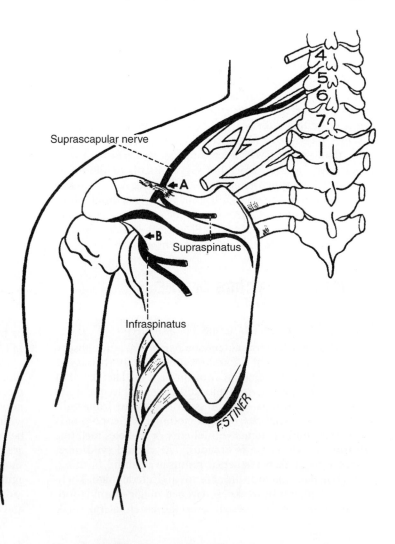

**FIGURE 19–9.** Anatomy of the suprascapular nerve. The suprascapular nerve originates from the upper trunk of the brachial plexus. The nerve first runs under the suprascapular notch (*A*) to innervate the supraspinatus muscle. Sensory fibers are then given to the shoulder joint before the nerve wraps around the spinoglenoid notch (*B*) to supply the infraspinatus muscle. (Adapted from Haymaker W, Woodhal B. *Peripheral Nerve Injuries.* Philadelphia: WB Saunders; 1953.)

trapezius and crosses the scapula via the scapular notch. The suprascapular notch is U-shaped, located along the superior border of the scapula, and covered by the transverse scapular ligament. The suprascapular nerve first supplies motor fibers to the supraspinatus muscle before proceeding laterally to supply deep sensory fibers to the glenoacromial and acromioclavicular joints. It then wraps around the spinoglenoid notch of the scapular spine to enter the infraspinous fossa, where it supplies motor fibers to the infraspinatus muscle. The most common site of entrapment is the suprascapular notch under the transverse scapular ligament. In that location, suprascapular neuropathy usually results in shoulder pain and weakness of the supraspinatus and infraspinatus muscles (abduction and external rotation of the arm). There is no associated cutaneous sensory loss. Less frequently, the nerve can also be entrapped distally at the spinoglenoid notch. In such a case there is no pain, only atrophy and weakness of the infraspinatus muscle. Less common causes of suprascapular neuropathy include forcible depression of the shoulder, such as in football injuries, and ganglionic cysts arising from the glenohumeral joint. The differential diagnosis includes C5-6 radiculopathy, upper trunk brachial plexopathy, brachial neuritis, bursitis, and tendinitis.

Diagnostic testing of suprascapular neuropathy involves imaging and electrophysiologic studies. MRI is useful in identifying structural mass lesions, especially ganglionic cysts and tumors. Otherwise, the diagnosis of suprascapular neuropathy is usually confirmed with electrophysiologic studies. In suprascapular neuropathy at the suprascapular notch, abnormalities detected on needle EMG are limited to the infraspinatus and supraspinatus muscles. In suprascapular neuropathy at the spinoglenoid notch, only the infraspinatus muscle is abnormal. In all cases of suspected suprascapular neuropathy, it is essential to check other C5-6 innervated muscles as well as the cervical paraspinal muscles to exclude either a cervical radiculopathy or an upper trunk brachial plexopathy. Nerve conduction studies are of less value than needle EMG. Recording can be performed with needle electrodes in either the supraspinatus or the infraspinatus stimulating the nerve at Erb's point. A side-to-side comparison may show a significantly prolonged distal motor latency and reduced CMAP amplitude on the affected side. This technique, in concert with EMG, may indicate the primary pathologic site (i.e., axonal or demyelinative).

## MONONEUROPATHIES OF THE LOWER EXTREMITY

### LATERAL FEMORAL CUTANEOUS NEUROPATHY

The lateral femoral cutaneous nerve is a pure sensory nerve derived from the L2 and L3 roots (Fig. 19–10). It enters the thigh by passing under or through the lateral end of the inguinal ligament. At that location the most frequent site of entrapment occurs. Compression may occur from tight girdles, belts or seatbelts, or tight clothing. The condition is most common in patients with obesity or diabetes mellitus. Occasionally, no cause is obvious. The clinical syndrome, known as meralgia paresthetica, results in a painful, burning, numb patch of skin over the anterior and lateral thigh. There are no complaints of weakness. On neurologic examination, sensory loss may be present over the anterolateral thigh

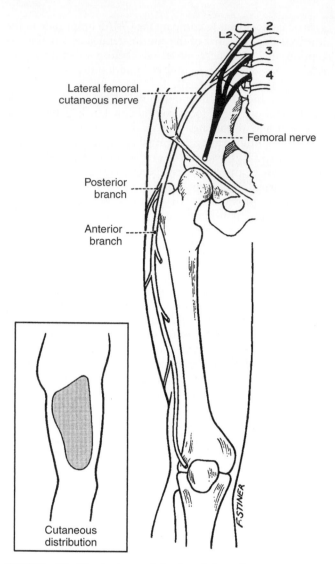

**FIGURE 19–10.** Anatomy of the lateral femoral cutaneous nerve. (Adapted from Haymaker W, Woodhal, B. *Peripheral Nerve Injuries.* Philadelphia: WB Saunders; 1953.)

without any weakness and reflex change. Tinel's sign may be elicited over the proximal portion of the nerve.

The differential diagnosis of lateral femoral cutaneous neuropathy (LFCN) includes femoral neuropathy, upper lumbar plexopathy, and L2-4 radiculopathy. Atrophy or weakness of proximal lower extremity muscles or a diminished patellar reflex distinguishes femoral neuropathy, plexopathy, and radiculopathy from LFCN. Significant low-back or buttock discomfort with radicular pain do not occur in LFCN.

Diagnosis is essentially clinical. Sensory nerve conduction studies of the lateral femoral cutaneous nerve are technically difficult but can be performed by recording a sensory nerve action potential (SNAP) and comparing the response with that of the contralateral side. Since these responses may be small or difficult to record in obese individuals, SNAPs are not a reliable tool for localizing the lesion. Needle EMG should be performed in any patient in whom the clinical diagnosis is not straightforward to exclude plexopathy or radiculopathy. The thigh adductors, quadriceps, iliopsoas, and lumbar paraspinals should be examined in such cases. In isolated LFCN the needle EMG examination is completely normal. Occasionally, pelvic imaging is indicated in patients with LFCN. Rare cases of LFCN have been described that are caused by intrapelvic mass lesions (e.g., tumors, abscess). Accordingly, in any patient with an atypical or progressive course, pelvic imaging (computed tomography [CT]/magnetic resonance imaging [MRI]) should be considered.

## FEMORAL NEUROPATHY (Fig. 19–11)

The femoral nerve is derived from the L2-L4 nerve roots and provides motor innervation to the hip flexors and knee extensors and sensory innervation to the anterior thigh and medial aspect of the lower leg and ankle. The saphenous nerve is the terminal sensory branch of the femoral nerve, accompanying the parent nerve between the vastus and adductor group before running along with the saphenous vein distal to the knee.

Lesions of the femoral nerve may occur in its proximal portion, causing partial paralysis of the iliopsoas. The paralysis is not complete since the muscle derives part of its innervation directly from the L2-3 portions of the plexus. After the takeoff of branches to the iliopsoas, femoral nerve lesions affect the quadriceps group. Knee extension will be weak and the patellar reflex may be absent or depressed. Common

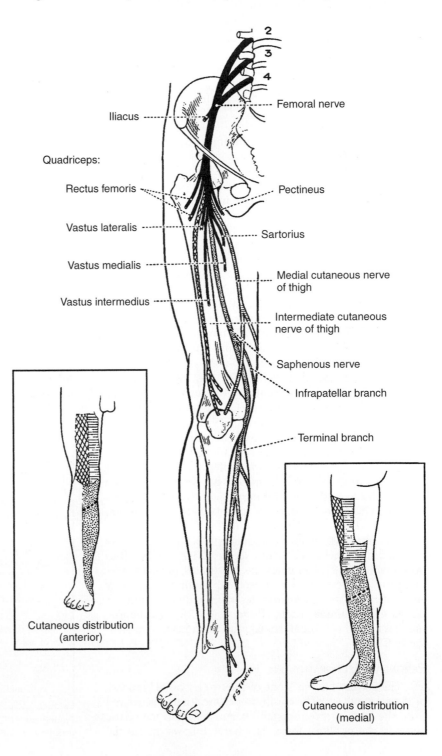

**FIGURE 19–11.** Anatomy of the femoral nerve. (From Haymaker W, Woodhal B. *Peripheral Nerve Injuries.* Philadelphia: WB Saunders; 1953.)

---

**PROTOCOL 19–4. Recommended Nerve Conduction Protocol for Femoral Neuropathy**

**Routine Studies**
1. Femoral motor study recording rectus femoris, stimulating femoral nerve below the inguinal ligament, bilateral studies
2. Saphenous sensory studies, recording medial ankle, stimulating medial calf, bilateral studies

To exclude a more generalized plexopathy or polyneuropathy:
3. Ipsilateral tibial motor study, recording abductor hallucis brevis, stimulating medial ankle and popliteal fossa
4. Ipsilateral peroneal motor study, recording extensor digitorum brevis, stimulating ankle, below fibular neck, and lateral popliteal fossa
5. Ipsilateral tibial and peroneal F responses
6. Ipsilateral sural sensory response, recording lateral ankle, stimulating lateral calf

---

From Preston DC, Shapiro BE. *Electromyography and Neuromuscular Disorders.* Boston: Butterworth-Heinemann; 1998. Reprinted with permission.

causes of femoral neuropathy include injury during lower abdominal surgery (either by compression and stretch from retractors or from compression from the lithotomy position), arteriography, aortofemoral bypass surgery, and, rarely, knee replacement.[1,4] The nerve may be injured directly or via stretching. Retroperitoneal hematomas, often secondary to anticoagulants, can preferentially affect femoral nerve fibers within the lumbosacral plexus. Femoral neuropathies also occur in diabetes mellitus, especially as part of a larger diabetic lumbar plexopathy (e.g., diabetic amyotrophy). The differential diagnosis includes lumbar radiculopathy, lumbar plexopathy, and diabetic amyotrophy.

The electrodiagnostic approach to femoral neuropathy focuses on differentiation from radiculopathy and plexopathy. The two key tests are the saphenous sensory conduction studies and needle EMG of nonfemoral L2-L4 muscles and the lumbar paraspinal muscles. One can perform motor nerve conduction studies recording one of the quadriceps muscles and compare the femoral CMAP amplitude to that of the asymptomatic side (Protocol 19–4). However, a reduced CMAP amplitude can be seen in femoral neuropathy, lumbar plexopathy, and lumbar radiculopathy. The presence of an abnormal saphenous sensory potential can localize the lesion as being distal to the dorsal root ganglion, either in the lumbar plexus or the femoral nerve. Unfortunately, saphenous SNAPs are often difficult to obtain, even in normal controls, and are considered most useful if they are normal or asymmetric. Many normal individuals older than 40 may have absent saphenous SNAPs. Needle EMG abnormalities in nonfemoral L2-L4 muscles (i.e., obturator, gluteal innervated muscles) can exclude an isolated femoral neuropathy and indicate a more proximal lesion in either the lumbar plexus or the lumbar roots (Protocol 19–5). EMG abnormalities in the lumbar paraspinal muscles indicate a lesion at the root level.

## PERONEAL NEUROPATHY (Fig. 19–12)

The peroneal nerve is one of the two terminal branches of the sciatic nerve. The common peroneal nerve is derived from the L4-S2 nerve roots and originates from the sciatic nerve in the popliteal fossa. The nerve follows the medial edge of the biceps femoris muscle to the fibular head and enters the peroneal compartment. At the fibular head the nerve is juxtaposed to the periosteum. It runs through a canal formed by the fibula and the peroneus longus muscle, whose origin is dually attached to the fibular head and the shaft of the fibula. The area between these two sites of origin forms a space where the nerve runs and divides into the deep and superficial branches. The superficial peroneal nerve gives off muscular branches to the peroneus longus and brevis muscles and supplies sensation to the lateral lower leg and the dorsum of the foot and toes. In about 25% of the population an accessory deep peroneal nerve, a branch of the superficial peroneal nerve, supplies one or both extensor digitorum muscles of the foot. The deep peroneal nerve supplies the extensor muscles of the ankle and toes. Its terminal branches supply sensation only to the skin between the dorsum of the first and second toes.

The most common symptoms of peroneal neuropathy are weakness of ankle dorsiflexion and numbness over the lateral calf and dorsum of the foot. Acute compressive lesions usually cause painless loss of motor function. The signs and symptoms depend on the location of the nerve lesion. If the lesion involves the deep and superficial branches, foot eversion and sensation over the dorsum of the foot will be involved in addition to ankle and toe dorsiflexion weakness. If only the deep branch is affected, altered sensation will be limited to the web space between the first and second toes and the strength of foot eversion will be normal.

The differential diagnosis of peroneal neuropathy includes sciatic neuropathy, lower lumbosacral plexopathy, and L5 radiculopathy. Lesions of the sciatic nerve, lumbosacral plexus, and L5 nerve root can often preferentially affect peroneal fibers more than tibial fibers.[25] Any weakness of tibial innervated muscles, especially the tibialis posterior and flexor digitorum longus, and sciatic innervated muscles in the thigh (e.g., biceps femoris) exclude an isolated peroneal neuropathy. In addition, assessment of the gluteal muscles (hip extension, abduction, and internal rotation) is key to helping exclude either a lower lumbosacral plexopathy or L5 radiculopathy.

---

**PROTOCOL 19–5. Recommended EMG Protocol for Femoral Neuropathy**

1. At least two heads of the quadriceps (e.g., vastus lateralis, vastus medialis, or rectus femoris)
2. Iliopsoas
3. At least one obturator innervated adductor muscle (e.g., adductor brevis, longus, or magnus)
4. Tibialis anterior
5. L2, L3, and L4 paraspinal muscles
6. At least two nonfemoral, non-L2-4 muscles to exclude a more generalized process (e.g., medial gastrocnemius, tibialis posterior, biceps femoris, gluteus maximus)

**Special Considerations**
- If any of the above muscles are equivocal, comparison to the contralateral side is useful.
- If the lesion is pure demyelination, the only abnormality on needle EMG will be decreased recruitment of normal configuration MUAPs in weak muscles.

---

From Preston DC, Shapiro BE. *Electromyography and Neuromuscular Disorders.* Boston: Butterworth-Heinemann; 1998. Reprinted with permission.

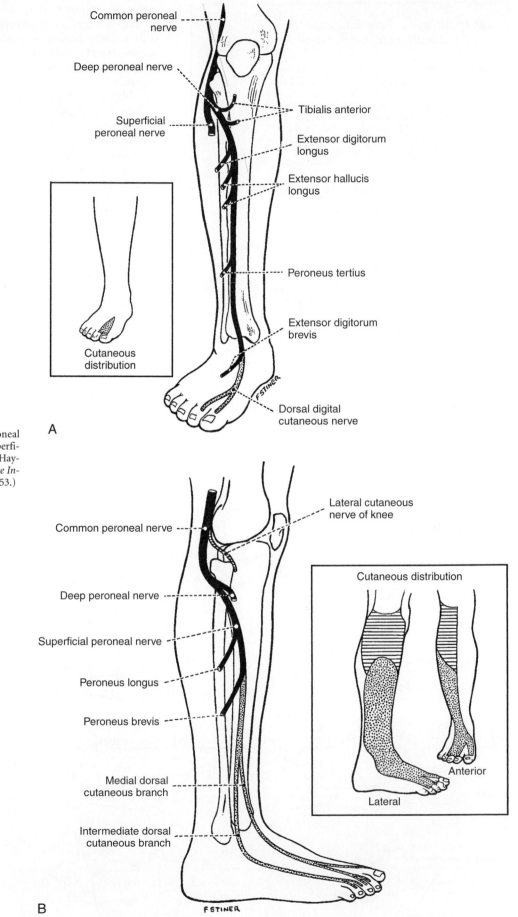

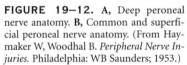

**FIGURE 19—12. A,** Deep peroneal nerve anatomy. **B,** Common and superficial peroneal nerve anatomy. (From Haymaker W, Woodhal B. *Peripheral Nerve Injuries.* Philadelphia: WB Saunders; 1953.)

From Preston DC, Shapiro BE. *Electromyography and Neuromuscular Disorders.* Boston: Butterworth-Heinemann; 1998. Reprinted with permission.

The most common compression site of the common peroneal nerve is at or near the fibular head, usually causing a neurapraxic lesion.[4] Compression may be secondary to tight plaster casts or bandages, but it is also common in cachectic or bed-bound patients. Less commonly, individuals who cross their legs on a long trip may compress the nerve at the fibular head. Peroneal neuropathy may also rarely develop from mass lesions (e.g., ganglia or tumors) or may be selectively involved in hereditary neuropathy with liability to pressure palsies (HNPP). The common peroneal nerve is also the most commonly affected nerve in multiple mononeuropathies secondary to vasculitic neuropathy.[22]

Diagnosis of peroneal neuropathy is made on clinical and electrophysiologic grounds (Protocol 19–6). Nerve conductions of the peroneal nerve typically use the extensor digitorum brevis (EDB) as the recording muscle. For recording done over the EDB, the peroneal nerve can be stimulated over the dorsum of the ankle, below the fibular head and in the lateral popliteal fossa to calculate conduction velocities in the leg and the across-fibular-head nerve segment. Key elements in this study include comparison of CMAP amplitude with stimulation below and above the fibular head, in a search for evidence of focal slowing or conduction block. In some patients, localization of peroneal neuropathy at the fibular neck cannot be made by recording the EDB, either because the fascicle to the EDB is relatively spared or because the response is very low or absent.[8,21] In cases where peroneal neuropathy cannot be localized by recording the EDB, it is essential to record the tibialis anterior, stimulating the peroneal nerve below the fibular neck and in the lateral popliteal fossa.[28] CMAP amplitude of the tibialis anterior can also be compared with the contralateral asymptomatic side to assess the amount of axonal loss. Recording the tibialis anterior has the main advantage of recording the muscle that is most significant clinically (most disability in peroneal neuropathy is secondary to foot drop).

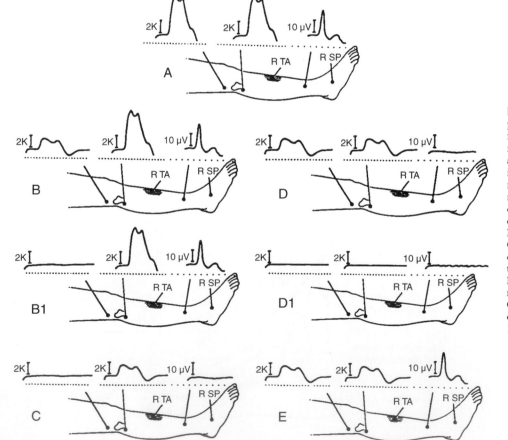

**FIGURE 19–13.** Nerve conduction patterns in peroneal neuropathy. Waveforms above each figure: *left:* peroneal motor, stimulating lateral popliteal fossa above fibular neck, recording (*R*) the tibialis anterior (*TA*); *middle:* peroneal motor, stimulating below fibular neck, recording tibialis anterior; *right:* superficial peroneal (*SP*) sensory, stimulating lateral calf, recording dorsum of the foot. **A,** Normal. **B,** Partial conduction block. **B1,** Complete conduction block. **C,** Complete conduction block with axonal loss. **D,** Partial axonal loss. **D1,** Complete axonal loss. **E,** Partial axonal lesion—deep peroneal nerve. (From Katirji MB, Wilbourn AJ. Common peroneal mononeuropathy: a clinical and electrophysiologic study of 116 lesions. *Neurology.* 1988;38:1723.)

Peroneal neuropathies at the fibular neck may be demyelinating, axonal, or a combination of the two. In 116 cases studied by Katirji and Wilbourn,[8] 64 were solely axonal, 52 had demyelinative and axonal features, and only 23 were purely demyelinative. In pure axonal lesions, all CMAP amplitudes are low, whereas in demyelinative lesions, CMAPs are normal below the lesion but fall on proximal stimulation (Fig. 19–13).

In addition to motor studies, superficial peroneal sensory nerve studies are important in assessing the peroneal nerve. This potential is commonly small, and a study of the contralateral leg is often necessary to compare SNAP amplitude. Abnormalities of the superficial peroneal nerve that are not caused by a coexistent polyneuropathy imply a lesion distal to the dorsal root ganglion, located in the peroneal nerve, sciatic nerve, or lower lumbosacral plexus, and argue strongly against L5 radiculopathy (although rare cases of very lateral disk herniations may diminish superficial peroneal sensory amplitudes).

Needle EMG is the key diagnostic test in differentiating peroneal neuropathy from other proximal lesions (Protocol 19–7). In all 116 of Katirji and Wilbourn's patients, abnormalities were present on needle EMG.[8] One should study (1) two muscles innervated by the deep peroneal nerve, with one always being the tibialis anterior; (2) one muscle innervated by the superficial peroneal nerve; (3) one tibial innervated L5 muscle, preferentially the tibialis posterior; (4) the short head of the biceps femoris; and (5) at least one proximal L5 nonsciatic muscle (e.g., gluteus medius or tensor fascia lata). If either of the last two muscles is abnormal, one should also examine the L5 paraspinal muscles.[28] The short head of the biceps femoris is a key muscle to study on needle EMG in suspected peroneal neuropathy. Although derived from the sciatic nerve, the short head of the biceps femoris is the only sciatic muscle derived from the peroneal division of the sciatic nerve. Some cases of sciatic neuropathy may mimic per-

oneal neuropathy at the fibular neck almost exactly, other than the presence of needle EMG abnormalities in the short head of the biceps femoris.

## TIBIAL NEUROPATHY

The tibial nerve is derived from the L4-S3 roots and runs essentially as a separate nerve trunk within the sciatic nerve high in the pelvis before separating in the popliteal fossa. The medial cutaneous sural nerve is given off in the proximal popliteal fossa and joins the lateral cutaneous sural nerve (branch of the peroneal) at the level of the Achilles tendon. The motor branches to the medial and lateral gastrocnemius and soleus depart in the distal popliteal fossa. Further distally, the nerve sends branches to the deep flexors and the invertor of the ankle and toes and then enters the

---

**PROTOCOL 19–7. Recommended EMG Protocol for Peroneal Neuropathy**

1. At least two muscles innervated by the deep peroneal nerve (e.g., tibialis anterior, extensor hallucis longus)
2. At least one muscle innervated by the superficial peroneal nerve (e.g., peroneus longus, peroneus brevis)
3. Tibialis posterior and at least one other tibial muscle (e.g., medial gastrocnemius, soleus, flexor digitorum longus)
4. Short head of the biceps femoris

**Special Considerations**
- If any muscle is borderline, compare to the contralateral side.
- If the short head of the biceps femoris or any tibial innervated muscle is abnormal, or if nerve conduction studies demonstrate a nonlocalizing peroneal neuropathy, then a more extensive needle exam of other sciatic, gluteal, and paraspinal muscles needs to be performed to identify the level of the lesion.

From Preston DC, Shapiro BE. *Electromyography and Neuromuscular Disorders.* Boston: Butterworth-Heinemann; 1998. Reprinted with permission.

---

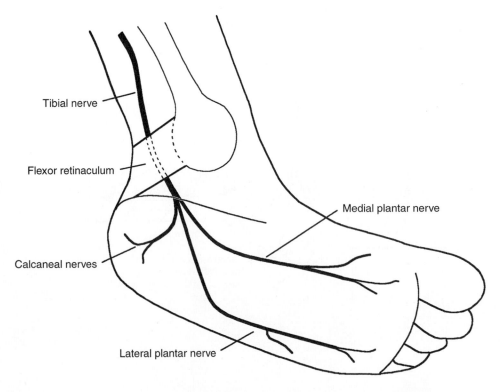

**FIGURE 19–14.** Anatomy of the distal tibial nerve at the ankle and sole of the foot. The distal tibial nerve runs posterior to the medial malleolus under the flexor retinaculum on the medial side of the ankle (the tarsal tunnel), before dividing into the medial plantar, lateral plantar, and calcaneal nerves. The calcaneal nerves are purely sensory and provide sensation to heel of the sole. The medial and lateral plantar branches both contain motor fibers to supply the foot intrinsics and sensory fibers to supply the medial and lateral sole, respectively. (From Preston DC, Shapiro BE. *Electromyography and Neuromuscular Disorders.* Boston: Butterworth-Heinemann; 1997.)

Tibial nerve

Flexor retinaculum

Medial plantar nerve

Calcaneal nerves

Lateral plantar nerve

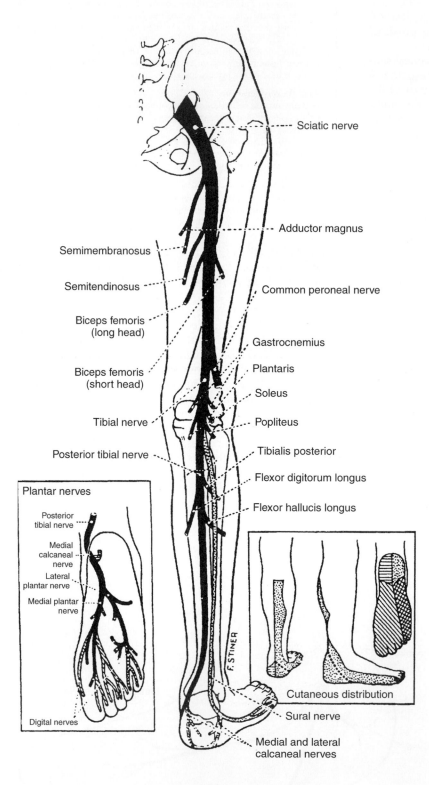

Sciatic nerve

Adductor magnus

Semimembranosus

Semitendinosus

Common peroneal nerve

Biceps femoris
(long head)

Gastrocnemius

Plantaris

Biceps femoris
(short head)

Soleus

Tibial nerve

Popliteus

Posterior tibial nerve

Tibialis posterior

Flexor digitorum longus

Flexor hallucis longus

Plantar nerves

Posterior
tibial nerve

Medial
calcaneal
nerve

Lateral
plantar nerve

Medial plantar
nerve

Digital nerves

Cutaneous distribution

Sural nerve

Medial and lateral
calcaneal nerves

F. STINER

**FIGURE 19–15.** Sciatic nerve anatomy. From Haymaker W, Woodhal B. *Peripheral Nerve Injuries.* Philadelphia: WB Saunders; 1953.)

malleolar canal (tarsal tunnel) (Fig. 19–14). The three terminal branches are the medial and lateral plantar nerves and the calcaneal nerve.

The tibial nerve may be injured in the popliteal fossa by trauma (e.g., gunshot wound, femur fracture). Dislocations of the knee, however, are much more likely to result in peroneal neuropathy. The tarsal tunnel syndrome usually follows trauma in the malleolar region, tenosynovitis, rheumatoid arthritis, or an ankle sprain. In this syndrome, pain and dysesthesias are prominent and may be present during walking or at rest. There is often objective sensory loss and weakness of intrinsic foot muscles. There may be a Tinel's sign over the tibial nerve in the region of the medial malleolus. In many of these cases, symptoms are present without neurologic signs.

Electrodiagnostic testing in proximal tibial neuropathies may show reduced distal tibial CMAP amplitudes. Careful attention must be taken to not overcall conduction block with stimulation of the tibial nerve in the popliteal fossa, where a 40% reduction in CMAP amplitude, compared with stimulation at the ankle, is not uncommon in normals. The sural sensory response may show a reduction in amplitude as well in tibial neuropathies proximal to the ankle. Needle EMG can be used to distinguish tibial neuropathy from more proximal lesions of the sciatic neuropathy, lumbosacral plexopathy, and S1-S2 roots. In cases of suspected tarsal tunnel syndrome, one can record CMAPs from the abductor hallucis muscle and the abductor digiti quinti and stimulate the tibial nerve at the ankle (posterior to the medial malleolus). Mixed nerve potentials can also be obtained by stimulating the medial and lateral plantar nerves in the sole with recording over the tibial nerve at the ankle, in a search for slowing of conduction velocity across the ankle.[17] Near-nerve recording electrodes may increase the sensitivity of detecting focal slowing across the tarsal tunnel. Needle EMG of distal foot muscles is often employed but is of questionable value. Intrinsic foot muscles are prone to trauma. EMG abnormalities are often present in normal controls without any symptoms.

## SCIATIC NEUROPATHY (Fig. 19–15)

The sciatic nerve is composed of fibers from the L4-S3 nerve roots. The nerve leaves the pelvis through the sciatic notch (greater sciatic foramen) under the piriformis muscle. It then takes a lateral course, running beneath the gluteus maximus muscle before descending into the thigh to supply motor innervation to the hamstrings. In the popliteal fossa the sciatic nerve bifurcates into the common peroneal and posterior tibial nerves. These nerves, as mentioned previously, run as separate bundles within the sciatic nerve course proximal to the bifurcation in the popliteal fossa. The sciatic nerve proper innervates the hamstrings and, via its terminal branches, all the muscles of the lower leg and foot. The sensory distribution includes the lateral leg and the entire foot, except for the area supplied on the medial ankle by the saphenous nerve.

Common causes of sciatic neuropathy include tumors (e.g., neurofibroma, lymphoma, sarcoma), penetrating injuries (e.g., gunshot and knife wounds, misplaced intramuscular injections), fractures of the pelvis and femur, posterior dislocation of the hip, and perioperative retraction injuries (i.e., total hip replacement, surgical repair of femoral neck

fractures). Hematomas in anticoagulated patients and, rarely, those caused by trauma may result in sciatic neuropathy. The sciatic nerve is also subject to compression in the gluteal region in cachectic individuals or chronically hospitalized patients.[4] Last is the issue of the controversial piriformis syndrome. Theoretically, a hypertrophied piriformis muscle can entrap the sciatic nerve. However, the existence of a true piriformis syndrome is widely debated. Few cases have been reported that meet the following criteria for definite piriformis syndrome: sciatic neuropathy clinically, electrophysiologic evidence of sciatic neuropathy, surgical exploration showing entrapment of the sciatic nerve within a hypertrophied piriformis muscle, and subsequent improvement following surgical decompression.

The differential diagnosis of sciatic neuropathy includes peroneal neuropathy, lumbosacral plexopathy, and lumbosacral radiculopathy. Diagnostic testing relies on nerve conduction and EMG studies; in many cases, imaging of the sciatic nerve is also necessary. In suspected sciatic neuropathy, nerve conduction testing should include peroneal and tibial motor nerve conduction studies, superficial peroneal and sural sensory nerve conduction studies, and careful attention to F- and H-wave latencies (Protocol 19–8). The classic electrophysiologic picture of sciatic neuropathy is one of reduced tibial and peroneal motor amplitudes compared with those of the contralateral side, with normal or slightly prolonged distal motor latencies and normal or slightly slowed conduction velocities. The tibial and peroneal F responses are prolonged or absent on the symptomatic side, with similar findings for the H reflexes. Both the sural and superficial peroneal sensory nerves are reduced in amplitude or absent, with normal potentials on the contralateral asymptomatic side.

It is well appreciated that sciatic neuropathy may preferentially affect peroneal nerve fibers. Thus, to differentiate sciatic neuropathy from peroneal neuropathy, the key muscles to examine on needle EMG are the tibial innervated muscles in the lower leg and sciatic innervated muscles in the thigh (Protocol 19–9). If the peroneal muscles are ab-

---

### PROTOCOL 19–8. Recommended Nerve Conduction Protocol for Sciatic Neuropathy

**Routine Studies**
1. Tibial motor study, recording abductor hallucis brevis, stimulating medial ankle and popliteal fossa, bilateral studies
2. Peroneal motor study, recording extensor digitorum brevis, stimulating ankle, below fibular neck and lateral popliteal fossa, bilateral studies. In patients with an isolated foot drop and clinical findings limited to the distribution of the peroneal nerve, recording the tibialis anterior, stimulating below fibular neck and lateral popliteal fossa, should be performed to increase the yield of demonstrating conduction block or focal slowing across the fibular neck
3. Sural sensory study, stimulating posterior calf, recording lateral ankle, bilateral studies
4. Superficial peroneal sensory study, stimulating lateral calf, recording ankle, bilateral studies
5. Tibial and peroneal F responses, bilateral studies
6. H reflex, bilateral studies

From Preston DC, Shapiro BE. *Electromyography and Neuromuscular Disorders.* Boston: Butterworth-Heinemann; 1998. Reprinted with permission.

**PROTOCOL 19–9. Recommended EMG Protocol for Sciatic Neuropathy**

1. At least two peroneal muscles (e.g., tibialis anterior, extensor hallucis longus, peroneus longus)
2. At least two tibial muscles (e.g., medial gastrocnemius, tibialis posterior, flexor digitorum longus)
3. Short and long heads of the biceps femoris
4. At least one superior gluteal muscle (e.g., gluteus medius, tensor fascia latae)
5. At least one inferior gluteal muscle (e.g., gluteus maximus)
6. L5 and S1 paraspinal muscles
7. At least two nonsciatic, non-L5/S1 innervated muscles (e.g., vastus lateralis, iliopsoas, adductor longus) to exclude a more widespread lesion

**Special Considerations**
If MUAP abnormalities are borderline or equivocal, comparison should be made to the contralateral side.

From Preston DC, Shapiro BE. *Electromyography and Neuromuscular Disorders.* Boston: Butterworth-Heinemann; 1998. Reprinted with permission.

normal and the tibial muscles are normal, one should sample the short and long heads of the biceps femoris to rule out peroneal neuropathy at the fibular head. If abnormalities are found in sciatic innervated muscles, the muscles supplied by the inferior and superior gluteal muscles should also be examined along with the L5 and S1 paraspinals in order to exclude a lower lumbosacral plexopathy or radiculopathy.

Sciatic neuropathies from trauma, surgery, or prolonged immobility present acutely and can usually be recognized in a straightforward manner. However, sciatic neuropathies that present in a slow and progressive manner may indicate a mass lesion. In those cases, imaging studies of the lower pelvis and thigh (MRI or CT) are indicated.

## REFERENCES

1. Al Hakim M, Katirji MB. Femoral mononeuropathy induced by the lithotomy position: a report of 5 cases and a review of the literature. *Muscle Nerve.* 1993;16:891.
2. Benecke R, Conrad B. The value of electrophysiological examination of the flexor carpi ulnaris muscle in the diagnosis of ulnar nerve lesions at the elbow. *J Neurol.* 1980;223:207-217.
3. Brown WF, Watson BV. *AAEM Case Report #27. Acute Retrohumeral Radial Neuropathies.* Rochester, Minn: American Association of Electrodiagnostic Medicine; 1993.
4. Dawson DM, Hallett M, Millender LH. *Entrapment Neuropathies.* 2nd ed. Boston: Little, Brown; 1990.
5. Hartz CR, Linscheid RL, Gramse RR, Daube JR. The pronator teres syndrome: compressive neuropathy of the median nerve. *J Bone Joint Surg.* 1981;63A:885.
6. Hill NA, Howard FM, Huffer BR. The incomplete anterior interosseous nerve syndrome. *J Hand Surg.* 1985;10A:4-16.
7. Johnson RK, Spinner M, Shrewsbury MM. Median nerve entrapment syndrome in the proximal forearm. *J Hand Surg.* 1979;4:48.
8. Katirji MB, Wilbourn AJ. Common peroneal mononeuropathy: a clinical and electrophysiologic study of 116 lesions. *Neurology.* 1988;38:1723.
9. Kiloh LG, Nevin S. Isolated neuritis of the anterior interosseous nerve. *BMJ.* 1952;1:850-851.
10. Kimura J. The carpal tunnel syndrome: localization of conduction abnormalities within the distal segment of the median nerve. *Brain.* 1979;102:619-635.
11. Kincaid JC. AAEE Minimonograph #31. The electrodiagnosis of ulnar neuropathy at the elbow. *Muscle Nerve.* 1988;11:1005-1015.
12. Kothari MJ, Preston DC. Comparison of the flexed and extended elbow positions in localizing ulnar neuropathy at the elbow. *Muscle Nerve.* 1995;18:336-340.
13. Lesser EA, Venkatesh S, Preston DC, Logigian EL. Stimulation distal to the lesion in patients with carpal tunnel syndrome. *Muscle Nerve.* 1995;18:503.
14. Maeda K, Miura T, Komada T, Chiba A. Anterior interosseous nerve paralysis. *Hand.* 1977;9:165-171.
15. Martinez Cruz A. Diagnostic yield of different electrophysiological methods in carpal tunnel syndrome. *Muscle Nerve.* 1991;14:183-184.
16. Mumemthaler M, Schliack H, eds. *Peripheral Nerve Lesions: Diagnosis and Therapy.* New York: Thieme Medical Publishers; 1991.
17. Oh SJ, Sarala PK, Kuba T, Elmore RS. Tarsal tunnel syndrome: electrophysiological study. *Ann Neurol.* 1979;5:327-330.
18. Payan J. Electrophysiological localization of ulnar nerve lesions. *J Neurol Neurosurg Psychiatry.* 1969;32:208-220.
19. Preston DC, Logigian EL. Lumbrical and interossei recording in carpal tunnel syndrome. *Muscle Nerve.* 1992;15:1253-1257.
20. Raynor EM, Shefner JM, Preston DC, Logigian EL. Sensory and mixed nerve conduction studies in the evaluation of ulnar neuropathy at the elbow. *Muscle Nerve.* 1994;17:785-792.
21. Redford JB. Nerve conduction in motor fibers to the anterior tibial muscle in peroneal neuropathy. *Arch Phys Med Rehabil.* 1964;45:500.
22. Said G. Vasculitis and the nervous system: necrotizing peripheral nerve vasculitis. *Neurol Clin.* 1997;15:835-848.
23. Spinner M. The anterior interosseous syndrome. *J Bone Joint Surg.* 1970;52A:84-94.
24. Stoehr M, Petruch F, Scheglmann K, Schilling K. Retrograde changes of nerve fibers with the carpal tunnel syndrome: an electroneurographic investigation. *J Neurol.* 1978;218:287-292.
25. Sunderland S. *Nerves and Nerve Injuries.* 2nd ed. London: Churchill-Livingstone; 1978.
26. Thomas JE, Lambert EH, Cseuz KA. Electrodiagnostic aspects of the carpal tunnel syndrome. *Arch Neurol.* 1967;16:635-641.
27. Uncini A, Lange DJ, Solomon M, Soliven B, Meer J, Lovelace RE. Ring finger testing in carpal tunnel syndrome: a comparative study of diagnostic utility. *Muscle Nerve.* 1989;12:735-741.
28. Wilbourn AJ. AAEM Case Report 12. Common peroneal neuropathy at the fibular head. *Muscle Nerve.* 1986;9:825-836.

# 20

# Neuromuscular Diseases

*David S. Younger*

The diagnosis of neuromuscular disorders is an art that depends upon experience and logical reasoning. This chapter reviews aspects of neuromuscular diagnosis as a background for the chapters that will follow, emphasizing the unique contributions of the neurologic history and examination; electrodiagnostic, neuroimaging, and molecular genetic studies; and muscle and nerve biopsy analysis.[44]

## HISTORY

The neurologic history and examination are important first steps in the diagnosis of a neuromuscular disorder.[42] The goal is to establish the neurologic symptoms and signs, their temporal progression, and associated findings and to formulate a categorical diagnosis and localize the disease process along the motor unit.

Patients should be asked about specific motor and sensory symptoms. Some patients may not use the term *weakness* but will instead give an equivalent history of difficulty in combing hair, brushing teeth, rising out of a chair, or going upstairs, which are indicative of proximal weakness. Problems in buttoning a shirt or stepping over a curb point to predominant distal involvement. Progressive proximal weakness is the presenting symptom of polymyositis (PM), dermatomyositis (DM); mitochondrial, glycolytic, or lipid storage myopathy; and the Lambert-Eaton myasthenic syndrome (LEMS). Proximal weakness and prominent wasting are seen in facioscapulohumeral (FSH) and limb-girdle muscular dystrophy, Duchenne's muscular dystrophy (DMD), and Becker's muscular dystrophy (BMD), which are further separable by clinical and molecular genetic studies. Myotonic dystrophy, scapuloperoneal dystrophy, distal myopathy, amyotrophic lateral sclerosis (ALS) and spinal muscular atrophy (SMA) are all associated with predominant distal weakness.

Patients should also be asked about sensory symptoms, and the responses should be recorded in the patients' own words. If there is sensory loss, there is more than a myopathy, and the cause should be sought in the peripheral nerves, dorsal root ganglia (DRG), or dorsal columns of the spinal cord. Symptoms of autonomic insufficiency such as erectile failure in men, light-headedness, diarrhea, constipation,

bladder fullness, anhidrosis or hyperhidrosis, venous congestion, and reflex pain may be the first clue to a peripheral nervous system (PNS) disorder, and can accompany diabetic, amyloid, and alcoholic neuropathy, acute intermittent porphyria, Guillain-Barré syndrome (GBS), or botulism.

The tempo and distribution of symptoms may provide important clues to the underlying diagnosis. Weakness and sensory loss that evolves over several weeks while the patient is in the intensive care unit strongly suggest critical illness polyneuropathy. Fluctuating cranial and limb weakness over the course of a day, with exacerbations and remissions for months or years in an otherwise healthy patient, is likely due to myasthenia gravis (MG). The distribution of weakness in MG is characteristic, affecting ocular, facial, limb, oropharyngeal, and respiratory muscles, and is confirmed by unequivocal and reproducible improvement after the intravenous injection of 10 mg of edrophonium chloride (Tensilon), a rapidly acting acetylcholinesterase (AChE) inhibitor. Precipitous weakness follows myoglobinuria, suggested by dark coloration of the urine, transient worsening over days, and a high serum creatine kinase (CK) level. In most cases there is a heritable enzymatic defect in muscle glycogenolysis, glycolysis, or mitochondrial metabolism. Recurrent attacks of slight to severe weakness lasting a few hours upon awakening that spare oropharyngeal and respiratory muscles usually are due to periodic paralysis. Weakness of the legs that evolves over years and progresses from the thighs to the rest of the legs is likely due to DMD in boys and to inclusion body myositis (IBM) in older adults of either gender. The cause of an acute paralytic disorder such as GBS may lie in a forgotten or overlooked viral illness, immunization, new medication, or potentially toxic exposure.

Selective weakness of extensor neck muscles defines the "floppy" or "drooped" head syndrome, which most often proves to be due to FSH dystrophy, myotonic dystrophy, sclerodermatomyositis, ALS, or severe cervical spondylosis. Painless wasting of the hand is often the first clue to ALS or syringomyelia; however, associated radiating pain should lead to consideration of cervical root compression. Although frank enlargement of calf muscles in DMD is due to replacement of muscle by fat and connective tissue, the diffuse hypertrophy of myotonia congenita results from continuous muscle contraction. A painful muscle mass can develop as a consequence of rupture of a tendon or muscle belly, tumor, infection, or focal muscle infarction, the latter typically in a diabetic.[3]

Fatigue, cramps, myalgia, fasciculation, stiffness, and spasms are nonspecific symptoms but may also be useful clues. Although it is often stated that fatigue is never the solitary finding of MG, it can accompany true weakness and may worsen with repetitive contraction. Frequent cramping with myalgia is seen in myoadenylate deaminase deficiency. There is a syndrome of benign fasciculation and cramps.[2] Muscle contractures are separated from true cramps, dystonic postures, and spasms by the absence of electrical activity in the EMG. Stiffness is exquisitely painful in stiff-man syndrome.

Clues to the cause of muscular weakness may be obtained in a pedigree, which should include the names, sex, age, and specific symptoms and physical characteristics of affected family members. The pedigree is an essential part of the neurologic history to indicate the pattern of inheritance. However, it may not be informative if the patient is an index case or if failure of expressivity of the gene defect leads to a phenotypically normal heterozygote. The possible modes of single-gene inheritance include autosomal dominant (AD), autosomal recessive (AR), and X-linked dominant transmission. DNA analysis has revealed new insights into single-gene disorders and has allowed more precise diagnosis and genetic counseling through improved carrier detection and prenatal screening. Possibly affected relatives should be examined and photographed, and the records of deceased family members with neurologic illnesses should be reviewed closely.

The distinctive biologic nature of mitochondrial DNA (mtDNA) has added new concepts and terminology to classic mendelian genetics.[8] Several biologic factors explain the heterogeneity of human mitochondria disease. Each cell has multiple mitochondrial genomes, with the absolute number depending upon the requirement for oxidative energy. Some organs, such as the brain, heart, and skeletal muscle, have lower thresholds for mitochondrial dysfunction. A mutation can affect some or all of the mtDNA, leading to varying proportions of mutant mtDNA among tissues over the lifetime of the patient, explaining the appearance of particular syndromes at different ages. Virtually all mtDNA derives from the oocyte; therefore a mother transmits mutant mtDNA to all her children, but only the females pass it on to their offspring.

## EXAMINATION

A detailed but targeted neurologic examination is the next step in the diagnosis of a neuromuscular disorder. Examination of the cranial nerves includes assessment of ocular motility, lid position, facial motor strength, auditory and vestibular function, appearance of the tongue, and extensor and flexor neck strength. Individual muscles should be graded on a scale of 0 to 5, according to criteria of the Medical Research Council (MRC).[28] It is useful to observe the patient rising from a low chair or a deep squat, with arms folded on the chest. Focal wasting and fasciculation are best appreciated with the patient sitting or lying quietly with eyes closed to avoid the perception of staring. The patient should be observed erect with eyes open and closed. Gait should be assessed with the patient on toes, heels, or tandem and after hopping on either foot. Sensation is tested by using thermal, light-touch, proprioceptive, and vibratory stimuli and is graded from the feet and along the leg to the hands. Tendon reflexes are best tested in the seated position with the hands folded in the lap and the legs dangling. Knee jerks are considered absent only after reinforcement, as are ankle reflexes in the kneeling position.

The pattern of neurologic signs may be crucial to the diagnosis and may direct further specific evaluation. For example, focal limb weakness, wasting, fasciculation, and tendon areflexia without sensory loss—the essential pattern of lower motor neuron (LMN) or anterior horn cell involvement—suggests motor neuron disease (singular) (MND).[49] When the Hoffmann sign, the Babinski sign, and clonus—the unequivocal signs of upper motor neuron (UMN) or corticospinal tract involvement—are combined with LMN signs in a clinically compatible patient, the diagnosis of ALS is virtually "inescapable." Another example is the combination of glove or stocking sensory loss, ataxia, and areflexia, which are indicative of DRG involvement. When these signs are combined with cortical, cerebellar, brainstem, and spinal cord anterior horn cell signs, paraneoplastic encephalomyelitis and sensory neuronopathy (PEM-SN) are likely, and further evaluation for anti-Hu seropositivity is called for; and if the test result is positive, a search for occult small-cell lung cancer (SCLC) is initiated.[41]

## LABORATORY EVALUATION

The choice of laboratory studies in a given patient with a neuromuscular disorder depends upon the presumed etiologic and differential diagnosis. It may include one or more of the following: electromyography (EMG) and nerve conduction studies (NCS), neuroradiologic studies, autoantibody serology, lumbar cerebrospinal fluid (CSF) analysis, muscle and nerve biopsy, and genetic analysis.

### NEUROPHYSIOLOGIC STUDIES

Electrodiagnostic studies are necessary in the investigation of suspected myopathy, disorders of the neuromuscular junction (NMJ), peripheral neuropathy, entrapment neuropathy, plexopathy, radiculopathy, and MND. The electrodiagnostic features of myopathy include normal NCS and short-duration, low-amplitude motor unit potentials (MUP), with excessive polyphasia best appreciated on quantitative MUP analysis and a full recruitment pattern at the onset of a forceful contraction in clinically weak muscles. In myopathy, MUPs are reduced in duration because of loss of slow initial and terminal components, with reduction in the temporal dispersion of surviving muscle fibers along the end-plate region. These findings correlate with the pattern of myofiber involvement in the muscle biopsies of affected patients.[4]

Demyelinating neuropathy is distinguished by slow nerve conduction velocity (NCV), prolongation of distal and F-wave latencies, motor conduction block (MCB), and absence of spontaneous activity in affected muscles. A drop of 50% or more of the proximal compound muscle action potential (CMAP) at sites not prone to compression is indicative of MCB, whereas a reduction of 20% of the CMAP in the absence of abnormal temporal dispersion is strongly suggestive of a block. Although MCB and focal amplitude and waveform and velocity changes of the CMAP are all potentially indicative of focal demyelination, only MCB results in focal weakness. Axonal neuropathy, or axonopathy, is recognized by normal or mildly slow NCV, reduced CMAP, and sensory nerve action potential (SNAP) amplitudes, normal distal latencies, and mildly prolonged F wave responses in addition to variable active and chronic distal spontaneous activity, long-duration MUPs, and a reduced recruitment pattern in weak muscles.

The NMJ disorders MG and LEMS are clinically, electrophysiologically, and pathogenically heterogenous. They have in common loss of the safety factor for NMJ transmission, with an abnormal response to repetitive nerve stimulation. The safety factor for neuromuscular transmission depends on the amount of ACh released from the nerve terminal, the number of ACh receptors (AChR), and the concentration of sodium channels at the endplate.[21] A decremental response of 12% to 15% or more of successive CMAP after 3 Hz stimulation and aggravation of the block for several minutes after brief exercise are indicative of a postsynaptic defect typical of MG. Maximal exercise for 15 seconds transiently improves the decrement, termed *postactivation facilitation*, as does injection of edrophonium chloride. Prolonged exercise for 1 minute followed by repetitive trains of nerve stimulation at 1-minute intervals worsens the block, resulting in *postactivation exhaustion*. Movement of the recording or stimulating electrode can lead to an apparent decremental response, whereas cooler temperatures can reduce or normalize an abnormal study. Once used as a provocative test for MG, the injection of 1/16 of the normal dose of curare in a patient with MG leads to further impairment of the safety factor for neuromuscular transmission, with aggravation of the clinical weakness and accentuation of the decremental response to repetitive stimulation. LEMS is due to the action of antibodies directed against presynaptic P/Q-type voltage-gated calcium channels. The diagnosis is usually first suggested by the finding of low CMAP amplitudes on conventional NCS, which increase by 100% to 200% following repetitive stimulation at rates of 20 Hz or more, a change that is indicative of the underlying presynaptic defect.

Single fiber electromyography (SFEMG) supplements repetitive nerve stimulation by quantifying transmission at individual end plates while the patient voluntarily activates the muscle fiber under examination. However, it requires strict patient cooperation and examiner proficiency. Action potentials are recorded from two muscle fibers in the same motor unit near the single fiber electrode. The variability in the time between consecutively recorded potentials is termed *jitter*. Blocking is recognized by consecutive impulses that do follow one another. The expected finding in MG is normal jitter in some potential pairs and increased jitter in others. As a rule, 20 potential pairs are studied in each muscle. Up to 85% of patients with generalized MG have abnormal decrement in a hand or shoulder muscle with repetitive nerve stimulation, whereas 86% of patients with generalized myasthenia and 65% of those with ocular involvement reveal abnormalities on SFEMG studies. With the addition of a second muscle, jitter is seen in 99% of patients with generalized MG, making it a more sensitive method of analysis.[36]

Electrodiagnostic studies can provide useful information in the differentiation of axillary, suprascapular, and musculocutaneous neuropathies from a C5 root or upper trunk lesion; radial neuropathy from a C7 root, middle trunk, or posterior cord lesion; or combined median and ulnar neuropathies from a C8 root, lower trunk, or medial cord lesion. In idiopathic brachial neuritis, NCS show a reduction in CMAP and SNAP amplitudes that parallels the severity of the illness, often in association with active spontaneous activity in muscles innervated by proximal and distal motor nerve branches. Radiculopathy, or a root lesion, leads to peripheral motor deficits in a myotomal distribution. They most often occur in association with acute or chronic disc disease and degenerative arthritis with narrowing of the lateral recess and impingement of the exiting root. Since root lesions occur proximal to DRG, the SNAP of the corresponding spinal segment remains normal. The one exception is herpes zoster virus infection because of concomitant involvement of the DRG. Motor NCS are generally normal because the studied segments are distal to the site of involvement; however, F-wave latencies along named nerves with a known root innervation can be delayed, with abnormal impersistence and reduced amplitude, duration, or asymmetry in side-to-side comparisons. H responses are more sensitive, but they are generally restricted to abnormality of the S1 segment. EMG is performed in muscles sharing the same or different peripheral innervation and myotomal segments to establish the pattern of involvement. Fibrillation, positive sharp waves, fasciculation, and complex repetitive discharges may be delayed for weeks in the legs, but these signs are usually evident in paraspinal muscles 10 days after the initial injury and are clear evidence of a lesion proximal to the DRG. Fibrillation may be absent in chronic lesions if reinnervation has kept pace with denervation; then excessive polyphasia of MUPs will be present. Some muscles are useful to study by needle EMG because they derive their innervation from single roots, such as the rhomboids with involvement of the C5 root; the pronator teres and triceps in C6 and C7 segments, respectively; and the extensor carpi ulnaris in C8 radiculopathy. The distinction of an L5 root lesion from a peroneal or sciatic neuropathy requires examination of the tibialis posterior, tensor fascia lata, and gluteus medius muscles. The gluteus maximus is abnormal in S1 radiculopathy but is typically spared in high sciatic lesions.

Electrodiagnostic studies are imperative in the diagnosis and prognosis of ALS, especially to demonstrate normality of sensory responses, to search for MCB, and to estimate the degree of motor axon loss. Motor velocities may be slightly slowed and F-wave and distal motor latencies may be mildly prolonged owing to loss of the fastest conducting fibers, usually in proportion to the reduction in CMAP amplitude. Even before a muscle fibrillates electrically, the degeneration of a population of anterior horn cells leads to loss of innervation of muscle fibers in the respective motor units while the remaining cells sprout collateral fibers. The reinnervated fibers generate motor units, first with a variation in their configuration owing to conduction block and reduced synchrony of nerve terminal conduction. The inclusion of other fibers into the motor unit leads to motor units of longer mean duration, higher amplitude, and increased fiber density. The reduction in the number of motor neurons that can be activated leads to reduced recruitment upon voluntary contraction and, with increasing effort, an abnormally high firing rate of individual motor units and an increased ratio of the number of motor units to the firing rate. Although many parameters correlate with prognosis, severe disease, older age, and the presence of widespread low CMAP amplitudes with reduced velocities are associated with a poorer prognosis.

In carefully selected patients autonomic studies have an important role in management. Autonomic neuropathy contributes to the risk of malignant ventricular arrhythmia because of prolongation of the QTc interval of the resting electrocardiogram (ECG) and to sudden cardiorespiratory arrest following general anesthesia or the use of medications that suppress baroreceptor responses. Noninvasive quantitative autonomic tests include studies of cardiovagal function, such as heart rate response to deep breathing, Valsalva maneuver, and standing upright; sympathetic tests of blood pressure control to standing, tilting, or sustained handgrip; sudomotor control to thermally and chemically induced sweating; and the assessment of sphincter and erectile dysfunction.[1]

Somatosensory evoked responses (SSER) are useful in evaluating sensory symptoms that may be related to a central nervous system (CNS) lesion. They are elicited by stimulation of an accessible sensory or mixed nerve, but the median and posterior tibial nerves are the ones most commonly chosen. The responses are generated by impulse traffic along proximal peripheral nerve pathways from the popliteal fossa or clavicle to the dorsal horn along the posterior columns to the contralateral thalamus and cortex. The respective waveforms are displayed by electrode montages or combinations placed at various locations over the lumbar and cervical enlargements of the cord and on the scalp, corresponding to local synaptic activity (*near-field potentials*) or synchronous depolarizations along white-matter fiber tracts at a distance from the recording electrodes (*far-field potentials*).

Transcranial magnetic stimulation has been used in the evaluation of patients with ALS, particularly in those with equivocal UMN signs. Circular high-power coils are positioned on the scalp with the center over the vertex to record compound muscle action potentials and distal latencies in the arms and over Fz (i.e., frontal midline placement) for the legs. The motor roots are stimulated with the cathode positioned over C7 or L1. A central motor conduction time is calculated by subtracting the distal motor latencies obtained after nerve root stimulation from those obtained by cortical stimulation. The CMAP amplitudes recorded after cortical stimulation are expressed as a percentage of those obtained from root stimulation. An abnormally prolonged central motor conduction time and reduced CMAP amplitude correlates with the presence of corticospinal tract involvement.

## NEUROIMAGING STUDIES

Radiologic studies can be useful in selected patients with neuromuscular diseases. Magnetic resonance imaging (MRI) is probably the most widely used neuroimaging study for CNS disorders, and it is preferred over computed tomography (CT) of the brain. The intravenous contrast agent gadopentetate dimeglumine crosses the blood-brain barrier and is associated with few side effects. It shortens T1 and T2 relaxation times of spin-echo images and accumulates in lesions as areas of increased signal intensity compared to precontrast images. In selected patients with symptomatic mitochondrial encephalomyopathy, MRI can show white-matter degeneration resembling leukodystrophy and cortical lesions simulating vascular infarction. Functional neuroimaging employing positron emission tomography (PET) complements MRI in such patients. MRI can also be used to image the cross-sectional planes of individual limbs at sites of focal muscle wasting or inflammation due to myopathy and nerves enlarged by lymphomatous infiltrates. Phosphorus-31 MR spectroscopy is useful in the evaluation of muscle glycogenolysis.

## BLOOD TESTS AND AUTOANTIBODY ASSAYS

Blood can be processed for a variety of diagnostic studies depending upon the presumptive diagnosis. A serum creatine kinase (CK) of more than 10 times normal suggests myopathy. It is the earliest detected laboratory abnormality in myopathy and is always accompanied by increased levels of aspartate aminotransferase (AST; formerly serum glutamic-oxaloacetic transaminase [SGOT]), alanine aminotransferase (ALT; formerly glutamic-pyruvic transaminase [SGPT]), and lactate dehydrogenase (LDH). The highest CK levels, in the tens to hundreds of thousands, are found in attacks of myoglobulinuria; and in the thousands of units in DMD. Lesser magnitudes of up to three times normal can be seen in chronic myopathic or neurogenic disorders. Properly performed, a forearm ischemic test with simultaneous measurement of serum CK, venous lactate, and ammonia levels is the most widely employed means of assessing muscle anaerobic metabolism, whereas cyclic exercise protocols are useful in the evaluation of muscle oxidative metabolism.

The specific blood studies that should be performed in patients with peripheral neuropathy should be guided by the clinical presentation and the postulated etiologic diagnosis. Tests for diabetes, renal and hepatic disease, vitamin $B_{12}$ deficiency, thyroid and parathyroid disease, monoclonal paraproteinemia, selective immunoglobulin elevation, peripheral T-cell subset abnormalities; infectious etiologic disorders such as Lyme neuroborreliosis, syphilis, and human immunodeficiency virus (HIV) infection are relatively inexpensive and may reveal important information at the outset of the evaluation in selected patients.

The serologic evaluation of Lyme neuroborreliosis is especially challenging and requires integration of the clinical history, examination, and pertinent laboratory data.[31] A two-step testing scheme using an immunofluorescence assay or enzyme-linked immunosorbent assay (ELISA), followed by an immunoblot or Western blot, should be employed. The immunofluorescence assay is better suited for low-volume testing because false-positives can be easily recognized by the pattern of immunofluorescence. The ELISA method, however, is most often chosen by commercial and research laboratories because, compared to the immunofluorescence assay, there are fewer deficiencies or failures of diagnosis. The occasional failures of diagnosis when ELISA is used are generally related to laboratory performance and experience issues. An immunoglobulin M (IgM) immunoblot is considered positive when it exhibits reactivity against two of the following three kDa bands: 23, 39, 41; and, similarly, when the IgG component exhibits reactivity against five of the following 10 kDa bands: 18, 23, 28, 30, 39, 41, 45, 58, 66, and 93. Both IgM and immunoglobulin G (IgG) immunoblots should be used in the serodiagnosis of Lyme neuroborreliosis in the first 4 weeks of disease, but only the IgG should be used in late disease.

Patients with mononeuritis multiplex or distal symmetrical polyneuropathy and stigmata of a specific underlying connective tissue disorder, such as polyarteritis nodosa, rheumatoid arthritis, Wegener's granulomatosis, or systemic lupus erythematosus, are at increased risk for vasculitic neuropathy and should have blood analysis for erythrocyte sedimentation rate (ESR), p- and c-type antineutrophil cytoplasmic antibodies (p- and c-ANCA), hepatitis B and C serologic values, cryoglobulins, rheumatoid factor, antinuclear antibody (ANA) and double-stranded (ds) DNA antibody detection, as clinically indicated.[43] Patients with subacute sensory neuropathy should be screened for Sjögren's syndrome with Ro/SS-A and La/SS-B serologic values.

The neuropathies associated with monoclonal paraproteinemia are clinically and pathogenically heterogenous. Immunofixation electrophoresis is the most sensitive study for monoclonal paraproteinemia. The nonmalignant IgM monoclonal paraproteins, once called *gammopathies of unknown significance* (MGUS),[22,23] are now better understood for their potential autoreactive specificities to peripheral nerve. Whereas MGUS generally results from nonmalignant B-cell proliferation, monoclonal paraproteinemia may also be the first clue to possible underlying multiple myeloma, cryoglobulinemia, amyloidosis, chronic lymphocytic leukemia (CLL), or lymphocytic lymphoma resulting from malignant B-cell proliferation, further detectable in a bone marrow aspirate and biopsy.

The past decade has witnessed tremendous progress in the elucidation of several antinerve antibody syndromes with serologically specific assays (Table 20–1). However, the use of commercially available "panels" or "batteries" should probably be discouraged for several reasons. First, they are extremely expensive and often are not reimbursed by third-party payers. Second, they combine antibodies with widely divergent antigen reactivities, each relating to a different clinical neuropathic syndrome. Third, they test for relatively rare disorders; therefore only a minority of sera will ever have pathogenically high titers. Moreover, screening panels can yield spurious low titer results. Immunofluorescent studies performed on a nerve biopsy specimen should be offered to patients with potentially false-positive serologic findings who might otherwise receive toxic empiric immunosuppressive therapy.[40]

Autoimmune serologic values also play a pivotal role in the diagnosis of NMJ disorders. The serologic studies for MG include binding, blocking, and modulating AChR antibodies (Ab), which together assay the most important pos-

## SEROLOGICAL TEST PRIORITIES
### History & Exam Suggest MG

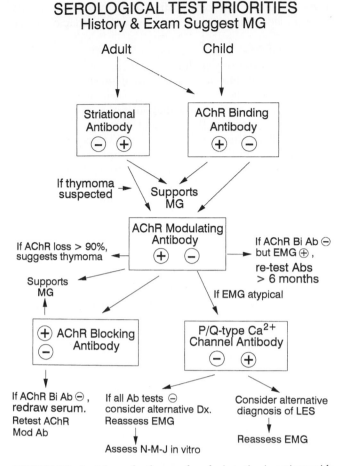

**FIGURE 20–1.** Scheme for the use of serologic testing in patients with myasthenia gravis and Lambert-Eaton myasthenic syndrome. (From Younger DS. Peripheral nerve pathology. In: Younger DS, ed. *Motor Disorders.* Philadelphia: Lippincott–Williams & Wilkins; 1999.)

tulated disturbances of AChR function (Fig. 20–1): accelerated degradation and endocytosis (AChR-binding Ab), cross-linking of ACh receptor antibodies (AChR-modulating Abs), and functional blockade (AChR-blocking Ab). The binding assay, expressed in nmol/L of bound AChR, is positive in up to 90% of patients with generalized MG[26] and is the preferred screening test. Striational antibodies are found in 80% of patients with MG and a thymoma and in a quarter of those with thymoma without clinically apparent MG.[26] Many of those patients will have electrophysiologic evidence of MG and will develop frank clinical signs of MG later in their course, sometimes even after thymectomy. Although it is useful to obtain thyroid function tests in all patients with MG, there is probably little urgency in ordering testing for antibodies to thyroid microsomes, thyroglobulin, and gastric parietal cells in the absence of Graves' disease or pernicious anemia. Patients with the LEMS should be studied, in addition, for antibodies to P/Q and N-type calcium channels. P/Q channels initiate the presynaptic release of acetylcholine and are the target antigens in the LEMS. N-type channels are widely distributed in the CNS and may be a target antigen in rubrocortical, spinal, and autonomic syndromes in association with LEMS. High titers of either type of antibody should raise suspicion of a primary lung cancer. Fewer than 5% of patients with MG have calcium channel antibodies, making it a useful assay to distinguish the two.[26]

| TABLE 20–1. Neuropathic Autoantibody Syndromes | | |
|---|---|---|
| **SYNDROME** | **ANTIGEN** | **ANTIBODY** |
| Chronic motor neuropathy | GM1 | |
| | GD1b | Monoclonal or polyclonal IgM |
| Acute motor axonal neuropathy | GD1a | Polyclonal IgG, IgA |
| Miller Fisher syndrome | GQ1b | Polyclonal IgG |
| Anti-MAG neuropathy | MAG | Monoclonal IgM |
| Predominantly sensory neuropathy | GD1b | Monoclonal IgM |
| | Sulfatide | Monoclonal or polyclonal IgM |
| Paraneoplastic sensory neuropathy | Hu | Polyclonal IgG |

Ig, Immunoglobulin; MAG, myelin-associated glycoprotein.

Even though the serologic profiles of the two disorders may occasionally overlap, these disorders rarely overlap clinically.

## CEREBROSPINAL FLUID

Properly performed, lumbar puncture is a safe and informative procedure in a variety of neuromuscular disorders. Acellular CSF with a raised protein content of 100 mg/dl or higher supports the diagnosis of Kearns-Sayre syndrome (KSS), and both GBS and chronic inflammatory polyradiculoneuropathy (CIDP). Pleocytosis and a mild protein elevation that varies with the severity of the paralysis occurs in poliomyelitis, with a shift from polymorphonuclear to mononuclear cells over several days.

Virtually all patients with acute meningitis, cranial neuritis, and radiculitis caused by Lyme neuroborreliosis show evidence of CSF lymphocytosis, intrathecal production of *Borrelia burgdorferi*–specific antibodies and, in some cases, demonstration of the organism by culture or polymerase chain reaction (PCR). In such patients the presence of CSF inflammation is only one element of a more disseminated process affecting the peripheral nerve, subarachnoid space, and corresponding levels of the spinal cord.[16]

Most patients with ALS have a normal CSF profile, but a protein content of 75 mg/dl or more, oligoclonal bands, and serum monoclonal paraproteinemia, especially in those with a syndrome of SMA or subacute motor neuronopathy clinically, indicate the need for further studies for occult lymphoproliferative cancer.[48]

## MUSCLE AND NERVE BIOPSY: INDICATIONS AND TECHNIQUE

The indications for nerve and muscle biopsy have continued to expand as the evaluative process has improved[17] (Table 20–2). Practically, muscle and nerve biopsy should be

---

**TABLE 20–2. Indications for Nerve and Muscle Biopsy**

**Nerve Biopsy**
Peripheral nerve vasculitis*
Amyloid neuropathy*
Polyglucosan body disease
Cholesterol emboli syndrome*
Sarcoid neuropathy*
Leprosy
Neurolymphomatosis
Anti-MAG neuropathy
Chronic inflammatory demyelinating polyneuropathy
Diabetic neuropathy
Motor neuropathy
CMT-1A, 1B, and 3; HNPP-A
Critical illness polyneuropathy

**Muscle Biopsy**
Polymyositis
Inclusion body myositis
Dermatomyositis
Metabolic myopathy due to glycogenolytic, glycolytic, and oxidative enzyme defects
Progressive muscular dystrophy
Cholesterol emboli syndrome
Diabetic muscle infarction
Limb-girdle syndrome

---

*Muscle biopsy should also be performed to increase yield of diagnostic lesions.

CMT, Charcot-Marie-Tooth neuropathy; HNPP, hereditary neuropathy with pressure palsies; MAG, myelin-associated glycoprotein.

---

considered only after the formulation of a preliminary diagnosis. Biopsy can be approached with confidence by the patient and the referring neurologist when the procedure is in the hands of a neurologist or surgeon skilled in biopsy techniques and is performed at a center with a neuropathologist who has been trained to process and examine the specimens for all the diagnostic possibilities. The nerve and muscle chosen for biopsy should be clinically and electrophysiologically affected; however, the muscle should not be so affected, or end-stage, as to preclude interpretation. A segment of the sural, superficial peroneal sensory, and femoral cutaneous nerves can be surgically removed, depending upon the clinical circumstances, without incurring a serious deficit; each has the advantage of allowing for biopsy of underlying muscle, respectively, from the soleus, peroneus brevis, and rectus femoris (Fig. 20–2). Obtaining a specimen of muscle for microscopic analysis can provide useful information about the severity of underlying neuropathy, and it increases the yield of diagnosis in vasculitis. There is a technique for biopsy of the motor and sensory nerve branches of the anterior obturator nerve and gracilis muscle in the medial thigh that does lead to a noticeable deficit[5]; however, it entails a deeper dissection and has a higher risk of postoperative complications. The overall estimated risk of residual pain, paresthesia, analgesia, and anesthesia from a nerve biopsy is approximately 5%.[17]

## INSIGHTS INTO IMMUNOPATHOGENESIS

Tremendous progress has been made in the inflammatory myopathies, which include PM, IBM, and DM and are further separable from one another by distinct clinical, morphologic, immunohistochemical, and immunophenotypic features. PM occurs alone or in association with systemic autoimmune or connective tissue diseases and viral or bacterial infections. The essential clinical features are myalgia, cranial and proximal limb weakness, and an elevated CK level. Biopsy of an affected muscle shows myofiber necrosis, regeneration, lymphocytic infiltration, and variable fibrosis (Fig. 20–3); cytotoxic CD8$^+$ cells surround healthy endomysial myofibers leading to phagocytosis and necrosis. IBM is distinguished by the finding of rimmed vacuoles and eosinophilic inclusions that strongly react with ubiquitin, Congo red, and crystal violet in histochemistry studies (Fig. 20–4). Patients with DM have a characteristic violaceous, shiny rash of the upper eyelids, face, neck, trunk, elbows, knuckles, and nail beds and variable proximal weakness. B cells and CD4$^+$ cells invade the endomysium and surround blood vessels, without significant lymphocytic invasion of nonnecrotic muscle fibers (Fig. 20–5). The disorder frequently overlaps with systemic sclerosis, mixed connective tissue disease, and systemic malignancy. It is not known whether patients with dermatomyositis are a greater risk for an underlying malignancy. Nevertheless, it is still reasonable to include CT of the chest, abdomen, and pelvis; manual rectal and pelvic examination; mammogram; and tumor markers in older patients, who may be at greater risk for occult malignancy.

MG is probably the best known autoimmune disorder. Our present understanding of the disorder followed a series of historic achievements.[50] An autoimmune cause was postulated more than three decades ago but awaited contemporary advances, first by electrophysiology and ultrastructure of the

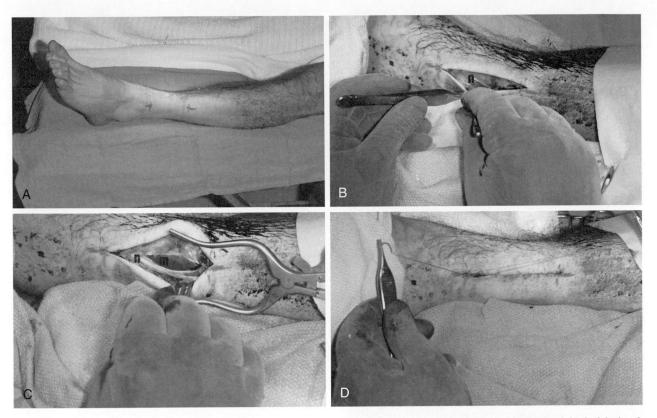

**FIGURE 20–2.** Technique of superficial peroneal sensory nerve and peroneus brevis muscle. **A,** The nerve is palpated in the distal third of the leg along a line between the fibular head and lateral malleolus, providing the markings for the incision. **B,** Under monitored anesthesia care, an incision is made and the area is dissected, revealing the nerve (*n*) obliquely traversing the field. **C,** Incising the aponeurosis reveals muscle (*m*) available for biopsy. **D,** After the specimens are removed and the site is irrigated, a subcuticular closure is performed with absorbable sutures. (From Younger DS. Peripheral nerve pathology. In: Younger DS, ed. *Motor Disorders*. Philadelphia: Lippincott–Williams & Wilkins; 1999.)

**FIGURE 20–3.** Muscle biopsy findings in polymyositis. **A,** A longitudinal section of skeletal muscle stained with hematoxylin and eosin reveals lymphocytic infiltration. **B,** Immunocytochemistry reveals that the majority of infiltrating cells are CD8[+]. (From Younger DS. Peripheral nerve pathology. In: Younger DS, ed. *Motor Disorders*. Philadelphia: Lippincott–Williams & Wilkins; 1999.)

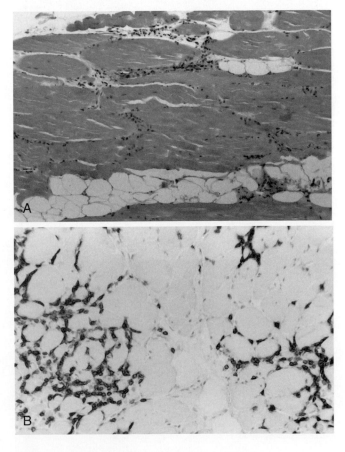

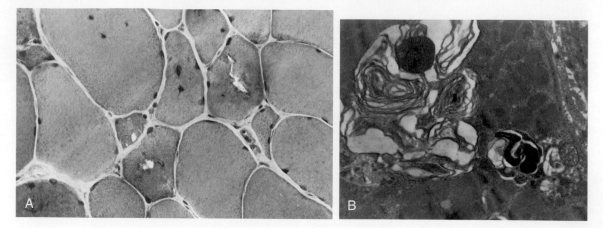

**FIGURE 20–4.** Muscle biopsy findings in inclusion body myositis. **A,** Rimmed vacuoles are visualized in trichrome-stained fresh-frozen cross sections. The vacuoles vary in shape, size, number, and location and are generally bordered by dark-staining material that extends to nearby fiber regions. **B,** Ultrastructurally, vacuoles contain multilaminated membranous structures accompanied by glycogen granules, dense bodies, and amorphous granulofibrillar material. (From Younger DS. Peripheral nerve pathology. In: Younger DS, ed. *Motor Disorders.* Philadelphia: Lippincott–Williams & Wilkins; 1999.)

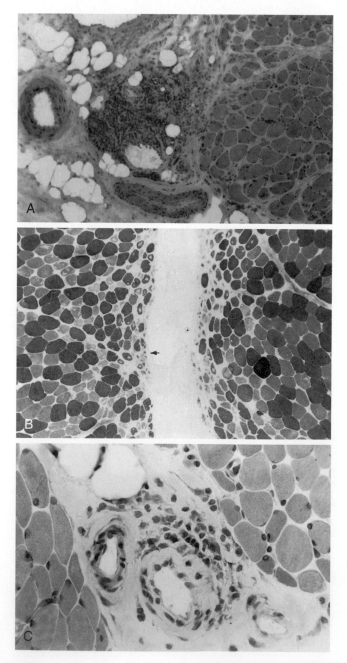

**FIGURE 20–5.** Muscle biopsy findings in dermatomyositis. **A,** There is a prominence of lymphocytes in the perimysial connective tissue in a cross section of muscle stained with hematoxylin and eosin. **B,** Perifascicular atrophy is seen in cross section of muscle stained with ATPase (*arrow*). **C,** A collection of lymphocytes is noted in and around a perimysial vein stained with hematoxylin and eosin. (From Younger DS. Peripheral nerve pathology. In: Younger DS, ed. *Motor Disorders.* Philadelphia: Lippincott–Williams & Wilkins; 1999.)

AChR and later with the investigation of experimental animal models and motor point biopsies in affected patients. Nature provided two gifts that facilitated characterization of the nicotinic AChR: (1) bungarotoxin (BuTx) from krait snakes and (2) the electric organs of the torpedo eel, a rich reservoir of AChRs. Investigators intending to make antibodies against AChRs in rabbits immunized with purified receptors from the electric organ of eels instead gave rise to experimental autoimmune MG as a result of an autoimmune attack against native AChRs. Later, investigators applied BuTx to muscle motor point biopsies from patients with MG and found a marked reduction in the number of AChRs, averaging 20% of that of controls. The essential clinical and morphologic correlates of human MG in animals was finally established by passive transfer of human myasthenic syndrome and with AChR-specific monoclonal antibodies.

Significant advances have also been achieved in our recognition of basic immune reactions of the peripheral nerves,[6] which in turn, were applied to the understanding of such diverse neuropathic disorders as vasculitis and diabetic neuropathy. Under normal circumstances the PNS is protected from the immune reactions by the blood-nerve barrier, which consists of perineurial and endoneurial vascular tight junctions. In the early phases of inflammation there is enhancement of vascular permeability by vasoactive substances, complement activation, and cytokine secretion. These alterations lead to leakage of inflammatory mediators and immigration of lymphocytes and macrophages to the endoneurial space. Local immune activation requires the interaction of a specific autoantigen, a main histocompatibility (MHC) class II antigen-presenting cell (APC), and antigen-specific T cells in the trimolecular complex. This interaction leads to proliferation of specific helper (CD4) and cytotoxic (CD8) T cells, with expression of human leukocyte antigen (HLA)-DR, interleukin (IL)-2 receptor, and the secretion of tumor necrosis factor (TNF)-$\alpha$ and other interleukins. Macrophages are the primary APC of the PNS.[14] They appear as immunoreactive CD68$^+$ cells with elongated or cylindrical cell bodies, scattered in the endoneurium often in proximity to blood vessels. Intensely stained MHC class II–positive macrophages appear in excessive numbers at foci of wallerian degeneration and in primary immune-mediated neuropathy. The complement system also contributes to vascular and neural injury. Activation of the classical or alternative pathways leads to cleavage of C3 to C3d, which then results in activation of the terminal lytic sequence C5b-9, membrane attack complex (MAC). Commercially available monoclonal and polyclonal antibodies directed against T- and B-cell subsets, macrophages, immunoglobulins, complement proteins, cytokines and other inflammatory mediators, and MHC class I and II antigens can be easily applied to clinical and research protocols for the evaluation of patients with various immune-mediated neuropathies[46] (Table 20–3).

Vascular endothelial cells appear to have a prominent role in the pathobiologic process of vascular inflammation in peripheral nerve vasculitis because of their postulated interactions with the immune system, supporting their active role, not simply as targets of injury.[43] The functions of these cells are regulated by interleukins, TNF, and endotoxins derived from immigrant or resident mononuclear cells. Their action, by virtue of binding to specific receptors, appears to

**TABLE 20–3. Nerve Biopsy: Immunohistochemistry Protocol**

| ANTIBODY SPECIFICITY | ANTIGEN | SOURCE | DILUTION |
|---|---|---|---|
| Macrophage | CD68 | Dako | 1:100 |
| HLA class II | HLA-DR | BD | 1:100 |
| HLA class I | HLA-ABC | Dako | 1:100 |
| T cell/pan T | CD3 | Dako | 1:100 |
| Helper T cell | CD4 | Dako | 1:20 |
| Cytotoxic T cell | CD8 | Dako | 1:20 |
| LCA | CD45 | Dako | 1:40 |
| TNF | TNF | ABT | 1:40 |
| IL-1 | IL-a | Olympus | 1:40 |
| IL-1 | IL-b | UBI | 1:50 |
| IL-6 | IL-6 | Genzyme | 1:20 |
| B cell | CD20 | Dako | 1:40 |
| IgG | $\gamma$-chain | Sigma | 1:100 |
| IgA | $\alpha$-chain | Sigma | 1:20 |
| IgM | $\mu$-chain | Sigma | 1:20 |
| C5b-9 | C5b-9 neoantigen | Quidel | 1:100 |
| C3d | C3d | Quidel | 1:300 |
| C4d | C4d | Quidel | 1:300 |
| Albumin | Albumin | Dako | 1:50 |
| Fibrinogen | Fibrinogen | Dako | 1:50 |

HLA, Human leukocyte antigen; Ig, immunoglobulin; IL, interleukin; LCA, leukocyte common antigen; TNF, tumor necrosis factor.

be alteration of the transcription of an array of endothelial genes that program cellular inflammatory mediator secretion, local expression of leukocyte adhesion molecules, and other inflammatory intermediaries.

Microangiopathy is the most common cause of diabetic neuropathy, associated with potentially reversible metabolic, ischemic, and immunologic mechanisms of injury.[46] A lymphocytic microvasculitis that comprises activated CD8$^+$ cells and, to a lesser extent, CD4$^+$ cells was found in 60% of sural nerve biopsies of severely affected patients with proximal and distal diabetic polyneuropathy and mononeuropathy multiplex (Fig. 20–6A). Associated immunologic findings also included C3d, C4d, and activated MAC deposits along microvessel walls, not simply at sites of inflammation (Fig. 20–6B), with local expression of IL-2 receptor and MHC class I and II determinants. Whether the T cells are directed at an antigen (or antigens) that is specific for the peripheral nerve or is shared by the pancreas and nerve is not yet understood. The initiating factor in the complement activation is still speculative, but one possibility is a defect in the expression of one or more regulatory membrane proteins. Microvessel alterations, once thought to include early closure of capillaries, and intraluminal platelet thrombi related to the severity of neuropathy were not confirmed in later ultrastructural studies by the same authors.[11,39] With immunohistochemistry, the density of microvessels is increased in nerves of patients with diabetes compared with those of controls.[33]

Significant achievements have also been made in the elucidation of the humoral and cell-mediated mechanisms underlying anti-Hu–associated paraneoplastic sensory neuropathy (PSN)-EM. Perivascular and interstitial Hu-sensitized T cells infiltrate regions of the CNS and DRG that also bind anti-Hu–IgG. In addition, epineurial and perimysial lymphocytic microvasculitis (MV) composed of CD8+ cells was found in a patient with PSN-EM and high serum anti-Hu antibody titers.[47] That patient improved with treatment

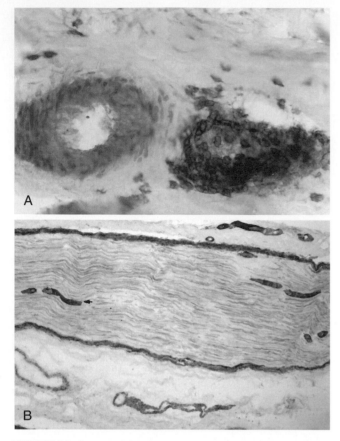

**FIGURE 20–6.** **A,** Peripheral nerve microvasculitis in diabetic polyneuropathy. The sural nerve has been cross-sectioned and stained with immunoperoxidase, revealing CD8$^+$ T cell–mediated microvasculitis of an endoneurial microvessel, and counterstained with anti–smooth muscle actin antibody to highlight the vessel wall. **B,** Complement activation in diabetic polyneuropathy. The sural nerve has been sectioned longitudinally and stained with a monoclonal antibody to C5b-9 neoantigen to show deposits along the perineurium and walls of microvessels. (From Younger DS, Rosoklija G, Hays AP. Diabetic peripheral neuropathy. *Semin Neurol.* 1998; 18:95-104.)

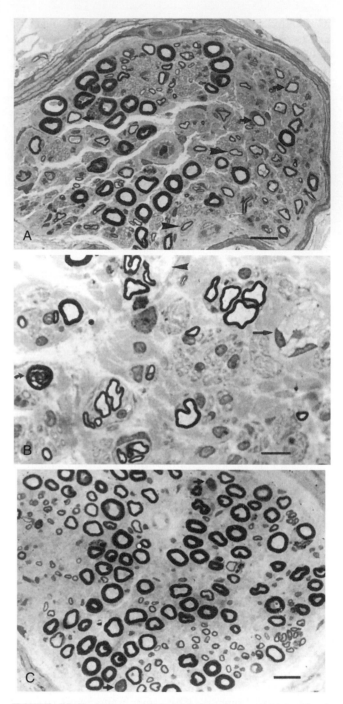

**FIGURE 20–7.** Motor nerve biopsy findings in motor neuropathy. **A,** Semithin sections of a motor nerve fascicle from the anterior obturator nerve reveal many thinly myelinated fibers (*arrows*) and small onion bulbs (*arrowheads*). **B,** At higher magnification, a motor fascicle also shows four regenerative clusters of small myelinated fibers, band of Büngner (*arrow*), demyelinated axon (*arrowhead*), and myelin ovoid (*curved arrow*). **C,** Motor nerve biopsy findings in motor neuron disease. Semithin sections of the anterior obturator nerve show a reduction in myelinated nerve fibers and a few foci of myelin debris (*arrows*). (From Corbo M, Abouzhahr MK, Latov N, et al. Motor nerve biopsy studies in motor neuropathy and motor neuron disease. *Muscle Nerve.* 1997;20:15-21. Reprinted by permission of John Wiley & Sons, Inc.)

of the underlying small cell lung carcinoma, an outcome that is consistent with the premise that the MV was paraneoplastic in its etiologic complex.

Highly suspected cases of motor neuropathy can be confirmed histologically in a motor nerve biopsy by the presence of large-caliber thinly myelinated fibers, onion bulbs, and, frequently, regenerative clusters of small myelinated fibers (Fig. 20–7*A* and *B*) in contrast to cases of ALS, in which regeneration is rarely, if at all, present (Fig. 20–7*C*).[5] There is generally little justification for the routine performance of a nerve biopsy in patients with ALS in the absence of MCB on electrophysiologic studies or elevated titers of GM$_1$ or other autoantibodies. Direct immunofluorescence of nerve biopsy tissues in more than 50 cases of ALS generally showed no differences compared to normal controls.[17] However, several reported patients indeed had exceptional findings, revealed on morphologic studies, supporting the importance of a thorough analysis to identify a potentially treatable concurrent underlying disorder in all patients if possible. One patient was a 73-year-old woman with typical ALS, prior breast cancer, and a monoclonal IgA serum paraprotein. Sural nerve biopsy showed deposits of IgA and lambda light chains along axons. At postmortem examina-

tion, indirect immunofluorescence also revealed binding of the IgA to spinal anterior horn cells and specificity for the high-molecular-weight subunit of neurofilament protein and a neuronal surface antigen.[18,35] The second patient was a 38-year-old woman with ALS, multifocal motor conduction blocks on electrodiagnostic studies, and a high serum IgM GM$_1$ titer.[37] Sural nerve biopsy showed granular deposits of IgM at nodal and paranodal regions of myelinated nerve fibers. When the patient's serum was injected into rat sciatic nerve, the serum IgM bound at the nodes of Ranvier, and this binding activity was removed by preincubation with GM1.[38] Further, among 26 reported patients with motor neuron disease and lymphoproliferative disorders seen over the past two decades at the Columbia-Presbyterian Medical Center in New York City, all three with pure LMN syndromes had monoclonal paraproteins and improved with treatment of the underlying malignancy. One patient had an IgM paraprotein with motor conduction block and CLL.[48] A second patient had high titers of GM1 and GD1b antibodies and myeloma; sural nerve biopsy in this patient showed focal demyelination and increased numbers of regenerative clusters.[24] The third had IgA monoclonal paraproteinemia and Waldenström's macroglobulinemia.[13]

## GENETIC ANALYSIS

The genetic analysis of neuromuscular disorders has witnessed unprecedented progress in the past two decades. Neuromuscular disorders of known transmission are summarized in Tables 20–4 and 20–5. The DNA analysis of primary myopathies, congenital MG, hereditary neuropathies, and inherited MND has revealed new insights into single-gene disorders and allowed more precise diagnosis and genetic counseling through improved carrier detection and

### TABLE 20–4. Neuromuscular Diseases of Known Transmission

| DISEASE | MIM | MODE OF INHERITANCE | GENE LOCATION | GENE PRODUCT |
|---|---|---|---|---|
| **Muscular Dystrophies** | | | | |
| DMD | 310200 | XR | Xp21.2 | Dystrophin |
| BMD | 310200 | XR | Xp21.2 | Dystrophin |
| EDMD | 310300 | XR | Xq28 | Emerin |
| FSH | 158900 | AD | 4q35 | |
| LGMD | 253600 | AR | 15q | LGMD2 |
| | 253600 | AR | 2p | LGMD3 |
| | 159000 | AD | 5q | LGMD1 |
| Severe childhood | 253700 | AR | 13q12 | SCARMD1 |
| DM | 160900 | AD | 19q13 | Protein kinase |
| **Congenital Myopathies** | | | | |
| Myotubular | 310400 | XR | Xq28 | MTM1 |
| Central core | 117000 | AD | 19q13.1 | Ryanodine receptor |
| Nemaine | 161800 | AD | 1q21-q23 | NEM1 |
| Fukuyama | 253800 | AR | 9q31-q33 | FCMD |
| Merosin deficiency | | AR | 6q2 | Merosin |
| **Other Myotonic Disorders** | | | | |
| Hyperkalemic period paralysis | 170500 | AD | 17q13.1-q13.3 | Sodium channel |
| Paramyotonic congenita | 168300 | AD | 17q13.1-q13.2 | Sodium channel |
| Hypokalemic period paralysis | 170400 | AD | 1q31-q32 | Calcium channel (dihydropyridine receptor) |
| **Metabolic Myopathies** | | | | |
| *Glycogenoses* | | | | |
| Type II-Pompe's disease | 232300 | AR | 17q23 | GAA |
| Type IV-McArdle's disease | 232600 | AR | 11q13 | Muscle phosphorylase |
| Type VII-Tarui disease | 232800 | AR | 1ccnq32 | Muscle phosphofructokinase |
| Type IX | 311800 | XR | Xq13 | Phosphoglycerate kinase |
| Type X | 261670 | AR | 7p12-p13 | Phosphoglycerate mutase |
| Type XI | 150000 | AR | 11p15.4 | Lactate dehydrogenase |
| *Lipidoses* | | | | |
| Carnitine palmitoyltransferase deficiency | 255110 | AR | 11p11-p13 | Carnitine palmitoyltransferase |
| **Congenital Myasthenic Syndromes** | | | | |
| Familial infantile | 259210 | AR | | |
| Paucity of synaptic vesicles | | AR | | |
| AChE deficiency | | AR | | |
| AChR deficiency | | AR | | |
| Paucity of synaptic folds | | AR | | |
| Abnormal ACh-AChR interaction | | | | |
| Slow channel | | | | |
| Fast channel | | | | |

ACh, Acetylcholine; AChE, acetylcholinesterase; AChR, ACh receptor; AD, autosomal dominant; ALD, adrenoleukodystrophy; ALS, amyotrophic lateral sclerosis; AR, autosomal recessive; BMD, Becker's muscular dystrophy; CMT, Charcot-Marie-Tooth disease; DM, dystrophica myotonica (myotonic muscular dystrophy); DMD, Duchenne's muscular dystrophy; EDMD, Emery-Dreifuss muscular dystrophy; FAP, familial amyloid polyneuropathy; FSH, fascioscapulohumeral; GKB1, gene of uncertain function; Hex, hexosaminidase; HNPP, hereditary neuropathy with pressure palsies; HSMN, hereditary sensorimotor neuropathy; KSS, Kearns-Sayre syndrome; LGMD, limb-girdle muscular dystrophy; MIM, *Mendelian Inheritance in Man* (McKusick[27]); MLD, metachromatic leukodystrophy; MNGIE, mitochondrial neuropathy, gastrointestinal disorder, and encephalopathy; P, peripheral nerve protein; PBG, porphobilinogen; PMP, peripheral myelin protein; SMA, spinal muscular atrophy; SOD, superoxide dismutase; TTR, transthyretin; XR, X-linked recessive.

*Table continued on following page*

**TABLE 20–4. Neuromuscular Diseases of Known Transmission** *Continued*

| DISEASE | MIM | MODE OF INHERITANCE | GENE LOCATION | GENE PRODUCT |
|---|---|---|---|---|
| **Hereditary Sensorimotor Neuropathy** | | | | |
| Type 1a | 118220 | AD | 17p12-p11.2 | PMP22 |
| Type 1b | 159440 | AD | 1q21.1-q23.3 | $P_0$ |
| Type 11a | 118210 | AD | 1p35-p36 | |
| Type 11b | | | 3q | |
| Type 111 | 145900 | AD | 17p11.2 | PMP22 |
| | | AD | 1q21-q23 | Phytanic acid D-hydroxylase |
| Type IV | 214400 | AR | 8q13-q21.1 | TTR |
| CMT $X_1$ | 302800 | XD | Xq13.1 | GKB1 encoding connexin-32 |
| CMT $X_2$ | 382801 | XR | Xp22.2;Xq2 | |
| HNPP | 162500 | AD | 17p11.2 | PMP22 |
| Refsum's disease | 266500 | AR | | Phytanic acid α-hydroxylase |
| FAP | 176300 | AD | 18q11.2-q12.1 | TTR |
| Friedreich's ataxia | 229300 | AR | 9q13-q21.1 | |
| Acute intermittent porphyria | 176000 | AD | 11q24.1-q24.2 | PGB deaminase |
| Familial dysautonomia | 223900 | AR | 9q31-q33 | |
| Tangier disease | 205400 | AR | | |
| MLD | 250100 | AR | 22q1331-qter | Arylsulfatase A |
| ALD | 300100 | XR | Xq28 | ALD protein (peroxisomal transporter protein) |
| Fabry's disease | 301500 | X-linked | X chromosome | α-galactosidase |
| Multiple sulfatase deficiency | 272200 | AR | | Arylsulfatase A, B, and C |
| Krabbe's disease | 245200 | AR | 12q21-q31 | Galactocerebrosidase |
| **Motor Neuron Diseases** | | | | |
| Werdnig-Hoffman syndrome | 253300 | AR | 5q11-q13 | SMA |
| Kugelberg-Welander syndrome | 253400 | AR | 5q11-q13 | SMA |
| Familial ALS | 105400 | AD | 21q22 | SOD |
| | 205100 | AR | 2q33-q35 | ALS2 |
| Kennedy syndrome | 313200 | XR | Xq21-22 | Androgen receptor |
| Late-onset Tay-Sachs disease | 27800 | | 15q23-24 | Hexosaminidase A deficiency |
| Sandhoff's disease | 268800 | | 5q11.2-13.6 | Hexosaminidase A & B deficiency |
| AB variant disease | 272750 | | 5q | $GM_2$ activator protein deficiency |

prenatal screening. The defective gene in DMD was identified along several independent lines of investigation with the use of restriction fragment length polymorphisms and the process of "reverse genetics."[15] Out-of-frame deletions in a band near the middle of the short arm of the X chromosome, designated Xp21, in two clusters or "hot spots" results in DMD, whereas in-frame deletions result in BMD. In the latter the related dystrophin protein is altered in size or reduced in quantity but not altogether lost from the muscle. The application of DNA probes and antidystrophin antibodies to muscle biopsy specimens, in turn, resulted in a refinement in the diagnosis and expansion of the recognized Xp21 myopathies or dystrophinopathies. They include BMD variants such as those with atypical distribution (e.g., quadriceps or distal myopathies) and others with minimal weakness or idiopathic elevations of the CK level.

Currently, mitochondrial disorders can be classified according to whether the gene defect lies in nuclear (nDNA) or mtDNA or in the faulty communication between the two genomes.[7] The historical term *mitochondrial myopathy* has been replaced by the more appropriate designation, *mitochondrial encephalomyopathy,* emphasizing the more common widespread systemic and CNS involvement. Deletions or point mutations of mtDNA lead to two distinctive neurologic syndromes, progressive external ophthalmoplegia (PEO) and KSS. In purely clinical terms, PEO is characterized by the slow, steady progression of ptosis and ophthalmoparesis beginning in childhood or young adulthood.

Strictly defined, KSS includes PEO, with onset before age 20 years, and pigmentary retinopathy, with at least one of the following: heart block, cerebellar syndrome, and CSF protein content above 100 mg/dl. There may also be associated dementia, sensorineural hearing loss, short stature, diabetes mellitus, and hypoparathyroidism. The essential gene product in KSS is still unknown. Skeletal muscle biopsy in mitochondrial encephalomyopathy shows myofibers with accumulation of mitochondria along their borders. The proliferation of mitochondria in "ragged red" fibers (RRF), so named for their appearance with Gomori trichrome staining, appears to be a compensatory mechanism for the imbalance between energy requirements and the oxidative phosphorylation capabilities of affected myofibers. Ultrastructural analysis, when performed, shows densely packed cristae with rodlike inclusions. Two other multisystem mitochondrial disorders, myoclonic epilepsy with RRF (MERRF) and mitochondrial myopathy with encephalopathy, lactic acidosis, and strokelike episodes (MELAS), have the additional distinctive features of seizures, exercise intolerance, dementia, retardation with normal early development, and onset before age 40 years. Another category of mitochondrial gene defects includes those caused by faulty communication between nDNA and mtDNA. These disorders are transmitted by mendelian inheritance because the primary genetic error often resides in nDNA. There is a late-onset progressive myopathy associated with multiple mtDNA deletions, in which exaggerated age-related abnormalities in mitochondrial function embody the presumed pathogenesis of the disorder and muscle biopsy shows RRF (Fig. 20–8).[20]

Current understanding of the congenital myasthenic syndromes and ion channel abnormalities has been achieved by the application of molecular genetics to the detection of mutations in AChR subunit genes, accompanied by sophisticated morphologic and electrophysiologic studies of the NMJ.[9] Symptomatic congenital MG results from the loss of the safety factor for normal NMJ transmission and can be divided into presynaptic, synaptic, and postsynaptic disorders. Two presynaptic disorders are due to defects in ACh resynthesis or to a paucity of synaptic vesicles with reduced quantal release of ACh. End-plate AChE deficiency causes a synaptically mediated disorder. The postsynaptic form of congenital MG is generally associated with a kinetic abnormality of AChR, with or without receptor deficiency, or it is related to a AChR deficiency without a primary kinetic abnormality. Conditions associated with AChR and a kinetic abnormality include ion channel disorders due to short open time, a slow-channel syndrome associated with prolonged open time due to delayed channel closure, a slow-channel syndrome due to increased affinity of the receptor for ACh causing repeated openings during prolonged acetylcholine occupancy; and another syndrome in which the nature of the kinetic abnormality has not yet been elucidated. Conditions associated with ACh deficiency include the low-affinity fast-channel syndrome and the high-conductance fast-channel syndrome. Conditions associated with ACh deficiency without a primary kinetic abnormality are caused by nonsense mutations in the e subunit gene of the receptor complex. Motor point biopsy can add precision to the diagnosis of congenital myasthenia in suspected patients, but it should be performed at centers with a genuine interest in the disorder because of the necessary detailed studies. The muscle tissue should first be processed for routine studies and then for cytochemical localization of acetylcholinesterase and immune deposits at end-plates. Electron microscopic and immunocytochemical studies are necessary to determine the size and density of synaptic vesicles and the morphologic features of nerve terminals and postsynaptic membranes. Quantitative assessment of acetylcholine receptor binding can be performed by using peroxidase-labeled $\alpha$-bungarotoxin. In vitro microelectrode studies, including noise analysis and patch-clamp recordings, provide additional information about the kinetic properties of abnormal acetylcholine receptor channels.

New insights gained through molecular genetics have also influenced the classification of the Charcot-Marie-Tooth (CMT) or hereditary sensorimotor neuropathies (HSMN).[30] First categorized phenotypically by common clinical, electrophysiologic, and histopathologic nerve findings and patterns of inheritance, three genes have since been identified: peripheral myelin protein 22 (*PMP22*), peripheral nerve protein ($P_0$), and *connexin 32*, located on chromosomes 17, 1, and the X-chromosome, respectively. Others have yet to be defined on chromosome 3 and 8. Locus heterogeneity resulting from defects in either the *PMP22* or $P_0$ gene leads to phenotypic differences due to the involvement of different gene products. Different point mutations in the *PMP22* gene likewise accord phenotypic heterogeneity

---

**TABLE 20–5. Mitochondrial Encephalomyopathies of Known Transmission**

| DISEASE | mtDNA MUTATION | MODE OF INHERITANCE | DNA DEFECT |
|---------|----------------|---------------------|------------|
| Kearns-Sayre syndrome | Deletion | Sporadic | |
| PEO | Deletion | Sporadic | |
| | Point mutation | Maternal | tRNA$^{\text{Leu (UUR)}}$ |
| | | | tRNA$^{\text{Asn}}$ |
| | Multiple deletions | AD | tRNA$^{\text{Leu}}$ |
| PEO, myopathy, sudden death | Point mutation | Maternal | tRNA$^{\text{Leu}}$ |
| MELAS | Point mutation | Maternal | tRNA$^{\text{Lys}}$ |
| MERRF | Point mutation | Maternal | tRNA$^{\text{Lys}}$ |
| MERRF/MELAS | Point mutation | Maternal | ATPase6 |
| NARP | Point mutation | Maternal | ATPase6 |
| MILS | Point mutation | Maternal | tRNA$^{\text{Leu}}$ |
| Myopathy | Duplication | Sporadic | tRNA$^{\text{Pro}}$ |
| | Multiple deletions | AR, AD | |
| MIMyCa | Point mutation A-G | Maternal | tRNA$^{\text{Leu}}$ |
| Multisystem cardiomyopathy | Point mutation | Maternal | tRNA$^{\text{Ile}}$ |
| Fatal congenital multisystem | Point mutation | Maternal | tRNA$^{\text{Thr}}$ |
| LHON | Point mutation T-C, G-A, A-G | Maternal | ND1, ND2, III, ND4, ND5, ND6, Cytb |
| DAD | Point mutation A-G | Maternal | Cox1, Cox |
| | Duplication | Maternal | |
| Progressive encephalomyopathy | Multiple deletions | AD | tRNA$^{\text{Leu}}$ |
| Familial recurrent myoglobinuria | Multiple deletions | AR | |
| MEPOP or MNGIE | Multiple deletions | AR | |
| Fatal infantile myopathy | Severe depletion | | |
| Myopathy of childhood | Partial depletion | | |

AD, Autosomal dominant; AR, autosomal recessive; DAD, diabetes and deafness; LHON, Leber's hereditary optic neuropathy; MELAS, mitochondrial myopathy with lactic acidosis and strokelike episodes; MEPOP, mitochondrial encephalomyopathy, polyneuropathy, ophthalmoplegia, and pseudoobstruction; MERRF, myoclonic epilepsy with ragged-red fibers; MILS, maternally inherited Leigh syndrome; MIMyCa, maternally inherited myopathy and cardiomyopathy; MNGIE, mitochondrial neuropathy, gastrointestinal disorder, and encephalopathy; NARP, neuropathy, ataxia, retinitis pigmentosa; PEO, progressive external ophthalmoplegia.

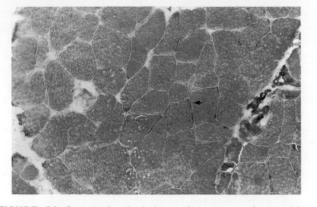

**FIGURE 20–8.** Mitochondrial abnormalities in a syndrome of late-onset mitochondrial myopathy presenting with progressive proximal weakness and wasting. A Gomori trichrome-stained section shows ragged red fibers recognized by myofibers with increased subsarcolemmal and intermyofibrillar membrane material (*arrow*).

within CMT-1A, as does the dosage of the gene—for example, when two copies of the *PMP22* result in the normal state and a triple dose leads to expression of the abnormal phenotype. Sporadic cases of either CMT-1A or CMT-1B usually prove to be due to new mutations in their respective genes.

A decade of intense research in molecular genetics has also begun to unravel the nature of the clinical diversity of familial MND. There are several different types of progressive SMA, classified clinically as types 1 to 3 by virtue of the age at onset, with the most lethal forms in early infancy (type 1 or Wernig-Hoffman syndrome). All demonstrate linkage to chromosome 5q, with differences in age of onset and distribution of weakness ascribed to allelic heterogeneity. Linkage of autosomal recessive (AR)-SMA was ascribed to chromosome 5q11.2-13.3, with major deletions in patients with SMA type 1 and no deletions or smaller deletions in patients with mild SMA (Kugelberg-Welander syndrome).[25] Two novel genes, also at 5q13, called the neuronal apoptosis inhibitory protein (NAIP) and the survival motor neuron gene (SMN), contain deletions in the majority of patients with SMA.[29,34] There are also three forms of adult-onset $GM_2$ gangliosidosis that can have a clinical phenotype similar to that of SMA: (1) late-onset Tay-Sachs disease, caused by deficiency of the alpha subunit of Hex A; (2) Sandhoff's disease, caused by deficiency of the Hex A and B beta subunits; and (3) AB variant syndrome, caused by deficiency in $GM_2$ protein activation. Two disorders, one that appears in childhood, Fazio-Londe syndrome, and the other seen in midlife, X-linked recessive bulbospinal muscular atrophy (Kennedy disease) are associated with prominent bulbar weakness. Approximately 10% of cases of ALS demonstrate autosomal dominant (AD) inheritance. Familial ALS (FALS-AD) is indistinguishable from sporadic ALS. The gene locus for FALS-AD has been identified on chromosome 21q, and several mutations have also been reported in the gene for Cu/Zn superoxide dismutase that are coinherited with FALS-AD in several families.[32]

## REFERENCES

1. American Academy of Neurology. Clinical autonomic testing: reports of the Therapeutics and Technology Assessment Subcommittee of the American Academy of Neurology. *Neurology.* 1996;46:873-880.
2. Blexrud MD, Windebank AL, Daube JR. Long-term follow-up of 121 patients with benign fasciculations. *Ann Neurol.* 1993;34:622-625.
3. Bodner R, Younger DS. Diabetic muscle infarction. *Muscle Nerve.* 1994; 17:949-950.
4. Buchtal F, Rosenflack P, Erminio F. Motor unit territory and fiber density in myopathies. *Neurology.* 1960;10:398-408.
5. Corbo M, Abouzhahr MK, Latov N, et al. Motor nerve biopsy studies in motor neuropathy and motor neuron disease. *Muscle Nerve.* 1997;20: 15-21.
6. Dalakas MC. Basic aspects of neuroimmunology as they relate to immunotherapeutic targets: present and future prospects. *Ann Neurol.* 1995;37(suppl 1):S2-S8.
7. DiMauro S, Moraes CT. Mitochondrial encephalomyopathies. *Arch Neurol.* 1993;50:1197-1208.
8. DiMauro S, Wallace DS, eds. *Mitochondrial DNA in Human Pathology.* New York: Raven Press; 1993.
9. Engel AG, Ohno K, Milone M, Sine SM. Congenital myasthenic syndromes caused by mutations in acetylcholine receptor genes. *Neurology.* 1997;48(suppl 5):S28-S36.
10. Fetell MR, Younger DS. Neurologic paraneoplastic syndromes. In: Rowland LP, ed. *Merritt's Textbook of Neurology.* Baltimore: Williams & Wilkins; 1995:935-945.
11. Giannini C, Dyck PJ. Ultrastructural morphometric features of human sural nerve endoneurial microvessels. *Ann Neurol.* 1994;36:408-415.
12. Gilliam TC, Brzustowicz LM, Castilla LH, et al. Genetic heterogeneity between acute and chronic forms of spinal muscular atrophy. *Nature.* 1990;345:823-825.
13. Gordon PH, Rowland LP, Younger DS, et al. Lymphoproliferative disorders and motor neuron disease: an update. *Neurology.* 1997;48:1671-1678.
14. Griffin JW, George R, Ho T. Macrophage systems in peripheral nerves: a review. *J Neuropathol Exp Neurol.* 1993;52:553-560.
15. Griggs RC, Fischbeck KH. X-linked muscular dystrophies. In: Rowland LP, DiMauro S, eds. *Handbook of Clinical Neurology.* Amsterdam: Elsevier; 1992;62:117-143.
16. Halperin J, Logigian E, Finkel M, et al. Practice parameters for the diagnosis of patients with Lyme borreliosis (Lyme disease). *Neurology.* 1996; 46:619-627.
17. Hays AP. Separation of motor neuron diseases from pure motor neuropathies: pathology. *Adv Neurol.* 1991;56:385-398.
18. Hays AP, Roxas A, Sadiq SA, et al. A monoclonal IgA in a patient with amyotrophic lateral sclerosis reacts with neurofilaments and surface antigen on neuroblastoma cells. *J Neuropathol Exp Neurol.* 1990;49:383-398.
19. Hays AP, Younger DS. Muscle and nerve biopsy. In: Rowland LP, ed. *Merritt's Textbook of Neurology.* Baltimore: Williams & Wilkins; 1995: 97-100.
20. Johnston W, Karpati G, Carpenter S, et al. Late-onset mitochondrial myopathy. *Ann Neurol.* 1995;37:16-23.
21. Kaminski HJ, Suarez JI, Ruff RL. Neuromuscular junction physiology in myasthenia gravis: isoforms of the acetylcholine receptor in extraocular muscle and the contribution of sodium channels to the safety factor. *Neurology.* 1997;48(suppl 5):S8-S17.
22. Kyle RA. Monoclonal gammopathy of undetermined significance: natural history in 24 cases. *Am J Med.* 1978;64:814-826.
23. Latov NL. Pathogenesis and therapy of neuropathies associated with monoclonal gammopathies. *Ann Neurol.* 1995;37(suppl 1):S32-S42.
24. Latov N, Hays AP, Donofrio PD, et al. Monoclonal IgM with unique specificity to gangliosides $GM_1$ and to lactose-N-tetrose associated with human motor neuron disease. *Neurology.* 1990;38:763-768.
25. Lefebvre S, Burglen L, Reboullet S, et al. Identification and characterization of a spinal muscular atrophy determining gene. *Cell.* 1995;80: 155-165.
26. Lennon VA. Serologic profile of myasthenia gravis and distinction from the Lambert-Eaton myasthenic syndrome. *Neurology.* 1997;48:S23-S27.
27. McKusick VA. *Mendelian Inheritance in Man.* 10th ed. Baltimore: Johns Hopkins University Press; 1992.
28. Medical Research Council of the United Kingdom. *Aids to the Examination of the Nervous System.* United Kingdom: Pendragon; 1978.
29. Melki J, Abdelhak S, Burglen L, et al. De novo and inherited deletions of the 5q13 region in spinal muscular atrophy. *Science.* 1990;264:1474-1477.
30. Mendell JR. Charcot-Marie-Tooth neuropathies and related disorders. *Semin Neurol.* 1998;18:41-62.
31. Prasad A, Younger DS. Lyme neuroborreliosis. *Drugs for Today.* 1998;34: 537-540.

32. Rosen DR, Siddique T, Patterson D, et al. Mutations in Cu/Zn superoxide dismutase gene are associated with familial amyotrophic lateral sclerosis. *Nature.* 1993;362:59-62.

33. Rosoklija G, Dwork AJ, Younger DS, et al. Local activation of the complement system in endoneurial microvessels of diabetic neuropathy. In preparation.

34. Roy N, Mahadevan MS, McLean M, et al. The gene for neuronal apoptosis inhibitory protein is partially deleted in individuals with spinal muscular atrophy. *Cell.* 1995;80:167-178.

35. Sadiq SA, van den Berg LH, Kilidireas K, et al. Human monoclonal antineurofilament antibody cross-reacts with a neuronal surface protein. *J Neurosci Res.* 1991;29:319-325.

36. Sanders DB. The electrodiagnosis of myasthenia gravis. *Ann N Y Acad Sci.* 1987;505:539-555.

37. Santoro M, Thomas FP, Fink ME, et al. IgM deposits at nodes of Ranvier in a patient with amyotrophic lateral sclerosis, anti-GM₁ antibodies and multifocal motor conduction block. *Ann Neurol.* 1990;28:373-377.

38. Santoro M, Uncini A, Corbo M, et al. Conduction abnormalities induced by sera of patients with multifocal motor neuropathy and anti-GM₁ antibodies. *Muscle Nerve.* 1993;16:610-615.

39. Yasuda H, Dyck PJ. Abnormalities of endoneurial microvessels and sural nerve pathology in diabetic neuropathy. *Neurology.* 1987;37:20-28.

40. Younger DS. Historical notes: nerve models, role models, reminiscences, and a tribute to Robert E. Lovelace, MD, FRCP. *Semin Neurol.* 1998;18:145-149.

41. Younger DS, Dalmau J, Inghirami G, et al. Anti-Hu associated peripheral nerve and muscle microvasculitis. *Neurology.* 1994;44:181-183.

42. Younger DS, Gordon PH. Diagnosis in neuromuscular diseases. *Neurol Clin.* 1996;14:135-168.

43. Younger DS, Kass RM. Vasculitis and the nervous system. *Neurol Clin.* 1997;15(4):737-758.

44. Younger DS, Leung DK. Neuromuscular diseases, 1: overview. *Drugs for Today.* 1996;32:501-507.

45. Younger DS, Rosoklija G, Hays AP. Peripheral nerve immunohistochemistry in diabetic neuropathy. *Semin Neurol.* 1996;16:139-142.

46. Younger DS, Rosoklija G, Hays AP. Diabetic peripheral neuropathy. *Semin Neurol.* 1998;18:95-104.

47. Younger DS, Rosoklija G, Hays AP, Latov N. Diabetic peripheral neuropathy: a clinicopathologic and immunohistochemical analysis of sural nerve biopsies. *Muscle Nerve.* 1996;19:722-727.

48. Younger DS, Rowland LP, Hays AP, et al. Lymphoma, motor neuron disease, and amyotrophic lateral sclerosis. *Ann Neurol.* 1991;29:78-86.

49. Younger DS, Rowland LP, Latov N, et al. Motor neuron diseases and ALS: relation of high CSF protein content to paraproteinemia and clinical syndromes. *Neurology.* 1990;40:595-599.

50. Younger DS, Worrall BB, Penn AS. Myasthenia gravis: historical perspective and overview. *Neurology.* 1997;48(suppl 5):S1-S7.

# 21

# Electromyography Waveform Analysis

*Barbara E. Shapiro and David C. Preston*

Nerve conduction studies and needle electromyography (EMG) play a pivotal role in the evaluation of patients with neuromuscular disorders.[29] This chapter provides an overview of the needle EMG study, including analysis of insertional and spontaneous activity with the muscle at rest and voluntary motor unit action potential (MUAP) morphology and firing patterns with the muscle contracted. Nearly all spontaneous waveforms and voluntary MUAPs can be properly identified by defining the morphology, stability, and firing pattern of the waveform.[29]

## OVERVIEW OF ELECTROMYOGRAPHY

### PHYSIOLOGY

The basic component of the peripheral nervous system is the motor unit, defined as a motor neuron, its axon, and associated neuromuscular junctions (NMJs) and muscle fibers[23] (Fig. 21–1). The extracellular needle EMG recording of a motor unit is the MUAP.[2] Under normal circumstances, when an axon is depolarized, all muscle fibers of the motor unit depolarize more or less simultaneously, with any variability due to differences in the length of the terminal axons and NMJ transmission times.

During the needle EMG examination, each MUAP recorded represents the extracellular compound potential of the muscle fibers of a motor unit, weighted heavily toward the fibers nearest to the needle.[18] This extracellular potential is $\frac{1}{10}$ to $\frac{1}{100}$ the amplitude of the actual transmembrane potential and falls off rapidly as the distance between the needle and the membrane increases.[30]

The "size principle" governs many of the properties of motor units.[20] The size of the motor neuron is directly related to (1) the size of the axon, (2) the thickness of the myelin sheath, (3) the conduction velocity of the axon, (4) the threshold to depolarization, and (5) the metabolic type of muscle fibers that are innervated. With voluntary contraction, the smallest type I motor units with the lower thresholds and connections to type I, slow-twitch muscle fibers fire first.[20] As contraction increases, progressively larger motor units begin to fire until the largest type II motor units with connections to type II, fast-twitch muscle fibers fire, with maximum contraction. During routine needle EMG, most MUAPs analyzed are thus the smaller motor units that innervate type I muscle fibers.

### TECHNICAL FACTORS

Various technical factors should be kept in mind when needle EMG studies are performed. Cool limb temperature can result in longer duration and higher amplitude MUAPs and a corresponding increase in the number of phases.[8] Age also affects many parameters on the needle EMG study, most prominently MUAP duration.[2] As an individual ages, MUAP duration increases. In childhood this increase in duration is due to the physiologic increase of muscle fiber and motor unit size as the child grows. In later life the normal aging process results in a drop-out of motor units, with compensatory reinnervation, which results in prolongation of the motor unit.[2] Finally, standardized filter settings should always be used, with results compared only to normal values based on studies using the same filter settings.[4,33]

## NEEDLE ELECTROMYOGRAPHY EXAMINATION

Once a muscle has been selected for study and the needle insertion point has been located, the needle is quickly inserted into the muscle in a relaxed state. The patient then briefly activates the muscle to confirm that the placement is correct, resulting in sharp MUAPs with minimal activation. If the MUAPs do not sound sharp, the needle placement is slightly adjusted.

## BASIC ELECTROMYOGRAPHY: ANALYSIS OF INSERTIONAL AND SPONTANEOUS ACTIVITY

The needle examination begins with assessment of insertional and spontaneous activity with the muscle at rest, after which voluntary contraction of MUAPs and their firing pattern is assessed. To assess insertional activity, the sweep speed is set at 10 ms per division and the sensitivity is set at 50 μV per division. In general, all four quadrants are sampled with each needle insertion. When a quick needle movement is made through muscle, there is a brief burst of mus-

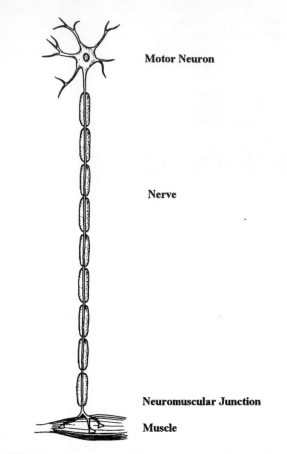

**FIGURE 21–1.** Motor unit. The basic component of the peripheral nervous system is the motor unit, which includes the individual motor neuron, its axon, and associated neuromuscular junctions and muscle fibers.

cle fiber depolarizations, usually lasting no more than 300 ms after needle movement ceases, known as *normal insertional activity*. If the activity lasts longer than 300 ms, *increased insertional activity* is present. If potentials persist longer than 3 seconds, this is considered *spontaneous activity*. Increased insertional and spontaneous activity may be seen in both neurogenic and myopathic disorders. Rarely, insertional activity is decreased, when muscle has been replaced by fat or connective tissue. Spontaneous activity is always abnormal, except when the needle is inserted near the NMJ. In the end-plate zone, end-plate potentials are normally present as long as the needle remains in this position.

The ability to identify abnormal spontaneous activity is one of the most crucial aspects of the needle EMG examination. When a spontaneous waveform is encountered on the needle EMG study, it can usually be correctly identified when analyzed along three major dimensions: morphology, stability, and firing characteristics.

## MORPHOLOGY AND SOURCE GENERATORS

The morphology of a waveform refers to its size, shape (amplitude, duration, number of phases), and initial deflection. By characterizing the morphology of the potential, one can usually identify its source generator (Fig. 21–2).[29] Several source generators can be distinguished, including (1) the NMJ (end-plate zone), (2) a single muscle fiber, (3) the terminal axon twig, (4) a motor neuron or axon, and (5) multiple muscle fibers linked together. Once the source gen-

erator is identified, along with the stability and the firing characteristics of the potential, the type of spontaneous discharge can usually be determined.

## Neuromuscular Junction

Potentials that arise at the NMJ (end-plate zone) are miniature end-plate potentials (mepps).[3,16] They are small in amplitude and monophasic, with an initial negative deflection (Fig. 21–2A). These potentials result from the spontaneous exocytosis of individual quanta of acetylcholine that traverse the NMJ, resulting in subthreshold end-plate potentials. They are recorded when the EMG needle is placed near the end-plate zone and are normal spontaneous discharges referred to as *end-plate noise*.

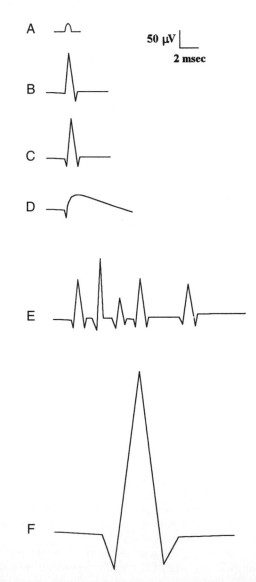

**FIGURE 21–2.** Spontaneous waveform morphologies (*top to bottom*). **A,** Miniature end-plate potential (monophasic negative); **B,** muscle fiber action potential, brief spike morphology (initial negative, diphasic); **C,** muscle fiber action potential, brief spike morphology (initial positive, triphasic); **D,** muscle fiber action potential, positive wave morphology (initial positive, slow negative); **E,** multiple different muscle fiber action potentials linked together; **F,** motor unit action potential (note the longer duration and higher amplitude compared to muscle fiber action potentials above). (From Preston DC, Shapiro BE. *Electromyography and Neuromuscular Disorders: Clinical-Electrophysiologic Correlations.* Boston: Butterworth-Heinemann; 1998.)

## Single Muscle Fiber or Terminal Axon Twig

When a single muscle fiber depolarizes to threshold, a muscle fiber action potential (MFAP) is generated. *The potential from a single muscle fiber can take on only one of two shapes, either a brief spike or a positive wave morphology.* Two types of brief spike morphologies are recognized: (1) a biphasic spike with an initial negative deflection and (2) a triphasic spike with an initial positive deflection, depending on where the depolarization begins. If the depolarization begins under the recording needle electrode, the potential is biphasic, with an initial negative deflection followed by a short positive phase (Fig. 21–2B). This occurs when the EMG needle irritates the terminal axon twigs near the end-plate zone, causing a nerve twig action potential to depolarize and propagate across the NMJ, resulting in a single MFAP. This potential, known as an end-plate spike,[9] is the normal result of irritation of the terminal axon twig near the end-plate zone. Note the initial negative deflection of this potential as well as mepps, both of which are recorded with the needle at or near the end-plate zone.

The other type of brief spike, a triphasic potential with an initial positive deflection, occurs when a muscle fiber depolarizes spontaneously at a distance from the needle. In this case the waveform has an initial positive deflection as the depolarization moves toward the needle, followed by a negative phase as it passes beneath the needle, and then a final positive deflection as it moves away from the needle (Fig. 21–2C). This type of brief spike, known as a fibrillation potential,[13] is low in amplitude (10 to 100 μV) and brief in duration (1 to 5 ms).

Depending on needle position to a muscle fiber, a single MFAP can also assume a positive wave morphology. These positive waves are biphasic potentials with an initial brief positive phase followed by a long negative phase (Fig. 21–2D).

## Motor Neuron or Axon

Spontaneous discharges that arise from motor neurons or their axons have the morphology of a MUAP, although they arise spontaneously (Fig. 21–2F). These potentials include fasciculations, tetany, myokymic discharges, neuromyotonic discharges, and cramps. It is important to note that although these potentials have the morphology of MUAPs, they are not under voluntary control. They are best thought of as lying along a spectrum of abnormal spontaneous MUAPs, differentiated from one another by differences in their stability and firing patterns.[29] The actual morphology of the MUAP depends on whether the underlying motor unit is normal or pathologic. If normal, the MUAP typically has between 2 and 4 phases, a duration of 5 to 15 ms, and a variable amplitude, depending on the proximity of the needle to the motor unit. The initial phase is usually positive. If the motor unit is pathologic, the number of phases, duration, and amplitude may be abnormal. In general, MUAPs are easily differentiated from single MFAPs by the longer duration and generally larger amplitude of MUAPs.

## Multiple Muscle Fibers Linked Together

The last waveform morphology to recognize is that of individual muscle fibers that are time-linked together, such as occurs in complex repetitive discharges.[14,15,31] Although a MUAP also represents many muscle fibers linked together, muscle fibers in a motor unit fire more or less synchronously and summate to create a potential that is 5 to 15 ms in duration. In contrast, the multiple muscle fibers in a complex repetitive discharge fire consecutively. This creates a distinctive morphology: individual spikes that are time-linked together (Fig. 21–2E). These abnormal spontaneous discharges occur in chronic denervating conditions, either neurogenic or myopathic.

### STABILITY

Assessing the stability of a spontaneous potential can be very helpful in identifying the waveform. Most spontaneous discharges have a relatively stable morphology. However, in some potentials the morphology changes between potentials. For example, they may wax and wane, decrement, or abruptly change. Myotonic discharges are MFAPs that wax and wane in amplitude, whereas fibrillations and positive waves are MFAPs that fire regularly. In contrast, neuromyotonic discharges are MUAPs that distinctly decrement in amplitude. Although complex repetitive discharges are generally completely stable, they may occasionally change abruptly in morphology.

### FIRING CHARACTERISTICS

A spontaneous potential can often be identified by its firing characteristics, including both its firing pattern and firing rate. For example, the firing pattern may be regular or irregular. If regular, it can be perfectly regular (as in complex repetitive discharges) or predominantly regular (as in fibrillations and positive waves). If the firing pattern is irregular, it may take on a waxing and waning quality (as in myotonic discharges), a sputtering quality (as in end-plate spikes), or a decremental quality (as in neuromyotonic discharges). The firing pattern can also take on a bursting pattern—relative electrical silence between groups of discharges. This pattern can be seen in myokymic discharges and tremor. The firing rate is also important. If the firing rate is very slow (<4 to 5 Hz), the discharge must be spontaneous rather than voluntary since one cannot activate a motor unit slower than 4 to 5 Hz. On the other hand, if the firing rate is very fast (150 to 250 Hz), only certain types of spontaneous discharges can fire this quickly, such as cramps or neuromyotonic discharges.[21,32]

Once the morphology, stability, and firing characteristics of a spontaneous waveform are analyzed, the potential can usually be identified. Table 21–1 summarizes the morphology, stability, and firing characteristics of the common spontaneous potentials seen during the needle EMG.

### NORMAL SPONTANEOUS ACTIVITY

Potentials that occur at the NMJ (i.e., in the end-plate zone) constitute normal spontaneous activity. Two types of potentials are seen: end-plate noise and end-plate spikes. These potentials are generally found near the center of the muscle belly. The patient often experiences pain when the needle is in the end-plate zone. It is crucial to be able to distinguish these potentials, which are normal, from all other forms of spontaneous activity encountered on the EMG, which are abnormal.

### End-Plate Noise

These are low-amplitude, monophasic, negative potentials that fire irregularly at 20 to 40 Hz (Fig. 21–3A).

**TABLE 21–1. Spontaneous Activity**

| POTENTIAL | SOURCE GENERATOR/MORPHOLOGY | STABILITY | FIRING RATE | FIRING PATTERN |
|---|---|---|---|---|
| End-plate noise | Miniature end-plate potential (monophasic negative) | | 20–40 Hz | Irregular (hissing) |
| End-plate spike | Muscle fiber initiated by terminal axonal twig (brief spike, diphasic, initial negative) | | 5–50 Hz | Irregular (sputtering) |
| Fibrillation | Muscle fiber (brief spike, diphasic or triphasic, initial positive) | Stable | 0.5–10 Hz (occas. up to 30 Hz) | Regular |
| Positive wave | Muscle fiber (diphasic, initial positive, slow negative) | Stable | 0.5–10 Hz (occas. up to 30 Hz) | Regular |
| Myotonia | Muscle fiber (brief spike, initial positive, or positive wave) | Waxing and waning amplitude | 20–150 Hz | Waxing and waning |
| Complex repetitive discharge | Multiple muscle fibers time-linked together | Usually stable; may change in discrete jumps | 5–100 Hz | Perfectly regular (unless overdriven) |
| Fasciculation | Motor unit (motor neuron/axon) | | Low (0.1–10 Hz) | Irregular |
| Myokymia | Motor unit (motor neuron/axon) | | 1–5 Hz (interburst) 5–60 Hz (intraburst) | Bursting |
| Cramp | Motor unit (motor neuron/axon) | | High (20–150 Hz) | Interference pattern or several individual units |
| Neuromyotonia | Motor unit (motor neuron/axon) | Decrementing amplitude | Very high (150–250 Hz) | Waning |

From Preston DC, Shapiro BE. *Electromyography and Neuromuscular Disorders: Clinical-Electrophysiologic Correlations.* Boston: Butterworth-Heinemann; 1998.

Their distinctive morphology identifies their source generator as the NMJ. They are recognized not only by their morphology and firing pattern but also by their characteristic "seashell" sound on EMG. These potentials represent mepps and are frequently seen in association with end-plate spikes.

### End-Plate Spikes ("Nerve Potentials")

These are low-amplitude, biphasic, initially negative MFAPs that fire irregularly up to 50 Hz (Fig. 21–3B). They have a characteristic "sputtering" or "crackling" sound on EMG. These potentials are thought to occur secondary to irritation of the terminal axon twig by the EMG needle, inducing a nerve action potential that generates a MFAP. They are commonly seen in association with end-plate noise. Note that end-plate spikes are differentiated from fibrillation potentials (which are also brief spikes) by their initial negative deflection and their irregular firing rate.

### ABNORMAL SPONTANEOUS ACTIVITY: MUSCLE FIBER ACTION POTENTIALS

Any spontaneous activity outside of the end-plate zone that lasts longer than 3 seconds is abnormal. Such activity may be seen at rest, or it may be induced by needle movement, muscle contraction, muscle percussion, or electrical stimulation.

### Fibrillation Potentials

These are low-amplitude (typically 10 to 100 μV), initially positive, brief spike potentials, typically 1 to 5 ms in duration (Fig. 21–4A). They represent the spontaneous depolarizations of single muscle fibers, derived from the extracellular recording of a single muscle fiber. Their firing pattern is regular, usually at a rate of 0.5 to 10 Hz but occasionally up to 30 Hz. These potentials often slow down just before stopping. They have a distinctive sound, like "rain on a roof," on EMG. Fibrillations are electrophysiologic

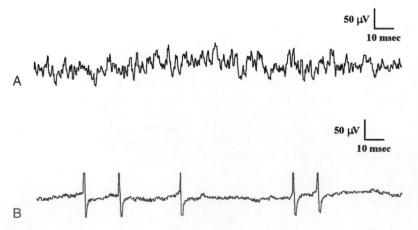

50 μV | 10 msec

50 μV | 10 msec

**FIGURE 21–3.** **A,** End-plate noise. These low-amplitude, high-frequency, predominantly monophasic negative potentials are the EMG correlate of miniature end-plate potentials. **B,** End-plate spikes. These are muscle fiber potentials that result from needle-induced irritation of the terminal axon twigs near the end-plate. Their initial negative deflection, brief duration, biphasic morphology, and irregular, sputtering firing pattern differentiate them from fibrillation potentials.

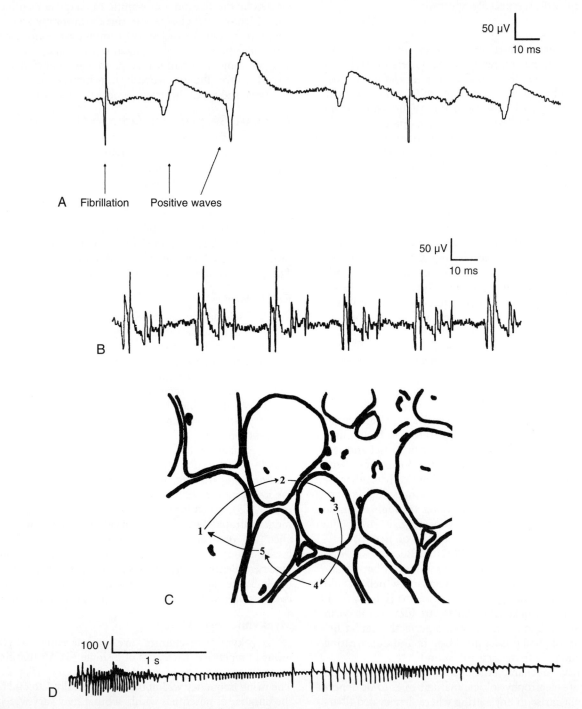

**FIGURE 21—4.** **A,** Fibrillations and positive waves. These are spontaneous depolarizations of single muscle fibers. Note the initial positive deflection, brief duration, and triphasic morphology of fibrillations. Note also the initial positive deflection and the slow negative phase of positive waves. **B,** Complex repetitive discharges. Note the multiple spikes within the complex, each of which represents a different single muscle fiber. These potentials fire in a perfectly repetitive manner. **C,** Pathophysiology of a complex repetitive discharge. Ephaptic transmission occurs from one denervated muscle fiber to an adjacent one. If the original pacemaker is reactivated, a circus movement is formed without an intervening synapse. **D,** Myotonic discharges. These result from the spontaneous depolarization of a single muscle fiber. Note the waxing and waning of both amplitude and frequency. (*B* and *C* from Preston DC, Shapiro BE. *Electromyography and Neuromuscular Disorders: Clinical-Electrophysiologic Correlations.* Boston: Butterworth-Heinemann; 1998. *D* from Sethi RK, Thompson LL. *The Electromyographer's Handbook.* 2nd ed. Boston: Little, Brown; 1989.)

markers of denervation. They can be seen in both neurogenic and some myopathic disorders (especially toxic, inflammatory, and some dystrophic myopathies) and rarely in severe NMJ disorders, especially botulism.

## Positive Waves

Positive waves, like fibrillations, are also markers of denervation; likewise, they represent the spontaneous depolarization of a single muscle fiber. They have a brief initial positivity followed by a long negative phase (Fig. 21–4A). The amplitude is variable (usually 10 to 100 μV, occasionally up to 3 mV), and, like fibrillations, their firing pattern is regular, usually with a rate of 0.5 to 10 Hz but occasionally up to 30 Hz. Their slow negative phase and long duration confer a distinguishing "dull pop" sound on EMG. Although MUAPs recorded at a distance will occasionally have a positive wave morphology, their firing pattern is irregular. Positive waves and fibrillations usually occur together, although occasionally positive waves are seen in isolation, early in denervation.

Whether a single MFAP assumes a brief spike (i.e., fibrillation) or a positive wave morphology depends on the position of the needle in relationship to the muscle fiber. Positive waves are thought to be generated when the EMG needle deforms an irritable muscle fiber, inducing a denervating potential at a distance down the fiber, which propagates to the area of the needle but not beyond. This might explain why positive waves are occasionally seen earlier than fibrillations: the presence of the needle is required to help generate these potentials.

## Complex Repetitive Discharges

Complex repetitive discharges (CRDs) are recognized on EMG as high-frequency (typically 20 to 150 Hz), multiserrated repetitive discharges with an abrupt onset and termination (Fig. 21–4B). They occur when a single denervated muscle fiber depolarizes and spreads ephaptically to adjacent denervated fibers. If the original depolarizing muscle fiber (the pacemaker cell) is then reactivated through ephaptic spread, a recurrent discharge develops (Fig. 21–4C). The pacemaker may be a fibrillation potential or may be activated by needle movement or a MUAP. Because the discharge spreads ephaptically from one muscle fiber to another, there is no intervening synapse, which would normally give rise to some jitter and thereby variability from one potential to the next. Thus CRDs are identical in form from one discharge to the next, with a perfectly regular firing pattern. Individual phases may drop in and out, creating an abrupt change in frequency and sound.

CRDs have a characteristic "machinelike" sound on EMG. They are electrophysiologic markers of chronic denervation and may arise in any setting where denervated fibers lie adjacent to other denervated fibers. In neuropathic diseases, CRDs occur where denervation is followed by reinnervation, with subsequent denervation (i.e., grouped atrophy). In myopathic disorders, CRDs occur where there is inflammation or muscle fiber splitting.

## Myotonic Discharges

A myotonic discharge is the spontaneous discharge of a single muscle fiber, just as are fibrillations and positive waves (Fig. 21–4D). As such, the morphology is either a brief spike or a positive wave. In contrast, however, there is a character-

istic waxing and waning of both amplitude and frequency.[34] The firing rate is generally between 20 and 150 Hz. Myotonic discharges have a distinctive "dive-bomber" sound on EMG, created by the waxing and waning of frequency and amplitude. Myotonic discharges are most commonly seen in the myotonic muscle disorders (myotonic dystrophy, myotonia congenita, paramyotonia congenita), but they can also be seen in some myopathies (acid maltase deficiency, polymyositis, myotubular myopathy), in hyperkalemic periodic paralysis, and rarely in severe denervation as brief runs.

## ABNORMAL SPONTANEOUS ACTIVITY: MOTOR UNIT ACTION POTENTIALS

Abnormal spontaneous activity may also occur in the form of motor unit (as opposed to muscle fiber) action potentials. In each case the source generator is the motor neuron or its axon, and the potential is an involuntary firing MUAP. These potentials can be thought of as occurring along a spectrum, from MUAPs firing singly, as in fasciculations, to those firing repetitively as in doublets or triplets, to those firing in a bursting pattern, as in myokymic discharges. The disorders they accompany are neurogenic.

## Fasciculations

A fasciculation is the spontaneous, involuntary discharge of a single motor unit[12] (Fig. 21–5A). The source generator is the motor neuron or its axon up to the point where its terminal branches begin. These motor units are not under voluntary control, and unlike voluntary MUAPs, they tend to fire slowly and irregularly, generally between 0.1 and 10 Hz. They usually have the morphology of a simple MUAP, but they can be large and complex if they represent a pathologic motor unit.

Fasciculations are recognized clinically as individual brief muscle twitches. Pathologic fasciculations, associated with weakness and wasting, are seen in several disorders affecting the lower motor neuron, including amyotrophic lateral sclerosis (ALS), radiculopathies, polyneuropathies, and entrapment neuropathies. Although most individuals will experience an occasional fasciculation, known as "benign" fasciculations, these are not associated with muscle wasting or weakness. Benign fasciculations tend to fire quickly and repetitively at the same site, as opposed to fasciculations seen in disease states, which tend to fire more slowly and randomly.

## Myokymic Discharges

Myokymic discharges are spontaneous, rhythmic, grouped repetitive discharges of a single MUAP that fire in a bursting pattern (i.e., grouped fasciculations)[27] (Fig. 21–5B). The firing frequency within bursts is typically 5 to 60 Hz, and the number of potentials within a burst may vary widely and change from burst to burst. The firing frequency between bursts is much slower (typically <2 Hz). Myokymic discharges are recognized on EMG by their distinctive bursting pattern of MUAPs that produce a characteristic "marching" sound on EMG. It is best to use a long sweep speed to appreciate their bursting pattern. Myokymic discharges are thought to originate from spontaneous depolarization or ephaptic transmission along segments of demyelinated nerve.

Clinically, myokymia is recognized as the continuous, involuntary, rippling or undulating movement of muscle. On EMG, limb myokymia may be seen in radiculopathy, en-

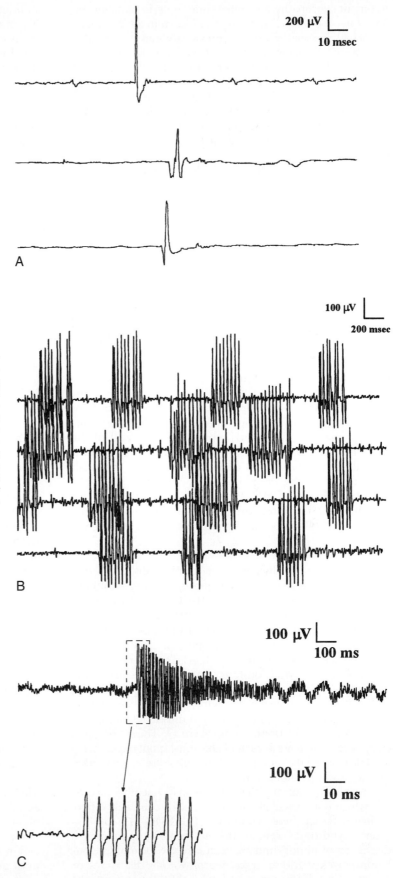

**FIGURE 21–5.** **A,** Fasciculations (*rastered traces*). Each potential has the morphology of a single MUAP. Fasciculations are recognized by their motor unit morphology and irregular, slow firing pattern. **B,** Myokymic discharges. These are involuntary grouped repetitive discharges of a single MUAP. Note the fast firing frequency within each burst and the slow firing frequency between bursts. Myokymia produces a marching sound on EMG. **C,** Neuromyotonic discharges. These are the spontaneous repetitive discharges of a single motor unit that fire at very high frequencies (150 to 250 Hz). Note the decrementing response. *Inset:* Change in sweep speed identifies each potential as the same MUAP. (From Preston DC, Shapiro BE. *Electromyography and Neuromuscular Disorders: Clinical-Electrophysiologic Correlations.* Boston: Butterworth-Heinemann; 1998.)

trapment neuropathy, and, most commonly, in radiation-induced nerve damage.[1] If myokymia is seen in a patient with a brachial plexopathy who has previously undergone radiation therapy for cancer, the myokymia strongly suggests the diagnosis of radiation-induced plexitis rather than recurrent cancer. Facial myokymia may be seen in brainstem lesions (e.g., multiple sclerosis or pontine glioma) or following radiation. A small percent of patients with Guillain-Barré syndrome may have facial myokymia. Administration of calcium can transiently decrease the generation of myokymic discharges.

Spontaneous grouped repetitive discharges can be seen in any condition associated with hypocalcemia. These discharges tend to occur in bursts of twos or threes (doublets, triplets) and are known as tetany. Distal muscles are most affected, resulting in involuntary spasms of the hands and feet (carpopedal spasms).

### Cramps

Cramps are high-frequency discharges of motor axons, resulting in painful, involuntary muscle contractions.[28] They tend to occur when a muscle is in the shortened, contracted position. They are recognized on EMG either as a full interference pattern of MUAPs with a normal morphology or as several motor units firing repetitively and sometimes irregularly at high frequencies (usually 40 to 60 Hz). They may occur as benign nocturnal or postexercise cramps or can be associated with a wide number of metabolic, endocrinologic, and neuropathic conditions. Although superficially cramps may resemble contractures seen in several of the metabolic muscle diseases, the needle EMG of a cramp is quite different from that of a contracture. Cramp potentials are generated along the motor axon, resulting in high-frequency discharges of MUAPs, and as such are nerve potentials. In contrast, contractures, a primary muscle phenomenon, are typically associated with complete electrical silence.

### Neuromyotonic Discharges

Neuromyotonic discharges are repetitive discharges of a single MUAP that fire at a high frequency (150 to 250 Hz) in a decrementing firing pattern[24] (Fig. 21–5C). They have a characteristic "pinging" sound on EMG. These are a very rare phenomenon, seen either in chronic neuropathic diseases (e.g., old polio or adult spinal muscular atrophy) or in syndromes of continuous motor unit activity (CMUA). The latter syndromes have been described variously as Isaacs' syndrome, neuromyotonia, pseudomyotonia, neurotonia, normocalcemic tetany, and continuous muscle fiber activity.[21] Affected patients present with generalized stiffness, delayed muscle relaxation, hyperhidrosis, fasciculations, and myokymia.[17] The stiffness and delay in relaxation are a result of abnormal spontaneous firing of MUAPs along the motor axon. Thus these are a nerve, rather than a muscle, phenomenon.

Although clinically the stiffness may resemble myotonia, which is a muscle phenomenon, EMG can easily differentiate between these syndromes. The EMG in neuromyotonic syndromes reveals the involuntary spontaneous discharges of motor units that can take the form of fasciculations, myokymic discharges, neuromyotonic discharges, or complete interference patterns of MUAPs. By contrast, the EMG in myotonic syndromes reveals the spontaneous discharges of muscle fibers that take the form of positive waves

or brief spike potentials. Since neuromyotonic discharges are generated along peripheral motor axons, they persist during sleep and spinal or general anesthesia. They can be diminished with distal nerve blocks and are abolished by curare. Treatment consists of phenytoin or carbamazepine. Note that neuromyotonic discharges are not seen in stiff-man syndrome, which is a disorder of spinal interneurons, that frequently is treated with diazepam. Most cases of neuromyotonia or CMUA are sporadic and are thought to have an autoimmune etiology, with antibodies directed at peripheral nerve potassium channels. Some of these cases have been reported to improve with immunosuppressive therapy. Some cases are familial, rarely with a coexistent peripheral neuropathy.

## BASIC ELECTROMYOGRAPHY: ANALYSIS OF VOLUNTARY MOTOR UNIT ACTION POTENTIALS

Once insertional and spontaneous activity have been characterized, the analysis turns to the evaluation of voluntary MUAPs. The sensitivity is changed to 200 μV per division since MUAPs are generally much larger than abnormal spontaneous waveforms, and the sweep speed is left at 10 ms per division. The patient is asked to slowly contract the muscle. With the patient minimally contracting the muscle, the needle is slightly moved until the MUAPs sound loud and crisp. The closer the needle is to the motor unit, the less intervening tissue there is to attenuate the potential, resulting in a MUAP with a higher amplitude and shorter major spike rise time.

It is only when the MUAP comes into sharp focus that its morphology can be properly evaluated. In addition, the stability and firing characteristics are also assessed. As the patient slowly increases force, both the number of MUAPs and the firing rate should increase. The number of MUAPs and their relationship to the firing rate (recruitment and activation pattern) can also be determined. After the MUAPs are assessed at one location, the needle is moved slightly within the muscle to a different site until more MUAPs come into sharp focus. Approximately 10 to 20 different MUAPs per muscle should be studied. Classifying a MUAP as normal, neuropathic, or myopathic rests on several findings, including its morphology (duration, polyphasia, amplitude), stability, and firing characteristics.

### MORPHOLOGY

MUAP morphology can be determined either quantitatively or qualitatively. Each muscle contains a range of large and small motor units. For quantitative analysis, the duration, amplitude, and number of phases are measured in 20 different MUAPs from each muscle. A mean is then computed for each measurement, and it is compared to normal control values for that particular muscle and age group. Most EMG machines currently have programs that greatly automate quantitative assessment of MUAP duration, amplitude, and phases. In general, MUAPs tend to be longer in duration in more distal muscles than in proximal muscles and in adults as opposed to children. Therefore comparison must always be made with normal control values for that particular muscle and age group. Well-trained, experienced electromyographers can usually accurately assess these MUAP parameters qualitatively by visual estimation. As the needle is moved to several locations within the muscle, approximately 20 different MUAPs are examined and qualitatively analyzed, with the findings compared to the expected normal values for that particular muscle and age group.

## Duration

MUAP duration is the parameter that best reflects the number of muscle fibers within a motor unit and is the most reliable measure to use when judging MUAP morphology.[8] It is defined as the time from the initial deflection from baseline to the final return of the MUAP to baseline (Fig. 21–6). Typical MUAP duration is between 5 and 15 ms and depends primarily on the number of muscle fibers within the motor unit and the dispersion of their depolarizations over time. Duration increases with age and also in cold temperature. In general, proximal muscles have shorter duration motor units than distal ones have. On EMG, duration correlates well with pitch. Long-duration MUAPs sound dull and thuddy, whereas short-duration MUAPs sound crisp and sharp. With experience, the sound of a long-duration vs. a short-duration MUAP is unmistakable on EMG.

## Polyphasia/Serrations/Satellite Potentials

Polyphasia is a measure of the extent to which muscle fibers within a motor unit fire synchronously.[2] The number of phases is calculated by counting the number of baseline crossings of the MUAP and adding 1 (Fig. 21–6). Normally, MUAPs have two to four phases, although up to 5% to 10% of the MUAPs in a muscle may be polyphasic. It is considered abnormal for more than 10% of the MUAPs in a muscle to be polyphasic, except in the deltoid, where up to 25% polyphasia is considered normal. Increased polyphasia is a nonspecific finding that can be seen in myopathic and neuropathic disorders. Polyphasic MUAPs have a high-frequency clicking sound on EMG.

Serrations (turns) are changes in the direction of the motor unit potential that do not cross the baseline. They have the same implication as polyphasia, indicating less synchronous firing of muscle fibers within a motor unit. Often, a serration can be changed into an additional phase with needle movement.

Satellite potentials (linked potentials, parasite potentials) are seen in early reinnervation, when muscle fibers are reinnervated by collateral sprouts from adjacent intact motor units (see Fig. 21–6). These newly formed sprouts conduct slowly, creating satellite potentials that trail behind the main MUAP. They are extremely unstable and may vary slightly in their firing rate or may block and not fire at all. As the sprout matures, the conduction velocity increases and the satellite potential fires more closely to the main potential, eventually becoming an additional phase or serration within the main MUAP complex. Satellite potentials are best appreciated when the main MUAP is put on a delay line to demonstrate that it is time-locked to the main potential.

## Amplitude

MUAP amplitude is generally measured from peak to peak of the MUAP and is usually >100 μV and <2 mV (see Fig. 21–6). Since MUAP amplitude reflects only those few fibers nearest to the needle, it varies widely among normals and is the least reliable measure of MUAP morphology.[35] MUAP amplitude depends on the proximity of the needle to the motor unit, the number of muscle fibers in a motor unit, the diameter of the muscle fibers (i.e., muscle fiber hypertrophy), and how synchronously the muscle fibers fire.[10,30] On EMG, the amplitude of MUAPs is correlated with volume.

## Major Spike

The major spike, the largest positive-to-negative component of the MUAP, usually occurs after the first positive peak (see Fig. 21–6). As the needle is moved closer to the MUAP, the major spike increases in amplitude and its rise time shortens, indicating that the needle is close to the motor unit. A sharp MUAP sound and a major spike rise time <500 μs in-

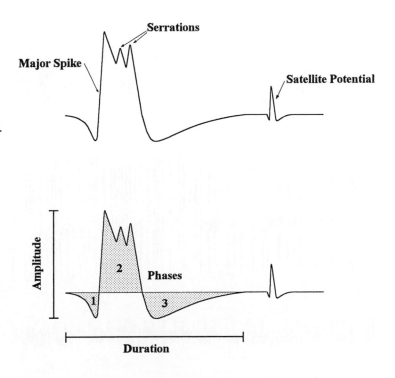

**FIGURE 21–6.** Motor unit action potential measurements. Duration is measured as the time from the initial MUAP deflection from the baseline to its final return to baseline. Amplitude is measured from peak to peak. Phases (*shaded areas*) are determined by counting the number of baseline crossings and adding 1. MUAPs are generally triphasic. Serrations are changes in the direction of the potentials that do not cross the baseline. The major spike is the largest positive-to-negative deflection and usually occurs after the first positive peak. Satellite, or linked, potentials occur following the main potential and usually denote early reinnervated muscle fibers. (From Preston DC, Shapiro BE. *Electromyography and Neuromuscular Disorders: Clinical-Electrophysiologic Correlations.* Boston: Butterworth-Heinemann; 1998.)

dicate proper needle placement. This sharp sound represents the high frequency component of the major spike, which is the highest frequency component of the MUAP.

### STABILITY

MUAPs are usually stable in morphology from potential to potential. However, if individual muscle fibers are either blocked or come to action potential at varying times, the MUAP will change in configuration with each impulse, resulting in an unstable MUAP. This may cause a change in the amplitude or number of phases between potentials. Unstable MUAPs may be seen not only in disorders of the NMJ such as myasthenia gravis but also in neuropathic and myopathic disorders accompanied by denervation. During early reinnervation, immature NMJs often fail to conduct NMJ transmission consistently, resulting in variability in end-plate transmission or intermittent blocking of transmission across some of the muscle fibers within a motor unit.

### FIRING PATTERN (ACTIVATION, RECRUITMENT, INTERFERENCE PATTERN)

One of the most important tasks for the electromyographer is to assess the number of different MUAPs firing and their relationship to the firing rate, which determines the firing pattern. Voluntary MUAPs normally fire in a semirhythmic pattern, with slight variation in the time interval between consecutive firings of the same MUAP. This is in distinct contrast to potentials that fire in a regular pattern (e.g., fibrillations and positive waves), to those with a waxing and waning quality (e.g., myotonic discharges), to those that fire in a bursting pattern (e.g., myokymic discharges), and finally to fasciculations, which have an irregular firing pattern.

In analyzing the firing pattern of MUAPs, it is important to keep in mind that there are only two ways for an individual to increase muscle force—either to increase the firing rate or to fire additional MUAPs. The ability to increase firing rate is called *activation* and is mediated through central mechanisms. Poor activation may be seen in diseases of the central nervous system (CNS) or as a manifestation of pain, poor cooperation, or functional disorders. The ability to add motor units as the firing rate increases is called *recruitment* and is mediated through peripheral mechanisms. Reduced recruitment is seen primarily in neurogenic disorders, although rarely severe end-stage myopathy may result in reduced recruitment (Fig. 21–7). In neurogenic disorders, reduced recruitment is due to loss of MUAPs, usually through axonal loss or conduction block. In end-stage myopathy, if every muscle fiber of a MUAP is lost, the number of MUAPs will also effectively decrease, leading to reduced recruitment.

Normally, one uses a combination of activation and recruitment to increase force.[22] A single motor unit begins firing semirhythmically at 4 to 5 Hz, the onset firing frequency of a motor unit under voluntary control.[25,26] As one attempts to increase force, two things take place: the first motor unit increases its firing rate to approximately 10 Hz, and then a second motor unit begins to fire. This process continues, with additional motor units being recruited about every 5 Hz as the firing rate increases, up to tetanic fusion frequency of about 50 Hz. Thus the ratio of firing frequency to the number of different MUAPs firing is approximately 5:1.[11] Accordingly, by the time the first MUAP reaches a firing frequency of 10 Hz, a second MUAP should begin to fire, and by 15 Hz, a third unit should fire, maintaining an approximate 5:1 ratio of firing rate to the number of different MUAPs firing. When MUAPs fire at maximal contraction, several MUAPs overlap to create an *interference pattern* in which no single potential can be distinguished. For most

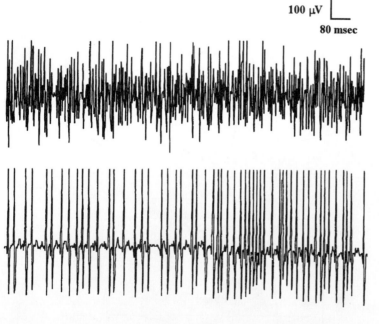

100 μV

80 msec

**FIGURE 21–7.** Interference patterns. *Top trace:* normal; *middle trace:* neurogenic; *bottom trace:* myopathic. In each case the patient is asked to maximally contract. In normals, multiple MUAPs fire during maximal contraction so that individual units are difficult to differentiate. In neurogenic recruitment, a decreased number of MUAPs fire at a high frequency, creating an incomplete interference pattern. In myopathic recruitment, a normal number of MUAPs fire, but the interference pattern consists of short-duration, small-amplitude MUAPs. (From Preston DC, Shapiro BE. *Electromyography and Neuromuscular Disorders: Clinical-Electrophysiologic Correlations.* Boston: Butterworth-Heinemann; 1998.)

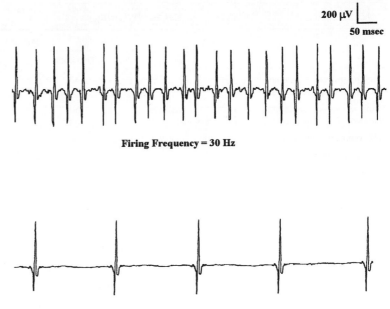

**FIGURE 21–8.** Incomplete interference patterns. In both traces, the patient is asked to maximally contract. The top trace demonstrates an incomplete interference pattern due to reduced recruitment (fast firing rate). The bottom trace demonstrates an incomplete interference pattern due to reduced activation (slow firing rate). (From Preston DC, Shapiro BE. *Electromyography and Neuromuscular Disorders: Clinical-Electrophysiologic Correlations.* Boston: Butterworth-Heinemann; 1998.)

muscles, the maximal firing frequency is 30 to 50 Hz. Some muscles, such as the soleus, are predominantly slow twitch, with a much lower maximal firing frequency of approximately 15 Hz.

When an interference pattern is being assessed, the major question to ask is whether the number of different MUAPs firing is appropriate for the firing rate. An incomplete interference pattern may be due to either poor activation or poor recruitment of motor units. Consider the two different incomplete interference patterns in Figure 21–8. In the first case (*top trace*) the patient has been asked to maximally contract the muscle, resulting in a single MUAP firing rapidly at 30 Hz. Thus, at a maximal firing rate of 30 Hz, only one MUAP fires, or a 30:1 ratio, far greater than the expected normal ratio of 5:1. This reflects a drop-out of MUAPs. In this first case the interference pattern is reduced because of decreased recruitment (30:1 ratio), and activation (firing rate of 30 Hz) is normal.

In the second patient (*bottom trace*), one also sees a single MUAP firing when the patient is asked to maximally contract the muscle. In this case, however, the single MUAP is firing at 5 Hz, a 5:1 ratio, which is normal. The major problem here is the reduced firing rate of 5 Hz (activation), although the number of MUAPs firing (recruitment) is appropriate for the firing rate (approximate 5:1 ratio). Thus poor activation has resulted in a decreased interference pattern, but recruitment is normal. This pattern can be seen if a patient cannot fully cooperate, perhaps because of pain or a CNS lesion (e.g., stroke, multiple sclerosis).

Although there is a single motor unit interference pattern in both cases, the cause is different. Note that occasionally both decreased activation and recruitment are seen in the same patient. For example, this can be seen in ALS, in which both upper and lower motor neurons are involved.

The last concept to understand is that of *early recruitment.* In myopathies and severe disorders of the NMJ, motor units may lose individual muscle fibers, resulting in a smaller motor unit. These smaller motor units cannot generate as much force as a normal motor unit, thus requiring many motor units to fire to generate small amounts of force. This phenomenon is known as early recruitment, meaning the inappropriate firing of many motor units to generate only a small amount of force. This pattern is recognized on EMG when many MUAPs appear to fire almost simultaneously, with small amounts of force (see Fig. 21–7, *bottom trace*). Usually only the electromyographer holding the needle can assess early recruitment since one must be able to judge how much force is being generated. An early recruitment pattern can be seen in muscle disorders and some disorders of the NMJ. Note that the number of MUAPs firing remains normal for the level of activation.

Although it may seem preferable to judge recruitment during maximum contraction, by examining the interference pattern, recruitment is actually more easily evaluated during moderate levels of contraction. At moderate levels of contraction one can more easily judge whether the number of different MUAPs firing (recruitment) is appropriate for the level of activation (firing rate). For example, if only one MUAP is seen firing at 15 Hz, then recruitment is reduced, even at this low level of activation. One does not need to increase the firing rate to maximal contraction to make this determination. Not only is maximal contraction painful with the EMG needle in the muscle, but judging the relationship between the number of MUAPs firing and the firing rate can actually be more difficult.

## PATTERNS OF MOTOR UNIT ACTION POTENTIAL ABNORMALITIES

Once the needle examination is completed, one can generally determine if there is a lesion. If a lesion is present, one can also usually determine the severity and chronicity of the lesion and whether the primary problem is neuropathic or myopathic. The distribution and pattern of abnormalities along with the clinical data should allow one to formulate an electrophysiologic diagnosis. It is important to remember

## TABLE 21–2. MUAP Patterns and Pathophysiology

| | MUAP Morphology | | | MUAP Firing Pattern | |
|---|---|---|---|---|---|
| | Duration | Amplitude | Phases | Activation | Recruitment |
| Acute neuropathic—axonal | NL | NL | NL | NL | ↓ |
| Chronic neuropathic—axonal | ↑ | ↑ | ↑ | NL | ↓ |
| Neuropathic—demyelinating (conduction velocity slowing) | NL | NL | NL | NL | NL |
| Neuropathic—demyelinating (conduction block) | NL | NL | NL | NL | ↓ |
| Early reinnervation after severe denervation (nascent units) | ↓ | ↓ | ↑ | NL | ↓↓ |
| Acute myopathic | ↓ | ↓ | ↑ | NL | NL/early |
| Chronic myopathic | ↓/↑ | ↓/↑ | ↑ | NL | NL/early |
| Myopathic—end stage | ↓/↑ | ↓/↑ | ↑ | NL | ↓↓ |
| NMJ disorders—increased jitter | NL | NL | NL | NL | NL |
| NMJ disorders—intermittent block | NL/↓* | NL/↓* | NL/↑* | NL | NL/early |
| NMJ disorders—severe block | ↓ | ↓ | ↑ | NL | ↓↓ |
| CNS disorders | NL | NL | NL | ↓↓ | NL |

NL, Normal; ↑, increased; ↓, decreased; ↓/↑, may be decreased and/or increased; ↓↓, usually markedly decreased.

*May vary from potential to potential (unstable MUAPs).

From Preston DC, Shapiro BE. *Electromyography and Neuromuscular Disorders. Clinical-Electrophysiologic Correlations.* Boston: Butterworth-Heinemann; 1998.

that no single parameter identifies a MUAP as myopathic, neuropathic, or associated with a NMJ disorder. Rather, specific patterns of abnormalities in MUAP morphology and firing rate indicate whether the underlying disorder is (1) acute, chronic, or end stage; (2) neuropathic, myopathic, or associated with an NMJ transmission defect; and (3) if neuropathic, whether the primary pathophysiology is axonal loss or demyelination (Table 21–2). Some of the more common patterns are described in the following discussions.

### ACUTE NEUROPATHIC—AXONAL LOSS

Following an acute axonal nerve injury, wallerian degeneration occurs within 4 to 7 days.[13] Eventually, the distal muscle fibers of the involved motor units become denervated. On EMG, the only abnormality seen in an acute neuropathic lesion is decreased recruitment of MUAPs in weak muscles; MUAP morphology remains normal. Decreased recruitment is due to the loss of motor units. This pattern is usually seen acutely after trauma, compression, or nerve infarction. A similar pattern may be seen in pure demyelinating lesions with conduction block.

### CHRONIC NEUROPATHIC—AXONAL LOSS

Following axonal loss and denervation, reinnervation takes place by one of two mechanisms. After complete denervation, reinnervation must occur by axonal regrowth from the site of injury; it occurs slowly, approximately 1 mm/d (see later discussion of early reinnervation following severe or complete denervation). For this type of regrowth to occur, the anterior horn cells must remain intact. In contrast, if the denervation is partial or has occurred gradually, reinnervation occurs through collateral sprouting by adjacent surviving motor units (Fig. 21–9). In this case, the number of muscle fibers per motor unit increases, and MUAPs become prolonged, high in amplitude, and polyphasic (Fig. 21–10). These MUAP changes in conjunction with decreased recruitment are the hallmarks of reinnervated motor units and nearly always imply chronic neuropathic disease (i.e., disorders of the anterior horn cell, nerve root, or peripheral nerve). Such MUAP changes are never seen acutely, and they

imply that the process has been present for several weeks, if not months or years. This is a common pattern seen in the EMG laboratory, where patients present with slowly progressive or chronic conditions, such as polyneuropathies.

### NEUROPATHIC—DEMYELINATING LESIONS

With purely or predominantly demyelinating lesions, the underlying axon remains intact. Neither denervation nor subsequent reinnervation occurs. Therefore in pure demyelinating lesions MUAP morphology remains normal. If demyelination results only in conduction velocity slowing, the nerve action potential still reaches the muscle, and the number of functioning motor units remains normal. Accordingly, the recruitment pattern remains normal. If demyelination results in conduction block, the number of available MUAPs effectively decreases, resulting in decreased recruitment. This pattern can be seen, for example, in Guillain-Barré syndrome or carpal tunnel syndrome, but it is also seen in acute axonal loss lesions.

### ACUTE MYOPATHIES

In myopathies the number of functioning muscle fibers in a motor unit decreases (see Fig. 21–10).[5] Because each motor unit contains fewer muscle fibers, the resultant MUAPs are shorter in duration and smaller in amplitude than normal (Fig. 21–11).[6,19] In addition, the muscle fibers fire less synchronously, resulting in polyphasic MUAPs. The actual number of functioning motor units remains normal, and thus the recruitment pattern remains normal for the level of activation. However, since each motor unit contains fewer muscle fibers, it cannot generate as much force as a normal motor unit. More MUAPs will fire than normally are needed for a certain level of force, resulting in early recruitment. Thus the pattern associated with an acute myopathy is short duration, small amplitude, and polyphasic MUAPs with normal or early recruitment.

### CHRONIC MYOPATHIES

In chronic myopathies, especially those with necrotic or inflammatory features (e.g., polymyositis, muscular dystrophies), there is often some denervation and subsequent reinnervation. This may result in long-duration, high-amplitude, polyphasic MUAPs, more commonly seen in chronic neuropathic disease. Two populations of MUAPs may be seen in chronic myopathies—long-duration, high-amplitude, polyphasic MUAPs and short-duration, small-amplitude, polyphasic MUAPs, often in the same muscle. Rarely, long-duration, large-amplitude, polyphasic MUAPs alone are seen. In

such cases the assessment of the recruitment pattern is key to differentiating chronic myopathic from chronic neuropathic MUAPs. In chronic myopathies, recruitment is usually normal or early, even if the MUAPs are large. Occasionally, a slightly reduced recruitment pattern is seen, but one that is still better than would be expected from the chronic MUAP changes. In some very chronic myopathies, especially inclusion body myositis, the EMG may resemble that of active

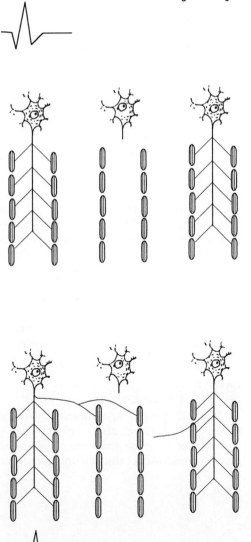

NORMAL

PARTIAL DENERVATION

EARLY REINNERVATION

**FIGURE 21–9.** Collateral sprouting and satellite potentials. Following partial denervation (*middle trace*), reinnervation commonly occurs by sprouting from adjacent intact axons. These sprouts are initially small and thinly myelinated and conduct slowly. The slow conduction time and increased distance of these reinnervated fibers cause them to initially occur as time-locked potentials that trail the main MUAP (*bottom trace*). As these sprouts mature, they conduct more quickly, allowing these time-locked (satellite) potentials to eventually incorporate into the main MUAP. This results in a MUAP with increased amplitude, duration, and phases. (From Preston DC, Shapiro BE. *Electromyography and Neuromuscular Disorders: Clinical-Electrophysiologic Correlations.* Boston: Butterworth-Heinemann; 1998.)

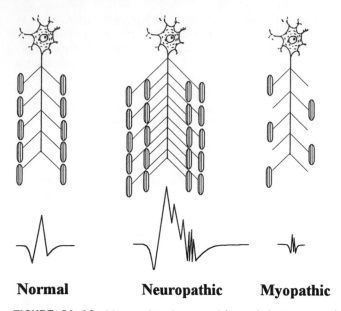

**Normal**          **Neuropathic**          **Myopathic**

**FIGURE 21–10.** Motor unit action potential morphologies. Normal MUAPs have two to four phases. In chronic neurogenic lesions following reinnervation, the number of muscle fibers per motor unit increases. This results in long-duration, high-amplitude, polyphasic MUAPs. In myopathies or in neuromuscular junction disorders with block, the number of functional muscle fibers per motor unit decreases. This results in short-duration, small-amplitude, polyphasic MUAPs. (From Preston DC, Shapiro BE. *Electromyography and Neuromuscular Disorders: Clinical-Electrophysiologic Correlations.* Boston: Butterworth-Heinemann; 1998.)

motor neuron disease—fibrillations with long-duration, high-amplitude, polyphasic MUAPs. In this situation only the recruitment pattern may differentiate the two.

## END-STAGE MYOPATHIES

In the very late stages of some muscular dystrophies, periodic paralysis disorders, and very chronic inflammatory myopathies (e.g., inclusion body myositis), end-stage muscle disease may occur. In these situations, if every muscle fiber of some motor units dies or becomes dysfunctional, there may actually be a reduction in the number of motor units. In such cases, one sees reduced recruitment of MUAPs, as motor units drop out. The MUAPs are usually short duration, small amplitude, and polyphasic, but long-duration, high-amplitude, polyphasic MUAPs may also be seen. Although decreased recruitment nearly always implies a neurogenic disorder, this rare exception arises in end-stage muscle from myopathy.

## EARLY REINNERVATION FOLLOWING SEVERE OR COMPLETE DENERVATION

Following severe or complete denervation, if there are no surviving adjacent axons, reinnervation must occur by regrowth of the axon from the site of injury. In the early phase the regrowing axon will only reinnervate a fraction of

the original muscle fibers. This results in short-duration, small-amplitude, polyphasic MUAPs, like those seen in acute myopathies. These early reinnervated motor units are known as nascent motor units (Fig. 21–12). However, one can easily differentiate nascent motor units from myopathic motor units by the recruitment pattern. Nascent MUAPs always occur in the setting of markedly reduced recruitment, whereas small MUAPs in myopathies are seen in the context of normal or early recruitment. Thus not all short-duration, small-amplitude, polyphasic MUAPs are myopathic.

## NEUROMUSCULAR JUNCTION DISORDERS

The MUAP morphology and firing patterns seen in NMJ disorders depend on the severity of the disorder. In mild disorders, with only slight variation of muscle fiber firing within the motor unit, the morphology and recruitment pattern of the MUAP are normal. In more severe disorders there may be intermittent blocking of some muscle fibers within the motor unit, making the MUAP unstable. In this situation the morphology will vary from potential to potential. With more persistent blocking, individual muscle fibers are effectively lost from a motor unit, and the MUAP becomes short, small, and polyphasic, similar to those seen in myopathy. Similarly, recruitment may be normal or early. If the NMJ block is severe, as in botulism, all the fibers in some motor units may be blocked, effectively resulting in loss of motor units. This leads to reduced recruitment, reflecting the reduced number of available motor units, with the remaining MUAPs being short, small, and polyphasic. This unusual pattern can also be seen in end-stage myopathy and in nascent motor units.

## CENTRAL NERVOUS SYSTEM DISORDERS

The EMG pattern generally seen in CNS disorders is an incomplete interference pattern because of reduced activation—the inability to fire motor units rapidly. Although the interference pattern is incomplete, the actual number of motor units firing (i.e., recruitment) is appropriate for the reduced level of activation. MUAP morphology and recruitment remain normal.

Other patterns may also be seen with CNS disorders. In spinal cord lesions, segmental loss of anterior horn cells may result in loss of motor units at the level of the lesion. Although denervation, reinnervation, and decreased recruitment may be seen at that segment, only decreased activation may be seen below the lesion. Some patients with multiple sclerosis may have denervation and reinnervation, presumably from involvement of motor fibers as they leave the anterior horn cells, prior to exiting and becoming motor roots. Whether EMG abnormalities are seen in other CNS disorders, such as stroke, remains controversial. Poor mobility leaves such patients prone to entrapments and external compressive lesions, which more often explain any EMG abnormalities.

**200 µV** ⌐
**10 msec**

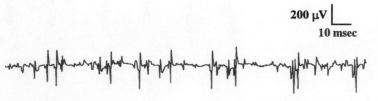

**FIGURE 21–11.** Myopathic motor unit action potentials. These MUAPs are usually short duration, small amplitude, and polyphasic. There is a characteristic early recruitment pattern in which a small amount of force causes many small polyphasic MUAPs that cannot be differentiated from one another to fill the screen.

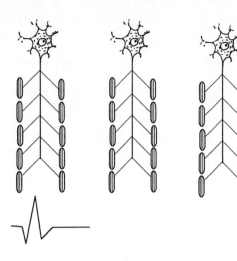

**NORMAL**

**FIGURE 21–12.** Nascent motor units. Following a severe axonal lesion, wallerian degeneration occurs distal to the injury, resulting in denervation (*middle trace*). If there are no intact axons nearby, reinnervation must occur by regrowth of the axon from the terminal stump. Early in this process, there is a point at which some (but not all) the muscle fibers will be reinnervated (*bottom trace*). It is at this point, early in the reinnervation process, that MUAPs will be short duration, small amplitude, and polyphasic, resembling myopathic units. These are known as nascent motor units. (From Preston DC, Shapiro BE. *Electromyography and Neuromuscular Disorders: Clinical-Electrophysiologic Correlations.* Boston: Butterworth-Heinemann; 1998.)

**SEVERE DENERVATION**

**EARLY REINNERVATION**

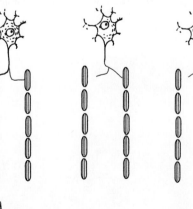

Last, tremor may be seen in some patients with CNS disorders. Tremor is recognized as a bursting pattern of voluntary MUAPs separated by relative silence. As multiple MUAPs fire simultaneously, it may be difficult to assess individual MUAP morphology, and polyphasia appears increased. If tremor occurs at rest, as in Parkinson's disease, the bursting discharge of MUAPs may be mistaken for myokymia. However, although both tremor and myokymia result in a bursting pattern of MUAPs, in myokymia the burst is composed of a single MUAP that fires repetitively, whereas in tremor the burst is composed of many different MUAPs. Furthermore, myokymia is a spontaneous phenomenon that cannot be voluntarily influenced by the patient, whereas most patients can alter their tremor voluntarily by changing their limb position or action.

## REFERENCES

1. Albers JW, Allen AA, Bastron JA, et al. Limb myokymia. *Muscle Nerve.* 1981;4:494.
2. Brown WF. *The Physiological and Technical Basis of Electromyography.* Boston: Butterworth; 1984.
3. Brown WF, Varkey GP. The origin of spontaneous electrical activity at the end-plate zone. *Ann Neurol.* 1981;10:557.
4. Buchthal F. *An Introduction to Electromyography.* Copenhagen: Scandinavian University Books; 1957.
5. Buchthal F. Diagnostic significance of the myopathic EMG. In: Rowland LP, ed. *Pathogenesis of Human Muscular Dystrophies.* Proceedings of the Fifth International Scientific Conference of the Muscular Dystrophy Association; June 1976; Durango, Colo. Amsterdam: Excerpta Medica; 1977:205.
6. Buchthal F. Electrophysiologic signs of myopathy as related with muscle biopsy. *Acta Neurol (Napoli).* 1977;32:1.
7. Buchthal F. Fibrillations: clinical electrophysiology. In: Culp WJ, Ochoa J, eds. *Abnormal Nerves and Muscles as Impulse Generators.* Oxford: Oxford University Press; 1982:632.
8. Buchthal F, Pinelli P, Rosenfalck P. Action potential parameters in normal human muscle and their physiologic determinants. *Acta Physiol Scand.* 1954;32:219.
9. Buchthal F, Rosenfalck P. Spontaneous electrical activity of human muscle. *Electroencephalogr Clin Neurophysiol.* 1966;20:321.
10. Buchthal F, Schmalbruch H. Motor unit of mammalian muscle. *Physiol Rev.* 1980;60:90.
11. Daube JR. *Needle Examination in Electromyography.* Minimonograph No. 11, Rochester, Minn: American Association of Electromyography and Electrodiagnosis; 1979.
12. Denny-Brown D, Pennybacker JB. Fibrillation and fasciculation in voluntary muscle. *Brain.* 1938;61:311.
13. Donat JR, Wisniewski HM. The spatio-temporal pattern of Wallerian degeneration in mammalian peripheral nerves. *Brain Res.* 1973;53:41.
14. Emeryk B, Hausmanowa-Petrusewicz I, Nowak T. Spontaneous volleys of bizarre high frequency potentials in neuromuscular diseases, I: occurrence of spontaneous volleys of bizarre high frequency potentials in neuromuscular diseases. *Electromyogr Clin Neurophysiol.* 1974;14:303.
15. Emeryk B, Hausmanowa-Petrusewicz I, Nowak T. Spontaneous volleys of bizarre high frequency potentials in neuromuscular diseases, II: an analysis of the morphology of spontaneous volleys of bizarre high frequency potentials in neuromuscular diseases. *Electromyogr Clin Neurophysiol.* 1974;14:339.
16. Fatt P, Katz B. Spontaneous subthreshold activity at motor nerve endings. *J Physiol (Lond).* 1952;117:109.
17. Gamstorp I, Wohlfart G. A syndrome characterized by myokymia, myotonia, muscular wasting and increased perspiration. *Acta Psych Neurol Scand.* 1959;34:181.
18. Gath I, Stålberg E. The calculated radial decline of the extracellular action potential compared with in situ measurements in the human brachial biceps. *Electroencephalogr Clin Neurophysiol.* 1978;44:547.
19. Hausmanowa-Petrusewicz I, Emeryk B, Wasowicz B, et al. Electromyography in neuromuscular diagnostics. *Electromyography.* 1967;7:203.
20. Henneman E. Relation between size of neurons and their susceptibility to discharge. *Science.* 1957;126:1345.
21. Isaacs H. A syndrome of continuous muscle-fibre activity. *J Neurol Neurosurg Psychiatry.* 1961;24:319.
22. Kimura J. *Electrodiagnosis in Diseases of Nerve and Muscle: Principles and Practice.* 2nd ed. Philadelphia: FA Davis; 1989.
23. Liddell EGT, Sherrington CS. Recruitment and some other features of reflex inhibition. *Proc R Soc Lond Biol.* 1925;97:488.
24. Mertens HG, Zschocke S. Neuromyotonie. *Klin Wochenschr.* 1965;43:917.
25. Milner-Brown HS, Stein RB, Yemm R. Changes in firing rate of human motor units during linearly changing voluntary isometric contraction. *J Physiol (Lond).* 1973;230:371.
26. Milner-Brown HS, Stein RB, Yemm R. The contractile properties of human motor units during voluntary isometric contractions. *J Physiol (Lond).* 1973;228:285.
27. Norris FH, Jr. Myokymia (corres.). *Arch Neurol.* 1977;34:133.
28. Norris FH, Jr., Gasteiger EL, Chatfield PO. An electromyographic study of induced and spontaneous muscle cramps. *Electroencephalogr Clin Neurophysiol.* 1957;9:139.
29. Preston DC, Shapiro BE. *Electromyography and Neuromuscular Disorders: Clinical-Electrophysiologic Correlations.* Boston, Butterworth-Heinemann; 1998.
30. Rosenfalck P. Intra- and extracellular potential fields of active nerve and muscle fibers. *Acta Physiol Scan.* 1969;75(suppl 321):1.
31. Stålberg E, Trontelj JV. Abnormal discharges generated within the motor unit as observed with single-fiber electromyography. In: Culp WJ, Ochoa J, eds. *Abnormal Nerves and Muscles as Impulse Generators.* Oxford: Oxford University Press; 1982:443.
32. Stohr M. Repetitive impulse-induced EMG discharges in neuromuscular diseases. *Ann Neurol.* 1981;9:204.
33. Stolov W. *Instrumentation and Measurement in Electrodiagnosis.* Minimonograph No. 16, Rochester, Minn: American Association of Electromyography and Electrodiagnosis; 1981.
34. Streib EW. *Differential Diagnosis of Myotonic Syndromes.* Minimonograph No. 27. Rochester, Minn: American Association of Electromyography and Electrodiagnosis; 1987.
35. Thiele B, Bohle A. Number of spike-components contributing to the motor unit potential. *Z EEG-EMG.* 1978;9:125.

# 22

# Autonomic Function

*Louis H. Weimer*

## CONSIDERATIONS IN TESTING

Formal laboratory evaluation of autonomic disorders is becoming more widely available, in part because of the evolution and validation of reliable noninvasive techniques. Unlike other anatomic systems, such as the somatic peripheral nervous system, autonomic function cannot be assessed directly. However, the responses of complex overlapping reflex loops can be measured after controlled perturbations. Numerous techniques to evaluate autonomic function have been described, but only a minority are considered suitable for routine clinical application.[8] Tests of cardiovagal, adrenergic, and sudomotor function are the most commonly performed and were formally recognized for their usefulness in 1997 with dedicated Current Procedural Terminology codes.

Suspicion of possible autonomic dysfunction rests on the clinician, and includes the neurologist but also spans numerous other specialties. Autonomically mediated symptoms may go underrecognized because of involvement of seemingly unrelated systems, for example, distal limb vasomotor complaints with postprandial fullness. Additionally, early symptoms of the most characteristic finding, orthostatic hypotension, may appear as nonspecific fatigue, cognitive change, anxiety, or vertigo.[135] A chronic decline in standing blood pressure (BP) is often asymptomatic, especially in elderly patients with chronically adapted cerebral autoregulation. Approximately half of the patients older than 60 have initial postural cognitive changes prior to the development of dizziness,[121] which can progress to sudden syncope. Some patients may develop neck heaviness or headache as a prominent sign of postural intolerance.[162] Often more dramatic and advanced symptoms of severe dizziness, impending syncope, or, rarely, frank syncope may be necessary before autonomic failure is suspected. The frequency of reported postural complaints is listed in Table 22–1.[118] Many of the other common autonomic complaints listed in a review of autonomic systems (Table 22–2) may appear nonspecific and lead to an evaluation restricted to the system in question aimed at evaluating end-organ damage.

A general neurologic history and examination with attention to an autonomic review of systems is a useful screening tool. The history should include specific questions for each category listed in Table 22–2 because many patients do not volunteer these complaints unless the questions are directly posed. The patient may also have overlooked some physical changes even when asked about them, for example, reduced distal sweating or sweating after exercise or a hot shower. The clinical history also may gather information not amenable to formal testing, such as the time course of evolution, paroxysmal patterns, exacerbating factors, symptoms referable to areas unable to be reliably tested, and the impact on overall function.[118] The physical examination should include particular attention to pupillary size, shape, and reactivity and skin properties, including texture and skin and mucous membrane moisture. Orthostatic BP measurement is vital and should be performed lying to standing, preferably after a short supine period. Measurements of both BP and heart rate (HR) should be checked at 1 and 2 minutes after standing, with attention given to induced symptoms. More prolonged measurement of 5 or even 10 minutes is indicated in cases with postural complaints without a significant fall in BP to screen for postural tachycardia as seen in mild forms of autonomic failure and syndromes of orthostatic intolerance. In some instances further formal evaluation in a dedicated laboratory is desirable. Additional bedside screening tests complement a clinical evaluation, and several measures (discussed later) can be performed with limited equipment, such as an electrocardiograph (ECG) or electromyograph (EMG) machine, if a formal laboratory is

### TABLE 22–1. Symptoms of Orthostatic Intolerance

| SYMPTOM | % REPORTED |
|---|---|
| Light-headedness (dizziness) | 88 |
| Weakness or tiredness | 72 |
| Cognitive (thinking/concentrating) | 47 |
| Blurred vision | 47 |
| Tremulousness | 38 |
| Vertigo | 37 |
| Pallor | 31 |
| Anxiety | 29 |
| Tachycardia or palpitations | 26 |
| Clammy feeling | 19 |
| Nausea | 18 |

Modified from Low PA, ed. *Clinical Autonomic Disorders.* 2nd ed. Philadelphia: Lippincott-Raven; 1997:8.

## TABLE 22–2.  Autonomic Review of Symptoms

*Secretomotor:* Dry eyes and mouth
*Orthostatic:* Dizziness, weakness, fatigue, cognitive changes, visual disturbance, vertigo, anxiety, palpitations, pallor, nausea, syncope
*Exacerbating factors:* Prolonged standing, exercise, meals, warm environment, early morning, prolonged recumbency, physical countermaneuvers, speed of postural change, medication effects
*Postprandial:* Bloating, fullness, nausea, dizziness, sweating, orthostatic hypotension
*Gastrointestinal:* Constipation, nocturnal or intermittent diarrhea
*Genitourinary:* Urinary retention, difficulty with initiation, incomplete emptying, incontinence
*Sexual:* Erectile failure, ejaculatory dysfunction, retrograde ejaculation into bladder
*Visual:* Blurred vision, sensitivity to light/glare, reduced night vision
*Sudomotor:* Reduced or loss of sweating ability (distally in polyneuropathies); excessive, paroxysmal, or inappropriate sweating; mixed pattern of loss and excessive areas; heat intolerance
*Vasomotor:* Distal color changes, change in skin appearance, persistently cold extremities, Raynaud's phenomenon, loss of skin wrinkling in water, heat intolerance
*Other:* Unexplained syncope

unavailable. However, because of technical limitations and pitfalls, the general consensus is to recommend the use of a standardized battery of measures under controlled settings as a more reliable approach.[5] Low has outlined the prime indications for formal testing (Table 22–3).

### INDICATIONS FOR LABORATORY EVALUATION

The primary goal of testing is to determine whether autonomic failure is present and to assess and quantify the severity of involvement. If abnormalities are reliably detected, further characterization is possible to determine the systems involved, such as parasympathetic, sympathetic, or panautonomic. A pattern of distribution or selective or regional involvement may be discerned. In some instances information on central, preganglionic, or postganglionic localization is possible.

Confirmation with formal testing is especially valuable when involvement is suspected, but overt clinical signs such as orthostatic hypotension are not evident, as seen with early stages of progressive disorders, syndromes with primarily cholinergic involvement that do not demonstrate orthostatic hypotension, and disorders restricted to specific systems. This point is not trivial because, despite a pattern of symptoms, objective support for autonomic involvement on examination may be lacking, leaving only a presumptive diagnosis. This presumption may not be valid if the pathology lies with the end organ in question and not with autonomic control. Testing is valuable to confirm that an isolated finding or syndrome is not part of a progressive and generalized syndrome of autonomic failure, which may carry a poor prognosis. If a generalized progressive syndrome is present, confirmation is key for prognosis and institution of symptomatic treatment. Prognosis is also less favorable in certain settings if autonomic changes are evident. Increased mortality rates have been described in patients with diabetes who have autonomic neuropathy,[22,23,45] following myocardial infarction,[19,94,218] and with Guillain-Barré syndrome[217] in association with certain testing abnormalities. Testing is instrumental in defining and characterizing a separate but possibly related group of disorders of orthostatic intolerance as well

as patients with delayed or paroxysmal phenomena (discussed later). Testing is potentially useful in distinguishing between static and progressive disorders when quantitative measures are used over time. Recognition is important for the initiation of treatment. Although underutilized, multiple symptomatic treatments are available for neurogenic orthostatic hypotension and many of the other involved systems.[61,160] In addition, there is growing evidence that autonomic function can improve with specific treatment in certain cases, for example, in diabetic neuropathy,[34,76] amyloid polyneuropathy,[17] and Lambert-Eaton myasthenic syndrome.[136] As additional treatment options become available, current and evolving techniques will aid in tailoring appropriate therapy based on the underlying physiologic mechanisms rather than simple empiric symptomatic treatment.

Autonomically mediated effects are ubiquitous in neurologic disease, in part because of the far-ranging anatomic structures and extensive interactions with other portions of the nervous system. Such factors as structural lesions, pressure effects, seizures, and inflammatory and infectious processes affect autonomic physiology and somatic systems. Less commonly, autonomic function is specifically or predominantly compromised. Lesions are not restricted to peripheral autonomic fibers. Processes affecting the cortex, hypothalamus, limbic system, cerebellum, brainstem, and spinal cord can also disturb autonomic pathways or physiology. Table 22–4 lists selected prominent entities. A more comprehensive classification scheme has been proposed.[118]

### ANATOMY

A brief review of autonomic anatomy and physiology is necessary to understand the rationale of the tests described in the following sections. The autonomic system traditionally is divided into the thoracolumbar sympathetic nervous system (SNS) and the craniosacral parasympathetic nervous system (PNS).[175] Langley[101] coined the term *autonomic nervous system* (ANS) before the turn of the century to describe portions of the nervous system controlling "automatic," or unconscious, functions. He subdivided the major components as sympathetic and craniosacral (later called parasympathetic). He also acknowledged an independent nervous system of the gut as a third system largely ignored until years later, when its significance as a system capable of autonomous neural programming was rediscovered.

Preganglionic cell bodies of the sympathetic and parasympathetic systems are located in the brainstem and spinal

## TABLE 22–3.  Indications for Laboratory Evaluation

1. Diagnosis of generalized autonomic failure
2. Diagnosis of benign autonomic disorders that may mimic life-threatening disorders
3. Diagnosis of distal small-fiber neuropathy
4. Evaluation of orthostatic intolerance
5. Evaluation of the course of the autonomic disorder
6. Evaluation of the response to therapy
7. Evaluation of autonomic involvement in the peripheral neuropathies
8. Detection of sympathetic dysfunction in sympathetically maintained pain
9. Research questions

From Low PA, ed. *Clinical Autonomic Disorders.* 2nd ed. Philadelphia: Lippincott-Raven; 1997:12.

## TABLE 22–4. Selected Disorders of Autonomic Function

**Pure Autonomic Failure (PAF)***

**Multisystem Disorders**
Multiple system atrophy (MSA)*
• Shy-Drager syndrome
• Striatonigral degeneration
• Sporadic olivopontocerebellar atrophy
Parkinson's disease with autonomic failure*
Idiopathic Parkinson's disease
Machado-Joseph disease (spinocerebellar atrophy [SCA] III)
Progressive supranuclear palsy
Diffuse Lewy body disease

**Central Disorders**
Brain tumors (posterior fossa, third ventricle, hypothalamus),
syringobulbia, multiple sclerosis, tetanus, fatal familial insomnia,*
Wernicke-Korsakoff syndrome

**Spinal Cord Disorders**
Multiple sclerosis, syringomyelia, transverse myelitis, transection/trauma,
tumor

**Peripheral Disorders**
*Immune mediated:* Guillain-Barré syndrome,* acute and subacute
pandysautonomia,* acute cholinergic neuropathy,* Sjögren's disease,
systemic lupus erythematosus, rheumatoid arthritis, Holmes-Adie
syndrome
*Metabolic:* Diabetes mellitus,* vitamin $B_{12}$ and thiamine deficiency, uremia
*Paraneoplastic:* Paraneoplastic autonomic neuropathy,* sensory
neuronopathy with autonomic failure (ANNA antibodies), enteric
neuronopathy,* Lambert-Eaton myasthenic syndrome (cholinergic)
*Infectious:* Chagas' disease (cholinergic),* human immunodeficiency virus,
tabes, leprosy, Lyme disease, diphtheria
*Hereditary:* Familial amyloidosis,* hereditary sensory and autonomic
neuropathies I-V (type III: familial dysautonomia*), dopamine beta-
hydroxylase deficiency,* porphyria, Fabry's disease,* Navajo neuropathy
*Toxins:* Botulism, vincristine, cis-platin, paclitaxel, amiodarone, vacor,
hexacarbon, carbon disulfide, thallium, arsenic, inorganic mercury,
acrylamide, podophyllin,* alcohol

**Other Disorders**
Acquired amyloidosis, chronic idiopathic autonomic neuropathies,*
idiopathic small-fiber neuropathy, idiopathic hyperhidrosis,* idiopathic
anhidrosis,* Horner's syndrome, Ross syndrome*

**Reduced Orthostatic Tolerance**
Neurocardiogenic syncope, postural orthostatic tachycardia syndrome,*
mitral valve prolapse syndrome,* prolonged bedrest or weightlessness*

**Drug and Medication Effects**

---

*Autonomic dysfunction is typically clinically important.

cord. Axons leave the central nervous system (CNS) and synapse in specialized ganglia. Second-order (postganglionic) neurons directly innervate smooth and cardiac muscle as well as secretory glands. Both afferent and efferent functions are part of the ANS. Higher CNS centers comprising the central autonomic network reside mainly in the hypothalamus, brainstem, and limbic system and have vital connections with the preganglionic neurons to integrate and regulate visceral function in order to maintain homeostasis. Most viscera have dual sympathetic and parasympathetic innervation with a few notable exceptions. In nearly all organs these effects are antagonistic, producing a resting tone between the two systems. Although this description is an oversimplification with certain exceptions, the concept is a useful framework in most organs. Acetylcholine is the primary neurotransmitter in ganglia and effector sites of the parasympathetic system, sympathetic ganglia, and sudomotor ef-

fector sites. Norepinephrine is the primary neurotransmitter in other sympathetic end-organ targets with two main subtypes of alpha and beta receptors. However, multiple other neurotransmitters and peptides also play important roles. Nonadrenergic, noncholinergic cells are found in sympathetic ganglia. Many other substances have vital neuromodulatory or cotransmitter roles. Most prominent among these are vasoactive intestinal polypeptide (VIP), neuropeptide Y (NPY), enkephalins, substance P, and nitric oxide. The added complexity in part allows for peripheral integration not available with somatic anatomy.

### Sympathetic Nervous System

The SNS is designed to rapidly respond to emergent stressful changes in the internal or external environment with a widespread activation of the heart and other organs, leading to increased cardiac output, BP, HR, temperature, sweating for cooling, blood glucose for quick energy, and pupil dilation. Preganglionic neuronal cell bodies are located in the intermediolateral (IML) and intermediomedial (IMM) cell columns of the spinal cord from T1 to L2 (thoracolumbar outflow). These neurons slowly decline with age at approximately 8% per year.[124] Exiting fibers are small (2 to 5 μm) myelinated fibers (white rami) that pass via the ventral root. Fibers typically synapse (nicotinic acetylcholine) in various paravertebral ganglia located from cervical to sacral regions. However, there is not a simple one-to-one innervation ratio. Preganglionic fibers typically send axons up or down the sympathetic chain, innervating neurons at other levels in an approximate 1:10 to 1:20 ratio of preganglionic to postganglionic neurons, enabling the system to provide a broad amplified response. In contrast, the PNS has a much lower innervation ratio (1:3) to produce a more focused response. Other fibers do not synapse in these ganglia but pass through forming splanchnic nerves that synapse in the prevertebral celiac, superior mesenteric, or inferior mesenteric ganglia. Second-order postganglionic fibers (gray rami) travel as thin unmyelinated fibers and innervate various organs, blood vessels, sweat glands, and other structures. The adrenal medulla is a unique case, innervated directly by splanchnic nerves.

### Parasympathetic Nervous System

Efferent cell bodies are located with various cranial nerve nuclei and in a less distinct IML cell column of the sacral spinal cord (craniosacral outflow). Unlike sympathetic peripheral pathways, preganglionic parasympathetic fibers travel with various cranial or sacral nerves and synapse at ganglia near the end organ. Cranial nerves III (oculomotor), VII (facial), IX (glossopharyngeal), and X (vagus) all carry efferent fibers originating from the brainstem nuclei as well as important afferent connections, most destined for the nucleus of the solitary tract. Functions include pupillary constriction, accommodation, stimulation of tears and saliva, HR slowing, and inhibition of gastrointestinal (GI) peristalsis. One vital pathway includes cells in the ventrolateral nucleus ambiguus and dorsal motor nucleus of the vagus nerve that project to cardiac ganglia instrumental in all cardiovagal tests to be discussed. Important afferent information is supplied from baroreceptors located in the carotid sinus, aortic arch, and other large vessels as well as input from pulmonary stretch and cardiac mechanoreceptors. Negative feedback loops linking these circuits are so finely controlled that a change in rate is evident to many perturbations on the following heartbeat.

### Central Autonomic Network

The supraspinal integration of autonomic function involves a complex interaction of multiple brainstem, mesencephalic, subcortical, and cortical areas.[14] Critical sites include the hypothalamus, nucleus of the solitary tract (NTS), insular cortex, amygdala, periaqueductal gray matter, and ventrolateral medulla. The hypothalamus has traditionally been viewed as the most important central center. It receives input from diffuse areas, including the limbic system, brainstem, and sensorimotor cortex, and influences many of the first-order neurons secondarily through descending reticulospinal pathways from the pons and medulla, which synapse on spinal cord interneurons that modulate preganglionic neurons. The descending axons are not in discrete pathways and may be dispersed through the cord. There is no neat tract to the lesion as in other systems; however, an extensive cord lesion effectively interrupts autonomic fibers. Stimulating the lateral hypothalamus leads to general sympathetic activation, including piloerection, increases in BP and HR, sweating, and pupil dilatation. The hypothalamus also can uniquely influence a large territory of end organs through its influence over pituitary neuroendocrine outflow. However, most functions do not require this hypothalamic influence to function. Transection models and brain injury patients without an acting hypothalamus still have functional respiration, cardiac output, and visceral function, indicating that the brainstem also is capable of functional integration. The most important afferent brainstem center, especially in the rat and likely also in the human, is the nucleus of the solitary tract. In the rat it is viscerotopically organized to receive afferent input from virtually every organ acting as an important integration and relay station.

The NTS also projects to other brainstem nuclei, which directly influence preganglionic nuclei. These input-output loops enable sets of reflex circuits that affect the heart, lungs, vasomotor control, GI tract, and multiple other homeostatic mechanisms. Other major areas of influence include the ventromedial prefrontal cortex, anterior cingulate gyrus, amygdala, bed nucleus of the stria terminalis, and portions of the thalamus, basal ganglia, and reticular formation. Many act through the hypothalamus, which integrates the signals into a more coherent pattern. Afferent information from humoral and environmental signals is integrated in addition to visceral input. The ventrolateral medulla is integral in cardiovascular outflow, vasopressin release, and cardiorespiratory interactions involved in many of the adrenergic measures. This area has been confirmed to be depleted of tyrosine hydroxylase neurons in patients with multiple system atrophy (MSA).[16]

### Physiology

The ANS subserves an extensive array of regulatory and homeostatic mechanisms, many of which have antagonistic parasympathetic and sympathetic influence. Notable exceptions of organs without significant parasympathetic innervation are seen, including sweat glands, piloerector muscles, and many small blood vessels. Some organs, such as the lacrimal and salivary glands, are dually stimulated by the sympathetic and parasympathetic systems, although with somewhat different stimulation products. Knowledge of the basic mechanisms of each test performed is helpful for meaningful interpretation of results. For example, baroreflex effects are an important mechanism underlying many of the cardiovascular tests (carotid sinus reflex). A change in systemic BP (e.g., acute BP increase) leads to stimulation of baroreceptor afferents. This activity is transmitted to the nucleus of the solitary tract for integration, which projects to several other centers. The motor nucleus of the vagus and cells in the nucleus ambiguus are stimulated to increase cardiovagal tone and slow HR. Neurons in the ventrolateral medulla project to sympathetic cells in the spinal cord, inhibiting peripheral vasomotor tone and reducing cardiac rate and force of contraction, all serving to return BP to baseline values. Autonomic screening tests attempt to harness specific, reproducible reflexes such as these for quantitation. However, the underlying physiology can be quite complex, with multiple potentially confounding factors. For this reason, test reliability and controlled examination conditions are vitally important if meaningful information is to be gathered. Despite the ubiquitous nature of autonomic control in the body and a multitude of described testing methods, only a handful of systems and measures are generally agreed to be sensitive and reproducible enough for routine and common application.[8]

### PATIENT PREPARATION

Many endogenous and environmental factors can confound autonomic testing and need to be controlled as much as feasible. The patient should be normovolemic, comfortable, without significant anxiety, and recuperated from any recent acute illness or period of prolonged bedrest. Compressive garments should be removed. Caffeine, nicotine, and alcohol should be avoided on the day of testing. Vigorous exercise should be avoided on the day prior to examination. The testing room should have a controlled, comfortable temperature. Medications with any sympathetic or parasympathetic activity or BP modulation should be discontinued, ideally 24 to 48 hours prior to testing, unless the referring physician deems it medically unsafe to interrupt taking them. These drugs include, but are not limited to, over-the-counter cold remedies, antidepressants with anticholinergic activity, diuretics, alpha- or beta-blockers or agonists, mineralocorticoids, and antihistamines (Table 22–5). Movement toward more noninvasive testing methods has helped to minimize patient anxiety and improve testing time duration. Photoplethysmographic devices (e.g., Finapres) have enabled beat-to-beat BP recordings without the need for invasive lines.[80,148] New instruments are no longer commercially sold, but other similar devices have been developed and are available (e.g., Colin Pilot).

Patient safety during testing is always of concern, especially because syncope is a potential risk during tilt-table testing and intrathoracic and intraocular pressure is raised with the Valsalva maneuver. In one large trial of 1441 consecutive studies, the Mayo Clinic experience with more than 20,000 cardiovascular tests, and approximately 100 additional studies, no complications with sequelae have been ascribed to cardiovascular tests.[34,37,113] Infrequent asymptomatic dysrhythmias (premature ventricular contractions [PVCs]) were detected in a review of 925 subjects.[153] Inci-

*Anticholinergics:* Tricyclic antidepressants, atropine, probanthine, oxybutynin
*Cholinomimetics:* Pilocarpine, bethanechol, muscarine
*Anticholinesterases:* Pyridostigmine, neostigmine, organophosphates
*Beta-adrenergic blockers:* Propranolol and others
*Alpha-adrenergic agonists:* Phenylpropanolamine, ephedrine (including over-the-counter cold remedies), midodrine, ergot alkaloids
*Ganglionic blockers:* Guanethidine, hexamethonium
*Alpha$_1$ antagonists:* Phentolamine, phenoxybenzamine, guanabenz
*Alpha$_2$ activity:* Clonidine, prazosin, alpha-methyldopa, terazosin, yohimbine
*Antihistamines:* Benadryl and others
*Other blood pressure–lowering agents:* Hydralazine, nitroglycerin, diuretics, angiotensin-converting enzyme inhibitors
*Other:* Neuroleptics, nonsteroidal antiinflammatory drugs (NSAIDs), carbidopa/levodopa (Sinemet), tyramine, disopyramide, fludrocortisone, monoamine oxidase inhibitors, combination medications

dence was significantly higher in patients with prior myocardial infarction, but none required medical intervention. Skin irritation or minor injury can be associated with a small percentage of sudomotor tests and are discussed further in those sections.

## VALSALVA MANEUVER

The Valsalva maneuver is a reliable and reproducible method that can provide information for both parasympathetic (Valsalva ratio) and sympathetic function if simultaneous HR and BP beat-to-beat data are recorded. Traditionally, the BP has been measured with intraarterial lines or HR data are solely used; however, in recent years photoplethysmographic devices such as the Finapres have enabled data to be gathered without invasive techniques.[15,79] Finapres signals have correlated well with arterial transducers in most studies and have produced acceptable reliability under various conditions, such as on a tilt table or during a Valsalva maneuver. Careful attention to finger cuff application and temperature is vital. Reliability may break down with temperature extremes or marked vascular disease.

### Procedure

Typically, the subject blows into a closed tube connected to a pressure monitor. The tube has a small leak to prevent the subject from falsely maintaining apparent pressure with a closed glottis. A half breath is taken prior to blowing and 40 mm Hg of pressure is ideally maintained for 15 seconds. This level of effort appears to yield the most reproducible results.[97,113] Two to four efforts are measured; they are either averaged or the best effort is taken. A number of variations have been used. The maneuver causes a cascade of events, as outlined in Table 22–6 and Figure 22–1.

### Responses

Four distinct BP phases comprise a normal Valsalva response (Table 22–6). Phase I is induced by the initial strain and causes a rapid rise in intrathoracic and intraabdominal pressure, resulting in a mechanical acute increase in systolic BP. Soon thereafter the increased pressure of continued effort causes a decline in venous return and a drop in stroke volume, cardiac output, and therefore BP. This drop marks the onset of the early phase II (II$_e$). After several seconds the BP normally begins to recover, marking the onset of late phase II (II$_l$). The BP recovery is predominantly due to sympathetically mediated vasoconstriction triggered by the baroreceptor mediated initial BP fall with an associated rise in muscle sympathetic nerve traffic[32] and a rise in peripheral vascular resistance.[97] This effect is blunted or lost with alpha-adrenergic receptor blockade (phentolamine) or autonomic failure.[169] The partial recovery is accompanied by a steady increase in HR. The HR increase initially is due to vagal withdrawal and later to continued sympathetic influence. The HR response can be blunted both with atropine and beta-blockade. The peak HR (shortest RR interval) during this period is taken for the Valsalva ratio calculation.[10] This recovery from the BP fall in phase II is normally highly efficient, often producing a return to baseline levels prior to the onset of phase III. Phase III is the counterpart of phase I; BP drops acutely with the release of effort. Immediately thereafter the BP begins to rise again, marking phase IV onset. The BP slowly increases, overshoots, and gradually returns to baseline levels. Simultaneously the HR progressively declines, partly because of baroreceptor inhibition, and undershoots below baseline values. The HR nadir (longest RR interval) is recorded, and the Valsalva ratio is calculated from this value divided by the peak HR value. In pharmacologic dissection studies the HR drop in phase IV is lost with beta-blockade but not with atropine and is enhanced with phentolamine.[169]

Several trials may be needed to ensure reproducibility of the BP waveform. Critical portions of the BP wave for interpretation include the degree of decline during phase II, the presence and degree of partial recovery in the late portion prior to release, and the presence of the phase IV overshoot. Examples of responses from different subjects are shown in Figure 22–1. Most, but not all, series have found a decline in Valsalva ratio with age. An accepted set of normal values for the Valsalva ratio[113,120] are age 10 to 40 years (>1.5), 41 to 60 years (>1.45), and 61 to 70 years (>1.35). Some studies require a value <1.2 to be considered clearly abnormal.[10,104]

An alternate HR measure is the tachycardia ratio. In this ratio the longest baseline RR interval is used in place of the postmaneuver bradycardic value. The shortest (peak HR) value is used as the denominator. This measure reportedly is more reproducible than the Valsalva ratio, but it is more dependent on resting HR.[10]

**TABLE 22–6. Valsalva Maneuver Phases**

| PHASE | BP | HR | PROBABLE MECHANISM |
|---|---|---|---|
| I | Increase | Unchanged | Mechanical increase in pressure |
| II$_e$ (early) | Fall | Unchanged | Fall in venous return, SV, and CO |
| II$_l$ (late) | Recovery | Increase | Vagal withdrawal, peripheral vasoconstriction |
| III | Fall | Increase | Mechanical decrease in pressure |
| IV | Slow increase | Fall | Vagal, sympathetic overshoot |

CO, cardiac output; HR, heart rate; BP, blood pressure; SV, stroke volume.

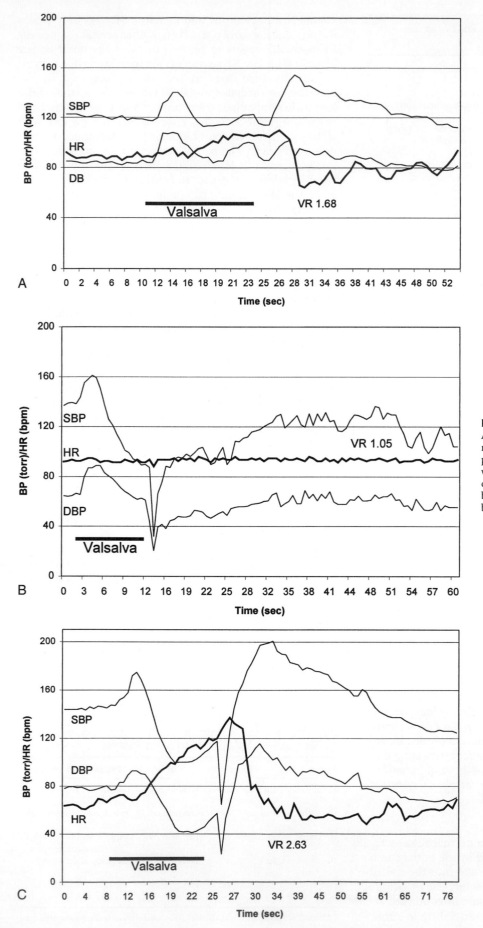

**FIGURE 22–1.** Valsalva maneuver patterns. **A,** Normal control. **B,** Autonomic failure from familial amyloidosis. Note lack of phase II recovery, phase IV overshoot, and HR response. **C,** Patient with POTS. Note blunted phase II, large phase IV overshoot, and HR response. *DBP,* Diastolic blood pressure; *HR,* heart rate; *SBP,* systolic blood pressure; *VR,* Valsalva ratio.

## Confounding Factors

The Valsalva ratio can be measured simply with an ECG tracing and a method of measuring the degree of strain, for example, a large syringe or tube connected to a sphygmomanometer or other pressure monitor. This method has been used in countless studies as a screening tool. However, a number of factors can confound results. The HR change is largely a baroreflex response. A falsely normal Valsalva ratio can result if sympathetic (baroreflex) failure is present, providing an enhanced BP drop as the stimulus to increase HR. Also, lack of the phase IV overshoot produces a reduced baroreflex-mediated bradycardia, which may spuriously reduce the Valsalva ratio.[15,205] For these reasons, as well as the added information, it is desirable to have simultaneous beat-to-beat BP recordings in addition to the ECG. Other factors that need standardization include the angle of recline (0 vs. 30 degrees) and the degree and length of effort. Other variables include age (which affects the Valsalva ratio and the magnitude of phase II), minor gender differences, inspiratory volume, and improper patient preparation (which also affect results).[113] Most patients are able to perform the task adequately; however, some debilitated or demented subjects are unable to provide sufficient force or duration of effort during the maneuver for meaningful interpretation.

## Clinical Applications

The Valsalva maneuver is fast, reproducible, quantitative, and sensitive. Valsalva ratio recording needs minimal equipment, but much more information is gathered with less chance of spurious results if the BP waveform is simultaneously recorded. Abnormalities have been detected in a wide variety of disorders and are part of most current autonomic screening batteries. The consensus committee has deemed that the combined test enhances the sensitivity and specificity of the evaluation of adrenergic function and is an established test.[8] Sensitivity for the detection of adrenergic dysfunction is higher than with standing or tilt-table studies. This measure is especially valuable, therefore, in lesser degrees of adrenergic failure without a diagnostic degree of orthostatic hypotension. Characteristic changes are valuable in certain syndromes of orthostatic intolerance that have distal vasoconstrictor insufficiency but intact cardiovagal and sympathetic cardiac responses. These changes are readily apparent in the BP waveform with an enlarged phase II with blunted recovery and an augmented phase IV and Valsalva ratio (Fig. 22–1). Other patterns described are the following[113]:

- Purely vagal: minimal phase II decline and reduced Valsalva ratio
- Mild sympathetic: augmented phase II with reduced or absent late phase II with other portions and Valsalva ratio normal
- Moderate to severe sympathetic: progressively larger phase II without recovery, reduction, or elimination of phase IV

Panautonomic failure produces loss of phase II recovery, phase IV, and reduced Valsalva ratio (see Fig. 22–1). Abnormalities have been described in 90% of patients with MSA and pure autonomic failure (PAF).[28,159] Abnormalities in patients with diabetes mellitus correlate with the severity of autonomic neuropathy and disease duration.[46,193]

# HEART RATE VARIABILITY

Measures of HR variability in response to cyclic deep breathing are among the simplest to record and the most sensitive indicators of parasympathetic function. Both afferent and efferent pathways are vagally mediated,[63,113] although underlying sympathetic tone can affect responses.[150] The response is not a single feedback loop but the effect of multiple overlapping reflex circuits involving the medullary respiratory center, baroreflex input, and pulmonary and cardiac stretch receptors and the effects of small relative changes in central venous volume.[60] The response is abolished by atropine. A number of other factors influence response magnitude, but they are well described and can be relatively well controlled[113,150,157] (Table 22–7). Most commonly, beat-to-beat HR recordings are obtained with an ECG machine or with an EMG machine set with a wide filter band. RR intervals or sequential HR data are measured while the subject continually breathes deeply in a cyclic sinusoidal pattern. Maximal changes in HR are seen at 6 breaths per minute (5 seconds for each expiratory and inspiratory phase). Numerous methods of analyzing the magnitude of the resultant enhanced sinus arrhythmia have been described.[38,44,60,70,113,142] The simplest method involves measuring the magnitude of HR change over each cycle (I-E difference) and averaging several cycles (4 to 5 cycles) after premature ventricular contractions (PVCs) and other confounding signals have been discarded. Some investigators also discard the initial cycle, which tends to be larger than average subsequent cycles. Additional recordings above 5 to 6 cycles tend to dampen the response range, likely because of the eventual development of hypocarbia, which leads to vagal suppression. Another simple measure is a ratio of the longest RR interval in expiration to the shortest inspiratory one (E:I ratio).[177] Multiple other statistical techniques have been employed to minimize the effects of resting HR, ectopic beats, and drift of the underlying HR over the time of the recording. The mean circular resultant employs complex vector analysis to minimize the effects of drift. Other commonly employed techniques include the mean consecutive difference, root mean square of consecutive differences (RMSCD), coefficient of variation, and power spectral analysis. Ziegler et al[222,223] examined eight different techniques, including power spectral analysis, in 120 healthy controls and later in patients to assess sensitivity data and day-to-day test variability. All techniques showed acceptable reproducibility with the lowest on Valsalva ratio measures. I-E difference, 30:15 ratio, and RMSCD were found to be less reliable, mainly because of the confounding effects of the resting HR.

---

**TABLE 22–7. Factors That Affect Heart-Rate (Diastolic Pressure) Variability**

1. Age
2. Depth of breathing
3. Rate of breathing
4. Hypocapnia/hyperventilation
5. Increased sympathetic tone/anxiety
6. Position
7. Anticholinergic medications
8. Statistical techniques used in analysis
9. Increased body surface area
10. Resting heart rate
11. Underlying cardiac, pulmonary, or central nervous system disease

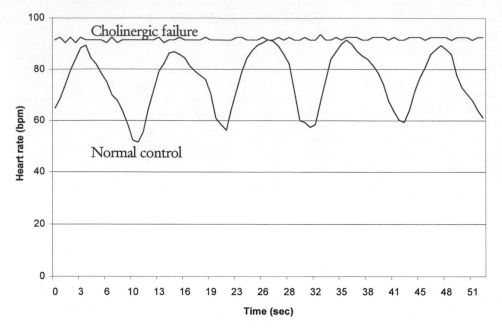
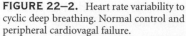

**FIGURE 22–2.** Heart rate variability to cyclic deep breathing. Normal control and peripheral cardiovagal failure.

## Responses

Data are gathered as a series of RR intervals or sequential HR points. The sinusoidal pattern is generally clearly visible when graphed unless it is severely attenuated, as seen with severe parasympathetic failure. Examples are shown in Figure 22–2. Once the time series is manually or digitally recorded and ectopic beats are eliminated, any of the statistical methods can be applied. Computerized methods have greatly simplified additional analysis. Age-dependent normal ranges have been reported for the HR range and E:I ratios.[120] Values reported for each age range of HR change in beats per minute are: 10 to 40 years, >18; 41 to 50 years, >16; 51 to 60 years, >12; 61 to 70 years, >8.

## Pitfalls

These techniques are fast, reproducible, and quantitative. They can be performed without extensive specialized equipment, other than the computerized methods for data manipulation. All the analytic techniques described are applicable, but there is no general consensus as to which is the best or ideal calculation. The factors listed in Table 22–7 can confound results if they are not controlled. Some coaching is necessary for the subject to perform the breathing task optimally. Some laboratories employ a metronome to ensure exactly six phases per minute and record respiratory excursions to correlate. Power spectral analysis is increasingly used as a sensitive method of analyzing BP and HR signals during deep breathing as well as rest, standing, and tilt and over longer time periods.[62,170] A reliable high-frequency signal is seen at the same rate as the paced breathing (0.1 Hz), which has been determined to be predominantly parasympathetic but is highly affected by the breathing depth and consistency. Despite promising prospects of these powerful techniques and valuable investigational contributions, no standardization of the acquisition algorithms or analytic methods has been agreed on to date. A task force has issued recommendations that may improve this problem in the future.[71] However, there are currently no definitive guidelines for clinical application of power spectral analysis in routine screening batteries.[108]

## Clinical Applications

HR variability to deep breathing employing one or more statistical methods is the most commonly used test and is part of most autonomic screening batteries; it is currently the closest to an optimal cardiovagal measure available.[8,63] It has been examined in diverse conditions and is a sensitive marker for diabetic autonomic neuropathy (DAN).[177] Since many neuropathies affect nerves in a length-dependent manner, distal sudomotor and vasomotor fibers are often affected early, with the long vagal fibers destined for the heart another early target, often showing abnormalities prior to clinical manifestations. The cardiovagal changes may be the earliest abnormality in certain neuropathies, such as DAN and Chagas' disease,[63,185] although distal sympathetic failure appears to occur with equal frequency in DAN.[127]

## OTHER PARASYMPATHETIC TESTS OF HEART RATE CHANGE

Numerous other cardiovagal reflexes have been adapted as clinical measures, but none are well established enough for routine clinical use. Notable examples include HR variability at rest, changes with coughing, the diving reflex, squatting, and lying down.

### COUGH

Coughing generates a large increase in intrathoracic pressure that leads to a decrease in BP and an increase in HR. This phenomenon is one of multiple potential triggers of vasodepressor syncope. The degree of HR increase has been adapted as a clinical measure,[210,211] although its clinical utility has been questioned.[203]

### FACIAL IMMERSION/COLD FACE TEST

Facial cooling triggers the diving reflex, consisting of bradycardia, apnea, reduced cardiac output, and peripheral vasoconstriction.[56,91] This reflex is believed to be an adaptation to reduce metabolic demand under special adverse conditions. The degree of HR decrease can be quantified. The test can be performed in an uncooperative or unconscious patient, unlike many of the other cardiovagal indexes.[91] Reflex pathways uniquely bypass the baroreflex peripheral and central connections, but they involve somatic trigeminal sensory as well as cardiovagal and sympathetic pathways.[39] The magnitude of the bradycardia is attenuated in a variety of conditions compromising cardiovagal responses. Further refinement and validation are needed before this measure can be considered well established.

### SQUATTING

Marfella et al[130,131] described a protocol for testing the effects of squatting. They measured responses in controls and patients with diabetes. Subjects stood for 3 minutes, squatted for 1 minute, then stood again during inspiration. A resultant bradycardia ensues with squatting that is blocked by atropine. The HR increases again with subsequent standing and is blocked by beta-blockade. A ratio of the extremes is used as the calculation. Values were abnormal in 40% of patients with diabetes and <1% of controls and are suggested as a measure of both parasympathetic and sympathetic integrity.[130,131]

## TESTS OF THERMOREGULATION

Regulation of thermal homeostasis is carried out primarily by sweating and vasomotor changes for heat dissipation and by shivering and nonshivering mechanisms for heat production and conservation. The hypothalamus is the main integration and control center. Afferent signals are relayed through the preoptic and anterior hypothalamic nuclei, where warm- and cold-sensitive neurons reside. However, temperature-sensitive sites are present in other areas, such as the medullary reticular formation and the spinal cord.[146] Warm-sensitive neurons are approximately fourfold more abundant than cold ones. Relative activities likely determine a "set-point," deviation from which induces effector mechanisms to alter body temperature. Sweating, the primary mechanism for heat dissipation, is mainly sympathetic, providing a useful system for testing peripheral sympathetic function. Measurement of sweat gland activity is the most commonly performed and most reliable effector mechanism evaluated, with several techniques discussed here. Unlike other sympathetic systems, both preganglionic and postganglionic neurons are cholinergic. Two main types of sweat glands are present in humans. First, *apocrine glands* open directly into hair follicle lumens (epitrichial). These glands are relatively unimportant and are found in limited areas, such as the axilla, perineum, and areola. Second, *eccrine glands* open directly onto the skin (atrichial) and are the primary source of sweat for evaporative heat loss. This gland type is found throughout the body with varying densities and capabilities. The environment during the developmental period influences sweat gland density with more abundant glands in hot climates.[145]

Most sweat glands are activated in response to signals to dissipate heat, such as a temperature increase. These glands are the basis of measurements in response to chemical and thermal stimuli. Other sweat glands in the palms and soles respond little to temperature signals but instead are activated in response to stressful and emotional triggers. These

sites are the basis of part of the waveform generated in sympathetic skin response recordings. Numerous factors can influence sweat gland activation and output volume in response to stimuli, and they can hamper laboratory measurements if they are not controlled.[146] Most important is the underlying state of hydration. Hypovolemia and hyperosmolality inhibit sweat output and lead to a rise in core temperature.[58,59,146] Hypocapnia, such as that induced by hyperventilation, typically leads to reduced sweat output, peripheral vasoconstriction, and a consequential rise in body temperature. Hypercapnia has the opposite effect. Emotional stress, sleep, and hormonal factors also may alter sweat output.

## QSART

The quantitative sudomotor axon reflex test (QSART) records chemically induced dynamic sweat output. Unlike most autonomic measures, these responses assess postganglionic function and can be of potential localizing value, especially when combined with other sudomotor tests, such as the thermoregulatory sweat test (TST), that assess the integrity of the entire sudomotor pathway. The basis of testing is an axon reflex induced by stimulating the muscarinic receptors of eccrine sweat glands. This activation induces an antidromic response up the postganglionic cholinergic axon. When a branch point is reached, an orthodromic signal propagates down to another sweat gland isolated from the chemical stimulus. The sweat produced is measured over time.[113] Testing is reproducible in controls with a coefficient of variation <20%.[120]

### Procedure

Testing involves measuring sweat output induced by the axon reflexes by chemically stimulating one population of glands and recording from a contiguous but isolated area. Important components are a compartmentalized sweat capsule that separates patches of skin into discrete zones and a sudrometer that assesses minute changes in relative humidity. Ten percent acetylcholine is iontophoresed into one compartment in a standardized fashion via a constant current generator. Low-humidity nitrogen gas is pumped into the contiguous but chemically isolated chamber and read by a sudrometer. As sweating is induced, a change in relative humidity is recorded, converted to sweat volume, and displayed as a continuous readout over time. Numerous proximal and distal sites have been tested and standardized.[115] Typically, several sites in the arm and leg are studied to provide some degree of topographic information.

### Responses

Several types of responses have been described and are displayed in Figure 22–3. Normally, a rise in sweat volume is detectable within 2 minutes and returns to baseline levels by 5 minutes. Onset latency is primarily determined by the speed of acetylcholine diffusion. Abnormal patterns include an overall reduced or absent response. Volumes are normally higher in men and are variably reduced with age, depending on the anatomic site. Other abnormal patterns include a response that fails to return to baseline levels (persistent sweat activity) or a response with an abnormally short onset latency, which may reflect altered excitability of the pathways involved.[113] Response at rest (resting sweat activity) or sweat

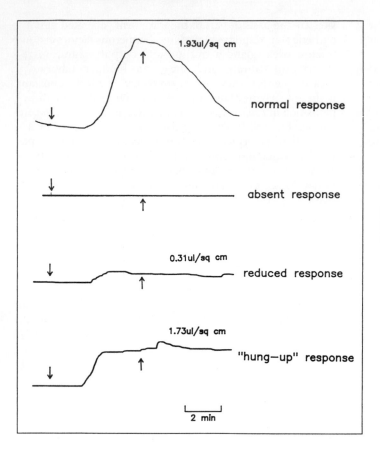

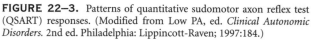

**FIGURE 22–3.** Patterns of quantitative sudomotor axon reflex test (QSART) responses. (Modified from Low PA, ed. *Clinical Autonomic Disorders.* 2nd ed. Philadelphia: Lippincott-Raven; 1997:184.)

activity at temperatures not expected to induce a response may also be seen.

### Pitfalls

Testing is time-consuming and requires extensive specialized equipment currently available in only a handful of centers. Individual components are commercially available and can be assembled. A complete unit is under commercial development and is projected to be available soon. Responses are affected by factors that inhibit sweating, including hypovolemia and anticholinergic medications. Undue anxiety and low temperature in the limbs may also affect results. A small risk of local skin injury is present from the electrical current delivered. Low has reported minor local injuries in some of the 40,000 studies performed,[4] but no injuries have been reported in the last 3000 tests after minor procedural modifications.[113]

### Applications

The QSART has been used in a wide range of causes of sympathetic dysfunction. A reduced or absent response implies postganglionic sudomotor failure. The topographic information gained, employing both distal and proximal recordings, is useful in neuropathies with autonomic involvement, including small-fiber neuropathy. Especially in the early stages only distal sites may be involved. Responses should be unaffected with central or preganglionic lesions; however, response reduction may be seen in later stages of more central dysfunction, suggesting a transsynaptic defect.[113] QSART abnormalities have been found in 58% of diabetics, 83% of patients with various causes of peripheral neuropathy,[115] and 80% of patients with small-fiber neu-

ropathy (SFN).[188] Testing is especially valuable in SFN when conventional tests, such as electrodiagnostic studies and nerve biopsy, are unrevealing.

Persistent sweat activity or a delayed return to baseline levels may be seen in painful neuropathies or other causes of hyperalgesia, for example, complex regional pain disorder (reflex sympathetic dystrophy). The resting sweat activity associated with neuropathies is most commonly found when causalgia, vasomotor changes, and excessive sweating (hyperhidrosis) are present and may coexist with the persistent sweat response pattern. It has been suggested that the mechanism involves repetitive firing of the sympathetic sudomotor axons. QSART with measurement of resting sweat activity has been suggested to be predictive of reflex sympathetic dystrophy response to sympathetic block; however, this assertion has been challenged.[24,144]

### THERMOREGULATORY SWEAT TEST

The TST provides a method of assessing sweat output over the entire body (or anterior surface) in response to a thermal stimulus. This approach has the advantages of a physiologic stimulus (a rise in core temperature) and simultaneous assessment of wide areas of skin. The distribution of anhidrotic areas is readily noted. Testing is sensitive, well standardized, and often clinically relevant, providing a visible map of the areas deficient in sweating. Abnormalities have been described in a broad range of causes of sympathetic dysfunction.[8,53]

### Procedure

The subject (except the head) is placed in a chamber with tightly controlled baseline temperature and humidity.

Prior to entering, an indicator dye, such as a mixture with alizarin red, is applied to the anterior body surface area. This dye is an improvement over earlier preparations, such as iodine solution or quinizarin, which caused prolonged staining and skin irritation, respectively. Alizarin is said to cause skin irritation in only 0.1% of subjects.[53] Core body temperature is warmed to a predetermined degree, for example, a 1° C rise or an absolute level above 38° C to ensure an adequate thermal stimulus. After 30 to 45 minutes the response, noted as a color change, is recorded. A qualitative impression or photograph may be taken. Newer digital cameras have paved the way for semiquantitative assessments, reported as percent anhidrosis.[53]

## Results

Normal sweating patterns reflected in the indicator color change produce a generalized pattern. Normal variants include a variable response in proximal limbs or proximal arms as well as entire lower extremity[54] and could lead to false-positive results. Abnormal patterns are consistent with expected clinical distributions in sweat impairment. Fealey[53] has described seven patterns (Table 22–8), with examples shown in Figure 22–4.[116]

## Applications

The TST is applicable in a broad range of central and peripheral causes of sympathetic dysfunction. In conjunction with the QSART or sweat imprint techniques, localization of a deficit as a probable preganglionic or postganglionic lesion is possible. Since denervation supersensitivity is not manifest in the sudomotor system with loss of innervation (exception to Hering's law), abnormal areas on both the TST and the QSART imply a postganglionic lesion.

## Pitfalls

Testing is somewhat messy, uncomfortable, and time-consuming. Indicator dyes rinse off well, but rinsing may be incomplete in some patches. Results are affected by factors that reduce sweat production, including dehydration and anticholinergic medications. Topical lotions and pressure wraps may hamper assessment in the focal areas administered.[53] There remains some controversy as to whether sweat output is age dependent, hampering interpretation in the elderly. If not accounted for, several normal variant patterns can be misdiagnosed as abnormalities. As with the majority of measures, specificity is limited as a stand-alone test.

---

**TABLE 22–8. Sweat Distribution Patterns With the Thermoregulatory Sweat Test**

1. *Distal* in a length-dependent pattern
2. *Segmental* with large zones of anhidrosis, borderline normal zones in sympathetic dermatomal patterns
3. *Focal* in peripheral nerve, root, or small skin patch distributions; focal patterns also with local dermatologic disorders or radiation effects
4. *Global* defined as >80% of body surface area
5. *Regional* large anhidrotic areas that blend into contiguous areas
6. *Mixed* patterns
7. *Normal* patterns

From Fealey RD. Thermoregulatory sweat test. In: Low PA, ed. *Clinical Autonomic Disorders.* 2nd ed. Philadelphia: Lippincott-Raven; 1997:248.

## SWEAT IMPRINT TECHNIQUES

Sweat imprint techniques are additional methods of assessing sudomotor function. As noted earlier, eccrine sweat glands are more readily accessible than other sympathetically innervated sites, and they provide a useful system to stimulate directly. A variety of methods have been described, all relying on inducing sudomotor outflow using heat or cholinergic agents and recording the resultant sweat output on a recording medium. It is possible to quantify both the number and water output of secreting glands by analyzing the image or impression in the recording media. Heat stimulation has been accomplished with regional or generalized warming or with exercise.[87] The entire circuit of thermoregulatory function is employed; thus abnormalities may result from preganglionic, postganglionic, or central dysfunction. Direct chemical induction with the use of iontophoresed cholinergic agents such as acetylcholine, methacholine, or pilocarpine is the most commonly employed, best tolerated, and most uniform method, although direct injection and even direct electrical stimulation have been used. Acetylcholine is a less ideal agent because, unlike the others, it is deactivated by acetylcholinesterase, shortening the period of stimulation. Directly stimulating sweat glands in this way has the advantage of testing only the postganglionic arm of the pathway. Since sweat glands do not demonstrate denervation supersensitivity,[87] a reduction in chemically induced stimulation is a direct reflection of sympathetic denervation. Each sweat gland, however, is innervated by more than one cholinergic axon and may continue to respond after partial, but not complete, denervation.[88]

## Techniques

A number of indicator dyes, applied to a test area of skin to visualize the individual sweat droplets, have been tried in addition to Minor's original iodine-starch method. Dyes can also be excreted after subcutaneous or intravenous administration. Stopcock grease has been used to limit the problem of sweat droplets coalescing and obscuring accurate droplet counts.[69] However, impressions of the skin made with plastic or silicone materials that record skin markings and sweat output have the highest resolution.[87] In a direct comparison of various techniques, colloidal graphite plastic imprints yielded an average of 55% more droplets than bromphenol blue plus grease and 107% more droplets that Wada's starch-iodine method.[69] Silicone imprints yielded 11% higher counts than the plastic mixture, but the results were not statistically significant. Superior sensitivity and lack of skin irritation make the silicone mold imprints currently the best overall method. Based on the silicone methods, this test has been deemed to be sensitive and well established for inclusion as part of a clinical battery.[8]

## Procedure

Kennedy's protocol involves stimulating a 1 cm² area, typically at two sites by iontophoresis (2 mA direct current for 5 minutes) of a 1% pilocarpine nitrate solution. The silicon elastomer (Silastic) material is applied after 5 minutes and again at 20 minutes. The material hardens within 3 minutes, and an impression of skin markings and emerging sweat droplets is made in the material.[87] The analysis involves counting the number of impressions by using a dissecting microscope while transilluminating the mold. An es-

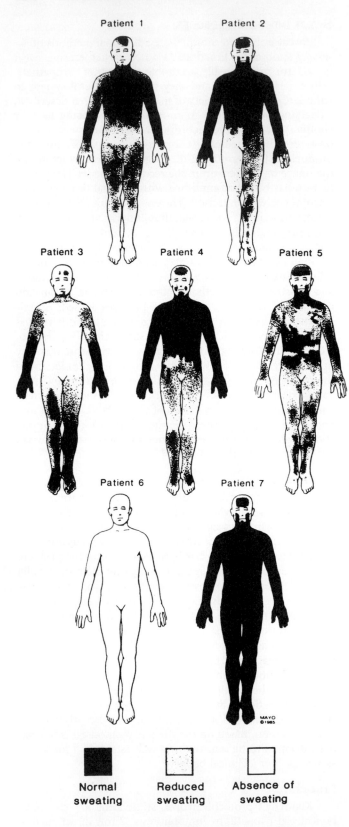

**FIGURE 22–4.** Examples of sweat distribution patterns in patients with diabetes mellitus. Descriptions correspond to list in Table 22–8. (Modified from Low and Fealey[116] with permission.)

timate of sweat volume is obtained by projecting a photographic negative onto a digitizer pad and outlining the drops.[89] A more recent semiautomated computerized system that uses a video camera and special computer software has been described and correlated with other methods.[86] Direct macrophotography has been demonstrated to be as sensitive

as counting methods, but it requires extensive expertise in advanced photographic techniques.

**Responses**

Ranges of normal values of sweat gland density and sweat droplet size have been published.[139] Values for sweat gland density are higher in the hand dorsum in comparison to the foot with similar normal droplet size. An age-related decline in density has been reported, with sex and body surface area as covariant factors.[55]

### Pitfalls

Silastic imprint techniques are time-consuming and require some specialized equipment; however, the imprint materials involved are relatively inexpensive. Currently, these studies are performed only in a few centers. The dynamic components measured with the QSART are not evaluated. With the direct stimulation methods, postganglionic dysfunction can be localized; however, preganglionic causes of hypohidrosis are not evaluated. This limitation can be overcome if the Silastic imprint technique is combined with tests that use central stimulation such as heat. Only a small number of anatomic sites, typically the dorsum of the hand and foot, are usually studied, providing little topographic information. Nonneurologic conditions can lead to abnormal results, including congenital absence of sweat glands,[100] Sjögren's syndrome, occlusion of skin pores, and several dermatologic conditions.

### Applications

These techniques have been applied to a variety of conditions, but they are used most extensively in patients with peripheral neuropathy. As part of an autonomic screening battery, they are a sensitive and reproducible component. Kennedy[86] found reduced numbers of activated glands by using the Silastic mold technique in 24% of hands and 56% of feet in a population of patients with type I diabetes. Percentages rose to 36% and 60%, respectively, if sweat volume data were also considered. Abnormalities were found in roughly a third of diabetic patients with a normal neurologic examination and a third with normal electrophysiologic studies, as would be expected from a process with early involvement of unmyelinated fibers, such as diabetic polyneuropathy. These abnormalities were correlated with abnormalities of other small-fiber functions, such as quantitative thermal sensory threshold testing, but not with vibratory thresholds or nerve conduction studies.[139] Many of the abnormalities were symptomatically subclinical in this population, however. In a population of 30 chronic alcoholics, Navarro et al[140] found abnormal responses in 7 hands and 18 feet. A slightly lower percentage of sympathetic skin response abnormalities was found, but the two populations did not correlate well with each other, with cardiovagal reflexes, or with nerve conduction study abnormalities. In a comparison of direct vs. axon reflex stimulation, Stewart et al[189] found a slight increase in sensitivity with direct techniques.

## SYMPATHETIC SKIN RESPONSE

The phenomenon of movement of a galvanometer needle in response to physical or emotional stimuli while connected to the body has been known for well over 100 years (Féré). The sympathetic skin response (SSR) is a related phenomenon mediated by the same afferent and efferent pathways.[174] Recent interest has renewed the popularity of recording this complex reflex as a measure of sudomotor activity. The interest stems primarily from the relative simplic-

ity of recording and the lack of need for the specialized equipment necessary for other sudomotor tests. A conventional EMG machine, preferably with multichannel recording capability, is the only equipment necessary.

SSRs are a type of *evoked* electrodermal activity, as distinguished from *spontaneous* discharges or *direct* electrodermal stimulation, which is impractical to elicit in humans. The electrodermal activity originates from sweat glands and surrounding epidermal and dermal structures. The recorded SSR is a summation of the multiple waveforms generated by the various structures. The reflex is highly complex and appears to be multisynaptic, based in part on the variability of responses and a tendency to habituate. Efferent pathways are sympathetic and cholinergic. Microneurographic studies have confirmed that the SSR activity is synchronous with traffic in small unmyelinated fibers[52,206] and is abolished by sympathectomy, atropine, and nerve transection.[95,99,102,149] In fact, studies have proposed using the SSR as a gauge of the adequacy of surgical sympathectomy for conditions such as idiopathic hyperhidrosis.[102]

Afferent pathways appear to be large-diameter sensory fibers. Central pathways have not been clearly defined, but multiple areas have been suggested by animal studies; these include the posterior hypothalamus, mesencephalic reticular formation, and cortical and subcortical areas. Thus the SSR is of potential interest in both central and peripheral causes of sympathetic dysfunction. Recordings are made over the prime sites of emotional sweating, namely, the palms and soles.

### Protocol

Multiple protocols have been used with various methods of eliciting a response. A noxious electrical stimulus is the most commonly employed technique. Other stimuli include an inspiratory gasp or cough, auditory stimulus or startling sound, and magnetic stimulation. Response amplitude varies depending on the technique. Our method involves recording simultaneously over each palmar and plantar area with Ag/AgCl electrodes referenced to the dorsum of the hand or foot, respectively. Recording sites are cleaned but not abraded. Ideally, recording is done on all four limbs simultaneously with a four-channel preamplifier to maximize information and limit the number of stimuli. A ground is applied to the stimulated arm. An electrical stimulating electrode is taped over the median nerve at the elbow, and the patient is allowed to relax in a supine position in a quiet, darkened, temperature-controlled room for at least 15 minutes. The patient is not permitted to drift into sleep, however. Low-frequency (high-pass) filters are set at 0.2 Hz (or as low as available). A long sweep speed such as 500 ms per division with a gain at 500 μV is used and adjusted as necessary. Baseline recordings without stimulation are monitored to prevent stimulation in proximity to a spontaneous discharge. Stimulation strength beginning at 50 mA (0.2 ms duration) is used and delivered without prompting. Subsequent stimulations are delivered at irregular intervals, but at least 60 seconds after the previous stimulus, with monitoring done for spontaneous discharges. The patient is warned of the procedure in general, but care must be taken not to cue actual responses. Several responses are recorded, and latency and amplitude are measured if waveforms are reproducible. The best four responses are averaged. Responses after an alternate method, such as deep inspiratory gasp or a startling sound, are also recorded to provide information on both afferent and efferent function. Electrical stimulation may need to be increased in patients with significant sensory neuropathy to ensure an adequately noxious stimulus.

### Responses

In general, the SSR is recordable in all normal controls,[9,95] except in the feet of half of individuals over age 60.[35] The waveform is most commonly biphasic with an initial negative deflection. Approximately 30% have a second negative phase of unclear clinical significance. The initial negative portion appears to arise directly from sweat gland activity and is absent in cases with congenital absence of sweat glands.[100] Other components appear to arise from other dermal and epidermal sources. An example of a control set of waveforms is seen in Figure 22–5.

The latency is the most reliable measure but unfortunately is highly insensitive. Abnormalities of onset latency have been reported in a number of conditions, including multiple sclerosis (MS); however, most were not subsequently reproduced. The evoked amplitude is a more sensitive indicator but is variable in response. Hoeldtke et al[75] examined SSR reproducibility and found a high degree of variability in amplitude within a single day or on consecutive days. Latency measures were much less variable. The range of normal values in reported series is correspondingly wide. Mean values in reported series range from 180 µV ± 90 to 5530 ± 3.24 in the palm and 80 µV ± 50 to 2170 ± 1620 in the sole of the foot.[95,141,172,184,199,201,220] These extreme differences are likely in part a result of technical differences (e.g., the low filter settings used), but they underscore why many investigators require a response to be unrecordable to be considered abnormal, limiting testing sensitivity and eliminating the quantitative aspects of testing.

### Pitfalls

Numerous pitfalls hamper meaningful SSR interpretation, especially if the response amplitude is the measure of abnormality. One of the prime limitations for universal clinical application is that no consensus has yet been reached as to what constitutes an abnormal response. Determining control values for a particular laboratory setup is recommended, especially if latency and amplitude measurements are used to determine abnormality. However, the most prominent pitfall is habituation. Reduction of response amplitude can be influenced by previous responses, extraneous stimuli such as stray sounds, and spontaneous discharges of various causes. Recording simultaneously from multiple limbs to reduce the number of trials needed and waiting an adequate interval between stimuli and after a spontaneous discharge can reduce, but not eliminate, this phenomenon.

Filter settings are another important variable. Since the response is a very low frequency waveform, small alterations in the low-frequency filters modify the size of the recorded response considerably. Lack of a standard low filter setting explains in part the marked range between control series.

Neuropathies impairing the large afferent sensory fibers also impede SSR recordings. Levy et al[105] were able to record the SSR in only half of patients with obvious diabetic neuropathy through electrical stimulation. It is interesting that the SSR evoked by deep inspiration, which bypasses the large-fiber afferent loop used with an electrical stimulus, was recordable in 96% of 68 patients with diabetic neuropathy, many of whom had symptoms of autonomic neuropathy. Uncini et al[199] also found this pattern with a selective ischemic block of large afferent fibers but not sudomotor fibers. In this setting the SSR was recordable with inspiratory gasp and with a contralateral electrical stimulus but not with ipsilateral stimulation. Thus interpretation becomes problematic in patients with significant large-fiber sensory loss.

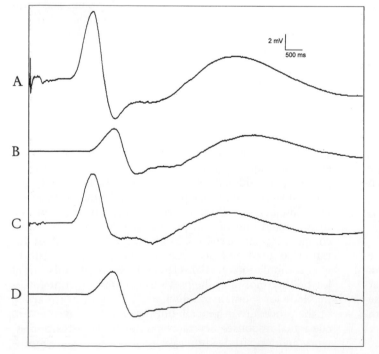

**FIGURE 22–5.** Sympathetic skin responses from normal control. Simultaneous four-channel recording after 50 mA stimulation of the left median nerve. Recording sites: *A*, left palm; *B*, left sole; *C*, right palm; *D*, right sole.

Other important variables include the limb temperature, the size and type of electrodes, and the patient's emotional state, age, and height.[7,171]

Latency abnormalities have been reported in some studies,[201] but, in general, latency prolongation caused by peripheral effects would not be expected in pathways involving unmyelinated fibers. Correspondingly, in studies including both axonal and demyelinating neuropathies, no differences in onset latency were found.[52,95,174,184] In one study of patients with multiple sclerosis, a delay in latency with normal evoked amplitude was noted in 85% of patients.[40] Other studies have found similar results, suggesting a possible delay in central, and not peripheral, pathways.[109,220] Currently, this finding has not been validated for diagnostic purposes.

### Clinical Applications

Due to the technical limitations discussed above, the SSR is not recommended in isolation as a useful test of sudomotor or sympathetic function. The consensus committee on autonomic testing of the American Academy of Neurology (AAN) determined that it is an established test but of limited reproducibility.[8] Other tests of sympathetic and sudomotor function are preferable if available. Some direct comparisons, however, with the Silastic imprint test and the QSART have yielded similar sensitivities; thus this measure can be a useful adjunct to a screening battery, as long as it is not the sole adrenergic measure.[134]

The SSR has been examined in numerous series of potential causes of peripheral sudomotor loss and also some possible central ones. By far the largest experience is with diabetes mellitus. In series of patients with diabetes not selected for the presence of neuropathy, absent SSRs were found in 4.4%[105] to 9%[209] of patients, and amplitude reductions were noted in an additional 16% to 35%. In the largest series of diabetic patients with clinical polyneuropathy, absent SSRs were found in 20% to 46% in the hand and 59% to 83% in the foot.[134,141,184] In one of these series of 47 patients with diabetic neuropathy, Soliven et al[184] found 31 cases with absent plantar SSRs, 90% of whom displayed signs and symptoms of autonomic dysfunction. However, only 80% with autonomic signs concomitantly showed an absent plantar SSR. In the Niaken and Harati series of 72 patients with diabetic neuropathy in which 83% showed a loss of one or both SSRs, a high percentage had indications of autonomic dysfunction.[141] SSR abnormalities have shown variable correlation with other measures of autonomic or somatic fiber neuropathy. Positive correlations have been seen with the E:I ratio (cardiovagal),[134,184,209] QSART,[134] and diabetes duration.[105] Responses have inconsistently correlated with nerve conduction findings.[184,209] Absent SSRs have been demonstrated in variable percentages in a variety of other neuropathies, both with and without prominent autonomic dysfunction, including chronic renal failure, Guillain-Barré syndrome, alcoholic neuropathy, and several others.[140,200,208]

Limited work is available on the application of the SSR in disorders affecting central pathways. Abnormalities have been described in spinal cord injuries, amyotrophic lateral sclerosis (ALS), selected stroke patients, idiopathic Parkinson's disease, MSA, pure autonomic failure, and others.[95,158,219] Abnormalities in the SSR amplitude or latency have been found in 59% of patients with clinically definite MS and have even been suggested as an adjunct diagnostic tool in equivocal cases.[220]

Abnormalities of SSR latency or amplitude have been reported in a majority of limbs affected with complex regional pain disorder; however, this finding is of unclear diagnostic or prognostic utility.[36,165] The SSR has been suggested as an easily obtained marker for assessing the adequacy of surgical sympathectomy performed for an increasingly recognized number of cases of idiopathic essential hyperhidrosis. Notably in this benign but disruptive or even disabling condition, many cases appear to have baseline SSR abnormalities. These include absent palmar responses in 20% in one series[107] and may show excessively inconsistent amplitude and additional elicited waveforms that may stem from excessive background sympathetic tone[98,102] (also noted by personal observation).

In sum, an undue amount of attention has been given to this complex response, mostly because of the ease in recording. Other measures of sudomotor function may eventually supplant the SSR if they become less cumbersome and more widely available.

## ORTHOSTATIC TESTING

### STANDING AND THE 30:15 RATIO

The simple act of standing initiates a coordinated sequence of reflexes to maintain BP, cardiac output, and therefore cerebral perfusion. The mechanical pumping action of muscular contraction compresses capacitance and resistance vessels, offsetting the gravitational shift of approximately 300 to 800 ml of volume to dependent regions. The muscular contraction thereby initiates an exercise reflex. Baroreflexes are stimulated to lower BP by decreasing sympathetic outflow, vasomotor tone, and peripheral resistance, leading to a transient drop in BP.[157] The degree of BP drop is more substantial than that seen with passive tilting, which lacks a significant exercise reflex phenomenon. The HR abruptly increases over several seconds and then more slowly and progressively rises until a peak occurs near beat 15.[20] The initial changes are related to parasympathetic withdrawal followed by the addition of baroreflex-mediated sympathetic activation. Subsequently the pattern is reversed by this reflexive BP fall, and the opposite effects ensue to restore the BP to baseline levels. Vasoconstriction of splanchnic beds is an important component of the compensatory response, explaining in part why compressive stockings often fail to be effective without some degree of abdominal compression.[33] A subsequent reflexive drop in HR occurs with a nadir around beat 30 in response to the compensatory overshoot in BP. This HR effect is blocked by atropine. Pharmacologic dissection suggests that the HR changes are primarily parasympathetically mediated and have been applied as a test of cardiovagal function (30:15 ratio).[47] After stabilization within 1 to 2 minutes, continued BP maintenance is influenced not only by autonomic systems but also by humoral, renal, fluid shifts, and other factors, involving catecholamines, renin-angiotensin, vasopressin, neuropeptide Y, and atriopeptin.

### Responses

Simple HR and BP responses to standing are important bedside markers of autonomic integrity, but further information is gained by laboratory testing in a more controlled setting with continuous monitoring. Most laboratories, however, currently use passive tilting in place or in addition to simple standing. Responses are best measured after a supine rest period of 15 to 30 minutes. Baseline values are recorded, and readings are taken at least every minute for 3 to 5 minutes. An ECG or other beat-to-beat HR recording enables calculation of the 30:15 ratio, the predominantly parasympathetically mediated changes discussed earlier. The calculation employs the longest RR interval (HR nadir) around beat 30 (after standing) divided by the shortest (HR peak) near beat 15. Ewing[47] required a ratio <1 to be considered abnormal. Age-related norms have been described and are reported for ages 10 to 29 (>1.17), 30 to 49 (>1.09), and 50 to 65 (>1.03).[214] There is some disagreement on methodology and how literally to take the exact fifteenth and thirtieth beats for calculation. Most centers use the peaks close to those reference points. A reduced ratio is a marker for the lack of parasympathetic withdrawal expected with the orthostatic changes.

There is some disagreement on the degree of BP drop considered to be abnormal. Most commonly, a systolic decrease of 20 to 30 mm Hg or 10 to 20 diastolic within 3 minutes is considered significant.[30,138] In 1996 an AAN consensus committee defined orthostatic hypotension as a systolic drop of ≥20 mm Hg or ≥10 diastolic within 3 minutes of standing or on at least 60 degrees of passive tilt with attention to symptoms induced.[30] The committee also noted that repeated measures may be necessary in some patients and that, rarely, the decline may be delayed for up to 10 minutes. More recently, examination of other markers, such as BP recovery from the initial drop, suggests that this approach may be a more valuable indicator of vasoconstrictor insufficiency.[187] Orthostatic tachycardia of more than 30 beats per minute or an absolute level over 120 is also considered significant.

A related response to active lying down has been described with an acute increase in HR over several beats followed by a reflex bradycardia that is maximal around beat 25 to 30.[12,13] This finding, in association with monitoring the degree of excessive passive overshoot of BP, is of potential value. However, the results have not yet been sufficiently characterized to be considered a test for routine clinical application.

### Pitfalls

Testing is simple, requires little special equipment, and yields quantitative results in response to an everyday physiologic event. However, multiple confounding factors can hamper interpretation if they are not controlled. The physiology is quite complex, and a normal response relies on intact sympathetic, cardiovagal, and afferent baroreflex systems. Given this complex set of interactions, there is concern about using the 30:15 ratio as a pure parasympathetic marker. Moreover, the magnitude of HR change is dependent on the duration of the preceding rest,[196] which is difficult to control in an office setting. In fact, a low correlation of the 30:15 ratio with measures of HR variability to deep breathing suggest that different mechanisms may be involved.[215] In isolated cases with sympathetic vasomotor failure but intact cardiovagal function, the reflex bradycardia is lost not from cardiovagal failure, but from a lack of stimulus, leading to a spuriously reduced 30:15 ratio.[47,48,147,205] As

with the Valsalva maneuver, isolated HR or BP measurement can be problematic to interpret in certain circumstances. Despite these concerns, the 30:15 ratio is used as a test of cardiovagal function, but it is not believed to be the most sensitive or reproducible measure in comparison to HR variability measures or the Valsalva ratio.[222] Confounding variables are not as extensively described as with other common cardiovagal tests; however, the 30:15 ratio is considered a sufficiently reproducible and well-established test.[8]

Although most patients are able to perform the task of standing adequately, patients with neurologic impairment, such as parkinsonism or cerebellar dysfunction, may not be able to stand quickly or smoothly enough for determination of the initial HR changes or to stand quietly enough to prevent repeated influences of muscular contraction.

Some additional signs discernible in the BP waveform that are reported as early or milder indicators of orthostatic intolerance are more easily determined on a tilt table with beat-to-beat HR and BP values, such as excessive BP oscillations. Standing is also less practical when a prolonged orthostatic challenge is needed or a delay in BP drop is suspected. As with other measures, important factors that must be excluded before meaningful interpretation can be performed include hypovolemia from various causes, prolonged bedrest with deconditioning, autonomically active medications, adrenal insufficiency, acute illness or sepsis, and hypothyroidism. An orthostatic drop in BP is also described in a minority of subjects over age 70,[81,164,180] but this condition is usually mild or asymptomatic.[31,163,164] Orthostatic hypotension is seen in approximately 14% to 20% of patients over age 75.[112,180] Often the changes are seen only under conditions of enhanced orthostatic stress, such as brief bedrest of several days, postprandial period, acute volume depletion, and medication effects. The phenomenon is likely multifactorial.

### Clinical Applications

Most laboratories prefer orthostatic testing done in the more controlled setting of a tilt table, but response to standing remains a valuable bedside screening tool if properly performed. Some laboratories use both methods because of the differing initial physiologic manifestations over the first 1 to 2 minutes. Many of the abnormal patterns that are also evident with tilt testing are described in more detail in the next section. However, responses to standing have been used in a wide variety of disorders and are suitable as part of a battery that measures both cardiovagal and adrenergic function. This type of bedside testing is vital in patients with known autonomic failure, especially for continual monitoring of responses to specific treatments, because serial formal tilt tests are usually impractical. Notable examples include response to medications for treatment of symptomatic orthostasis, detecting an exacerbation by concomitant treatments such as levodopa, and monitoring the effects of autonomically active medications needed for other indications (e.g., antidepressants). In general, symptomatic orthostatic hypotension to standing is a less sensitive marker of autonomic failure, especially in length-dependent neuropathies.

### TILT-TABLE STUDIES

Orthostatic challenge with passive upright tilting is currently the standard method used in most autonomic laboratories and nearly all cardiologic laboratories. Passive tilting does not employ the identical physiologic mechanisms as active standing. However, testing is more easily controllable with standardized tilting angles, is simpler to maintain the point of BP monitoring at heart level, and is easier for patients who are slowed by neurologic impairment. Otherwise, the physiologic reflexes are similar to those of standing. The tilt table is used somewhat differently in the autonomic laboratory, which is concerned with neurogenic autonomic failure or dysregulation, vs. in a cardiologic examination, which is more concerned with unexplained syncope, most commonly neurocardiogenic (vasovagal) syncope.[2,83,166] Neurogenic orthostatic hypotension due to autonomic failure or HR changes characteristic of the postural orthostatic tachycardia syndrome (POTS) generally are evident within the first 5 to 10 minutes of tilting, in contrast to studies needed to demonstrate a syncopal pattern, which may not appear for up to an hour.

## Procedure

ECG recordings are continuously monitored, and serial BP measurements are recorded manually or with an automated sphygmomanometer. Ideally a continuous BP monitoring device (e.g., Finapres or similar device) is used, obviating the need for invasive arterial catheters. Additional measures can be monitored simultaneously, such as respiration, transcranial Doppler signals, EEG, carbon dioxide expiration, and noninvasive cardiac impedance plethysmography (for cardiac output and peripheral vascular resistance determinations). As with standing, a supine rest period precedes tilting. The subject is secured to the tilt table, and the arm used for BP measurements is placed on an arm board that will maintain the measuring point at or just below heart level irrespective of the tilt angle. In autonomic laboratories the subject is tilted, typically to 60 to 90 degrees, depending on the center, for at least 5 to 10 minutes unless syncope ensues or is imminent. Both motorized and manual tables are used. Studies assessing the speed of tilt have questioned the need for rapid posture change over several seconds, although a rapid speed is typical.[113] For unexplained syncope, tilting angles are more variable. Prolonged tilt of 40 to 60 minutes or pharmacologic challenge with isoproterenol infusion[3] after a shorter interval of simple tilt is used.

## Responses

Normally, a small decline in systolic BP is seen immediately on tilting, but it is less marked than with active standing,[78,186] with recovery within 1 to 2 minutes. With marked autonomic failure the decline is persistent and continuous, often stabilizing at a lower level or progressing until syncope ensues (Fig. 22–6). In chronic cases with preserved cerebral autoregulation, a relatively low BP may be asymptomatic. An increase in HR in compensation for the fall in BP typically is attenuated in autonomic failure; however, in cases with preserved cardiovagal function, the HR responses may be robust because of the strong stimulus of the BP fall. This pattern appears indistinguishable from simple hypovolemia and other secondary causes, which must be carefully excluded before a conclusion of autonomic failure is reached. Low[113] has described a grading system of orthostatic intolerance that includes measures in addition to simple decline in BP. The scale, from 0 to 4, is outlined in Table 22–9. In addi-

tion to the severity, persistence, and symptoms associated with the BP fall, more sensitive indicators, such as excessive BP oscillations, pulse pressure narrowing, and HR changes, are included in grade I. The value obtained is one facet of a composite autonomic scoring scale.[111]

### Clinical Applications

Tilt testing has been studied in a wide variety of conditions and is of value in testing both vasoconstrictor integrity and compensatory cardiovagal HR responses. Orthostatic hypotension and other patterns of orthostatic intolerance can be documented in a controlled setting. Orthostatic hypotension in and of itself, however, is a sign and not a disease.[30] Further correlation with other measures and with the clinical syndrome is necessary for meaningful application of the findings.

Testing is fundamental in diagnosing the causes of orthostatic intolerance, especially in cases without hypotensive changes. POTS has been defined as a symptomatic 30 beats per minute increment in HR or an absolute level >120 in response to tilt or standing without secondary causes or other evident autonomic failure syndromes. Half of these cases appear to have evidence of a more generalized autonomic neuropathy (discussed later).[173] Tilt studies in combination with more advanced monitoring techniques attempt to identify possible underlying mechanisms.

Confirmation of neurocardiogenic syncope, which comprises the majority of cases of unexplained recurrent syncopal episodes, currently is probably the most common use of tilt table testing. Studies suggest that predisposition to this exaggerated response when the Bezold-Jarisch reflex is invoked may be common in certain disorders, such as chronic fatigue syndrome and some cases of mitral valve prolapse and may overlap with other syndromes of orthostatic intolerance and mild forms of autonomic failure. Neurocardiogenic syncope is reportedly responsible for 50% to 75% of unexplained syncope,[83,166] 67% of recurrent unexplained seizurelike episodes not responsive to anticonvulsants,[67] and 71% of vertigo with near or frank syncope.[68]

### Pitfalls

Although the degree of orthostatic stress is more controllable with consistent speed and angle of tilting, the physiology invoked is not identical to the changes with standing. Special relatively expensive equipment is needed, including a tilt table with arm board (requiring considerable space) plus

---

**TABLE 22–9. Orthostatic Tolerance Grade to Tilt-up**

Grade 0: Normal
Grade 1: Any of the following changes:
    Excessive BP oscillations
    Pulse pressure reduction (≥50%)
    HR increment (≥30 beats/min)
Grade 2: Transient OH with recovery
Grade 3: Sustained asymptomatic OH
    Systolic BP >30 mm Hg
    Diastolic BP >15 mm Hg
    Mean BP >20 mm Hg
Grade 4: Sustained symptomatic OH

BP, blood pressure; HR, heart rate; OH, orthostatic hypotension.
Modified from Low PA, ed. *Clinical Autonomic Disorders.* 2nd ed. Philadelphia: Lippincott-Raven; 1997:191.

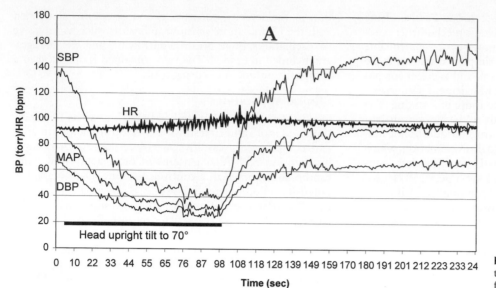

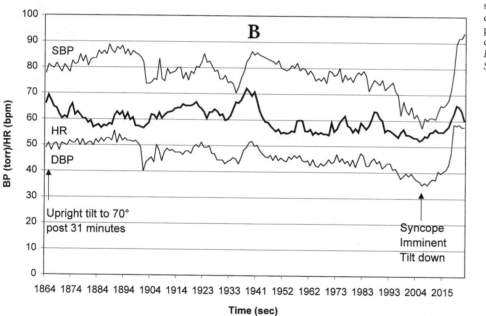

**FIGURE 22–6.** Abnormal upright-tilt test patterns. **A,** Panautonomic failure from familial amyloidosis. **B,** Neurocardiogenic syncope associated with chronic fatigue syndrome. Terminal portion of tracing is displayed. Note inappropriate fall in HR with drop in BP. *DBP,* Diastolic blood pressure; *HR,* heart rate; *MAP,* mean arterial pressure; *SBP,* systolic blood pressure.

other monitoring equipment. If drug infusions or more extensive monitoring is used, the testing becomes minimally invasive. False-positive responses for neurocardiogenic syncope occur in approximately 4% to 5% of control subjects.[83,85] This value increases significantly to 20%[82] or higher, if isoproterenol challenge is added. For this reason many laboratories have opted for simple but prolonged tilt studies for high specificity at the price of lower sensitivity. Care must be taken to minimize extraneous movements or stressors, which may lower sensitivity, by periodically augmenting venous return or other mechanisms to raise the BP. This produces a long, monotonous procedure but is nonetheless well tolerated by most patients.

## OTHER SELECTED ADRENERGIC TESTS

Multiple other techniques that stress the adrenergic system in addition to tilt testing and simple standing have been devised. Some have been insufficiently validated to be considered suitable for routine clinical application but are used in certain settings or for investigational purposes. A few noteworthy examples are discussed further.

### Orthostatic Stressors

Orthostatic hypotension with only passive upright tilt or standing is often an advanced development in the progression of autonomic failure. Tests that provide an augmented orthostatic stress theoretically detect abnormalities at an earlier stage or in milder forms. All methods challenge compensatory mechanisms by increasing peripheral vasodilation. Notable examples include lower body negative pressure, a quantified meal, nitroglycerin infusion, warm bath, and exercise.

***Lower Body Negative Pressure.*** This measure has been used in place of or in addition to upright tilt as a provocative orthostatic stressor. A vacuum pump applied to the abdomen and lower extremities causes augmented venous pooling, functionally reducing the available blood for circulation. Normal subjects eventually undergo syncope when the negative pressure is sufficiently increased.

***Sustained Handgrip Test.*** Sustained muscle contraction, as provided in the sustained handgrip test, induces an exercise reflex similar to that initiated by active standing. The reflex causes parasympathetic withdrawal and an increase in sympathetic vascular tone, resulting in an increase in cardiac output, HR, and BP. In the typical procedure, maximal handgrip strength is assessed, and at a later point the subject is asked to maintain 30% of that maximal force for 3 to 5 minutes. The rise in diastolic BP is frequently monitored as the test result. A rise of >15 mm Hg has traditionally been reported as normal, with 11 to 15 mm Hg considered borderline.[49] More recent control series have challenged these values, reporting a much lower limit of normal.[223] No clear decline of this reflex with age has been found; however, factors affecting sensitivity and specificity have not been extensively studied, making this measure currently less well accepted. Response reductions have been reported with a number of causes of sympathetic dysfunction, including diabetic and other autonomic neuropathies. Minimal equipment is required other that a gauge to measure grip force and a BP cuff. Many patients find the procedure uncomfortable or are unable to maintain the necessary effort for an adequate period.

## Mental Stress

Sympathetic outflow can be augmented with various mental stressors such as serial sevens, loud noises, or stressful emotional conditions. Maneuvers have been adapted as clinical measures of sympathetic outflow.[72,128] Confounding factors have not been well studied; moreover, these measures are not generally believed to be well-established or sensitive indicators of sympathetic failure.

## Cold Pressor Test

This measure is an older test of sympathetic outflow. Typically the subject's hand is immersed in a container of ice water, which predictably leads to a measurable rise in BP. This technique is currently not in wide usage for several reasons. The process is notably uncomfortable for the subject, who frequently prematurely aborts the test. The sensitivity appears to be relatively low, with overlap with control subjects who manifest minimal BP increases. Confounding variables are not well studied, and this measure is not considered a well-established test.

## Plasma Catecholamine Levels

Measurement of supine and standing levels of plasma norepinephrine and other catecholamines is a useful but less sensitive adjunctive marker of adrenergic function. Supine norepinephrine is an index of net sympathetic activity.[154,207] In the advent of diffuse postganglionic adrenergic failure, supine norepinephrine levels are reduced. Conversely, levels are preserved in predominantly preganglionic processes. Additional standing levels improve sensitivity.[113] Levels fail to rise sufficiently in both preganglionic and postganglionic failure and excessively with certain processes, such as pheochromocytoma.[191] Further improvement of sensitivity has been attempted by factoring in additional metabolite concentrations to the indexes.[27,73] These preganglionic and

postganglionic effects are illustrated by studies used to differentiate PAF from MSA.[28] In the predominantly postganglionic failure of PAF, supine norepinephrine and epinephrine levels are low and fail to rise normally on standing. In the mostly preganglionic failure of MSA, supine levels are normal or mildly depressed and again rise less than normal on standing. There remains sufficient overlap between these two groups, however, limiting specificity and making this measure of limited diagnostic use in an individual patient.[28] Catecholamine measures are instrumental in the diagnosis of a rare entity with a specific defect of the enzyme dopamine beta-hydroxylase. In such cases both norepinephrine and epinephrine are unrecordable; however, serum and cerebrospinal fluid dopamine levels are excessive because of the enzymatic defect.[18,161]

## Skin Vasomotor Reflexes

Skin blood flow can be assessed by using laser Doppler flowmeters or plethysmography as a measure of reflexive vasoconstriction. Recordings are typically made on fingerpads and toepads, where sympathetic vascular responses are purely vasoconstrictory. Responses to challenges such as inspiratory gasp, standing, Valsalva maneuver, and contralateral cold have been studied.[119] The venoarteriolar reflex measures changes in blood flow, inferring changes in vasomotor tone in response to a standardized change in limb position. Meaningful interpretation has been criticized because of the complex pathways involved and numerous confounding variables, many of which are problematic to control. Distal vasomotor fibers are highly sensitive to small temperature or emotional changes, leading to marked response variability. Some studies have reported reasonable reproducibility in highly controlled settings[1,50] and the ability of these techniques to separate controls from neuropathic conditions. In general, however, these measures are still considered investigational, with questionable sensitivity and specificity in comparison to other measures, and their use is currently considered premature for routine clinical application.

## Microneurography

Direct recording of sympathetic nerve impulses can be accomplished from human peripheral nerve. Insertion of a tungsten microelectrode through the perineurium directly into a nerve fascicle enables recording of muscle or skin sympathetic impulses if all somatic traffic is suppressed. This powerful technique has played an important investigational role in clarifying physiologic control mechanisms, but it currently has limited clinical utility. The technique requires considerable expertise and experience to gather reliable information and minimize numerous technical constraints.

## Pupillary Responses

Tests of pupillary function have been used as indexes of both parasympathetic and sympathetic function. Traditionally, pharmacologic challenges have been the mainstay of testing, especially in diagnosing focal or regional processes, such as Horner's syndrome, Adie's tonic pupil, and other causes of anisocoria. Sympathetic activation causes pupil dilation and contraction of Müller's muscle in the eyelid. Parasympathetic activity leads to constriction and controls accommodation. Dilute parasympathomimetic agents such as pilocarpine normally induce minimal constriction except when denervation supersensitivity is present. Similarly, dilute sympathomimetics such as epinephrine cause dilation only if they are sympathetically denervated. Cocaine causes dilation by blocking norepinephrine reuptake. If there are insufficient terminals to produce norepinephrine, this effect is lost and dilation fails to occur. Likewise, hydroxyamphetamine induces release of norepinephrine. If no effect is produced, a postganglionic defect is implied.

More recently, noninvasive pupillometry without medication challenge has renewed interest in measuring pupillary response as a marker of more general autonomic function.[77,133,151,152,179,181] Constriction is parasympathetically mediated, but experimental data have raised the question of whether active dilation is purely sympathetic or primarily parasympathetic withdrawal. Dark-adapted pupil diameter is a measure of sympathetic tone that can be tested with an infrared pupillometer or a specialized Polaroid camera[179] to precisely measure the resting size of the dark-adapted pupil. Testing is reported to have high sensitivity, specificity, and reproducibility,[151,183] which is further augmented by parasympathetic blockade.[151] Measurements are strongly age dependent in most series.[179,183,194] With a sufficient pupillometer, several other measurements also can be taken, including pupillary dilation and constriction rates, relative size changes, and latencies. The amplitude change on light-induced constriction depends on the resting pupil size but not on age when corrected for size.[182] The velocity of pupillary redilation is independent of diameter but appears to involve both parasympathetic inhibition and adrenergic drive.[178] Thus neither is an ideal test in isolation. Associations of abnormalities on these tests have been made in diabetic patients with isolated abnormalities of quantitative vibratory perception, HR variability, and sudomotor function, but this has not been found consistently across different protocols. Piha and Halonen[152] used a portable pupillometer to assess a variety of measures, including relative reflex amplitude, time to minimum diameter, and maximal velocities of constriction and redilation. They found abnormalities in 25% of diabetic patients without autonomic neuropathy and in 50% of those with autonomic neuropathy. The data did not correlate with HR variability or the Valsalva ratio. The presence of autonomic neuropathy was based on abnormalities on two of five tests in a conventional battery, which raises the question of the sensitivity of portable pupillometry for routine testing. Testing has not gained wide usage thus far, limiting experience and the validation needed for a well-established test. Some specialized equipment is needed, and the parasympathetic block reduces the noninvasiveness of the test.

Pupil cycle time involves shining a small spot of light at the edge of the pupil through to the retina. Reflex iris constriction is induced, thereby blocking light transmission, resulting in dilatation. The cycle is then perpetually repeated. The efferent arm is primarily parasympathetic, and the test has been proposed as a general measure of parasympathetic function.[133] However, responses are modulated by the degree of underlying sympathetic tone. Parasympathetic lesions slow cycle time, but sympathetic, combined, or even optic nerve lesions may also affect results, limiting specificity. This measure is still considered investigational.

## Other Organ- or System-Specific Tests

Cardiovascular and sudomotor function measures comprise the bulk of testing in most autonomic batteries, primarily because of the standardization and validation described earlier. However, testing involving multiple other systems can be performed. Many of these measures are either less reliable or more difficult to perform, require additional expertise, or need further evaluation. Certain disorders are not generalized or limited to predominantly parasympathetic or sympathetic involvement; they disproportionately or solely affect one organ system or function. When the function involved can be tested with conventional, well-validated methods, such as sweating loss with isolated idiopathic hypohidrosis, test results can support the diagnosis and exclude a more generalized process. In other instances, such as those restricted to GI, genitourinary, pupillary, or sexual function, routine batteries may not provide support for a diagnosis, other than excluding more generalized subclinical autonomic involvement. Many of these tests are also important in excluding primary failure of the end organ, not primary autonomic dysfunction. A number of additional tests are available, but most do not isolate autonomic physiology and are generally performed by specialists in the field and not in most autonomic laboratories. Detailed descriptions of the extensive anatomic and physiologic control mechanisms are beyond the scope of this chapter, but these tests are among those listed in Table 22–10. Some examples are discussed in the following sections.

*Gastrointestinal System.* The enteric nervous system comprises a complex network of sensory neurons, motor neurons, and interneurons in the wall of the GI tract that are capable of autonomous local control of peristalsis, fluid transport, vascular tone, absorption, gastric secretion, and sphincter coordination.[65] Parasympathetic and sympathetic outflow regulate motility and other functions and can override local activity under emergent conditions but are not required for most basic functions. Symptoms of dysphagia, gastroparesis, recurrent pseudoobstruction, and severe constipation are common testing indications. Techniques such as videofluoroscopy, gastric emptying times, colonic transit times, and gastroduodenal and anorectal manometry are helpful in detecting and localizing alterations in normal peristalsis, but they do not highlight autonomic control mechanisms. Abnormalities are common in patients with autonomic failure, including asymptomatic gastric retention in 20% to 30% of a population of diabetic patients in one study based on delayed motility and transit time.[84]

*Genitourinary System.* The most important central sites of bladder control hierarchy include the frontal cortex, medullary micturition center (Barrington's nucleus in the cat), and multiple amplified efferent and afferent spinal pathways. Parasympathetic efferents from the sacral cord stimulate bladder contraction and inhibit detrusor muscle tone. Sympathetic functions have antagonistic but less prominent effects. Local reflex loops are normally partially inhibited by supraspinal input under most circumstances. Bladder dysfunction can occur at any of these anatomic levels. Cystometric studies are one vital aspect in testing algorithms for the evaluation of urinary dysfunction. Results can be an aid in localization, but they do not isolate autonomic reflexes. Infusions of bethanechol may augment autonomic assessment by attempting to detect parasympathetic denervation supersensitivity.

| TABLE 22–10.  Selected Tests of Autonomic Function |
|---|

**Cardiovagal Tests**
*Well-Established*
HR variability to cyclic deep breathing
HR response to Valsalva maneuver (Valsalva ratio)
HR response to standing (30:15 ratio)

*Other*
Diving reflex/cold face test
HR variability at rest
HR response to cough
Spectral analysis of HR signals (frequency domain)
Transfer function analysis (nonlinear dynamics)

**Adrenergic Tests**
*Well-Established*
BP response to Valsalva maneuver (phases IV and late II)
BP response to orthostatic stress
    Head-up tilt
    Standing

*Other*
Sustained hand-grip test
Squat test
BP response to alternate stressors
    Lower body negative pressure
    Neck suction
    Lying down
    Liquid meal
Plasma catecholamine levels (supine/standing)
Microneurography
Mental stress tests
Cold pressor test
Spectral and transfer function BP analysis

**Sudomotor Tests**
*Well-Established*
Sympathetic skin response (SSR)
Quantitative sudomotor axon reflex test (QSART)
Thermoregulatory sweat test (TST)
Silastic sweat imprint testing

**Additional or Investigational Methods**
Pharmacologic challenges
Vasomotor testing (venoarteriolar reflex)
Pupillary testing (pharmacologic)
Pupillometry (pupil cycle time, dark-adapted pupil size, others)
Urodynamics/cystometrogram with bethanechol
GI motility studies
GI manometry
Salivary testing/Schirmer's test
Penile plethysmography, papaverine injection
Neuroendocrine tests
Neurogenic flare test

BP, Blood pressure; GI, gastrointestinal; HR, heart rate.

***Sexual Dysfunction.*** As part of the workup for male sexual dysfunction, intracavernosal injections of vasoactive compounds (e.g., papaverine, phentolamine, and prostaglandin $E_1$) are used to exclude vascular causes. Nocturnal penile tumescence and rigidity studies, usually conducted in a dedicated sleep laboratory, can be performed. SSRs have been recorded from the perineum,[42] and these are reportedly absent in a high percentage of patients with diabetes.[41]

***Lacrimation.*** Tear production can be assessed with Schirmer's test and tear osmolarity.[11] Filter paper is placed behind the lower lid, and the length of wetting at 5 minutes is measured. Sensitivity is reported to be 90% and the specificity 85% in detecting dry eyes but not the underlying responsible defect.[11]

# APPLICATIONS OF TESTS IN SELECTED CLINICAL PRESENTATIONS

Tests of autonomic function have been applied to a wide variety of clinical situations. In most settings a battery of measures are recorded, usually standardized for a specific laboratory. Ideally, multiple systems are examined in a noninvasive manner, with discrete evaluation of parasympathetic and sympathetic functions. In practical terms the best-validated, simplest, and most sensitive tests are typically employed. However, a regimented battery applied uniformly to all patients may not lead to optimal usefulness. Testing remains an extension of the clinical and bedside evaluation, and some degree of tailoring of testing choices to the clinical situation is needed.[118] The greater the number and variety of established tests available, the better the individual fit for each patient. The measures most commonly performed include HR variability to cyclic deep breathing and HR and BP responses to Valsalva maneuver and tilt plus some form of sudomotor testing. It has been recommended that abnormalities be noted on at least two separate measures to decrease the likelihood of false-positive results.[5] A scoring system of abnormalities has been developed and applied to better quantitate resultant data.[111] This type of battery works well with generalized autonomic failure and most autonomic neuropathies; however, it may fall short in cases when noncardiovascular or sudomotor systems are selectively involved. In these cases additional testing aimed at the symptomatic system or organ is appropriate, although in some instances historical information may prove to be a more useful diagnostic tool. Specific approaches have been applied in certain situations, such as selective SFN, sympathetically mediated pain, unexplained syncope, and POTS. More advanced and more invasive studies are employed at some large research centers to determine the underlying physiologic mechanisms in complex individual situations, for example, in idiopathic orthostatic intolerance, in part to provide a more rational approach to therapy.

## CHRONIC AUTONOMIC NEUROPATHY

A multitude of peripheral neuropathies have demonstrable autonomic involvement on formal testing. Most are limited to distal changes in sudomotor and vasomotor function and are asymptomatic or minimally bothersome. McLeod and Tuck[137] designated many as clinically important or usually unimportant. This breakdown is used in Table 22–4. Testing in causes typically deemed unimportant is discretionary. A minority of these cause more widespread clinically relevant changes, which can lead to frank autonomic failure with symptomatic orthostatic hypotension. Particularly noteworthy causes include diabetes mellitus, amyloidosis, paraneoplastic syndromes, selected hereditary and toxic neuropathies, and dopamine beta-hydroxylase deficiency.

Diabetic autonomic neuropathy (DAN) is the most important and prevalent type in the United States; it is also the most extensively examined, including abnormalities in the majority of the tests described earlier as well as many others still considered investigational. Documenting DAN is clinically relevant for several reasons in addition to simply establishing a diagnosis. Diabetics with DAN have a less favorable long-term prognosis.[23,46,155,167] Ewing et al[46] found that 56% of 73 patients with DAN died within 5 years, but many of these deaths were due to other diabetic complications, such as renal failure. Other studies have shown an increased but less ominous mortality rate in younger diabetic subjects without initial renal failure (25% by 10 years).[167] A lone abnormality in HR testing did not predict increased mortality, supporting the need for more than one abnormality to conclude that autonomic dysfunction is present. Recognition of DAN can lead to better symptomatic treatment and increased symptom awareness. Also, recognition of denervation supersensitivity, present in approximately 25% of cases, can lead to avoidance of potentially harmful but usually innocuous treatments.[114,126] For example, small doses of the over-the-counter adrenergic agonists contained in cold preparations can lead to a dangerous increase in BP.[114] BP instability and perioperative mortality are also increased.[22,96]

Because of the probable length-dependent nature of DAN, distal vasomotor and sudomotor functions are affected early or more severely, along with cardiovagal function, partly because of the protracted course of the vagus nerve, supporting HR variability as a sensitive marker of involvement.

Familial amyloidotic neuropathy is noteworthy because of the severity of autonomic involvement. Early recognition of cases and family members is important so that evolving treatment modalities (e.g., hepatic transplantation) can be considered.[17]

Dopamine beta-hydroxylase deficiency is a rare but important entity to recognize so that treatment with the norepinephrine precursor L-DOPS can be instituted.[80,161] Numerous additional entities are listed in Table 22–4.

### ACUTE AUTONOMIC NEUROPATHY

The Guillain-Barré syndrome commonly affects autonomic peripheral pathways and is an important cause of cardiovascular disturbances, tachyarrhythmias and bradyarrhythmias, and sudden death.[224] Involvement has been reported in one third to two thirds of cases[106,176,198] and can affect both afferent and efferent fibers. Dysfunction may present as failure or overactivity. Findings correlate with the severity of weakness, elevated serum and urinary catecholamine levels, and respiratory failure. Excessive sympathetic discharges have been documented with microneurography in three cases during hypertensive episodes.[51] Recognition of these phenomena is vital so that appropriate intensive monitoring and intervention can be provided as necessary. Paroxysmal sweating bursts, episodic hypertensive episodes, and the characteristic resting tachycardia in part are due to autonomic overactivity. Failure of function is also common with clinical and laboratory evidence of orthostatic hypotension, although the bedridden state is an exacerbating factor that complicates testing. Anhidrosis, reduced HR variability, vasomotor changes, and abnormalities on most of the tests described earlier can be found in specific cases. The reduced HR variability is notable because of work done in post–myocardial infarction patients. Patients with reduced HR variability reportedly are predisposed to arrhythmogenic complications, thought to be secondary to an imbalance created by reduced vagal and increased sympathetic tone.[19,94,218] Recognition of this altered balance may prove to be a clinical application of power spectral analysis. Urinary retention is traditionally considered rare, but many series have found abnormalities to be not uncommon.[213]

Ileus and GI dysmotility, incontinence, and pupillary changes are less common but described.

A rare but notable acute entity is acute autonomic neuropathy, or pandysautonomia, which is primarily, but not exclusively, restricted to peripheral autonomic involvement. Half of the cases are preceded by a viral syndrome similar to that of Guillain-Barré syndrome, but at a lower percentage. Patients develop generalized autonomic failure, including orthostatic hypotension. Abnormalities on general autonomic screening are diffuse and marked. An attenuated form of this disorder has been proposed to underlie many cases of orthostatic intolerance.[173] Roughly 25% of patients have a restricted cholinergic form with dry eyes and mouth, ileus, hypohidrosis, and sexual dysfunction without significant orthostatic hypotension, making laboratory confirmation extremely valuable. A paraneoplastic form can also be seen and is indistinguishable on clinical or laboratory grounds. Botulism (cholinergic) and acute intermittent porphyria are also part of the acute-onset differential diagnosis.

### Paraneoplastic Syndromes

Although paraneoplastic syndromes are rare, their recognition is crucial to detection of the underlying tumor. Several syndromes have prominent autonomic involvement that may benefit from confirmation with autonomic testing. Approximately 80% of the cases of Lambert-Eaton myasthenic syndrome have parasympathetic or sympathetic involvement, which may benefit from drug therapy.[90] However, Lambert-Eaton syndrome is usually confirmed by other means, such as repetitive stimulation or $Ca^{2+}$ channel antibodies. Sensory neuronopathy may have prominent autonomic features that often precede tumor detection (most commonly small cell lung cancer (SCLC) and can be demonstrated on formal testing.[93] ANNA antibodies (anti-HU) are often detected as well. Enteric neuronopathy causes intestinal pseudoobstruction and marked derangement of function on gastric and intestinal motility studies. When formally examined, many patients show widespread evidence of autonomic dysfunction, supporting the underlying autonomic basis. An immune-mediated attack of enteric neurons of the myenteric and submucosal plexi is presumed,[103] most often in association with SCLC, which typically precedes tumor detection.[26] The GI manifestations may be present in isolation[29] or with more extensive autonomic or somatic findings. A subacute autonomic neuropathy can also be seen with SCLC in isolation or with some degree of somatic neuropathy and has been described with pancreatic adenocarcinoma[197] and Hodgkin's disease.[204]

### PARKINSONISM AND AUTONOMIC FAILURE

Marked autonomic failure is pervasive in patients with MSA, Shy-Drager syndrome, and MSA with parkinsonian or cerebellar onset.[28,159,168] Lesser degrees of dysautonomia appear to be present in a significant number of patients with idiopathic Parkinson's disease (IPD) when subjected to formal testing.[6,132] This finding is not surprising because Lewy bodies can be found neuropathologically in enteric motor neurons, the intermediolateral cell column of the spinal cord, sympathetic ganglia, and other areas of autonomic control at autopsy. However, formal autonomic testing remains helpful as an extension of the clinical examination to identify the presence and severity of dysautonomia and as an aid in differentiating MSA from idiopathic Parkinson's disease (PD). Many cases clinically diagnosed as idiopathic PD were later neuropathologically proven to be MSA-based through demonstration of characteristic glial cytoplasmic inclusions and a lack of Lewy bodies.[129] Up to 97% of MSA cases eventually show significant autonomic abnormalities, irrespective of whether they have initial or predominant autonomic, parkinsonian, or cerebellar signs.[212] To complicate matters, many patients with IPD have potentially autonomically mediated complaints, most commonly constipation. Patients may show mild-to-moderate abnormalities on formal testing. However, orthostatic hypotension is rare unless it is pharmacologically induced, for example, with levodopa.

A small subset of patients with IPD have more severe signs of autonomic failure and are separately designated as having PD with autonomic failure. Whether this is an overlap form with pure autonomic failure or diffuse Lewy body disease or is simply a more widespread manifestation of the neurodegenerative process is not clear at this point. Evidence of autonomic failure has been seen with diffuse Lewy body disease[221] and in isolated cases of progressive supranuclear palsy.[202] In general, however, marked autonomic failure that includes symptomatic neurogenic orthostatic hypotension with parkinsonism is most likely due to MSA. For diagnosis, the clinical syndrome and lack of significant response to levodopa are primary components. Other ancillary tests, such as positron emission tomography (PET) scan, motor neuron disease changes on sphincter EMG, growth hormone response to clonidine,[92] and sleep studies, may also be helpful for antemortem diagnosis of MSA.

The clinically distinct but possibly related disorder of PAF is a rare, slowly progressive, but profound disorder with disabling orthostatic hypotension. Testing abnormalities on screening tests are marked, with orthostatic hypotension and failure on other adrenergic measures. Cardiovagal and other parasympathetic measures are generally not as severe as with MSA. The plasma norepinephrine level is low at baseline in contrast to the normal or mildly decreased values in MSA. On tilt or standing, the response in PAF is blunted.[28] The complete lack of other somatic involvement, including parkinsonism, is mandatory (as the name implies) for diagnosis. In fact, most centers require a period of 3 to 5 years without multisystem involvement before a firm clinical diagnosis is reached.

## SYNCOPE

Tilt-table testing has become a prime method of evaluation of cryptogenic and noncardiogenic syncope.[25,57,83,85,156,190] Most notable of these disorders is neurocardiogenic syncope (vasovagal syncope, simple faint), which may be more prevalent than previously realized. If structural cardiac disease and dysrhythmia are excluded, the majority of cases prove to be neurocardiogenic syncope, but this process cannot always be accurately distinguished from other causes purely on clinical grounds. The phenomenon is a paradoxical reflex activation, causing a sudden withdrawal of vasomotor tone and a vagally mediated drop in HR. The effect can be triggered spontaneously or with afferent discharges from various organs or processes, including cough, swallow, micturition, defecation, anxiety, fear, and needle phobia. Under certain environmental conditions, upright posture may spontaneously trigger the effect by increasing venous pooling. This reduces available blood for pumping (decreased preload) and increases sympathetic augmentation of the force of cardiac contraction. This added force stimulates ventricular mechanoreceptors, which can trigger the Bezold-Jarisch reflex. This paradoxical reflex induces a sudden and dramatic fall in sympathetic outflow, producing relative vasodilation and vagally mediated relative bradycardia, which often progresses to imminent or frank syncope. Tilt studies can reproduce this spontaneous effect with acceptable specificity and sensitivity.[3,25] The true sensitivity and specificity are variable and depend on the center and protocol employed. Recognition leads to confirmation of a relatively benign disorder and justifies instituting one of the evolving treatments. None of the current treatments, however, have been scrutinized with double-blinded controlled series to date. Vulnerability to neurocardiogenic syncope with prolonged tilt testing is seen in a small percentage of normal subjects and in an apparently high percentage of patients with chronic fatigue syndrome, raising the possibility of numerous aborted or subclinical manifestations short of frank syncope as a contributory cause of the disabling fatigue.[21] This phenomenon has been duplicated by several centers; moreover, conventional neurocardiogenic syncope treatments have been reported to improve chronic fatigue symptoms independent of baseline activity levels.[21] However, concerns that this effect may be a nonspecific secondary complication have not been erased.

Syncope from marked orthostatic hypotension is not uncommon in advanced cases of autonomic failure and is a potentially life-threatening complication. Detection is vital, and multiple treatment options, both pharmacologic and nonpharmacologic, are available.[61,160] Tilt-table assessment can be an important aid in initial diagnosis, treatment response, and progression monitoring over time. Syncope is especially common in elderly patients with preserved cerebral autoregulatory capabilities. Patients may have few or no recognizable symptoms, or they may simply have vague difficulty with cognitive abilities or concentration immediately before frank syncope. The process may develop with enough rapidity to be considered as part of the differential of drop attacks. Less commonly the progressive orthostatic decline in BP is delayed for 5 or rarely 10 minutes and may be missed on routine bedside orthostatic BP measurements.

## BENIGN CONDITIONS

Some disorders may be restricted to a single system but raise suspicions of more ominous and generalized autonomic failure, loosely analogous to benign fasciculations and ALS. In such a case the syndrome of benign fasciculations may be clinically suspected, yet formal electrodiagnostic testing to confirm the lack of motor neuron disease is important for confirmation. Similarly, in conditions such as chronic idiopathic anhidrosis with isolated sudomotor failure, documenting normal function in other systems is reassuring and critical for accurate diagnosis.[117]

## ORTHOSTATIC INTOLERANCE AND POTS

Development of orthostatic symptoms without a concomitant drop in systemic BP is increasingly recognized and considered as a separate category of disorders that includes POTS.[123] Orthostatic tachycardia may be the earliest finding in many cases of orthostatic intolerance,[192] but it is also seen in secondary causes, such as hypovolemia, deconditioning, and spaceflight as well as milder stages of autonomic failure. These conditions must be excluded for a primary diagnosis of POTS, defined as an increment of ≥30 beats per minute in HR on tilt or standing or an absolute value ≥120 beats per minute with development of orthostatic complaints within 5 minutes. Alternate names for this condition have included sympathotonic orthostatic hypotension, idiopathic hypovolemia, neurasthenia, and the effort syndrome. Additionally, overlap of complaints exists with chronic fatigue syndrome, mitral valve prolapse syndrome, and panic and anxiety disorders. Complaints may also be cyclic or catamenial (5:1 female predominance). Despite the "benign" designation, patients often become severely disabled by the symptoms, which interfere with routine daily activities.

Roughly one half of POTS cases involve an antecedent viral syndrome, and one half to two thirds show laboratory evidence of a length-dependent autonomic neuropathy.[122,123,173] Formal autonomic testing is instrumental for initial diagnosis and separating out problematic overlapping cases of chronic fatigue syndrome and panic disorder after adequate exclusion of secondary and cardiogenic causes. Patterns of tilt abnormalities and more advanced testing may provide guidance in the multiple treatment options in the heterogeneous group of underlying mechanisms.[123] Patients characteristically have the postural increase in HR with a normotensive or hypertensive BP response. Symptoms are referable to those of sympathetic activation and reduced cerebral perfusion with hypoxia. Abnormalities on sudomotor testing include decreased sweat volumes on QSART,[123,173] a peripheral pattern of sweat loss on TST, and reduced or absent skin potentials.[74] Sudomotor abnormalities appear to be overrepresented in cases with a postviral onset. In turn, an association with idiopathic acute autonomic neuropathy has been proposed.[173] Valsalva maneuver shows changes in two thirds of cases with an excessive BP drop in phase II with insufficient recovery and an excessive phase IV overshoot, as demonstrated in Figure 22–1. HR variability measures are normal or enhanced with a normal or increased Valsalva ratio. Cases with excessive venous pooling reportedly demonstrate marked drops in pulse pressure and a normal-to-excessive rise in diastolic blood pressure. Cases associated with peripheral sudomotor abnormalities are associated with the Valsalva maneuver changes.[125] More advanced experimental techniques use simultaneous transcranial Doppler and EEG recordings to look for paradoxical cerebral vasoconstriction to tilt[66] and signs of hypoxia as well as alterations in spectral power in the recorded transcranial Doppler and EEG signals.[143] Challenges with pharmacologic infusions to tilt and the Valsalva maneuver studies have attempted to identify the underlying physiologic mechanisms. These mechanisms appear to be heterogeneous[123] and include excessive venous pooling, possibly related to a distal vasomotor neuropathy. Generalized hypovolemia, as implied by the term *idiopathic hypovolemia,* has been demonstrated in only a small percentage of cases. Moreover, formal plasma volume tests are cumbersome and expensive. Beta-adrenergic receptor supersensitivity, altered alpha-receptor sensitivity, disturbed sympathetic-parasympathetic balance, and primary central dysregulation at the brainstem level have all been suggested by specific cases.[123]

Other "benign" disturbances of orthostatic tolerance include neurocardiogenic syncope, deconditioning, and prolonged weightlessness. Significant overlap in symptoms and laboratory findings is found in a percentage of patients with echocardiographic mitral valve prolapse.[195]

## SMALL-FIBER NEUROPATHY

A subset of patients with neuropathy have predominate or exclusive affection of small-diameter fibers. Cases often come to attention because of bothersome distal dysesthetic complaints that frequently are associated with a decrease in distal pinprick and temperature perception. Minor degrees of light touch and vibration are sometimes present, but marked vibratory loss, proprioceptive defect, or motor signs are absent. Electrodiagnostic studies, which test only the largest-diameter fibers, are typically normal, leaving scant objective evidence for the neuropathy. Autonomic signs are typically restricted to distal sudomotor and vasomotor changes with uncommon bowel, bladder, or erectile dysfunction.[188] Frank autonomic failure with orthostatic hypotension in not generally seen. Moreover, bedside confirmation of the sudomotor and vasomotor loss is difficult and inexact. Formal autonomic studies have been examined in affected patients and appear to be valuable in support of the diagnosis. Stewart et al[188] reported sudomotor abnormalities in 32 of 40 (80%) cases with QSART and 18 of 25 (72%) on TST. When the results were combined, abnormalities were found in 90% of suspected patients. In the same cohort 28% had minor changes of HR variability on deep breathing or the Valsalva ratio, consistent with a length-dependent process. None had orthostatic hypotension. Giuliani et al[64] reported 39 cases demonstrating a similar percentage of sudomotor abnormalities but a somewhat higher percentage of cardiovagal abnormalities (23 of 36 or 66%) in a tertiary selection of patients. Yield of the SSR is low in isolated SFN, revealing abnormal results in only 10% of suspected SFN patients with concomitantly normal nerve conduction and EMG studies.[43]

Quantitative sensory testing of somatic thermal and pain thresholds are also useful in assessing small-fiber function. These methods are currently undergoing a formal review process by the AAN to determine suitability for routine clinical application, but they have been used in numerous patient series and clinical trials to date.

## COMPLEX REGIONAL PAIN SYNDROME

Reflex sympathetic dystrophy has been designated as type I complex regional pain syndrome under International Association for Study of Pain task force nomenclature. Sympathetically mediated pain symptoms may or may not, however, be evident in an individual case and may be coincident with sympathetically independent pain not benefited by sympathetic blockade.[216] Sympathetically mediated symptoms include alterations in perceived temperature, swelling, skin color changes, and an alteration in sweat output (usually increased). Exaggerated findings in the hand are not unexpected based on the much denser distal sympathetic innervation in the arm compared with more proximal areas. Autonomic testing has been applied, and correlation with clinical profiles assessed. Low and associates[24] have used a battery of tests to measure alterations in sudomotor and vasomotor function. Testing included resting sweat output with the QSART technology and traditional QSART. Abnormalities included excessive resting sweat output and reduced

QSART amplitude or ultrashort-onset latency. Temperature asymmetry was assessed with telethermography by charting multiple sites on affected and contralateral limbs, but it can also be measured using local infrared thermometry. In 1990 an AAN consensus committee gave thermography an unfavorable assessment for use in radiculopathies; however, sympathetically mediated pain appears to be one of the justifiable applications of this previously abused technology.[4] Local blood flow was assessed by laser Doppler techniques. Resting sweat output plus QSART had the highest correlation with clinical profiles, whereas skin blood flow was abnormal in less than half of suspected cases. None of the tests except local skin temperature measurements are widely available, making other ancillary procedures, such as three-phase bone scan and empiric response to sympathetic blockade, more commonly used in addition to detailed clinical profiles.[216]

## CONCLUSION

Current autonomic testing batteries have multiple well-validated, sensitive, and noninvasive tests available that can help confirm, localize, quantify, and characterize clinical autonomic disorders. Resultant data, however, are limited by the necessity of performing indirect measures from controlled perturbations. Numerous confounding factors also hamper results and must be carefully controlled as much as feasible. Multiple clinical syndromes can benefit from testing to institute symptom- and disease-specific therapy and to aid with diagnosis and management. Valuable information on prognosis and severity is applicable in certain cases. Laboratories of varying levels of sophistication and test availability are present in most large cities in the United States and Europe. Confirmation of autonomic dysfunction will likely become increasingly important as awareness of clinical syndromes and available treatment options increases.

## REFERENCES

1. Abbot NC, Beck JS, Wilson SB, Khan F. Vasomotor reflexes in the fingertip skin of patients with type I diabetes mellitus and leprosy. *Clin Auton Res.* 1993;3:189-193.
2. Abboud FM. Neurocardiogenic syncope. *N Engl J Med.* 1993;328:1117-1120.
3. Almquist A, Goldenberg IF, Milstein S, et al. Provocation of bradycardia and hypotension by isoproterenol and upright posture in patients with unexplained syncope. *N Engl J Med.* 1989;320:346-351.
4. American Academy of Neurology, Therapeutics and Technology Assessment Subcommittee. Assessment: thermography in neurologic practice. *Neurology.* 1990;40:523-525.
5. American Diabetes Association/American Academy of Neurology. Consensus statement: report and recommendations of the San Antonio Conference on Diabetic Neuropathy. *Diabetes Care.* 1988;11:592-597.
6. Appenzeller O, Goss JE. Autonomic deficits in Parkinson's syndrome. *Arch Neurol.* 1971;24:50-57.
7. Arunodaya GR, Taly AB. Sympathetic skin response: a decade later. *J Neurol Sci.* 1995;129:81-89.
8. Assessment: clinical autonomic testing report of the Therapeutics and Technology Assessment Subcommittee of the American Academy of Neurology. *Neurology.* 1996;46:873-880.
9. Baba M, Watahiki Y, Matsunaga M, Takebe K. Sympathetic skin response in healthy man. *Electromyogr Clin Neurophysiol.* 1988;28:277-283.
10. Baldwa VS, Ewing DJ. Heart rate response to Valsalva manœuvre: reproducibility in normals, and relation to variation in resting heart rate in diabetics. *Br Heart J.* 1977;39:641-644.
11. Baum J. Discussion of Farris RL, Stuchell RN, Mandel ID. Basal and reflex human tear analysis. *Ophthalmology.* 1981;88:862.
12. Bellavere F, Cardone C, Ferri M, et al. Standing to lying heart rate variation: a new simple test in the diagnosis of diabetic autonomic neuropathy. *Diabet Med.* 1987;4:41-43.
13. Bellavere F, Ewing DJ. Autonomic control of the immediate heart rate response to lying down. *Clin Sci.* 1982;62:57-64.
14. Benarroch EE. The central autonomic network: functional organization, dysfunction and perspective. *Mayo Clin Proc.* 1993;68:988-1001.
15. Benarroch EE, Opfer-Gehrking TL, Low PA. Use of the photoplethysmographic technique to analyze the Valsalva maneuver in normal man. *Muscle Nerve.* 1991;14:1165-1172.
16. Benarroch EE, Smithson IL, Low PA, Parisi JE. Depletion of catecholaminergic neurons of the rostral ventrolateral medulla in multiple system atrophy with autonomic failure. *Ann Neurol.* 1998;43:156-163.
17. Bergethon PR, Sabin TD, Lewis D. Improvement in the polyneuropathy associated with familial amyloid polyneuropathy after liver transplantation. *Neurology.* 1996;47:944-951.
18. Biaggioni I, Hollister AS, Robertson D. Dopamine in dopamine-beta-hydroxylase deficiency. *N Engl J Med.* 1987;317:1415-1416.
19. Bigger JR Jr, Fleiss JL, Steinman RC, et al. Frequency domain measures of heart period variability and mortality after myocardial infarction. *Circulation.* 1992;85:164-171.
20. Borst C, Wieling W, van Brederode JF, et al. Mechanisms of initial heart rate response to postural change. *Am J Physiol.* 1982;243:H676-H681.
21. Bou-Holaigah I, Rowe PC, Kan J, Calkins H. The relationship between neurally mediated hypotension and the chronic fatigue syndrome. *JAMA.* 1995;274:961-967.
22. Burgos LG, Ebert RJ, Asiddao C, et al. Increased intraoperative cardiovascular morbidity in diabetics with autonomic neuropathy. *Anesthesiology.* 1989;70:591-597.
23. Chambers JB, Sampson MJ, Sprigings DC, Jackson G. QT prolongation on the electrocardiogram in diabetic autonomic neuropathy. *Diabet Med.* 1990;7:105-110.
24. Chelimsky TC, Low PA, Naessens JM, et al. Value of autonomic testing in reflex sympathetic dystrophy. *Mayo Clin Proc.* 1995;70:1029-1040.
25. Chen MY, Goldenberg IF, Milstein S, et al. Cardiac electrophysiologic and hemodynamic correlates of neurally mediated syncope. *Am J Cardiol.* 1989;63:66-72.
26. Chinn JS, Schuffler MD. Paraneoplastic visceral neuropathy as a cause of severe gastrointestinal motor dysfunction. *Gastroenterology.* 1988;95:1279-1286.
27. Christensen NJ, Dejgaard A, Hilsted J. Plasma dihydroxyphenylglycol (DHPG) as an index of diabetic autonomic neuropathy. *Clin Physiol.* 1988;8:577-580.
28. Cohen J, Low P, Fealey R, et al. Somatic and autonomic function in progressive autonomic failure and multiple system atrophy. *Ann Neurol.* 1987;22:692-699.
29. Colombel JF, Parent M, Lescut D, et al. Paraneoplastic intestinal pseudo-obstruction as the presenting feature of small-cell lung cancer. *Gastroenterol Clin Biol.* 1988;12:394-396.
30. The Consensus Committee of the American Autonomic Society and the American Academy of Neurology. Consensus statement on the definition of orthostatic hypotension, pure autonomic failure, and multiple system atrophy. *Neurology.* 1996;46:1470.
31. Dambrink JH, Wieling W. Circulatory response to postural change in healthy male subjects in relation to age. *Clin Sci.* 1987;72:335-341.
32. Delius W, Hagbarth KE, Hongell A, Wallin BG. General characteristics of sympathetic activity in human muscle nerves. *Acta Physiol Scand.* 1972;84:65-81.
33. Denq JC, Opfer-Gehrking TL, Giuliani M, et al. Efficacy of compression of different capacitance beds in the amelioration of orthostatic hypotension. *Clin Auton Res.* 1997;7:321-326.
34. The Diabetes Control and Complications Trial Research Group. The effect of intensive diabetes therapy on the development and progression of neuropathy. *Ann Intern Med.* 1995;122:561-568.
35. Drory VE, Korczyn AD. Sympathetic skin response: age effect. *Neurology.* 1993;43:1818-1820.
36. Drory VE, Korczyn AD. The sympathetic skin response in reflex sympathetic dystrophy. *J Neurol Sci.* 1995;128:92-95.
37. Dyck PJ, Karnes JL, O'Brien PC, et al. The Rochester diabetic neuropathy study: reassessment of tests and criteria for diagnosis and stages severity. *Neurology.* 1992;42:1164-1170.
38. Eckberg DL. Parasympathetic cardiovascular control in human disease: a critical review of methods and results. *Am J Physiol.* 1980;239:H581-H593.

39. Eckberg DL, Mohanty SK, Raczkowska M. Trigeminal-baroreceptor reflex interactions modulate human cardiac vagal efferent activity. *J Physiol (Lond)*. 1984;347:75-83.

40. Elie B, Louboutin JP. Sympathetic skin response (SSR) is abnormal in multiple sclerosis. *Muscle Nerve*. 1995;18:185-189.

41. Ertekin C, Ertekin N, Almis S. Autonomic sympathetic nerve involvement in diabetic impotence. *Neurourol Urodyn*. 1989;8:589-598.

42. Ertekin C, Ertekin N, Mutlu S, et al. Skin potentials (SP) recorded from the extremities and genital regions in normal and impotent subjects. *Acta Neurol Scand*. 1987;76:28-36.

43. Evans BA, Lussky D, Knezevic W. The peripheral autonomic surface potential in suspected small-fiber neuropathy. *Muscle Nerve*. 1988;11: 982.

44. Ewing DJ, Borsey DQ, Bellavere F, Clarke BF. Cardiac autonomic neuropathy in diabetes: comparison of measures of R-R interval variation. *Diabetologia*. 1981;21:18-24.

45. Ewing DJ, Campbell IW, Clarke BF. Assessment of cardiovascular effects in diabetic autonomic neuropathy and prognostic implications. *Ann Intern Med*. 1980;92:308-311.

46. Ewing DJ, Campbell IW, Clarke BF. The natural history of diabetic autonomic neuropathy. *QJM*. 1980;49:95-108.

47. Ewing DJ, Campbell IW, Murray H, et al. Immediate heart-rate response to standing: simple test for autonomic neuropathy in diabetes. *BMJ*. 1978;1:145-147.

48. Ewing DJ, Hume L, Campbell IW, et al. Autonomic mechanisms in the initial heart rate response to standing. *J Appl Physiol*. 1980;49:809-814.

49. Ewing DJ, Irving JB, Kerr F, et al. Cardiovascular responses to sustained handgrip in normal subjects and in patients with diabetes mellitus: a test of autonomic function. *Clin Sci Mol Med*. 1974;46:295-306.

50. Faes TJ, Wagemans MF, Cillekens JM, et al. The validity and reproducibility of the skin vasomotor test: studies in normal subjects, after spinal anaesthesia, and in diabetes mellitus. *Clin Auton Res*. 1993;3: 319-324.

51. Fagius J, Wallin BG. Microneurographic evidence of excessive sympathetic outflow in the Guillain-Barré syndrome. *Brain*. 1983;106:589-600.

52. Fagius J, Wallin BG. Sympathetic reflex latencies and conduction velocities in normal man. *J Neurol Sci*. 1980;47:433-448.

53. Fealey RD. Thermoregulatory sweat test. In: Low PA, ed. *Clinical Autonomic Disorders*. 2nd ed. Philadelphia: Lippincott-Raven; 1997:245-257.

54. Fealey RD, Low PA, Thomas JE. Thermoregulatory sweating abnormalities in diabetes mellitus. *Mayo Clin Proc*. 1989;64:617-628.

55. Ferrer T, Ramos MJ, Perez-Sales P, Perez-Jimenez A, Alvarez E. Sympathetic sudomotor function and aging. *Muscle Nerve*. 1995;18:395-401.

56. Finley JP, Bonet JF, Waxman MB. Autonomic pathways responsible for bradycardia on facial immersion. *J Appl Physiol*. 1979;47:1218-1222.

57. Fitzpatrick A, Sutton R. Tilting towards a diagnosis in recurrent unexplained syncope. *Lancet*. 1989;1:658-660.

58. Fortney SM, Nadel ER, Wenger CB, Bove JR. Effect of blood volume on sweating rate and body fluids in exercising humans. *J Appl Physiol*. 1981;51:1594-1600.

59. Fortney SM, Wenger CB, Bove JR, Nadel ER. Effect of hyperosmolarity on control of blood flow and sweating. *J Appl Physiol*. 1984;57: 1688-1695.

60. Freeman R. Noninvasive evaluation of heart rate variability. In: Low PA, ed. *Clinical Autonomic Disorders*. 2nd ed. Philadelphia: Lippincott-Raven; 1997:297-307.

61. Freeman R, Miyawaki E. The treatment of autonomic dysfunction. *J Clin Neurophysiol*. 1993;10:61-82.

62. Freeman R, Saul JP, Roberts MS, et al. Spectral analysis of heart rate in diabetic autonomic neuropathy: a comparison with standard tests of autonomic function. *Arch Neurol*. 1991;48:185-190.

63. Genovely H, Pfeifer MA. RR-variation: the autonomic test of choice in diabetes. *Diabetes Metab Rev*. 1988;4:255-271.

64. Giuliani MJ, Stewart JD, Low PA. Distal small-fiber neuropathy. In: Low PA, ed. *Clinical Autonomic Disorders*. 2nd ed. Philadelphia: Lippincott-Raven; 1997:699-714.

65. Goyal RK, Hirano I. The enteric nervous system. *N Engl J Med*. 1996; 334:1106-1115.

66. Grubb BP, Gerard G, Roush K, et al. Cerebral vasoconstriction during head-upright tilt-induced vasovagal syncope: a paradoxic and unexpected response. *Circulation*. 1991;84:1157-1164.

67. Grubb BP, Gerard G, Roush K, et al. Differentiation of convulsive syncope and epilepsy with head-up tilt testing. *Ann Intern Med*. 1991;115: 871-876.

68. Grubb BP, Rubin AM, Wolfe D, et al. Head-upright tilt-table testing: a useful tool in the evaluation and management of recurrent vertigo of unknown origin associated with near-syncope or syncope. *Otolaryngol Head Neck Surg*. 1992;107:570-576.

69. Harris DR, Polk BF, Willis I. Evaluating sweat gland activity with imprint techniques. *J Invest Dermatol*. 1972;58:78-84.

70. Harry JD, Freeman R. Determining heart-rate variability: comparing methodologies using computer simulations. *Muscle Nerve*. 1993;16: 267-277.

71. Heart rate variability: standards of measurement, physiological interpretation, and clinical use. Task Force of the European Society of Cardiology and the North American Society of Pacing and Electrophysiology. *Circulation*. 1996;93:1043-1065.

72. Hjemdahl P, Freyschuss U, Juhlin-Dannfelt A, Linde B. Differentiated sympathetic activation during mental stress evoked by the Stroop test. *Acta Physiol Scand Suppl*. 1984;527:25-29.

73. Hoeldtke RD, Cilmi KM, Reichard GA Jr, et al. Assessment of norepinephrine secretion and production. *J Lab Clin Med*. 1983;101:772-782.

74. Hoeldtke RD, Davis KM. The orthostatic tachycardia syndrome: evaluation of autonomic function and treatment with octreotide and ergot alkaloids. *J Clin Endocrinol Metab*. 1991;73:132-139.

75. Hoeldtke RD, Davis KM, Hshieh PB, et al. Autonomic surface potential analysis: assessment of reproducibility and sensitivity. *Muscle Nerve*. 1992;15:926-931.

76. Hreidarsson AB. Pupil motility in long-term diabetes. *Diabetologia*. 1979;17:145-150.

77. Hreidarsson AB, Gundersen HJ. The pupillary response to light in type I (insulin dependent) diabetes. *Diabetologia*. 1985;28:815-821.

78. Imholz BPM, Dambrink JHA, Karemaker JM. Orthostatic circulatory control in the elderly evaluated by noninvasive continuous blood pressure measurement. *Clin Sci*. 1990;79:73-79.

79. Imholz BP, van Montfrans GA, Settels JJ, et al. Continuous non-invasive blood pressure monitoring: reliability of Finapres device during the Valsalva manœuvre. *Cardiovasc Res*. 1988;22:390-397.

80. Imholz BP, Wieling W, Langewouters GJ, van Montfrans GA. Continuous finger arterial pressure: utility in the cardiovascular laboratory. *Clin Auton Res*. 1991;1:43-53.

81. Johnson RH, Smith AC, Spalding JMK, Wollner L. Effect of posture on blood pressure in elderly patients. *Lancet*. 1965;1:731-733.

82. Kapoor WN, Brant N. Evaluation of syncope by upright tilt testing with isoproterenol: a nonspecific test. *Ann Intern Med*. 1992;116:358-363.

83. Kapoor WN, Smith MA, Miller NL. Upright tilt testing in evaluating syncope: a comprehensive literature review. *Am J Med*. 1994;97:78-88.

84. Kassander P. Asymptomatic gastric retention in diabetics (gastroparesis diabeticorum). *Ann Intern Med*. 1958;48:797-812.

85. Kaufmann H. Neurally mediated syncope: pathogenesis, diagnosis, and treatment. *Neurology*. 1995;45(suppl 5):S12-S18.

86. Kennedy WR, Navarro X. Sympathetic sudomotor function in diabetic neuropathy. *Arch Neurol*. 1989;46:1182-1186.

87. Kennedy WR, Navarro X. Evaluation of sudomotor function by sweat imprint methods. In: Low PA, ed. *Clinical Autonomic Disorders*. Boston: Little Brown; 1993:253-261.

88. Kennedy WR, Sakuta M, Quick DC. Rodent eccrine sweat glands: a case of multiple efferent innervation. *Neuroscience*. 1984;11:741-749.

89. Kennedy WR, Sakuta M, Sutherland D, Goetz FC. Quantitation of the sweating deficiency in diabetes mellitus. *Ann Neurol*. 1984;15:482-488.

90. Khurana RK. Paraneoplastic autonomic dysfunction. In: Low PA, ed. *Clinical Autonomic Disorders*. 2nd ed. Philadelphia: Lippincott-Raven; 1997:545-554.

91. Khurana RK, Watabiki S, Hebel JR, et al. Cold face test in the assessment of trigeminal-brainstem-vagal function in humans. *Ann Neurol*. 1980;7:144-149.

92. Kimber JR, Watson L, Mathias CJ. Distinction of idiopathic Parkinson's disease from multiple-system atrophy by stimulation of growth-hormone with clonidine. *Lancet*. 1997;349:1877-1881.

93. Kimmel DW, O'Neill BP, Lennon VA. Subacute sensory neuronopathy associated with small cell lung carcinoma: diagnosis aided by autoimmune serology. *Mayo Clin Proc*. 1988;63:29-32.

94. Kleiger RE, Miller JP, Bigger JT Jr, Moss AJ. Decreased heart rate variability and its association with increased mortality after acute myocardial infarction. *Am J Cardiol*. 1987;59:256-262.

95. Knezevic W, Bajada S. Peripheral autonomic surface potential: a quantitative technique for recording sympathetic conduction in man. *J Neurol Sci*. 1985;67:239-251.

96. Knuttgen D, Weidemann D, Doehn M. Diabetic autonomic neuropathy: abnormal cardiovascular reactions under general anesthesia. *Klin Wochenschr.* 1990;68:1168-1172.

97. Korner PI, Tonkin AM, Uther JB. Reflex and mechanical circulatory effects of graded Valsalva maneuvers in normal man. *J Appl Physiol.* 1976;40:434-440.

98. Kunimoto M, Kirno K, Elam M, Karlsson T, Wallin BG. Neuro-effector characteristics of sweat glands in the human hand activated by irregular stimuli. *Acta Physiol Scand.* 1992;146:261-269.

99. Lader MH, Montagu JD. The psycho-galvanic reflex: a pharmacological study of the peripheral mechanism. *J Neurol Neurosurg Psychiatry.* 1962;25:126-133.

100. Lambert WC, Bilinski DL. Diagnostic pitfalls in anhidrotic ectodermal dysplasia: indications for palmar skin biopsy. *Cutis.* 1983;31:182-187.

101. Langley JN. On the union of cranial autonomic (visceral) fibres with the nerve cells of the superior cervical ganglion. *J Physiol (Lond).* 1898; 23:240-270.

102. Lefaucher JP, Fitoussi M, Becquemin JP. Abolition of sympathetic skin responses following endoscopic thoracic sympathectomy. *Muscle Nerve.* 1996;19:581-586.

103. Lennon VA, Sas DF, Busk MF, et al. Enteric neuronal autoantibodies in pseudoobstruction with small cell lung carcinoma. *Gastroenterology.* 1991;100:137-142.

104. Levin AB. A simple test of cardiac function based upon the heart rate changes induced by the Valsalva maneuver. *Am J Cardiol.* 1966;18:90-99.

105. Levy DM, Reid G, Rowley DA, Abraham RR. Quantitative measures of sympathetic skin response in diabetes: relation to sudomotor and neurological function. *J Neurol Neurosurg Psychiatry.* 1992;55:902-908.

106. Lichtenfeld P. Autonomic dysfunction in the Guillain-Barré syndrome. *Am J Med.* 1971;50:772-780.

107. Lin TK, Chee ECY, Chen HJ, Cheng MH. Abnormal sympathetic skin response in patients with palmar hyperhidrosis. *Muscle Nerve.* 1995; 18:917-919.

108. Linden D, Diehl RR. Comparison of standard autonomic tests and power spectral analysis in normal adults. *Muscle Nerve.* 1996;19:556-562.

109. Linden D, Diehl RR, Berlit P. Subclinical autonomic disturbances in multiple sclerosis. *J Neurol.* 1995;242:374-378.

110. Low PA. Autonomic neuropathy. *Semin Neurol.* 1987;7:49-57.

111. Low PA. Composite autonomic scoring scale for laboratory quantification of generalized autonomic failure. *Mayo Clin Proc.* 1993;68:748-752.

112. Low PA. The effect of aging on the autonomic nervous system. In: Low PA, ed. *Clinical Autonomic Disorders.* 2nd ed. Philadelphia: Lippincott-Raven; 1997:161-175.

113. Low PA. Laboratory evaluation of autonomic function. In: Low PA, ed. *Clinical Autonomic Disorders.* 2nd ed. Philadelphia: Lippincott-Raven; 1997:179-208.

114. Low PA. Standardization of autonomic function. In: Low PA, ed. *Clinical Autonomic Disorders.* 2nd ed. Philadelphia: Lippincott-Raven; 1997:287-295.

115. Low PA, Caskey PE, Tuck RR, Fealey RD, Dyck PJ. Quantitative sudomotor axon reflex test in normal and neuropathic subjects. *Ann Neurol.* 1983;14:573-580.

116. Low PA, Fealey RD. Sudomotor neuropathy. In: Dyck PJ, Thomas PK, Asbury AK, Winegrad AI, Porte D Jr, eds. *Diabetic Neuropathy.* Philadelphia: WB Saunders; 1987:140-145.

117. Low PA, Fealey RD, Sheps SG, et al. Chronic idiopathic anhidrosis. *Ann Neurol.* 1985;18:344-348.

118. Low PA, Guillermo SA, Benarroch EE. Clinical autonomic disorders: classification and clinical evaluation. In: Low PA, ed. *Clinical Autonomic Disorders.* 2nd ed. Philadelphia: Lippincott-Raven; 1997:3-15.

119. Low PA, Neumann C, Dyck PJ, et al. Evaluation of skin vasomotor reflexes by using laser Doppler velocimetry. *Mayo Clin Proc.* 1983;58:583-592.

120. Low PA, Opfer-Gehrking RL, Proper CJ, Zimmerman I. The effect of aging on cardiac autonomic and postganglionic sudomotor function. *Muscle Nerve.* 1990;13:152-157.

121. Low PA, Opfer-Gehrking TL, McPhee BR, et al. Prospective evaluation of clinical characteristics of orthostatic hypotension. *Mayo Clin Proc.* 1995;70:617-622.

122. Low PA, Opfer-Gehrking TL, Textor SC, et al. Comparison of the postural tachycardia syndrome (POTS) with orthostatic hypotension due to autonomic failure. *J Auton Nerv Syst.* 1994;50:181-188.

123. Low PA, Opfer-Gehrking TL, Textor SC, et al. Postural tachycardia syndrome (POTS). *Neurology.* 1995;45(suppl 5):S19-S25.

124. Low PA, Okazaki H, Dyck PJ. Splanchnic preganglionic neurons in man. I. Morphometry of preganglionic cytons. *Acta Neuropathol.* 1977;40:55-61.

125. Low PA, Schondorf R, Novak V, et al. Postural tachycardia syndrome. In: Low PA, ed. *Clinical Autonomic Disorders.* 2nd ed. Philadelphia: Lippincott-Raven; 1997:681-697.

126. Low PA, Walsh JC, Huang CY, McLeod JG. The sympathetic nervous system in diabetic neuropathy: a clinical and pathological study. *Brain.* 1975;98:341-356.

127. Low PA, Zimmerman BR, Dyck PJ. Comparison of distal sympathetic with vagal function in diabetic neuropathy. *Muscle Nerve.* 1986;9:592-596.

128. Ludbrook J, Vincent A, Walsh JA. Effects of mental arithmetic on arterial pressure and hand blood flow. *Clin Exp Pharmacol Physiol.* 1975; 2(suppl):67-70.

129. Magalhães M, Wenning GK, Daniel SE, Quinn NP. Autonomic dysfunction in pathologically confirmed multiple system atrophy and idiopathic Parkinson's disease: a retrospective comparison. *Acta Neurol Scand.* 1995;91:98-102.

130. Marfella R, Guigliano D, di Maro G, et al. The squatting test: a useful tool to assess both parasympathetic and sympathetic involvement of the cardiovascular autonomic neuropathy in diabetes. *Diabetes.* 1994; 43:607-612.

131. Marfella R, Salvatore T, Guigliano D, et al. Detection of early sympathetic cardiovascular neuropathy by squatting test in NIDDM. *Diabetes Care.* 1994;17:149-151.

132. Martignoni E, Pacchetti C, Godi L, Micieli G, Nappi G. Autonomic disorders in Parkinson's disease. *J Neurol Transm.* 1995;45(suppl):11-19.

133. Martyn CN, Ewing DJ. Pupil cycle time: a simple way of measuring an autonomic reflex. *J Neurol Neurosurg Psychiatry.* 1986;49:771-774.

134. Maselli RA, Jaspan JB, Soliven BC, Green AJ, Spire JP, Arnason BGW. Comparison of sympathetic skin response with quantitative sudomotor axon reflex test in diabetic neuropathy. *Muscle Nerve.* 1989;12:420-423.

135. Mathias CJ. Orthostatic hypotension: causes, mechanisms, and influencing factors. *Neurology.* 1995;45(suppl 5):S6-S11.

136. McEvoy KM, Windebank AJ, Daube JR, Low PA. 3,4-Diaminopyridine in the treatment of Lambert-Eaton myasthenic syndrome. *N Engl J Med.* 1989;321:1567-1571.

137. McLeod JG, Tuck RR. Disorders of the autonomic nervous system. 1. Pathophysiology and clinical features. *Ann Neurol.* 1987;21:419-530.

138. McLeod JG, Tuck RR. Disorders of the autonomic nervous system. 2. Investigation and treatment. *Ann Neurol.* 1987;21:519-529.

139. Navarro X, Kennedy WR, Fries TJ. Small nerve fiber dysfunction in diabetic neuropathy. *Muscle Nerve.* 1989;12:498-507.

140. Navarro X, Miralles R, Espadaler JM, Rubiés-Prat J. Comparison of sympathetic sudomotor and skin responses in alcoholic neuropathy. *Muscle Nerve.* 1993;16:404-407.

141. Niakan E, Harati Y. Sympathetic skin response in diabetic peripheral neuropathy. *Muscle Nerve.* 1988;11:261-264.

142. Norgués MA, Stålberg EV. Automatic analysis of heart rate variation. II. Findings in patients attending an EMG laboratory. *Muscle Nerve.* 1989;12:1001-1008.

143. Novak P, Novak V, Low PA, et al. Transcranial Doppler evaluation in disorders of reduced orthostatic tolerance. In: Low PA, ed. *Clinical Autonomic Disorders.* 2nd ed. Philadelphia: Lippincott-Raven; 1997:349-368.

144. Ochoa JL. Reflex? Sympathetic? Dystrophy? Triple questioned again. *Mayo Clin Proc.* 1995;70:1124-1126.

145. Ogawa T, Asayama M, Sugenoya J, et al. Temperature regulation in hot-humid environments, with special reference to the significance of hidromeiosis. *J Therm Biol.* 1984;9:121-125.

146. Ogawa T, Low PA. Autonomic regulation of temperature and sweating. In: Low PA, ed. *Clinical Autonomic Disorders.* 2nd ed. Philadelphia: Lippincott-Raven; 1997:83-96.

147. Opfer-Gehrking TL, Low PA. Impaired respiratory sinus arrhythmia with paradoxically normal Valsalva ratio indicates combined cardiovagal and peripheral adrenergic failure. *Clin Auton Res.* 1993;3:169-173.

148. Parati G, Casadei R, Groppelli A, Di Rienzo M, Mancia G. Comparison of finger and intra-arterial blood pressure monitoring at rest and during laboratory testing. *Hypertension.* 1989;13:647-655.

149. Pavesi G, Medici D, Gemignani F, et al. Sympathetic skin response (SSR) in the foot after sural nerve biopsy. *Muscle Nerve.* 1995;18:1326-1328.

150. Pfeifer MA, Cook D, Brodsky J, et al. Quantitative evaluation of cardiac parasympathetic activity in normal and diabetic man. *Diabetes.* 1982;31:339-345.

151. Pfeifer MA, Cook D, Brodsky J, et al. Quantitative evaluation of sympathetic and parasympathetic control of iris function. *Diabetes Care.* 1982;5:518-528.

152. Piha SJ, Halonen JP. Infrared pupillometry in the assessment of autonomic function. *Diabetes Res Clin Pract.* 1994;26:61-66.

153. Piha SJ, Voipio-Pulkki LM. Cardiac dysrhythmias during cardiovascular autonomic reflex tests. *Clin Auton Res.* 1993;3:183-187.

154. Polinsky RJ, Kopin IJ, Ebert MH, Weise V. Pharmacologic distinction of different orthostatic hypotension syndromes. *Neurology.* 1981;31:1-7.

155. Rathmann W, Ziegler D, Jahnke M, et al. Mortality in diabetic patients with cardiovascular autonomic neuropathy. *Diabet Med.* 1993;10:820-824.

156. Raviele A, Gasparini G, Di Pede F, et al. Usefulness of head-up tilt test in evaluating patients with syncope of unknown origin and negative electrophysiologic study. *Am J Cardiol.* 1990;65:1322-1327.

157. Ravits JM. AAEM Minimonograph No. 48. Autonomic nervous system testing. *Muscle Nerve.* 1997;20:919-937.

158. Ravits JM, Baker M, Hallet M, et al. A comparative study of electrophysiologic tests of autonomic function in patients with autonomic failure. *Muscle Nerve.* 1986;9:657.

159. Ravits J, Hallett M, Nilsson J, Polinsky R, Dambrosia J. Electrophysiological tests of autonomic function in patients with idiopathic autonomic failure syndromes. *Muscle Nerve.* 1996;19:758-763.

160. Robertson D, Davis TL. Recent advances in the treatment of orthostatic hypotension. *Neurology.* 1995;45(suppl 5):S26-S32.

161. Robertson D, Goldberg MR, Onrot J, et al. Isolated failure of autonomic noradrenergic neurotransmission: evidence for impaired beta-hydroxylation of dopamine. *N Engl J Med.* 1986;314:1494-1497.

162. Robertson D, Kincaid DW, Haile V, Robertson RM. The head and neck discomfort of autonomic failure: an unrecognized ætiology of headache. *Clin Auton Res.* 1994;4:99-103.

163. Robinson BJ, Johnson RH, Lambie DG, Palmer KT. Do elderly patients with an excessive fall in blood pressure on standing have evidence of autonomic failure? *Clin Sci.* 1983;64:587-591.

164. Rodstein M, Neman FD. Postural blood pressure changes in the elderly. *J Chronic Dis.* 1957;6:581-588.

165. Rommel O, Tegenthoff M, Pern U, et al. Sympathetic skin response in patients with reflex sympathetic dystrophy. *Clin Auton Res.* 1995;5:205-210.

166. Samoil D, Grubb BP. Head-upright tilt testing for recurrent, unexplained syncope. *Clin Cardiol.* 1993;16:763-766.

167. Sampson MJ, Wilson S, Karagiannis P, et al. Progression of diabetic autonomic neuropathy over a decade in insulin-dependent diabetics. *QJM.* 1990;75:635-646.

168. Sandroni P, Ahlskog JE, Fealey RD, Low PA. Autonomic involvement in extrapyramidal and cerebellar disorders. *Clin Auton Res.* 1991;1:147-155.

169. Sandroni P, Benarroch EE, Low PA. Pharmacological dissection of components of the Valsalva maneuver in adrenergic failure. *J Appl Physiol.* 1991;71:1563-1567.

170. Schondorf R. New investigations of autonomic nervous system function. *J Clin Neurophysiol.* 1993;10:28-38.

171. Schondorf R. Skin potentials: normal and abnormal. In Low PA, ed. *Clinical Autonomic Disorders.* 2nd ed. Philadelphia: Lippincott-Raven; 1997:221-231.

172. Schondorf R, Gendron D. Evaluation of sudomotor function in patients with peripheral neuropathy. *Neurology.* 1990;40(suppl 1):386.

173. Schondorf R, Low PA. Idiopathic postural orthostatic tachycardia syndrome: an attenuated form of acute pandysautonomia? *Neurology.* 1993;43:132-137.

174. Shanahi BT, Halperin JJ, Boulu P, Cohen J. Sympathetic skin response: a method of assessing unmyelinated axon dysfunction in peripheral neuropathies. *J Neurol Neurosurg Psychiatry.* 1984;47:536-542.

175. Shields RW Jr. Functional anatomy of the autonomic nervous system. *J Clin Neurophysiol.* 1993;10:2-13.

176. Singh NK, Jaiswal AK, Misra S, Srivastava PK. Assessment of autonomic dysfunction in Guillain-Barré syndrome and its prognostic implications. *Acta Neurol Scand.* 1987;75:101-105.

177. Smith SA. Reduced sinus arrhythmia in diabetic autonomic neuropathy: diagnostic value of an age-related normal range. *BMJ.* 1982;285:1599-1601.

178. Smith SA. Pupillary function in autonomic failure. In: Bannister R, ed. *Autonomic Failure.* 2nd ed. Oxford: Oxford University Press; 1988:393-412.

179. Smith SA, Dewhirst RR. A simple diagnostic test for pupillary abnormality in diabetic autonomic neuropathy. *Diabet Med.* 1986;3:38-41.

180. Smith JJ, Porth CM, Erickson M. Hemodynamic response to the upright posture. *J Clin Pharmacol.* 1994;34:375-386.

181. Smith SA, Smith SE. Reduced pupillary light reflexes in diabetic autonomic neuropathy. *Diabetologia.* 1983;24:330-332.

182. Smith SA, Smith SE. Assessment of pupillary function in diabetic neuropathy. In: Dyck PJ, Thomas PK, Asbury AK, Winegrad AI, Porte E, eds. *Diabetic Neuropathy.* Philadelphia: WB Saunders; 1987:134-139.

183. Smith SE, Smith SA, Brown PM, et al. Pupillary signs in diabetic autonomic neuropathy. *BMJ.* 1978;2:924-927.

184. Soliven B, Maselli R, Jaspan J, et al. Sympathetic skin response in diabetic neuropathy. *Muscle Nerve.* 1987;10:711-716.

185. Sousa AC, Marin-Neto JA, Maciel BC, et al. Cardiac parasympathetic impairment in gastrointestinal Chagas' disease. *Lancet.* 1987;1:985.

186. Sprangers RL, Veerman DP, Karemaker JM, Wieling W. Initial circulatory responses to changes in posture: influence of the angle and speed of tilt. *Clin Physiol.* 1991;11:211-220.

187. Stewart JD, Abrahamowicz M, Du Berger R, Bartlett-Esquilant B. Testing for sympathetic vasoconstrictor dysfunction: recovery rate of blood pressure is a better diagnostic measure than the drop itself. *Clin Auton Res.* 1998;8:294.

188. Stewart JD, Low PA, Fealey RD. Distal small-fiber neuropathy: results of tests of sweating and autonomic cardiovascular reflexes. *Muscle Nerve.* 1992;15:661-665.

189. Stewart JD, Nguyen DM, Abrahamowicz M. Quantitative sweat testing using acetylcholine for direct and axon reflex mediated stimulation with silicone mold recording: controls versus neuropathic diabetics. *Muscle Nerve.* 1994;17:1370-1377.

190. Strasberg B, Rechavia E, Sagie A, et al. The head-up tilt-table test in patients with syncope of unknown origin. *Am Heart J.* 1989;118:923-927.

191. Streeten DH, Anderson GH Jr. Mechanisms of orthostatic hypotension and tachycardia in patients with pheochromocytoma. *Am J Hypertens.* 1996;9:760-769.

192. Streeten DH, Anderson GH Jr, Richardson R, Thomas FD. Abnormal orthostatic changes in blood pressure and heart rate in subjects with intact sympathetic nervous function: evidence for excessive venous pooling. *J Lab Clin Med.* 1988;111:326-335.

193. Sundkvist G, Lilja B. Autonomic neuropathy in diabetes mellitus: a follow-up study. *Diabetes Care.* 1985;8:129-133.

194. Tan ET, Lambie DG, Johnson RH, Whiteside EA. Parasympathetic denervation of the iris in alcoholics with vagal neuropathy. *J Neurol Neurosurg Psychiatry.* 1984;47:61-64.

195. Taylor AA, Davies AO, Mares A, et al. Spectrum of dysautonomia in mitral valve prolapse. *Am J Med.* 1989;86:267-274.

196. Ten Harkel AD, van Lieshout JJ, van Lieshout EJ, Wieling W. Assessment of cardiovascular reflexes: influence of posture and period of preceding rest. *J Appl Physiol.* 1990;68:147-153.

197. Thomas JP, Shields R. Associated autonomic dysfunction and carcinoma of the pancreas. *BMJ.* 1970;4:32.

198. Truax BT. Autonomic disturbances in Guillain-Barré syndrome. *Semin Neurol.* 1984;4:462-468.

199. Uncini A, Pullman SL, Lovelace RE, Gambi D. The sympathetic skin response: normal values, elucidation of afferent components and application limits. *J Neurol Sci.* 1988;87:299-306.

200. Valls-Sole J, Monforte R, Estruch R. Abnormal sympathetic skin response in alcoholic subjects. *J Neurol Sci.* 1991;102:233-237.

201. Van den Bergh P, Kelly JJ. The evoked electrodermal response in peripheral neuropathies. *Muscle Nerve.* 1986;9:656-657.

202. van Dijk JG, Haan J, Koenderink M, Roos RAC. Autonomic nervous function in progressive supranuclear palsy. *Arch Neurol.* 1991;48:1083-1084.

203. van Lieshout EJ, van Lieshout JJ, ten Harkel AD, Wieling W. Cardiovascular response to coughing: its value in the assessment of autonomic nervous control. *Clin Sci.* 1989;77:305-310.

204. van Lieshout JJ, Wieling W, van Montfrans GA, et al. Acute dysautonomia associated with Hodgkin's disease. *J Neurol Neurosurg Psychiatry.* 1986;49:830-832.

205. van Lieshout JJ, Wieling W, Wesseling KH, Karemaker JM. Pitfalls in the assessment of cardiovascular reflexes in patients with sympathetic failure but intact vagal control. *Clin Sci.* 1989;76:523-528.

206. Wallin BG. Sympathetic nerve activity underlying electrodermal and cardiovascular reactions in man. *Psychophysiology.* 1980;18:470-476.

207. Wallin BG, Sundlof G, Eriksson BM, et al. Plasma noradrenaline correlates to sympathetic muscle nerve activity in normotensive man. *Acta Physiol Scand.* 1981;111:69-73.

208. Wang SJ, Liao KK, Liou HH, et al. Sympathetic skin response and R-R interval variation in chronic uremic patients. *Muscle Nerve.* 1994;17:411-418.

209. Watahiki Y, Baba M, Matsunaga M, et al. Sympathetic skin response in diabetic neuropathy. *Electromyogr Clin Neurophysiol.* 1989;29:155-157.

210. Wei JY, Harris WS. Heart rate response to cough. *J Appl Physiol.* 1982;53:1039-1043.

211. Wei JY, Rowe JW, Kestenbaum AD, Ben-Haim S. Post-cough heart rate response: influence of age, sex, and basal blood pressure. *Am J Physiol.* 1983;245:R18-R24.

212. Wenning GK, Ben Shlomo Y, Magalhães M, et al. Clinical features and natural history of multiple system atrophy: an analysis of 100 cases. *Brain.* 1994;117:835-845.

213. Wheeler JS Jr, Siroky MB, Pavlakis A, Krane RJ. The urodynamic aspects of the Guillain-Barré syndrome. *J Urol.* 1984;131:917-919.

214. Wheeler T, Watkins PJ. Cardiac denervation in diabetes. *BMJ.* 1973;4:584-586.

215. Wieling W, van Brederode JFM, de Rijk LG, et al. Reflex control of heart rate in normal subjects in relation to age: a database for cardiac vagal neuropathy. *Diabetologia.* 1982;22:163-166.

216. Wilson PR. Reflex sympathetic dystrophy. In: Low PA, ed. *Clinical Autonomic Disorders.* 2nd ed. Philadelphia: Lippincott-Raven; 1997:537-543.

217. Winer JB, Hughes RAC. Identification of patients at risk of arrhythmia in the Guillain-Barré syndrome. *QJM.* 1988;68:735-739.

218. Wolf MM, Varigos GA, Hunt D, Sloman JG. Sinus arrhythmia in acute myocardial infarction. *Med J Aust.* 1978;2:52-53.

219. Yokota T, Hayashi M, Tanabe H, Tsukagoshi H. Sympathetic skin response in patients with cerebellar degeneration. *Arch Neurol.* 1993;50:422-427.

220. Yokota T, Matsunaga T, Okiyama R, et al. Sympathetic skin response in patients with multiple sclerosis compared with patients with spinal cord transection and normal controls. *Brain.* 1991;114:1381-1394.

221. Yoshimura M. Diffuse Lewy body disease. *Rinsho Shinkeigaku.* 1997;37:1134-1136.

222. Ziegler D, Dannehl K, Mühlen H, et al. Prevalence of cardiovascular autonomic dysfunction assessed by spectral analysis, vector analysis, and standard tests of heart rate variation and blood pressure responses at various stages of diabetic neuropathy. *Diabet Med.* 1992;9:806-814.

223. Ziegler D, Laux G, Dannehl K, et al. Assessment of cardiovascular autonomic function: age-related normal ranges and reproducibility of spectral analysis, vector analysis, and standard tests of heart rate variation and blood pressure responses. *Diabet Med.* 1992;9:166-175.

224. Zochodne DW. Autonomic involvement in Guillain-Barré syndrome: a review. *Muscle Nerve.* 1994;17:1145-1155.

# 23

# Micturition and Sexual Disorders

*George D. Baquis*

Disorders affecting micturition and sexual function are common and can result from a large number of diseases affecting the central and peripheral nervous system. Urinary incontinence affects approximately 13 million Americans, and the prevalence of urinary incontinence ranges from 15% to 35% of noninstitutionalized persons older than 60 years of age.[3] This increases to approximately 40% of hospitalized patients and over 50% of nursing home patients.[257] In the Massachusetts Male Aging Study,[112] a community-based survey of 40- to 70-year-old men, the prevalence of impotence was 52%. With aging, the probability of complete impotence tripled from 5% to 15% and that of moderate impotence doubled from 17% to 34%.[112] Although many causes of erectile dysfunction are not neurologic, a cross-sectional study of aged impotent men revealed coexistence of neurologic and vascular disorders (30.3%) and diabetic neuropathy (17.1%) to be frequent causes of erectile dysfunction.[220]

Since the peripheral neural anatomic pathways and the organs responsible for micturition and sexual function are physically close to each other, diseases of micturition and sexual function have traditionally been grouped together. However, although disturbances of these functions may occur simultaneously as a result of shared disease, they may also be affected separately and result from different pathophysiologies. The laboratory diagnostic studies also differ for each of these categories. Despite the large number of different etiologies, the repertoire of clinical responses to disease is limited. Therefore a careful history and physical examination are essential to guide the remainder of the diagnostic evaluation. Some of the examination techniques and diagnostic studies may be unfamiliar to neurologists and require expertise outside the realm of a traditional neurologic diagnostic evaluation. A multidisciplinary approach is needed, one that emphasizes close cooperation between urologists, gynecologists, physiatrists, and general medical practitioners, who traditionally have directed the diagnostic evaluation.

This chapter reviews basic principles of clinical micturition and sexual function, urodynamic studies, diagnostic tests for impotence, and specialized neurologic diagnostic studies and then addresses the application of these tests to specific neurologic disorders.

## GENERAL CONSIDERATIONS

The bladder and urethra function as both a reservoir (during filling) and as a pump (during voiding) that store urine without leakage and periodically expel it. The smooth muscle and striated muscle urethral sphincters relax during voiding.[71] Preganglionic efferent parasympathetic neurons originate in the intermediolateral cell column of the S2 to S4 spinal cord and supply the bladder detrusor muscle through the pelvic nerves. The preganglionic fibers synapse on cholinergic postganglionic neurons within the pelvic plexus or on intramural ganglia within the bladder.[60] Sympathetic efferent nerves arise from preganglionic neurons within the intermediolateral cell column from the T11 to L2 spinal cord and supply the bladder via the inferior hypogastric nerves. These cholinergic preganglionic neurons synapse on noradrenergic postganglionic neurons within the sympathetic chain, pelvic plexus, bladder, and urethra.[60] They activate beta receptors of the bladder dome, alpha receptors at the bladder base (trigone), and alpha receptors of urethral smooth muscle fibers.[71] They terminate as the cavernous nerves of the penis.[132] The striated muscle of the external urethral sphincter is supplied by pudendal nerve branches originating from the nucleus of Onufrowicz in the anterior horn of sacral spinal cord segments S1 to S3.[239] The pelvic floor striated muscles, including the puborectalis muscle and the perivaginal striated muscle in females, are supplied directly by pelvic nerve branches.[312] The afferent limb of the bladder parasympathetic pathway originates in the S2 to S4 dorsal root ganglia, and the afferent sympathetic neurons reside in T11 to L2 dorsal root ganglia.[60] The external urethral afferents travel in the pudendal nerve.[60] Sensory fibers from the glans penis travel in the dorsal nerve to join the pudendal nerve and reach the spinal cord via S2 to S4 dorsal root ganglia. Fine neural fibers connecting the cavernous nerves and dorsal nerve of the penis have been identified in human cadaver dissections.[48]

Penile erection is mediated via parasympathetic neural pathway activation and probably by simultaneous sympathetic outflow inhibition.[132] In men, sympathetic efferents close the bladder neck to retrograde flow and induce the emission of semen through rhythmic smooth muscle contraction; in women, they induce contraction of genital smooth muscle during orgasm. Parasympathetic activity in women increases vaginal secretions in association with clitoral swelling.[189] Central nervous system (CNS) integration of the peripheral and somatic nervous systems is accomplished at neural centers within the spinal cord, pons, midbrain, and subcortical and cortical structures.[60,71,132]

## CLASSIFICATION

Multiple classification systems of bladder dysfunction have been developed based upon anatomic localization of nervous system lesions (Bradley neurologic classification), traumatic spinal cord injury (Bors and Comarr), functional bladder emptying (Wein), urologic symptoms (Agency for Health Care Policy and Research), and urodynamic findings (Lapides, Krane, and Siroky).[3,40] Neurogenic disturbances of male sexual function include both erectile and ejaculatory dysfunction, and in females disturbances are related to vaginal lubrication and orgasm. Causes contributing to erectile dysfunction have been broadly classified as "organic and psychological."[227] The evaluation of erectile dysfunction represents the preponderance of published information on diagnostic testing of male sexual function. Relatively little information exists on the neuropathophysiology of female sexual dysfunction associated with neurologic diseases.

## CLINICAL HISTORY AND PHYSICAL EXAMINATION

Patients generally present to neurologists in three contexts. The first are those who present with a history of a known neurological disease with symptoms of bladder or sexual dysfunction. A second group has symptoms of neurologic disease, as well as bladder or sexual dysfunction, without a well-established diagnosis of either condition. The third group has symptoms of bladder or sexual dysfunction in the absence of any clinical neurologic disease. This group includes patients referred for evaluation of abnormal urodynamic tests. The approach to each of these groups differs.[272]

It is initially necessary to establish whether the symptoms and signs of bladder and sexual dysfunction are neurologic. The first group of patients need to know whether their symptoms are consistent with their known neurologic condition or whether other etiologies need to be considered. Establishment of a diagnosis of both urogenital and neurologic disease is the focus for those patients in the second and third groups. Clinical neurologic abnormalities, when present, may direct the neurologic assessment. Patients in the third group are clinically challenging because (1) their symptoms may be similar to those associated with nonneurologic diseases, (2) the underlying neurologic disease may be occult and only become apparent with laboratory diagnostic testing, and (3) neurourologic abnormalities may be neuroanatomically nonlocalizing.[272]

This initial history of micturition dysfunction should include inquiry about urinary voiding habits (frequency, urgency, initiation and termination of stream, quality of stream, nighttime and daytime pattern), dysuria, hematuria, sensation of bladder or pelvic fullness, episodes of incontinence, relationship to fluid intake, and association with physical activities such as those that alter intraabdominal pressure. The temporal profile of symptoms and clinical progression should be carefully noted. Completion of a daily diary by the patient can facilitate information gathering and provide a useful baseline for future comparison. Inquiry should be made about any history of urinary tract infections, pelvic infections, abdominopelvic surgery, renal insufficiency, or renal calculi. All medications should be recorded. A careful obstetric history should be recorded for all women and should include the birth weight of children, mode of delivery, use of forceps, and performance of episiotomy.

The sexual history should include inquiry about libido, symptoms of erectile dysfunction or ejaculatory dysfunction, penile and perineal skin sensation, orgasm, menstrual history, and a description of the situational circumstances of occurrence. A full psychiatric history and social history, including alcohol and drug use, should be obtained.[183]

The neurologic history should be directed toward the associated neurologic symptoms (when these are present) or an assessment of specific neurologic diseases known to complicate bladder and sexual function. The medical history may include systemic illnesses known to affect the neural control of micturition or sexual function. Since the number of candidate diseases may be large, the initial inquiry should attempt to distinguish possible peripheral from CNS disease. A refined history regarding specific neurologic diseases may then be more easily obtained.

In addition to the classic neurologic examination, the clinical examination should incorporate a careful abdominal examination, assessment for bladder fullness, assessment of the appearance of the external genitalia, palpation of the extremity pulses, and evaluation for hernias. A rectal examination should include notation of anal sphincter tone and strength of contraction. The prostate of males should be examined. A female gynecologic examination is necessary to assess for cystoceles or rectoceles and to examine pelvic muscle tone and strength. Superficial skin sensation should be evaluated over the abdomen, pelvis, buttocks, inner thighs, and external genitalia.[183]

Several superficial skin reflexes have been described.[73] The absence of superficial abdominal skin reflexes can be helpful, but these reflexes fatigue with repeated elicitation. They may be absent after abdominal surgery and childbirth, in the elderly, and in the setting of abdominal or bladder distention. The cutaneous anal reflex consists of contraction of the anal sphincter after stroking or pricking the perianal skin; it is mediated through the inferior hemorrhoidal nerve (S2 to S5 segments). The cremasteric reflex consists of contraction of the cremasteric muscle with elevation of the homologous testicle after stroking or pinching of the inner thigh; it is felt to assess innervation of the ilioinguinal and genitofemoral nerves (L1 and L2 segments). The bulbocavernosus reflex is elicited by squeezing, stroking, or pricking the dorsum of the penis (or clitoris) to evoke contraction of the external anal sphincter (S3 and S4 segments).

## DIAGNOSTIC TESTING

The specialized diagnostic tests performed for evaluation of disturbances of micturition and sexual dysfunction fall into two groups. The first group consists of studies that are often performed predominantly by urologists or gynecologists. These studies directly assess the function of the organs supplied by the nerves of concern and provide indirect information regarding neurogenic function. They include urodynamic studies, tests of penile tumescence and rigidity, penile vascular studies, and tests of erectile capacity. When these test results are abnormal, neurologists may be asked to evaluate patients for the presence of neurologic disease. Many of these studies will have been completed prior to the request for neurologic consultation. The second group of studies directly assess peripheral and CNS function. They include peripheral nerve conduction testing of penile and pudendal nerves, needle EMG of the urethral sphincter and pelvic floor muscles, pudendal nerve and bladder evoked responses, bulbocavernosus reflex testing, other sacral reflex electrodiagnostic tests, sympathetic skin response, and electrical or magnetic stimulation of the brain and spinal cord. These studies are best performed as an extension of the clinical neurologic examination, and neurologists are well suited to provide the specialized expertise needed for their performance and interpretation. Each of these tests has different advantages and disadvantages (Table 23–1).

## DIAGNOSTIC TESTS: GROUP 1

### Urodynamic Testing

Urodynamic testing is a cornerstone in the evaluation of patients with disturbances of micturition. This evaluation usually begins with measurement of postvoid residual urine, which can be accomplished by catheterization or pelvic ultrasonography. Ultrasound of residual urine volumes of 24 men with neurogenic bladder dysfunction detected urine volumes of $\geq 100$ ml, with a sensitivity of 90% and a specificity of 81% when compared to catheterized volumes.[259] Urinalysis is performed to detect hematuria, pyuria, glucosuria, bacteriuria, and proteinuria.[112]

The urodynamic evaluation consists of several different complementary tests performed to classify the type of voiding dysfunction. These include cystometry, uroflowmetry, urethral pressure profilometry, videourodynamics, and ambulatory urodynamics.[171] Cystometry evaluates bladder filling through a catheter. It is usually performed with sterile water or normal saline and can be done with varying degrees of sophistication. Single-channel devices measure only bladder pressure. Multichannel instruments can simultaneously measure total bladder pressure, abdominal (rectal) pressure (which can be subtracted from total bladder pressure to calculate detrusor pressure), and the striated urethral sphincter EMG signal.[88] During testing the patient should be questioned regarding sensation of filling, pain, and urgency. Sensation, capacity, and the presence of involuntary detrusor contractions are recorded. The normal adult bladder capacity is 300 to 500 ml.[18] Although any bladder contraction during filling is abnormal, the International Bladder Continence Society has established a minimum criteria of 15 cm $H_2O$ for an unstable or hyperreflexic detrusor contraction.[2,88] Compliance, the relationship of pressure to volume, is measured during the filling phase. Normal compliance has been arbitrarily defined as <12.5 ml/cm $H_2O$.[321] However, compliance is a dynamic entity that is not reflected by this single measure, and it can also be described by changes in slope or area of the pressure volume curve.[88]

Uroflowmetry is the measurement of urine volume passed per unit of time by using a uroflowmeter. It is an easily performed noninvasive test. Measured values include the maximum flow rate, time to reach maximum flow, and time to void. Maximum flow rate declines with age and has been described in normal populations of varying age.[159] However, there is no universally agreed upon nomogram of normal values, and patient straining can introduce artifacts.[166] The test is difficult to perform in patients with Parkinson's disease, dementia, and other severe neurologic diseases; it does not reliably distinguish between outlet obstruction and diminished detrusor contractility.[166]

Micturitional urethral pressure profilometry (UPP) is the measurement of the pressure profile along the length of the urethra performed with a triple-lumen catheter containing pressure transducers that simultaneously measure vesical and vesicourethral pressure. Rectal pressure should also be measured. Pressures are recorded as the catheter is slowly withdrawn. This technique would appear to be ideal for defining the pathophysiology of bladder outlet obstruction, stress incontinence, and bladder sphincter dyssynergia.[309] However, discriminant analysis of UPP for the diagnosis of stress incontinence has revealed a significant overlap between patients with stress incontinence and normal patients, which limits the diagnostic usefulness of this test.[328] When performed by experienced investigators, evaluation of males with symptoms of bladder outlet obstruction has demonstrated a sensitivity of 83% and a specificity of 82% for UPP as compared to pressure flow determination. Since, unlike pressure flow studies, UPP does not measure detrusor contractility, these tests are complementary.[91] Videofluoroscopy of the lower urinary tract after introduction of contrast material into the bladder and synchronous multichannel urodynamic monitoring can better define disorders of impaired detrusor contractility, detrusor instability, and sensory urgency, as well as facilitate precise localization of bladder outlet obstruction.[166,281]

Videourodynamic studies can be used to (1) identify upper urinary tract dilation, which can result from detrusor hyperreflexia with detrusor external sphincter dyssynergia, (2) visualize trabeculation of the inner bladder wall, and (3) demonstrate the relationship of involuntary bladder contraction to bladder neck and urethral contraction.[11]

Urodynamic testing is routinely performed for evaluation and management of bladder dysfunction, but conventional urodynamic testing has shortcomings. The testing circumstances are nonphysiologic, studies are performed over a short time, urinary incontinence is often not noted, and treatment of abnormalities present on testing do not always restore effective bladder function.[151] Ambulatory urodynamics can record bladder functioning under normal conditions and during the circumstances that evoke clinical symptoms. Information is acquired through a portable monitor attached to bladder and rectal pressure transducers, which simultaneously measure bladder and abdominal pressure. Involuntary urine leakage is quantified by using absorbent pads or a pad containing strip recording electrodes.[151] Observed differences, as compared to conventional urodynamics on examination of healthy volunteers, include the absence of bladder pressure rise with natural filling, decrease in mean voided volume, increased maximal detrusor pressure with micturition, and presence of detrusor instability.[261] This testing is labor intensive, requires the patient to conscientiously complete a diary, and is subject to data collection artifacts. Until the methods and terminology of ambulatory

## TABLE 23–1. Diagnostic Tests for Micturition and Sexual Disorders

| PROCEDURE | ADVANTAGES | DISADVANTAGES |
|---|---|---|
| **Vascular** | | |
| Penile brachial blood pressure index | Noninvasive blood pressure measurement using cuff | Lack of standardization, with high intraobserver and interobserver variability |
| Doppler ultrasound | Noninvasive measure of penile arterial and venous anatomy and blood flow; can assess for cavernous venous leakage | Should be performed after injection of pharmacologic vasodilatory agent |
| | | Not all studies strongly correlate results with arteriography |
| Iliac and pudendal arteriography | Definitive evaluation of venous and arterial anatomy | Invasive procedure that does not quantitate blood flow |
| | | Anatomic variability of internal pudendal artery exists |
| | | Lack of consensus regarding what constitutes significant anatomic vascular disease sufficient to result in erectile dysfunction |
| Cavernosometry and cavernosography | Identifies presence of and sites of cavernous venous leakage | Erectile dysfunction may persist despite surgery with correction of venous leakage on postoperative studies |
| Pharmacologic penile erection | Usually abnormal when patients have severe cavernous venous leakage or severe penile arterial insufficiency | Not useful for distinguishing between different causes of organic erectile dysfunction |
| | | Does not distinguish between arterial and venous disease |
| | | Subjectivity exists regarding what constitutes positive or negative test |
| **Penile Tumescence and Rigidity** | | |
| Stamp and snap-gauge tests | Easily performed and inexpensive | Neither sensitive nor specific measure of erectile dysfunction |
| | | Does not measure frequency or duration of erections or degree of penile rigidity |
| Home nocturnal portable monitoring devices | Records number and magnitude of penile erections during sleep | May fail to identify patients with mild degrees of erectile dysfunction or those with diminished REM sleep |
| | Results are reproducible in same patient over time | Normal NPT study may not correlate with ability to achieve vaginal penetration during sexual intercourse |
| | Good correlation with results from technician observations in sleep laboratories | Normal values for different age ranges are not well established |
| **Urodynamics** | | |
| Postvoid residual | Easily measured by catheterization or ultrasound | Does not distinguish between obstructive and nonobstructive causes of micturition dysfunction associated with increased postvoiding residual urine |
| Cystometry, uroflowmetry, urethral pressure profilometry, videourodynamics, ambulatory urodynamics | Variety of tests that measure bladder filling, capacity, compliance, and sensation | Conventional testing is nonphysiologic, obtained over short time, and treatment of urodynamic abnormalities does not always restore normal micturition function |
| | Useful for identifying structural nonneurologic diseases | Ambulatory testing records data under normal conditions that evoke clinical symptoms, but labor-intensive procedure is subject to data collection artifacts and requires patient to keep diary |
| | Assesses both upper and lower urinary tract | |
| **Electrodiagnosis*** | | |
| Pudendal nerve terminal motor latency | Direct neural measure of motor function to urinary striated muscle sphincter | Requires placement of Foley catheter–mounted recording electrode |
| | | Normal values for compound muscle action potential amplitude are lacking |
| Penile dorsal nerve conduction | Direct neural measure of primarily sensory function | Some of reported values are derived from indirect measures |
| | | Problem of standardization of technique for penile length measurement exists |
| Needle electromyography (EMG) | Direct quantitative measure of striated muscle function | Procedure can be painful and technically difficult to perform |
| | Can assess muscles that are not accessible for clinical examination or surface electrodes | |
| Pudendal nerve evoked potentials | Direct measure of both central nervous system and peripheral nervous system somatosensory function | Only limited information exists regarding test sensitivity and specificity for evaluation of disease conditions |
| Posterior urethral and bladder evoked potentials | Procedure with potential to provide direct neurophysiologic information about visceral afferent nerve function | Limited information exists based on reports from studies performed on small number of patients |
| Bulbocavernosus reflex (BCR) and other sacral reflexes | Direct quantitative measurement of sacral spinal cord oligosynaptic neurophysiologic function | Absence of BCR in males is indicative (in females suggestive) of sacral spinal cord disease (see text for limitations) |
| | | Although widely used for evaluation of male penile erectile dysfunction, clinical usefulness has been questioned |
| Sympathetic skin response | Direct measure of genital autonomic neurophysiologic function | Clinical usefulness for evaluation of micturition and sexual dysfunction has not been determined |
| Transcranial and spinal magnetic and electrical stimulation | Direct quantitative measurement of central nervous system motor pathway conduction | Promising techniques that are currently considered investigational |

*These tests require additional special expertise, and many require additional equipment, to perform and interpret.

testing are standardized, conventional urodynamic testing remains the "gold standard."[270,324]

## Penile Tumescence and Rigidity

Tests of nocturnal penile tumescence (NPT) and rigidity have been used to distinguish psychogenic from organic erectile dysfunction. NPT, which occurs during normal sleep, is associated with the rapid eye movement (REM) period. Testing assumes that the same physiologic mechanisms are responsible for both nocturnal and sexually stimulated penile erections.[191] Monitoring with NPT stamps was developed to detect nocturnal erections from breakage of stamps placed around the base of penis.[24] However, although this method is easily and inexpensively performed, significant problems include false-positive and false-negative results due to stamp slippage and incidental stamp tearing in the absence of erection.[207]

The snap-gauge test measures penile rigidity during sleep through the patient's ability to break three snap gauges with different release-force constants.[96] The number of gauges broken is related to the amount of pressure exerted by the engorged penis, and this measurement has been reported to correlate well with full NPT laboratory evaluations having a sensitivity of 70% and a specificity of 80%, with correct diagnosis of 77.5% of patients.[6,100] However, this approach does not provide a measure of the frequency, duration, and degree of rigidity, and not all patients will break all three snap gauges, even when a satisfactory erection occurs.[191,217]

The Rigiscan is a home nocturnal monitoring device that records the number and magnitude of penile erectile events during sleep.[47,161] A loop fitted around the tip and base of the penis samples penile tumescence and rigidity throughout the night. The data are recorded in an ambulatory unit strapped to the patient's inner thigh and are downloaded into a computer for processing after completion of the session.[217] The frequency and duration of recorded NPT episodes in healthy males decreases with age.[260,282] Overall, Rigiscan-measured radial rigidity through home testing correlates well with technician observations and tonometric measurements of axial rigidity performed in a sleep laboratory, and the results are reproducible in the same patient over time.[9,23,138] However, the Rigiscan may fail to identify patients with mild degrees of erectile dysfunction.[9] Normal values for different age ranges have not been well established, and although men older than 60 may not have measured full erections during NPT sleep evaluation, they and their partners may report regular normal sexual intercourse.[282] Since erectile activity is associated with REM sleep, diminished REM sleep may alter NPT recorded activity. Other problems include the absence of a gold standard for the diagnosis of organic vs. psychogenic erectile dysfunction against which to validate NPT testing.[340]

## Vascular Testing

Ultrasonic Doppler imaging is a noninvasive technique for evaluation of penile venous and arterial anatomy and blood flow. Since the diameter of the cavernosal arteries in the flaccid state is not considered to be a good indicator of potential blood flow during penile erection, it is measured again after injection into the corpus cavernosum of a vasodilating agent (e.g., papaverine, phentolamine, or prostaglandin $E_1$). The Doppler spectral waveform of cavernous artery systolic and diastolic blood flow, the blood flow velocity, and the direction of blood flow are recorded and correlated with the status of the erection. The presence of cavernous venous leakage, a potentially treatable cause of impotence, can also be assessed.[145] Cavernosal pressure and the cavernosal blood flow changes that occur in response to papaverine injection have been correlated with phases of penile erection.[286]

Iliac and pudendal arteriography definitively evaluates the iliac and pudendal vasculature, describes collateral blood flow, and can provide precise localization of vascular occlusions.[136] Significant disease more commonly tends to involve the more distal cavernosal arteries, but more proximal disease is also described. Anatomic variability of the origin of the internal pudendal artery exists.[323] However, angiography, an invasive method, is a major undertaking and does not provide quantitative blood flow information.[252]

Several studies have shown that penile Doppler ultrasound examination correlates well with the results of elective arteriography in 90% to 95% of cases, but not all studies report a strong correlation.[64,219,253,326] Some of this discrepancy may reflect technical considerations in performance of the ultrasound examination.[253] Although some reports have quantitated the sites and degree of vascular narrowings, the criteria for what constitutes significant vascular disease on angiography that is sufficient to result in erectile dysfunction have not been defined.[323] Some investigators have correlated the degree of vessel narrowing detected by angiography with cavernosal artery peak systolic velocities through ultrasound investigation. Although peak velocities of <25 cm/s are generally considered to be abnormal, definitions of normality differ among studies.[32,186,252,323]

Abnormal drainage of the corpus cavernosum has also been associated with erectile dysfunction.[75] Cavernosal venous sinusoidal leakage can be measured by techniques of cavernosometry and cavernosography. Cavernosometry measures pressure within the cavernous bodies during simultaneous infusion of saline. Cavernosal artery occlusion pressure (CAOP), noted during erection when cavernosal artery pressure disappears on Doppler ultrasonography, can be measured.[81] The lowest rate of saline infusion needed to induce an erection, termed the *induction flow,* and the lowest rate needed to maintain an erection, termed the *maintenance flow,* and the amount of pressure decrease from 150 mm Hg in 30 seconds represent other measured parameters.[185] Excessive venous outflow (venous leakage) prevents the development of pressure sufficient to initiate and maintain an adequate erection.[185] Performance of the study after the administration of vasodilators increases test reliability and reduces the number of false-positive (6%) and false-negative (16%) results, compared to performance of the test without pharmacotherapy.[185] Cavernosography is the radiologic imaging of the corpus cavernosum after injection of a contrast agent. It is performed to identify corpus cavernosal venous leakage through abnormally opacifying veins. The most common sites of leakage are the deep dorsal and cavernous veins.[81,274] The study is performed after administration of a pharmacologic vasodilator because, in the penile flaccid state, superficial veins may fill normally.[206] The frequency of abnormal cavernosography in large series of patients with erectile dysfunction of varying causes has been reported as >80%.[122,169,199,255] However, surgical correction of venous leakage by vein ligation has been reported with variable results.[80,254,353] Erectile dysfunction can persist despite adequate surgical correction of venous leakage on postoperative cavernosography, suggesting that venous leakage is associated with other factors responsible for erectile dysfunction.[353] Therefore, although these tests do provide physiologic diagnostic information, they are not routinely performed for the evaluation of erectile dysfunction.

The penile brachial blood pressure index (PBI) is the ratio of penile arterial pressure to brachial artery arterial pressure. Measurement is performed with blood pressure cuffs and a Doppler probe. A ratio below 0.6 is suggested as correlating with erectile dysfunction, and a ratio above 0.75 suggests absence of an arterial obstacle between the aorta and the penile artery measurement point.[81] However, no reported standardized technique exists for performance of PBI, the study can be technically difficult to perform, and intraobserver and interobserver variation of measured PBI is high. The test is limited by lack of accuracy and reproducibility.[5]

### Pharmacologic Penile Erection

The diagnostic intracavernous injection of pharmacologic vasodilators has been investigated for differentiation of psychogenic, vascular, and neurogenic causes of erectile dysfunction. The intracavernous injection of papaverine, phentolamine, or prostaglandin $E_1$ is considered to "bypass neurogenic influences" and relax cavernous and arteriolar smooth muscle through direct local actions.[200] Evocation of a normal erection implies normal penile vascular function, and failure of normal erection indicates venous or arterial insufficiency.[218] The response of males with organic erectile dysfunction has been compared to that of both normal volunteers and patients with psychogenic erectile dysfunction. Since no single set of criteria defines organic impotence, these patients have been identified by combining the results of other tests, including NPT, neurologic electrodiagnostic tests, arterial and venous vascular studies, and psychologic evaluations.[43,56,154,262,330] The response of control patients has not differed from that of patients with psychogenic dysfunction.[330] The test is not useful for differentiating among different causes of organic erectile dysfunction because the response rate among all patients with erectile dysfunction has been as high as 97%.[262] Although the test result can be normal in patients with mild or moderate vascular abnormalities, it is virtually always abnormal in patients with severe arterial lesions or venous leakage.[43,56] Intracavernous papaverine has been compared to NPT as having a reported sensitivity of 100% but a specificity of only 25%.[56] However, in an NPT study of 37 impotent males, 12% of those with psychogenic impotence by NPT evaluation failed to respond to intracorporeal papaverine and phentolamine.[8] The hypothesis that stress and anxiety increase adrenergic vasoconstrictor input to the penis and may explain the lack of response in some patients otherwise considered to have psychogenic erectile dysfunction has not been supported by studies of peripheral cortisol and catecholamine levels.[135,305] The addition of self-stimulation has been reported to improve the response to intracavernous prostaglandin $E_1$ injection by 74% in patients who initially fail to obtain a complete erection.[89] Limitations of pharmacologic testing include its inability to differentiate between arterial and ve-

nous system disease and observer subjectivity regarding what constitutes a positive or negative erectile response.

## DIAGNOSTIC TESTS: GROUP 2

### Penile Dorsal Nerve Conduction

Several techniques have been described for measurement of nerve conduction of the dorsal nerve of the penis. Tactile stimulation and sensory input play an important role in erectile and sexual function. The dorsal nerve contains sensory nerve fibers, and measurement of dorsal nerve conduction provides a direct quantitative measure of peripheral nerve function. The initial report[128] described stimulation of the dorsal nerve at two separate locations, the tip and the base, while the penis was affixed to a tongue depressor.[128] The averaged evoked response from the bulbocavernosus muscle (referred to the iliac crest) was recorded.[128] The latency difference between the two sites was divided by the measured penile distance for calculation of velocity, with a mean of 23.8 m/s (range 21.4 to 29.1 m/s). Subsequently, 27 normal men were studied by using an orthodromic technique of penile stimulation at the dorsum of the penis while recording was done from disks at the penile base.[46] The penile glans was attached to a traction apparatus. Distance and calculated conduction velocity were functions of the weight applied to the apparatus. Nerve conduction velocity measured to the peak of the evoked action potential was calculated as 27.4 m/s (range 21 to 36 m/s), and amplitude was measured as 12 µV (range 1.9 to 25 µV). The same investigator reported a third study evaluating orthodromic nerve conduction of 23 normal men and calculated conduction velocities with 0-, 1-, and 2-pound weights for traction. Results for nerve conduction varied based upon measured penile length, and the need for standardization of penile length measurement was emphasized.[193] A study of subjects with diabetes described normal values for penile nerve conduction velocity by calculation of the bulbocavernosus reflex latency difference divided by the distance between stimulation sites. Normal conduction velocity to curve onset was 45 m/s ± 6 m/s; to curve peak, 34 m/s ± 4 m/s.[162]

The dorsal nerve can be stimulated and recorded orthodromically using a simple orthoplast traction device. Normal values from 20 subjects were 36.2 m/s ± 3.2 m/s (1 SD) and 2.29 µV ± 1.08 µV (1 SD).[63] Nerve conduction has been compared in the flaccid, stretched, and erect penis. The calculated conduction velocity varies with the different measured distances obtained for dorsal nerve length.[349] In our own laboratory we use an antidromic technique of dorsal nerve stimulation at the penile base and record with a disk electrode placed over the distal penile shaft just proximal to the glans, referenced to a disk over the glans. The penis is stretched taut to measure dorsal nerve length. This technique generates larger amplitude potentials, is not painful, and is easily performed. Since the dorsal nerves are paired structures, electrodes are applied separately to each side of the penis, and separate responses are easily obtained from the right and left nerves. (Normal values from nine subjects were as follows: Nerve conduction velocity to curve onset: 49.9 ± 4.2 m/s right side and 47.7 ± 6.5 m/s left side. Amplitude: 6.4 ± 2.93 µV right side and 6.03 ± 3.59 µV left side.) There have been no published studies evaluating peripheral nerve conduction of the clitoral nerve in women.

## Pudendal Nerve Conduction (Pudendal Nerve Terminal Motor Latency)

The pudendal nerve supplies motor axons to the striated urinary sphincter.[160,308] It can be stimulated at the ischial spine, and the response can be recorded from the striated sphincter muscle by using a Foley catheter–mounted electrode within the urethra or from the anal sphincter. The nerve is stimulated transrectally by the St. Mark's electrode, a disposable electrode printed on a flexible circuitboard that adheres to an examining glove.[266] Normal values for distal latency in women, the "perineal nerve terminal motor latency," have been determined as 2.4 m/s ± 0.2 (1 SD).[296–298] The distance from the site of stimulation to the recording electrode cannot be directly measured, the recording and reference electrodes lie near each other on the Foley catheter and may both be active, and normal values for amplitude have not been reported. If one is familiar with pelvic anatomy, the procedure is not difficult to perform and is usually well tolerated by the patient.

## Needle Electromyography

Needle electromyography (EMG) of the striated urethral sphincter and of pelvic floor muscles complements pudendal nerve conduction testing, and provides information about muscle denervation or reinnervation after axonal injury. EMG quantitative information can be useful for establishing a neurogenic or myogenic basis for disease and for determining the timing, degree (axonal or demyelinating), and anatomic distribution of peripheral nerve injury. Since normal urethral sphincter motor unit potentials (MUPs) are of shorter duration than those observed in extremity muscles, a myopathy may be more difficult to discern than a neuropathy. As with the examination of extremity muscles, a qualitative examination is often sufficient. However, quantitative MUP duration is a more precise value that can be used to follow the course of disease.[52] Prolonged EMG recordings have been performed without complication from thin intramuscular wire electrodes placed in the pubococcygeus muscle of women with stress incontinence.[72] Advantages over surface electrode recording include the ability to record from muscles that are inaccessible to surface electrodes and the increased anatomic precision of recording. The potential exists to perform multichannel simultaneous recordings from several muscles in conjunction with the urodynamic evaluation.[72]

Several techniques have been used for needle placement. Men lie in the lateral decubitus position and a needle is introduced at the midline perineum with the needle tip directed at the prostate apex and guided by a finger in the rectum. Women lie supine with legs abducted and the needle is inserted 1 cm lateral to the urethral meatus.[120] In men a transrectal approach using a specially designed concentric needle passed through a transrectal ultrasound probe allows precise localization within the striated sphincter and has been described as less uncomfortable than other methods.[144] A transvaginal approach in women appears to be well tolerated.[197] Topical placement of anesthetic cream containing 2.5% lidocaine and 2.5% prilocaine over the vaginal or perineal mucosa reduces discomfort during the examination.[238] It has been suggested that placement of a Foley catheter prior to needle placement facilitates examination of the sphincter at rest and defines the urethral axis.[238] Normal values for urethral and pubococcygeal MUP duration are well described, but determinations have not been carefully age-stratified, and technical information, such as filter settings, is sometimes lacking.[1,7,94,95,196,238] Normal values for the bulbocavernosus muscle are described in a single report.[109] The urethral sphincter diminishes in size with age, and in older individuals it may be difficult to localize for EMG testing.[234,235]

Single-fiber EMG (SFEMG) is a needle EMG technique used for recording action potentials from single muscle fibers within a motor unit. Fiber density is the average number of synchronously firing MUPs in the vicinity of the single-fiber needle recording surface.[302] SFEMG fiber density measurements of the pubococcygeus, puborectalis, and external anal sphincter muscles have been reported for evaluation of urinary incontinence, and age-stratified normal values have been described.[13,208,225,293,296,299] Increased fiber density has been assumed to reflect reinnervation from collateral nerve terminal sprouting.[13,208,225,293,296,299] However, none of the control patients have undergone simultaneous routine needle EMG testing. Since increased fiber density can also be present with myopathies and can reflect selective muscle fiber type of atrophy and shrinkage in the vicinity of the recording electrode, other causes of increased fiber density need to be considered.[302]

EMG recordings of cavernous smooth muscle have been recorded from needle electrodes inserted into the cavernous bodies at the midpenile site and have been compared to simultaneous surface recordings.[213,306,338] Needle-recorded potentials were sharper and did not always accompany surface-recorded potentials. Although changes were present in patients with erectile dysfunction, as compared to control subjects, the significance of these changes is unclear.

## Pudendal Somatosensory Evoked Potentials

Pudendal somatosensory evoked potentials (PSEPs) are easily obtained in men and women by stimulation of the dorsal penile and dorsal clitoral nerves. Assessment of central somatosensory conduction is obtained by recording averaged responses over the spine or scalp with surface electrodes. Stimuli are usually evoked electrically at an intensity below pain threshold, recorded from scalp electrodes placed at Cz' referenced to Fz or Fpz, and averaged over several trials. The elicited cortical waves have a W-shape configuration, and latency is usually reported for the onset, P1 (initial positive peak), and N1 (initial negative peak) waves.[141] PSEPs recorded over the spine have been reported, but they are of lower amplitude and can be technically difficult to obtain.[141] Absence of technique uniformity precludes direct comparison between studies, but values for neurologically normal individuals have been reported.* Several studies describe data normalized for height.[84,228,250,316] PSEPs elicited by mechanical stimulation have been evaluated in children.[249] Although PSEPs are safe and effective for evaluation of the somatosensory pathways and have been used for the evaluation of the neurologic basis of erectile dysfunction and micturition disturbances, the sensitivity and specificity of these tests has not been determined.[319] When used for the evaluation of 280 impotent men, delay or absence of the P1 latency was present in

---

*References 74, 84, 102, 139, 141, 143, 163, 228, 240, 240, 248, 250, 280, 316, 331.

36%.[248] Since 72% of those subjects with abnormal PSEPs had a history of neurologic dysfunction and 40% had associated signs on neurologic physical examination or cystometrogram, most of the abnormal results could be predicted by clinical factors.[248] PSEPs have been normal in 12 neurologically normal women with detrusor instability.[74] PSEPs were abnormal in 8% of 126 patients with a variety of urogenital complaints; however, all but one had clinical evidence of neurologic disease.[77] In the absence of a neurologic clinical or physical examination abnormality, the likelihood of establishment by PSEP of a neurologic basis for urogenital dysfunction was thought to be small.[77]

Unlike SSEPs elicited over extremity nerves, all pudendal studies report PSEPs to simultaneous bilateral clitoral or dorsal nerve stimulation, and this could contribute to decreased test sensitivity.[77] It is possible to obtain PSEP responses to unilateral stimulation, and the unilaterality of stimulation can be confirmed in men by simultaneously recording the peripheral dorsal nerve response while separately stimulating the right and left dorsal nerves (personal observation).

## Bladder and Posterior Urethral Evoked Potentials

Bladder evoked responses have been recorded over the scalp from stimulation of the bladder with needle bipolar electrodes inserted through a cystoscope into the dorsal bladder wall just above the trigone and to stimulation from monopolar needle electrodes inserted in the bladder wall referenced to the thigh.[21,22,79] The bipolar stimulation technique evokes a scalp vertex negative wave with a peak latency of approximately 100 ms.[79] Use of monopolar stimulation evokes additional waves, which may reflect simultaneous stimulation of anatomic structures outside the bladder.[21,22,79] Values have been reported from a small number of normal individuals and from patients with neurogenic micturition disorders.

Cortical responses have also been obtained to urethral stimulation.[22,125,142,143,278,280] Responses are recorded from the scalp to bipolar stimulation from catheter-mounted ring electrodes within the urethra. Monopolar stimulation evokes additional waves, which may reflect stimulation of other anatomic structures, as described for bladder stimulation. Stimulation from the posterior urethra and the distal urethra evoke different waveforms, which may reflect excitation of different nerve fiber populations.[278] The peak latencies and wave shapes vary among individuals, and stimulation of the vesicourethral junction may elicit a sensation of burning or a desire to void.[125,142] The configuration of the evoked response is related to the intensity of stimulus strength and to the state of bladder filling.[142]

Unlike somatosensory evoked responses, these tests have the potential to provide information about visceral afferent nerves. However, they are not easily performed, and their clinical usefulness has not been established.

## Sacral Reflexes

Electrical or mechanical stimulation of genital and perineal structures evokes reflex muscular contraction of pelvic floor and sphincter muscles. The bulbocavernosus reflex, urethroanal reflex, bladder (vesicoanal) anal reflex, and cutaneoanal reflex are electrodiagnostically measurable responses.

The bulbocavernosus reflex (BCR) is a sacral segmental response obtained by electrical stimulation of the penile dorsal nerve or the clitoral nerve and recorded from needle electrodes placed in the bulbocavernosus muscle.[256] Unilateral simulation evokes a bilateral response that is felt to reflect crossed spinal cord pathways.[256] The response may have several components, and single motor neuron studies suggest that the early component is generated through a sacral spinal cord oligosynaptic pathway.[334] Suprasegmental modulation is demonstrated by complete reflex suppression during voiding.[289] Reflex suppression may be absent in the presence of upper motor neuron lesions.[289] In a study of 33 patients with upper motor neuron lesions, all experienced loss of normal BCR inhibition during voiding, 39% had detrusor–external sphincter dyssynergia (none with a purely cerebral lesion), and 61% had uninhibited bladder contractions, suggesting that loss of BCR inhibition may be a more sensitive indicator of upper motor neuron micturition dysfunction than these other measures.[289] The reflex latency is the only parameter reported in most studies, but this measure lacks sensitivity for assessment of axonal nerve injuries.[333] The response can be recorded from several sites, including the anal sphincter and urethra, and is usually obtainable in healthy men when sufficiently strong stimuli are used but is not always obtainable in healthy women.[331,332] The BCR can be reliably obtained intraoperatively without habituation from adults and children receiving general anesthesia.[76]

The BCR has been reported for the evaluation of patients with sacral spinal cord disease and has been widely studied for evaluation of erectile dysfunction, with well-described normal values.* Evaluation of 73 patients with sacral spinal cord lesions, taken from a group of 299 patients prospectively evaluated with urodynamic testing, revealed absence of the BCR by both clinical and EMG testing in all patients with complete lesions.[41] Of patients with incomplete lesions, 44% had an intact BCR clinically, and 78% electrodiagnostically. Of the 99 patients with lesions of the suprasacral spinal cord, 90% had an intact clinical BCR, and 93% electrodiagnostically. Of the 127 patients who clinically were neurologically normal, 98% of males and 81% of females had a normal BCR clinically. Although a normal BCR does not exclude a clinically significant lesion, absence of the BCR in a male is indicative of, and in a female suggestive of, sacral spinal cord disease.[41]

The diagnostic usefulness and validity of the BCR for the evaluation of impotence has been questioned.[83,153,188] Evaluation of the BCR in 18 patients with diabetes and neurogenic erectile dysfunction was compared to that in 15 diabetic patients with psychogenic erectile dysfunction.[83] The sensitivity of the pudendoanal and pudendourethral latency (onset value) responses was 27.8%, and the specificity was 100%.[83] In a study of 90 patients evaluated for impotence, 19 had prolonged or absent BCR latencies; of these 19 patients, 8 had normal nocturnal erections by NPT testing.[188] Another study,[153] which evaluated 268 patients seen for impotence, revealed a trend toward increased BCR latency with

---

*References 18, 36, 65, 83, 86, 106, 124, 143, 173, 184, 216, 230, 231, 250, 279, 316, 325, 336.

age and a greater proportion of abnormal BCR latency studies in men with diabetes.[153] However, the proportion of men with abnormal BCR tests was not different in men with and without impotence, and no significant correlation between BCR latency and impotence was present in the diabetic group.[153]

The urethroanal reflex (UAR) measures the reflex muscular contraction of the anal striated sphincter to stimulation of the urethra. Urethral stimulation is accomplished from catheter ring electrodes placed within the proximal urethra and recorded from surface or needle anal sphincter electrodes.* It has been suggested that the latency, which is in the 60- to 80-ms range and is longer than the BCR, reflects conduction through slower conducting autonomic fibers, but it is also possible that this response subserves a different reflex arc.[132,279] Stimulation of the bladder mucosa from electrodes placed through a cystoscope elicits an anal sphincter striated muscle contraction with a latency similar to that of the UAR.[205,265] The response is reproducible, but it has been studied in only a small number of patients.[205,265] Although these tests have been used for evaluation of patients with erectile dysfunction and disturbed micturition, their diagnostic usefulness is unclear.[28,29,82,113,180,241,265]

The cutaneoanal reflex (CAR) can be elicited by pinprick or by electrical stimulation of the perianal skin; it can be visually observed, palpated from a finger within the anal sphincter, or recorded from bipolar or concentric needle electrodes in the anal sphincter.[25,149,245,246,316,335] The latency decreases with increasing stimulus intensity and is recordable simultaneously from the right and left anal sphincter to unilateral stimulation.[245] The latency changes in patients with leg spasticity and can be absent after sacral nerve blockade or in cauda equina syndrome.[245] Several response components have been observed. The first two (early components) are thought to represent direct stimulation since they are unaffected by epidural anesthesia.[25] Later components have a wide range of latencies of approximately 30 to 60 ms, consistent with oligosynaptic or polysynaptic spinal reflexes.[246,311,335] This test is well described, but its clinical usefulness has not yet been determined.

## Sympathetic Skin Response

The sympathetic skin response (SSR) is the electrodermal activity evoked from the sweat glands and adjacent epidermal and dermal tissues; it can be elicited by electrical stimulation of peripheral skin afferents and recorded with skin surface electrodes.[284] This response has been recorded from the peripheral skin and from the genital region of individuals with erectile dysfunction, ejaculatory dysfunction, and neurologic disorders.[84,103,104,187,192,350,352,354] It can be elicited by both genital and extremity stimulation.[104,352] The activity recorded from extremity surface electrodes has been compared to the spontaneous electrical activity recorded from needle electrodes within corpus cavernosum smooth muscle.[350] Electrical stimulation and deep breathing have elicited simultaneous responses from both areas; however, spontaneous electrical activity recorded from intracavernous needle electrodes has not been associated with ex-

tremity skin responses, suggesting that two different types of activity exist that may originate from separate electrical generators.[350] The SSR was absent over the genital skin in 47% of 49 patients with diabetes and erectile dysfunction, absent over extremity skin to peripheral stimulation in 53% of another series of 30 men with erectile dysfunction, and absent in one of five patients with traumatic cauda equina lesions and detrusor areflexia with bladder neck incompetence.[192] The SSR was recordable in 100% of 60 normal subjects with a coefficient of variance for repeated tests of 10%.[84] In a series of 20 patients diagnosed with neurogenic erectile dysfunction, the sensitivity of the SSR was 45%, compared to 70% for BCR and 60% for pudendal SSEP.[84] This test is intriguing because it directly measures genital autonomic function; however, it has been evaluated in only a small number of patients with micturition or sexual dysfunction.

## Cranial and Spinal Stimulation

The EMG response of the urethral sphincter, bulbocavernosus muscle, external anal sphincter, and other perineal musculature can be recorded to electrical and magnetic transcutaneous stimulation of the brain and spinal cord.

Electrical stimulation is performed with a special high-voltage stimulator placed over the cortex and at the L1 and L4 levels with responses recorded from surface or intramuscular needle electrodes.[105,313,320] Stimulation-evoked bursts of activity in multiple muscle groups can be confusing unless electrodes are used that allow precise muscle sampling. During micturition, an increase in the motor evoked response latency or EMG silence has been observed.[320] This technique has been used to calculate motor conduction in the cauda equina by examining the latency ratio of conduction time from stimulation at L1 and L4 vertebral levels to the anal sphincter and puborectalis muscles.[313] Prolonged cauda equina conduction time has been described in patients with spinal stenosis, tumor, arachnoiditis, and trauma to the cauda equina, and prolonged central conduction time has been recorded in patients with multiple sclerosis.[208,313,314] Cauda equina conduction time was normal in 12 patients with genuine stress incontinence without described neurologic disease.[296]

Magnetic stimulation can also be performed transcutaneously over the scalp and spine.[94,105,130,131,247] Voluntary contraction of the anal sphincter shortens response latency, increases response amplitude, and decreases threshold to stimulation.[93,105] This technique has been limited by uncertainty regarding the precise site of neural stimulation, by the volume conduction from surface electrode–recorded adjacent muscles, and by the ability to position the coil to optimally stimulate the areas of interest in the medial brain cortex.[93] Central conduction time can be calculated from the difference of latencies to transcranial and lumbar stimulation.[129] Small numbers of normal subjects have been studied by recording from different muscles.[129,130,247] Magnetic stimulation has also been used to evaluate patients with multiple sclerosis and disturbances of micturition and sexual function, patients with tropical spastic paraplegia and urinary symptoms, and female patients with idiopathic detrusor instability.[74,92,94,132] At present, this remains a promising but investigational technique.

---

*References 1, 24, 29, 45, 82, 83, 113, 124, 180, 264, 279, 325.

# DIAGNOSIS OF SPECIFIC NEUROLOGIC DISEASES

## STROKE

The complexities of continence, which include awareness, control, mobility, and dexterity, are vulnerable to the direct and indirect effects of cerebrovascular disease.[68] The incidence of poststroke urinary incontinence ranges from 57% to 83% in the early stages and gradually subsides over the following year.[54] In a series of 135 stroke patients, 51% were acutely incontinent.[50] In 41% the urinary incontinence had cleared by 2 weeks, and at 1 year only 15% of the survivors were incontinent.[50] Since both stroke and incontinence are common in the elderly, it is likely that stroke will occur in some previously incontinent patients.[50] In a prospective study of 151 stroke patients, 17% had preexisting urinary incontinence.[44] Mechanisms of urinary incontinence include disruption of micturition pathways, stroke-related cognitive dysfunction and language deficits, concurrent neuropathy, and medication effects.[127] The effect of a stroke on micturition depends on the degree, size, and location of the lesion.[17] Urinary retention may be present initially, and over time symptoms of urgency, frequency, dysuria, and incontinence can appear.[17,322]

Urodynamic testing after stroke reveals a variable pattern. A study of 33 stroke patients at differing times after their stroke showed involuntary detrusor muscle contractions in 26 patients.[175] The majority of those with internal capsule or cortical lesions had uninhibited sphincter relaxation with bladder contraction; however, those with lesions confined to the thalamus or basal ganglia had normal sphincter function.[175] Cystometry of 39 patients examined at a mean of 19 months after stroke revealed bladder hyperactivity in 10 of 11 patients with frontal lobe or internal capsule lesions of whom 6 had uninhibited sphincter relaxation.[322] Although 8 of 11 patients with putamenal lesions experienced bladder hyperactivity, none showed uninhibited sphincter relaxation.[322] Incomplete bladder emptying was evaluated through measurement of postvoid residual (PVR) urine volume in 85 stroke patients admitted to a rehabilitation center.[126] Incomplete bladder emptying was initially present in 48 patients, was sustained in 28 patients, and was associated with a significantly higher rate of urinary tract infections.[126] In general, larger-sized infarctions, regardless of hemispheral location on computed tomography (CT) scan, have been associated with abnormal bladder cystometrograms, and the pattern of abnormality has been variable, including both areflexia and hyperreflexia.[20,110,172] The pattern of urodynamic findings may reflect timing after the stroke or the presence of concurrent conditions. Urinary incontinence is a common feature of multiinfarction dementia (MID) and is often present early in the course.[182,268] In a series of 84 outpatients with MID, urinary abnormalities were present in 66% of men and 30% of women, often prior to the diagnosis of MID or a documented stroke.[182]

Stroke may interfere with sexual activity through direct injury of neural structures important to sexual function and through paralysis, sensory loss, spasticity, communication difficulty, personality change, and depression, which interfere with the formation and maintenance of interpersonal relationships.[223] The frequency and duration of sexual intercourse is reduced in men and women after stroke, but occasionally stroke results in an increase in sexual interest and activity.[215,292] The most common problem encountered by men is difficulty with erection and ejaculation; women with hemiplegic strokes report problems with vaginal lubrication and orgasm.[214] The prevalence of major sexual dysfunction in a study of 26 men with unilateral stroke was greater after right-hemisphere stroke (9 of 12 subjects) than after left-hemisphere stroke (4 of 14 subjects), consistent with a hypothesis that the right hemisphere is dominant for activation and that this capacity is important for normal sexual function.[66]

## DEMENTIA

Brain positron emission tomography (PET) has demonstrated decreased anterior cingulate gyrus blood flow during withholding of urine and increased blood flow in the right dorsomedial pontine tegmentum, periaqueductal gray matter, hypothalamus, and right inferior frontal gyrus during micturition, favoring a specific role for these brain regions in micturition control.[42] Disturbances of micturition can occur with lesions of the anteromedial frontal lobe that include the genu of the corpus callosum and the anterior part of the cingulate gyrus.[14] Although lesions of these areas may cause general indifference, symptoms of bladder dysfunction may be present in patients who are socially aware and not demented.[14,155]

The presence of periventricular high-signal and subcortical white-matter lesions in patients with Alzheimer's disease, selected for absence of risk factors for cerebrovascular disease, is associated with an increased frequency of urinary incontinence.[31] Urinary incontinence is a frequent accompaniment of Alzheimer's disease, vascular dementia, and Binswanger's disease, and it may be an earlier feature of vascular dementia than of Alzheimer's disease.[267,268,318] Although low-volume urinary incontinence has been described, careful clinical and urodynamic studies are lacking.[90] A longitudinal prospective study of patients with confirmed diagnoses at autopsy demonstrated a significantly earlier onset of incontinence in patients with diffuse Lewy body disease as compared to patients with Alzheimer's disease.[78] Early symptoms of micturition dysfunction in normal pressure hydrocephalus (NPH) consist of urgency and frequency, which later may advance to urge incontinence.[114,158] Cystometrograms demonstrate involuntary bladder contractions at low volumes.[114,158] Bladder hyperactivity on cystometrogram can be temporarily improved after lumbar puncture and can be abolished by shunt placement.[4] Rarely, a patient with hydrocephalus due to aqueductal obstruction may present with chronic bladder and bowel incontinence and improve after shunting, in the absence of any clinical symptoms or neurologic signs.[329] Sexual disinhibition has been described in 7% of 178 patients diagnosed with Alzheimer's disease.[55] There is little published information on sexual dysfunction in patients with Alzheimer's disease.

## PARKINSONISM

Urinary incontinence can complicate the care of patients with Parkinson's disease, multiple system atrophy (MSA), and Shy-Drager syndrome. The incidence ranges from 37% to 71% of patients diagnosed with Parkinson's disease.[243] The majority of patients with Parkinson's disease and micturition dysfunction describe frequency, urgency, and urge incontinence (57% to 83%), and the remainder describe hesitancy, decreased force of stream, retention, or a combination of irritative and obstructive symptoms.[33,243]

Urodynamic findings in separate studies of 30 subjects and 29 subjects revealed detrusor hyperreflexia in 75% of patients and in 83% of those undergoing cystometrograms.[33,243] Sporadic involuntary activity of the external sphincter during involuntary detrusor contractions was present in 61% of subjects in the former series but in only 18% of those in the latter series.[33,243] In the latter group, detrusor hyperreflexia with sphincter relaxation was the most common pattern.[243] Involuntary sphincter activity could represent pseudodyssynergia, a voluntary contraction in an attempt to prevent urine leakage, or a manifestation of increased striated muscle tone in Parkinson's disease.[243] The risk of incontinence was increased after transurethral prostatectomy if voluntary sphincter control was absent during preoperative urodynamic evaluation (incontinence present in 5 of 6 patients without preoperative voluntary control compared to 1 of 24 patients with voluntary control).[304] Urodynamic studies obtained on 10 patients with long-standing Parkinson's disease before levodopa therapy and several hours after stopping levodopa treatment revealed both improvement and worsening of bladder hyperreflexia.[115] A difference was present after medication stoppage, but the changes were not predictable.[115] Although stress incontinence is the most common cause of micturition dysfunction in women, urodynamic evaluation of 17 women with Parkinson's disease revealed 70.6% with detrusor instability.[174] Of 8 patients with stress incontinence, 3 had detrusor instability, 3 had a hyporeflexic bladder, and 2 had stable bladders.[174] Sexual dysfunction in 41 married men with Parkinson's disease was compared to sexual activity in 29 married men with arthritis. Although sexual dysfunction was common in both groups, no significant difference in sexual dysfunction was noted between them, suggesting a possible role for the comorbid effects of age, disease severity, and depression.[195]

In a study of 100 patients with MSA, 71% experienced urinary incontinence with symptoms of urgency, urge incontinence, hesitancy, retention, double micturition, nocturia, and persistent daytime frequency; 90% of the men experienced erectile dysfunction, and 2 women described anorgasmia.[343] Erectile dysfunction may be the earliest symptom; it was the first symptom alone in 37% of a series of 62 patients with this condition.[27] Urodynamic findings in patients with MSA and Parkinson's disease are similar, with bladder hyperreflexia noted in conjunction with vesicosphincteric synergy and incomplete pelvic floor relaxation.[307] However, urodynamic abnormalities in Parkinson's disease correlated with overall disease duration and severity, but, in patients with MSA urodynamic abnormalities could be prominent early in the illness and did not correlate with disease severity or duration.[307] Urethral and anal sphincter EMG, with individual motor unit analysis, reveals abnormalities consistent with denervation and chronic reinnervation in patients with MSA but not in patients with Parkinson's disease. Studies report abnormal sphincter EMG findings in 75% to 100% of patients with MSA and only rarely in patients with Parkinson's disease; the BCR latency is normal in both diseases.[27,95,115,172,251,307] This could reflect selective degeneration of anterior horn cells within Onuf's nucleus of the sacral spinal cord.[177,251] In a series of 54 patients presenting with parkinsonism, urethral sphincter EMG was abnormal in 16 of 26 patients with probable MSA, 5 of 15 with possible MSA, and in only 1 of 13 with idiopathic Parkinson's disease, suggesting that EMG is a useful diagnostic test for distinguishing between these diseases.[95]

Clinical features may also be helpful. In a study of 52 patients with probable MSA and 41 with idiopathic Parkinson's disease, 94% of the patients with Parkinson's disease carried their neurologic diagnosis prior to the onset of urogenital symptoms, but 60% of the patients with MSA had urinary symptoms preceding their diagnosis.[62] Most of the patients with MSA (73%) experienced urinary incontinence, and 85% of the patients with idiopathic Parkinson's disease had urgency or frequency but were not incontinent. A significant postvoid residual volume was present in 66% of patients with MSA and in 16% of patients with idiopathic Parkinson's disease. All patients with MSA who underwent transurethral resection of the prostate were incontinent postoperatively.[62]

Urodynamic and sphincter EMG testing of 9 patients with the clinical diagnosis of Shy-Drager syndrome revealed detrusor areflexia in 6 patients, detrusor hyperreflexia in 3, findings consistent with denervation and reinnervation of the urethral striated sphincter in all 9, and an open bladder neck in 5 patients who underwent voiding cystourethrography.[276] Similar findings have been described in other clinical case reports.[344]

A report of 9 patients with progressive supranuclear palsy described urinary incontinence in 8 patients, increased postvoid residual urine in 3 of 6 patients evaluated (4 with detrusor hyperreflexia, 1 with a low compliance cystometrogram, and 1 with detrusor sphincter dyssynergia), and neurogenic changes on external urethral sphincter EMG in 2 of 4 patients.[275]

## MULTIPLE SCLEROSIS

Micturition dysfunction occurs in 50% to 80% of patients with multiple sclerosis (MS) at some point during their illness.[15] Common symptoms include urgency, urge incontinence, urinary frequency, hesitancy, voiding of small volumes with a staccato pattern, and a sense of incomplete bladder emptying.[15] Detrusor hyperreflexia is the most common abnormal urodynamic voiding pattern.[39,133] Other urodynamic abnormalities include detrusor sphincter dyssynergia, detrusor hypocontractility, detrusor areflexia, and vesicoureteral reflux.[10,12,38,39,133,134,210] Voiding symptoms alone do not correlate well with the findings on urodynamic evaluation.[39,133,134]

In a series of 41 patients with MS evaluated with cystometrograms, only 63% with symptoms of urgency, frequency, and urge incontinence had uninhibited bladder contractions, and 73% with obstructive symptoms had detrusor areflexia.[39] The presence of detrusor external sphincter dyssynergia in a selected series of 18 men was correlated with an increased risk of urosepsis, vesicoureteral reflux, and urolithiasis (observed in 50% of these patients).[38] The urodynamic findings of patients with MS can change over time.[39] Repeated urodynamic testing of 10 men and 18 women revealed new changes in 55%.[39] Development of detrusor sphincter dyssynergia was the predominant pattern on reevaluation, but those with this pattern at initial evaluation maintained it, suggesting that detrusor sphincter dyssynergia may be a urodynamic indicator of progression of disease.[345] Disease duration correlates with the presence of urinary symptoms, and a positive clinical correlation has been described between pyramidal dysfunction on the Kurtzke neurologic assessment and detrusor hyperreflexia or areflexia, and between cerebellar dysfunction and detrusor areflexia.[19] In a study of 149 patients with MS who had vesicourethral dysfunction evaluated urodynamically, low maximal urethral pressure in women was associated with incontinence (69% of these patients).[123] Pyelonephritis was more common in males and was associated with a postvoid residual urine volume of >30% of functional detrusor capacity.[123] A retrospective review of 90 patients with MS who had voiding complaints and underwent cranial MRI and urodyamic evaluations revealed no correlation between cranial magnetic resonance imaging (MRI) and urodynamic abnormalities.[176]

Urodynamic abnormalities can be present in the absence of symptoms of micturition dysfunction and were present in 52% of a series of 27 patients with MS who were without symptoms.[28] Evaluation of 24 patients with MS who had urinary symptoms and underwent neurophysiologic testing revealed prolongation or absence of the motor response to cortical magnetic stimulation in 7 of 10 studied patients, prolongation of the cortical motor response in 2 of 4 patients undergoing spinal magnetic stimulation, an increased number of polyphasic MUPs in 22 patients undergoing urethral sphincter EMG, absence or prolongation of the PSEP P1 response in 88% of patients, and no significant difference on sacral reflex latency testing compared to a control group.[94] Urodynamic abnormalities were noted in 83% of patients with abnormal PSEP studies, and abnormal motor conduction times were related to functional motor disability.[94] The 6 patients in this study with urinary symptoms in the absence of urodynamic abnormalities had no neurophysiologic study abnormalities. Other studies have been performed that have demonstrated abnormal sacral reflex latency or PSEP results in patients with MS.[133,141,316] Although the presence of abnormality on electrodiagnostic electrophysiologic tests corroborates the clinical impression of neurologic micturition dysfunction and further characterizes the dysfunction, it is unclear whether these studies provide additional diagnostic information.

Sexual dysfunction is common in patients with MS. In a series of 65 women and 36 men, 78% of men and 45% of women experienced sexual dysfunction, which was associated with urinary problems and with a history of depression. Men experienced erectile dysfunction, women noticed abnormal vaginal lubrication, and both groups experienced problems with decreased sensation and achieving orgasm.[209] A study of 41 men with MS who had erectile dysfunction demonstrated a relationship between the presence of impotence and bladder dysfunction, with impotence usually appearing after the onset of bladder dysfunction.[35] None of the men presented with impotence alone as an initial symptom of MS, and only a small percentage spontaneously recovered erectile function. All the men with clinical erectile dysfunction had marked leg pyramidal findings and on cystometry had bladder hyperreflexia.[35] Recording the PSEP provided no more information than did the tibial SSEP.[35] Another study evaluating 29 men with MS and erectile dysfunction revealed normal penile arterial inflow and venous outflow by PBI and infusion caversonometry.[35] The PSEP was abnormal

in 26 patients, and 8 of these patients had an abnormal BCR.[262] A group of 6 patients with MS without erectile dysfunction revealed normal electrodiagnostic test results.[35] Nocturnal erectile activity, measured by nocturnal penile tumescence and rigidity (NPTR) recordings, was normal in 11 patients, of whom 9 had abnormal PSEP or BCR studies.[178] A study of NPTR, PSEPs, motor evoked potentials, and BCRs of 34 men with definite or possible MS revealed delayed responses in 26, 20, and 3, respectively.[131] However, no relationship was found between the abnormalities and the severity of erectile dysfunction (abnormal PSEP studies were present in 5 of 6 patients with MS without erectile dysfunction), all the patients with BCR abnormalities had other neurophysiologic test abnormalities, and NPTR was normal in 10 of 14 patients, including 3 with severe paraplegia.[131]

## SPINAL CORD DISEASE

Micturition and sexual dysfunction can result from congenital and acquired myelopathies. An acontractile bladder is generally present initially after a traumatic suprasacral spinal cord injury and later gradually evolves to a hyperreflexic bladder, which may be accompanied by sphincter dyssynergia.[346] Disease at or below the sacral level usually results in bladder areflexia.[164] However, this correlation is not absolute or specific. In a series of 489 patients with spinal cord disease undergoing clinical and videourodynamic evaluation, 20 of 117 patients with cervical cord lesions had detrusor areflexia, 42 of 156 with lumbar cord lesions had detrusor external sphincter dyssynergia, and 26 of 84 with sacral cord lesions had either detrusor hyperreflexia or detrusor external sphincter dyssynergia.[164] The positive predictive value of positive sacral cord signs on clinical examination and detrusor areflexia was 87%, and the positive predictive value of negative sacral cord signs and detrusor hyperreflexia or detrusor external sphincter dyssynergia was 81%.[164] An evaluation of 70 patients with incomplete spinal cord and cauda equina lesions revealed 14% with clinically silent bladder and sphincter dysfunction.[140] Symptoms such as urgency, incontinence, and nocturnal incontinence were associated with detrusor hyperactivity, and urinary retention was associated with urethral overactivity and dyssynergia.[140] Of 44 consecutive patients evaluated clinically and by videourodynamic testing within 72 hours of thoracolumbar vertebral fracture, lower urinary tract dysfunction was present in 41% of clinically neurologically normal patients, and 62% with intact pinprick sensation and 59% with intact BCR had lower urinary tract dysfunction.[341] These studies suggest that urodynamic testing of patients with spinal cord injury is necessary to provide a precise diagnosis.[140,164,341]

Sacral electrodiagnostic reflex latency measurements were correlated with serial videourodynamic studies of 20 patients with complete acute suprasacral spinal cord lesions.[198] Reproducibility of sacral reflex latencies was poor (mean variation from initial measurements of 21%); reflex latencies were normal in 84% to 93% of recordings, and they did not correlate with urodynamic findings.[198] A comparison of BCR and UAR latency with detrusor function on urodynamic study was performed on 73 patients with chronic cervical and thoracic spinal cord injuries.[180] The BCR was abnormal in 47%, and urodynamic evaluation showed bladder hyperreflexia in 84% of patients, of whom 75% had associated detrusor-sphincter dyssynergia.[180] A correlation was present between BCR and UAR with detrusor hyperreflexia.[180] A normal sacral reflex latency was often present with detrusor hyperreflexia, and an unobtainable reflex was present in patients with detrusor hyporeflexia.[180] A correlation was also noted between the presence of reflex penile erections (present in 77%) and the presence of the BCR or detrusor hyperreflexia.[180] PSEPs and urethrovesical junction evoked potentials have been evaluated in small numbers of patients and may be absent, but their diagnostic usefulness is unclear.[69,125,141]

After trauma to the spinal cord and cauda equina, erectile and ejaculatory function are lost during the period of spinal shock, with gradual recovery of function over the following year.[30,295] Approximately 54% to 82% of affected patients regain erectile function (reflexogenic and psychogenic), and 3% to 15% regain ejaculatory function.[30] Those with lower motor neuron lesions are less likely to achieve erections than those with upper motor neuron lesions.[295]

In a group of 30 consecutive patients with symptoms of radiculopathy or myelopathy and spinal cord compression by myelography, cervical spondylosis with spinal stenosis was associated with symptoms of frequency, urgency, and urge incontinence in 61% of patients.[317] Urodynamic testing revealed detrusor hyperreflexia in 46%, but detrusor hypotonia was present in 11%. Tibial SSEP abnormalities were more prominent in patients with clinically more severe myelopathy but did not correlate with the presence of detrusor hyperactivity.

Myelodysplasia is the most common cause of neuropathic bladder in children, occurring in 1 in 1000 births, and urodynamic studies are performed as part of the routine evaluation of these children.[287] Urodynamic evaluation has revealed detrusor hyperreflexia in 62% and detrusor areflexia in 38%.[342] It has been determined that bladder leak pressure (the detrusor pressure at which urinary leakage occurs) >40 cm $H_2O$ and detrusor sphincter dyssynergia are strong risk factors for upper urinary tract deterioration from complications of vesicoureteral reflux.[287] The neurophysiologic evaluation of 51 patients with thoracolumbar myelodysplasia revealed a variable pattern of upper and lower motor neuron involvement, with imprecise correlation between clinical and neurophysiologic findings.[327] Of 36 patients with clinical signs suggesting a complete lower motor neuron lesion, only 64% had complete lower motor neuron lesions noted by using a combination of tests, including BCR, CAR, and Valsalva reflexes, pelvic floor EMG, and urodynamic studies. Of 14 patients with a clinically mixed pattern of upper and lower motor neuron dysfunction, 50% had upper motor neuron abnormalities only, and 28% had lower motor neuron abnormalities only on urodynamic and neurophysiologic studies.[327] The pattern of abnormality changes over time and may include improvement of external urethral sphincter innervation or evidence of further denervation.[301] Detrusor sphincter dyssynergy may develop, but it can also convert to a pattern of synergy.[301] Infants were found to have a 32% chance of such change in the first year, 6% in the second year, and 2% during the third year.[301] The preoperative assessment of 40 children with occult spinal lesions revealed normal urodynamic studies in 64% of infants but in only 8% of older children. Of 10 infants with abnormal studies, 8 returned to normal or improved, but only 3 of 11 older children returned to

normal, emphasizing the importance of early detection and intervention.[170]

Tethered spinal cord syndrome symptoms include difficulty with urination, incontinence, sensation of incomplete voiding, urgency, and impotence.[181] Urodynamic findings in a series of 15 adults included detrusor areflexia in 9, hyperreflexia in 1, a mixed lesion in 2, and a stable bladder in 3 patients.[181] Recognition is important because neurogenic bladder abnormalities are potentially reversible with early surgical intervention.[148,165,181]

Neurourologic abnormalities described in 6 men and 2 women with a history of transverse myelitis included detrusor sphincter dyssynergia in 6 subjects, detrusor hyperreflexia in 2, and an incompetent urinary sphincter in 1.[34] Erectile or ejaculatory dysfunction was described by 3 men.[34] The BCR was clinically absent in 2 men.[34]

Symptoms of micturition dysfunction in 6 boys and 1 girl (mean age 4 years) after spinal cord arterial ischemia included urge incontinence, stress incontinence, frequency, and retention.[26] Bladder areflexia with EMG lower motor neuron signs was present on urodynamic testing of 3 subjects, detrusor hyperreflexia with detrusor sphincter dyssynergia was present in 1, and the others had a mixed pattern.[26] Complete urinary retention was present acutely in 10 adult patients with anterior spinal artery syndrome, and it resolved by 120 days in all but 1 patient.[351] Cystometry of 3 patients during the acute stage revealed detrusor areflexia, and in 2 of 3 patients the condition later evolved to hyperreflexia. Urodynamic studies during a neurologically stable phase revealed 8 patients with detrusor hyperreflexia.[351] Detrusor sphincter dyssynergia was present in 4 patients.[351] Subjective sensation of bladder fullness, a function often lost after traumatic spinal cord injury, was present in all patients.[351] This finding is consistent with the hypothesis that at least some bladder sensation is mediated through the relatively preserved dorsal columns within the posterior third of the spinal cord.[351]

## CAUDA EQUINA SYNDROME

Injury to the cauda equina from disk herniation, trauma, and neoplasm can cause urinary incontinence.[16] Although 70% of patients with disk lesions have a history of chronic back pain, 30% of patients may present with cauda equina syndrome as an initial manifestation of lumbar disk herniation.[290] In a series of 14 patients, all had radiating back pain with signs of lower extremity weakness, and the level of herniation was L4-L5 in 3 patients, L5-S1 in 3, and L3-L4 in 2. Urinary or stool incontinence was present in 93%.[290] However, urinary retention secondary to lumbar disk herniation with cauda equina compression was described in a report of 5 women without neurologic symptoms.[101] Preexisting spinal stenosis, tethered cord, and arachnoidal adhesions may predispose to cauda equina syndrome if disk herniation occurs.[290] Reports of prognosis for recovery of micturition function are variable. In a series of 29 men and women, 18 of 29 subjects regained full control of micturition and defecation.[237] However, in another series of 30 patients, only 1 patient regained normal function.[236] This difference could reflect patient selection and timing of surgery.

Neurogenic micturition dysfunction can occur in the setting of degenerative lumbar spondylosis with spinal stenosis in the absence of disk herniation.[291] The neurologic examination may be normal, and symptoms may be limited to backache. Urinary symptoms may be intermittent and include poor stream, incontinence, retention, frequency, and frequent urinary tract infections.[291]

Urodynamic testing after disk herniation usually reveals detrusor areflexia with incomplete bladder emptying, but detrusor hyperreflexia is described in a small percentage of patients.[147,236,291] Detrusor compliance may be normal or decreased.[192]

Needle EMG of the urethral sphincter may reveal evidence of denervation or chronic reinnervation with complex repetitive discharges, fibrillation potentials, positive waves, and prolonged-duration polyphasic MUPs.[119,192,242,277] The BCR was clinically absent in 84% of patients in a series of 57 patients with varying underlying causes of cauda equina syndrome.[242] It was absent in all 13 patients with cauda equina syndrome in a series of 80 patients with neurologic bladder dysfunction or impotence.[106] The loss of the BCR acutely after traumatic cauda equina lesions was a poor prognostic sign for recovery of bladder and sexual function in a study of 40 patients with traumatic or slowly compressive lesions.[107] Slowly progressive lesions were associated with BCR delay, which could improve after surgical correction of the underlying lesion.[107] The vesicoanal reflex may be absent or delayed.[264,265] Cortical responses to stimulation of the vesicourethral junction or pudendal nerve may be absent.[125]

Sacral myeloradiculitis is associated with a cerebrospinal fluid (CSF) pleocytosis and may result in transient urinary retention. The BCR latency was normal in a report of 5 patients.[150] The PSEP P1 latency was delayed in 1 patient, and polyphasic or prolonged-duration polyphasic MUPs were present on external sphincter needle EMG study of 2 patients.[150]

## PERIPHERAL NEUROPATHY

Micturition and sexual dysfunction can be manifestations of a generalized polyneuropathy and are common complications of diabetic polyneuropathy. Although bladder dysfunction is a common complication of diabetes mellitus, the problem may remain asymptomatic until decompensation occurs.[98,226] Performance of a 3-hour oral glucose tolerance test on 58 patients with erectile dysfunction revealed 12.1% with unsuspected diabetes mellitus.[85] In a series of 70 men evaluated at a center for sexual dysfunction, 15 patients had impaired glucose intolerance or overt diabetes.[212] The prevalence of impotence in diabetic men is approximately 50%.[99]

Diabetic cystopathy is present in 43% to 87% of insulin-dependent diabetics, and the prevalence in patients with diabetic polyneuropathy is 75% to 100%.[121] Of 182 diabetic patients undergoing videourodynamic study, 55% had bladder hyperreflexia, 23% had impaired detrusor contractility, and 19% had detrusor areflexia.[167] Bladder outlet obstruction was present in 36% (all men).[167] The most common symptoms were nocturia (more than two times per night), frequency, hesitancy, decreased stream, and sensation of incomplete bladder emptying.[167] In a group of 23 elderly diabetic patients in a nursing home who presented with symptoms of urinary dysfunction, 17 patients were incontinent, and urodynamic testing revealed involuntary bladder contractions in 61%, reduced magnitude of voluntary contractions in 17%, and absence of voluntary contractions in 9%.[303] These findings could reflect coexistent neurologic conditions (e.g.,

stroke or prior spinal trauma) and emphasize the importance of urodynamic testing for the evaluation of diabetic patients with symptoms of micturition dysfunction.[303]

Electrodiagnostic studies have been described primarily for the evaluation of male erectile dysfunction. The penile dorsal nerve conduction velocity is slowed in diabetics with erectile dysfunction, as compared to nondiabetic healthy men; however, the BCR latency was not significantly different between the groups.[162,193] Of 22 patients with polyneuropathy of various causes from a series of 80 patients selected for evaluation of neurogenic bladder or erectile dysfunction, all had prolonged BCR latencies.[242] The diagnostic usefulness of the BCR latency for evaluation of erectile dysfunction has been investigated in several studies.[70,83,118,216,241,279,337] Responses in diabetic men with impotence have been compared to those of normal controls,[279] patients with psychogenic impotence,[83] and nonimpotent diabetic subjects.[70] Prolongation or absence of the response in diabetic patients with erectile dysfunction has been described, but the percentage of abnormal patients is variable, ranging from approximately 20% to 83%.[70,216] In a study of 45 men with erectile dysfunction, the sensitivity (22.2%), specificity (46.7%), and positive predictive values of a positive (33.3%) and negative (33.3%) test were low.[83] A retrospective review of 300 men revealed a trend to increasing BCR latency with age and an increased likelihood of a prolonged BCR latency in diabetic men, but no significant correlation between BCR latency and impotence.[153]

In a group of 27 diabetic men evaluated with papaverine injections, 24 had poor or absent erections, suggesting that vascular factors may play a role.[263] Several series of men with diabetic impotence have revealed small percentages with abnormal testosterone and prolactin levels.[117,168,190] Despite the high incidence of neurologic, vascular, and endocrine complications that result in impotence, psychiatric illness may be an important contributor to impotence in diabetic men.[57,97,202] In a study of 100 diabetic men and 400 nondiabetic men with erectile dysfunction who underwent polysomnography in a sleep laboratory, men with diabetes had fewer sleep-related erections, shorter tumescence time, diminished penile circumference increase, and lower penile rigidity than nondiabetic men.[283] The diabetic men had lower penile brachial blood pressure values.[152] NPT sleep laboratory polysomnographic studies of diabetic men without sexual dysfunction, as compared to healthy control subjects, have revealed diminished NPT profiles in the diabetic patients, despite descriptions of clinically satisfactory sexual function.[58,157] Therefore the finding of an NPT abnormality should not necessarily be interpreted as evidence of irreversible erectile dysfunction; NPT abnormalities should be interpreted cautiously in diabetic patients.[229,283]

Sexual dysfunction in women with diabetes includes decreased libido, slow arousal, inadequate lubrication, anorgasmia, and dyspareunia and is present at the onset of the illness in the majority of those affected.[58,157] The incidence of abnormality does not appear to differ from that of healthy controls, and it is possible that sexual dysfunction is one measure of overall psychologic coping with disease.[58,157] Studies are limited by the absence of direct clinical physiologic measures of sexual function in women.

Toxic and metabolic polyneuropathies that can cause urinary retention include pernicious anemia, hypothyroidism, alcohol-related conditions, vitamin E deficiency, and porphyria.[226] Bladder involvement can also occur in Guillain-Barré syndrome (GBS).[269] The incidence of urinary retention in the Massachusetts General Hospital retrospective GBS series was 27%, and in the prospective series it was 14%; cystometrograms of 3 patients revealed flaccid paralytic bladders.[269] A report of 3 patients with GBS and nerve root enhancement on MRI scan described urinary incontinence and retention in 2 patients, which gradually resolved at 2 to 4 weeks.[67] Both obstructive and irritative symptoms have been described in 8 patients with urinary dysfunction due to tabes dorsalis, including urinary retention, frequency, and urgency with urge incontinence.[146] Patients may have normal or increased bladder capacity at first desire to void, and detrusor sphincter dyssynergia may be present.[146]

## PELVIC PLEXOPATHY

Injury to the pelvic plexus may be a consequence of major pelvic surgery, such as abdominoperineal resection or radical hysterectomy.[51] Radical hysterectomy may be accompanied by micturition dysfunction, including prolonged postoperative urinary retention or incomplete voiding, increase in bladder volume required to elicit the urge sensation associated with lower abdominal bloating and fullness, stress incontinence, and hypertonic cystometric findings.[37] In a series of 22 patients undergoing radical hysterectomy, these features were less prominent in patients with incomplete transection of the cardinal ligaments.[37] The diminished bladder capacity with high filling pressure may reflect unopposed parasympathetic tone or an intrinsic increase in myogenic tone of the detrusor muscle secondary to perivesical dissection and the presence of an indwelling Foley catheter during surgery.[288]

Tumor invasion of the pelvic plexus with deficits of parasympathetic, sympathetic, and somatic innervation of the bladder and urethra can result in impotence and an atonic bladder, with reduced urethral sphincter pressure and incontinence.[156,347] This is usually associated with large tumor masses and should raise concern about epidural extension.[156,347] A videourodynamic study of 13 patients with urinary symptoms after abdominoperineal rectal resection revealed diminished urethral pressure suggestive of sympathetic denervation in all patients and incomplete bladder emptying in 38%.[37] Small-capacity bladders with involuntary detrusor contractions and an open bladder neck were present in 3 patients.[37] Similar abnormalities have been described after proctocolectomy and anterior resection of the rectum.[348] The presence of prior damage to the pelvic plexus, characterized by denervation and reinnervation of the pelvic floor striated muscles (e.g., pubococcygeus and striated anal sphincter) is associated with lack of improvement after the Burch colposuspension surgical procedure for treatment of female stress incontinence.[179] Removal of the cardinal ligaments or a long cuff of the upper vagina during hysterectomy may increase the likelihood of a plexus neuropathy, and the posterior pelvic plexus and parasympathetic nerves may be damaged during mobilization of the rectum during abdominoperineal resection.[221] Sexual dysfunction in a series of 221 patients undergoing abdominoperineal resection or anterior resection included erectile dysfunction in 60% and 57%, respectively, in men, and diminished vaginal lubrication, dyspareunia, and diminished orgasm in women.[111]

Up to 30% of patients undergoing prostatectomy are left with residual symptoms of frequency, nocturia, urgency, loin or perineal pain, or incontinence, and these symptoms may be difficult to explain.[211] A series of 42 neurologically normal patients had hypocontractile or acontractile bladders on urodynamic testing.[211] Seven patients had "poor compliance," and the others had normal filling cystometrograms; all but 8 patients had normal postvoiding residual urine volumes.[211] Detrusor instability was the cause of incontinence in a series of 63 men with postprostatectomy urinary incontinence (only 6 of whom had known neurologic disease) who underwent uroflowmetry, cystometrogram, videocystourethrography, cystourethroscopy, and striated urethral sphincter EMG.[173] Damage to the striated sphincter was present in only 47% of patients, and 53% had concomitant detrusor instability.[173] It has been suggested that careful dissection of the apical prostate with sparing of the striated sphincter and laterally placed neurovascular bundles may decrease the risk of postoperative micturition dysfunction.[222] The external urethral sphincter also receives innervation from nerve branches of the dorsal nerve of the penis near the prostate apex, which are susceptible to injury during surgery.[224] Prospective comparison of 10 patients who had undergone nerve-sparing radical prostatectomy for prostate carcinoma, 10 patients who had undergone radical cystoprostatectomy for bladder carcinoma, and a normal control group did not reveal any significant differences in PSEP or BCR latencies.[196] MUP duration was similarly prolonged in both surgical groups compared to the control subjects, consistent with subclinical axonal injury to nerves supplying the striated external urethral sphincter.[196] However, postoperative erectile dysfunction was present in 2 of 10 prostatectomy patients and 10 of 10 cystoprostatectomy patients.[196]

Quantitative needle EMG measurement of MUP duration was performed on 9 patients with benign prostatic hyperplasia (BPH) and on 13 patients without disturbance of micturition.[1] Although MUP duration was increased in the BPH group, this was explainable by an age difference between the groups.[1] The BCR obtained to the bulbocavernosus and striated urethral sphincter muscles in patients with BPH was not prolonged preoperatively in 47 patients; it remained normal in 30 patients who underwent repeated postoperative study.[108] In a series of 11 patients with MSA undergoing transurethral resection of the prostate (TURP), all patients failed to improve postoperatively.[62] The incidence of postoperative incontinence after TURP was significantly increased in patients with Parkinson's disease who lacked voluntary sphincter control on preoperative urodynamic testing.[304] Urinary incontinence was present in 50% of patients undergoing prostate surgery after a stroke, and a poorer result was associated with age >70 years, surgery performed less than 12 months after stroke, bilateral hemispheral involvement, and right-hemisphere stroke. The results of urodynamic testing, which revealed detrusor instability in the few patients studied, did not correlate with outcome.[201]

## PUDENDAL NEUROPATHY

Pudendal nerve conduction studies on women with stress incontinence and genitourinary prolapse reveal prolongation of the PNTML.[294,296] SFEMG studies of the pubococcygeus and anal sphincter muscles in women with genitourinary prolapse show increased fiber density consistent with neurogenic axonal injury and subsequent reinnervation.[13,293] Pubococcygeus muscle quantitative MUP duration measurement in 75 nulliparous women, performed before and after delivery, revealed prolongation of MUP duration after delivery in 80% of those studied.[7] This is consistent with reinnervation and suggests that delivery causes partial denervation of the pelvic floor muscles in women undergoing a first vaginal delivery, even in the absence of prolapse or stress incontinence.[7] Vaginal delivery in another group of 128 unselected pregnant women was associated with prolongation of the mean PNTML.[310] The presence of abnormality has been associated with prolongation of the second stage of labor, increased birth weight, multiparity, forceps delivery, and third-degree perineal tear, and it could reflect stretching of the pudendal nerve or a direct pressure effect of the fetal head on small nerve branches.[7,310] Abnormal descent of the pelvic floor was associated with prolongation of the terminal motor latencies of the pudendal and perineal nerves and with increased fiber density on SFEMG of the striated anal sphincter in a study of 40 women with idiopathic fecal incontinence, of whom 20 also had stress urinary incontinence.[297]

Kinesiologic EMG studies of the right and left pubococcygeus muscles with intramuscular wire electrodes in 8 parous women with stress urinary incontinence were compared to those of 10 nulliparous continent women, and they revealed asymmetric and uncoordinated levator muscle activation patterns.[72] In a prospective study of 24 multiparous women, followed up for 5 years and with reevaluation of 14, mean SFEMG fiber density and PNTML measurements persisted or worsened, and 5 of 14 women developed stress urinary incontinence.[300] These studies suggest that (1) denervation of pelvic floor and sphincter muscles is a feature of pelvic floor disorders, (2) it can be accompanied by stress incontinence, (3) it can be quantified and followed by nerve conduction and EMG studies, (4) it may be initiated by subclinical damage during childbirth, and (5) for unclear reasons it may progress later in life, resulting in stress urinary incontinence.[315]

Pudendal neuropathy has also been described after trauma. Penile skin insensitivity was described in two bicyclists after prolonged bicycle riding; it was associated with erectile dysfunction and resolved after 4 and 7 weeks, respectively. A detailed evaluation, including urodynamic studies, bone x-ray studies of the pelvis, MRI scan of the spine and pelvis, investigation for an underlying polyneuropathy with nerve conduction testing, and extensive blood work for metabolic, endocrinologic, and toxic conditions, was normal.[232] Traction of the perineum on the fracture post, in patients undergoing surgery on a fracture table, may be associated with transient urinary incontinence, impotence, penile and scrotal numbness, and perineal numbness in women.[194,203,285] However, although the majority of patients fully recover, return of normal sexual function is unpredictable, and symptoms of erectile dysfunction may persist.[203]

## MYOPATHY

Myopathies are rarely associated with disturbances of micturition. A study of 6 patients with myotonic dystrophy described 1 patient with hesitancy and prolonged urination and 1 patient who noticed frequency, hesitancy, and stress incontinence.[273] Urodynamic studies revealed low maximum urethral pressure in 2 patients, 3 with large bladder capacity, 2 with small bladder capacity, 1 with detrusor hyperreflexia, and 1 with an atonic cystometrogram. The BCR was absent in 1 patient, and anal reflex was absent in 1.[273] EMG of the external urethral sphincter in 1 patient revealed polyphasic MUPs.[273] Evaluation of 7 patients with Duchenne's muscular dystrophy revealed 5 patients with abnormal urodynamic studies, consisting of uninhibited bladder contractions or bladder sphincter dyssynergia, and 1 patient with a lower motor neuron lesion, consisting of prolonged-duration pelvic floor muscle MUPs, but no evidence of a myopathy of pelvic floor muscles.[59] The reflex response of the pelvic floor muscles on BCR and CAR testing was normal.[59] It was suggested that incontinence in this group of patients was most likely secondary to upper motor neuron dysfunction rather than a direct consequence of the myopathy.[59]

Stress incontinence in a 48-year-old woman with limb-girdle muscular dystrophy, with symptoms first present at age 12, was associated with marked bladder base descent on videourodynamic testing and with a pelvic floor muscle biopsy consistent with a muscular dystrophy.[87] A case report of a 68-year-old man with acid maltase deficiency describes urinary incontinence, occurring without warning only after walking for a minimum of 20 minutes, as a feature of the presenting symptom complex.[61] Videocystometrogram revealed gross detrusor instability, and the patient's incontinence responded to anticholinergic medication.[61] It was suggested that the incontinence may have resulted from the inability of striated muscles to augment sphincter closure pressure during exercise-induced muscle fatigue or that detrusor overactivity reflected an unidentified neurogenic component.[61]

## ELDERLY PATIENTS: SPECIAL CONSIDERATIONS

The etiology of voiding dysfunction in elderly patients is complex and differs from that of younger patients. Detrusor hyperactivity with impaired contractile function was present in 33% of 32 elderly patients in a chronic care facility who were evaluated for urinary incontinence.[258] Diminished bladder contractile function was associated with bladder trabeculation, a slow velocity of bladder contraction, and a significant postvoid residual volume.[257] Patients with this pattern are predisposed to developing urinary retention in response to an added insult, such as fecal impaction or medication, and symptoms need to be distinguished from those of bladder hyporeflexia, detrusor sphincter dyssynergia, and bladder outlet obstruction.[258] A study of 73 elderly incontinent patients (mean age 79) and 27 continent subjects (mean age 78) demonstrated urge incontinence with normal bladder sensation in 20 patients, urge incontinence with decreased bladder sensation in 14, and 39 patients with other types of incontinence.[137] Those with urge incontinence and reduced bladder sensation had a significantly lower Mini-Mental Status Exam score, significantly poorer perfusion of the frontal cortex than other continent and incontinent groups, and significantly poorer global cortical perfusion than the other incontinent groups.[137] A comparative study of urodynamic parameters of 253 men and 183 women revealed significant changes with age. With increasing age, postvoid residual volume increased, peak and average flow rate decreased, bladder capacity decreased, and voided volume decreased.[204] In women, functional urethral length and maximal urethral closing pressure decreased with age, and in men, prostate volume increased. Detrusor instability increased from 23.4% for men age 40 to 60 years to 46.7% for men older than 80 years; it did not change with age in women.[204]

These studies suggest that detrusor overactivity is an important component of micturition dysfunction and incontinence in elderly patients and that men and women experience many of the same changes in bladder function with aging and suggest the possibility that a gender nonspecific primary aging process affects the bladder.[233] These studies also emphasize the importance of urodynamic studies for determining the etiologic basis of the condition and for planning therapeutic management of elderly patients with micturition dysfunction.[233]

## CONCLUSION

The key to effective care of patients with micturition dysfunction is formulation of a correct diagnosis. The initial evaluation of micturition dysfunction or incontinence should include a complete history that characterizes the type, frequency, pattern, and associated symptoms. Inquiry should be made regarding all medications taken. Specific inquiry should be directed toward those neurologic diseases known to be associated with disturbances of micturition. Symptoms of urgency and urge incontinence are associated with bladder hyperreflexia, failure to adequately store urine, bladder hypertonicity, and uninhibited bladder contractions. Symptoms of diminished urinary stream and urinary retention are associated with bladder hypocontractility or sphincter obstruction. Unfortunately, none of these symptoms is specific for neurologic disease. A general physical and neurologic examination, a rectal examination, and a pelvic examination of all women should be performed. The pelvic examination should incorporate an assessment of pelvic floor muscle function.

A urinalysis and assessment of postvoiding residual urine represent the initial step of the laboratory evaluation. Formal urodynamic testing can more accurately and precisely evaluate for bladder and urinary sphincter functional abnormalities, exclude concurrent nonneurologic disease, and assess for illness complications. A uroflow study and cystometry with simultaneous bladder, intraabdominal, and striated urinary sphincter EMG monitoring provides useful information for the majority of patients. Other sophisticated urodynamic tests can characterize micturition function of patients with more complex problems. Electrodiagnostic tests, including PSEP, BCR, and other sacral latency studies, are safe and directly measure neurologic function. However, these studies require special expertise to perform and interpret, and they have not been demonstrated to be useful screening tests for neurologically normal patients with micturition dysfunction. Urethral sphincter EMG abnormalities can help distinguish patients with MSA or Shy-Drager syndrome from those with Alzheimer's or Parkinson's disease.

The historical information obtained for patients with sexual dysfunction should include a psychologic and social assessment. Inquiry should be made about bladder and bowel dysfunction, endocrine diseases, and neurologic diseases known to affect sexual function. The standard evaluation of male sexual dysfunction includes a complete blood count, testosterone level, prolactin level, serum glucose, urinalysis, serum creatinine, blood urea nitrogen, FSH and LH serum levels, and thyroid function tests. Screening tests of nocturnal tumescence, such as the postage-stamp and snap-gauge tests, can provide evidence for organic impotence. However, these studies are not sensitive measures of the frequency and quality of erections. Testing of NPT with the Rigiscan or similar devices can quantitate the frequency and quality of erections and can be performed at home. However, normative data are limited, both false-negative (spinal cord injury patients) and false-positive (diabetic patients without symptoms of sexual dysfunction) results have been described, and the presence of a normal NPT study may not correlate with the ability to achieve vaginal penetration during sexual activity. Erectile failure after intracorporeal injection of vasoactive medication supports the diagnosis of vascular insufficiency but does not distinguish between arterial and venous insufficiency. An abnormal study can also reflect anxiety or discomfort, and a normal erection can occur with both psychogenic and neurogenic disease. In the absence of any clinical general medical or neurologic disease, a patient with a satisfactory pharmacologic response to locally injectable or oral medication may prefer to be treated symptomatically and not undergo further diagnostic testing.

Penile ultrasonography can better define vascular disorders. Measurement of venoocclusive function with cavernosometry and cavernosography provides anatomic information used to guide vascular surgical therapy. However, surgical results have been mixed and unpredictable. Electrodiagnostic techniques that measure penile dorsal nerve conduction, BCR, and other sacral reflex latencies and central pudendal SSEPs provide a direct measure of neurologic function. However, the sensitivity and specificity of these studies for the diagnosis of neurogenic sexual dysfunction is unclear.

Unfortunately, there is no diagnostic "gold standard" that distinguishes psychogenic from neurogenic sexual dysfunction. The diagnosis of sexual dysfunction in women is limited by the absence of direct quantitative physiologic measures and remains an unexplored area. Since the presentation of patients with micturition and sexual dysfunction is nonspecific and may reflect many different diseases, clinical clarification often requires additional diagnostic testing. Urinary incontinence imposes a significant financial burden upon individuals, families, and health care organizations.[339] The annual societal cost of urinary incontinence for individuals over the age of 65 years was estimated at $26.3 billion in 1995, of which 97% represented the direct cost of treatment and its effects.[339] Urinary incontinence also imposes a significant social burden, impairing the quality of life of affected individuals.[244] The cost of diagnostic testing for the evaluation of incontinence is not insignificant, but it represents only a small fraction of the overall cost of patient care.[339] Close cooperation among the members of a multidisciplinary team, which may include a general internist, a neurologist, a urologist, a gynecologist, and a psychiatrist, ultimately contributes to optimal patient care.

## REFERENCES

1. Abe S, Kawabe K, Niijima T, Shimada Y. Electromyography of the external urethral sphincter in patients with prostatic hyperplasia. *J Urol.* 1984;132:510-512.

2. Abrams P, Blaivas JG, Stanton SL, et al. Standardization of terminology of lower urinary tract function. *Scand J Urol Nephrol.* 1988; 114(suppl):5-19.

3. AHCPR Guideline. In: Fantl JA, Newman DK, Colling J, et al. *Urinary Incontinence in Adults: Acute and Chronic Management.* Clinical Practice Guideline No. 2 (1996 update). Rockville, MD: US Depart of Health and Human Services, Agency for Health Care Policy and Research. AHCPR Publication No. 96-0682, March 1996.

4. Ahlberg J, Norlen L, Blomstrand C, Wikkelso C. Outcome of shunt operation on urinary incontinence in normal pressure hydrocephalus predicted by lumbar puncture. *J Neurol Neurosurg Psychiatry.* 1988;51: 105-108.

5. Aitchison M, Aitchison J, Carter R. Is the penile brachial index a reproducible and useful measurement? *Br J Urol.* 1990;66:202-204.

6. Allen RP, Brendler CB. Nocturnal penile tumescence predicting response to intracorporeal pharmacological erection testing. *J Urol.* 1988;140:518-522.

7. Allen R, Brendler CB. Snap-gauge compared to a full nocturnal penile tumescence study for evaluation of patients with erectile impotence. *J Urol.* 1990;143:51-54.

8. Allen RE, Hosker GL, Smith ARB, Warrell DW. Pelvic floor damage and childbirth: a neurophysiological study. *Br J Obstet Gynaecol.* 1990; 97:770-779.

9. Allen RP, Smolev JK, Engel RM, Brendler CB. Comparison of Rigiscan and formal nocturnal penile tumescence testing in the evaluation of erectile rigidity. *J Urol.* 1993;149:1265-1268.

10. Amarenco G, Kerdraon J, Denys P. Les troubles vesico-sphincteriens de la sclérose en plaques étude clinique, urodynamique et neurophysiologique de 225 cas. *Rev Neurol (Paris).* 1995;151:722-730.

11. Amis ES, Blaivas JG. The role of the radiologist in evaluating voiding dysfunction. *Radiology.* 1990;175:317-318.

12. Andersen JT, Bradley WE. Abnormalities of detrusor and sphincter function in multiple sclerosis. *Br J Urol.* 1976;48:193-198.

13. Anderson RS. A neurogenic element to urinary genuine stress incontinence. *Br J Obstet Gynaecol.* 1984;91:41-45.

14. Andrew J, Nathan PW. Lesions of the anterior frontal lobes and disturbances of micturition and defaecation. *Brain.* 1964;87:233-265.

15. Andrews KL, Husmann DA. Bladder dysfunction and management in multiple sclerosis. *Mayo Clin Proc.* 1997;72:1176-1183.

16. Appell RA. Voiding dysfunction and lumbar disc disorders. *Probl Urol.* 1993;7:35-40.

17. Arunabh MB, Badlani G. Urologic problems in cerebrovascular accidents. *Probl Urol.* 1993;7:41-53.

18. Awad SA, Gajewski JB, Sogbein SK, et al. Relationship between neurological and urological status in patients with multiple sclerosis. *J Urol.* 1984;132:499-502.

19. Awad EA, Smith A, Bilkey W, Agre J. Bulbo-sphincteric reflex latency: technique. *Prog Clin Biol Res.* 1981;78:145-156.

20. Badlani GH, Vohra S, Motola JA. Detrusor behavior in patients with dominant hemispheric strokes. *Neurourol Urodyn.* 1991;10:119-123.

21. Badr G, Carlsson CA, Fall M, et al. Cortical evoked potentials following stimulation of the urinary bladder in man. *Electroencephalogr Clin Neurophysiol.* 1982;54:494-498.

22. Badr GG, Fall M, Carlsson CA, et al. Cortical evoked potentials obtained after stimulation of the lower urinary tract. *J Urol.* 1984;131: 306-309.

23. Bain CL, Guay AW. Reproducibility in monitoring nocturnal penile tumescence and rigidity. *J Urol.* 1991;148:811-814.

24. Barry JM, Blank B, Boileau M. Nocturnal penile tumescence monitoring with stamps. *Urology.* 1980;15:171-172.

25. Bartolo DCC, Jarratt JA, Read NW. The cutaneo-anal reflex: a useful index of neuropathy? *Br J Surg.* 1983;70:660-663.

26. Batista J-E, Bauer SB, Shefner JM, et al. Urodynamic findings in children with spinal cord ischemia. *J Urol.* 1995;154:1183-1187.

27. Beck RO, Betts CD, Fowler CJ. Genitourinary dysfunction in multiple system atrophy: clinical features and treatment in 62 cases. *J Urol.* 1994;151:1336-1341.

28. Bemelmans BLH, Hommes OR, Van Kerrebroeck PEV, et al. Evidence for early lower urinary tract dysfunction in clinically silent multiple sclerosis. *J Urol.* 1991;145:1219-1224.

29. Bemelmans BLH, Meuleman EJH, Anten BWM, et al. Penile sensory disorders in erectile dysfunction: results of a comprehensive neurourophysiological diagnostic evaluation in 123 patients. *J Urol.* 1991; 146:777-782.

30. Bennett CJ, Seager SW, Vasher EA, McGuire E. Sexual dysfunction and electroejaculation in men with spinal cord injury: a review. *J Urol.* 1988;139:453-457.

31. Bennett DA, Gilley DW, Wilson RS, et al. Clinical correlates of high signal lesions on magnetic resonance imaging in Alzheimer's disease. *J Neurol.* 1992;239:186-190.

32. Benson CB, Aruny JE, Vickers MA. Correlation of duplex sonography with arteriography in patients with erectile dysfunction. *AJR.* 1993; 160:71-73.

33. Berger Y, Blaivas JG, DeLarocha, Salinas JM. Urodynamic findings in Parkinson's disease. *J Urol.* 1987;138:836-838.

34. Berger Y, Blaivas JG, Oliver L. Urinary dysfunction in transverse myelitis. *J Urol.* 1990;144:103-105.

35. Betts CD, Jones SJ, Fowler CG, Fowler CJ. Erectile dysfunction in multiple sclerosis: associated neurological and neurophysiological deficits, and treatment of the condition. *Brain.* 1994;117:1303-1310.

36. Bilkey WJ, Awad EA, Smith AD. Clinical application of sacral reflex latency. *J Urol.* 1983;129:1187-1189.

37. Blaivas JG, Barbalias GA. Characteristics of neural injury after abdomino-perineal resection. *J Urol.* 1983;129:84-87.

38. Blaivas JG, Barbalias GA. Detrusor–external sphincter dyssynergia in men with multiple sclerosis: an ominous urologic condition. *J Urol.* 1984;131:91-94.

39. Blaivas JG, Bhimani G, Labib KB. Vesicourethral dysfunction in multiple sclerosis. *J Urol.* 1979;122:342-347.

40. Blaivas JG, Chancellor MB. Classification of neurogenic bladder disease. In: Chancellor MB, Blaivas JG, eds. *Practical Neuro-urology: Genitourinary Complications in Neurologic Disease.* Boston: Butterworth-Heinemann; 1995:25-32.

41. Blaivas JG, Zayed AAH, Labib KB. The bulbocavernosus reflex in urology: a prospective study of 299 patients. *J Urol.* 1981;126:197-199.

42. Blok BFM, Willemsen ATM, Holstege G. A PET study on brain control of micturition in humans. *Brain.* 1997;120:111-121.

43. Blum MD, Bahnson RR, Porter TN, Carter MF. Effect of local alpha-adrenergic blockade on human penile erection. *J Urol.* 1985;134:479-481.

44. Borrie MJ, Campbell AJ, Caradoc-Davies TH, Spears GFS. Urinary incontinence after stroke: a prospective study. *Age Ageing.* 1986;15:177-181.

45. Bradley WE. Urethral electromyography. *J Urol.* 1972;108:563-564.

46. Bradley WE, Lin JTY, Johnson B. Measurement of the conduction velocity of the dorsal nerve of the penis. *J Urol.* 1984;131:1127-1129.

47. Bradley WE, Timm GW, Gallagher JM, Johnson BK. New method for continuous measurement of nocturnal penile tumescence and rigidity. *Urology.* 1986;26:4-9.

48. Breza J, Aboseif SR, Orvis BR, et al. Detailed anatomy of penile neurovascular structures: surgical significance. *J Urol.* 1989;141:437-443.

49. Brittain KR, Peet SM, Castleden CM. Stroke and incontinence. *Stroke.* 1998;29:524-528.

50. Brocklehurst JC, Andrews K, Richards B, Laycock PJ. Incidence and correlates of incontinence in stroke patients. *J Am Geriatr Soc.* 1985;33: 540-542.

51. Brown JS, Seeley DG, Fong J, et al. Urinary incontinence in older women: who is at risk? *Obstet Gynecol.* 1996;87:715-721.

52. Brown WF. *The Physiological and Technical Basis of Electromyography.* Boston: Butterworth Publishers; 1984:317-338.

53. Brumback RJ, Ellison TS, Molligan H, et al. Pudendal nerve palsy complicating intramedullary nailing of the femur. *J Bone Joint Surg.* 1992; 74:1450-1455.

54. Burney TL, Senapati M, Desai S, et al. Effect of cerebrovascular accident on micturition. *Urol Clin North Am.* 1996;23:483-490.

55. Burns A, Jacoby R, Levy R. Psychiatric phenomena in Alzheimer's disease, IV: disorders of behavior. *J Psychiatry.* 1990;157:86-94.

56. Buvat J, Buvat-Herbaut M, Dehaene JL, Lemaire A. Is intracavernous injection of papaverine a reliable screening test for vascular impotence? *J Urol.* 1986;135:476-478.

57. Buvat J, Lemaire A, Buvat-Herbaut M, et al. Comparative investigations in 26 impotent and 26 nonimpotent diabetic patients. *J Urol.* 1985;133:34-38.

58. Campbell LV, Redelman MJ, Borkman M, et al. Factors in sexual dysfunction in diabetic female volunteer subjects. *Med J Aust.* 1989;151: 550-552.

59. Caress JB, Kothari MJ, Bauer SB, Shefner JM. Urinary dysfunction in Duchenne muscular dystrophy. *Muscle Nerve.* 1996;19:819-822.

60. Chai TC, Steers WD. Neurophysiology of micturition and continence. *Urol Clin North Am.* 1996;23:221-236.

61. Chancellor AM, Webb JN, Lucas MG, et al. Acid maltase deficiency presenting with a myopathy and exercise induced urinary incontinence in a 68-year-old male. *J Neurol Neurosurg Psychiatry.* 1991;54: 659-660. Letter.

62. Chandiramani VA, Palace J, Fowler CJ. How to recognize patients with parkinsonism who should not have urological surgery. *Br J Urol.* 1997; 80:100-104.

63. Clawson DR, Cardenas DD. Dorsal nerve of the penis nerve conduction velocity: a new technique. *Muscle Nerve.* 1991;14:845-849.

64. Collins JP, Lewandowski BJ. Experience with intracorporeal injection of papaverine and duplex ultrasound scanning for assessment of arteriogenic impotence. *Br J Urol.* 1987;59:84-88.

65. Colpi GM, Fanciullacci F, Beretta G, et al. Evoked sacral potentials in subjects with true premature ejaculation. *Andrologia.* 1986;18:583-586.

66. Coslett HB, Heilman KM. Male sexual function: impairment after right hemisphere stroke. *Arch Neurol.* 1986;43:1036-1039.

67. Crino PB, Zimmerman R, Laskowitz D, et al. Magnetic resonance imaging of the cauda equina in Guillain-Barré syndrome. *Neurology.* 1994;44:1334-1336.

68. Currie CT. Urinary incontinence after stroke. *BMJ.* 1986;293:1322-1323.

69. D'Alpa F, Ventimiglia B, Scrofani A, Grasso A. Pudendal nerve SEPs in myelopathies. *Acta Neurol.* 1987;9:139-146.

70. Daniels JS. Abnormal nerve conduction in impotent patients with diabetes mellitus. *Diabetes Care.* 1989;7:449-454.

71. de Groat WC. Anatomy and physiology of the lower urinary tract. *Urol Clin North Am.* 1993;20:383-401.

72. Deindl FM, Vodusek DB, Hesse U, Schussler B. Pelvic floor activity patterns: comparison of nulliparous continent and parous urinary stress incontinent women: a kinesiological EMG study. *Br J Urol.* 1994; 73:413-417.

73. DeJong RN. *The Neurological Examination.* 3rd ed. New York: Harper & Row, Publishers; 1970:609-613, 700-701.

74. Del Carro U, Riva D, Comi GC, et al. Neurophysiological evaluation in detrusor instability. *Neurourol Urodyn.* 1993;12:455-462.

75. Delcour C, Wespes E, Vandenbosch G, et al. Impotence: evaluation with cavernosography. *Radiology.* 1986;161:803-806.

76. Deletis V, Vodusek DB. Intraoperative recording of the bulbocavernosus reflex. *Neurosurgery.* 1997;40:88-93.

77. Delodovici ML, Fowler CJ. Clinical value of the pudendal somatosensory evoked potential. *Electroencephalogr Clin Neurophysiol.* 1995;96: 509-515.

78. Del-Ser T, Munoz DG, Hachinski V. Temporal pattern of cognitive decline and incontinence is different in Alzheimer's disease and diffuse Lewy body disease. *Neurology.* 1996;46:682-686.

79. Deltenre PF, Thiry AJ. Urinary bladder cortical evoked potentials in man: suitable stimulation techniques. *Br J Urol.* 1989;64:381-384.

80. DePalma RG, Olding M, Yu GW, et al. Vascular interventions for impotence: lessons learned. *J Vasc Surg.* 1995;21:576-585.

81. DePalma RG, Schwab FJ, Emsellem HA, et al. Noninvasive assessment of impotence. *Surg Clin North Am.* 1990;70:119-133.

82. DeRidder PA, Dauben RD. Electromyelography, a useful test for evaluation of the sacral spinal cord. *J Urol.* 1981;125:835-838.

83. Desai KM, Dembny K, Morgan H. et al. Neurophysiological investigation of diabetic impotence: are sacral response studies of value? *Br J Urol.* 1988;61:68-73.

84. Dettmers C, Van Ahlen H, Faust H, et al. Evaluation of erectile dysfunction with the sympathetic skin response in comparison to bulbocavernosus reflex and somatosensory evoked potentials of the pudendal nerve. *Electromyogr Clin Neurophysiol.* 1994;34:437-444.

85. Deutsch S, Sherman L. Previously unrecognized diabetes mellitus in sexually impotent men. *JAMA.* 1980;244:2430-2432.

86. Dick HC, Bradley WE, Scott FB, Timm GW. Pudendal sexual reflexes. electrophysiologic investigations. *Urology.* 1974;3:376-379.

87. Dixon PJ, Christmas TJ, Chapple CR. Stress incontinence due to pelvic floor muscle involvement in limb-girdle muscular dystrophy. *Br J Urol.* 1990;65:653-660.

88. Dmochowski R. Cystometry. *Urol Clin North Am.* 1996;23:243-252.

89. Donatucci CF, Lue TF. The combined intracavernous injection and stimulation test: diagnostic accuracy. *J Urol.* 1992;148:61-62.

90. Dougherty JH, Simmons JD, Parker J. Subcortical ischemic disease: clinical spectrum and MRI correlation. *Stroke.* 1986;17:146.

91. DuBeau CE, Sullivan MP, Cravalho E, et al. Correlation between micturitional urethral pressure profile and pressure-flow criteria in bladder outlet obstruction. *J Urol.* 1995;154:498-503.

92. Eardley I, Fowler CJ, Nagendran K, et al. The neurourology of tropical spastic paraparesis. *Br J Urol.* 1991;68:598-603.

93. Eardley I, Nagendran K, Kirby RS, Fowler CJ. A new technique for assessing the efferent innervation of the human striated urethral sphincter. *J Urol.* 1990;144:948-951.

94. Eardley I, Nagendran K, Lecky B, et al. Neurophysiology of the striated urethral sphincter in multiple sclerosis. *Br J Urol.* 1991;68:81-88.

95. Eardley I, Quinn NP, Fowler CJ, et al. The value of urethral sphincter electromyography in the differential diagnosis of Parkinsonism. *Br J Urol.* 1989;64:360-362.

96. Ek A, Bradley WE, Krane RJ. Nocturnal penile rigidity measured by the snap-gauge band. *J Urol.* 1983;129:964-966.

97. El-Bayoumi M, El-Sherbini O, Mostafa M. Impotence in diabetics: organic versus psychogenic factors. *Urology.* 1984;24:459-463.

98. Ellenberg M. Development of urinary bladder dysfunction in diabetes mellitus. *Ann Intern Med.* 1980;92:321-323.

99. Ellenberg M. Sexual function in diabetic patients. *Ann Intern Med.* 1980;92:331-333.

100. Ellis DJ, Doghramji K, Bagley DH. Snap-gauge band versus penile rigidity in impotence assessment. *J Urol.* 1988;140:61-63.

101. Emmett JL, Love JG. Urinary retention in women caused by asymptomatic protruded lumbar disk: report of 5 cases. *J Urol.* 1968;99:597-606.

102. Ertekin G, Akyurekli O, Gurses AN, Turgut H. The value of somatosensory-evoked potentials and bulbocavernosus reflex in patients with impotence. *Acta Neurol Scand.* 1985;71:48-53.

103. Ertekin C, Ertekin N, Almis S. Autonomic sympathetic nerve involvement in diabetic impotence. *Neurol Urodyn.* 1989;8:589-598.

104. Ertekin C, Ertekin N, Mutlu S, et al. Skin potentials (SP) recorded from the extremities and genital regions in normal and impotent subjects. *Acta Neurol Scand.* 1987;76:28-36.

105. Ertekin C, Hansen MV, Larsson L-E, Sjodahl R. Examination of the descending pathway to the external anal sphincter and pelvic floor muscles by transcranial cortical stimulation. *Electroencephalogr Clin Neurophysiol.* 1990;75:500-510.

106. Ertekin C, Reel F. Bulbocavernosus reflex in normal men and in patients with neurogenic bladder and/or impotence. *J Neuro Sci.* 1976; 28:1-15.

107. Ertekin C, Reel F, Mutlu R, Kerkuklu I. Bulbocavernosus reflex in patients with conus medullaris and cauda equina lesions. *J Neuro Sci.* 1979;41:175-181.

108. Ertekin C, Yurtseven O, Reel F. Bulbocavernosus reflex in benign hypertrophy of the prostate. *Int Urol Nephrol.* 1981;13:69-76.

109. Fanciullacci F, Kokodoko A, Garavaglia PF, et al. Comparative study of the motor unit potentials of the external urethral sphincter, anal sphincter, and bulbocavernosus muscle in normal men. *Neurourol Urodyn.* 1987;6:65-69.

110. Feder M, Heller L, Tadmar R, et al. Urinary continence after stroke: association with cystometric profile and computerised tomography findings. *Eur Neurol.* 1987;27:101-105.

111. Fegiz G, Trenti A, Bezzi M, et al. Sexual and bladder dysfunctions following surgery for rectal carcinoma. *Ital J Surg Sci.* 1986;16:103-109.

112. Feldman HA, Goldstein I, Hatzichristou DG, et al. Impotence and its medical and psychosocial correlates: results of the Massachusetts Male Aging Study. *J Urol.* 1994;151:54-61.

113. Fidas A, Elton RA, McInnes A, Chisholm GD. Neurophysiological measurement of voiding reflex arcs in patients with functional disorders of the lower urinary tract. *Br J Urol.* 1987;60:205-211.

114. Fisher CM. Hydrocephalus as a cause of disturbances of gait in the elderly. *Neurology.* 1982;32:1358-1363.

115. Fitzmaurice H, Fowler CJ, Rickards D, et al. Micturition disturbance in Parkinson's disease. *Br J Urol.* 1985;57:652-656.

116. Forney JP. The effect of radical hysterectomy on bladder physiology. *Am J Obstet Gynecol.* 1980;138:374-382.

117. Forsberg L, Hojerback T, Olsson AM, Rosen I. Etiologic aspects of impotence in diabetes. *Scand J Urol Nephrol.* 1989;23:173-175.

118. Fowler CJ, Ali Z, Kirby RS, Pryor JP. The value of testing for unmyelinated fibre: sensory neuropathy in diabetic impotence. *Br J Urol.* 1988; 61:63-67.

119. Fowler CJ, Kirby RS. Electromyography of urethral sphincter in women with urinary retention. *Lancet.* 1986;I:1455-1456.

120. Fowler CJ, Kirby MJ, Harrison MJG, et al. Individual motor unit analysis in the diagnosis of disorders of urethral sphincter innervation. *J Neurol Neurosurg Psychiatry.* 1984;47:637-641.

121. Frimodt-Moller C. Diabetic cystopathy: epidemiology and related disorders. *Ann Intern Med.* 1980;92:318-321.

122. Fuchs AM, Mehringer CM, Rajfer J. Anatomy of penile venous drainage in potent and impotent men during cavernosography. *J Urol.* 1989;141:1353-1356.

123. Gallien P, Robineau S, Nicolas B, et al. Vesicourethral dysfunction and urodynamic findings in multiple sclerosis: a study of 149 cases. *Arch Phys Med Rehabil.* 1998;79:255-257.

124. Galloway NTM, Chisholm GD, McInnes A. Patterns and significance of the sacral evoked response (the urologist's knee jerk). *Br J Urol.* 1985;57:145-147.

125. Ganzer H, Madersbacher H, Rumpl E. Cortical evoked potentials by stimulation of the vesicourethral junction: clinical value and neurophysiological considerations. *J Urol.* 1991;146:118-123.

126. Garrett VE, Scott JA, Costich J, et al. Bladder emptying assessment in stroke patients. *Arch Phys Med Rehabil.* 1989;70:41-43.

127. Gelber DA, Good DC, Laven LJ, Verhulst SJ. Causes of urinary incontinence after acute hemispheric stroke. *Stroke.* 1993;24:378-382.

128. Gerstenberg TC, Bradley WE. Nerve conduction velocity measurement of dorsal nerve of penis in normal and impotent males. *Urology.* 1983;21:90-92.

129. Ghezzi A, Callea L, Zaffaroni M, et al. Motor potentials of bulbocavernosus muscle after transcranial and lumbar magnetic stimulation: comparative study with bulbocavernosus reflex and pudendal evoked potentials. *J Neurol Neurosurg Psychiatry.* 1991;54:524-526.

130. Ghezzi A, Callea L, Zaffaroni M, et al. Perineal motor potentials to magnetic stimulation, pudendal evoked potentials and perineal reflex in women. *Neurophysiol Clin.* 1992;22:321-326.

131. Ghezzi A, Malvestiti GM, Baldini S, et al. Erectile impotence in multiple sclerosis: a neurophysiological study. *J Neurol.* 1995;242:123-126.

132. Giuliano FA, Rampin O, Benoit G, Jardin A. Neural control of penile erection. *Urol Clin North Am.* 1995;22:747-766.

133. Goldstein I, Siroky MB, Sax DS, Krane RJ. Neurourologic abnormalities in multiple sclerosis. *J Urol.* 1982;128:541-545.

134. Gonor SE, Carroll DJ, Metcalfe JB. Vesical dysfunction in multiple sclerosis. *Urology.* 1985;25:429-431.

135. Granata A, Bancroft J, Del Rio G. Stress and erectile response to intracavernosal prostaglandin E$_1$ in men with erectile dysfunction. *Psychosom Med.* 1995;57:336-344.

136. Gray RR, Keresteci AG, St. Louis EL. Investigation of impotence by internal pudendal angiography: experience with 73 cases. *Radiology.* 1982;144:773-780.

137. Griffiths DJ, McCracken PN, Harrison GM, et al. Cerebral aetiology of urinary urge incontinence in elderly people. *Age Ageing.* 1994;23:246-250.

138. Guay AT, Heatley GJ, Murray FT. Comparison of results of nocturnal tumescence and rigidity in a sleep laboratory versus a portable home monitor. *Urology.* 1996;48:912-916.

139. Guerit JM, Opsomer RJ. Bit-mapped imaging of somatosensory evoked potentials after stimulation of the posterior tibial nerves and dorsal nerve of the penis. *Electroencephalogr Clin Neurophysiol.* 1991;80:228-237.

140. Gunasekera WSL, Richardson AE, Seneviratne KN, Eversden ID. Clinical correlation of urodynamic findings in patients with localized partial lesions of the spinal cord and cauda equina. *Surg Neurol.* 1984;21:148-154.

141. Haldeman S, Bradley WE, Bhatia N. Evoked responses from the pudendal nerve. *J Urol.* 1982;128:974-980.

142. Hansen MV, Ertekin C, Larsson L-E. Cerebral evoked potentials after stimulation of the posterior urethra in man. *Electroencephalogr Clin Neurophysiol.* 1990;77:52-58.

143. Hansen MV, Ertekin C, Larsson L-E, Pedersen K. A neurophysiological study of patients undergoing radical prostatectomy. *Scand J Urol Nephrol.* 1989;23:267-273.

144. Hasan ST, Hamdy FC, Schofield IS, Neal DE. Transrectal ultrasound guided needle electromyography of the urethral sphincter in males. *Neurourol Urodyn.* 1995;14:359-363.

145. Hattery RR, King KB, Lewis RW, et al. Vasculogenic impotence: duplex and color Doppler imaging. *Radiol Clin North Am.* 1991;29:629-645.

146. Hattori T, Yasuda K, Kita K, Hirayama K. Disorders of micturition in tabes dorsalis. *Br J Urol.* 1990;65:497-499.

147. Hellstrom WJG, Edwards MSB, Kogan BA. Urological aspects of the tethered cord syndrome. *J Urol.* 1986;135:317-320.

148. Hellstrom P, Kortelainen P, Kontturi M. Late urodynamic findings after surgery for cauda equina syndrome caused by a prolapsed lumbar intervertebral disk. *J Urol.* 1986;135:308-312.

149. Henry MM, Swash M. Assessment of pelvic-floor disorders and incontinence by electrophysiological recording of the anal reflex. *Lancet.* 1978;1:1290-1291.

150. Herbaut AG, Nogueira MC, Wespes E. Urinary retention due to sacral myeloradiculitis: a clinical and neurophysiological study. *J Urol.* 1990;144:1206-1208.

151. Heslington K, Hilton P. Ambulatory urodynamic monitoring. *Br J Obstet Gynaecol.* 1996;103:393-399.

152. Hirshkowitz M, Karacan I, Rando KC, et al. Diabetes, erectile dysfunction, and sleep-related erections. *Sleep.* 1990;13:53-68.

153. Ho KH, Ong BKC, Chong PN, Teo WL. The bulbocavernosus reflex in the assessment of neurogenic impotence in diabetic and non-diabetic men. *Ann Acad Med Singapore.* 1996;25:558-561.

154. Hwang TI, Yang C, Wang S, et al. Impotence evaluated by the use of prostaglandin E$_1$. *J Urol.* 1989;141:1357-1359.

155. Ishii N, Nishihara Y, Imamura T. Why do frontal lobe symptoms predominate in vascular dementia with lacunes? *Neurology.* 1986;36:340-345.

156. Jaeckle KA, Young DF, Foley KM. The natural history of lumbosacral plexopathy in cancer. *Neurology.* 1985;35:8-15.

157. Jensen SB. The natural history of sexual dysfunction in diabetic women: a 6-year follow-up study. *Acta Med Scand.* 1986;219:73-78.

158. Jonas S, Brown J. Neurogenic bladder in normal pressure hydrocephalus. *Urology.* 1975;5:44-50.

159. Jorgensen JB, Jensen KME. Uroflowmetry. *Urol Clin North Am.* 1996;23:237-241.

160. Juenemann KP, Schmidt RA, Melchior H, Tanagho EA. Neuroanatomy and clinical significance of the urethral sphincter. *Urol Int.* 1987;42:132-136.

161. Kaneko S, Bradley WE. Evaluation of erectile dysfunction with continuous monitoring of penile rigidity. *J Urol.* 1986;136:1026-1029.

162. Kaneko S, Bradley WE. Penile electrodiagnosis value of bulbocavernosus reflex latency versus nerve conduction velocity of the dorsal nerve of the penis in diagnosis of diabetic impotence. *J Urol.* 1987;137:933-935.

163. Kaneko S, Park YC, Yachiku S, Kurita T. Evoked central somatosensory potentials after penile stimulation in man. *Urology.* 1983;21:58-59.

164. Kaplan SA, Chancellor MB, Blaivas JG. Bladder and sphincter behavior in patients with spinal cord lesions. *J Urol.* 1991;146:113-117.

165. Kaplan WE, McLone DG, Richards I. The urological manifestations of the tethered spinal cord. *J Urol.* 1988;140(2):1285-1288.

166. Kaplan SA, Te AE. Uroflowmetry and urodynamics. *Urol Clin North Am.* 1995;22:309-320.

167. Kaplan SA, Te AE, Blaivis JG. Urodynamic findings in patients with diabetic cystopathy. *J Urol.* 1995;153:342-344.

168. Karacan I. Diagnosis of erectile impotence in diabetes mellitus. *Ann Intern Med.* 1980;92:334-337.

169. Kaufman JM, Borges FD, Fitch WP, et al. Evaluation of erectile dysfunction by dynamic infusion cavernosometry and cavernosography (DICC): multi-institutional study. *Urology.* 1993;41:445-451.

170. Keating MA, Rink RC, Bauer SB, et al. Neurourological implications of the changing approach in management of occult spinal lesions. *J Urol.* 1988;140:1299-1301.

171. Kelleher CJ, Cardozo L: Urodynamic assessment. In: Rushton DN, ed. *Handbook of Neuro-urology.* New York: Marcel Dekker; 1994:129-149.

172. Kim YH, Goodman C, Omessi E, et al. The correlation of urodynamic findings with cranial magnetic resonance imaging findings in multiple sclerosis. *J Urol.* 1998;159:972-976.

173. Kirkeby HJ, Poulsen EU, Petersen T, Dorup J. Erectile dysfunction in multiple sclerosis. *Neurology.* 1988;38:1366-1371.

174. Khan Z, Hertanu J, Yang WC, et al. Predictive correlation of urodynamic dysfunction brain injury after cerebrovascular accident. *J Urol.* 1981;86-88.

175. Khan Z, Mieza M, Starer P, Singh VK. Post-prostatectomy incontinence: a urodynamic and fluoroscopic point of view. *Urology.* 1991;38:483-488.

176. Khan Z, Starer P, Bhola A. Urinary incontinence in female Parkinson disease patients. *Urology.* 1989;33:486-489.

177. Khan Z, Starer P, Yang WC, Bhola A. Analysis of voiding disorders in patients with cerebrovascular accidents. *Urology.* 1990;35:265-270.

178. Kirby R, Fowler C, Gosling J, Bannister R. Urethro-vesical dysfunction in progressive autonomic failure with multiple system atrophy. *J Neurol Neurosurg Psychiatry.* 1986;49:554-562.

179. Kjolhede P, Lindehammar H. Pelvic floor neuropathy in relation to the outcome of Burch colposuspension. *Int Urogynecol J.* 1997;8:61-65.

180. Koldewijn EL, Van Kerrebroeck PEV, Bemelmans BLH, et al. Use of sacral reflex latency measurements in the evaluation of neural function of spinal cord injury patients: a comparison of neuro-urophysiological testing and urodynamic investigations. *J Urol.* 1994;152:463-467.

181. Kondo A, Kato K, Kanai S, Sakakibara T. Bladder dysfunction second-

ary to tethered cord syndrome in adults: is it curable? *J Urol.* 1986;135: 313-316.

182. Kotsoris H, Barclay LL, Kheyfets S, et al. Urinary and gait disturbances as markers for early multi-infarct dementia. *Stroke.* 1987;18:138-141.

183. Krane RJ, Goldstein I, de Tejada IS. Impotence. *N Engl J Med.* 1989; 321:1648-1659.

184. Krane RJ, Siroky MB. Studies on sacral-evoked potentials. *J Urol.* 1980; 124:872-876.

185. Kromann-Andersen B, Nielsen KK, Nordling J. Cavernosometry: methodology and reproducibility with and without pharmacological agents in the evaluation of venous impotence. *Br J Urol.* 1991;67:517-521.

186. Krysiewicz S, Mellinger BC. The role of imaging in the diagnostic evaluation of impotence. *AJR.* 1989;153:1133-1139.

187. Kunesch E, Reiners K, Muller-Mattheis V, et al. Neurological risk profile in organic erectile impotence. *J Neurol Neurosurg Psychiatry.* 1992; 55:275-281.

188. Lavoisier P, Proulx J, Courtois F, De Carufel F. Bulbocavernosus reflex: its validity as a diagnostic test of neurogenic impotence. *J Urol.* 1989; 141:311-314.

189. Lechtenberg R, Ohl DA. *Sexual Dysfunction.* Philadelphia: Lea & Febiger; 1994:29-34.

190. Lehman TP, Jacobs JA. Etiology of diabetic impotence. *J Urol.* 1983; 129:291-294.

191. Levine LA, Lenting EL. Use of nocturnal penile tumescence and rigidity in the evaluation of male erectile dysfunction. *Urol Clin North Am.* 1995;22:775-787.

192. Light KJ, Beric A, Petronic I. Detrusor function with lesions of the cauda equina, with special emphasis on the bladder neck. *J Urol.* 1993; 149:539-542.

193. Lin JT, Bradley WE. Penile neuropathy in insulin-dependent diabetes mellitus. *J Urol.* 133;1985:213-215.

194. Lindenbaum SD, Fleming LL, Smith DW. Pudendal-nerve palsies associated with closed intramedullary femoral fixation. *J Bone Joint Surg.* 1982;64:934-938.

195. Lipe H, Longstreth WT, Bird TD, Linde M. Sexual function in married men with Parkinson's disease compared to married men with arthritis. *Neurology.* 1990;40:1347-1349.

196. Liu S, Christmas J, Nagendran K, Kirby RS. Sphincter electromyography in patients after radical prostatectomy and cystoprostatectomy. *Br J Urol.* 1992;69:397-403.

197. Lowe EM, Fowler CJ, Osborne JL, DeLancey JOL. Improved method for electromyography of the urethral sphincter in women. *Neurol Urodyn.* 1994;13:29-33.

198. Lucas MG, Thomas DG. Lack of relationship of conus reflexes to bladder function after spinal cord injury. *Br J Urol.* 1989;63:24-27.

199. Lue TP, Hricak H, Schmidt RA, Tanagho EA. Functional evaluation of penile veins by cavernosography in papaverine-induced erection. *J Urol.* 1986;135:479-482.

200. Lue TF, Tanagho EA. Physiology of erection and pharmacological management of impotence. *J Urol.* 1987;137:829-836.

201. Lum SK, Marshall VR. Results of prostatectomy in patients following a cerebrovascular accident. *Br J Urol.* 1982;54:186-189.

202. Lustman PJ, Clouse RE. Relationship of psychiatric illness to impotence in men with diabetes. *Diabetes Care.* 1990;13:893-895.

203. Lyon T, Koval KJ, Kummer F, Zuckerman JD. Pudendal nerve palsy induced by fracture table. *Orthop Rev.* 1993;22:521-525.

204. Madersbacher S, Pycha A, Schatzl G, et al. The aging lower urinary tract: a comparative urodynamic study of men and women. *Urology.* 1998;51:206-212.

205. Maiden C, Benson JT, McClellan E. Bladder-anal reflex. In: *American Association of Electrodiagnostic Medicine Continuing Education Course: The Electrophysiologic Evaluation of Bladder and Bowel Dysfunction.* Rochester, NY: Johnson Printing; 1997:25-31.

206. Malhotra CM, Balko A, Wincze JP, et al. Cavernosography in conjunction with artificial erection for evaluation of venous leakage in impotent men. *Radiology.* 1986;161:799-802.

207. Marshall P, Earls C, Morales A, Surridge D. Nocturnal penile tumescence recording with stamps: a validity study. *J Urol.* 1982;128:946.

208. Mathers SE, Ingram DA, Swash M. Electrophysiology of motor pathways for sphincter control in multiple sclerosis. *J Neurol Neurosurg Psychiatry.* 1990;53:955-960.

209. Mattson D, Petrie M, Srivastava DK, McDermott M. Multiple sclerosis: sexual dysfunction and its response to medications. *Arch Neurol.* 1995;52:862-868.

210. Mayo ME, Chetner MP. Lower urinary tract dysfunction in multiple sclerosis. *Urology.* 1992;34:67-70.

211. McInerney PD, Robinson LQ, Weston PMT, et al. Assessment of the poorly contractile or acontractile bladder in the older male in the absence of neuropathy. *Br J Urol.* 1990;65:161-163.

212. Melman A, Kaplan D, Redfield J. Evaluation of the first 70 patients in the Center for Male Sexual Dysfunction. *J Urol.* 1984;131:53-55.

213. Merckx LA, De Bruyne RM, Keuppens FI. Electromyography of cavernous smooth muscle during flaccidity: evaluation of technique and normal values. *Br J Urol.* 1993;72:353-358.

214. Monga TN, Lawson JS, Inglis J. Sexual dysfunction in stroke patients. *Arch Phys Med Rehabil.* 1986;67:19-22.

215. Monga TN, Monga M, Raina MS, Hardjasudarma M. Hypersexuality in stroke. *Arch Phys Med Rehabil.* 1986;67:415-417.

216. Moon JH, Kang SW, Chun SI. Pudendal somatosensory evoked potential and bulbocavernosus reflex testing in erectile dysfunction. *Yonsei Med J.* 1993;34:71-77.

217. Morales A, Condra M, Reid K. The role of nocturnal penile tumescence monitoring in the diagnosis of impotence: a review. *J Urol.* 1990; 143:441-446.

218. Mouritsen L, Lyngdorf P, Frimodt-Moller C. The intracavernous injection of papaverine as a diagnostic procedure in patients with erectile dysfunction. *Scand J Urol Nephrol.* 1988;22:161-163.

219. Mueller SC, Wallenberg-Pachaly H, Voges GE, Schild HH. Comparison of selective internal iliac pharmacoangiography, penile brachial index and duplex sonography with pulsed Doppler analysis for the evaluation of vasculogenic (arteriogenic) impotence. *J Urol.* 1990;143:928-932.

220. Mulligan T, Katz G. Why aged men become impotent. *Arch Intern Med.* 1989;149:1365-1366.

221. Mundy AR. An anatomical explanation for bladder dysfunction following rectal and uterine surgery. *Br J Urol.* 1982;54:501-504.

222. Myers RP, Goellner JR, Cahill DR. Prostate shape, external striated urethral sphincter and radical prostatectomy: the apical dissection. *J Urol.* 1987;138:543-550.

223. Nankervis A. Sexual function in chronic disease. *Med J Aust.* 1989; 151:548-549.

224. Narayan P, Konety B, Aslam K, et al. Neuroanatomy of the external urethral sphincter: implications for urinary continence preservation during radical prostate surgery. *J Urol.* 1995;153:337-341.

225. Neill ME, Swash M. Increased motor unit fibre density in the external anal sphincter muscle in ano-rectal incontinence: a single fiber EMG study. *J Neurol Neurosurg Psychiatry.* 1980;43:343-347.

226. Nickell K, Boone TB. Peripheral neuropathy and peripheral nerve injury. *Urol Clin North Am.* 1996;23:491-500.

227. NIH consensus conference (NIH Consensus Development Panel on Impotence). Impotence. *JAMA.* 1993;270:83-90.

228. Nikiforidis G, Koutsojannis C, Giannoulis S, Barbalias G. Reduced variance of latencies in pudendal evoked potentials after normalization for body height. *Neurourol Urodyn.* 1995;14:239-251.

229. Nofzinger EA, Reynolds CF, Jennings R, et al. Results of nocturnal penile tumescence studies are abnormal in sexually functional diabetic men. *Arch Intern Med.* 1992;152:114-118.

230. Nogueira MC, Herbaut AG, Wespes E. Neurophysiological investigations of two hundred men with erectile dysfunction. *Eur Urol.* 1990; 18:37-41.

231. Nogues MA, Starkstein S, Davalos M, et al. Cardiovascular reflexes and pudendal evoked responses in chronic haemodialysis patients. *Funct Neurol.* 1991;6:359-365.

232. Oberpenning F, Roth S, Leusmann DB, et al. The Alcock syndrome: temporary penile insensitivity due to compression of the pudendal nerve within the Alcock canal. *J Urol.* 1994;151:423-425.

233. O'Donnell PD. Special considerations in elderly individuals with urinary incontinence. *Urology.* 1998;51(suppl 2A):20-23.

234. Oelrich TM. The urethral sphincter muscle in the male. *Am J Anat.* 1980;158:229-246.

235. Oelrich TM. The striated urogenital sphincter muscle in the female. *Anat Rec.* 1983;205:223-232.

236. O'Flynn KJ, Murphy R, Thomas DG. Neurogenic bladder dysfunction in lumbar intervertebral disc prolapse. *Br J Urol.* 1992;69:38-40.

237. O'Laoire SA, Crockard HA, Thomas DG. Prognosis for sphincter recovery after operation for cauda equina compression owing to lumbar disc prolapse. *BMJ.* 1981;282:1852-1854.

238. Olsen AL. Methodology of urethral needle EMG in women. In: *American Association of Electrodiagnostic Medicine Continuing Education Course: The Electrophysiologic Evaluation of Bladder and Bowel Dysfunction.* Rochester, NY: Johnson Printing; 1997:21-24.

239. Onufrowicz B. On the arrangements and function of the cell groups of the sacral region of the spinal cord in man. *Arch Neurol.* 1901;3:387-417.

240. Opsomer RJ, Guerit JM, Wese FX, Van Cangh PJ. Pudendal cortical somatosensory evoked potentials. *J Urol.* 1986;135:1216-1218.

241. Parys BT, Evan CM, Parsons KF. Bulbocavernosus reflex latency in the investigation of diabetic impotence. *Br J Urol.* 1988;61:59-62.

242. Pavlakis AJ, Siroky MB, Goldstein I, Krane RJ. Neurourologic findings in conus medullaris and cauda equina injury. *Arch Neurol.* 1983;40:570-573.

243. Pavlakis AJ, Siroky MB, Goldstein I, Krane RJ. Neurourologic findings in Parkinson's disease. *J Urol.* 1983;129:80-83.

244. Payne CK. Epidemiology, pathophysiology, and evaluation of urinary incontinence and overactive bladder. *Urology.* 1998;51(suppl 2A):3-10.

245. Pedersen E, Harving H, Kemar B, Torring J. Human anal reflexes. *J Neurol Neurosurg Psychiatry.* 1978;41:813-818.

246. Pedersen E, Klemar B, Schroder HDAA, Torring J. Anal sphincter responses after perianal electrical stimulation. *J Neurol Neurosurg Psychiatry.* 1982;45:770-773.

247. Pelliccioni G, Scarpino O, Piloni V. Motor evoked potentials recorded from external anal sphincter by cortical and lumbo-sacral magnetic stimulation: normative data. *J Neurol Sci.* 1997;149:69-72.

248. Pickard RS, Powell PH, Schofield IS. The clinical application of dorsal penile nerve cerebral-evoked response recording in the investigation of impotence. *Br J Urol.* 1994;74:231-235.

249. Podnar S, Vodusek DB, Trsinar B, Rodi Z. A method of uroneurophysiological investigation in children. *Electroencephalogr Clin Neurophysiol.* 1997;104:389-392.

250. Porst H, Tackmann W, Van Ahlen H. Neurophysiological investigations in potent and impotent men. *Br J Urol.* 1988;61:445-450.

251. Pramstaller PP, Wenning GK, Smith SJM, et al. Nerve conduction studies, skeletal muscle EMG, and sphincter EMG in multiple system atrophy. *J Neurol Neurosurg Psychiatry.* 1995;58:618-621.

252. Quam FP, King BF, James EM, et al. Duplex and color Doppler sonographic evaluation of vasculogenic impotence. *AJR.* 1989;153:1141-1147.

253. Rajfer J, Canan V, Dorey FJ, Mehringer CM. Correlation between penile angiography and duplex scanning of cavernous arteries in impotent men. *J Urol.* 1990;143:1128-1130.

254. Rajfer J, Mehringer M. Cavernosography following clinical failure of penile vein ligation for erectile dysfunction. *J Urol.* 1990;143:514-517.

255. Rajfer J, Rosciszewski, Mehringer M. Prevalence of corporeal venous leakage in impotent men. *J Urol.* 1988;140:69-71.

256. Rechthand E. Bilateral bulbocavernosus reflexes: crossing of nerve pathways or artifact? *Muscle Nerve.* 1997;20:616-618.

257. Resnick NM, Yalla SV. Management of urinary incontinence in the elderly. *N Engl J Med.* 1985;313:800-805.

258. Resnick NM, Yalla SV. Detrusor hyperactivity with impaired contractile function: an unrecognized but common cause of incontinence in elderly patients. *JAMA.* 1987;257:3076-3081.

259. Revord JP, Opitz JL, Murtaugh P, Harrison J. Determining residual urine volumes using a portable ultrasonographic device. *Arch Phys Med Rehabil.* 1993;74:457-462.

260. Reynolds CF, Thase ME, Jennings JR, et al. Nocturnal penile tumescence in healthy 20- to 59-year-olds: a revisit. *Sleep.* 1989;12:368-373.

261. Robertson AS, Griffiths CJ, Ramsden PD, Neal DE. Bladder function in healthy volunteers: ambulatory monitoring and conventional urodynamic studies. *Br J Urol.* 1994;73:242-249.

262. Robinette MA, Moffat MJ. Intracorporeal injection of papaverine and phentolamine in the management of impotence. *Br J Urol.* 1986;58:692-695.

263. Robinson LQ, Woodcock JP, Stephenson TP. Results of investigation of impotence in patients with overt or probable neuropathy. *Br J Urol.* 1987;60:583-587.

264. Rockswold GL, Bradley WE. The use of evoked electromyographic responses in diagnosing lesions of the cauda equina. *J Urol.* 1977;118:629-631.

265. Rockswold GL, Bradley WE, Timm GW, Chou SN. Electrophysiological technique for evaluating lesions of the conus medullaris and cauda equina. *J Neurosurg.* 1976;45:321-326.

266. Rogers J, Henry MM, Misiewicz JJ. Disposable pudendal nerve stimulator: evaluation of the standard instrument and new device. *Gut.* 1988;29:1131-1133.

267. Roman GC. Senile dementia of the Binswanger type: a vascular form of dementia in the elderly. *JAMA.* 1987;258:1782-1788.

268. Roman GC, Tatemichi TK, Erkinjuntti T, et al. Vascular dementia: diagnostic criteria for research studies: report of the INIDS-AIREN International Workshop. *Neurology.* 1993;43:250-260.

269. Ropper AH, Wijdicks EFM, Truax AT. *Guillain-Barré Syndrome.* Philadelphia: FA Davis; 1991:102.

270. Rosario DJ, Potts KL, Chapple CR. Ambulatory urodynamic monitoring. *Br J Urol.* 1996;78:964-966.

271. Rosen MP, Greenfield AJ, Walker TG, et al. Arteriogenic impotence: findings in 195 impotent men examined with selective internal pudendal angiography. *Radiology.* 1990;174:1043-1048.

272. Rushton DN. Neuro-urological history and examination. In: Rushton DN, ed. *Handbook of Neuro-urology.* New York: Marcel Dekker; 1994:117-128.

273. Sakakibara R, Hattori T, Tojo M, et al. Micturitional disturbance in progressive supranuclear palsy. *J Auton Nerv Syst.* 1993;45:101-106.

274. Sakakibara R, Hattori T, Tojo M, et al. Micturitional disturbance in myotonic dystrophy. *J Auton Nerv Syst.* 1995;52:17-21.

275. Salinas JM, Berger Y, De L Rocha RE, Blaivas JG. Urological evaluation in the Shy-Drager syndrome. *J Urol.* 1986;135:741-743.

276. Sandri SD, Fanciullacci F, Politi P, Zanollo A. Urinary disorders in intervertebral disc prolapse. *Neurourol Urodyn.* 1987;6:11-19.

277. Sarica Y, Karacan I. Cervical responses evoked by stimulation of the vesicourethral junction in normal subjects. *Electroencephalogr Clin Neurophysiol.* 1986;65:440-446.

278. Sarica Y, Karacan I. Bulbocavernosus reflex to somatic and visceral nerve stimulation in normal subjects and in diabetics with erectile impotence. *J Urol.* 1987;138:55-58.

279. Sarica Y, Karacan I, Thornby JI, Hirshkowitz M. Cerebral responses evoked by stimulation of vesico-urethral junction in man: methodological evaluation of monopolar stimulation. *Electroencephalogr Clin Neurophysiol.* 1986;65:130-135.

280. Saxton HM. Urodynamics: the appropriate modality for the investigation of frequency, urgency, incontinence, and voiding difficulties. *Radiology.* 1990;175:307-316.

281. Schiavi RC, Schreiner-Engle P. Nocturnal penile tumescence in healthy aging men. *J Gerontol.* 1988;43:M146-M150.

282. Schiavi RC, Stimmel BB, Mandeli J, Rayfield EJ. Diabetes mellitus and male sexual function: a controlled study. *Diabetologia.* 1993;36:745-751.

283. Schondorf R: The role of the sympathetic skin response in the assessment of autonomic function. In: Low P, ed. *Clinical Autonomic Disorders.* Boston: Little, Brown; 1993:231-241.

284. Schulak DJ, Bear TF, Summers JL. Transient impotence from positioning on the fracture table. *J Trauma.* 1980;20:420-421.

285. Schwartz AN, Wang KY, Mack LA, et al. Evaluation of normal erectile function with color flow Doppler sonography. *AJR.* 1989;153:1155-1160.

286. Selzman AA, Elder JS, Mapstone TB. Urologic consequences of myelodysplasia and other congenital abnormalities of the spinal cord. *Urol Clin North Am.* 1993;20:485-504.

287. Seski JC, Diokno AC. Bladder dysfunction after radical abdominal hysterectomy. *Am J Obstet Gynecol.* 1977;128:643-651.

288. Sethi RK, Bauer SB, Dyro FM, Krarup C. Modulation of the bulbocavernosus reflex during voiding: loss of inhibition in upper motor neuron lesions. *Muscle Nerve.* 1989;12:892-897.

289. Shabsigh R, Fishman IJ, Toombs BD, Skolkin M. Venous leaks: anatomical and physiological observations. *J Urol.* 1991;146:1260-1265.

290. Shapiro S. Cauda equina syndrome secondary to lumbar disc herniation. *Neurosurgery.* 1993;32:743-747.

291. Sharr MM, Garfield JS, Jenkins JD. The association of bladder dysfunction with degenerative lumbar spondylosis. *Br J Urol.* 1973;45:616-620.

292. Sjögren K, Damber JE, Liliequist B. Sexuality after stroke with hemiplegia, I: aspects of sexual function. *Scand J Rehabil Med.* 1983;15:55-61.

293. Smith ARB, Hosker GL, Warrell DW. The role of partial denervation of the pelvic floor in the aetiology of genitourinary prolapse and stress incontinence of urine: a neurophysiological study. *Br J Obstet Gynaecol.* 1989;96:24-28.

294. Smith ARB, Hosker GL, Warrell DW. The role of pudendal nerve damage in the aetiology of genuine stress incontinence in women. *Br J Obstet Gynaecol.* 1989;96:29-32.

295. Smith EM, Bodner DR. Sexual dysfunction after spinal cord injury. *Urol Clin North Am.* 1993;20:535-542.

296. Snooks SJ, Badenock DR, Tiptaft RC, Swash M. Perineal nerve damage in genuine stress urinary incontinence: an electrophysiological study. *Br J Urol.* 1985;57:422-426.

297. Snooks SJ, Barnes PRH, Swash M. Damage to the innervation of the voluntary anal and periurethral sphincter musculature in inconti-

nence: an electrophysiological study. *J Neurol Neurosurg Psychiatry.* 1984;47:1269-1273.

298. Snooks SJ, Swash M. Perineal nerve and transcutaneous spinal stimulation: new methods for investigation of the urethral striated sphincter musculature. *Br J Urol.* 1984;56:406-409.

299. Snooks SJ, Swash M, Henry MM, Setchell M. Risk factors in childbirth causing damage to the pelvic floor innervation. *Int J Colorectal Dis.* 1986;1:20-24.

300. Snooks SJ, Swash M, Mathers SE, Henry MM. Effect of vaginal delivery on the pelvic floor: a 5-year follow-up. *Br J Surg.* 1990;77:1358-1360.

301. Spindel MR, Bauer S, Dyro F, et al. The changing neurourologic lesion in myelodysplasia. *JAMA.* 1987;258:1630-1633.

302. Stalberg E, Trontelj JV. *Single Fiber Electromyography.* New York: Raven Press; 1994:45-90.

303. Starer P, Libow L. Cystometric evaluation of bladder dysfunction in elderly diabetic patients. *Arch Intern Med.* 1990;150:810-813.

304. Staskin DS, Vardi Y, Siroky MB. Post-prostatectomy continence in the Parkinsonian patient: the significance of poor voluntary sphincter control. *J Urol.* 1988;140:117-118.

305. Steers WD. Impotence evaluation. *J Urol.* 1993;149:1284. Editorial.

306. Stief CG, Djamilian M, Anton P, et al. Single potential analysis of cavernous electrical activity in impotent patients: a possible diagnostic method for autonomic cavernous dysfunction and cavernous smooth muscle degeneration. *J Urol.* 1991;146:771-776.

307. Stocchi F, Carbone A, Inghilleri M, et al. Urodynamic and neurophysiological evaluation in Parkinson's disease and multiple system atrophy. *J Neurol Neurosurg Psychiatry.* 1997;62:507-511.

308. Strasser H, Klima G, Poisel S, Horninger W, Bartsch G. Anatomy and innervation of the rhabdosphincter of the male urethra. *Prostate.* 1996;28:24-31.

309. Sullivan MP, Comiter C, Yalla SV. Micturitional urethral pressure profilometry. *Urol Clin North Am.* 1996;23:263-278.

310. Sultan AH, Kamm MA, Hudson CN. Pudendal nerve damage during labour: prospective study before and after childbirth. *Br J Obstet Gynaecol.* 1994;101:22-28.

311. Swash M. Early and late components in the human anal reflex. *J Neurol Neurosurg Psychiatry.* 1982;45:767-769.

312. Swash M. Pelvic floor incompetence. In: Rushton DN, ed. *Handbook of Neuro-urology.* New York: Marcel Dekker; 1994:303-327.

313. Swash M, Snooks SJ. Slowed motor conduction in lumbosacral nerve roots in cauda equina lesions: a new diagnostic technique. *J Neurol Neurosurg Psychiatry.* 1986;49:808-816.

314. Swash M, Snooks SJ, Charmers DHK. Parity as a factor in incontinence in multiple sclerosis. *Arch Neurol.* 1987;44:504-508.

315. Swash M, Snooks SJ, Henry MM. Unifying concept of pelvic floor disorders and incontinence. *J R Soc Med.* 1985;78:906-911.

316. Tackmann W, Porst H, Van Ahlen H. Bulbocavernosus reflex latencies and somatosensory evoked potentials after pudendal nerve stimulation in the diagnosis of impotence. *J Neurol.* 1988;235:219-225.

317. Tammela TLJ, Heiskari MJ, Lukkarinen OA. Voiding dysfunction and urodynamic findings in patients with cervical spondylotic spinal stenosis compared with severity of the disease. *Br J Urol.* 1992;70:144-148.

318. Thal LJ, Grundman M, Klauber MR. Dementia: characteristics of a referral population and factors associated with progression. *Neurology.* 1988;38:1083-1090.

319. Therapeutics and Technology Assessment Subcommittee of the American Academy of Neurology. Assessment: neurological evaluation of male sexual dysfunction. *Neurology.* 1995;45:2287-2292.

320. Thiry AJ, Deltenre PF. Neurophysiological assessment of the central motor pathway to the external urethral sphincter in man. *Br J Urol.* 1989;63:515-519.

321. Toppercer A, Tetreault JP. Compliance of the bladder: an attempt to establish normal values. *Urology.* 1979;14:204.

322. Tsuchida S, Noto H, Yamaguchi O, Itoh M. Urodynamic studies on hemiplegic patients after cerebrovascular accident. *Urology.* 1983;21:315-318.

323. Valji K, Bookstein JJ. Diagnosis of arteriogenic impotence: efficacy of duplex sonography as a screening tool. *AJR.* 1993;160:65-69.

324. van Waalwijk van Doorn ES, Gommer ED. Ambulatory urodynamics. *Curr Opin Obstet Gynecol.* 1995;7:378-381.

325. Varma JS, Fidas A, McInnes A, et al. Neurophysiological abnormalities in genuine female stress urinary incontinence. *Br J Obstet Gynaecol.* 1988;95:705-710.

326. Velcek D, Sniderman KW, Vaughan ED, et al. Penile flow index utilizing a Doppler pulse wave analysis to identify penile vascular insufficiency. *J Urol.* 1980;123:669-673.

327. Venkatesh S, Bauer SB, Dyro FM, Shefner JM. Spared sacral function in patients with complete thoracolumbar myelodysplasia. *Muscle Nerve.* 1994;17:1213-1214.

328. Versi E. Discriminant analysis of urethral pressure profilometry data for the diagnosis of genuine stress incontinence. *Br J Obstet Gynaecol.* 1990;97:251-259.

329. Vertosick F Jr, Sekhar L. Adult aqueductal stenosis presenting as double incontinence: a case report with magnetic resonance imaging. *Surg Neurol.* 1989;31:387-389.

330. Virag R, Frydman D, Legnam M, Virag H. Intracavernous injection of papaverine as a diagnostic and therapeutic method in erectile failure. *Angiology.* 1984;35:79-87.

331. Vodusek DB. Pudendal SEP and bulbocavernosus reflex in women. *Electroencephalogr Clin Neurophysiol.* 1990;77:134-136.

332. Vodusek DB. Evoked potential testing. *Urol Clin North Am.* 1996;23:427-446.

333. Vodusek DB. Electromyogram: evoked sensory and motor potentials in neurourology. *Neurophysiol Clin.* 1997;27:204-210.

334. Vodusek DB, Janko M. The bulbocavernosus reflex: a single motor neuron study. *Brain.* 1990;113:813-820.

335. Vodusek DB, Janko M, Lokar J. Direct and reflex responses in perineal muscles on electrical stimulation. *J Neurol Neurosurg Psychiatry.* 1983;46:67-71.

336. Vodusek DB, Light KL. The "external urethral sphincter." *Neurol Urodyn.* 1983;2:193-200.

337. Vodusek DB, Ravnik-Oblak M, Oblak C. Pudendal versus limb nerve electrophysiological abnormalities in diabetics with erectile dysfunction. *Int J Impot Res.* 1993;5:37-42.

338. Wagner G, Gerstenberg T, Levin RJ. Electrical activity of corpus cavernosum during flaccidity and erection of the human penis: a new diagnostic method? *J Urol.* 1989;142:723-725.

339. Wagner TH, Hu T-W. Economic costs of urinary incontinence in 1995. *Urology.* 1998;51:355-361.

340. Wasserman MD, Pollack CP, Spielman AJ, Weitzman ED. Theoretical and technical problems in the measurement of nocturnal penile tumescence for the differential diagnosis of impotence. *Psychosom Med.* 1980;42:575-585.

341. Watanabe T, Vaccaro AR, Kumon H, et al. High incidence of occult neurogenic bladder dysfunction in neurologically intact patients with thoracolumbar spinal injuries. *J Urol.* 1998;159:965-968.

342. Webster GD, El-Mahroudy A, Stone AR, et al. The urological evaluation and management of patients with myelodysplasia. *Br J Urol.* 1986;58:205-209.

343. Wenning GK, Shlomo YB, Magalhaes M, et al. Clinical features and natural history of multiple system atrophy. *Brain.* 1994;117:835-845.

344. Wheeler JS, Canning JR. Voiding dysfunction in Shy-Drager syndrome. *J Urol.* 1985;134:362-363.

345. Wheeler JS, Siroky MB, Pavlakis AJ, et al. The changing neurourologic pattern of multiple sclerosis. *J Urol.* 1983;130:1123-1126.

346. Wheeler JS, Walter JW. Acute urologic management of the patient with spinal cord injury. *Urol Clin North Am.* 1993;20:403-411.

347. Woodside JR, Crawford ED. Urodynamic features of pelvic plexus injury. *J Urol.* 1980;124:657-658.

348. Yalla SV, Andriole GL. Vesicourethral dysfunction following pelvic visceral ablative surgery. *J Urol.* 1984;132:503-509.

349. Yang CC, Bradley WE, Berger RE. The effect of pharmacologic erection on the dorsal nerve of the penis. *Muscle Nerve.* 1997;20:1439-1444.

350. Yarnitsky D, Sprecher E, Barilan Y, Vardi Y. Corpus cavernosum electromyogram: spontaneous and evoked electrical activities. *J Urol.* 1995;153:653-654.

351. Yasuda K, Yamanishi T, Hattori T, et al. Lower urinary tract dysfunction in the anterior spinal artery syndrome. *J Urol.* 1993;150:1182-1184.

352. Young-Chol P, Esa A, Sugiyama T, et al. Sympathetic skin response: a new test to diagnose ejaculatory dysfunction. *J Urol.* 1988;139:539-541.

353. Yu GW, Schwab FJ, Melograna FS, et al. Preoperative and postoperative dynamic cavernosography and cavernosometry: objective assessment of venous ligation for impotence. *J Urol.* 1992;147:618-622.

354. Zarola F, Bernardi G, Traversa R, et al. Analysis of sympathetic skin responses in a group of health subjects and in patients affected by sphincter disorders and impotence. *Funct Neurol.* 1991;6:293-298.

# Section V

# NEUROMEDICAL DISORDERS

# 24

# Syncope

*David G. Benditt*

Syncope is a syndrome, the defining clinical characteristics of which are a relatively sudden transient loss of both consciousness and postural tone, with subsequent spontaneous, complete, and usually prompt recovery.[16,86] Pathophysiologically, syncope results from a self-limited diminution of cerebral nutrient flow, most often the direct result of a temporary loss of systemic arterial perfusion pressure.[16] Typically, syncopal episodes are brief. Complete loss of consciousness rarely lasts longer than 10 or 20 seconds. In some forms of syncope there may be an extended premonitory period in which various symptoms (e.g., lightheadedness, weakness, visual disturbance) offer warning of an impending syncopal event. Often, however, loss of consciousness seems to occur without warning. Recovery from syncope is generally accompanied by almost immediate restoration of appropriate behavior and orientation. Retrograde amnesia has been thought to be uncommon, although loss of recollection of immediate preceding symptoms may be more common than previously believed, especially in older individuals. Furthermore, particularly in the case of vasovagal faints, the postrecovery period may be marked by an extended period of fatigue or listlessness lasting many hours.

It is crucial that true syncope be differentiated from other conditions that may be associated with real or apparent loss of consciousness, such as seizures, sleep disturbances, accidents, and some psychiatric conditions. Nevertheless, syncope alone is an inadequate diagnosis. Establishing the underlying cause of syncope is critical in order to provide direction for effective treatment and offering prognostic insight for patients and their families. The physician must always address this question: "Is the diagnosis sufficiently certain to permit confident and effective treatment, whether by reassurance, drugs, devices, or combinations of all of these?"[12]

This chapter provides an overview of (1) the principal clinical conditions associated with syncope, (2) a strategy for evaluation of the patient with syncope, and (3) appropriate directions for treatment of the most important conditions causing syncope. The primary focus is the neurally mediated syncopal syndromes, syncope associated with orthostatic and dysautonomic disturbances of blood pressure control, syncope resulting from various bradyarrhythmias and tachyarrhythmias, and syncope associated with structural cardiac and cardiovascular disease. Syncopal and syncope-like conditions associated with cerebrovascular, neurologic, and psychiatric conditions are also noted but are not treated in detail.

## CAUSES OF SYNCOPE

Most studies examining the frequency with which syncope occurs have comprised relatively small numbers of subjects and have focused on select populations, such as the military or patients referred to tertiary care medical centers for evaluation. Consequently, the true incidence of syncope in the general population remains uncertain. Nevertheless, it is commonly stated that syncope accounts for approximately 3% of emergency department visits and from 1% to 6% of general hospital admissions in the United States.[39,62,102] In the Framingham study[90] the occurrence of at least one syncopal event was reported to have occurred in approximately 3% of men and 3.5% of women, with the prevalence of syncope increasing in older age groups. Additionally, among patients who have experienced syncope, recurrence of symptoms was reported to be very common. Several reports suggest that syncope recurrences are to be expected in about 30% of individuals.[11,51,90]

There are many potential causes of syncope, and the diagnostic problem in a given patient may be complicated by the fact that more than one cause often contributes to the clinical picture. For example, in patients with valvular aortic stenosis, transient systemic hypotension may be due to any combination of the following conditions: restriction of cardiac output by a narrowed orifice, inappropriate or inadequate vascular reflex responsiveness, increased tendency to cardiac arrhythmias, and poor left ventricular function. Similarly, in individuals with paroxysmal tachyarrhythmias (e.g., paroxysmal supraventricular tachycardia, paroxysmal atrial fibrillation), vascular reflex responsiveness may be as critical as heart rate and the status of left ventricular function are in determining susceptibility to syncope. Nevertheless, to derive a manageable strategy for evaluation of the syncope patient, it is helpful to categorize the apparent causes of syncope into a number of major diagnostic groups. These groups are based on what appears to be the most relevant clinical finding in each patient. To this end, the following discussion provides a working classification of the causes of syncope, with prioritization based on the approximate frequency with which they occur in clinical practice (Table 24–1).

---

**TABLE 24–1. Syncope: Diagnostic Classification**

**Neurally Mediated Syncopal Syndromes**
Vasovagal faint
Carotid sinus syncope
Cough syncope and related disorders
Gastrointestinal, pelvic, or urologic origin

**Orthostatic, Dysautonomic, and Drug-Induced Conditions**
Idiopathic orthostatic hypotension
Shy-Drager syndrome
Diabetic neuropathy
Drug-induced orthostasis

**Primary Cardiac Arrhythmias**
Sinus node dysfunction (including bradycardia/tachycardia syndrome)
Atrioventricular (AV) conduction system disease
   Drug-induced AV block
Paroxysmal supraventricular and ventricular tachycardias
   Drug-induced tachyarrhythmias (proarrhythmia)
Implanted device (pacemaker, implantable cardioverter-defibrillators [ICD]) malfunction

**Structural Cardiovascular or Cardiopulmonary Disease**
Cardiac valvular disease/ischemia
Acute myocardial infarction
Obstructive cardiomyopathy
Subclavian steal syndrome
Pericardial disease/tamponade
Pulmonary embolus
Pulmonary hypertension

**Cerebrovascular, Neurologic, and Psychiatric Disturbances (Syncope or Syncope-Like)**
Vascular steal syndromes
Seizure disorders
Panic attacks
Hysteria

**Miscellaneous Syncope-Like Conditions**
Hyperventilation (hypocapnia)
Hypoglycemia
Volume depletion (Addison's disease)
Hypoxemia

---

**TABLE 24–2. Neurally Mediated Syncopal Syndromes**

Emotional syncope (common or vasovagal faint, malignant vasovagal faint)
Carotid sinus syncope
Cough, sneeze syncope
Exercise, postexercise variant
Gastrointestinal stimulation swallow syncope, defecation syncope
Glossopharyngeal neuralgia
Postmicturition syncope
Raised intrathoracic pressure, airway stimulation, brass wind instrument
   playing, weight lifting

---

## NEURALLY MEDIATED SYNCOPE

The neurally mediated syncopal syndromes (Table 24–2) refer to a group of apparently related disorders in which symptomatic systemic hypotension is principally the result of inappropriate neural reflex activity. In some cases syncope is the result of severe parasympathetically induced cardioinhibition (i.e., heart rate slowing) (Fig. 24–1). The outcome may be prolonged asystole, marked sinus or junctional bradycardia, or even paroxysmal atrioventricular (AV) block (see Fig. 24–1). In others, vascular dilation, believed to be primarily due to inappropriate withdrawal of sympathetic neural constrictor tone (i.e., vasodepressor component), is the prime mover causing systemic hypotension and loss of consciousness. In most cases, however, both bradycardia and vascular dilatation contribute in some measure to the hypotension and inadequate cerebral blood flow.[3,16,52,99]

Vasovagal faint and carotid sinus syndromes are the best known forms of neurally mediated syncope. Vasovagal faint is generally considered to be the most frequent of all causes of syncope in humans. Carotid sinus syndrome, although a well-known condition for many years,[4,104] possibly has been underappreciated as a cause of syncope and falls in older individuals.[84] Postmicturition syncope and cough syncope are probably the next most common forms of neurally mediated faints.

The vasovagal faint (also known as the common faint) may be triggered by any of a variety of factors. In the classic vasovagal faint, these include unpleasant sights, pain, extreme emotion, and prolonged standing. Consequently, circumstances surrounding a faint may lead to suspicion of vasovagal syncope as the cause. However, most informed practitioners have come to realize that the so-called classic features of vasovagal faint are often either absent or not recollected. Therefore even a detailed medical history undertaken by an experienced professional may not provide a definitive diagnosis. In such cases additional testing is prudent. Tilt-table testing is the most important readily available supportive test.[3,15,16,52,99]

Carotid sinus syndrome is the second most common form of the neurally mediated syncopal syndromes.[4,104] However, it is often overlooked in clinical practice.[84] The occurrence of syncope or unexplained falls, especially in older persons, should lead to consideration of carotid sinus syndrome. From a diagnostic perspective, the condition is considered to be confirmed when firm linear carotid sinus massage (one side at a time) reproduces symptoms in conjunction with a period of asystole, paroxysmal AV block, or a marked drop (usually >50 mm Hg systolic) in systemic arterial pressure.[4]

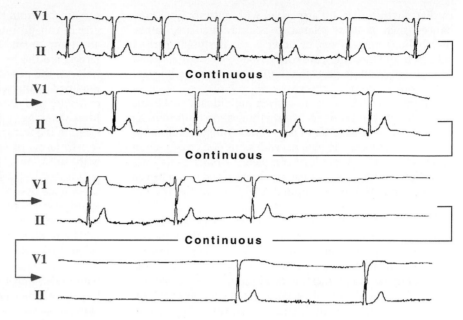

**FIGURE 24–1.** ECG tracings depicting onset of vasovagal spell in a 20-year-old young woman. Recording shows patient to be in sinus rhythm (*top panel*). Progressive sinus bradycardia ensues followed by a prolonged asystolic spell. Return of heart rhythm is noted as a junctional rhythm (*bottom panel*). Patient recovered spontaneously.

The carotid sinus massage procedure is best undertaken with the patient in the upright position and gently secured to a tilt table. Continuous arterial pressure (not sphygmomanometer measurements) and electrocardiographic (ECG) recordings should be obtained throughout the procedure. The test is usually contraindicated if a carotid bruit is present or if the patient has symptoms suggestive of transient ischemic attacks. In the absence of symptom reproduction, a pause in the cardiac rhythm of 5 seconds or longer is generally accepted as sufficient to support the diagnosis.

Postmicturition syncope and cough syncope are the next most frequently encountered forms of the neurally mediated faint. They are usually diagnosed by history alone. However, individuals with susceptibility to cough syncope may be identified in the laboratory. Such cases tend to be characterized not only by the magnitude of cough-induced blood pressure decline but also by the subsequent delayed blood pressure recovery after cough.

## ORTHOSTATIC, DYSAUTONOMIC, AND DRUG-INDUCED CAUSES OF SYNCOPE

Movement from the supine or sitting position to the standing position is often accompanied by a transient sensation of light-headedness and near-faint, even in entirely healthy individuals. The more abrupt the postural change, especially if it occurs in the setting of a concomitant illness or relative dehydration, the more likely the development of syncopal symptoms. Most often, the tendency to faintness passes and no problems arise. Occasionally, however, frank syncope may occur. The elderly or less physically fit person or those who are volume depleted because of exposure to hot environments or inadequate fluid intake are at greatest risk. Iatrogenic factors are also important contributors to the tendency for postural faints. Diuretics, angiotensin-converting enzyme (ACE) inhibitors, nitrates, vasodilators, sympatholytic antihypertensives, and beta-adrenergic blockers are among the most commonly prescribed offending agents. Careful documentation of the patient's drug history is an important aspect of the syncope evaluation.

Neuropathies associated with certain chronic diseases (e.g., diabetes) or certain commonly abused "toxic" agents (e.g., alcohol) are among the more common identifiable contributing factors in patients with recurrent orthostatic dizziness and syncope. Other forms of autonomic nervous system dysfunction are perhaps less common, but their importance may be underappreciated because they are readily overlooked by nonspecialists. Some of the more important of these conditions include acute sympathetic neural dysfunction following infection (e.g., Guillain-Barré syndrome), multiple system atrophy (e.g., Shy-Drager syndrome), and familial dysautonomia (Riley-Day syndrome).[9,58,59,103] In this regard, Low et al[59] reviewed their experience with 155 patients referred for assessment of suspected orthostatic hypotension. Findings revealed that among the most severely affected symptomatic patients (n = 90, mean age 64 years), pure autonomic failure accounted for 33%; multisystem atrophy, 26%; and autonomic/diabetic neuropathy, 31%.

Tilt-table testing may be helpful for identifying patients susceptible to syncope associated with orthostatic hypotension. However, protocols for such testing and diagnostic laboratory criteria have not yet been established. Further, the specific identification of various forms of autonomic failure requires a level of expertise beyond those available in most tilt-table testing laboratories. Greater routine collaboration between those physicians engaged in routine tilt-table testing and neurologists knowledgeable in autonomic function studies would seem to be essential for establishing testing protocols.

## PRIMARY CARDIAC ARRHYTHMIAS

Primary cardiac arrhythmias are those heart rhythm disturbances that occur as a consequence of underlying cardiac conduction system disease, anomalous electrical connections (e.g., Wolff-Parkinson-White syndrome), or myocardial disease of any cause. Arrhythmias initiated by or aggravated by commonly used drugs are often included in this category as a matter of convenience, although they may well merit a separate category. Conversely, abnormalities of cardiac rhythm that are associated with autonomic disturbances, such as those related to neurally mediated faints, metabolic derangements, or other organ dysfunction (e.g., subarachnoid bleeding), are considered to be secondary and are incorporated as part of the discussion of the relevant condition.

Loss of consciousness in a given individual may be due to bradyarrhythmias or tachyarrhythmias, or both. Among the bradyarrhythmias, the most common offenders are sinus arrest or sinus pauses in patients with sinus node dysfunction and new-onset, high-grade or complete AV block in individuals with disease of the cardiac conduction system. In regard to tachyarrhythmias, sustained hypotensive ventricular tachycardia is the greatest threat. This condition tends to occur most often in the setting of a new myocardial ischemic event. However, it is also frequently a recurrent phenomenon in patients with chronic ischemic heart disease or cardiomyopathy. If sustained and unstable, ventricular tachycardia can rapidly and unpredictably evolve into a life-threatening situation. Consequently, although affected patients may from time to time present with dizziness or syncope, they need to be evaluated as potential candidates for cardiac arrest. Less common, although not to be disregarded, abrupt onset of paroxysmal supraventricular tachycardia or atrial fibrillation can also be associated with syncope. In these cases, symptoms are typically manifest at the onset of the arrhythmia, before there has been adequate time for vascular tone to adjust to the new circumstance. Once again, elderly and infirm patients are at greatest risk.

Sinus node dysfunction, or sick sinus syndrome, is common, especially among the elderly.[19,49,88] The clinical picture may range from the patient being essentially asymptomatic to having life-threatening bradyarrhythmias or tachyarrhythmias (Fig. 24–2). Often, however, the patient's complaints are relatively nonspecific (e.g., fatigue, light-headedness). A high level of clinical suspicion is necessary to identify the real cause of symptoms in such patients. In terms of the relationship between arrhythmic manifestations and patient complaints, it is often impossible to ascertain by clinical judgment alone whether the problem is due to excessively slow (sinus bradycardia, sinus pauses, sinoatrial exit block) or fast (most often paroxysmal or persistent atrial fibrillation or atrial flutter) heart beating. In fact, many times both kinds of arrhythmias are participating.

The syndrome of sinus node dysfunction also places patients at higher risk of systemic embolism. Emboli, derived presumably from stasis and perhaps a greater than usual degree of clot-promoting endocardial disease in the atria, can affect any organ. The most frequently recognized embolic targets are the heart (e.g., coronary artery embolism), the kidneys, the peripheral vascular tree, and the brain. When the brain is affected, the complications may be overt stroke or subtle and slowly progressive disturbances of cerebral function, or both. Embolism is a special concern if atrial fibrillation is a feature of the arrhythmic picture.

In terms of syncope, the bradyarrhythmias associated with sinus node dysfunction appear to play the larger causative role. For instance, among 56 patients with manifest sinus node dysfunction in the report by Rubenstein et al,[88] syncope was a principal finding in 25 patients (45%) and presyncopal symptoms were present in an additional 15 (27%). In 80% of the patients, bradyarrhythmias were considered to be the responsible rhythm disturbance.

Sinus node dysfunction is most often closely associated with underlying structural disturbances in the atria (e.g., fibrosis, chamber enlargement). However, other factors, including autonomic nervous system influences, cardioactive drugs, and metabolic disturbances, also often contribute. Drug effects are particularly important to consider when evaluating such patients. Beta-adrenergic receptor blockers, calcium channel blockers, membrane-active antiarrhythmics, the antiepileptic drug carbamazepine (Tegretol), and less commonly used agents such as lithium are well known to impair sinus node function.[14,19,56] With regard to antiarrhythmic agents, class 1C drugs (e.g., flecainide, encainide) and amiodarone exert powerful effects on slowing the rate of sinus node depolarization, especially in the setting of preexisting disease. Thus marked sinus bradycardia and sinus pauses should be looked for when these drugs are used. Similarly, in the setting of an already diseased conduction system, these drugs may induce transient or complete AV block. If the bradyarrhythmia is sufficiently severe, syncope may be the presenting feature.

Disturbances of cardiac conduction are widely recognized as being among the more common causes of syncope and dizziness. These disturbances may range from relatively innocent prolongation of the time it takes for the atrial electrical impulse to reach the ventricle (PR interval >200 ms, first-degree AV block), to intermittent conduction block (second-degree AV block), to complete conduction failure (third-degree AV block).[65,78,87] A complete review of these disturbances and their implications is beyond the scope of

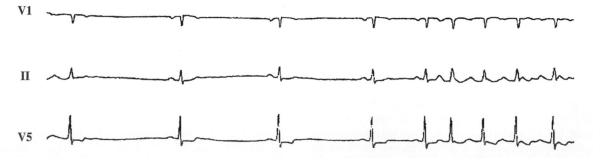

**FIGURE 24–2.** ECG recordings $V_1$, II, and $V_5$ from an elderly patient with sinus node dysfunction. Patient presented with spells of light-headedness. ECG recording shows transition from marked sinus bradycardia to primary atrial tachycardia. In such a patient, symptoms of light-headedness could be due to either of these dysrhythmias.

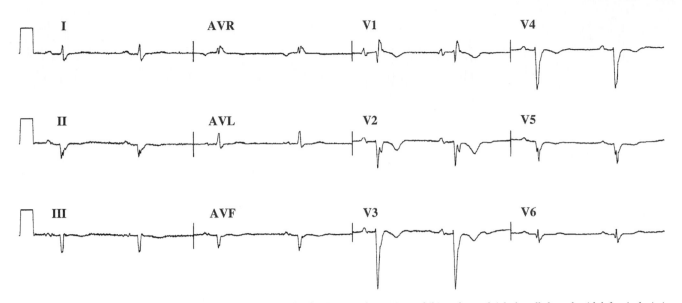

**FIGURE 24–3.** This 12-lead ECG reveals a long PR interval and wide QRS complex. Patient exhibits a form of right bundle branch with left axis deviation, indicating bifascicular block. Patients who present with syncope or dizziness and ECGs of this type may be experiencing either transient high-grade AV block or ventricular tachycardia due to severe underlying structural heart disease. Unless ECG documentation is obtained while symptoms are present, an invasive electrophysiologic study may be required.

this discussion, but a few key points are worthy of attention here. Isolated first-degree AV block is not usually associated with sufficient hemodynamic compromise to cause syncope. However, in the presence of a wide QRS complex, first-degree AV block may be a clue to the presence of far more severe underlying conduction system disease (Fig. 24–3). Similarly, second-degree AV block of the Wenckebach type (Mobitz type I) would not be expected to cause syncope since only one cardiac cycle is "dropped" every so often. Once again, however, if Wenckebach block occurs in the setting of a wide QRS complex, it should raise suspicion that more severe conduction system may be present. In general, it is the more severe forms of acquired AV block (i.e., Mobitz type II block, high-grade, and complete AV block) that are likely to result in syncopal symptoms. These rhythms tend to be associated with prolonged periods of bradycardia and cause the heart to become dependent on exceedingly slow and unreliable subsidiary pacemaker sites. The outcome is a variable period of diminished cardiac output that leads to inadequate cerebral blood flow.

Syncope in patients with various forms of bundle-branch block or fascicular blocks on their ECG presents a special problem. In such cases, one should not simply assume that transient high-grade AV block is at fault. Ventricular tachycardia is also an important concern. Electrophysiologic studies of the heart can help to identify the relative likelihood of conduction failure vs. susceptibility to ventricular tachyarrhythmias (Fig. 24–4). Specifically, the risk of conduction block as the cause increases the longer the duration of the HV interval (normal range 35 to 55 ms) and is particularly great for HV intervals >100 ms.[31,91] On the other hand, if cardiac stimulation reproducibly initiates a monomorphic ventricular tachycardia, the role of tachyarrhythmia as a cause of symptoms increases in likelihood.[31] Consequently, invasive electrophysiologic testing is probably indicated to address this concern in individual patients.

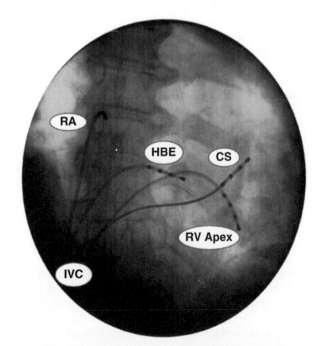

**FIGURE 24–4.** Fluoroscopy image depicting typical positioning of electrode catheters in a patient undergoing invasive cardiac electrophysiologic study. Spine is in center of the image posteriorly. Right ventricular apex is at right side of image at approximately 5 o'clock. Right atrium is on left side of the image at approximately 10 o'clock. An electrode catheter with multiple poles is placed in right atrium for pacing and recording. A second electrode catheter can be seen at approximately the right ventricular apex. A third catheter (approximately 3 o'clock) is within the coronary sinus. (NOTE: this image has been enhanced.) A fourth electrode catheter with four electrodes is positioned in middle of image at approximately the position of the His bundle for recording signals from the cardiac conduction system. Positioning of electrode catheters for electrophysiologic study varies, depending upon the specific objectives of the study. Nonetheless this image represents a relatively typical scenario.

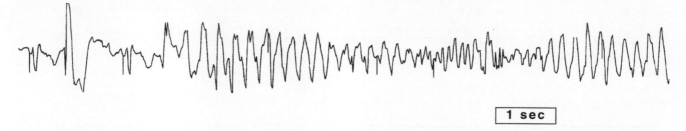

1 sec

**FIGURE 24–5.** ECG tracing depicts typical example of torsades de pointes ventricular tachycardia. This condition may be associated with congenital long QT syndrome or, more commonly, drug-induced long QT syndrome. Patients frequently present with dizziness or syncope. Life-threatening ventricular fibrillation can also occur.

Sustained ventricular tachyarrhythmias have been reported to be responsible for syncope in up to 20% of patients referred for electrophysiologic assessment.[26,67,100] Risk factors favoring ventricular tachyarrhythmias as the cause of syncope include underlying structural heart disease, evident conduction system disease, and congenital or drug-induced long QT syndrome. The tachycardia rate, status of left ventricular function, and the efficiency of peripheral vascular reactivity determine whether the arrhythmia is of sufficient severity to account for syncopal symptoms. Nonsustained ventricular tachycardia, on the other hand, presents a more challenging diagnostic problem in assessing the patient with syncope. Such a finding is common during ambulatory ECG monitoring, especially in patients with structural heart disease. As a result, documentation of nonsustained ventricular tachycardia in the absence of symptoms is not usually very helpful. Often, invasive electrophysiologic testing is recommended to determine whether the individual is susceptible to sustained tachycardia episodes and whether he or she can tolerate them hemodynamically.

Drug-induced symptomatic bradyarrhythmias were alluded to earlier as potential, and all too common, causes of syncope. However, drug-induced tachycardias, especially ventricular tachyarrhythmias, are perhaps even more common and more serious. Virtually all antiarrhythmic agents can result in unfortunate proarrhythmic effects. Perhaps the best-known example of this phenomenon is syncope due to torsades de pointes in the setting of class 1A antiarrhythmics (Fig. 24–5), especially quinidine (formerly known as "quinidine syncope").[46,92] Class 1A antiarrhythmics (e.g., quinidine, disopyramide) and class 3 agents (sotalol, N-acetyl procainamide) tend to prolong ventricular repolarization (usually recognized in terms of prolongation of the QT interval on the ECG). This pharmacologic action is well known to increase the propensity for inducing torsades de pointes (an important cause of syncope but also a rhythm that can induce ventricular fibrillation). However, many other drugs have a similar propensity (Table 24–3). Further, induction of sustained monomorphic ventricular tachycardia is also a well-recognized proarrhythmic phenomenon, especially with drugs that markedly slow cardiac conduction, such as class 1C agents (e.g., flecainide, encainide). Drug-induced aggravation of atrial arrhythmias probably also occurs but is less readily recognized.

The supraventricular tachycardias have been reported to be the cause of syncope in approximately 15% of patients referred for electrophysiologic evaluation[26] (Fig. 24–6). The rate of the tachycardia, the volume status and posture of the patient at onset of the arrhythmia, the presence of associated or structural cardiopulmonary disease, and the integrity of reflex peripheral vascular compensation are key factors determining whether hypotension of sufficient severity to cause syncope occurs.[55]

## STRUCTURAL CARDIOVASCULAR OR CARDIOPULMONARY DISEASE

A medical history and physical examination, augmented by a chest x-ray examination and echocardiographic assessment, are usually sufficient to determine the presence of clinically important structural heart or cardiopulmonary disease. In such cases the most common cause of syncope is that which occurs in conjunction with acute myocardial ischemia or infarction. Other acute med-

**TABLE 24–3. Selected Common Pharmacologic Agents Associated With Torsades de Pointes Ventricular Tachycardia**

**Antiarrhythmic Drugs (Prolongation of the QT Interval)**
Quinidine
Procainamide
Disopyramide
N-Acetyl procainamide
Sotalol
Amiodarone

**Vasodilators**
Bepridil
Lidoflazine

**Antipsychotic and Tricyclic Antidepressant Drugs**
Chlorpromazine
Thioridazine
Haloperidol
Imipramine
Amitriptyline
Nortriptyline

**Antibiotics**
Erythromycin
Pentamidine

**Antihistamines (Used in Conjunction With Hepatic Disease or Ketoconazole Therapy)**
Terfenadine
Astemizole

**Serotonin Antagonists (Usually Used in Conjunction With Hypokalemia or Bradycardia)**
Ketanserin
Zimeldine

**Poisons**
Arsenic
Organophosphorous insecticides

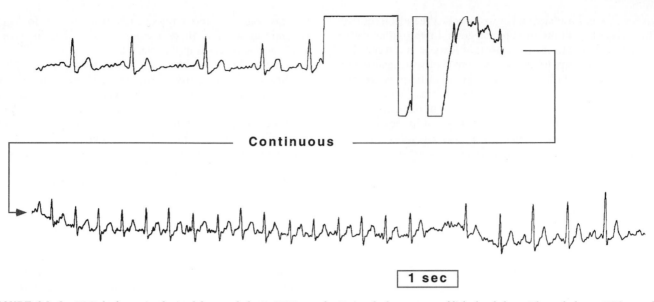

**Continuous**

**1 sec**

**FIGURE 24–6.** ECG rhythm strip obtained from ambulatory ECG recorder. Patient had symptoms of light-headedness. The ambulatory ECG recorder shows transition from sinus rhythm (*top strip at left*) to rapid narrow QRS tachycardia. Later electrophysiologic study demonstrated this patient to be susceptible to paroxysmal supraventricular tachycardia due to reentry within atrioventricular node.

ical conditions associated with syncope include pulmonary embolism and pericardial tamponade. As noted earlier, however, the basis of syncope in these conditions is multifactorial, including both the hemodynamic impact of the specific lesion and the neurally mediated reflex effects (the latter being especially important in the setting of acute ischemic events).[16]

Syncope may also occur and be a presenting feature in conditions in which there is fixed or dynamic obstruction to ventricular outflow (e.g., aortic stenosis, hypertrophic obstructive cardiomyopathy, pulmonary hypertension) or inflow (e.g., atrial myxoma, severe myocardial restriction).[16] In such cases symptoms are often provoked by physical exertion, but they may also develop if an otherwise benign arrhythmia should occur (e.g., atrial fibrillation). The basis for the faint may be in part inadequate blood flow due to the mechanical obstruction. However, especially in the case of valvular aortic stenosis, ventricular mechanoreceptor-mediated bradycardia and vasodilatation are thought to be important contributors.[16,48] Other structural disturbances that on rare occasion precipitate syncope include subclavian steal syndrome, severe carotid artery disease, left ventricular inflow obstruction in patients with mitral stenosis, right ventricular outflow obstruction, and right-to-left shunting secondary to pulmonic stenosis or pulmonary hypertension.

Occasionally, primary transient disturbances of cerebrovascular blood flow may initiate a true syncopal spell. For example, it is thought, based on transcranial echo Doppler studies, that cerebrovascular spasm could initiate a sufficiently long period of cerebral hypoperfusion to cause syncope.[42,77] If this were in fact to occur, certain individuals would experience true syncope despite being normotensive in the systemic circulation. Currently, patients who appear to faint in the absence of systemic hypotension (and in whom seizures or severe metabolic disturbances are not thought to be relevant) are currently more often than not classified as psychogenic fainters.

## CEREBROVASCULAR, NEUROLOGIC, AND PSYCHIATRIC DISTURBANCES

Cerebrovascular disease and neurologic disturbances (e.g., seizure disorders) are rarely the cause of true syncope.[50,86] More often these conditions result in a clinical picture that may be mistaken for syncope. However, on rare occasions certain seizure types (particularly temporal lobe seizures) may so closely mimic (or induce) neurally mediated reflex bradycardia and hypotension that differentiation from true syncope is difficult. Nonneurologic specialists are usually ill equipped to make such a distinction, and diagnostic testing must revert to the neurologist.

A number of important features may help the practitioner differentiate seizures from true syncope: (1) seizures tend to be positionally independent, whereas syncope is most commonly associated with upright posture; (2) many seizures are preceded by an aura that, if present, tends to be distinctly different from the premonitory symptoms accompanying some forms of syncope; (3) seizures are more often immediately accompanied by convulsive activity and incontinence, whereas abnormal motor activity, if present in the patient with syncope, is less severe, and incontinence is unusual[41]; and (4) seizures are typically followed by a confusional state, whereas relatively prompt restoration of mental state is more common with syncope.

Syncope may also be mimicked by anxiety attacks, hysteria, or other psychiatric disturbances.[57] Anxiety attacks are frequently associated with hyperventilation and hypocapnia. Hysteria, however, characteristically occurs in the presence of onlookers with no marked alterations of heart rate, systemic pressure, or skin color noted. Currently, however, despite the apparent frequency of these conditions in patients referred for evaluation of syncope,[57] they must be considered only after other conditions have been carefully excluded.

## MISCELLANEOUS CAUSES

Metabolic and endocrine abnormalities are rarely the cause of true syncope. Severe hyperventilation resulting in hypocapnia and transient alkalosis may be the most frequent syncopelike condition in this category. In the latter case, marked anxiety is likely an important feature, and it may be difficult to differentiate from some types of vasovagal faint. More often, metabolic and endocrine disturbances are responsible for confusional states or behavioral disturbances. Retrospectively, however, making a clear-cut distinction between such symptoms and syncope may not be possible by history alone. As a rule, unlike true syncope, conditions such as diabetic coma or severe hypoxia or hypercapnia do not resolve in the absence of active therapeutic intervention.

## DIAGNOSTIC EVALUATION OF THE PATIENT WITH SYNCOPE

The ultimate objective of diagnostic testing in the patient with syncope is establishment of a strong correlation between symptoms and detected abnormalities. Specific goals are to obtain

1. A confident assessment of the basis of the faint
2. An estimation of the likelihood of symptom recurrence
3. An understanding of the patient's overall prognosis (including potential for injury, economic loss, and mortality)

Obtaining a detailed medical history, including as much information from bystander witnesses as possible, is always the first step in the diagnostic evaluation. Thereafter the physical examination and certain basic screening tests (ECG,

echocardiogram, chest x-ray examination) should focus on ascertaining whether there is evidence of underlying structural cardiac or cardiopulmonary disease. At that stage the need for further specialized diagnostic testing will vary, depending on the certainty of the initial clinical impression, the number and frequency of syncopal events reported, the occurrence of injury or accident, family history of syncope or sudden death, and potential risks associated with the individual's occupation (e.g., pilot, commercial vehicle driver, sign painter) or avocation (e.g., mountain climber, skier, swimmer) (Fig. 24–7).

As a rule, if structural heart disease is deemed to be absent by the initial screening evaluation outlined earlier, selected autonomic function assessment (in particular, tilt-table testing and evaluation of response to carotid sinus massage and, possibly, induced cough) is the most productive next step. On the other hand, if abnormal cardiac findings are identified, their functional significance should be characterized by hemodynamic or angiographic assessment. Furthermore, since cardiac arrhythmias are a common cause of syncope in patients with structural cardiac disease, it is appropriate to assess the patient's susceptibility to tachyarrhythmias and bradyarrhythmias by selected noninvasive studies, such as ambulatory heart rhythm recordings, signal-averaged ECG (SAECG), and possibly heart rate variability analysis. If necessary, invasive electrophysiologic testing may also be appropriate. If at this stage the diagnosis remains in doubt, assessment of autonomic function, including tilt-table testing, would follow. Only infrequently should specialized neurologic studies be ordered early in the evaluation

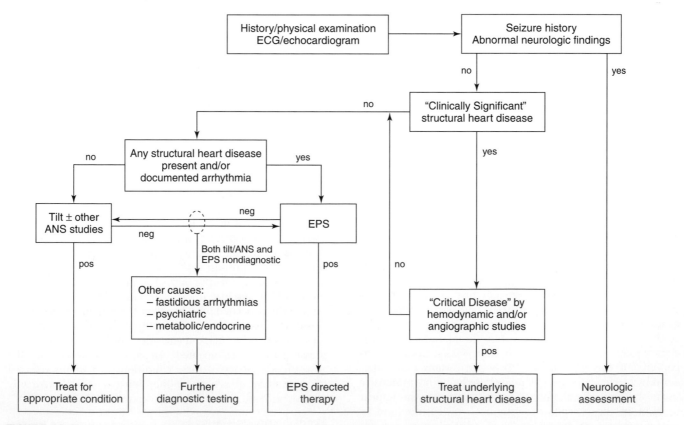

**FIGURE 24–7.** A strategy for evaluation of patients with syncope and dizziness. Presence of structural heart disease represents an important factor in determining the direction of subsequent diagnostic studies.

for syncope. Indications for such testing would include a medical history suggestive of a seizure disorder or evidence that the patient had exhibited fixed or transient abnormal neurologic signs.[41,50]

## NONINVASIVE CARDIOVASCULAR STUDIES

Cardiac arrhythmias are not only a frequent cause of syncope, but their importance is magnified by virtue of both their potential adverse prognosis and their ability to be cured or effectively suppressed by modern treatment techniques (e.g., antiarrhythmic drug therapy, transcatheter ablation, implantable pacing and defibrillation systems). Consequently, it is incumbent upon the physician to undertake a thorough search for symptomatic arrhythmia as part of syncope assessment, especially in patients with demonstrable structural heart disease.

Documentation of the cardiac rhythm during a spontaneous syncopal event is perhaps the most highly desirable evidence. If feasible at all, however, obtaining such documentation often necessitates prolonged ambulatory ECG monitoring by Holter or event recorders. In the most difficult cases, the use of a recently approved implantable monitor (Reveal; Medtronic, Inc.) may permit extended cardiac monitoring to be undertaken much more conveniently (Fig. 24–8). Exercise testing is usually of limited use unless the syncopal events are clearly exertionally related by the history. However, in rare instances, exercise testing may permit detection of rate-dependent AV block, exertionally related tachyarrhythmias, or the exercise-associated variant of neurally mediated syncope.[16,25,89] Finally, although SAECG cannot provide direct evidence for the cause of syncope, such testing may be helpful if the result is "normal" because it tends to exclude susceptibility to ventricular tachyarrhythmias in patients with ischemic heart disease.[53] A positive SAECG, on the other hand, does not necessarily indicate that ventricular tachycardia is the cause of symptoms. In such cases, invasive cardiac electrophysiologic testing may be warranted.[1,29,32,46,53,57,69,97]

The echocardiogram, a mainstay of the contemporary cardiac evaluation, is a crucial part of the search for underlying structural heart disease in patients with syncope. Although it rarely provides a definitive basis for syncope, the echocardiogram may in some cases provide important clues. For example, hypertrophic obstructive cardiomyopathy, severe valvular aortic stenosis, an atrial myxoma, or anomalous origin of one or more coronary arteries may be detected. The history and physical examination alone might have missed these diagnoses entirely or underestimated their potential hemodynamic significance. Ultrasound techniques are also appropriately used to assess suspected vascular disturbances. Thus assessment of the carotid or subclavian system or of both may be appropriate in selected individuals presenting with syncopal symptoms.

## INVASIVE CLINICAL ELECTROPHYSIOLOGIC TESTING

Invasive electrophysiologic testing consists of the use of cardiac catheterization laboratory techniques to place specialized pacing and recording catheters at various sites within the cardiac chambers (see Fig. 24–4). Intracardiac recordings are used to assess the integrity of sinus node function and AV conduction. Pacing methods (including in-

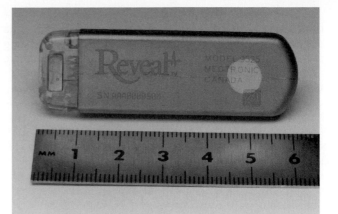

**FIGURE 24–8.** A small implantable event recorder for diagnosing difficult-to-detect rhythm disturbances. The device is placed under the skin in much the same way that a conventional pacemaker is implanted. A telemetry system is used to access the device memory and thereby retrieve stored ECG recordings. (Courtesy Medtronic Inc., Minneapolis, Minnesota.)

sertion of single or multiple timed premature beats) are used to evaluate susceptibility to atrial and ventricular tachyarrhythmias. In regard to arrhythmia induction, such studies exhibit a high specificity if the induced rhythm is reproducible, sustained, and monomorphic. Reproduction of patient symptoms is another key confirmatory step, although this may be achieved only if arrhythmia initiation is undertaken with the patient in an upright posture (usually using a tilt table during testing).

In the diagnostic assessment of the patient with syncope, invasive electrophysiologic studies are most helpful in individuals with underlying structural heart disease.[1,29,32,46,69,97] For example, in one review of the literature,[46] electrophysiologic testing was deemed to be successful in 71% of patients with structural cardiac disease, compared to 36% in patients without heart disease. However, care must be taken in interpreting the findings of these studies since both false-positive and false-negative results occur.[38]

## HEAD-UP TILT-TABLE TESTING, CAROTID SINUS MASSAGE, AND RELATED STUDIES

The neurally mediated syncopal syndromes, including the vasovagal faint, are often suspected based on presenting features of the faint or the circumstances in which it occurs. However, confirmation of the diagnosis may be valuable, especially when the history is not definitive. This is a particularly common problem in patients, particularly older ones, with vasovagal syncope.

To date, head-up tilt-table testing is the only diagnostic tool that has been subjected to sufficient clinical scrutiny to assess its effectiveness in the evaluation of susceptibility to vasovagal syncope. The methodology of the procedure is important and has been the subject of an American College of Cardiology–North American Society of Pacing and Electrophysiology expert consensus report.[15] In brief, testing should be carried out in a quiet, comfortable environment using continuous but unobtrusive heart rate and blood pressure monitoring. The preferred tilt angle is 70 to 80 degrees, using footboard support, for a maximum of 45 minutes.

Such testing, especially when undertaken in the absence of drugs, appears to discriminate well between symptomatic patients and asymptomatic control subjects.* When testing is undertaken with the aid of provocative pharmacologic agents (most often isoproterenol, but also edrophonium,[60] nitroglycerin,[83] or adenosine),[21,95] specificity is still quite acceptable and comparable to many other commonly used diagnostic tests in medicine and neurology. For example, Natale et al[76] found that tilt-table testing at 60, 70, and 80 degrees exhibited specificities of 92%, 92%, and 80%, respectively, when low doses of isoproterenol were used. In summary, there is very strong evidence to suggest that tilt-table testing at angles of 60 to 70 degrees, in the absence of pharmacological provocation, exhibits a specificity of approximately 90%. In the presence of pharmacologic provocation, test specificity may be reduced yet remain in a range that permits the test to be clinically useful. Quantitation of the sensitivity of tilt-table testing is more difficult since there is no independent diagnostic "gold standard." However, when tilt-table testing has been undertaken in patients with a classic history of vasovagal syncope, test sensitivity has been relatively good.

The combination of tilt-table testing and invasive electrophysiologic testing has substantially enhanced diagnostic capabilities in patients with syncope. Sra et al[97] reported results of electrophysiologic testing in conjunction with head-up tilt-table testing in 86 consecutive patients referred for evaluation of unexplained syncope. Electrophysiologic testing was abnormal in 29 patients (34%), with the majority of these (21 patients) having inducible sustained monomorphic ventricular tachycardia. Among the remaining patients, head-up tilt-table testing proved positive in 34 (40%) cases, whereas 23 patients (26%) remained undiagnosed. In general, patients exhibiting positive electrophysiologic findings were older, more frequently male, and exhibited lower left ventricular ejection fractions and higher frequency of evident heart disease than did patients with positive head-up tilt-table tests or patients in whom no diagnosis was determined.

In a further evaluation of the combined use of electrophysiologic testing and head-up tilt-table testing in assessment of syncope, Fitzpatrick et al[36] analyzed findings in 322 patients with syncope. Conventional electrophysiologic testing provided a basis for syncope in 229 of 322 cases (71%), with 93 patients having a normal electrophysiologic study. Among the patients with abnormal electrophysiologic findings, AV conduction disease was diagnosed in 34%, sinus node dysfunction in 21%, carotid sinus syndrome in 10%, and an inducible sustained tachyarrhythmia in 6%. Tilt-table testing was undertaken in 71 of the 93 patients with normal electrophysiologic studies and reproduced syncope consistent with a vasovagal faint in 53 of the 71 patients (75%).

### NEUROLOGIC STUDIES

Conventional neurologic laboratory studies (EEG, head CT and MRI) have had a relatively low yield in the patient with syncope. Among the 433 syncope evaluations reviewed by Kapoor,[50] the EEG proved helpful in only 3 cases. Consequently, as has been noted earlier, most neurologic labora-

tory studies should be restricted to those situations in which other clinical observations strongly suggest organic central nervous system disease.

## TREATMENT

An accurate etiologic diagnosis is the key to successful prevention of syncopal symptoms.

A wide range of pharmacologic and device therapy is available. The effectiveness of these therapies varies, however, depending on the specific diagnosis. For example, there is substantial evidence supporting the use of cardiac pacing for preventing carotid sinus syncope[23,30,71] and for ameliorating symptomatic bradycardias associated with sinus node dysfunction (sick sinus syndrome)[2,19,24,33] and acquired AV block.[24,33] Conversely, evidence supporting the effectiveness of currently favored pharmacologic interventions in vasovagal syncope is much more tenuous.

### NEURALLY MEDIATED SYNCOPE

In the case of neurally mediated syncopal syndromes (excluding for the most part carotid sinus syndrome), treatment strategies should address trigger factors (e.g., suppressing the cause of cough in cough syncope). However, in many conditions such an approach is not feasible. Thus, for patients with vasovagal syncope, a variety of pharmacologic approaches have been proposed when recurrent or severe symptoms demand more than reassurance. None of these, however, are unequivocally substantiated in terms of long-term benefit. Beta-adrenergic blocking drugs, disopyramide, and, to a lesser extent, vasoconstrictor agents (e.g., midodrine) have been the agents of principal interest. Volume expanders (e.g., fludrocortisone, salt tablets, sport drinks), anticholinergics, and serotonin-reuptake inhibitors have also been used in this setting. However, for any of these agents only a small experience currently exists.[22,37,61,70,73] The few small controlled studies that have been reported (atenolol, caffedrine, disopyramide, scopolamine, and etilefrine) all have methodologic problems. Nonetheless, only one of these (the beta-adrenergic blocker, atenolol) has shown a drug benefit during follow-up.[61]

Cardiac pacing has proved highly successful in carotid sinus syndrome and is acknowledged to be the treatment of choice when bradycardia has been documented.[18,23,30,71] In contrast, until very recently, experience with pacing in vasovagal syncope and other forms of neurally mediated syncope has been limited.[17,80] Three relatively recent reports address the latter issue.[80,93,94] In a retrospective study from the United Kingdom, Petersen et al[80] reported findings in 37 patients with pacing in whom vasovagal syncope appeared to exhibit a predominantly cardioinhibitory character during tilt-table testing. Implanted pacemaker pulse generators were programmed to detect vasovagal episodes when heart rates fell to the 40 to 50 beats per minute (bpm) range. Thereafter a period of pacing was initiated at rates of 80 to 90 bpm. During 39 ± 19 months of follow-up, symptomatic improvement was noted in 84% of cases, with complete resolution of symptoms in 35%. The annual syncope frequency was reported to have been reduced by tenfold (from approximately 126 to 13 episodes per year). Similar findings were noted in a prospective randomized controlled multicenter trial (North American Vasovagal Pacemaker Study).[94] Pre-

---

*References 25, 28, 35, 36, 43, 44, 76, 82, 89.

liminary results indicated that the annual actuarial rate of recurrent syncope was approximately 19% for patients with pacing and 60% in control subjects. Finally, Sheldon et al[93] recently reported outcomes, including quality-of-life indexes, in 12 patients with difficult-to-treat vasovagal syncope who were provided pacemaker therapy and followed for an average of 1 year. Compared to symptom status prior to pacemaker implantation, pacing was associated with a longer time to syncope recurrence (median values: no pacing, 7 days vs. pacing, 5.3 months), a marked reduction of fainting frequency, and a substantial increment in quality-of-life scores.

## ORTHOSTASIS AND DYSAUTONOMIAS

The treatment of patients with syncope due to orthostasis or dysautonomias bears a strong resemblance to that of the neurally mediated syncopal syndromes, with perhaps greater emphasis on physical maneuvers (e.g., support stockings, elevation of the head of the bed at night, intake of electrolyte containing beverages).[10] The mainstay of pharmacologic treatment has been attempts at chronic expansion of central circulating volume. To this end, increased salt in the diet or the use of salt-retaining steroids (i.e., principally fludrocortisone) is usually the first step. Additional benefit has been reported with the use of agents such as erythropoietin or fludrocortisone, which act to increase circulating volume, in conjunction with physical maneuvers such as elevating the head of the bed at night.[101] A second element in the strategy is reduction of the tendency for central volume to be displaced to the lower extremities with upright posture. To this end, vasoconstrictors have been employed, although with limited success because of the tendency for tachyphylaxis to develop. Of greatest current interest is midodrine, an agent that has prominent venoconstrictor properties and good overall tolerance.[47,96] Physical rehabilitation (gentle progressive increments of exercise) with enforced periods of increasing exposure to upright posture is also advisable. Cardiac pacing at relatively rapid rates may prove valuable in certain very difficult cases. However, tolerance to rapid pacing rates and long-term adverse effects on left ventricular function are a concern.

## PRIMARY CARDIAC ARRHYTHMIAS

In the treatment of primary cardiac arrhythmias, especially the bradycardias and hypotensive tachyarrhythmias, effective treatment interventions are readily available. The evidence unquestionably supports the importance of cardiac pacemaker therapy in patients with syncope due to bradyarrhythmias, whether resulting from sinus node dysfunction or AV conduction disturbances.[5,79,85,98] In the case of paroxysmal supraventricular tachyarrhythmias causing syncope, the efficacy of conventional antiarrhythmic drug treatment is not well studied but is likely to be good if the drugs are tolerated and compliance is maintained. However, at present patients thus affected are more often considered for curative transcatheter ablation techniques.[75] In brief, invasive electrophysiologic study is used to define the tachyarrhythmia mechanism, and radiofrequency energy is then applied in a very localized region to modify the arrhythmia substrate and eliminate susceptibility. On the other hand, although preliminary attempts have been quite encouraging, transcatheter curative ablation is not yet widely available for

treating atrial fibrillation. The latter patients, especially those who are importantly symptomatic as a consequence of the tachyarrhythmia, are increasingly being treated with low-dose amiodarone as long-term therapy.[40,68] Amiodarone is even finding increasing application in prevention of atrial fibrillation in high-risk settings such as cardiac surgery.[27] Other drugs, such as flecainide and propafenone, are also highly effective in selected individuals with symptomatic atrial fibrillation, although there are generally greater safety concerns with these agents than with amiodarone in patients with demonstrable structural heart disease.[6,45,81] In the near future, implantable low-energy atrial cardioverters may prove beneficial in some of the most difficult to control cases of atrial fibrillation.[8,74,75]

In the case of syncope due to ventricular tachycardia, underlying left ventricular dysfunction is often present. In such settings the proarrhythmic risk associated with antiarrhythmic drug therapy is markedly increased. The risk has been reported to range from 5% to 15% with class 1 agents (e.g., quinidine, disopyramide). Consequently, pharmacologic therapeutic strategies in this setting often involve early introduction of class 3 agents (particularly amiodarone). However, several recent large studies suggest that even amiodarone may not provide optimal prophylaxis against sudden death, especially in the setting of poor left ventricular systolic function (i.e., ejection fraction <30%).[7,20,66,67,72] Consequently, implantable pacemaker cardioverter-defibrillators (ICDs) are being increasingly recommended for high-risk patients. These devices can be implanted in much the same manner as conventional pacemakers. The pulse generator is typically placed subcutaneously (occasionally submuscularly) in the infraclavicular prepectoral area, and the pacing defibrillation lead is advanced via percutaneous puncture of the ipsilateral subclavian vein to the right ventricle. Cardiac ablation techniques, on the other hand, are still evolving for most forms of ventricular tachycardia and are currently only the first-choice therapy in a few forms of ventricular tachycardia (i.e., right ventricular outflow tract tachycardia, bundle-branch reentry tachycardia).[13,20] However, as technology advances, transcatheter ablation may find a greater role in the control of ventricular tachyarrhythmias.[13]

## STRUCTURAL CARDIAC OR VASCULAR DISEASE

In patients in whom structural cardiovascular or cardiopulmonary disease is the cause of syncope, treatment must be directed at the specific structural lesion or its consequences. Thus, in syncope associated with myocardial ischemia, pharmacologic therapy or revascularization is clearly the appropriate strategy in most cases. Similarly, when syncope is closely associated with surgically addressable lesions (e.g., valvular aortic stenosis, pericardial disease, atrial myxoma, congenital cardiac anomaly), a direct corrective approach is often feasible. On the other hand, when syncope is caused by certain difficult to treat conditions, such as primary pulmonary hypertension or restrictive cardiomyopathy, it is often impossible to ameliorate the underlying problem adequately. Even modifying outflow gradients in hypertrophic obstructive cardiomyopathy (HOCM or idiopathic hypertrophic subaortic stenosis [IHSS]) is not readily achieved surgically. Recent success with cardiac pacing techniques may offer promise for certain symptomatic individuals.[63,64]

## SUMMARY

Syncope has many potential causes and a wide range of prognostic implications, depending on the patient, the circumstances, and the nature of the underlying disease substrate. In the absence of effective therapy, the recurrence rate following an initial syncopal event is excessive (estimated to be in the 30% range within a few years of the index event). Thus reassurance in the absence of both a well-defined cause for the symptoms and a well-considered treatment plan is an unwise strategy. The potential for physical injury (especially in the elderly), loss of employment, need for repetitive medical attention, and psychologic impact on the patient and family are real concerns. Further, as pointed out by Kapoor et al[51] and by Bass et al,[11] apart from the morbidity associated with syncope recurrences, mortality remains a substantial concern in the patient with syncope. Consequently, assessment of each patient must be thorough.

Some claim that medical history taking and physician experience are sufficient for diagnosing the cause of syncope in most cases.[34,54] However, this approach has never been rigorously tested. Further, published experience suggests that use of the experiential method, even in the best of hands, is associated with a disconcerting frequency of "no diagnosis" (approximately 40%). Consequently, reliance solely on clinical judgment alone is not a prudent course of action for responsible physicians. Conversely, indiscriminate laboratory testing is also to be discouraged because it is both unnecessary and expensive. Carefully selected use of laboratory studies is usually sufficient to confirm any initial clinical suspicions, assess prognostic implications, and direct treatment strategy. Cost-effectiveness lies not in making a diagnosis but in making the correct diagnosis, acknowledging that the physician's ability will always be limited by many factors, including experience and available technology. Only after establishing the basis for syncope as accurately as possible can one offer rational and, it is hoped, effective treatment options. Overall, current practice permits establishing a basis for syncopal symptoms in 80% to 85% of cases. This is a marked improvement over the standard of a decade ago, but it still leaves room for improvement.

## ACKNOWLEDGMENT

We would like to thank Wendy Markuson and Barry L.S. Detloff for assistance in preparation of the manuscript.

## REFERENCES

1. Akhtar M, Shenasa M, Denker S, et al. Role of cardiac electrophysiologic studies in patients with unexplained recurrent syncope. *PACE.* 1983;6:192-201.
2. Albin G, Hayes DL, Holmes DR. Sinus node dysfunction in pediatric and young adult patients: treatment by implantation of a permanent pacemaker in 39 cases. *Mayo Clin Proc.* 1985;60:667-672.
3. Almquist A, Goldenberg IF, Milstein S, et al. Provocation of bradycardia and hypotension by isoproterenol and upright posture in patients with unexplained syncope. *N Engl J Med.* 1989;320:346-351.
4. Almquist A, Gornick C, Benson DW Jr, et al. Carotid sinus hypersensitivity: evaluation of the vasodepressor component. *Circulation.* 1985; 71:927-936.
5. Andersen HR, Thuesen L, Bagger JP, et al. Prospective randomised trial of atrial versus ventricular pacing in sick-sinus syndrome. *Lancet.* 1994;344:1523-1528.
6. Anderson JL, Gilbert EM, Alpert BL, et al, and the Flecainide Supraventricular Tachycardia Study Group. Prevention of symptomatic re-currences of paroxysmal atrial fibrillation in patients tolerating antiarrhythmic therapy: a multicenter, double-blind, crossover study of flecainide and placebo with transtelephonic monitoring. *Circulation.* 1989;80:1557-1570.
7. The Antiarrhythmics versus Implantable Defibrillators (AVID) Investigators. A comparison of antiarrhythmic drug therapy with implantable defibrillators in patients resuscitated from near-fatal ventricular arrhythmias. *N Engl J Med.* 1997;337:1576-1583.
8. Ayers GM. Internal atrial defibrillation and implantable atrial defibrillators. In: Oto MA, ed. *Practice and Progress in Cardiac Pacing and Electrophysiology.* Dordrecht, The Netherlands: Kluwer Academic Publishers; 1996:309-316.
9. Bannister R. Chronic autonomic failure with postural hypotension. *Lancet.* 1979;2:404-406.
10. Bannister R, Mathias C. Management of postural hypotension. In: Bannister R, ed. *Autonomic Failure: A Textbook of Clinical Disorders of the Autonomic Nervous System.* Oxford: Oxford University Press; 1988: 569-595.
11. Bass EB, Elson JJ, Fogoros RN, et al. Long-term prognosis of patients undergoing electrophysiologic studies for syncope of unknown origin. *Am J Cardiol.* 1988;62:1186-1191.
12. Benditt DG. Letter to the Editor. *Neurology.* 1997;49:901-902.
13. Benditt DG, Adler SW, Beatty G, et al. Advances in transcatheter endocardial mapping and radiofrequency ablation of ventricular arrhythmias. In: Oto MA, ed. *Practice and Progress in Cardiac Pacing and Electrophysiology.* Dordrecht, The Netherlands: Kluwer Academic Publishers; 1996:277-287.
14. Benditt DG, Benson DW Jr, Dunnigan A, et al. Drug therapy in sinus node dysfunction. In: Rapaport E, ed. *Cardiology Update–1984.* New York: Elsevier; 1984:79-101.
15. Benditt DG, Ferguson DW, Grubb BP, et al. Tilt-table testing for assessing syncope: an American College of Cardiology expert consensus document. *J Am Coll Cardiol.* 1996;28:263-275.
16. Benditt DG, Goldstein MA, Adler S, et al. Neurally mediated syncopal syndromes: pathophysiology and clinical evaluation. In: Mandel WJ, ed. *Cardiac Arrhythmias.* 3rd ed. Philadelphia: JB Lippincott; 1995: 879-906.
17. Benditt DG, Peterson M, Lurie K, et al. Cardiac pacing for prevention of recurrent vasovagal syncope. *Ann Intern Med.* 1995;122:204-209.
18. Benditt DG, Remole S, Asso A, et al. Cardiac pacing for carotid sinus syndrome and vasovagal syncope. In: Barold SS, Mugica J, eds. *New Perspectives in Cardiac Pacing.* 3rd ed. Mount Kisco, NY: Futura Publishing; 1993:15-28.
19. Benditt DG, Sakaguchi S, Goldstein MA, et al. Sinus node dysfunction: pathophysiology, clinical features, evaluation and treatment. In: Zipes DP, Jalife J, eds. *Cardiac Electrophysiology: From Cell to Bedside.* 2nd ed. Philadelphia: WB Saunders; 1995:1215-1246.
20. Bigger JT Jr, for the Coronary Artery Bypass Graft (CABG) Patch Trial Investigators. Prophylactic use of implanted cardiac defibrillators in patients at high risk for ventricular arrhythmias after coronary-artery bypass graft surgery. *N Engl J Med.* 1997;337:1569-1575.
21. Brignole M, Gaggioli G, Menozzi C, et al. Adenosine-induced atrioventricular block in patients with unexplained syncope: the diagnostic value of ATP testing. *Circulation.* 1997;96:3921-3927.
22. Brignole M, Menozzi C, Gianfranchi L, et al. A controlled trial of acute and long-term medical therapy in tilt-induced neurally mediated syncope. *Am J Cardiol.* 1992;70:339-342.
23. Brignole M, Sartore B, Barra M, et al. Ventricular and dual chamber pacing for treatment of carotid sinus syndrome. *PACE.* 1989;12:582-590.
24. British Pacing and Electrophysiology Group Working Party. Recommendations for pacemaker prescription for symptomatic bradycardia. *Br Heart J.* 1991;66:185-191.
25. Calkins H, Seifert M, Morady F. Clinical presentation and long-term follow-up of athletes with exercise-induced vasodepressor syncope. *Am Heart J.* 1995;129:1159-1164.
26. Camm AJ, Lau CP. Syncope of undetermined origin: diagnosis and management. *Prog Cardiol.* 1988;1:139-156.
27. Daoud EG, Srickberger A, Man C, et al. Preoperative amiodarone as prophylaxis against atrial fibrillation after heart surgery. *N Engl J Med.* 1997;337:1785-1791.
28. deMey C, Enterling D. Assessment of the hemodynamic responses to single passive head-up tilt by non-invasive methods in normotensive subjects. *Methods Find Exp Clin Pharmacol.* 1986;8:449-457.
29. Denes P, Ezri MD. The role of electrophysiologic studies in the management of patients with unexplained syncope. *PACE.* 1985;8:424-435.

30. Deschamps D, Richard A, Citron B, et al. Hypersensibilité sino-caroti-dienne: evolution à moyen et à long terme des patients traites par stimulation ventriculaire. *Arch Mal Coeur Vaiss.* 1990;83:63-67.

31. Dhingra RC, Denes P, Wu D, et al. Syncope in patients with chronic bi-fascicular block. *Ann Intern Med.* 1974;81:302-306.

32. DiMarco JB, Garan H, Hawthorne WJ, et al. Intracardiac electrophys-iologic techniques in recurrent syncope of unknown cause. *Ann Intern Med.* 1981;95:542-548.

33. Dreifus LS, Fisch C, Griffin JC, et al. Guidelines for implantation of cardiac pacemakers and antiarrhythmia devices: a report of the Amer-ican College of Cardiology/American Heart Association Task Force on Assessment of Diagnostic and Therapeutic Cardiovascular Proce-dures. *Circulation.* 1991;84:455-467.

34. Fetch MC. An accurate history tells all. *BMJ.* 1994;308:1251-1252.

35. Fitzpatrick A, Theodorakis G, Vardas P, et al. The incidence of malig-nant vasovagal syndrome in patients with recurrent syncope. *Eur Heart J.* 1991;12:389-394.

36. Fitzpatrick A, Theodorakis G, Vardas P, et al. Methodology of head-up tilt testing in patients with unexplained syncope. *J Am Coll Cardiol.* 1991;17:125-130.

37. Fitzpatrick AP, Ahmed R, Williams S, et al. A randomized trial of med-ical therapy in malignant vasovagal syndrome or neurally mediated bradycardia/hypotension syndrome. *Eur J Cardiac Pacing Electrophys-iol.* 1991;1:991-202.

38. Fujimura O, Yee R, Klein GJ, et al. The diagnostic sensitivity of elec-trophysiologic testing in patients with syncope caused by bradycardia. *N Engl J Med.* 1989;321:1703-1707.

39. Gendelman HE, Linzer M, Gabelman M, et al. Syncope in a general hospital population. *N Y State J Med.* 1983;83:116-165.

40. Gosselink ATM, Crijns HJGM, van Gelder IC, et al. Low-dose amio-darone for maintenance of sinus rhythm after cardioversion of atrial fibrillation or flutter. *JAMA.* 1992;267:3289-3293.

41. Grubb BP, Gerard G, Rousch K, et al. Differentiation of convulsive syn-cope and epilepsy with head up tilt table testing. *Ann Intern Med.* 1991;115:871-876.

42. Grubb BP, Gerard G, Roush K, et al. Cerebral vasoconstriction during head-upright tilt induced vasovagal syncope: a paradoxic and unex-pected response. *Circulation.* 1991;84:1157-1164.

43. Grubb BP, Temesy-Armos P, Hahn H, et al. Utility of upright tilt table testing in the evaluation and management of syncope of unknown ori-gin. *Am J Med.* 1991;90:6-10.

44. Grubb BP, Wolfe D, Samoil D, et al. Recurrent unexplained syncope in the elderly: the use of head-upright tilt table testing in evaluation and management. *J Am Geriatr Soc.* 1992;40:1123-1128.

45. Hammill S, Wood DL, Gersh BJ, et al. Propafenone for paroxysmal atrial fibrillation. *Am J Cardiol.* 1988;61:473-474.

46. Jackman WM, Friday KJ, Anderson JL, et al. The long QT syndromes: a critical review, new clinical observations, and a unifying hypothesis. *Prog Cardiovasc Dis.* 1988;31:115-172.

47. Jankovic J, Gilden JL, Hiner BC, et al. Neurogenic orthostatic hypo-tension: a double-blind placebo-controlled study with midodrine. *Am J Med.* 1993;95:38-48.

48. Johnson AM. Aortic stenosis, sudden death, and the left ventricular baroreceptors. *Br Heart J.* 1971;33:1-5.

49. Kaplan BM, Langendorf R, Lev M, et al. Tachycardia-bradycardia syn-drome (so-called "sick sinus syndrome"). *Am J Cardiol.* 1973;26:497-508.

50. Kapoor W. Evaluation and outcome of patients with syncope. *Medi-cine.* 1990;69:160-175.

51. Kapoor WN, Karpf M, Wieand S, et al. A prospective evaluation and follow-up of patients with syncope. *N Engl J Med.* 1983;309:197-204.

52. Kenny RA, Bayliss J, Ingram A, et al. Head up tilt: a useful test for in-vestigating unexplained syncope. *Lancet.* 1986;1:1352-1354.

53. Kuchar DL, Thorburn CW, Sammel NL. Signal-averaged electrocardio-gram for evaluation of recurrent syncope. *Am J Cardiol.* 1986;58:949-953.

54. Landau WM, Nelson DA. Clinical neuromythology XV: feinting sci-ence. *Neurology.* 1996;45:609-618.

55. Leitch JW, Klein GJ, Yee R, et al. Syncope associated with supraventric-ular tachycardia: an expression of tachycardia or vasomotor response. *Circulation.* 1992;85:1064-1071.

56. Linker NJ, Camm AJ. Drug effects on the sinus node: a clinical per-spective. *Cardiovasc Drugs Ther.* 1988;2:165-170.

57. Linzer M, Varia I, Pontinen M, et al: Medically unexplained syncope: relationship to psychiatric illness. *Am J Med.* 1992;92:18-25.

58. Low PA. Autonomic nervous system function. *J Clin Neurophysiol.* 1993;10:14-27.

59. Low PA, Opfer-Gherking TL, McPhee BR, et al. Prospective evaluation of clinical characteristics of orthostatic hypotension. *Mayo Clin Proc.* 1995;70:617-622.

60. Lurie KG, Dutton J, Mangat R, et al. Evaluation of edrophonium as a provocative agent for vasovagal syncope during head-up tilt table test-ing. *Am J Cardiol.* 1993;72:1286-1290.

61. Mahanonda N, Bhuripanyo K, Kangkagate C, et al. Randomized dou-ble-blind placebo-controlled trial of oral atenolol in patients with un-explained syncope and positive upright tilt table results. *Am Heart J.* 1995;130:1250-1253.

62. Martin GJ, Adams SL, Martin HG, et al. Prospective evaluation of syn-cope. *Ann Emerg Med.* 1984;13:499-504.

63. McAreavey D, Epstein ND, Fananapazir L. Dual chamber pacing is ef-fective therapy for hypertrophic cardiomyopathy patients with pro-vocable LV outflow tract obstruction and symptoms refractory to medical therapy. *J Am Coll Cardiol.* 1994;23:11. Abstract.

64. McKenna WJ, Deanfield J, Faruqui A, et al. Prognosis in hypertrophic cardiomyopathy: role of age and clinical electrocardiographic and he-modynamic features. *Am J Cardiol.* 1981;47:532-538.

65. Michaelsson M, Jonzon A, Riesenfeld T. Isolated congenital complete atrioventricular block in adult life. *Circulation.* 1995;92:442-449.

66. Middlekauff HR, Stevenson WG, Saxon LA. Prognosis after syncope: impact of left ventricular function. *Am Heart J.* 1993;125:121-127.

67. Middlekauff HR, Stevenson WG, Stevenson LW, et al. Syncope in ad-vanced heart failure: high risk of sudden death regardless of origin of syncope. *J Am Coll Cardiol.* 1993;21:110-116.

68. Middlekauff HR, Wiener I, Stevenson WG. Low-dose amiodarone for atrial fibrillation. *Am J Cardiol.* 1993;72:75F-81F.

69. Morady F, Shen E, Schwartz A, et al. Long-term follow-up of patients with recurrent unexplained syncope evaluated by electrophysiologic testing. *J Am Coll Cardiol.* 1983;2:1053-1059.

70. Morillo CA, Leitch JW, Yee R, et al. A placebo-controlled trial of intra-venous and oral disopyramide for prevention of neurally mediated syncope induced by head-up tilt. *J Am Coll Cardiol.* 1993;22:1843-1848.

71. Morley CA, Perrins EJ, Grant P, et al. Carotid sinus syncope treated by pacing: analysis of persistent symptoms and role of atrioventricular sequential pacing. *Br Heart J.* 1982;47:411-418.

72. Moss AJ, Hall WJ, Cannom DS, et al. Improved survival with an im-planted defibrillator in patients with coronary disease at high risk for ventricular arrhythmia. *N Engl J Med.* 1996;335:1933-1940.

73. Moya A, Permanyer-Miralda G, Sagrista-Sauleda J, et al. Limitations of head-up tilt test for evaluating the efficacy of therapeutic interven-tions in patients with vasovagal syncope: results of a controlled study of etilefrine versus placebo *J Am Coll Cardiol.* 1995;25:65-69.

74. Murgatroyd FD, Johnson EE, Cooper RAS, et al. Safety of low-energy transvenous atrial defibrillation: world experience. *Circulation.* 1994;90:1-14.

75. Naccarelli GV, Dougherty AH, Jalal S, et al. Paroxysmal supraventricu-lar tachycardia: comparative role of therapeutic methods—drugs, de-vices, and ablation. In: Saksena S, Luderitz B, eds. *Interventional Elec-trophysiology: A Textbook.* 2nd ed. Armonk, NY: Futura Publishing; 1996:461-470.

76. Natale A, Akhtar M, Jazayeri M, et al. Provocation of hypotension dur-ing head-up tilt testing in subjects with no history of syncope or pre-syncope. *Circulation.* 1995;92:54-58.

77. Njemanze PC. Cerebral circulation dysfunction and hemodynamic abnormalities in syncope during upright tilt test. *Can J Cardiol.* 1993;9:238-242.

78. Penton GB, Miller H, Levine SA. Some clinical features of complete heart block. *Circulation.* 1956;13:801-824.

79. Perrins EJ, Astridge PS. Clinical trials and experience. In: Ellenbogen KA, Kay GN, Wilkoff BL, eds. *Clinical Cardiac Pacing.* Philadelphia: WB Saunders; 1995:399-418.

80. Petersen MEV, Chamberlain-Webber R, Fitzpatrick AP, et al. Perma-nent pacing for cardioinhibitory malignant vasovagal syndrome. *Br Heart J.* 1994;71:274-281.

81. Porterfield JG, Porterfield LM. Therapeutic efficacy and safety of oral propafenone for atrial fibrillation. *Am J Cardiol.* 1989;63:114-116.

82. Raviele A, Gasparini G, DiPede F, et al. Usefulness of head-up tilt test in evaluating patients with syncope of unknown origin and negative electrophysiologic study. *Am J Cardiol.* 1990;65:1322-1327.

83. Raviele A, Menozzi C, Brignole M, et al. Value of head-up tilt testing

potentiated with sublingual nitroglycerin to assess the origin of unexplained syncope. *Am J Cardiol.* 1995;76:267-272.

84. Richardson DA, Bexton RS, Shaw FE, et al. Prevalence of cardioinhibitory carotid sinus hypersensitivity (CICSH) in accident and emergency attendances with falls or syncope. *PACE.* 1997;20:820-823.

85. Rosenqvist M, Brandt J, Schuller H. Long-term pacing in sick sinus node disease: effects of stimulation mode on cardiovascular morbidity and mortality. *Am Heart J.* 1988;116:16-22.

86. Ross RT. *Syncope.* London: WB Saunders; 1988.

87. Rowe JC, White PD. Complete heart block: a follow-up study. *Ann Intern Med.* 1958;49:260-270.

88. Rubenstein JJ, Schulman CL, Yurchak PM, et al. Clinical spectrum of the sick sinus syndrome. *Circulation.* 1972;46:5-13.

89. Sakaguchi S, Shultz J, Remole C, et al. Syncope associated with exercise, a manifestation of neurally mediated syncope. *Am J Cardiol.* 1995; 75:476-481.

90. Savage DD, Corwin L, McGee DL, et al. Epidemiologic features of isolated syncope: The Framingham Study. *Stroke.* 1985;16:626-629.

91. Scheinman MM, Peters RW, Sauve MJ, et al. Value of H-Q interval in patients with bundle branch block and the role of prophylactic permanent pacing. *Am J Cardiol.* 1982;50:1316-1322.

92. Selzer A, Wray HW. Quinidine syncope: paroxysmal ventricular fibrillation occurring during the treatment of chronic atrial tachyarrhythmias. *Circulation.* 1964;30:17-26.

93. Sheldon R, Koshman ML, Wilson W, et al. Effect of dual-chamber pacing with automatic rate-drop sensing on recurrent neurally mediated syncope. *Am J Cardiol.* 1998;81:158-162.

94. Sheldon RS, Gent M, Roberts RS, Connolly SJ, on behalf of the NAV-PAC Investigators. North American Vasovagal Pacemaker Study: study design and organization. *PACE.* 1997;20:844-848.

95. Shen WK, Hammill SC, Munger TM, et al. Usefulness of adenosine in evaluating vasovagal syncope: comparison to tilt test and isoproterenol test. *Circulation.* 1993;88(suppl I):398. Abstract.

96. Sra J, Maglio C, Biehl M, et al. Efficacy of midodrine hydrochloride in neurocardiogenic syncope refractory to standard therapy. *J Cardiovasc Electrophysiol.* 1997;8:42-46.

97. Sra JS, Anderson AJ, Sheikh SH, et al. Unexplained syncope evaluated by electrophysiologic studies and head-up tilt testing. *Ann Intern Med.* 1991;114:1013-1019.

98. Stangl K, Wirtzfeld A, Seitz K, et al. Atrial stimulation (AAI): long-term follow-up of 110 patients. In: Belhassen B, Feldman S, Copperman Y, eds. *Cardiac Pacing and Electrophysiology.* Proceedings of the Eighth World Symposium on Cardiac Pacing and Electrophysiology. Jerusalem: R & L Creative Communications; 1987:283-285.

99. Sutton R, Petersen M, Brignole M, et al. Proposed classification for tilt induced vasovagal syncope. *Eur J Cardiac Pacing Electrophysiol.* 1992;2: 180-183.

100. Swerdlow CD, Winkle RA, Mason JW. Determinants of survival in patients with ventricular tachyarrhythmias. *N Engl J Med.* 1983;308: 1436-1442.

101. Ten Harkel ADJ, van Lieshout JJ, Wieling W. Treatment of orthostatic hypotension with sleeping in the head-up position, alone and in combination with fludrocortisone. *J Intern Med.* 1992;232:139-145.

102. Wayne HH. Syncope: physiological considerations and an analysis of the clinical characteristics in 510 patients. *Am J Med.* 1961;30:418-438.

103. Wieling W, van Lieshout JJ. Investigation and treatment of autonomic circulatory failure. *Curr Opin Neurol Neurosurg.* 1993;6:537-543.

104. Weiss S, Baker JP. The carotid sinus reflex in health and disease: its role in the causation of fainting and convulsions. *Medicine.* 1933;12:297-354.

# 25

# Central Nervous System Infections

*Maria E. Carlini and Richard L. Harris*

Central nervous system (CNS) infections are a diagnostic challenge to clinicians because of the wide spectrum of presentations and the large number of possible infectious agents. This chapter provides an overview of the clinical presentations of the more common infections and diagnostic modalities. Traditional laboratory and imaging tests have been augmented by a number of molecular techniques (i.e., polymerase chain reaction [PCR] and nucleic acid probes) in recent years. Brief descriptions of newer laboratory techniques are provided at the conclusion of the chapter. Treatment issues are briefly reviewed.

## ACUTE VIRAL CENTRAL NERVOUS SYSTEM INFECTIONS

Many viral pathogens can cause CNS infections in humans. Most of these infections are mild, and patients may not seek medical treatment. Patients with serious infections present with fever, headache, photophobia, and neck stiffness consistent with meningitis. By definition, those with encephalitis also have altered mental status. Because of the large number of pathogens, a specific cause is often difficult to determine. This discussion focuses primarily on commonly diagnosed pathogens in the United States.[47,56,119,130]

Diagnosis is aided by the general history of the illness, as well as seasonal and geographic factors, since many medically important viruses are arthropod borne (insect-transmitted). Patients with suspected CNS viral infection should have complete blood counts, electrolyte levels, liver function tests, spinal tap for collection of cerebrospinal fluid (CSF), and imaging studies (i.e. computed tomography [CT] or magnetic resonance imaging [MRI]) when indicated. Laboratory studies of the CSF typically show an elevated white blood cell (WBC) count with a lymphocytic predominance (neutrophil predominance may be seen in the first 48 hours), relatively normal glucose level, and normal or mildly elevated total protein level. Specific findings for each etiology are discussed where they are clinically important.

Laboratory diagnosis may be made by direct detection of virus, evaluation of acute and convalescent serum antibody titers, enzyme-linked immunosorbent assay (ELISA), immunoglobulin M (IgM)–capture ELISA or PCR (Table 25–1). Virus is often difficult to isolate from CSF, and the newer ELISA methods for testing serum and CSF are very useful. An increasing number of PCR and molecular methods of diagnosis are available, but it is important for the clinician to remember that in many cases these are research tools and may not be standardized. Therefore the validity of the results is laboratory dependent.

### ARTHROPOD-BORNE VIRUSES

Arthropod-borne viruses, or arboviruses, are a common cause of CNS infection. More than 20 types of virus can cause disease worldwide, and only the most clinically important are discussed here. Alphaviruses cause eastern equine encephalitis (EEE), western equine encephalitis (WEE), and Venezuelan equine encephalitis (VEE). Flaviviruses cause Japanese B encephalitis, St. Louis encephalitis (SLE), dengue and yellow fever infections. The bunyaviruses cause California equine encephalitis (CEE, La Crosse strain).[26,47,56,119,130] In the United States the clinically important arboviruses are CEE, SLE, WEE, and EEE. Each of the viruses has a specific geographic distribution (often *not* in concordance with its name), which is a key point in diagnosis. Infections tend to occur in the warmer months when the vectors are active.[26,47,71] La Crosse encephalitis is the most commonly reported viral encephalitis in the United States, with 252 cases reported to the Centers for Disease Control and Prevention (CDC) in 1996–1997. Cases were reported in 12 states, mostly in West Virginia, Illinois, Ohio, and Wisconsin. It is most often seen in patients younger than 18 years and rarely causes serious outcomes. SLE is the most common cause of outbreaks of arboviral infection in the United States and has the greatest geographic distribution. Surveillance programs for the presence of the virus in mosquito populations helps prevent and contain epidemics. SLE is found in the United States throughout the central West and the South. It is most severe in older adults, and sequelae may occur in up to 20% of survivors. WEE occurs in the West and Midwest. Sequelae are highest in infants. No human cases of WEE in the United States have been reported since 1994. EEE, found in the East and Gulf Coast areas, is the most severe among the arboviral infections, with a high mortality and a high incidence of sequelae among survivors. In 1996–1997, 19 cases of EEE were reported.[14]

**TABLE 25–1. Diagnostic Testing for Viral Encephalitides**

| VIRUS | DIAGNOSTIC TESTING |
|---|---|
| Arboviruses | Acute and convalescent sera |
| | CSF viral culture (EEE) |
| | CSF virus-specific IgM |
| | Serum IgM |
| Enteroviruses | CSF viral culture |
| | CSF reverse-transcriptase PCR |
| | Acute and convalescent sera |
| | Throat and stool culture |
| Lymphocytic choriomenin- | Serology: IgM-capture ELISA |
| gitis | CSF reverse-transcriptase PCR |
| Herpes simplex virus | MRI of brain |
| | EEG |
| | CSF PCR |
| | CSF antibody titer (serum: CSF titers) |
| Rabies | Viral isolation from tissues or secretions |
| | Viral antigen in corneal smears or brain |
| | Serologic studies |
| | PCR |
| Measles postinfectious | Brain biopsy |
| encephalomyelitis | |
| HTLV-1 | Antibodies from serum or CSF |
| | CSF or serum PCR |
| JC virus | CSF PCR |
| | Brain biopsy |
| Subacute sclerosing panen- | CSF antibodies |
| cephalitis (measles virus) | CSF PCR |

CSF, Cerebrospinal fluid; EEE, eastern equine encephalitis; EEG, electroencephalography; HTLV, human T-cell lymphoma virus; Ig, immunoglobulin; MRI, magnetic resonance imaging; PCR, polymerase chain reaction.

Japanese B encephalitis is common in Asia and accounts for the greatest number of worldwide cases of arboviral encephalitis. It is rarely seen in the United States unless the patient has traveled to an endemic area, but given the increasing degree of travel exposure, the clinician must keep this condition in mind. A vaccine is available, and a history of its administration is helpful in excluding the diagnosis.[47,71]

Patients with arboviral encephalitis present with common signs, symptoms, and CSF findings, as discussed earlier. In EEE a predominance of polymorphonuclear leukocytes in the first 72 hours and a low glucose level in the CSF may help to distinguish it from others types of encephalitis in this class. Results of imaging studies are often normal or may show diffuse edema. Patients with EEE are more likely to show focal lesions in the basal ganglia and thalamus on imaging studies (more often present on MRI than CT scans) or electroencephalogram (EEG) and are more prone to seizures.[23]

Laboratory diagnosis of arboviral encephalitis is made primarily by serologic testing. Acute and convalescent blood samples (drawn 2 to 4 weeks after the onset of symptoms) may be tested by hemagglutination inhibition (HI) and complement fixation (CF). IgM capture ELISA of CSF is a newer technique that allows testing on a single specimen and has comparable sensitivity and specificity to HI and CF, with the added advantage of speed. Since IgM antibodies may persist for a prolonged period, resulting in false-positive results, it is preferable to confirm the diagnosis with a combination of methods. Cross-reactions between antigenically related viruses present a problem in interpreting test results. SLE, Japanese B encephalitis, dengue, and yellow fever are all antigenically related, as are WEE, EEE, and VEE. For this reason, travel and vaccination history (Japanese B encephalitis and yellow fever) are key components of the history.[9,10,14] Reverse transcriptase-PCR technology is available for some viruses, but it is still a research tool.[12,52]

According to 1998 CDC criteria for the diagnosis of arbovirus infection:

A confirmed case is defined as a febrile illness associated with neurologic manifestations ranging from headache to aseptic meningitis or encephalitis with onset during a period when arbovirus transmission is likely to occur, plus at least one of the following criteria: (1) fourfold or greater serial change in serum antibody titer; (2) isolation of virus from or demonstration of viral genomic sequences in tissue, blood, cerebrospinal fluid, or other body fluid; or (3) demonstration of specific immunoglobulin M (IgM) antibody in serum or cerebrospinal fluid by IgM-capture enzyme immunoassay with confirmation by demonstration of IgG antibodies by another serologic assay (e.g., neutralization or hemagglutination inhibition). A probable case is defined as compatible illness occurring during a period when arbovirus transmission is likely, plus an elevated but stable (twofold or less serial change) antibody titer to an arbovirus (e.g., greater than or equal to 320 by hemagglutination inhibition, greater than or equal to 120 by complement fixation, greater than or equal to 256 by immunofluorescence, greater than or equal to 160 by neutralization, or greater than or equal to 400 by IgM-capture enzyme immunoassay.[14]

Treatment is largely supportive because no effective antiviral drugs are currently available. Prognosis is dependent on the severity of illness and the specific virus causing the infection.

## ENTEROVIRUS INFECTIONS

Enteroviruses cause more than half the cases of CNS infection in which a cause is identified. The enterovirus genus includes coxsackieviruses, echoviruses, and polioviruses, among others. Signs and symptoms of infection are generally similar to those discussed for viral meningitis. A preceding respiratory or gastrointestinal constellation of symptoms is often present. Viral exanthems are common. Coxsackie B virus can be associated with concurrent pleurodynia, myocarditis, pericarditis, and orchitis. Coxsackie A virus infection may present with the vesicular exanthem and enanthem of hand-foot-and-mouth disease, with vesicles at those sites.[101] Echoviruses may cause progressive meningoencephalitis in patients with X-linked agammaglobulinemia.[82]

The CSF shows a lymphocytic pleocytosis with a mildly to moderately elevated protein concentration and a normal glucose concentration. Viral isolation from CSF is the gold standard of diagnosis but is too slow to be useful in acute diagnosis. Serologic studies should be performed on CSF or other sterile body fluids. Enzyme immunoassay is approximately 75% sensitive for IgM and 65% sensitive for IgG.[49,105] PCR techniques are under development but are not widely used.[93] Genetic probes for direct detection of viral RNA in specimens are a promising future technique.[133] MRI may demonstrate an area of focal cerebritis.

## LYMPHOCYTIC CHORIOMENINGITIS

Lymphocytic choriomeningitis (LCM) is an arenavirus that causes meningitis and encephalitis. Its most common reservoir is *Mus musculus*, the house mouse, and transmission to humans occurs via contaminated food and dust. It has also been associated with pet hamsters. This virus is seen principally in the northeastern United States.[47]

LCM presents as a nonspecific flulike illness occurring about 1 week after exposure, followed by signs of CNS infection 2 to 3 weeks later. Diagnosis can be made by history and appropriate serologic studies (i.e., IgM-capture ELISA). A reverse transcription–PCR technique for diagnosis has been reported.[67] Features that may help distinguish LCM from other viral CNS illnesses are the latent period between the flulike symptoms and CNS findings, low glucose concentration in the CSF, thrombocytopenia, and leukopenia. Hydrocephalus has been described as a complication.[92] Treatment is supportive.

## HERPES SIMPLEX

Herpes simplex virus (HSV) infection of the CNS can be a devastating and difficult to diagnose illness. It accounts for 10% to 20% of encephalitis cases and 0.5% to 3% of meningitis cases in the United States. HSV encephalitis is associated with a very high morbidity and mortality rate, but prompt initiation of antiviral treatment with acyclovir can reduce the severity of the illness.[111,122]

Clinical presentation may vary greatly, but it often includes fever, altered mental status (particularly personality changes), and seizures. In any patient with encephalitis, HSV should be strongly suspected if there is any evidence of focality by history, physical examination, EEG, or radiographic studies. In addition to HSV, the differential diagnosis of encephalitis with focal features includes enteroviruses, arboviruses, varicella zoster, human herpesvirus type 6, Epstein-Barr, cytomegalovirus (CMV), toxoplasmosis, subacute measles encephalitis, Powassan virus, Lyme disease, bacterial meningitis, brain abscess, subdural empyema, stroke, Rasmussen's syndrome, and postinfectious encephalomyelitis.

A variety of laboratory studies may be useful. CSF studies in HSV encephalitis are usually abnormal but nonspecific. Common findings are elevated opening pressure, mildly elevated protein concentration, WBC count of 5 to 500/mm³ with a lymphocytic predominance, and red blood cells (RBCs). Sensitivity and specificity of viral cultures from CSF is low. Serologic methods such as CSF antibody titers are available but are of little use in acute diagnosis. In the past, brain biopsy with pathologic examination of the tissue was considered the gold standard of diagnosis. However, PCR for HSV DNA in the CSF has been shown to be highly sensitive and specific.[99] Lakeman et al[65] and Lakeman and Whitley[66] report a sensitivity of 98% and a specificity of 94% for PCR compared with biopsy-proven HSV infection. PCR is less costly and far less invasive than brain biopsy; it is replacing brain biopsy as the test of choice when it is available. At present, testing is available through large research centers only. If possible, CSF PCR should be obtained before treatment is begun because the results may be negative once acyclovir therapy has been started. The EEG will be abnormal in up to 90% of cases. Unilateral temporal localization is the classic finding, but other focal abnormalities can be seen. In two thirds of pathologically proven cases, unilateral or bilateral periodic sharp-and-slow wave complexes occurring at regular intervals of 2 to 3 seconds are present, usually between day 2 and day 15 of the illness. MRI is the imaging test of choice because it is more sensitive than CT, particularly early in the illness. High signal intensity lesions may be seen in the medial and inferior temporal lobe extending up into the insula on T2-weighted images.

HSV (primarily type 2) may cause benign, recurrent lymphocytic meningitis (Mollaret's meningitis) due to reactivation of the virus.[118] This diagnosis should be considered in a patient who presents with recurrent symptoms of aseptic meningitis. These patients may or may not give a history of genital herpes and do not need to have active genital lesions in conjunction with CNS symptoms for this diagnosis to be valid. PCR amplification of HSV-2 from CSF may be present in some cases.

## RABIES

Rabies is a single-stranded RNA virus that is transmitted to humans by infected saliva from animals. In most areas of the world the dog is the most important animal source of rabies. In the United States, rabies is seen in different animals in various geographic areas. In the Northeast and Southeast, raccoons are the reservoir. Despite a tremendous number of rabid raccoons noted in the last two decades, human rabies contracted from raccoons has not been documented. Red and Arctic foxes in Alaska and gray foxes in Arizona and Texas can be infected. Skunks serve as the main reservoir in north central areas, south central areas, and California.[33,113] A recent outbreak has been traced to coyotes and dogs along the Texas-Mexico border.[100] Bats are the most important vector for the recently reported cases of human rabies in the United States.[13,15] Rabbits and rodents are rarely infected.

Successful treatment of rabies is possible only with early and appropriate postexposure intervention. Therefore, if the diagnosis is suspected, rapid treatment is essential. It is important to thoroughly cleanse the wound with soapy water. Postexposure prophylaxis must include both passive antibody administration and active vaccination (five injections over a 1-month period).[33]

A history that includes an animal bite or contact with saliva on an open wound or mucous membrane is a key feature in the diagnosis. However, not all cases include a history of animal exposure. Incubation ranges from days to several years. Signs and symptoms include fever, headache, autonomic nervous system dysfunction, and hyperesthesias or paresthesias around the site of the bite. The illness progresses to include profound disturbances in mental status and eventually coma and death due to dysfunction of central autonomic centers. Hydrophobia, which may be present in 50% of cases, is due to painful contractions of the laryngeal and pharyngeal muscles with attempted swallowing.[33,113]

Diagnosis is made by isolation of the virus from tissues or secretions, detection of viral antigen in tissue samples (corneal smears, brain, or, rarely, CSF), serologic evidence of acute infection, or molecular techniques such as PCR or genetic probes.[20,48,58,100] If possible, the animal should be observed and tested if warranted. Diagnosis is most commonly made with the direct immunofluorescent antibody (dIFA) test for rabies virus antigen in brain tissue. This test is rapid, sensitive, and widely available. Molecular techniques such as PCR and genetic probes are more expensive and may not be more sensitive than dIFA until later in the course of the illness. These molecular techniques do have a role in confirmatory testing if other techniques have failed or if specific characteristics of the virus strain are epidemiologically important. City and county health departments should be notified if the diagnosis of rabies is suspected and they can help with confirmatory studies and case management.

### POSTINFECTIOUS ENCEPHALOMYELITIS

Encephalitis can occur after infection with varicella, measles, and a variety of respiratory tract infections, especially influenza.[55,57] HSV can cause a late demyelinating syndrome.[61] The process is considered to have an autoimmune basis and is characterized by perivascular inflammation and demyelination. Measles is the most common cause worldwide. A similar syndrome may occur after vaccination for smallpox or with some rabies vaccines.[55–57,61]

The severity of this illness is variable. Onset is usually after the exanthem of the acute infection fades and may include altered mental status, meningismus, seizures, hemiparesis, and sensory loss. Laboratory studies of the CSF may show elevated protein levels and lymphocytic pleocytosis. MRI reveals extensive gadolinium-enhancing white-matter lesions.[55–57,61] The presence of measles can be demonstrated only by brain biopsy. History of recent illness or vaccination and usual young age of patients help to distinguish the process from similar entities such as multiple sclerosis (MS). Treatment is with intravenous steroids, and the prognosis depends on the severity of the disease.

## LATENT VIRUSES AND PRION DISEASES

Human T–lymphotrophic viruses (HTLV-1, HTLV-2) are retroviruses. HTLV-1 is endemic to southern Japan and the Caribbean. Infection has also been noted with increased prevalence in sub-Saharan Africa, Italy, Israel, and the southeastern part of the United States. Transmission occurs via blood products, sexual contact, and from mother to child. Adult T-cell lymphoma has been associated with HTLV-1. HTLV-1 also causes HTLV-associated myelopathy (HAM), which is also known as tropical spastic paraparesis. HAM is characterized by progressive motor weakness with spastic paraparesis or paraplegia accompanied by hyperreflexia. The disease may resemble multiple sclerosis (MS) but does not have remissions. HAM is more common in females than in males. Cranial nerve abnormalities are rare, and cognitive function is usually preserved. HAM develops in less than 5% of those infected and progresses over many years. The role of HTLV-2 in disease is still under investigation.[16,32,39,51]

HAM should be investigated as a possibility in a person with the preceding clinical findings who is from a known endemic area or who may have been exposed via blood transfusion, intravenous drug use, or sexual contact. MRI shows white-matter lesions in the cerebrum and spinal cord. HTLV-1 antibodies can be isolated from serum or CSF.[38,83] PCR techniques can detect the virus in CSF or serum.[1,59] Periventricular white-matter lesions similar to those seen in MS may be present. The spinal cord may show symmetrical lateral and posterior degeneration.

HAM has been treated successfully with corticosteroids. Physical therapy is an important component of management. Antiretrovirals have not shown clear benefit in treatment.

### PROGRESSIVE MULTIFOCAL LEUKOENCEPHALOPATHY

Progressive multifocal leukoencephalopathy (PML) is a demyelinating CNS infection seen most commonly in patients with underlying immunosuppression, such as human immunodeficiency virus (HIV), lymphoproliferative disorders, and chronic granulomatous diseases. The cause is a polyomavirus called JC virus (JCV). Patients present with progressive white-matter deficits: commonly, ataxia, cranial nerve deficits, and cerebellar findings. Visual symptoms are common.[35,76,103]

CT and MRI are important tools in diagnosis. Both studies show characteristic white-matter lesions in periventricular, parietal, and occipital lobes. MRI is more sensitive than CT scan, but MRI is not essential to diagnosis, given the characteristic patient population and physical findings. Pathologic examination of infected white matter shows characteristic inclusions in oligodendrocytes, atypical astrocytes, and foamy macrophages containing myelin debris. JCV particles can be visualized in the oligodendrocytes with electron microscopy.[85] Laboratory studies of the CSF are usually normal. EEG shows diffuse slowing or focal abnormalities corresponding to the areas of the lesions. PCR of CSF can identify the JCV, but false-positives do occur, and laboratory selection is crucial to ensure that proper technique is employed.[34,126] It appears that PML caused by the JCV, like many diseases now recognized in HIV-related illness, is due to reactivation of an agent that is benign in the immunocompetent host.

Treatment is largely supportive. Patients with acquired immunodeficiency syndrome (AIDS) may improve on highly active HIV-directed antiretrovirals, but no specific antiviral treatment for PML has been found to be uniformly effective.

### SUBACUTE SCLEROSING PANENCEPHALITIS

Caused by the measles virus, subacute sclerosing panencephalitis (SSPE) is a slowly progressive neurologic disorder. It presents in children and adolescents with a history of primary measles 6 years or more previously. It manifests with cognitive dysfunction, seizures, ataxia, and visual disturbances with a progression to coma and death within 1 to 2 years. EEG shows high-voltage, sharp, slow waves with a periodicity of 3 to 8 seconds and flattened background activity. CSF is notable for elevated gamma globulin level (>20% of total CSF protein). CSF also shows measles antibodies on serologic examination and measles DNA with PCR techniques. CT and MRI show multiple white-matter lesions. Treatment is largely supportive, although some benefits have been reported of treatment with inosine pranobex (Isoprinosine).[123]

### CREUTZFELDT-JAKOB DISEASE

Creutzfeldt-Jakob disease (CJD) is a spongiform encephalopathy that presents with rapidly progressive dementia. It is the best characterized human disease in the class referred to as prion diseases. Prions are proteinaceous infectious particles with latent periods in the host. The exact pathologic mechanism is still not well understood. An autosomal dominant pattern of inheritance has been noted in up to 15% of cases; the rest are sporadic. Transmission has occurred with corneal transplants and administration of cadaveric growth hormone.

CJD usually begins between 55 and 70 years of age but rarely has been described in teenagers and those over age 80. One third of cases begin with general fatigue, myalgia, decrease in appetite, and other systemic symptoms; another one third of them begin with cognitive abnormalities accompanied by forgetfulness, confusion, or uncharacteristic behavior; and the final one third of cases begin with focal neurologic symptoms such as ataxia, aphasia, or visual loss. Death occurs with a mean time of 5 months, and 80% of patients die within 12 months, although occasionally patients linger up to 8 years. The classic form of the disease appears in late middle age with dementia, myoclonus, ataxia, and emotional lability progressing to akinetic mutism. Patients infected from transplantation or hormone administration are younger and may have more prominent cerebellar abnormalities.[19,108]

Diagnosis is made by recognition of classic physical findings and laboratory and imaging studies. EEG shows a characteristic, periodic sharp-wave pattern with a slow background. The sharp-wave complexes occur at intervals of 0.5 to 2.5 seconds and last 200 to 600 ms. CT and MRI show generalized atrophy. The CSF may show a mildly elevated protein level but is otherwise nondiagnostic. Two proteins appear to be specific for CJD. These proteins are designated as 130 and 131. They seem to be similar to a protein designated as 14-3-3, which can be detected by immunoassay in >90% of sporadic cases of CJD, although it is also found in other dementias, stroke, and encephalitis. These assays currently are only research tools. Familial cases of CJD have a variety of mutations in the *PRNP* gene. Molecular techniques are not widely used for diagnosis at this point but may become increasingly available and valuable in the future. Pathologic changes are characterized by spongiform changes, which are most prominent in the cortex. There is little surrounding inflammation. There is no effective treatment for CJD at this time.[19,108]

## "MAD COW" DISEASE

In recent years a variant of CJD that appears to be related to bovine spongiform encephalopathy (BSE) has been identified in the United Kingdom. Current theories suggest that the bovine prion disease may have been spread to humans via ingestion of infected animals. Patients present with early ataxia and abnormal behavior. In contrast to CJD, in mad cow disease, dementia occurs later and the periodic EEG pattern is not seen. Prion protein plaques and spongiform changes are evident on pathologic examination of brain lesions. Strict beef control standards were put in place in the United Kingdom, and the scope of the problem remains under study. This disease is rare at present but is worthy of consideration if exposure to infected beef may have occurred or if a cluster of CJD-like cases is noted. As with CJD, the prognosis is poor and treatment is supportive only.[6,19,96]

## KURU

Kuru is a disease that is primarily of historical interest. It was once prevalent in central New Guinea, but new cases have not been reported since the abolishment of cannibalism. It is a reference model of spongiform encephalopathy and is characterized by cerebellar ataxia, tremors, dysarthria, and emotional lability.[123]

## ACUTE BACTERIAL MENINGITIS

Bacterial meningitis, an inflammatory process involving the pia, arachnoid, and CSF, results from infection with pyogenic bacteria. The three pathogens that account for approximately 80% of infections are *Streptococcus pneumoniae, Neisseria meningitidis,* and *Haemophilus influenzae* (type B). Other important pathogens are *Listeria monocytogenes,* gram-negative bacilli, *Staphylococcus aureus,* and group B streptococci (in neonates). The incidence of *H. influenzae* meningitis has decreased dramatically since the initiation of routine vaccination in infants and children.[110]

### CLINICAL PRESENTATION

Bacterial meningitis in adults classically presents with fever, headache, meningismus, and altered mental status. Nausea, vomiting, photophobia, and myalgias are also common. Kernig's or Brudzinski's sign or both are present in approximately half of the cases. Cranial nerve findings are found in less than 20% of cases.

### SPECIFIC PATHOGENS

Pneumococcal meningitis is the most common form of bacterial meningitis in adults in the United States. It is the most common cause of meningitis in patients with head trauma who have a CSF leak. Other systemic infections are often associated with pneumococcal meningitis, including sinusitis, otitis, pneumonia, and endocarditis.

*Neisseria meningitidis* infections occur most commonly in children and young adults. Epidemics occur with serogroups A and C. Infection is associated with nasopharyngeal carriage. Terminal complement deficiencies (C5-9) predispose a person to *Neisseria* infections.

Meningitis with *H. influenzae* occurs most commonly in children and in those with immunosuppression or another site of infection with *H. influenzae* (i.e., otitis). As noted earlier, vaccination with the polysaccharide-protein conjugate vaccine has decreased the incidence of this infection, and a history of adequate vaccination virtually excludes the diagnosis.

More unusual causes of meningitis include *Listeria* organisms and gram-negative bacilli. *Listeria* infection is usually seen in the very young, the elderly, the immunosuppressed, or those with underlying systemic illnesses such as diabetes. Outbreaks of *Listeria* infection have been reported in association with contaminated food products such as milk and cheese. Mortality is high. Gram-negative meningitis is rare, occurring primarily in infants, but is also seen as a cause of nosocomial meningitis in the elderly and immunosuppressed.[29,97,110,121]

### DIAGNOSIS

Diagnosis is based primarily on clinical presentation and CSF-derived information, although blood cultures may be positive in up to 50% of cases. Patients with focal neurologic findings should have imaging studies done prior to lumbar puncture. CT and MRI are usually not helpful in the specific diagnosis, although meningeal and ependymal enhancement and widened cisterns and sulci caused by the purulent exudate are suggestive findings. Neuroimaging can detect sequelae, including hydrocephalus, diffuse cerebral edema, cerebritis, abscess, subdural effusion, empyema, and stroke.

Specific CSF abnormalities are present. An elevated opening pressure, increased WBCs with neutrophilic predominance (1000 to 5000 cells/mm$^3$), increased protein level

(100 to 500 mg/dl) and low glucose level (<40 mg/dl or a CSF/serum ratio of <0.3) are the usual findings.[29,97,110,121] Approximately 90% of patients will have >100 WBCs/mm³, and 65% to 70% will have >1000 WBCs/mm³. Although the WBCs are predominantly neutrophils, initially 10% of patients may show mononuclear predominance (generally with cell counts <1000). CSF findings that have a very high predictive value for bacterial meningitis include the following: glucose <34 mg/dl; CSF/serum glucose <0.23; WBCs >2000/mm³; and neutrophils >1180/mm³. Gram's stain of the CSF, which is positive in 60% to 90% of patients, can help to identify pathogens. *Listeria* is often difficult to see on Gram's stain because of the low number of organisms and may be identified by inexperienced laboratory technicians as a contaminant because of its similarity to corynebacteria. The CSF culture is positive in at least 80% of cases.

Counterimmunoelectrophoresis (CIE) and latex agglutination tests are widely available to test for bacterial antigen in CSF.[44,69,104] Latex agglutination tests are more sensitive but have a wide range of variability, depending on the test and the laboratory. Agglutination tests are available for *S. pneumoniae, N. meningitidis, H. influenzae* type B, *Streptococcus agalactiae,* and *Escherichia coli*. PCR techniques have been developed but are expensive and are not sufficiently standardized to be clinically useful in this setting.[27,90,106] The rapid-detection tests noted earlier should be used only as adjuncts to standard CSF Gram's stain and culture techniques. They may be useful when there is a delay in obtaining CSF and presumptive antibiotics must be given. In such a situation, CSF cultures may be negative. Blood cultures should always be drawn prior to antibiotic therapy because they may be diagnostic.

## TREATMENT

Antibiotic treatment should be chosen to cover likely pathogens and should be initiated as soon as possible. A third-generation cephalosporin (e.g., ceftriaxone or cefotaxime) is the agent of choice for adults. To treat *Listeria* infection, ampicillin should be added if the patient is older than 50 or immunosuppressed. Vancomycin should be used if penicillin-resistant pneumococcus is endemic in the area or is suspected. After laboratory data are available to identify the likely pathogens, the antibiotics should be further tailored to the specific pathogen or pathogens.

Laboratory abnormalities change after incomplete antibiotic treatment. Patients with a partially treated meningitis will have a lower culture and Gram's stain yield and decreased neutrophil and protein abnormalities. CSF culture and Gram's stain become negative after appropriate intravenous antibiotic treatment for more than 24 hours. The CSF glucose level will approach normal in 80% of effectively treated patients at 3 days. The cell count will still be elevated in 50% of patients after 7 to 10 days of treatment but will be lower than the pretreatment count. Antigens remain positive 1 to 10 days after antibiotic treatment has been started.

## BRAIN ABSCESS

Brain abscess may be defined as a focal intracerebral infectious process. The most helpful classification system is based upon the site of origin of the infection. There are three primary causes of infection: (1) contiguous site of infection (i.e., otogenic, paranasal sinuses); (2) metastatic spread via hematogenous route (i.e., endocarditis, lung abscess, or intraabdominal infection); and (3) prior trauma or surgery (i.e., skull fracture, ventriculoperitoneal shunt). In 20% to 30% of cases, no predisposing condition is identified. The origin of the infection is often reflected in the microbiologic profile of the organisms isolated, and these data are invaluable in identifying other sources of infection.[79]

Signs and symptoms of brain abscess usually reflect the mass effect of the lesions. Headache is the most frequently reported symptom (70% of cases). Fever is more common in children and is present in about 50% of adult cases. Focal neurologic deficits reflect the site of the lesion, but they are present in less than half the cases.

Diagnosis is often challenging because of nonspecific initial signs and symptoms and must be aggressively pursued because of the high mortality associated with treatment delay. Laboratory data are rarely helpful in diagnosis. Blood cultures are positive in <10% of cases. Peripheral WBC counts may be elevated or normal. Erythrocyte sedimentation rate (ESR) is often elevated, but this is a nonspecific finding. Lumbar puncture is contraindicated if mass lesions are present because of risk of herniation; if obtained, CSF is rarely diagnostic unless the abscess has ruptured. The cornerstone of diagnosis is imaging with CT and MRI.[43,128] The classic finding of brain abscess by CT scan with contrast is a ring-enhancing lesion. The appearance varies based on the age and cause of the abscess. Early suppurative processes may not have organized sufficiently to display classic enhancement. Metastatic neoplastic lesions may be very difficult to distinguish from multiple brain abscesses. MRI is more sensitive than CT in detecting brain abscess because of greater soft tissue resolution. T1-weighted images show hypodense areas with ring enhancement after gadolinium is used. T2-weighted images show a hyperdense central area surrounded by a capsule. Surrounding edema is better visualized with MRI. Better imaging of the lesion allows more accurate estimates of its age and amenability to aspiration or drainage. Single photon emission computed tomography (SPECT) with thallium 201 is useful in delineating CNS lymphoma from toxoplasmosis, but its role in other forms of brain abscess is not yet fully delineated.[102]

Management of brain abscess is a challenging task that must be individualized for each specific clinical scenario and patient. Optimally, it involves the coordinated input of neurosurgical, neurologic, radiologic, and infectious disease clinicians. Aspiration is increasingly feasible with CT-guided and stereotactic needle techniques. These techniques allow drainage and provide material for microbiological studies to focus antibiotic therapy.[73,77,112]

Antibiotic therapy should be chosen to treat cultured pathogens or likely pathogens as indicated by the probable source of infection. Host factors often play a role in the etiology of infection and must be considered. Immunocompetent hosts are likely to have bacterial infections that originated from sources mentioned earlier, but travel history (i.e., travel to areas that make neurocysticercosis or amebic abscess possible) and history of prior CNS surgery or trauma are key features to be recorded. HIV-infected patients are more likely to have fungal or parasitic (e.g., toxoplasmosis) infections. Transplant or other immunosuppressed patients are prone to infections with fungal pathogens (e.g., *Asper-*

*gillus*) and unusual pathogens (e.g., *Nocardia*).[11,129] Infections in HIV-infected patients are discussed in greater detail in other sections of this chapter.

## CHRONIC (TUBERCULOUS) MENINGITIS

CNS infection with tuberculosis (TB) has two primary manifestations: tuberculomas of the brain parenchyma and meningitis. Immunosuppressed patients, such as those with HIV or a malignancy or those undergoing long-term therapy with immunosuppressive drugs are at higher risk for TB infection. CNS tuberculous infection is commonly a reactivation of prior disease. Therefore the history of a positive PPD (purified protein derivative [tuberculin]) or exposure to patients with active TB may be helpful.[124,125,132]

CNS tuberculomas may present as new-onset seizures or with signs of an enlarging cranial mass lesion. Neurologic deficits may be present corresponding to the location of the lesion or lesions. CT and MRI show enhancing lesions, often with surrounding calcifications. Edema around the lesions is variable. MRI provides greater resolution, but calcification may be more visible with CT.[64,117] The CSF usually is normal unless a tubercle has ruptured into the CSF, in which case the patient may present with signs and symptoms of meningitis (as discussed later). Diagnosis is based on a history of TB exposure, a positive PPD skin test, evidence of TB at other sites, and exclusion of other possible etiologies including malignancy and parasitic and fungal infection. Stereotactic biopsy of the lesion and isolation of acid-fast bacilli (AFB) is the gold standard of diagnosis, but isolation of TB from other tissue, such as that of lymph nodes, bone marrow, or liver, may be technically easier and, in conjunction with characteristic brain lesions, justifies treatment with antituberculous agents.[109] Presumptive treatment is indicated if clinical suspicion is high.

Tuberculous meningitis can be a devastating and difficult to diagnose illness. It usually presents as a subacute meningitis, with symptoms of fever, altered mental status, and the characteristic cranial nerve abnormalities developing over the course of a few weeks. It can also present acutely over the course of hours to days; in this form it is difficult to distinguish clinically from acute bacterial meningitis. Cranial nerve abnormalities caused by inflammation of the basilar meninges and diabetes insipidus resulting from hypothalamic dysfunction are nonspecific but should raise the suspicion of tuberculous meningitis. Presentation is similar in HIV-positive and non-HIV-positive patients.[124,125,132]

CT and MRI may show basilar enhancement, the presence of tuberculomas, enlargement of the ventricles, or areas of infarction, especially in the region of the basal ganglia. MRI is more sensitive in distinguishing areas of infarction.[117]

The CSF characteristically shows an elevated WBC count (100 to 500/mm³) with a lymphocytic predominance, protein elevation (100 to 500 mg/dl), and low glucose level (<45 mg/dl). Although the WBCs are usually lymphocytes, polymorphonuclear cells can predominate in up to 32% of cases. The presence of polymorphonuclear cells does not necessarily correlate with the acuteness of the clinical evolution of symptoms but does correlate with worse clinical signs. Although mean cell counts are in the range of 110 to 270/mm³, total cell counts can be as high as 4000/mm³. Approximately 8% of affected patients will have normal CSF cell counts. The CSF findings are similar in HIV-positive and HIV-negative patients. Mean protein concentrations range from 65 to 504 mg/dl with most in the 100 to 200 mg/dl range. In 10% to 38% of patients the protein content can be normal. In cases of marked exudation reaction and blockage of CSF pathways, especially at spinal levels, the protein concentration can be >1 g/dl.

CSF should be sent to the laboratory for AFB stains and culture. The sensitivity of AFB stains is variably reported as between 4% and 24%. Multiple high-volume samples may improve the yield. Cultures are not useful in the short term since growth often takes 2 to 6 weeks. PCR of CSF for *Mycobacterium tuberculosis* has shown high sensitivity (variably reported as 32% to 100%) and specificity (about 8% false-positives) for the diagnosis and should be obtained when available.[63,88] CSF will remain positive for mycobacterial DNA for weeks after treatment has been initiated and thus can be helpful even after initiation of therapy.[70] PCR techniques may also be useful in following the response to antibiotic therapy because studies have shown that patients who remain positive after many weeks of treatment may be nonresponders to therapy who have a poor prognosis. Nested PCR techniques (amplified twice) are 90% sensitive, but they are specialized and not widely available.[107] The Gen-Probe Amplified *Mycobacterium tuberculosis* Direct Test (MTD; a transcription-mediated amplification test), which is primarily used for sputum testing, has been applied to CSF with good sensitivity and specificity and may provide an alternative method of testing that is rapid and economical.[30,36] All patients should have CSF sent for culture, even if PCR or other molecular methods are done, because the organisms need to be isolated to obtain drug sensitivities.

Treatment should be initiated with a multidrug regimen as promptly as possible. Prognosis is most dependent upon the degree of illness at initial presentation, and recovery may be prolonged.

## SYPHILIS

Syphilis is a sexually transmitted disease caused by *Treponema pallidum* that results in chronic systemic infection. The initial exposure usually occurs during sexual contact. It results in the appearance of a primary lesion at the site of exposure and regional lymphadenopathy approximately 3 weeks later. Signs of secondary syphilis manifest about 6 to 8 weeks after the healing of the lesion and consist of maculopapular skin lesions, generalized nontender lymphadenopathy, and nonspecific constitutional symptoms, including low-grade fever, malaise, weight loss, pharyngitis, and arthralgias. CNS invasion at this stage occurs in up to 40% of cases and may be symptomatic or asymptomatic. Symptoms usually subside spontaneously, and the infection enters a latent period. Latency may last months to many years. The percentage of persons who subsequently develop tertiary syphilis is a controversial topic, but it is clearly lower in this era of modern medicine since many patients receive antibiotics for unrelated illnesses that eliminate the treponemal infection. Tertiary syphilis is traditionally discussed as three separate entities: meningovascular, parenchymatous, and tabes dorsalis. However, it is important to remember that a vast overlap of manifestations occurs. Meningovascular syphilis is the diffuse inflammation of the meninges with the development of endarteritis obliterans that results in multiple small infarctions in the brain and spinal cord. One classic presentation is that of a stroke in the middle cerebral artery area in a young person.[21,87]

Parenchymatous neurosyphilis results in the destruction of nerve cells and produces neurologic and psychiatric findings. The pneumonic *paresis* is useful in describing the key deficits: *P*ersonality, *A*ffect, *R*eflexes (hyperactive), *E*ye (Argyll Robertson pupil), *S*ensorium (hallucinations, delusions), *I*ntellect (poor memory and judgment), and *S*peech (slurred). *Tabes dorsalis* is the term used to describe demyelination of posterior columns, dorsal roots, and dorsal root ganglia that results in the characteristic lancinating pains, wide-based gait, and bowel and bladder dysfunction. Neurosyphilis occurs more commonly and may present much earlier in HIV-infected patients.[90]

## LABORATORY FINDINGS

A variety of serologic tests for syphilis are available, and an understanding of their intended uses and limitations is essential to make the diagnosis of neurosyphilis. Two general classes of laboratory tests are employed: nontreponemal antigen tests and treponemal tests. The nontreponemal tests use extracts of normal tissues (i.e., beef cardiolipin) as antigens to measure antibodies formed in the blood. The commonly used nontreponemal tests are the RPR (rapid plasma reagin) and the VDRL (Venereal Disease Research Laboratory Test). These tests show a positive result in the early stages of primary infection and are almost always positive by the secondary stage. Their positivity declines in later stages of the disease or after treatment. False-positive VDRL testing that is present for less than 6 months can be due to *Mycoplasma pneumoniae*, enterovirus infection, infectious mononucleosis, TB, viral pneumonia, leptospirosis, measles, or mumps. False-positives lasting longer than 6 months can be due to systemic lupus erythematosus and other connective tissue disorders, intravenous drug use, rheumatoid arthritis, reticuloendothelial malignancy, advanced age, or Hashimoto's thyroiditis. Because of the possible false-positive results, these tests should be used as screenings for the more specific treponemal tests. They also can be used to monitor the patient's response to treatment. When an HIV-1-positive patient is being screened for syphilis, a treponemal-specific test should be performed since the nontreponemal tests may be falsely negative. The specific treponemal tests use live or killed *T. pallidum* as antigen to directly detect treponemal antibody. The commonly used treponemal tests are the MHA-TP (microhemagglutination test for antibody to *T. pallidum*) and the FTA-ABS (fluorescent treponemal antibody absorption test). The FTA-ABS is the more sensitive of these two. These tests remain positive even after treatment.[68] A false-positive FTA-ABS test result may be due to technical error, Lyme borreliosis, genital herpes simplex, systemic lupus erythematosus, scleroderma, mixed connective tissue disease, cirrhosis, or nonvenereal treponematosis.

If a patient has a strongly positive serum RPR or VDRL and MHA-TP or FTA-ABS and symptoms or signs consistent with neurosyphilis, he or she should undergo lumbar puncture. The diagnosis is established based upon a CSF mononuclear pleocytosis or elevated protein concentration or reactive CSF VDRL. The glucose level is normal or slightly decreased. A nonreactive CSF VDRL does not exclude neurosyphilis. Al-

though the CSF may contain elevated IgG or oligoclonal bands, their presence alone is not diagnostic. The RPR has a high level of false-positives in the CSF and cannot be used. Contamination of the CSF with blood during lumbar puncture can also cause false-positive results for any of the tests. Although a nonreactive CSF FTA-ABS or MHA-TP excludes neurosyphilis, these studies, when reactive, do not establish the diagnosis. The sensitivity and specificity, respectively, of two key tests are as follows: CSF-VDRL, 50% and 100%; and CSF FTA-ABS, 100% and 30%. PCR methods, ELISA, and *T. pallidum*–specific IgG antibody tests have been developed, but their clinical utility is under investigation.[74]

Imaging studies may show evidence of vascular occlusive disease in the form of infarction or arteritis, meningeal enhancement, or white-matter changes. Gummas, which may be present, are very peripheral nodular enhancing lesions in the gray matter of the cerebral cortex surrounded by edema and associated with an adjacent area of meningeal enhancement. Imaging findings are nonspecific and must be interpreted within the constellation of signs and symptoms and laboratory studies.[5]

Regardless of the specific outcome of diagnostic tests, if the clinical suspicion is high enough, most clinicians begin treatment for neurosyphilis. Obtaining documentation of prior infection with or treatment for syphilis is important because it can shorten the evaluation considerably. Records are often available from city health departments, and women are routinely tested for seropositivity at the time of childbirth and during prenatal care. These are other sources of information that the clinician can use.

## TREATMENT

The standard treatment regimen is aqueous penicillin G (12 to 24 million U/d IV given in divided doses every 4 hours) for a total of 10 to 14 days. Alternative regimens are doxycycline (100 mg bid PO) for 21 days and procaine penicillin G (2.4 million U qd [IV or IM]) plus probenecid (1 g PO) daily for 10 days.

# LYME DISEASE

Lyme borreliosis, or Lyme disease, is a tick-transmitted illness caused by the spirochete *Borrelia burgdorferi*. The organism is carried by ticks of the *Ixodes* genus, and therefore it has the same geographic distribution as the tick vector—primarily the Northeast, upper Midwest, and Pacific coast areas of the United States. The disease is endemic in Europe, Asia, Russia, China, and Japan, but it often has a different clinical presentation from that seen in the United States.[54,114]

The first stage of the illness is localized skin infection. The classic skin lesion is erythema migrans (EM), which appears from several days to several weeks after the tick bite. EM begins as a macular or papular lesion that later becomes annular, with an area of central clearing. The lesion may eventually become indurated or necrotic. The most common sites for EM are the torso, thigh, groin, and axilla. The lesion may not occur in up to one fourth of infected patients. The second stage of the illness occurs several weeks to several months after the initial infection and may manifest as disseminated skin lesions, meningitis, Bell's palsy, peripheral neuropathy, myelitis, mononeuritis multiplex, myalgias, neuralgias, or cardiac involvement (e.g., pericarditis and dysrhythmias). The third stage of infection occurs months to years after infection and also presents with skin, neurologic, and musculoskeletal disease.[46,54] CNS and peripheral nervous system findings include subacute encephalopathy, axonal polyneuropathy, and leukoencephalitis. Leukoencephalitis is rare but presents with altered mental status, spastic paraparesis, ataxia, and bladder dysfunction.[45,46]

### DIAGNOSIS

Both clinical and laboratory findings are used to diagnose Lyme borreliosis. Because of the often confusing constellation of symptoms, specific criteria for the diagnosis have been adopted. To fulfill the diagnosis for Lyme disease established by the CDC criteria, the patient must have (1) exposure to the appropriate tick habitat, (2) EM diagnosed by a physician or one or more late manifestations of Lyme disease, and (3) laboratory confirmation of diagnosis.[120,127]

Laboratory diagnosis may be made by culture of the organism, detection of antibodies, or detection of DNA. Cultures have a low yield, require weeks to provide data, and therefore have little clinical value. Antibodies are detected by indirect immunofluorescence assay or ELISA. ELISA is more sensitive and more specific. Western blot, which can detect IgM and IgG, is used as a confirmatory test. Acute and convalescent-phase testing is desirable. False-negative results may be obtained in the first month of infection. The IgM Western blot is positive if two of three of the bands 23, 31, and 41 kDa are present. The IgG blot is positive if 5 of 10 of the bands 18, 23, 28, 30, 39, 41, 45, 58, 66, and 93 kDa are present. Serologic diagnosis may be problematic because antibodies may persist, making it difficult to delineate between acute and chronic infection. There is considerable variability in the reliability of testing among laboratories. Therefore it is important for the physician to interpret the results accordingly and to seek confirmation from the CDC in appropriate cases. False-positive results can occur as a result of cross-reactivity with other spirochetes (i.e., syphilis, *Borellia hermsii*) or with IgM rheumatoid factor. PCR methods for testing are available, but the results may remain positive even with appropriate treatment.[75,120]

The diagnosis of neuroborreliosis is particularly difficult. The diagnosis must be made based on clinical grounds, with supporting data from laboratory testing. Symptoms may be nonspecific and may include memory impairment and peripheral neuropathy. CSF may show a pleocytosis and elevated total protein level. Increased intrathecal production of IgG, IgM, and IgA has been found in neuroborreliosis. PCR detection of *Borrelia* DNA in the CSF can help to support the diagnosis in the correct clinical setting. Detection of intrathecal production of anti–*B. burgdorferi* antibody is a sensitive test and should be used when feasible.[45,46] Neuropsychologic testing and imaging with SPECT and positron emission tomography (PET) have been proposed as adjunct diagnostic modalities, but their use needs further investigation.[31]

### TREATMENT

Lyme borreliosis can be treated with doxycycline, tetracycline, ampicillin, amoxicillin, ceftriaxone, azithromycin, and imipenem. The most common treatment regimen for localized skin infection (EM) is doxycycline 100 mg PO bid for 10 days. Amoxicillin is used for children. CNS infection requires treatment for 3 to 4 weeks with intravenous antibi-

otics. Bell's palsy, arthritis, or minor cardiac dysfunction (first-degree AV block) may be treated with oral antibiotics for 1 month. Presumptive treatment for Lyme disease is warranted, but care must be taken not to use the diagnosis to account for symptoms, especially neurologic symptoms, unless the diagnostic criteria are met and other diagnoses are excluded.[98]

## HIV-ASSOCIATED CENTRAL NERVOUS SYSTEM INFECTIONS

HIV-infected patients are susceptible to all the previously mentioned CNS infections. The initial diagnosis of HIV infection is often made in the workup of acute illness. Initial screening for HIV is done with an ELISA test, which is about 99% specific and 98% sensitive when properly performed. False-positive results do occur, and therefore the diagnosis must be confirmed with more specific PCR or Western blot techniques.[53,89] The CD4 count of the patient can be used to help decide the patient's risk of having cryptococcosis, toxoplasmosis, PML, or CNS lymphoma since these generally occur only when the CD4 count is <200/μL. PML and primary CNS lymphoma are rarely seen when the CD4 count is >100/μL. AIDS-associated dementia may be seen at any time in the course of infection but is more common when the CD4 counts are <500/μL.

## AIDS DEMENTIA

Dementia due to HIV infection in the absence of other opportunistic infections is a diagnosis of exclusion. HIV-associated dementia is characterized by a subcortical pattern of dementia, manifesting as impaired functioning in concentration, motor speed, and information processing. Impairments in social function and fine motor skills may also be evident. Prevalence in the HIV-infected population is 4% to 7%.

The CSF typically reveals a pleocytosis in one third of patients, a mildly elevated protein level in two thirds, and oligoclonal bands in nearly one third. Direct markers of HIV-associated dementia have not been identified. Surrogate markers are beta-2-microglobulin, neopterin, and quinolinic acid. The amount of these markers in the CSF correlates with the degree of dementia. MRI and CT studies commonly reveal cortical atrophy, ventricular dilatation, and, less often, attenuation of the white matter. On MRI, white-matter abnormalities consist of either focal or diffuse increases in signal on T2-weighted images most often found in the centrum semiovale. Abnormalities noted on functional neuroimaging studies (PET, SPECT, proton magnetic resonance spectroscopy, and functional MRI imaging) are of research interest to study the natural history and response to new treatments.

EEG and imaging findings may be abnormal but are not specific to this disorder. No specific treatment is known, but many patients improve when the HIV infection is treated with antiretroviral agents.[62,80,95]

## CRYPTOCOCCOSIS

*Cryptococcus neoformans* is a saprophytic fungus that primarily causes pulmonary and CNS infections. In HIV-infected patients it is a common cause of meningoencephalitis.

The fungus is found worldwide in soil and in avian feces, especially pigeon droppings. Infection occurs via inhalation.

Clinical manifestations of meningoencephalitis in an HIV-infected patient are variable but characteristically consist of headache, altered mental status, and fever. Nuchal rigidity is not common in HIV-infected patients. Papilledema, blurred vision, and cranial nerve abnormalities may occur. Symptoms may progress over a few days or may be prolonged for weeks or even months prior to diagnosis.[25]

### DIAGNOSIS

CT and MRI are usually normal, although occasionally an obstructive cryptococcoma or dilated ventricles due to obstruction may be visualized. CSF typically shows increased opening pressure, elevated protein level, mildly decreased glucose level, and lymphocytic predominance. A WBC count of <20 in the CSF in conjunction with cryptococcal infection is a predictor of poor outcome because it signifies diminished inflammatory response. CSF parameters are often only minimally abnormal, increasing the need for more specific diagnostic tests. India ink stain of CSF is a rapid technique but is dependent upon the expertise of the laboratory for accuracy. Latex agglutination tests are the preferred method for diagnosis, and titers can be used to follow response to therapy. Serum antigen titers are usually positive and are useful as a screening test. False-negatives can occur as a result of immune complexes and prozones, and capsule-deficient isolates have been reported. False-positives may occur in the latex agglutination slide test with neurosyphilis, other fungi, or bacterial meningitis.[40,60] DNA probes for culture identification and PCR techniques are also available.[84,115] Culture confirmation is desirable in all cases, and is needed to determine resistance if this becomes important to treatment.

### TREATMENT

Initial treatment for patients with cryptococcal meningitis consists of intravenous amphotericin B (0.7 mg/kg/d) for 2 weeks. Some experts recommend the addition of flucytosine as adjunctive treatment. Initial treatment must be followed by treatment with oral fluconazole (400 mg PO qd for 8 weeks) and lifelong suppressive treatment with fluconazole (200 mg PO qd) to prevent relapses.

## TOXOPLASMOSIS

Toxoplasmosis is caused by infection with the intracellular parasite *Toxoplasma gondii.* The parasite's definitive host is the cat, and oocysts are shed in the feces. Human infection occurs with ingestion of oocysts in contaminated food or water. In HIV-infected persons, toxoplasmosis is a common cause of focal encephalitis.

Clinical presentation may include focal deficits, fever, altered mental status, and seizures. CSF is usually only minimally abnormal, with minimal pleocytosis and a mildly elevated protein level being the most common findings.[72] CT with contrast or MRI of the brain reveals single- or multiple-ring enhancing lesions. Lesions are most often seen in the basal ganglia and corticomedullary junction. MRI is more sensitive than CT and is the preferred test when available.[110] Serologic diagnosis is sensitive and specific. More than 90% of those patients with CNS toxoplasmosis have positive serum IgM titers for *Toxoplasma* organisms.[42] Direct detection of *Toxoplasma* DNA by CSF PCR is available in research centers but has little clinical utility at present.[28] The primary differential diagnosis is CNS lymphoma. A 201-SPECT scan can help to distinguish between CNS lymphoma and toxoplasmosis.[121]

Empiric treatment with sulfadiazine and pyrimethamine can also clarify the diagnosis, since up to 90% of patients with CNS toxoplasmosis will show clinical and radiographic response to treatment by day 14. Brain biopsy should be considered for those patients who do not respond to antibiotic therapy.

## CYTOMEGALOVIRUS

Cytomegalovirus (CMV) is a common opportunistic infection in patients with HIV. It has been shown to cause encephalitis, retinitis, polyneuropathy, and mononeuropathy multiplex. Focal findings and CSF pleocytosis help to distinguish CMV infection from HIV neurologic changes alone. CMV retinitis can usually be diagnosed by characteristic findings in funduscopic evaluation and has been shown to be a sensitive predictor of the presence of CNS CMV infection.[3,7,81]

### DIAGNOSIS

Patients with CNS CMV infection often have an elevated protein level and increased WBCs (sometimes with a neutrophilic predominance unusual for a viral infection) in the CSF, as well as a low glucose level.[22] CMV may be isolated from the CSF by traditional microbiologic techniques or by PCR. PCR has a sensitivity of 79% to 100% for detection in the CSF.[17,18,41,131] PCR positivity alone in CSF is not sufficient for the diagnosis of CNS disease because it may be present but not causative of disease. Therefore the entire constellation of findings must be considered. Serologic testing is helpful only if there is a fourfold or greater acute rise, since most adults are found to be positive for CMV by serologic testing without having active disease. CMV is characterized by the presence of cytomegalic cells with a large basophilic intranuclear inclusion, which has been likened to an "owl's eye."[2] CT or MRI may show focal enhancement of areas of the cerebrum or nerve roots (in the case of polyradiculopathy). MRI may show gadolinium enhancement of ependymal surfaces of the ventricular system.[50] Focal ring–enhancing lesions due to CMV have been reported.[86]

### TREATMENT

Treatment of CNS CMV infection is based on intravenous administration of ganciclovir or foscarnet. Newer agents such as cidofovir are under study as treatment agents.

## SELECTED LABORATORY TECHNIQUES

### POLYMERASE CHAIN REACTION

PCR is a technique that detects and amplifies target nucleic acid. First-generation systems amplified DNA only; however, RNA currently can be amplified by using a heat-stable reverse-transcriptase enzyme (RT-PCR). The process involves three basic steps: (1) heat denaturation to separate the two strands of target DNA, (2) annealing (attaching) of primers to the template DNA, and (3) extension of the sequences through incubation of the target DNA with a heat-stable DNA polymerase. The cycle is repeated 20 to 30 times over several hours, and the target DNA is amplified $10^5$ to $10^6$ times.[4,8,94] Various methods are used to detect amplification products. Two examples of detection methods are (1) an ELISA-like colorimetric system in microliter wells coated with appropriate oligonucleotide and (2) fluorescent dyes with different emission spectra for a multiplex system. Quantitative PCR (e.g., for HIV viral load) is performed by adding standards at a known copy number for comparison.

PCR is a sensitive detection method but is susceptible to interference from extraneous substances. Heme and metabolic products of heme in a variety of tissues, as well as acid polysaccharides in sputum, have been shown to inhibit the DNA polymerase enzymes used in PCR.[4] Consequently, serum or plasma is preferred over whole blood as the specimen to be tested. Such limitations are important to keep in mind because they affect the validity of the results obtained with PCR. For example, contamination with blood during a traumatic spinal tap will yield a sample that is not optimal for testing. Automated systems are designed to decrease the possibility of cross-contamination, a potential cause of false-positive results, given the high sensitivity of the technique.[24] PCR may be used to detect microbial nucleic acid, even in formalin-fixed tissue, and this method may provide valuable diagnostic information when other specimens are not available for evaluation.[91,116]

Two newer generation PCR techniques worthy of note are multiplex PCR and nested PCR.[37,94] The multiplex system amplifies two or more target nucleic acid sequences in a sample simultaneously. This technique has been applied to the diagnosis of sexually transmitted diseases and gastrointestinal pathogens. It is obviously advantageous to screen simultaneously for several organisms that could cause a constellation of symptoms. Nested PCR enhances the sensitivity of the process by reamplifying the product of an initial PCR with a second PCR. Because of the reamplification, nested PCR is extremely sensitive to cross-contamination.

The clinician must be aware that many research laboratories offer in-house PCR techniques. As with other diagnostic tests, it is important to inquire as to the sensitivity, specificity, and positive and negative predictive values of the methods used. The inclusion of an internal control to detect inhibitory substances is also an important issue, as are methods employed to prevent cross-contamination.

## ENZYME IMMUNOASSAY

In this technique, enzyme-labeled antigen or antibody is bound to a solid support (e.g., beads, tubes, microliter wells), patient sera and substrate are added, and products are detected by a color change indicating that the enzyme-substrate reaction has occurred. Direct ELISA measures antigen via competition for antibody binding sites between enzyme-labeled antigen and patient antigen. Indirect ELISA quantifies the binding of bound antigen to specimen antibodies. Indirect ELISA used for some IgM isotypes is prone to false-positive results because of the interaction of IgM rheumatoid factor with IgG-specific antibodies. IgM antibody–capture ELISA is a newer technique that achieves greater specificity. Microliter wells (or another solid support) coated with anti–human IgM antibodies bind all IgM isotype anti-

bodies present in the sample; reagent antigen and enzyme-labeled antigen specific antibodies are added; and the "sandwich" complex causes a quantifiable enzymatic color change.

## WESTERN BLOT

Western blot is often used to confirm the results of ELISA because of the former's greater specificity for antibodies. Electrophoresis separates purified HIV antigen into bands determined by molecular weight. The bands are blotted onto a nitrocellulose filter, and the patient's serum is reacted. If specific antibodies are present in the patient's serum, they bind to the antigenic bands. Enzyme-labeled antihuman immunoglobulin is then reacted with the complex, and a substrate that changes color in the presence of the positive reaction is added.

## REFERENCES

1. Aono Y, Imai J, Tominaga K, et al. Rapid, sensitive, specific, and quantitative detection of human T-cell leukemia virus type 1 sequence in peripheral blood mononuclear cells by an improved polymerase chain reaction method with nested primers. *Virus Genes.* 1992;6:159-171.
2. Arribas JR, Clifford DB, Fictenbaum CJ, et al. Level of cytomegalovirus DNA in cerebrospinal fluid of subjects with AIDS and CMV infection of the central nervous system. *J Infect Dis.* 1995;172:527-531.
3. Arribas JR, Storch GA, Clifford DB, et al. Cytomegalovirus encephalitis. *Ann Intern Med.* 1996;125:577-587.
4. Baselski VS. The role of molecular diagnostics in the clinical microbiology laboratory. *Clin Lab Med.* 1996;16:49-60.
5. Brightbill TC, Ihmeidan IH, Post MJ, et al. Neurosyphilis in HIV-positive and HIV-negative patients: neuroimaging findings. *Am J Neuroradiol.* 1995;16:703-711.
6. Brown P. The risk of bovine spongiform encephalopathy (mad cow disease) to human health. *JAMA.* 1997;278:1008-1011.
7. Bylsma SS, Achim CL, Wiley CL, et al. The predictive value of cytomegalovirus retinitis for cytomegalovirus encephalitis in acquired immunodeficiency syndrome. *Arch Opthalmol.* 1995;113:89-95.
8. Caliendo AM. Molecular diagnostics for infectious diseases. In: Pair JP, Remington JS, eds. *Mediguide to Infectious Disease.* New York: Lawrence DellaCorte Publications; 1997;17(2):1-7.
9. Calisher CH, Bernardi VP, Muth DJ, et al. Specificity of immunoglobulin M and G antibody responses in humans infected with Eastern and Western equine encephalitis viruses: applications to rapid serodiagnosis. *J Clin Microbiol.* 1986;233:69-72.
10. Calisher CH, Monath TP. Togaviridae and flaviviridae: the alphaviruses and flaviviruses. In: Lennette E, Halonen PE, Murphy FA, eds. *Laboratory Diagnosis of Infectious Diseases: Principles and Practices.* New York: Springer-Verlag; 1986:414-434.
11. Campbell S. Amebic brain abscess and meningoencephalitis. *Semin Neurol.* 1993;13:153-160.
12. Chang GJ, Trent DW, Vorndam V, et al. An integrated target sequence and signal amplification assay, reverse transcriptase-PCR-enzyme-linked immunosorbent assay, to detect and characterize flaviviruses. *J Clin Microbiol.* 1994;32:477-483.
13. Centers for Disease Control and Prevention. Human rabies—Kentucky and Montana, 1996. *MMWR.* 1997;46:397-400.
14. Centers for Disease Control and Prevention. Arboviral infections of the central nervous system—United States, 1996–97. *MMWR.* 1998; 47:517-522.
15. Centers for Disease Control and Prevention. Human rabies—Texas and New Jersey, 1997. *MMWR.* 1998;47:1-5.
16. Cereseto A, Mulloy JC, Franchini G. Insights on the pathogenicity of human T-lymphotropic/leukemia virus types I and II. *J Acquir Immune Defic Syndr Hum Retrovirol.* 1996;13(suppl 1):S69-S75.
17. Cinque P, Vago L, Brytting M, et al. Cytomegalovirus infection of the central nervous system in patients with AIDS: diagnosis by DNA amplification from cerebrospinal fluid. *J Infect Dis.* 1992;166:1408-1411.
18. Cinque P, Vago L, Terreni MR, et al. Diagnosis of cytomegalovirus infection of the nervous system in AIDS by polymerase chain reaction analysis of cerebrospinal fluid. *Scand J Infect Dis.* 1995;99:92-94.
19. Collinge J. Human prion diseases and bovine spongiform encephalopathy (BSE). *Hum Mol Genet.* 1997;6:1699-1705.

20. Crepin P, Audry L, Rotivel Y, et al. Intra vitam diagnosis of human rabies by PCR using saliva and cerebrospinal fluid. *J Clin Microbiol.* 1998;36:1117-1121.

21. Davis LE. Neurosyphilis. In: Feldman E, ed. *Current Diagnosis in Neurology.* St Louis: Mosby; 1994.

22. de Gans J, Tiessans G, Portegies P, et al. Predominance of polymorphonuclear leukocytes in cerebrospinal fluid of AIDS patients with cytomegalovirus polyradiculomyelitis. *J Acquir Immune Defic Syndr.* 1990; 3:1155-1158.

23. Deresiewicz RL, Thaler SJ, Hsu L, et al. Clinical and neuroradiographic manifestations of EEE. *N Engl J Med.* 1997;336:1867-1874.

24. DiDominico N, Link H, Knobel R, et al. Cobas Amplicor: fully automated RNA and DNA amplification and detection system for routine diagnostic PCR. *Clin Chem.* 1996;42:1915-1923.

25. Dismukes WE. Cryptococcal meningitis in patients with AIDS. *J Infect Dis.* 1988;157:624.

26. Dobler G. Arboviruses causing neurological disorders in the central nervous system. *Arch Virol.* 1996;11(suppl):33-40.

27. Du Plessis M, Smith AM, Klugman KP. Rapid detection of penicillin-resistant *Streptococcus pneumoniae* in cerebrospinal fluid by a semi-nested-PCR strategy. *J Clin Microbiol.* 1998;36:453-457.

28. Dupon M, Cazenave J, Pellegrin JL, et al. Detection of *Toxoplasma gondii* by PCR and tissue culture in cerebrospinal fluid and blood of human immunodeficiency virus seropositive patients. *J Clin Microbiol.* 1995;33:2421-2426.

29. Durand M, Calderwood SB, Weber DJ, et al. Acute bacterial meningitis in adults: a review of 493 episodes. *N Engl J Med.* 1993;328:21-28.

30. Ehlers S, Ignatius R, Regnath T, et al. Diagnosis of extrapulmonary tuberculosis by Gen-Probe Amplified *Mycobacterium tuberculosis* Direct Test. *J Clin Microbiol.* 1996;34:2275-2279.

31. Fallon BA, Das S, Plutchok JJ, et al. Functional brain imaging and neuropsychological testing in Lyme disease. *Clin Infect Dis.* 1997;25(suppl 1):S57-S63.

32. Ferreira OC Jr, Planelles V, Rosenblatt JD. Human T-cell leukemia viruses: epidemiology, biology, and pathogenesis. *Blood Rev.* 1997;11: 91-104.

33. Fishbein DB, Robinson LE. Rabies. *N Engl J Med.* 1993;329:1632.

34. Fong IW, Britton CB, Luinstra KE, et al. Diagnostic value of detecting JC virus DNA in cerebrospinal fluid of patients with progressive multifocal leukoencephalopathy. *J Clin Microbiol.* 1995;33:484-486.

35. Fong IW, Toma E. The natural history of progressive multifocal leukoencephalopathy in persons infected with AIDS. *Clin Infect Dis.* 1995; 20:1305.

36. Gamboa F, Manterola JM, Vinado B, et al. Direct detection of *Mycobacterium tuberculosis* complex in nonrespiratory specimens by Gen-Probe Amplified *Mycobacterium* Direct Test. *J Clin Microbiol.* 1997;35: 307-310.

37. Garcia-De Lomas J, Navarro D. New directions in diagnostics. *Pediatr Infect Dis.* 1997;16:543-548.

38. Gessain A, Caudie C, Gout O, et al. Intrathecal synthesis of antibodies to human T lymphotropic virus type I and the presence of IgG oligoclonal bands in the cerebrospinal fluid of patients with endemic tropical spastic paraparesis. *J Infect Dis.* 1988;157:1226-1234.

39. Gessain A, Gout O. Chronic myelopathy associated with human T-lymphotrophic virus type-1 (HTLV-1). *Ann Intern Med.* 1992;117:933.

40. Gordon MA, Vedder DK. Serologic tests in diagnosis and prognosis of cryptococcosis. *JAMA.* 1966;197:961-967.

41. Gozlan J, Salord J, Roullet E, et al. Rapid detection of cytomegalovirus DNA in cerebrospinal fluid of AIDS patients with neurologic disorder. *J Infect Dis.* 1992;166:1416-1421.

42. Grant IH, Gold JM, Rosenblum M, et al. *Toxoplasma gondii* serology in HIV-infected patients: the development of central nervous system toxoplasmosis in AIDS. *AIDS.* 1990;4:519-521.

43. Haimes AB, Zimmerman Morgello S, et al. MR imaging of brain abscesses. *AJR.* 1989;152:1073-1085.

44. Halloway Y, Boersam WG, Kuttschrutter H, et al. Minimum number of pneumococci required for capsular antigen to be detectable by latex agglutination. *J Clin Microbiol.* 1992;30:517-538.

45. Halperin JJ. Neuroborelliosis. *Am J Med.* 1995;98:525-565.

46. Halperin JJ. Nervous system Lyme disease. *J Neurol Sci.* 1998;153:182-191.

47. Hammer SM, Connolly KJ. Viral aseptic meningitis in the United States: clinical features, viral etiologies and differential diagnosis. *Curr Clin Top Infect Dis.* 1992;12:1-25.

48. Heaton PR, Johnstone P, McElhinney LM, et al. Hemi-nested PCR assay for detection of six genotypes of rabies and rabies-related viruses. *J Clin Microbiol.* 1997;35:2762-2766.

49. Hodgson J, Bendig J, Keeling P, et al. Comparison of two immunoassay procedures for detecting enterovirus IgM. *J Med Virol.* 1995;47:29-34.

50. Holland NR, Power C, Mathews VP, et al. Cytomegalovirus encephalitis in AIDS. *Neurology.* 1994;44:507-514.

51. Hollsberg P, Hafler DA. Pathogenesis of diseases induced by human lymphotrophic virus type I infection. *N Engl J Med.* 1993;328:1173.

52. Howe DK, Vodkin MH, Novak RJ, et al. Use of the polymerase chain reaction for the sensitive detection of St. Louis encephalitis viral RNA. *J Virol Methods.* 1992;26:101-110.

53. Hu DJ, Dondero TJ, Rayfield MA, et al. The emerging genetic diversity of HIV. *JAMA.* 1996;275:210-216.

54. Jacobs RA. Infectious diseases: spirochetal. In: Tierney LM, McPhee SJ, Papadakes MA, eds. *Current Medical Diagnosis and Treatment.* Stamford, CT: Appleton & Lange; 1998:1318.

55. Johnson RT. The pathogenesis of acute viral encephalitis and postinfectious encephalomyelitis. *J Infect Dis.* 1987;155:359-364.

56. Johnson RT. Acute encephalitis. *Clin Infect Dis.* 1996;23:219-226.

57. Johnson RT, Griffin DE, Gendelman HE. Postinfectious encephalomyelitis. *Semin Neurol.* 1985;5:180-190.

58. Kamolvarin N, Tirawatnpong T, Rattanasiwamoke R, et al. Diagnosis of rabies by polymerase chain reaction with nested primers. *J Infect Dis.* 1993;167:207-210.

59. Kira J, Itoyama Y, Koyanagi Y, et al. Presence of HTLV-I proviral DNA in central nervous system of patients with HTLV-I-associated myelopathy. *Ann Neurol.* 1992;31:39-45.

60. Kiska DL, Orkiszewski DR, Howell D, et al. Evaluation of new monoclonal antibody-based latex agglutination test for detection of cryptococcal polysaccharide antigen in serum and cerebrospinal fluid. *J Clin Microbiol.* 1994;32:2309-2311.

61. Koening H, Rabinowitz SG, Day E, et al. Post-infectious encephalomyelitis after successful treatment of herpes simplex encephalitis with adenine arabinoside: ultrastructural observations. *N Engl J Med.* 1979;300:1089-1093.

62. Kolson DL, Lave E, Gonzalez-Scarano F. The effects of human immunodeficiency virus in the central nervous system. *Adv Virus Res.* 1998;50:1-47.

63. Kox LF, Kuijper S, Kolk AH. Early diagnosis of tuberculous meningitis by polymerase chain reaction. *Neurology.* 1995;45:2228-2232.

64. Kumar R, Kohli N, Thavnani H, et al. Value of CT scan in the diagnosis of meningitis. *Indian Pediatr.* 1996;33:465-468.

65. Lakeman FD, Koga J, Whitley RJ. Detection of antigen to herpes simplex virus in cerebrospinal fluid from patients with herpes simplex encephalitis. *J Infect Dis.* 1987;155:1172-1178.

66. Lakeman FD, Whitley RJ. National Institute of Allergy and Infectious Diseases Collaborative Antiviral Study Group. Diagnosis of herpes simplex encephalitis by using Polymerase Chain Reaction assay of cerebrospinal fluid samples. *Clin Infect Dis.* 1995;25:86-91.

67. Larsen PD, Chartrand SA, Tomashek KM, et al. Hydrocephalus complicating lymphocytic choriomeningitis infection. *Pediatr Infect Dis J.* 1993;12:628-631.

68. Larsen SA, Steiner BM, Rudolph AH. Laboratory diagnosis and interpretation of tests for syphilis. *Clin Microbiol Rev.* 1995;8:1-21.

69. Lim LCL, Pennell DR, Schell RF. Rapid detection of bacteria in cerebrospinal fluid by immunofluorescence staining on membrane filters. *J Clin Microbiol.* 1990;28:670-675.

70. Lin JJ, Harn HJ. Application of the polymerase chain reaction to monitor *Mycobacterium tuberculosis* DNA in the CSF of patients with tuberculous meningitis after antibiotic treatment. *J Neurol Neurosurg Psychiatry.* 1995;59:175-177.

71. Lowry PW. Arbovirus encephalitis in the United States and Asia. *J Lab Clin Med.* 1997;129:405-411.

72. Luft BJ, Remington JS. Toxoplasmic encephalitis in AIDS. *Clin Infect Dis.* 1992;15:211-222.

73. Lunsford LD. Stereotactic drainage of brain abscess. *Neurol Res.* 1987; 9:270-274.

74. MacLean S, Luger A. Finding neurosyphilis without the VDRL. *Sex Transm Dis.* 1996;23:392-394.

75. Magnarelli LA, Anderson JF, Johnson RC. Cross-reactivity in serological tests for Lyme disease and other spirochetal infections. *J Infect Dis.* 1987;156:183-186.

76. Major EO, Ault GS. Progressive multifocal leukoencephalopathy: clinical and laboratory observations in a viral induced demyelinating disease in the immunodeficient patient. *Curr Opin Neurol.* 1995;8:184.

77. Mampalam TJ, Rosenblum ML. Trends in the management of bacterial brain abscesses: a review of 102 cases over 17 years. *Neurosurgery.* 1988;23:451-458.

78. Marra CM, Gary DW, Kuypers J, et al. Diagnosis of neurosyphilis in patients infected with human immunodeficiency virus type 1. *J Infect Dis.* 1996;174:219-221.

79. Mathisen GE, Johnson JP. Brain abscess. *Clin Infect Dis.* 1997;25:763-781.

80. McArthur JC, Hoover DR, Bacellar H, et al. Dementia in AIDS patients: incidence and risk factors. *Neurology.* 1993;43:2245-2252.

81. McCutchan JA. Cytomegalovirus infections of the nervous system in patients with AIDS. *Clin Infect Dis.* 1995;20:747-754.

82. McKinney RE, Katz SL, Wilfert CM. Chronic enteroviral meningoencephalitis in agammaglobulinemic patients. *Rev Infect Dis.* 1987;9:334-356.

83. McLean BN, Thompson EJ. Viral specific IgG and IgM antibodies in the CSF of patients with endemic tropical spastic paraparesis. *J Neurol.* 1989;236:351-352.

84. Mitchell TG, Freedman EZ, White TJ, et al. Unique oligonucleotide primers in PCR for identification of *Cryptococcus neoformans. J Clin Microbiol.* 1994;32:253-255.

85. Morris JH, Phil D. The nervous system. In: Cotran RS, Kumar V, Robbins SL, eds. *Robbins Pathologic Basis of Disease.* 4th ed. Philadelphia: WB Saunders; 1989:1400.

86. Mouligier A, Mikol J, Gonzalez-Canali G, et al. AIDS-associated cytomegalovirus infection mimicking central nervous system tumors: a diagnostic challenge. *Clin Infect Dis.* 1996;22:626-631.

87. Musher DM. Syphilis. In: Gorbach SL, Bartlett JG, Blacklow NR, eds. *Infectious Diseases.* Philadelphia: WB Saunders; 1992:822.

88. Nguyen LN, Kox LF, Pham LD, et al. The potential contribution of the polymerase chain reaction to the diagnosis of tuberculous meningitis. *Arch Neurol.* 1996;53:771-776.

89. Nuwayhid NF. Laboratory tests for detection of human immunodeficiency virus type I infection. *Clin Diagn Lab Immunol.* 1995;2:637-645.

90. Olcen P, Lantz PG, Backman A, et al. Rapid diagnosis of bacterial meningitis by seminested PCR strategy. *Scand J Infect Dis.* 1995;27:537-539.

91. Osaki M, Adachi H, Gomyo Y, et al. Detection of mycobacterial DNA in formalin fixed paraffin embedded tissue specimens by duplex PCR: application to histopathologic diagnosis. *Mod Pathol.* 1997;10:78-83.

92. Park JY, Peters CJ, Rollin PE, et al. Development of a reverse transcription-polymerase chain reaction assay for diagnosis of lymphocytic choriomeningitis virus infection and its use in a prospective surveillance study. *J Med Virol.* 1997;51:107-114.

93. Petijean J, Freymuth F, Kopecka H, et al. Detection of enteroviruses in cerebrospinal fluids: enzymatic amplification and hybridization with a biotinylated riboprobe. *Mol Cell Probes.* 1994;8:15-22.

94. Podzorski RP, Persing DH. Molecular detection and identification of microorganisms. In: Murray PR, Baron EJ, Pfaller M, et al, eds. *Manual of Clinical Microbiology.* 6th ed. Washington, DC: ASM Press; 1995:130-157.

95. Price RW, Brew B, Sidtis J, et al. The brain and AIDS: central nervous system HIV-1 infection and AIDS dementia complex. *Science.* 1988;239:586-592.

96. Prusiner SB. Prion diseases and the BSE crises. *Science.* 1997;278:245-251.

97. Quaglierello V, Scheld WM. Bacterial meningitis: pathogenesis, pathophysiology, and progress. *N Engl J Med.* 1992;327:864-872.

98. Reid MC, Schoen RT, Evans J, et al. The consequences of overdiagnosis and overtreatment of Lyme disease: an observational study. *Ann Intern Med.* 1998;128:354-362.

99. Revello MG, Manservigi R. Molecular diagnosis of herpes simplex encephalitis. *Intervirology.* 1996;39:185-192.

100. Rohde RE, Neill SU, Clark KA, et al. Molecular epidemiology of rabies epizootics in Texas. *Clin Diagn Virol.* 1997;8:209-217.

101. Rotbart HA, ed. *Human Enterovirus Infections.* Washington, DC: ASM Press; 1995.

102. Ruiz A, Gaaz WI, Post JD, et al. Use of thallium-201 brain SPECT to differentiate cerebral lymphoma from *Toxoplasma* encephalitis in AIDS patients. *Am J Neuroradiol.* 1994;15:1885-1894.

103. Sadler M. Progressive multifocal leukoencephalopathy in HIV. *Int J STD AIDS.* 1997;8:351.

104. Salih MA, Ahmed HS, Hofvander Y, et al. Rapid diagnosis of bacterial meningitis by an enzyme immunoassay of cerebrospinal fluid. *Epidemiol Infect.* 1989;103:301-310.

105. Samuelson A, Skoog E, Forsgren M. Aspects of the serodiagnosis of enterovirus infections by ELISA. *Serodiagn Immunother Infect Dis.* 1990;4:395-406.

106. Saruta K, Matsunga T, Kono M, et al. Simultaneous detection of *Streptococcus pneumoniae* and *Haemophilus influenzae* by nested PCR amplification from cerebrospinal fluid samples. *FEMS Immunol Med Microbiol.* 1997;19:151-157.

107. Scarpellini P, Racca S, Cinque P, et al. Nested polymerase chain reaction for diagnosis and monitoring treatment response in AIDS patients with tuberculous meningitis. *AIDS.* 1995;9:895-900.

108. Scheld WM. *Infections of the Central Nervous System.* 2nd ed. New York: Lippincott-Raven; 1997.

109. Schutte CM, Van der Meyden CH, Labuscagne JH, et al. Lymph node biopsy as an aid in the diagnosis of intracranial tuberculosis. *Tuber Lung Dis.* 1996;77:285.

110. Segreti J, Harris AA. Acute bacterial meningitis. *Infect Dis Clin North Am.* 1996;10:797-809.

111. Skoldenberg B. Herpes simplex encephalitis. *Scand J Infect Dis.*1996;100(suppl):8-13.

112. Skrap M, Melatini A, Vassallo A, Sidoti C. Stereotactic aspiration and drainage of brain abscesses: experience with 9 cases. *Minim Invasive Neurosurg.* 1996;39:108-112.

113. Smith JS. New aspects of rabies with emphasis on epidemiology, diagnosis, and prevention of the disease in the United States. *Clin Microbiol Rev.* 1996;9:166-176.

114. Steere AC. Lyme disease. *N Engl J Med.* 1989;321:586-596.

115. Stockman L, Clark KA, Hunt JM, et al. Evaluation of commercially available acridium ester labeled chemiluminescent DNA probes for culture identification of *Blastomyces dermatitidis, Coccidioides immitis, Cryptococcus neoformans,* and *Histoplasma capsulatum. J Clin Microbiol.* 1993;31:845-850.

116. Svoboda-Newman SM, Greenson JK, Singleton TP, et al. Detection of hepatitis C by RT-PCR in formalin fixed paraffin embedded tissue from liver transplant patients. *Diagn Mol Pathol.* 1997;6:123-129.

117. Tayfun C, Ucoz T, Tasar M, et al. Diagnostic value of MRI in tuberculous meningitis. *Eur Radiol.* 1996;6:380.

118. Tedder DG, Ashley R, Tyler KL, et al. Herpes simplex virus infection as a cause of benign recurrent lymphocytic meningitis. *Ann Intern Med.* 1994;121:334-338.

119. Toltzis P. Viral encephalitis. *Adv Pediatr Infect Dis.* 1991;6:111-136.

120. Tugwell P, Dennis DT, Weinstein A, et al. Laboratory evaluation in the diagnosis of Lyme disease. *Ann Intern Med.* 1997;127:1109-1123.

121. Tunkel AR, Scheld WM. Pathogenesis and pathophysiology of bacterial meningitis. *Clin Microbiol Rev.* 1993;6:118-136.

122. Tunkel AR, Scheld WM. Central nervous system infections. In: Reese RE, Betts RF, eds. *A Practical Approach to Infectious Diseases.* 4th ed. Boston: Little, Brown; 1996:133-183.

123. Tyler KL. Aseptic meningitis, viral encephalitis and prion diseases. In: Fauci AS, Braunwald E, Isselbacher KJ, et al, eds. *Harrison's Principles of Internal Medicine.* 14th ed. New York: McGraw-Hill; 1998:2439-2451.

124. Venna N, Sabin TD. Tuberculosis of the nervous system. In: Feldmann E, ed. *Current Diagnosis in Neurology.* St. Louis: Mosby; 1994:117.

125. Verdon R, Chevret S, Laissy JP, et al. Tuberculous meningitis in adults: review of 48 cases. *Clin Infect Dis.* 1996;22:982-988.

126. Weber T, Turner R, Frye S, et al. Specific diagnosis of progressive multifocal leukoencephalopathy by polymerase chain reaction. *J Infect Dis.* 1994;169:1138-1141.

127. Wharton M, Chorba TL, Vogt RL, et al. Case definitions for public health surveillance. *MMWR.* 1990;39(RR-13):1-43.

128. Whelan MA, Hilal SK. Computed tomography as a guide in the diagnosis of and follow-up of brain abscesses. *Radiology.* 1980;135:663-671.

129. White AC Jr. Neurocysticercosis: a major cause of neurological disease worldwide. *Clin Infect Dis.* 1997;24:101-115.

130. Whitley RJ. Viral encephalitis. *N Engl J Med.* 1990;323:242-250.

131. Wolf DG, Spector SA. Diagnosis of human cytomegalovirus central nervous system disease in AIDS patients by DNA amplification from cerebrospinal fluid. *J Infect Dis.* 1992;166:1412-1415.

132. Yechoor VK, Shandera WX, Rodriquez P, et al. Tuberculous meningitis among adults with and without HIV infection: experience in an urban public hospital. *Arch Intern Med.* 1996;157:1710.

133. Zoll GJ, Melchers JG, Kopecka H, et al. General primer-mediated polymerase chain reaction for detection of enteroviruses: application for diagnostic routine and persistent infections. *J Clin Microbiol.* 1992;30:160-165.

# 26

# Neuroendocrine Disorders

*A. Bernard Pleet*

Although endocrine disorders are not rare, initial presentation or referral to a neurologist because of neurologic signs and symptoms caused by an undiagnosed endocrine disturbance is distinctly uncommon. The practicing neurologist has a well-defined interest in the appropriate diagnosis on several levels: it is in the best interests of the patient to identify a treatable and potentially curable cause of disability; it establishes the reputation of the neurologist in the medical community as an astute diagnostician, more than does the diagnosis of an obscure neurologic disorder that only other neurologists can appreciate; and since many of these patients are referred by medical practitioners (internists and family practitioners), identification of a "missed" disorder in someone else's field of expertise has its own satisfactions. This chapter addresses the most common endocrine disturbances that a practicing neurologist is likely to see in a non-hospital-based practice. Cost-effective and efficient selection of diagnostic tests are stressed. The complete evaluation of many of these patients (including steps such as tumor localization) and long-term treatment and management are best left in the hands of the endocrinologist and internist, and therefore no attention is given to medical or surgical management of these diseases in this chapter.

## THE THYROID GLAND

Of the endocrinopathic disorders sought by the consulting neurologist, the most commonly tested for are diseases of the thyroid gland. In part this is because many of these patients will have disorders of consciousness (e.g., dementia, delirium, otherwise unexplained stupor and coma) that may be seen with thyroid dysfunction, in part because the neurologic manifestations of thyroid diseases are many, and in part because numerous tests for the diagnosis of thyroid dysfunction are readily available. In England and Wales the incidence of hyperthyroidism is 1.1 cases per 1000 per year and that of hypothyroidism is 1.7 cases per 1000 per year; in the United States the incidence of thyrotoxicosis was reported as 0.16 cases per 1000 per year and that of hypothyroidism as 0.13 cases per 1000 per year.[120] In a geriatric setting one may expect to see thyroid dysfunction in almost 5% of the population.[148]

## HYPERTHYROIDISM

The symptoms experienced by patients with hyperthyroidism in most cases are due to the metabolic consequences of oversecretion of thyroxine ($T_4$) and rarely are due to oversecretion of triiodothyronine ($T_3$) or a combination of the two. In elderly patients there may be few of the usual clinical signs of hyperthyroidism, and the presenting manifestations may be only atrial fibrillation or unexplained congestive heart failure. Thyroid enlargement is found in most patients with hyperthyroidism, but it may be absent in one third of geriatric patients.[84] In patients aged 61 to 80 years, no clinical feature other than goiter has a clinical sensitivity >60%.[215] Modest-sized goiters are notoriously difficult for nonendocrinologists to palpate, and it is easy to overlook adequate neck palpation on the routine neurologic examination.

Hyperthyroid patients may complain of weight loss (often despite increased appetite and caloric intake); they may feel nervous and often complain of an increased frequency of bowel movements (although actual diarrhea is uncommon).[84,169] Physical findings may include thyroid enlargement, "velvety" smooth and moist skin, onycholysis (separation of the distal margin of the fingernail from the nailbed), and tachycardia. Patients often look tense and anxious, and their speech may be rapid. Tremors may be found in the outstretched hands and in the tongue, and when the eyelids are gently closed, they too can exhibit pronounced tremors. The ocular globes may appear protuberant, but exophthalmos should not be diagnosed unless the globes are measured by exophthalmometry. Proptosis may be more apparent than real because of the hyperadrenergic state, causing upper lid retraction and a "stare." The symptoms of a hyper-beta-adrenergic state mimic those of a pheochromocytoma, except that the latter are frequently paroxysmal and those due to thyrotoxicosis are sustained.[167] On examination of the patient with a pheochromocytoma, the skin is often cool and pale because of vasoconstriction rather than warm and moist, as it is in thyrotoxicosis. Orthostatic hypotension is not uncommon with pheochromocytoma,[13,129,174,228] and some degree of retinal hypertensive change is often seen.[62,177]

Other physical findings in hyperthyroidism include lid lag (as the eyes slowly track a moving object downward, there is a lag in lid motion; if the object of pursuit is held too close to the face and moved quickly, a "pseudolag" may occur), absence of wrinkling of the forehead on up-gaze, and impaired movements of the ocular globes due to glycosaminoglycan infiltration of the ocular muscles ("infiltrative thyroid ophthalmopathy").[169] Diffuse hyperreflexia and headaches are common. Less frequently found are chorea, myalgias, muscle cramps, bulbar paralysis, flaccid paralysis of the legs (Basedow's disease), spasticity, Babinski's sign, spastic bladder, and periodic paralysis (predisposed to by depolarization of muscle fiber and impaired Na-K activity).[184] Thyrotoxic periodic paralysis is more common in Orientals than in Caucasians,[4] and more common in Asian men than in Asian women.[133] Proximal muscle weakness is common. Thyrotoxic myopathy may be caused by a combination of protein catabolism, accelerated metabolic rate, and impaired carbohydrate metabolism. Type II fibers are more affected than are type I. Reported shortening of muscle contraction time is probably caused by accelerated myosin adenosine triphosphatase (ATPase) activity and enhanced calcium uptake by the sarcoplasmic reticulum.

The incidence of myasthenia gravis in the course of thyrotoxicosis is low (0.2%), but the occurrence of thyrotoxicosis during the course of myasthenia gravis is substantially higher (3% to 10%).[117,173] Hyperthyroidism may worsen myasthenia gravis by its effect on the presynaptic membrane.[184]

In one study, thyrotoxicosis was the cause of seizures in a substantial number of patients,[106] but that situation is not commonly seen by most neurologists. Rarely, third-nerve palsies and optic neuropathy have been reported, although the relationship to thyrotoxicosis is not clear.[169]

Mental status changes, including emotional lability, irritability, euphoria, fatigue, mania, psychosis, and dementia have been seen in the hyperthyroid state.[27,48,119,204]

Subclinical hyperthyroidism has, at best, subtle clinical manifestations, and there is controversy regarding the importance of establishing the diagnosis.[46] This condition is diagnosed when the thyroid-stimulating hormone (TSH) level is depressed and the free $T_4$ and free $T_3$ levels are normal (in the absence of significant nonthyroidal illness).[98] Measurement of the free $T_3$ is necessary to exclude $T_3$ thyrotoxicosis.[80] Subclinical hyperthyroidism can progress to overt hyperthyroidism, contribute to osteoporosis, and cause atrial fibrillation,[98] which itself can predispose to cerebral embolization and infarction.* There are no data to suggest that subclinical hyperthyroidism leads directly to neurologic abnormalities, but this condition may do so indirectly through deleterious effects on the heart, which, in addition to atrial fibrillation, include an increased heart rate, more frequent premature atrial contractions, and increased left ventricular mass.[19,190]

There are several tests of thyroid function and structure offered by most clinical and hospital laboratories. The laboratory diagnosis of hyperthyroidism is based on a low TSH determination with elevation of the hormones $T_4$ and $T_3$.[98] Causes of a low TSH include Graves' disease, a solitary autonomous nodule, a multinodular goiter, various forms of self-limited thyrotoxicosis (e.g., postpartum, silent, and subacute thyroiditis and iodine-induced hyperthyroidism), central hypothyroidism, nonthyroidal systemic illnesses, and advanced age.[14,46,189] Total $T_4$ and $T_3$ determinations (bound

plus free fractions of the thyroid hormones) as well as unbound, or free, $T_4$ and $T_3$ levels ($fT_4$ and $fT_3$) are readily obtained. In some laboratories where free hormone levels cannot be obtained (and even in some where they can), a free thyroxine index (FTI) can be determined. The FTI is calculated from the total $T_4$ determination and a resin uptake of radiolabeled $T_3$. It is an estimate of the free $T_4$. When elevated, the FTI is diagnostic for hyperthyroidism, but it does not define hyperthyroidism resulting from rare TSH-secreting pituitary tumors ("central hyperthyroidism"), for which an accompanying TSH assay is required.[15] When the FTI is normal, a TSH assay is still required to exclude the possibility of $T_3$ thyrotoxicosis, subclinical hyperthyroidism, or thyroid hormone resistance.[15,46] The syndrome of thyroid hormone resistance (RTH) is characterized by elevated circulating thyroid hormones, unsuppressed TSH levels, and peripheral refractoriness to thyroid hormone action. Patients with RTH may have hyperthyroidism if the pituitary gland is more insensitive to thyroid hormones than other tissues. More often, patients have peripheral tissue resistance as well and are euthyroid. RTH is caused by point mutations in the $T_3$-binding domain of the beta-receptor gene.[75,178] For these reasons and because of the ready availability of thyrotropin (TSH) assays and unbound hormone levels, the FTI is used increasingly infrequently, but for detection of thyroidal disease, it has a reported sensitivity of nearly 100% and a specificity of 99.6%.[67] It adds little information when the TSH level is normal.[67,84,157,222]

Sensitive assays for the detection of TSH are easily obtained and are into the third and fourth generations. Second-generation TSH tests have a detection sensitivity of approximately 0.1 mU/L,[216] whereas third-generation assays can detect levels as low as 0.006 to 0.009 mU/L.[97,105] For the diagnosis of hyperthyroidism, TSH determinations have been reported to have a sensitivity of 90% to 100% (third generation) with a specificity of 91% to 99.3%.[6,22,58,140,193] In practical terms the sensitivity of the test depends not only on the ability of the assay to detect low levels of circulating TSH but also on the "cut points" selected by the individual laboratory based upon the receiver operating characteristic (ROC) curve of the test used.[86] Low levels of TSH do not always indicate hyperthyroidism. They are lower in an elderly population[189] and in nonthyroidal illness (NTI), such as trauma, renal disease, liver disease, and sepsis.* Low TSH levels may also be found in central hypothyroidism due to deficiencies of TSH or TRH.[25,44,64,89,183] For purposes of screening for hyperthyroidism, the TSH assay has few false-negative results.[148] A normal value excludes thyrotoxicosis, except in the rare cases of patients with TSH-secreting pituitary tumors and in those with selective pituitary resistance to thyroid hormone.[84]

When the TSH is lowered below the normal range and hyperthyroidism is suspected, the condition is best confirmed with an $fT_4$. The free hormone level obviates difficulties encountered from potential abnormalities of serum proteins and thyroid-binding globulin (TBG), which can be altered by nutritional status and concurrent illnesses. The $fT_4$ has good sensitivity and specificity, but the detection sensitivity is not as good as that of TSH.[205] An elevated $fT_4$

---

with a low TSH confirms thyrotoxicosis. When the $fT_4$ is normal, an $fT_3$ is necessary to exclude $T_3$-thyrotoxicosis.[84] When both $fT_3$ and $fT_4$ are normal (subclinical hyperthyroidism), there may be controversy with regard to the predictive value of the low TSH for ultimate development of overtly expressed thyrotoxicosis, but thyrotoxicosis will not be the cause of the patient's neurologic symptoms. The $fT_3$ has too low a sensitivity to be useful as the sole screening agent for thyrotoxicosis.[76] It is useful only when TSH is depressed and $fT_4$ is normal, to exclude $T_3$-thyrotoxicosis.

Imaging studies (radionuclide and ultrasound) are not useful for diagnosing thyrotoxicosis, but uptake studies assist with the correct diagnosis of unusual cases of hyperthyroidism, and imaging studies (including ultrasound) can help to define nodular disease.[217]

## HYPOTHYROIDISM

Hypothyroidism is most often due to failure of the thyroid gland (primary hypothyroidism).[227] Most cases are autoimmune and may occur with other autoimmune endocrine abnormalities, such as adrenal insufficiency (Schmidt's syndrome).[136] Up to 25% of cases are iatrogenic. Other causes include congenital hypoplasia, hereditary enzymatic defects of thyroid hormonogenesis, and pituitary gland dysfunction.[169] The subnormal concentrations of the thyroid hormones ($T_4$ and $T_3$) are responsible for the systemic and neurologic manifestations.

Patients with hypothyroidism, even in milder cases, report intolerance to cold, constipation, and impaired memory. In more advanced cases patients may appear dull and apathetic and have slowed speech. The voice is often hoarse, and articulated speech can be distorted from infiltration of the vocal cords and tongue with glycosaminoglycans.[169] For the same reason, the eyelids may appear puffy, facial lines may be flattened, and nonpitting peripheral edema may be detected. Fingernails may be brittle, and the skin is dry and thick. Excessive accumulation of carotene often gives the skin a yellowish tinge.[227] There may be bradycardia and chest roentgenography or echocardiography may disclose a pericardial effusion. Caution must be exercised in the evaluation of older patients (>70 years) since, as with hyperthyroidism, they tend to have fewer signs and symptoms and a diminished frequency of the classic signs.[69]

Muscle disorders are quite common in hypothyroidism but are usually limited to myalgias, stiffness, and cramps, often accompanied by a rise in the blood creatine kinase (CPK) level.[126] This constellation can be mistaken for polymyositis[43] or fibromyalgia.[36] Muscle weakness is less common but can be found in the shoulder and pelvic girdles.[43] Occasionally the myopathy can be sufficiently severe as to lead to rhabdomyolysis and renal failure.[126] In adults with hypothyroidism muscle weakness and elevated CPK may be associated with hypertrophy and pseudomyotonia, the Hoffman syndrome.[73] The hypothyroid state is thought to lead to (1) inhibition of the oxidative pathways of the mitochondrial respiratory chain (substrate incorporation and oxidation), (2) a transition in myosin isoforms, which express a slower ATPase, and (3) impairment of sarcolemic transport.[113] Muscle biopsies show atrophy of type II fibers and glycogen deposition with reduced activity of glycolytic and glycogenolytic enzymes.[141] Electron microscopy confirms abnormal mitochondrial and glycogen particle deposi-

tion in type I fibers.[61,104] Clinically, hypothyroid myopathy is best sought with assessment of the force of quadriceps contraction and ankle-jerk relaxation times.[116] The ankle-jerk reflex is nicely demonstrated with the patient kneeling on a chair, with the ankles extending beyond the edge of the seat. Caution must be exercised in the interpretation of delayed relaxation of the ankle-jerk reflex since it has been reported in association with hypothermia, leg edema, diabetes mellitus, parkinsonism, neurosyphilis, sarcoidosis, sprue, pernicious anemia, and with a number of pharmacologic agents.[169]

A small number of patients with myasthenia gravis have hypothyroidism,[55] frequently the consequence of an autoimmune thyroiditis.[1] There can be associated autoimmune disease of the adrenal gland (Schmidt's syndrome).[136] In a study of 27 patients with myasthenia gravis there was a surprising incidence of thyroid subnormality postulated as secondary hypothyroidism due to failure of the hypophysio-hypothalamic system, diagnosed by low thyroid hormone levels and their response to exogenous TSH.[94]

Cerebellar ataxia has been reported with hypothyroidism,[21] occasionally accompanied by dysarthric speech and nystagmus.[204] An ataxic gait has been noted in 5% to 32% of patients with hypothyroidism, and dysdiadochokinesia has been reported in 6% to 52%.[120] Newer studies have implicated vestibular system dysfunction (either central or peripheral)[185] or slowness of mechanical contraction related to an increase in muscle contraction time and the consequent excessive recruitment of antagonist muscles in the genesis of the hypothyroid "ataxic dysbasic" syndrome.[166]

Polyneuropathy and carpal tunnel syndrome can be seen in hypothyroidism.* Earlier studies suggested a demyelinative neuropathy,[72] but more recent reports suggest that hypothyroid neuropathy is axonal.[123,171] The most common symptom of polyneuropathy in hypothyroidism is paresthesias, and the most common site of electrophysiologic disturbance is the sensory nerves, especially the sural nerves.[16]

Hypothyroidism has long been known to lead to enlargement of the pituitary gland because of hyperplasia of the thyrotroph cells.[93,110,121,151,225] Prior to sophisticated imaging studies, the pituitary enlargement was on occasion of sufficient magnitude to lead to erosion and enlargement of the sella turcica on lateral skull roentgenograms.[121,225] With the advent of computed tomographic (CT) scanning and magnetic resonance imaging (MRI), secondary thyrotroph hyperplasia has been mistaken for pituitary tumor.[18,51] Such mistaken identity is compounded by associated endocrine disturbances in patients with hypothyroidism and thyrotroph hyperplasia, such as hyperprolactinemia with galactorrhea and amenorrhea,[90,156,214] excessive secretion of prolactin with growth hormone (GH),[231] blunting of GH secretion,[146] low basal cortisol levels,[156] and overt pituitary gland failure.[213] Hyperprolactinemia has also been found with subclinical hypothyroidism (elevated TSH with normal thyroid hormone levels).[153]

There is little doubt that thyrotroph hyperplasia due to hypothyroidism produces visual field defects, but there is debate about the frequency of the abnormality. Yamamoto et

---

*References 16, 24, 50, 107, 123, 131, 161, 169, 175.

al[231] determined abnormalities in 10 of 14 patients with hypothyroidism (71.4%) by using Goldmann's isopter perimetry, whereas Hallengren et al[96] found no defects in a series of 25 consecutive patients. The visual field defects usually regress with replacement therapy,[77,231] concordant with a regression in the size of the pituitary mass.[9,18,77,101,156,188] On occasion the pituitary mass actually increases in size once hormone replacement therapy has been initiated,[93] and visual field defects may appear where none had been noted, or the visual field deficits may worsen.[201,231]

Glaucoma may be caused or worsened by hypothyroidism,[23,40] and optic neuropathy may occur and can be mistaken for normal-tension glaucoma.[108] Other ophthalmic findings include ptosis due to diminished sympathetic tone and a tonic pupil.[169]

Trigeminal neuralgia and trigeminal pain syndromes, Bell's palsy, tinnitus, and hearing loss have all been accompaniments of the thyroprivic[201] state. Headaches are not specific to but are particularly common in hypothyroidism. Benign intracranial hypertension can develop, particularly during hormone replacement therapy.[34,59,128,172] Hypoxia has been seen in 69% of patients with hypothyroidism.[232] It is likely a result of depression of the respiratory center in the brain compounded by associated anemia. The hypoxia normalizes with hormone replacement. Its relation to obstructive and central sleep apnea syndromes seen in myxedematous patients is not clear.[169]

Mental abnormalities occur in about 3% to 5% of myxedematous patients. Changes cover a broad spectrum from mild dullness and memory defects to overt psychoses with delusions and hallucinations. Myxedema coma is rare[154,179] but may appear suddenly. There may be seizures, hypotension, bradycardia, a slow respiratory rate, and profound hypothermia.

The laboratory diagnosis of hypothyroidism depends upon the demonstration of an elevation of the TSH blood level with a subnormality of thyroid hormone, either total or free $T_4$. Subclinical hypothyroidism is defined by an elevated TSH level with normal thyroid hormones.[98] Elevated levels of TSH can be seen in three settings: with primary failure of the thyroid gland (primary hypothyroidism), with pituitary thyrotroph adenomas causing hyperthyroidism (central hyperthyroidism), and with nonneoplastic thyrotroph hyperplasia due to resistance to thyroid hormone. The latter two conditions belong to the category of inappropriate secretion of TSH (IST). The term *inappropriate* denotes the lack of anticipated suppression of TSH when thyroid hormone levels are elevated.[15] Conversely, TSH levels may be low in central hypothyroidism because of a deficit of TSH[25,44,64,89,183] or thyrotropin-releasing hormone (TRH).[52,85,142]

For the diagnosis of hypothyroidism, TSH has a sensitivity approaching 100% and a specificity of 94%, depending on test methodology.[67,192] Free $T_4$ has a reported sensitivity of 93.8% and a specificity of 99.3%.[22] $T_3$ concentrations are normal in as many as 30% of patients with hypothyroidism and when low may simply reflect a nonthyroidal illness that impairs peripheral $T_4$ 5'-monodeiodination to $T_3$.[227] The FTI, calculated from the total serum $T_4$ and the $T_3$ resin uptake, can be an excellent tool for the diagnosis of thyroid dysfunction, with a sensitivity approaching 100% and a specificity of 99.6%.[67,157]

## DIAGNOSTIC RECOMMENDATIONS

When screening for thyroid dysfunction, either hyperthyroidism or hypothyrodism, a TSH determination alone is sufficient. When the TSH is normal, the diagnosis of thyroid disease is virtually excluded.

When the TSH is low, determination of $fT_4$ is required. Although a low TSH suggests the hyperthyroid state, low levels may be seen in central hypothyroidism (due to a defect in TSH or TRH production) and with NTI. In these instances the $fT_4$ and $fT_3$ levels will be reduced accordingly. A low TSH level and an elevated $fT_4$ level are diagnostic for thyrotoxicosis. With a low TSH level and a normal $fT_4$, one must proceed to an $fT_3$ to exclude $T_3$ thyrotoxicosis.

When the TSH is low and both the $fT_4$ and the $fT_3$ levels are normal, the clinician is dealing with subclinical thyrotoxicosis. The appropriate management and follow-up of these patients is controversial because in some instances the TSH will return to normal, and it is not clear that treatment will alter the natural history of those who progress to overt hyperthyroidism.[46]

An elevated TSH level usually indicates hypothyroidism, but it may be seen with TSH-secreting pituitary tumors (central hyperthyroidism) and with thyroid hormone resistance. Both are rare disorders. In both diseases one is dealing with the inappropriate secretion of nonsuppressible TSH since in both conditions blood levels of thyroid hormones are elevated. The differentiation of IST syndromes[15] is best deferred to the endocrinologist.

When the TSH level is elevated and the $fT_4$ is normal, the clinician is faced with subclinical hypothyroidism. Following an extensive review of this variant of hypothyroidism, some authorities have concluded that there may be few, if any, symptoms and there is insufficient evidence to recommend for or against treatment.[98,99] Others have pointed out that these patients may have alterations in memory and mood, elevated intraocular pressure with reversal upon treatment, electrophysiologic changes in peripheral nerve function, and symptomatic abnormalities in skeletal muscle "energetics."[46] The symptoms enumerated in these reviews suggest that few neurologists would suspect a diagnosis of subclinical hypothyroidism on clinical grounds. It is more likely that this disorder will be encountered when thyroid function is included in a metabolic screen.

## THE PARATHYROID GLANDS

Disease of the parathyroid glands is defined by the level of the serum concentration of calcium. It must either be corrected for abnormalities of protein concentration (especially albumin) or measured directly as the ionized fraction.[70] In most hospital and commercial laboratories the upper limit of normal for serum calcium is 10.5 mg/dl. If an ionized serum calcium cannot be obtained and the serum albumin is low, the degree of ionized calcium can be estimated by adding 0.8 mg/dl for each 1 g/dl decrease in serum albumin below the normal limit (usually 4 g/dl).[70,211] Abnormalities of the parathyroid glands result in either high or low concentrations of calcium, and clinical phenomena are directly related to the level of the serum calcium.

## HYPERPARATHYROIDISM

Hyperparathyroidism results in hypercalcemia, but it is not the only cause of an elevated serum calcium concentration (see Table 26–1).

In an ambulatory setting primary hyperparathyroidism is the most common cause of hypercalcemia,[70] but in a hospital setting cancer is the most common cause.[169]

In hospitalized patients hypercalcemia is found in 0.3% of all admissions; 20% have malignancies, and 5% have hyperparathyroidism.[202] Hypercalcemia will evolve in 10% to 20% of patients with cancer.[150,169] The incidence of hyperparathyroidism in an unselected large screened population is between 0.1% and 0.2%, with most patients being asymptomatic.[70]

Hyperparathyroidism is due to adenomatous change in a single gland in 75% to 85% of cases; most other cases are due to hyperplasia in multiple glands; less than 1% are due to parathyroid carcinomas.[70] A subset of patients will have familial hypercalcemia associated with syndromes of multiple endocrine gland neoplasms. Multiple endocrine neoplasia type I is characterized by tumors of the parathyroid and pituitary glands and of the pancreatic islet cells; type IIa is characterized by medullary thyroid carcinoma, pheochromocytoma, and parathyroid adenomas and is known as Sipple's syndrome; type IIb (or III) has the features of IIa but includes mucosal neuromas, thickening of the corneal nerves, gastrointestinal ganglioneuromas, a marfanoid habitus, and pes cavus foot deformities.[167]

Hypercalcemia produces systemic, focal, and neurologic signs and symptoms. Calcium deposition in the tarsal plates and conjunctivae of the eye produces pain, burning, and redness. Slit-lamp examination may reveal a characteristic band keratopathy. The effect of hypercalcemia on the kidney is to produce a concentrating defect resulting in polyuria and polydipsia. Hypercalciuria and hyperphosphaturia lead to nephrolithiasis and recurrent episodes of acute renal colic.

---

### TABLE 26–1. Causes of Hypercalcemia

**Parathyroid Hormone–related Hypercalcemia**
Primary hyperparathyroidism
Ectopic production of parathyroid hormone
Familial hypocalciuric hypercalcemia
"Tertiary" hyperparathyroidism

**Hypercalcemia Not Mediated by Parathyroid Hormone**
Malignancy
  With bone metastasis
  Humoral hypercalcemia
Vitamin D intoxication
Sarcoidosis and other granulomatous diseases
Thyrotoxicosis
Immobilization
Milk-alkali syndrome
Acute renal failure and rhabdomyolysis
Vitamin A intoxication
Addison's disease

**Drugs**
Thiazides
Lithium

---

From Downs RW Jr. Hypercalcemia and hyperparathyroidism. In: Hurst WJ, ed. *Medicine for the Practicing Physician.* Stamford, CT: Appleton & Lange; 1996:656.

Reabsorption of bone predisposes to pathologic fractures. Gastrointestinal manifestations include constipation, anorexia, nausea, and dyspepsia.[70] Effects on the heart can sensitize it to the proarrhythmic effects of the cardiac glycosides and occasionally will lead to shortening of the QTc interval. Deposition of calcium in joints produces painful "pseudo-gout" (chondrocalcinosis). There may be calcification in soft tissues and in blood vessels.

Neurologic signs and symptoms usually are not sufficiently distinctive to suggest a diagnosis of hypercalcemia. Patients often complain of weakness and generalized malaise. A demonstrable myopathy with characteristic electromyographic changes or dysfunction of the myoneural junctions is uncommon.[169] The deep tendon reflexes are usually brisk to exaggerated, but Babinski's sign is not found. Mood and mental status changes are common and are seen in more than 50% of all patients with hypercalcemia.[163] Changes also include apathy, lethargy, depression, stupor, coma, paranoid psychoses, delirium, and dementia.[169] Changes in the mental state correlate well with the degree of elevation of the serum calcium: affective change and depression are seen at levels between 11 mg/dl and 16 mg/dl; alterations of consciousness and psychoses are usually seen with levels between 16 mg/dl and 19 mg/dl (levels in this range and above are life-threatening); somnolence, stupor, and coma occur when the calcium concentration exceeds 19 mg/dl.[169]

### Diagnostic Recommendations

The parathyroid hormone (PTH) level is an excellent test for initial evaluation of patients with hypercalcemia.[180] It is usually elevated in cases of primary hyperparathyroidism and is reliably depressed in patients who have hypercalcemia not mediated by PTH. One important caveat is that the neurologist recognize the confounding variable of renal insufficiency (which may occur as the result of nephrolithiasis and renal calculi from hypercalcemia). Some PTH assays recognize single midmolecule or carboxy-teminal antigenic sites, and even moderate renal insufficiency can delay renal clearance of these active parathyroid hormone fragments, giving an uninterpretable result.[70] Renal insufficiency may also cause secondary and tertiary hyperparathyroidism. Secondary hyperparathyroidism is characterized by an elevated PTH level in the presence of either normocalcemia or chronic hypocalcemia. Tertiary hyperparathyroidism occurs when hypocalcemia develops during the course of a disorder (e.g., malabsorption or chronic renal insufficiency) that produces secondary hyperparathyroidism and eventuates in autonomous function of the parathyroid glands.

Familial hypercalciuric hypercalcemia (FHH) may mimic primary hyperparathyroidism. FHH is characterized by a high serum calcium concentration, relatively low urine calcium excretion, and an inappropriately normal PTH concentration, although in some cases it may be high, giving the appearance of primary hyperparathyroidism.[70,147] It is an autosomal dominant disorder that is usually asymptomatic and discovered when a serum calcium determination is obtained for other reasons. When FHH is a diagnostic possibility (e.g., with family history of hypercalcemia or nephrolithiasis), and the multiple endocrine neoplasia syndromes are excluded, it may be tested for by determining the ratio of the calcium clearance to the creatinine clearance in a 24-

hour urine specimen. If $[U_{ca}/S_{ca}] \times [S_{cr}/U_{cr}] < 0.01$, FHH is possible.[70] For hypercalcemic states, current PTH assays have a sensitivity and specificity of >90%, being diagnostic for hyperparathyroidism in 90% of cases.[74,127,134] False-negative results may occur in cases of mild intermittent hypercalcemia.

Diagnostic localization procedures such as nuclide scans, ultrasonography, CT of the neck and mediastinum, and MRI are all available, but because of poor sensitivity and specificity, they are not used for the diagnosis of hyperparathyroidism. They may be used by surgeons and endocrinologists prior to exploration of the neck. Ancillary tests for patients with PTH-mediated hypercalcemia, such as creatinine clearance (for renal function), bone roentgenography, and bone mineral density are best left to the discretion of the primary care physician or endocrinologist, who will ultimately treat and follow the patient. In the patient with hypercalcemia not mediated by PTH, chest roentgenography (for tumor or sarcoidosis), bone scan (for osseous metastases), urine analysis (for evidence of a renal neoplasm), and stool for occult blood may be reasonable, but a more detailed search for metastatic disease or other causes of hypercalcemia can be more economically guided by an appropriate nonneurologic physician.

## HYPOPARATHYROIDISM

Hypoparathyroidism is suspected when the total concentration of serum calcium is below the lower limit of the normal range for calcium in a given laboratory, usually 8.5 mg/dl. When the serum albumin concentration is low, the same correction estimate for ionized serum calcium can be applied as described previously, or an ionized serum calcium can be directly measured. Practically, hypocalcemia is divided into states of PTH deficiency or a failure of PTH at its target tissues.[211] See Table 26–2 for causes of hypocalcemia.

There are few systemic manifestations of hypocalcemia, most resulting from the effect of low ionized calcium concentrations on the nervous system. When hypocalcemia has been chronic, patients may have subcapsular cataracts, which can cause decreased vision. In the early stages these are detectable only by slit-lamp examination and tend to evolve even after normalization of the serum calcium. There may be dental abnormalities, such as pitting of the enamel, dry skin, brittle nails, and patchy hair loss. Intestinal malabsorption can lead to weight loss and "greasy" stools.[169,211] Hypocalcemia, like hypomagnesemia, can lead to prolongation of the QTc electrocardiographic interval and predispose to a fatal polymorphic ventricular arrythmia (torsades de pointes).[3,31,54,109,135,158,233]

Increased neuromuscular irritability produces latent or overt tetany. Tetany or its equivalents, in the form of muscle and laryngeal spasm and acroparesthesias, are the most common manifestations of parathyroid deficiency. Clinically one may be able to elicit Trousseau's sign or Chvostek's sign. With Trousseau's sign the arm is compressed by squeezing it or compressing it with a tourniquet or sphygmomanometer cuff inflated just above systolic blood pressure for about 3 minutes. This is followed by carpal spasm of the hand, with resulting accoucheur's hand, often after a latency of 30 seconds to 4 minutes. Similar pressure over the leg or thigh will be followed by a pedal spasm. Although little used now, a more sensitive modification is the von Bonsdorff technique, in which the sphygmomanometer cuff is placed over the arm

| TABLE 26–2. Causes of Hypocalcemia |
|---|
| **Parathyroid Hormone Deficiency States** |
| Postsurgical |
| Idiopathic |
| Hypomagnesemia |
| **Failure of Parathyroid Hormone Action at Target Tissues** |
| Vitamin D deficiency or resistance |
| Pseudohypoparathyroidism |
| Renal failure |
| Hypomagnesemia |
| **Miscellaneous** |
| Acute pancreatitis |
| Osteoblastic metastasis |
| Rhabdomyolysis |
| Sepsis |
| Drugs |

From Umpierrez GW. Hypercalcemia and hyperparathyroidism. In: Hurst WJ, ed. *Medicine for the Practicing Physician.* Stamford, CT: Appleton & Lange; 1996:663.

and moderately inflated for about 10 minutes. It is then removed, and the patient is asked to hyperventilate. Typical tetanic spasm occurs far earlier in the previously ischemic limb in the presence of hypocalcemia. Chvostek's sign is elicited by tapping over the point of emergence or the division of the facial nerve just anterior to the ear, with either the finger or a percussion hammer. This action is followed by a spasm or tetanic contraction of some or all of the muscles supplied by the ipsilateral facial nerve. In some cases the response may be elicited by simple stroking of the skin in front of the ear. The sign is minimal if there is only a twitch at the angle of the mouth or the upper lip; moderate if there is movement of the ala nasi and the entire corner of the mouth; and maximal if the muscles of the forehead, eyelid, and cheek also contract.[60] Despite the irritability of the nerves, deep tendon reflexes are characteristically depressed or absent.[169]

Laryngeal spasm can be precipitated by cold and may be severe. It may be associated with diaphragmatic spasm and may cause death. Dysarthria and dysphagia may occur.

Muscles supplied by the autonomic nervous system may demonstrate irritability and spasm, including the gastrointestinal tract, the urinary bladder, the iris, and the ciliary muscles of the eyes. Rarely, there may be a myopathy.[169]

Seizures of many types, including tonic-clonic, partial motor, and complex partial seizures without and with secondary generalization, are seen in the setting of hypocalcemia. In most instances tetany precedes the seizures. Although the seizures respond to correction of the serum calcium, they are refractory to treatment with anticonvulsant drugs.[169]

There is a wide variety of alterations of the mental state, including confusion, excitation, emotional instability, delusions, hallucinations, dementia, and psychosis. A toxic delirium is most frequently encountered.

Intracranial pressure may be increased with papilledema and commonly is with headache. Hypoparathyrodism is a cause of pseudotumor cerebri.

Intracranial calcifications are well documented with hypocalcemia, and symmetric calcification of the basal ganglia is perhaps the most suggestive radiologic sign of hypoparathyroidism. Despite these concretions, chorea, pyramidal motor manifestations, and Parkinson's disease are not commonly encountered.

### Diagnostic Recommendations

Having defined and confirmed hypocalcemia, the clinician ascertains the level of the serum phosphate. In the absence of renal insufficiency, the finding of hypocalcemia and hyperphosphatemia is diagnostic for hypoparathyroidism. Renal insufficiency can be suggested by measurement of the serum creatinine. The glomerular filtration rate may be determined by any of several conventional methodologies. Hypomagnesemia must be sought since it is a cause of reversible hypoparathyroidism. To attribute hypocalcemia to hypomagnesemia, the serum magnesium must be below 1 mg/dl (0.4 mmol/L).[211] Definitive characterization of the form of hypoparathyroidism requires determination of the serum PTH and the response of urinary cyclic adenosine monophosphate (AMP) and urinary phosphate to administration of PTH. For the practicing neurologist the findings of hypocalcemia, hyperphosphatemia, and low PTH are sufficient to diagnose idiopathic hypoparathyroidism and refer the patient to an endocrinologist. A pattern of hypocalcemia, hyperphosphatemia, and elevated PTH suggest pseudohypoparathyroidism due to tissue resistance to PTH action. The proof and distinction between type I (receptor defect) and type II (defect distal to receptor-cyclase complex) pseudohypoparathyroidism is best left to the endocrinologist. Hypocalcemia, hypophosphatemia, and elevated PTH suggest deficiency or ineffectiveness of vitamin D and call for specialized laboratory testing, not usually available to or in the province of the clinical neurologist.

## THE ADRENAL GLANDS

The adrenal glands bear a close relationship to the nervous system. The adrenal medulla is derived from the embryologic central nervous system and maintains a generous nerve supply from the celiac sympathetic plexus. The adrenal medulla secretes the catecholamines epinephrine and norepinephrine; the adrenal cortex is the site of production of the adrenal steroids. Hyperfunction is common to both units, and hypofunction occurs in the cortex.

### PHEOCHROMOCYTOMA

This tumor arises from the chromaffin cells of the adrenal medulla. It is named for the color of its cut surface (from the Greek *phaios* for "dusky"). Functioning tumors derived from chromaffin cells have been found along the entire chain of the paraganglia: in the sympathetic chain in the neck; in the mediastinum; within the pericardium; along or near the aorta; in the organs of Zuckerkandl; in the pelvis; and in the urinary bladder. By far the most common location is the adrenal gland.[167] Many tumors are multiple, and approximately 10% are malignant. They may be familial and associated with multiple endocrine neoplasia (MEN) syndromes, with neurofibromatosis type I (with café au lait spots, axillary freckling, Lisch nodules, and neurofibromas), and with von Hippel-Lindau syndrome of retinal angiomas; cerebellar, spinal, and medullary hemagioblatomas; renal cell carcinoma; pancreatic cysts; and epididymal cystadenomas.

Tumors arising from the adrenal medulla most commonly secrete norepinephrine (NE) but can secrete a mixture of NE and epinephrine (EPI). Rarely, an adrenal pheochromocytoma may secrete only EPI. Extraadrenal tumors usually secrete only NE. Clinically, EPI is more apt to produce signs and symptoms of hypermetabolism, but either hormone may do so. Pheochromocytomas, being of neuroectodermal origin, elaborate active peptide hormones, including vasoactive intestinal peptide (which can cause diarrhea and hypokalemia), corticotropin-releasing hormone, adrenocorticotropic hormone (ACTH), substance P, neuropeptide Y, neurokinin B, pancreastatin, somatostatin, and calcitonin gene-related peptide (CGRP). The contribution of these hormones to the signs and symptoms of pheochromocytoma is not always clear.[167]

The most common symptom of a pheochromocytoma is headache, which is reported in 72% to 92% of all patients. Hypertension is the next most common symptom and is found in 90% of patients. It is paroxysmal in half of those affected and sustained in half. Signs of hypermetabolism are common, with sweating in up to 70%, palpitations in up to 73%, tachycardia with palpitations in 73%,[87] and hyperthermia and weight loss. Patients also complain of anxiety, warmth, abdominal pain, paresthesias, dizziness, and pallor.[167] Weakness has been reported in 38% of patients,[87] but it may be a manifestation of hypokalemia or another metabolic consequence of peptide production by the tumor.

The tumors have profound effects on the cardiovascular system. In addition to hypertension they may cause arrhythmias (sinus tachycardia or malignant ventricular arrhythmias). The hormones may result in focal myocardial necrosis, cardiac hypertrophy, congestive heart failure, angina pectoris (from either catechol excess or direct invasion of the tumor into the coronary arteries), and cardiomyopathy with pulmonary edema and cardiogenic shock. Hypertension may be of sufficient severity to evoke hypertensive encephalopathy and a stroke syndrome (either ischemic infarction or intraparenchymal hemorrhage).

Physical findings may include hypertension, hypertensive retinopathy (with the sustained form of hypertension), orthostatic hypotension, a paroxysm of hypertension during palpation of the abdomen, during flexing of the spine, or with twisting movements,[87] and there may be an accelerated pulse rate. Auscultation of the heart may reveal a fourth heart sound if there is cardiac hypertrophy or a third heart sound if there is a failing left ventricle.

### Diagnostic Recommendations

The most reliable test for the diagnosis of pheochromocytoma is determination of the plasma catecholamines in the fasting and resting state with the patient lying supine for 30 minutes after a needle has been inserted into the antecubital vein before blood is drawn.[87] Most patients with a pheochromocytoma will have plasma catecholamine levels >2000 ng/L even if they are normotensive and asymptomatic at the time. Patients with essential hypertension seldom have levels >1000 ng/L. If the patient is hypertensive and the plasma level is <500 ng/L, the diagnosis of pheochromocytoma is excluded.[87] The sensitivity of plasma catecholamines for the diagnosis of this tumor ranges from 83% to 94%.[17,35,125,143,160,165,170] When the results fall in the indeterminate range (500 ng/L to 2000 ng/L), pharmacologic tests beyond the purview of the neurologist are indicated.

When plasma catecholamines are not available, measurement of the 24-hour urinary excretion of metanephrines (metanephrine and normetanephrine) will do nicely, since the reported sensitivity is as high as 98%.[165] The sensitivity of the 24-hour collection of urinary vanillylmandelic acid (VMA) is only 60% to 70%,[143,165] and the sensitivity of the 24-hour urinary catecholamine excretion is only 60% to 79%.[87,125,143,165] The drawbacks to the determination of the 24-hour urinary excretion of metanephrines are the inconvenience to the patient and the adequacy of the complete collection.

Once the diagnosis of pheochromocytoma is chemically defined, the tumor needs to be localized. MRI is the technique of choice, offering a sensitivity of close to 100%.[87] It can be used for examining pregnant women, and it offers better sensitivity for determining cardiac localization of the tumor. If the MRI of the neck, thorax, abdomen, and pelvis fails to reveal the tumor, rescanning with CT is suggested. If the tumor still cannot be localized, nuclide scanning with [131]I-metaiodobenzylguanidine ([131]I-MIBG) may be employed.[170] [131]I-MIBG concentrates in pheochromocytomas, but nuclide scanning is expensive and not usually as sensitive as CT or MRI. It should be considered when multiple tumors are either identified or strongly suspected.[87]

## CUSHING'S DISEASE AND CUSHING'S SYNDROME

Both Cushing's disease and Cushing's syndrome are the result of excessive secretion of glucocorticoids from the adrenal cortex. Cushing's disease is the appropriate designation when the hypercortisolism is due to excessive secretion of ACTH by a pituitary tumor, most commonly a microadenoma. Cushing's syndrome is the appropriate terminology for hypercortisolism from all other causes, including glucocorticoid secretion by an adrenal neoplasm (adenoma or carcinoma), exogenous ingestion of glucocorticoids, or ectopic production of ACTH by a nonpituitary neoplasm. In rare instances the syndrome may be caused by ectopic secretion of corticotropin-releasing hormone (CRH).[168,169,223] Cushing's disease and Cushing's syndrome are relatively uncommon, with an incidence of 1 to 2 cases per million population, and a prevalence of 40 cases per million population.[223] These conditions are more common in women than in men.

A Cushing's disorder is usually suspected because of the peculiar body habitus. Most patients are aware of unexplained obesity, but it is the clinician who usually notes the odd distribution of fat, involving the upper third of the body, with the limbs remaining thin. Fat is thickened in the supraclavicular region and over the upper thoracic spine (the "dowager" or "buffalo" hump), and the face is often rounded and plethoric ("moon facies"). The abnormal fat distribution is found in more than 90% of patients with this disorder.[168] Cushing's syndrome due to ectopic ACTH secretion by malignant neoplasms does not usually produce the typical cushingoid truncal-obesity fat distribution, possibly because of the brevity of survival and tumor-associated cachexia.[202] The skin is thin and bruises easily, and striae (stretch marks from fat deposition) over the breasts, abdomen, and flanks have a purplish discoloration in about 80% of patients with this disorder. Scalp hair is thinned, but

increased facial hair may produce a hirsute appearance with masculinization of women, and amenorrhea, oligomenorrhea, or other menstrual irregularities may occur, possibly because of the excessive elaboration of 17-ketosteroids.[202] Hypertension is detected in more than 80% of patients. Myopathy involving the proximal limb-girdle musculature is common, and patients may complain of difficulty arising from a seated position and when climbing or descending stairs. Low back pain is common although not specific and may be a result of both osteoporosis and myopathic weakness. Occasionally it is due to pathologic compression fractures of the vertebrae. Pathologic fractures of the ribs are more common.

Generalized skin hyperpigmentation, peripheral edema, hyperglycemia, and hypokalemic alkalosis may all be present. Diffuse skin pigmentation indicates Cushing's disease rather than Cushing's syndrome[202] since it is found in the presence of excessive circulating ACTH and may be due to that molecule, to beta-melanocyte-stimulating hormone, or to the precursor molecule of ACTH, pro-opiomelanocortin (POMC). Of all the signs and symptoms, those with the highest discriminatory value in the diagnosis of Cushing's disease or syndrome are truncal obesity, hirsutism, menstrual irregularity, hypertension, diabetes mellitus, ecchymoses, and the symptoms and signs of a myopathy.[169]

Central nervous system abnormalities are frequently encountered but are not sufficiently characteristic to suggest hyperadrenalcortisolism. They include depression and psychoses. It is not certain if the mental aberrations are due solely to the effect of glucocorticoids on the nervous system or are aggravated by the accompanying salt retention and hypernatremia, producing a metabolic encephalopathy. Atrophy of the hippocampus has been described with Cushing's disease, is thought to be due to the glucocorticoid excess, and correlates with a decline in short-term verbal memory.[138,139]

### Diagnostic Recommendations

The best single test for the diagnosis of Cushing's disease or syndrome is measurement of the 24-hour urine free cortisol level. The test has a sensitivity of 93% to 100%, and false-negative results are rare, except in the presence of chronic alcoholism or stress.[32,33,223] In an unstressed patient the specificity also approaches 100%. While this may vary by laboratory, healthy persons will excrete <75 µg/24 h. Borderline values lie between 75 and 150 µg/24 h. Diagnostic levels exceed 150 µg/24 h.

The overnight dexamethasone suppression test (DST) is a satisfactory alternative to the 24-hour urine free cortisol test. Although convenient, measurement of plasma cortisol determines the total hormone rather than the free or unbound fraction, and the level is thus influenced by the vagaries of the plasma proteins in general and cortisol-binding globulin (CBG) in particular. Medications may also alter the results. False-positive results are more frequent than with the 24-hour urine free cortisol measurement, and they may occur in the context of stress (which overrides the negative feedback of dexamethasone), with the use of anticonvulsants (which accelerate the degradation of dexamethasone), with estrogen replacement therapy and the use of oral contraceptive agents (which increase CBG), and with depressive disorders (which can distort the hypothalamic-pituitary-adrenal axis).[223] The sensitivity of the DST approaches 100%,[11,32,33] but the specificity is 87%, less than that of the 24-hour urine free cortisol measurement.[11] A dose of 1 mg of dexamethasone is given orally at 11 PM, and the plasma cortisol is measured at 8 AM the following morning. A plasma cortisol level >10 μg/dl suggests Cushing's disease or syndrome, and one <2 μg/dl is considered a normal response,[223] although some authors consider a response of <5 μg/dl to still be normal.[168] Alternatively, plasma cortisol may be determined at 8 AM on the day dexamethasone is to be taken; 1 mg of dexamethasone is taken orally at 11 PM, and a second plasma cortisol level is determined at 8 AM the following morning. If the plasma cortisol level is <2 to 5 μg/dl or less than half of the baseline value, the test is considered negative for Cushing's disease or syndrome.[168]

Elevation of the urine free cortisol or an abnormal low dose (1 mg) of DST does not establish the cause of the hypercortisolism, and when the cortisol level is abnormal, a plasma ACTH level must be obtained. When ACTH is low to unmeasurable, the excess cortisol is due either to an adrenal tumor or to exogenous glucocorticoid ingestion. When the biochemical studies are indicative of an adrenal tumor (low ACTH), visualization of the adrenal glands with CT is recommended. When elevated to >400 pg/ml, ACTH is being produced by either a pituitary adenoma (Cushing's disease) or is being elaborated by a primary malignant or metastatic tumor.

When the urine free cortisol level is elevated or the DST is abnormal and the ACTH level is elevated, one should proceed to a high-dose overnight DST. A dose of 8 mg of dexamethasone is taken orally at 11 PM, and a plasma cortisol level is obtained at 8 AM the following day. If the plasma cortisol is <10 μg/dl, the ACTH is probably being produced by a pituitary tumor, and one should proceed with MRI of the pituitary gland. If the plasma cortisol level is >10 μg/dl, ectopic production of ACTH is likely, and the highest-yield follow-up study will be chest roentgenography and chest CT. Alternatively, as with the low-dose DST, a baseline plasma cortisol level may be obtained at 8 AM, 8 mg of dexamethasone taken by mouth at 11 PM, and plasma cortisol measured at 8 AM the following day. Suppression of the plasma cortisol by half (when compared to the baseline) suggests a pituitary tumor. Sensitivity of the high-dose DST has been reported from 81% to 92%, with a specificity of 57% to as high as 100%.[8,63,198,210]

## THE PITUITARY GLAND

Diseases of the pituitary gland produce symptoms because of abnormalities of hormone elaboration due to indirect changes in the target organs and their hormone secretions or to local pressure effects on contiguous structures and their blood supply. In a general way, hormonal imbalances produce more profound systemic effects than they do effects on the central or peripheral nervous systems, and therefore few of the hormonal imbalances will present initially to the neurologic specialist.

Pure prolactin-secreting tumors and those that produce ACTH are usually microadenomas, and pressure effects will be unlikely. Cushing's disease and hyperprolactinemia are most often suspected because of their changes to the outer aspect of the body, not the nervous system. Chromophobe adenomas and eosinophilic adenomas may produce pressure effects as a sole or dominant manifestation. The most important pressure effects are those involving the eyes and the hypothalamus. The pituitary tumor most likely to produce eye signs is the chromophobe adenoma. A substantial portion of these tumors are associated with hyperprolactinemia, but gynecomastia and galactorrhea are more common in women, with these features noted in only about 13% of men. Because of associated menstrual irregularities, amenorrhea, and anovulatory sterility, the diagnosis is more apt to be considered in women than in men before the tumor becomes large enough to produce pressure symptoms.[168,169] As a result, visual field defects due to pituitary adenomas are more likely to be seen in men.[199] The pituitary gland lies below the diaphragma sellae and a tumor must extend beyond this barrier and the cisterna chiasmatica before it produces pressure on the optic nerve or chiasm. Once it does, bitemporal hemianopia is the most common manifestation, although unilateral optic nerve abnormalities may be noted with eccentric tumor growth. Third, fourth, and sixth cranial nerve palsies are quite uncommon with primary pituitary tumors. The adenoma may cause atypical face pain[82] and rarely may invade the carotid artery, producing a stoke syndrome.[187] Pituitary tumors may undergo spontaneous necrosis with hemorrhage, producing the syndrome of "pituitary apoplexy,"[219] with headache, nausea, vomiting, vertigo, a diminished level of consciousness, alterations in visual acuity, ocular palsies, and evidence for a subarachnoid hemorrhage.[169]

### PROLACTINOMA

Numerous lesions arise from the pituitary gland or its neighboring structures. Of these, adenohypophyseal tumors are the most common. Pituitary adenomas account for 36% of sellar and juxtasellar lesions.[38] Prolactinoma is the most common type of secretory pituitary tumor.[194] Prolactin-secreting adenomas (prolactinomas) are classified by size: if they are ≤1 cm in diameter, they are classified as microadenomas; if >1 cm in diameter, they are macroadenomas. As a confounding variable, hyperprolactinemia is often seen with other pituitary neoplasms as a result of compression of prolactin-secreting cells or compression of the pituitary stalk, interfering with the infundibulohypophyseal dopaminergic pathways that are inhibitory to prolactin secretion. GH may be co-secreted from the same cells that secrete prolactin, and thus hyperprolactinemia may be seen with acromegaly, both from the "stalk effect" and as a direct result of tumorous prolactin secretion.[209] Dopaminergic inhibition of prolactin secretion may on rare occasions be interfered with by lesions that interfere with hypothalamic function, such as in a reported case of moyamoya disease.[7]

Many parasellar lesions including craniopharyngiomas and even carotid artery aneurysms can interfere with dopaminergic inhibitory pathways, leading to hyperprolactinemia.[112] In a fashion similar to cortisol, prolactin behaves as a "stress hormone"[2,79,169] and may even be elevated as a result of venipuncture.[38]

Hyperprolactinemia is seen in the setting of hypothyroidism, liver disease and alcohol abuse, and polycystic ovaries. Hyperprolactinemia is caused by a number of medications and drugs, including dopamine antagonists (psychotropic agents), monoamine oxidase (MAO) inhibitors, methyldopa, reserpine, verapamil, metoclopramide, domperidol, and H$_2$-receptor antagonists, and with the use or abuse of opiates and cocaine. It often rises transiently following a generalized convulsion, in which circumstance it may have diagnostic usefulness.[200]

In women, hyperprolactinemia is most likely to cause amenorrhea and galactorrhea, leading to early recognition. Amenorrhea may occur with prolactin levels >40 ng/ml and is almost always present with levels of ≥100 ng/ml.[200] Amenorrhea is thought to be due to suppression of luteinizing hormone–releasinbg hormone (LHRH) by prolactin. Other common complaints in women with hyperprolactinemia include headache, malaise, restlessness, and fatigue.[176] Headache is most likely to occur only if a prolactinoma is present, suggesting that it may not be the result of prolactin itself but rather a manifestation of the space-occupying mass effect of the prolactin-secreting adenoma.[203]

In men the literature suggests that prolactinomas present with the pressure effects of large pituitary tumors. In a more recent series the presenting symptoms in men were endocrine in 57% of the patients (the vast majority being loss of libido or potency).[220] In only 28% of the 53 patients reported were pressure effects of the tumor the presenting symptoms (with just under half complaining of headache and the rest describing a combination of visual loss or diplopia). Approximately 15% of the patients presented incidentally (pituitary "incidentalomas").[66,230] As in other series,[176] macroprolactinomas were the most common tumor type in men (70%), with just 15% having microadenomas and 15% having no detectable tumor.[220]

Otherwise unexplained weight gain and excessive body weight are associated with prolactinomas in both men and women and are not explained by a mass effect on the hypothalamus or by other abnormalities of pituitary function.[49,92] It has been suggested that the rapid weight gain is not due to a direct effect of prolactin but is part of a neuroendocrine response to environmental stimuli differing from the sympathoadrenal stress response because the prolactin level has a negative correlation to cortisol levels.[79]

Osteopenia is associated with prolactinomas and is due to the attendant hypogonadism, corresponding well with the duration.[114] Despite the stimulatory effect of prolactin on the breast, there is no increased incidence of breast malignancy with the hyperprolactinemic state in general or with prolactinomas in particular.[95,207]

Prolactinomas are found with an unusually high incidence in patients with multiple endocrine neoplasia type I (MEN I), and they are frequently the initial manifestation of that disorder.[47,149] Kindreds of MEN I report an incidence of pituitary adenomas from 9% to 65%.[29] Although most of the tumors are prolactinomas, 14% to 37% are somatotrophinomas, secreting GH.[29,137] Both GH and prolactin can be cosecreted from the same cell lineage. MEN I is due to a gene defect on chromosome 11q13[10] and may be the only inherited form of prolactinoma.

There is an interesting complication in the treatment of prolactinomas. In the case of pituitary tumors, cerebrospinal fluid (CSF) leakage may occur as a result of shunting between the subarachnoid and extradural spaces.[145] The communication may be "tamponaded" by the tumor mass. Most prolactinomas respond to treatment with bromocriptine by reduction in both prolactin levels and in tumor mass. When the tumor mass shrinks, the communication between the subarachnoid and extradural spaces may be unmasked, leading to CSF rhinorrhea, CSF otorrhea, pneumocephalus, and meningitis.[145,152,206]

## Diagnostic Recommendations

A prolactinoma is suspected only when the prolactin level exceeds 150 ng/ml. It is distinctly unusual for a neurologist to suspect a prolactin-secreting pituitary adenoma. Specific instances might include a woman referred for evaluation of headaches. If the history reveals amenorrhea or galactorrhea and there has been either recent weight gain or the patient appears obese, obtaining a prolactin level is worthwhile. Only if the prolactin level is ≥150 ng/ml is MRI of the pituitary gland reasonable, since below that level one will not find either a macroadenoma or a microadenoma. In a male patient with headaches, if there is a history of impotence or impaired libido (and especially if there is gynecomastia or galactorrhea), obtaining a prolactin level is a reasonable test for a suspected microprolactinoma. If there are associated visual complaints or a demonstrated visual field disturbance, it would be more reasonable to proceed to MRI to define the sellar and parasellar region. Determination of the tumor type then follows the diagnosis of a pituitary tumor and may best be left to the endocrinologist, just as the visual field determination will be left to the ophthalmologist.

For whatever reason, if the neurologist has found prolactin in excess of 150 ng/ml and if the MRI has demonstrated either a microadenoma or macroadenoma, further testing needs to be done. In the case of a macroadenoma, visual field determinations are mandatory. Further pituitary testing may be left to the endocrinologist but would include both a morning cortisol level for adequacy of the hypothalamic-pituitary-adrenal axis, sex hormone determination (estradiol in women, testosterone in men) for assessment of the hypothalamic-pituitary-gonadal axis, and TSH for assessment of the hypothalamic-pituitary-thyroid axis. Since prolactinomas may coexist with somatotrophinomas, the somatomedin C level (or, alternatively, a morning GH level) should be obtained. Because of the association of prolactinoma and MEN I and because 95% to 100% of patients with MEN I will have or will develop hyperparathyroidism, a serum calcium level is needed.[47]

## ACROMEGALY

Acromegaly is the disorder produced by chronic hypersecretion of GH. Usually the GH is secreted by an autonomous primary pituitary gland neoplasm, although very rarely it may result from ectopic production of growth hormone–releasing hormone (GH-RH) produced in a pancreatic islet cell tumor, from a carcinoid tumor of the lung or intestine, or from a central nervous system source (e.g., diencephalic hamartoma or gangliocytoma, pinealoma, craniopharyngioma, or optic glioma).[169,223]

If GH hypersecretion occurs in childhood before closure of the bony epiphyses, gigantism is the result. After epiphyseal closure, only limited bone growth occurs and is confined to the hands, feet, and skull. The hands and feet enlarge (increasing ring and shoe size), and thickening and tufting of the distal phalanges are visible radiographically. There may be frontal bossing as the skull grows, and the mandible enlarges, with widening of the space between the teeth and malocclusion due to an overbite. Enlargement of the ribs produces a "barrel chest." Thickening of subcutaneous tissues leads to coarsening of facial features. The skin feels thick; there are many skin tags; and there is excessive perspiration (60% to 80%),[168] which feels "oily" and has a foul odor.[224] Palpation of the neck often reveals a goiter. The lips are large, and the tongue appears to fill the mouth. More than half of the affected patients will complain of or admit to headache. Joint pain, aching, and stiffness are quite common. Hypertension is frequently present (30%), and there may be cardiac enlargement. Galactorrhea is seen in 25% of women with this disorder, and both men and women may admit to decreased libido. Men may become impotent, presumably from hyperprolactinemia. A third of GH-secreting tumors either co-secrete prolactin or are mixed tumors with prolactin-secreting cells added[224]; in other cases the bulk of the tumor may interrupt pituitary stalk dopaminergic pathways.[168] Insulin resistance and frank diabetes mellitus may be found.

Proximal muscle weakness can often be detected. Paresthesias of the hands due to carpal tunnel syndrome and ulnar entrapment neuropathies may occur. Visual field defects and cranial nerve palsies may be found with very large tumors.

### Diagnostic Recommendations

Although a morning basal GH level may be suggestive of acromegaly, values can be misleading because of the pulsatile nature of GH secretion. The sensitivity of a basal GH level for diagnosing acromegaly is only 70%.[65] For diagnostic purposes, random measurement of the serum level of somatomedin C (insulinlike growth factor I) is suggested. The protein is elaborated by the liver in response to the level of circulating GH, integrated over time. Elevated levels are consistent with acromegaly and call for further testing. An elevated somatomedin C level should be confirmed with a basal GH level. If the level is >10 ng/ml, 100 g of glucose is administered orally, and the GH level is obtained 1 hour later. If the level remains >10 ng/ml, the diagnosis of acromegaly is secure. If it is <2 ng/ml, the diagnosis is excluded.

MRI will demonstrate a tumor in the majority of cases of acromegaly, but its use should be restricted to instances with suggestive or diagnostic biochemical parameters.[224]

## THE PANCREAS: DIABETES MELLITUS

Diabetes mellitus is the most common endocrine disease, consuming almost 15% of the annual health care expenditures in the United States.[186] It is a chronic condition of hyperglycemia due either to a relative or absolute deficiency of insulin or to a deficiency of insulin action. The lack of insulin effect leads to alterations in the metabolism of glucose, fat, and protein. Over time, systemic complications arise involving the vascular system, the nervous system (both peripheral and central), and other specific organs. Diabetes mellitus is divided into two categories, type 1 (10% of patients) and type 2 (90% of patients).[186,196] Type 1 diabetes is further subdivided into two forms: immune-mediated diabetes mellitus and idiopathic diabetes mellitus.[5] A new stage of impaired glucose homeostasis has been defined and is called *impaired fasting glucose.* The definition is a fasting (no caloric intake for 8 hours) plasma glucose level ≥110 mg/dl and <126 mg/dl. The older term, *impaired glucose tolerance,*

has been retained and is defined as a 2-hour plasma glucose level ≥140 mg/dl and <200 mg/dl following ingestion of a 75 g glucose challenge.[5]

### TYPE 1 (INSULIN-DEPENDENT) DIABETES MELLITUS

Type 1 diabetes is the most common endocrinologic disease in children and adolescents and is usually a genetically linked autoimmune disease.[100] Type II major histocompatibility antigens (MHC-II) contribute to 48% of the incidence of the disease.[91] It is associated with other autoimmune diseases, most commonly autoimmune thyroiditis.[118] The disorder is also seen with the polyglandular autoimmune (PGA) syndromes, of which there are three types: PGA 1, PGA 2, and PGA 3. Type 1 diabetes mellitus is seen with all three of the disorders but is less common in type 1 (in which hypoparathyroidism, adrenal insufficiency, candidiasis, and ectodermal dystrophy may occur).[103] In patients with PGA 1, autoantibodies have been found against the enzyme aromatic L-amino acid decarboxylase of the pancreatic beta cells.[102]

A number of candidate autoantigens have been suggested as etiologic factors in type 1 diabetes, including the $GM_2$-1 pancreatic islet ganglioside,[68] glutamic acid decarboxylase 65 (GAD 65), GAD 67, heat-shock protein 65 (HSP 65), islet-cell antigen 69 (ICA 69), and insulin.[182] In patients with the necessary MHC-II genetic background, it is thought that viral infections may play a role in the induction of the autoimmune response. Viral infections frequently elicit strong cellular and humoral immune responses. Autoreactive lymphocytes may be coactivated through bystander activation by cytokines or through direct sharing of conformational determinants between self and virus (mimicry).[218] Viral infection of antigen-presenting cells can locally enhance inflammation and drive autoreactive lymphocytes.[218] Viral infections may produce superantigens (SAG). Expansion of the Vveta7 T-cell subset has been found in patients with the acute onset of type 1 diabetes mellitus, suggesting the presence of a surface membrane–bound SAG. A mouse mammary tumor virus–related human endogenous retrovirus has been isolated in which the N-terminal moiety of the envelope gene encodes an MHC-II-dependent SAG; the SAG encoded by the retrovirus is a candidate autoimmune gene for type 1 diabetes mellitus.[45]

Most patients with type I diabetes mellitus will develop the disease before age 30 years. The autoimmune process may begin several years before diagnosis and is expressed only when most of the pancreatic islet beta cells have been destroyed by an inflammatory process involving T lymphocytes, a process sometimes referred to as an "insulinitis."[196] Most patients will complain of polydipsia, polyuria, fatigue, and a variable degree of weight loss. Although polyphagia is classically described, at the time of presentation many of these patients are anorectic, possibly as a result of ketosis or acidosis. Approximately 20% will present with diabetic ketoacidosis.[196] In these patients the diagnosis is not difficult. The classic signs and symptoms associated with hyperglycemia—a random plasma glucose level of >200 mg/dl with glycosuria and with or without ketonemia and ketonuria—present little diagnostic challenge.

### TYPE 2 (INSULIN-INDEPENDENT) DIABETES MELLITUS

Type 2 diabetes mellitus does not require insulin to prevent death, ketoacidosis, or weight loss, although many affected patients will be given insulin to control hyperglycemia. The disorder is due to a combination of insulin resistance and insulin deficiency (relative or absolute).[20] The most common factor correlated with insulin resistance is obesity, and 80% of patients with type 2 diabetes in the United States are obese. Associated with the insulin resistance may be an inherited incapacity of the islet beta-cells to hypersecrete sufficient insulin to compensate for the resistance. A family history of diabetes is found in 25% to 30% of type 2 diabetics, and monozygotic twin studies disclose 80% to 100% concordance.[20] For a few variants of the rare monogenic form of non-insulin-dependent diabetes mellitus, specific genetic defects have been identified: for maturity-onset diabetes of the young (MODY), there are glucokinase defects in 40% of families; there are extreme insulin-resistance syndromes that often involve the insulin receptor; and there are diabetes-deafness syndromes in which mutations of mitochondrial genes have been identified.[111] Genes involved in the more common forms of type 2 diabetes have not been identified, but there is some evidence suggesting abnormalities of insulin-receptor-substrate 1 (IRS-1),[212] glycogen synthase,[155] the glucagon receptor, a ras-related protein (Rad),[111] histocompatibility antigens, PC-1, and fatty acid binding protein. It is speculated that the contributions of these genes to type 2 diabetes mellitus is probably small.[111]

The most common symptoms leading to a suspicion of type 2 diabetes are polyuria, polydipsia, and polyphagia. There is a tendency to develop monilial vaginitis and balanitis. Blurred vision caused by hyperglycemia-induced alterations in lens refraction is an additional common early complaint.[20] Occasionally, patients with type 2 diabetes will present with neurologic complaints.

Peripheral neuropathy is the most common neurologic disturbance in type 2 diabetes. It is usually a distal and often painful sensorimotor polyneuropathy, and EMG and nerve conduction studies may show predominantly axonal disease or axonal disease with a demyelinative component. Mononeuritis multiplex, radiculopathies (often truncal), femoral neuropathies, or lumbosacral plexopathies may be encountered. Autonomic neuropathy can occur in the form of gastroparesis diabeticorum, diarrhea, resting tachycardia, orthostatic hypotension, incomplete bladder emptying, impotence, pupillary changes, and a sudden death syndrome.[169]

Involvement of one or more of the cranial nerves may occasionally be the presenting complaint of a patient with type 2 diabetes. The third,[122,208] fourth,[28,229] fifth,[26,191] sixth,[124,181] seventh,[115,221] and eighth[169] cranial nerves have all been affected in type 2 disease. The mechanism may involve changes in small nutrient vessels to the nerves, or the third and sixth nerves may occasionally be subjected to pressure from atherosclerotic intracranial plaques. The diabetic third nerve palsy is characteristically painful and spares the pupil, presumably because of selective infarction of the nerve. Of the cranial nerves, the sixth is most frequently involved. Visual disturbances are common but are usually due to refractive lens errors consequent to hyperglycemia or to diabetic retinopathy. Ischemic optic neuropathy may be seen as a vascular complication of diabetes. Cataract and rubeosis iridis leading to neovascular glaucoma are other ocular complications of the diabetic state.[71]

Diabetic myelopathy is rarely considered, but plantar cutaneous responses,[37] dorsal column abnormalities, and other evidence of myelopathic change in patients with diabetes have been described,[88] and the presence of islet cell amylin (islet cell amyloid protein) in sensory neurons, perhaps mediating their function, lends theoretic support to the construct.[144]

## Diagnostic Recommendations

Diabetes mellitus is diagnosed when the fasting plasma glucose (FPG) level of ≥126 mg/dl (7 mmol/L) or the casual plasma glucose level of ≥200 mg/dl (11.1 mmol/L) is associated with the typical symptoms of polyuria, polydipsia, and unexplained weight loss. The abnormal result is best confirmed with a second determination. Previously the gold standard was the oral glucose tolerance test (OGTT).[162] The test has been retained, with diabetes mellitus diagnosed if the 2-hour plasma glucose level is ≥200 mg/dl. However, this test is not recommended for routine clinical use.[5] With the OGTT used as the defining standard, the fasting plasma glucose has a sensitivity of 78%.[226]

Glycosylated hemoglobin determinations are readily available and reflect glucose homeostasis over the preceding 2 months. At a cutoff point of 6.2% it is said to have a sensitivity of 41% with a specificity of 100%.[226] The sensitivity and specificity, however, were determined by considering the OGTT as the defining test for diabetes mellitus. There may be some improvement in diagnostic accuracy when the fasting glucose level is combined with the glycosylated hemoglobin level. A fasting blood glucose level of ≥120 mg/dl and a glycosylated hemoglobin level of >5.8% correlated with a 2-hour OGTT value ≥200 mg/dl (an accepted definition of diabetes mellitus) with a sensitivity of 64.7% and a specificity of 97.9%.[53] At this time the American Diabetes Association does not recommend use of the glycosylated hemoglobin (HbA$_{1c}$) level for diagnosis of diabetes mellitus.

When one is confronted with a neurologic disorder associated with diabetes mellitus it seems reasonable to obtain both a fasting plasma glucose level and an HbA$_{1c}$. If the FPG level is ≥126 mg/dl and the glycosylated hemoglobin is elevated, one may comfortably diagnose diabetes mellitus, since the glycosylated hemoglobin bears witness to a long-term abnormality in glucose metabolism. The FPG should be repeated, primarily to be certain that there has not been a mix-up of blood specimens (a rare but not impossible scenario). If both the FPG and the HbA$_{1c}$ levels are normal, diabetes mellitus as a cause for the neurologic disorder has been adequately excluded in most instances. If either test is abnormal but the FPG is in the "impaired fasting glucose" range (FPG ≥110 mg/dl but <126 mg/dl), one can proceed to an OGTT in those instances in which diabetes mellitus would be a strong candidate for the cause of the neurologic findings. If the test result is abnormal (showing either diabetes or "impaired glucose tolerance"), the abnormality in glucose homeostasis may tentatively be considered to be the cause of the disorder, provided all other reasonable causes have been excluded by adequate testing. If nothing else, the disorder is taken from the "idiopathic" and "cryptogenic" categories of illness.

## REFERENCES

1. Aarli JA, Thunold S, Heimann P. Thyroiditis in myasthenia gravis. *Acta Neurol Scand.* 1978;58:121-127.
2. Abraham RR, Dornhorst A, Wynn V, et al. Corticotrophin, cortisol, prolactin and growth hormone responses to insulin-induced hypogly-

caemia in normal subjects given sodium valproate. *Clin Endocrinol (Oxf).* 1985;22:639-644.

3. Akiyama T, Batchelder J, Worsman J, Moses HW, Jedlinski M. Hypocalcemic torsades de pointes. *J Electrocardiol.* 1989;22:89-92.

4. Ali AS, Akavaram NR. Neuromuscular disorders in thyrotoxicosis. *Am Fam Physician.* 1980;22:97-102.

5. American Diabetes Association. Clinical practice recommendations, 1997. *Diabetes Care.* 1997;20(suppl 1):S1-S70.

6. Arem R, Cusi K, Kiefe C. Value of sensitive thyrotropin measurement in ambulatory and hospitalized patients. *Clin Invest Med.* 1990;13:132-138.

7. Arita K, Uozumi T, Oki S, et al. Moyamoya disease associated with pituitary adenoma: report of two cases. *Neurol Med Chir (Tokyo).* 1992; 32:753-757.

8. Aron DC, Raff H, Findling JW. Effectiveness versus efficacy: the limited value in clinical practice of high dose dexamethasone suppression testing in the differential diagnosis of adrenocorticotropin-dependent Cushing's syndrome. *J Clin Endocrinol Metab.* 1997;82:1780-1785.

9. Atchison JA, Lee PA, Albright AL. Reversible suprasellar pituitary mass secondary to hypothyroidism. *JAMA.* 1989;262:3175-3177.

10. Bale SJ, Bale AE, Stewart K, et al. Linkage analysis of multiple endocrine neoplasia type 1 with INT2 and other markers on chromosome 11 [published erratum appears in *Genomics* 1989;5:166]. *Genomics.* 1989;4:320-322.

11. Barrou Z, Guiban D, Maroufi A, et al. Overnight dexamethasone suppression test: comparison of plasma and salivary cortisol measurement for the screening of Cushing's syndrome. *Eur J Endocrinol.* 1996; 134:93-96.

12. Bassett F, Eastman CJ, Ma G, Maberly GF, Smith HC. Diagnostic value of thyrotropin concentrations in serum as measured by a sensitive immunoradiometric assay. *Clin Chemistry.* 1986;32:461-464.

13. Baxter M, Hunter P, Thompson G, London D. Phaeochromocytomas as a cause of hypotension. *Clin Endocrinol (Oxf).* 1992;37:304-306.

14. Bayer MF, Kriss JP, McDougall IR. Clinical experience with sensitive thyrotropin measurements: diagnostic and therapeutic implications. *J Nucl Med.* 1985;26:1248-1256.

15. Beck-Peccoz P, Persani L, Asteria C, et al. Thyrotropin-secreting pituitary tumors in hyper- and hypothyroidism. *Acta Med Austriaca.* 1996;23:41-46.

16. Beghi E, Delodovici ML, Bogliun G, et al. Hypothyroidism and polyneuropathy. *J Neurol Neurosurg Psychiatry.* 1989;52:1420-1423.

17. Bernini GP, Vivaldi MS, Argenio GF, Moretti A, Sgro M, Salvetti A. Frequency of pheochromocytoma in adrenal incidentalomas and utility of the glucagon test for the diagnosis. *J Endocrinol Invest.* 1997;20:65-71.

18. Bilaniuk LT, Moshang T, Cara J, et al. Pituitary enlargement mimicking pituitary tumor. *J Neurosurg.* 1985;63:39-42.

19. Biondi B, Fazio S, Carella C, et al. Control of adrenergic overactivity by beta-blockade improves the quality of life in patients receiving long term suppressive therapy with levothyroxine. *J Clin Endocrinol Metab.* 1994;78:1028-1033.

20. Blackard WG. Type II (non-insulin-dependent) diabetes mellitus. In: Hurst JW, ed. *Medicine for the Practicing Physician.* 4th ed. Stamford, CT: Appleton & Lange; 1996:635-639.

21. Blume WT, Grabow JD. The "cerebellar" signs of myxedema. *Dis Nerv Syst.* 1969;30:55-57.

22. Bock JL, Morris D, Cheng J, Ehresman D. Evaluation of the Technicon Immuno 1 free thyroxine assay. *Am J Clin Pathol.* 1996;105:583-588.

23. Boles CB, Mignone U, Vadala G, Gastaldi C, Favero C, Brogliatti B. Glaucoma and hypothyroidism. *Acta Ophthalmol Scand Suppl.* 1997; 47-48.

24. Braund KG, Steinberg HS, Shores A, et al. Laryngeal paralysis in immature and mature dogs as one sign of a more diffuse polyneuropathy. *J Am Vet Med Assoc.* 1989;194:1735-1740.

25. Brown MR, Parks JS, Adess ME, et al. Central hypothyroidism reveals compound heterozygous mutations in the *Pit-1* gene. *Horm Res.* 1998; 49:98-102.

26. Bucher MB, Assal JP, Leuenberger PM. Optic neuropathy in diabetics. *Klin Monatsbl Augenheilkd.* 1980;176:711-717.

27. Bulens C. Neurologic complications of hyperthyroidism: remission of spastic paraplegia, dementia and optic neuropathy. *Arch Neurol.* 1981; 38:669-670.

28. Burger LJ, Kalvin NH, Smith JL. Acquired lesions of the fourth cranial nerve. *Brain.* 1970;93:567-574.

29. Burgess JR, Shepherd JJ, Parameswaran V, Hoffman L, Greenaway TM. Somatotrophinomas in multiple endocrine neoplasia type 1: a review of clinical phenotype and insulin-like growth factor-1 levels in a large

30. multiple endocrine neoplasia type 1 kindred. *Am J Med.* 1996;100:544-547.

31. Burra P, Franklyn JA, Ramsden DB, Elias E, Sheppard MC. Severity of alcoholic liver disease and markers of thyroid and steroid status. *Postgrad Med J.* 1992;68:804-810.

32. Buskila D, Sukenik S, Levene NA, et al. Hypocalcemia and QT interval prolongation during the acute phase of measles. *South Med J.* 1991; 84:675.

33. Caduff F, Staub JJ, Nordmann A, Radu EW, Landolt H. The diagnosis of Cushing's syndrome: results of diagnostic assessment of 20 patients with Cushing's syndrome of variable etiology (1979–1989). *Schweiz Med Wochenschr.* 1991;121:10-20.

34. Calvo RJ, Morales PF, Alvarez BJ, Diaz PDM. Cushing's syndrome: clinical study of fifteen cases. *An Med Interna.* 1998;15:237-240.

35. Campos SP, Olitsky S. Idiopathic intracranial hypertension after L-thyroxine therapy for acquired primary hypothyroidism. *Clin Pediatr (Phila).* 1995;34:334-337.

36. Canale MP, Bravo EL. Diagnostic specificity of serum chromogranin-A for pheochromocytoma in patients with renal dysfunction. *J Clin Endocrinol Metab.* 1994;78:1139-1144.

37. Carette S, Lefrancois L. Fibrositis and primary hypothyroidism. *J Rheumatol.* 1988;15:1418-1421.

38. Cassar J. Extensor plantar response in diabetic neuropathy. *Diabetes Care.* 1993;16:1048-1049.

39. Cawley CM, Tindall GT. Pituitary and neighboring tumors. In: Hurst JW, ed. *Medicine for the Practicing Physician.* 4th ed. Stamford, CT: Appleton & Lange; 1996:540-544.

40. Celani MF, Bonati ME, Stucci N. Prevalence of abnormal thyrotropin concentrations measured by a sensitive assay in patients with type 2 diabetes mellitus. *Diabetes Res.* 1994;27:15-25.

41. Centanni M, Cesareo R, Verallo O, et al. Reversible increase of intraocular pressure in subclinical hypothyroid patients. *Eur J Endocrinol.* 1997;136:595-598.

42. Chandramouli BV, Kotler MN. Atrial fibrillation: drug therapies for ventricular rate control and restoration of sinus rhythm. *Geriatrics.* 1998;53:46-52.

43. Chrzanowski DD. Managing atrial fibrillation to prevent its major complication: ischemic stroke. *Nurse Pract.* 1998;23:26-32.

44. Ciompi ML, Zuccotti M, Bazzichi L, Puccetti L. Polymyositis-like syndrome in hypothyroidism: report of two cases. *Thyroidology.* 1994;6:33-36.

45. Collu R, Tang J, Castagne J, et al. A novel mechanism for isolated central hypothyroidism: inactivating mutations in the thyrotropin-releasing hormone receptor gene. *J Clin Endocrinol Metab.* 1997;82:1561-1565.

46. Conrad B, Weissmahr RN, Boni J, Arcari R, Schupbach J, Mach B. A human endogenous retroviral superantigen as candidate autoimmune gene in type I diabetes. *Cell.* 1997;90:303-313.

47. Cooper D. Subclinical thyroid disease: a clinician's perspective. *Ann Intern Med.* 1998;129:135-137.

48. Corbetta S, Pizzocaro A, Peracchi M, Beck-Peccoz P, Faglia G, Spada A. Multiple endocrine neoplasia type 1 in patients with recognized pituitary tumours of different types. *Clin Endocrinol (Oxf).* 1997;47:507-512.

49. Corn T, Chekley S. A case of recurrent mania with recurrent hyperthyroidism. *Br J Psychiatry.* 1983;143:74-77.

50. Creemers LB, Zelissen PM, van Koppeschaar HP. Prolactinoma and body weight: a retrospective study. *Acta Endocrinol (Copenh).* 1991; 125:392-396.

51. Cruz MW, Tendrich M, Vaisman M, Novis SA. Electroneuromyography and neuromuscular findings in 16 primary hypothyroidism patients. *Arq Neuropsiquiatr.* 1996;54:12-18.

52. Dadachanji MC, Bharucha NE, Jhankaria BG. Pituitary hyperplasia mimicking pituitary tumor. *Surg Neurol.* 1994;42:397-399.

53. Dakshinamurti K, Paulose CS, Vriend J. Hypothyroidism of hypothalamic origin in pyridoxine-deficient rats. *J Endocrinol.* 1986;109:345-349.

54. D'Alessandro A, Simon D, Coignet MC, Cenee S, Giorgino R, Eschwege E. [Assessment of the use of hemoglobin A1c in diabetes mellitus screening]. *Diabete Metab.* 1990;16:213-219.

55. Davis TM, Singh B, Choo KE, Ibrahim J, Spencer JL, St John A. Dynamic assessment of the electrocardiographic QT interval during citrate infusion in healthy volunteers. *Br Heart J.* 1995;73:523-526.

56. De Assis JL, Scaff M, Zambon AA, Marchiori PE. Thyroid diseases and myasthenia gravis. *Arq Neuropsiquiatr.* 1984;42:226-231.

57. De Los S, Mazzaferri EL. Sensitive thyroid-stimulating hormone assays: clinical applications and limitations. *Compr Ther.* 1988;14:26-33.

57. De Los S, Starich GH, Mazzaferri EL. Sensitivity, specificity, and cost-effectiveness of the sensitive thyrotropin assay in the diagnosis of thyroid disease in ambulatory patients. *Arch Intern Med.* 1989;149:526-532.

58. De Rosa G, Testa A, Giacomini D, et al. Comparison between TRH-stimulated TSH and basal TSH measurement by a commercial immunoradiometric assay in the management of thyroid disease. *Q J Nucl Med.* 1996;40:182-187.

59. Deev AS, Chelnokova SN, Pchelintseva ZI, Gromyko LV, Zakharushkina IV, Karpikov AV. Benign intracranial hypertension syndrome. *Klin Med (Mosk).* 1990;68:41-43.

60. DeJong RN. *The Neurologic Examination.* 3rd ed. New York: Harper & Row; 1970:655-661.

61. del Palacio A, Trueba JL, Cabello A, et al. Thyroid myopathy: effect of treatment with thyroid hormones. *An Med Interna.* 1990;7:120-122.

62. DeQuattro V, Myers M, Campese V. Pheochromocytoma: diagnosis and therapy. In: DeGroot L, Besser G, Cahill G Jr, et al, eds. *Endocrinology.* 2nd ed. Philadelphia: WB Saunders; 1989:1780-1797.

63. Dichek HL, Nieman LK, Oldfield EH, Pass HI, Malley JD, Cutler GBJ. A comparison of the standard high dose dexamethasone suppression test and the overnight 8-mg dexamethasone suppression test for the differential diagnosis of adrenocorticotropin-dependent Cushing's syndrome. *J Clin Endocrinol Metab.* 1994;78:418-422.

64. Doeker BM, Pfaffle RW, Pohlenz J, Andler W. Congenital central hypothyroidism due to a homozygous mutation in the thyrotropin beta-subunit gene follows an autosomal recessive inheritance. *J Clin Endocrinol Metab.* 1998;83:1762-1765.

65. Dohan O, Goth M, Szabolcs I, Kovacs L, Kovacs Z, Szilagyi G. The place of insulin-like growth factor I in the diagnosis of acromegaly. *Orv Hetil.* 1993;134:2301-2303.

66. Dombrowski RC, Romeo JH, Aron DC. Verapamil-induced hyperprolactinemia complicated by a pituitary incidentaloma. *Ann Pharmacother.* 1995;29:999-1001.

67. dos Remedios LV, Weber PM, Feldman R, Schurr DA, Tsoi TG. Detecting unsuspected thyroid dysfunction by the free thyroxine index. *Arch Intern Med.* 1980;140:1045-1049.

68. Dotta F, Gianani R, Previti M, et al. Autoimmunity to the GM$_2$-1 islet ganglioside before and at the onset of type I diabetes. *Diabetes.* 1996;45:1193-1196.

69. Doucet J, Trivalle C, Chassagne P, et al. Does age play a role in clinical presentation of hypothyroidism? *J Am Geriatr Soc.* 1994;42:984-986.

70. Downs RWJ. Hypercalcemia and hyperparathyroidism. In: Hurst JW, ed. *Medicine for the Practicing Physician.* 4th ed. Stamford, CT: Appleton & Lange; 1996:655-659.

71. Ducrey N. Ocular lesions due to diabetes. *Schweiz Med Wochenschr.* 1996;126:1610-1612.

72. Dyck PJ, Lambert EH. Polyneuropathy associated with hypothyroidism. *J Neuropathol Exp Neurol.* 1970;29:631-658.

73. Emser W, Schimrigk K. Myxedema myopathy: a case report. *Eur Neurol.* 1977;16:286-291.

74. Endres DB, Villanueva R, Sharp CFJ, Singer FR. Measurement of parathyroid hormone. *Endocrinol Metab Clin North Am.* 1989;18:611-629.

75. Erichsen KE, Berg JP, Torjesen PA, Haug E, Johannesen O. Thyroid hormone resistance: clinical, biochemical and genetic study of a family. *Tidsskr Nor Laegeforen.* 1998;118:525-529.

76. Evered DC, Vice PA, Green E, Appleton D. Assessment of thyroid hormone assays. *J Clin Pathol.* 1976;29:1054-1059.

77. Farley JD, Toth EL, Ryan EA. Primary hypothyroidism presenting as growth delay and pituitary enlargement. *Can J Neurol Sci.* 1988;15:35-37.

78. Feldkamp CS, McKenna MJ. Contemporary approach to thyroid disease emphasizing use of high-sensitivity thyrotropin assays. *Henry Ford Hosp Med J.* 1991;39:25-29.

79. Ferreira MF, Sobrinho LG, Pires JS, Silva ME, Santos MA, Sousa MF. Endocrine and psychological evaluation of women with recent weight gain. *Psychoneuroendocrinology.* 1995;20:53-63.

80. Figge J, Leinung M, Goodman AD, et al. The clinical evaluation of patients with subclinical hyperthyroidism and the free triiodothyronine (free T$_3$) toxicosis. *Am J Med.* 1994;96:229-234.

81. Franklyn JA, Black EG, Betteridge J, Sheppard MC. Comparison of second and third generation methods for measurement of serum thyrotropin in patients with overt hyperthyroidism, patients receiving thyroxine therapy, and those with nonthyroidal illness. *J Clin Endocrinol Metab.* 1994;78:1368-1371.

82. Friedman AH, Wilkins RH, Kenan PD, Olanow CW, Dubois PJ. Pituitary adenoma presenting as facial pain: report of two cases and review of the literature. *Neurosurgery.* 1982;10:742-745.

83. Gage BF, Cardinalli AB, Owens DK. Cost-effectiveness of preference-based antithrombotic therapy for patients with nonvalvular atrial fibrillation. *Stroke.* 1998;29:1083-1091.

84. Gardner D. Hyperthyroidism. In: Hurst JW, ed. *Medicine for the Practicing Physician.* 4th ed. Stamford, CT: Appleton & Lange; 1996:593-597.

85. Gharib H, Abboud CF. Primary idiopathic hypothalamic hypothyroidism: report of four cases. *Am J Med.* 1987;83:171-174.

86. Gibold G, Liehn JC, Deltour G, Delisle MJ. Ultrasensitive TSH: a new diagnostic approach to hyperthyroidism. *An Endocrinologie.* 1986;47:415-419.

87. Gifford RWJ, Bravo EL, Manger WM. Pheochromocytoma. In: Hurst JW, ed. *Medicine for the Practicing Physician.* 4th ed. Stamford, CT: Appleton & Lange; 1996:1103-1107.

88. Giladi N, Turezkite T, Harel D. Myelopathy as a complication of diabetes mellitus. *Isr J Med Sci.* 1991;27:316-319.

89. Giroux B, Metz C, Giroux JD, de Parscau L. [Hypophyseal central hypothyroidism due to isolated TSH deficiency: apropos of a familial neonatal case (letter)]. *Arch Pediatr.* 1997;4:1146-1148.

90. Gomez F, Reyes FI, Faiman C. Nonpuerperal galactorrhea and hyperprolactinemia: clinical findings, endocrine features and therapeutic responses in 56 cases. *Am J Med.* 1977;62:648-660.

91. Gorodezky C, Olivo A, Alaez C, et al. High- and low-risk molecular sequences in autoimmune diseases: an analysis of type I diabetes in Latin America. *Gac Med Mex.* 1997;133(suppl 1):125-132.

92. Greenman Y, Tordjman K, Stern N. Increased body weight associated with prolactin secreting pituitary adenomas: weight loss with normalization of prolactin levels. *Clin Endocrinol (Oxf).* 1998;48:547-553.

93. Gup RS, Sheeler LR, Maeder MC, Tew JMJ. Pituitary enlargement and primary hypothyroidism: a report of two cases with sharply contrasting outcomes. *Neurosurgery.* 1982;11:792-794.

94. Guzowski K, Halawa B, Podemski R. Thyroid activity in patients with myasthenia. *Neurol Neurochir Pol.* 1977;11:201-204.

95. Haga S, Watanabe O, Shimizu T, et al. Breast cancer in a male patient with prolactinoma. *Surg Today.* 1993;23:251-255.

96. Hallengren B, Manhem P, Bramnert M, Redlund-Johnell I, Heijl A. Normal visual fields as assessed by computerized static threshold perimetry in patients with untreated primary hypothyroidism. *Acta Endocrinol (Copenh).* 1989;121:495-500.

97. Hashimoto T, Matsubara F, Nishibu M, Kawai K. Evaluation of a new chemiluminescence technique for human thyrotropin (BeriLux hTSH): diagnostic value of five immunometric assay methods. *Eur J Clin Chem Clin Biochem.* 1991;29:753-757.

98. Helfand M, Redfern CC. Clinical guideline, part 2. Screening for thyroid disease: an update. *Ann Intern Med.* 1998;129:144-158.

99. Helfand M, Redfern CC, Sox HCJ. Clinical guideline, part 1. Screening for thyroid disease. *Ann Intern Med.* 1998;129:141-143.

100. Herwig J. Type I diabetes mellitus in childhood and adolescence. *Z Arztl Fortbild Qualitatssich.* 1997;91:233-242.

101. Hung W, Fitz CR, Lee ED. Pituitary enlargement due to lingual thyroid gland and primary hypothyroidism. *Pediatr Neurol.* 1990;6:60-62.

102. Husebye ES, Gebre-Medhin G, Tuomi T, et al. Autoantibodies against aromatic L-amino acid decarboxylase in autoimmune polyendocrine syndrome type I. *J Clin Endocrinol Metab.* 1997;82:147-150.

103. Iannello S, Campanile E, Cipolli D, et al. A rare case of juvenile diabetes mellitus associated with APECED (autoimmune poly-endocrinopathy, candidiasis and ectodermal dystrophy) with strong X-linked familial inheritance. *Minerva Endocrinol.* 1997;22:51-59.

104. Ikeda M, Uchihara T, Tani N, Kanda T, Tsukagoshi H. A case of Hoffmann's syndrome with peripheral neuropathy and various pathological findings in muscle biopsy. *Rinsho Shinkeigaku.* 1990;30:548-552.

105. Ito M, Takamatsu J, Yoshida S, et al. Incomplete thyrotroph suppression determined by third generation thyrotropin assay in subacute thyroiditis compared to silent thyroiditis or hyperthyroid Graves' disease. *J Clin Endocrinol Metab.* 1997;82:616-619.

106. Jabbari B, Huott A. Seizures in thyrotoxicosis. *Epilepsia.* 1980;21:91-96.

107. Jaggy A, Oliver JE. Neurologic manifestations of thyroid disease. *Vet Clin North Am Small Anim Pract.* 1994;24:487-494.

108. Jamsen K. Thyroid disease, a risk factor for optic neuropathy mimicking normal-tension glaucoma. *Acta Ophthalmol Scand.* 1996;74:456-460.

109. Janeira LF. Torsades de pointes and long QT syndromes. *Am Fam Physician.* 1995;52:1447-1453.

110. Jawadi MH, Ballonoff LB, Stears JC, Katz FH. Primary hypothyroidism and pituitary enlargement: radiological evidence of pituitary regression. *Arch Intern Med.* 1978;138:1555-1557.

111. Kahn CR, Vicent D, Doria A. Genetics of non-insulin-dependent (type-II) diabetes mellitus. *Annu Rev Med.* 1996;47:509-531.

112. Kahn SR, Leblanc R, Sadikot AF, Fantus IG. Marked hyperprolactinemia caused by carotid aneurysm. *Can J Neurol Sci.* 1997;24:64-66.

113. Kaminsky P, Klein M, Duc M. Hypothyroid myopathy: physiopathological approach. *Ann Endocrinol (Paris).* 1992;53:125-132.

114. Kayath MJ, Lengyel AM, Vieira JG. Prevalence and magnitude of osteopenia in patients with prolactinoma. *Braz J Med Biol Res.* 1993;26:933-941.

115. Keane JR. Bilateral seventh nerve palsy: analysis of 43 cases and review of the literature. *Neurology.* 1994;44:1198-1202.

116. Khaleeli AA, Griffith DG, Edwards RH. The clinical presentation of hypothyroid myopathy and its relationship to abnormalities in structure and function of skeletal muscle. *Clin Endocrinol (Oxf).* 1983;19:365-376.

117. Kiessling WR, Pflughaupt KW, Haubitz I, Ricker K, Mertens HG. $T_3$, $T_4$, TSH and circulating antithyroglobulin antibodies in myasthenia gravis. *Endokrinologie.* 1981;78:67-72.

118. Kinova S, Payer J, Kalafutova I, Kucerova E. Autoimmune thyroid disease in patients with type I diabetes mellitus. *Bratisl Lek Listy.* 1998;99:23-25.

119. Kua E. Hyperthyroid psychosis. *Med J Malaysia.* 1982;37:60-61.

120. Kudrjavcev T. Neurologic complications of thyroid dysfunction. *Adv Neurol.* 1978;19:619-636.

121. Kurnick JE, Hartman CR, Lufkin EG, Hofeldt FD. Abnormal sella turcica: a tumor board review of the clinical significance. *Arch Intern Med.* 1977;137:111-117.

122. Kwan ES, Laucella M, Hedges TR, Wolpert SM. A cliniconeuroradiologic approach to third cranial nerve palsies. *AJNR Am J Neuroradiol.* 1987;8:459-468.

123. Lagueny A, Manciet G, Vital A, Ferrer X, Julien J. Hypothyroid neuropathy. *Rev Neurol (Paris).* 1990;146:205-210.

124. Lazzaroni F, Laffi GL, Galuppi V, Scorolli L. Paralysis of oculomotor nerves in diabetes mellitus: a retrospective study of 44 cases. *Rev Neurol (Paris).* 1993;149:571-573.

125. Lenders JW, Keiser HR, Goldstein DS, et al. Plasma metanephrines in the diagnosis of pheochromocytoma. *Ann Intern Med.* 1995;123:101-109.

126. Leonetti F, Dussol B, Berland Y. Rhabdomyolysis and kidney failure in hypothyroidism. *Presse Med.* 1992;21:31-32.

127. Lepage R, D'Amour P, Boucher A, Hamel L, Demontigny C, Labelle F. Clinical performance of a parathyrin immunoassay with dynamically determined reference values. *Clin Chem.* 1988;34:2439-2443.

128. Lessell S. Pediatric pseudotumor cerebri (idiopathic intracranial hypertension). *Surv Ophthalmol.* 1992;37:155-166.

129. Levenson J, Safar M, London G, Simon A. Haemodynamics in patients with phaeochromocytoma. *Clin Sci.* 1980;58:349-356.

130. Li H, Easley A, Barrington W, Windle J. Evaluation and management of atrial fibrillation in the emergency department. *Emerg Med Clin North Am.* 1998;16:389-403.

131. Lin KP, Kwan SY, Chen SY, et al. Generalized neuropathy in Taiwan: an etiologic survey. *Neuroepidemiology.* 1993;12:257-261.

132. Loewen P, Sunderji R, Gin K. The efficacy and safety of combination warfarin and ASA therapy: a systematic review of the literature and update of guidelines. *Can J Cardiol.* 1998;14:717-726.

133. LoVecchio F, Jacobson S. Approach to generalized weakness and peripheral neuromuscular disease. *Emerg Med Clin North Am.* 1997;15:605-623.

134. Marcus R. Laboratory diagnosis of primary hyperparathyroidism. *Endocrinol Metab Clin North Am.* 1989;18:647-658.

135. Martinez-Lopez JI. ECG of the month: on the QT—hypocalcemia. *J La State Med Soc.* 1992;144:3-6.

136. McAlpine JK, Thomson JE. Myasthenia gravis and Schmidt syndrome. *Postgrad Med J.* 1988;64:787-788.

137. McCutcheon IE. Management of individual tumor syndromes: pituitary neoplasia. *Endocrinol Metab Clin North Am.* 1994;23:37-51.

138. McEwen BS, Conrad CD, Kuroda Y, Frankfurt M, Magarinos AM, McKittrick C. Prevention of stress-induced morphological and cognitive consequences. *Eur Neuropsychopharmacol.* 1997;7(suppl 3):S323-S328.

139. McEwen BS, Magarinos AM. Stress effects on morphology and function of the hippocampus. *Ann N Y Acad Sci.* 1997;821:271-284.

140. Miller AB, Nelson RW, Scott-Moncrieff JC, Neal L, Bottoms GD. Serial thyroid hormone concentrations in healthy euthyroid dogs, dogs with hypothyroidism, and euthyroid dogs with atopic dermatitis. *Br Vet J.* 1992;148:451-458.

141. Monforte R, Fernandez-Sola J, Casademont J, Vernet M, Grau JM, Urbano-Marquez A. Hypothyroid myopathy: a clinical and histologic prospective study of 19 patients. *Med Clin (Barc).* 1990;95:126-129.

142. Mori M, Shoda Y, Yamada M, et al. Central hypothyroidism due to isolated TRH deficiency in a depressive man. *J Intern Med.* 1991;229:285-288.

143. Mornex R, Peyrin L. The biological diagnosis of pheochromocytoma. *Bull Mem Acad R Med Belg.* 1996;151:269-277.

144. Mulder H, Leckstrom A, Uddman R, Ekblad E, Westermark P, Sundler F. Islet amyloid polypeptide (amylin) is expressed in sensory neurons. *J Neurosci.* 1995;15:7625-7632.

145. Nakajima T, Tamura T, Kuroki M, Tanaka R, Hayashi H. [A case of prolactinoma presenting with CSF rhinorrhea and CSF otorrhea during bromocriptine therapy]. *No Shinkei Geka.* 1992;20:1091-1095.

146. Nishi Y, Hamamoto K, Kajiyama M, et al. Pituitary enlargement, hypertrichosis and blunted growth hormone secretion in primary hypothyroidism. *Acta Paediatr Scand.* 1989;78:136-140.

147. Nishiyama S. Hypercalcemia in children: an overview. *Acta Paediatr Jpn.* 1997;39:479-484.

148. Nuutila P, Irjala K, Viikari J, Prinssi VP, Kaihola HL. Comparative evaluation of serum thyroxine, free thyroxine and thyrotropin determinations in screening of thyroid function. *Ann Clin Res.* 1988;20:158-163.

149. O'Brien T, O'Riordan DS, Gharib H, Scheithauer BW, Ebersold MJ, van Heerden JA. Results of treatment of pituitary disease in multiple endocrine neoplasia, type I. *Neurosurgery.* 1996;39:273-278.

150. Odell WD, Wolfsen AR. Humoral syndromes associated with cancer. *Annu Rev Med.* 1978;29:379-406.

151. Okuno T, Sudo M, Momoi T, et al. Pituitary hyperplasia due to hypothyroidism. *J Comput Assist Tomogr.* 1980;4:600-602.

152. Okuyama T, Sato O, Daibo M, Niwa J. Cessation of cerebrospinal fluid rhinorrhea by bromocriptine treatment of a patient with invasive prolactinoma. *No Shinkei Geka.* 1984;12:319-323.

153. Olive KE, Hennessey JV. Marked hyperprolactinemia in subclinical hypothyroidism. *Arch Intern Med.* 1988;148:2278-2279.

154. Olsen CG. Myxedema coma in the elderly [published errata appear in J Am Board Fam Pract. 1995;8:502 and 1996;9:63]. *J Am Board Fam Pract.* 1995;8:376-383.

155. Orho M, Nikula-Ijas P, Schalin-Jantti C, Permutt MA, Groop LC. Isolated and characterization of the human muscle glycogen synthase gene. *Diabetes.* 1995;44:1099-1105.

156. Ozbey N, Sariyildiz E, Yilmaz L, Orhan Y, Sencer E, Molvalilar S. Primary hypothyroidism with hyperprolactinaemia and pituitary enlargement mimicking a pituitary macroadenoma. *Int J Clin Pract.* 1997;51:409-411.

157. Pannall PR. Free thyroxine index or effective thyroxine ratio? *S Afr Med J.* 1977;51:163-164.

158. Papaceit J, Moral V, Recio J, de Ferrer JM, Riva J, Bayes dL. Severe heart arrhythmia secondary to magnesium depletion: torsades de pointes. *Rev Esp Anestesiol Reanim.* 1990;37:28-31.

159. Parle JV, Franklyn JA, Cross KW, Jones SC, Sheppard MC. Prevalence and follow-up of abnormal thyrotrophin (TSH) concentrations in the elderly in the United Kingdom. *Clin Endocrinol.* 1991;34:77-83.

160. Peaston RT, Lennard TW, Lai LC. Overnight excretion of urinary catecholamines and metabolites in the detection of pheochromocytoma. *J Clin Endocrinol Metab.* 1996;81:1378-1384.

161. Perkins AT, Morgenlander JC. Endocrinologic causes of peripheral neuropathy: pins and needles in a stocking-and-glove pattern and other symptoms. *Postgrad Med.* 1997;102:81-82.

162. Peters AL, Davidson MB, Schriger DL, Hasselblad V. A clinical approach for the diagnosis of diabetes mellitus: an analysis using glycosylated hemoglobin levels. Meta-analysis Research Group on the Diagnosis of Diabetes Using Glycated Hemoglobin Levels [see comments] [published erratum appears in JAMA. 1997;277:1125]. *JAMA.* 1996;276:1246-1252.

163. Petersen P. Psychiatric disorders in primary hyperparathyroidism. *J Clin Endocrinol Metab.* 1968;28:1491-1495.

164. Petty GW, Brown RDJ, Whisnant JP, Sicks JD, O'Fallon WM, Wiebers DO. Ischemic stroke: outcomes, patient mix, and practice variation for neurologists and generalists in a community. *Neurology.* 1998;50:1669-1678.

165. Peyrin L, Mornex R. Biological diagnosis of pheochromocytoma: im-

pact of technological improvement. *Ann Biol Clin (Paris).* 1993;51:835-865.

166. Pinelli P, Pisano F, Miscio G. Ataxia in myxoedema: a neurophysiological reassessment. *J Neurol.* 1990;237:405-409.

167. Pleet AB. Funny spells in neuroendocrine disorders. *Semin Neurol.* 1995;15:133-150.

168. Pleet AB. Neuroendocrine disorders as viewed by a neurologist. In: Hurst JW, ed. *Medicine for the Practicing Physician.* 4th ed. Stamford, CT: Appleton & Lange; 1996:1814-1822.

169. Pleet AB, Saphier DJ. Neurologic aspects of endocrine disturbances. In: Joynt RH, ed. *Clinical Neurology.* Philadelphia: Harper & Row; 1992:1-57.

170. Plewe G, Beyer J, Krause U, Cordes U, Eissner D, Hahn K. Comparison of $^{131}$I-metaiodobenzylguanidine scintigraphy with urinary and plasma catecholamine determinations in the diagnosis of pheochromocytoma. *Klin Wochenschr.* 1985;63:627-630.

171. Pollard JD, McLeod JG, Honnibal TG, Verheijden MA. Hypothyroid polyneuropathy: clinical, electrophysiological and nerve biopsy findings in two cases. *J Neurol Sci.* 1982;53:461-471.

172. Press OW, Ladenson PW. Pseudotumor cerebri and hypothyroidism. *Arch Intern Med.* 1983;143:167-168.

173. Puvanendran K, Cheah JS, Naganathan N, Yeo PP, Wong PK. Neuromuscular transmission in thyrotoxicosis. *J Neurol Sci.* 1979;43:47-57.

174. Ram C, Engelman K. Pheochromocytoma: recognition and management. *Curr Probl Cardiol.* 1979;4:1-37.

175. Ramos-Remus C, Sahagun RM, Perla-Navarro AV. Endocrine disorders and musculoskeletal diseases. *Curr Opin Rheumatol.* 1996;8:77-84.

176. Ramot Y, Rapoport MJ, Hagag P, Wysenbeek AJ. A study of the clinical differences between women and men with hyperprolactinemia. *Gynecol Endocrinol.* 1996;10:397-400.

177. Raper A, Jessee E, Texter J Jr, et al. Pheochromocytoma of the urinary bladder: a broad clinical spectrum. *Am J Cardiol.* 1977;40:820-824.

178. Reinhardt W, Jockenhovel F, Deuble J, Chatterjee VK, Reinwein D, Mann K. Thyroid hormone resistance: variable clinical manifestations in five patients. *Nuklearmedizin.* 1997;36:250-255.

179. Reinhardt W, Mann K. Incidence, clinical picture and treatment of hypothyroid coma: results of a survey. *Med Klin.* 1997;92:521-524.

180. Rizzoli R, Vadas L, Bonjour JP. Determination of circulating parathyroid hormone levels and differential diagnosis of hypercalcemia. *Nucl Med Biol.* 1994;21:337-347.

181. Rocha G, Garza G, Font RL. Orbital pathology associated with diabetes mellitus. *Int Ophthalmol Clin.* 1998;38:169-179.

182. Roep BO. T-cell responses to autoantigens in IDDM: the search for the Holy Grail. *Diabetes.* 1996;45:1147-1156.

183. Rose SR. Isolated central hypothyroidism in short stature. *Pediatr Res.* 1995;38:967-973.

184. Ruff RL, Weissmann J. Endocrine myopathies. *Neurol Clin.* 1988;6:575-592.

185. Rybak LP. Metabolic disorders of the vestibular system. *Otolaryngol Head Neck Surg.* 1995;112:128-132.

186. Sacks DB, McDonald JM. The pathogenesis of type II diabetes mellitus: a polygenic disease. *Am J Clin Pathol.* 1996;105:149-156.

187. Salomez JL, Jomin M, Petit H, Combelles M, Decaudaveine B. Cerebral ischaemic accident revealing the presence of a large pituitary adenoma. *Rev Otoneuroophtalmol.* 1981;53:249-253.

188. Sarlis NJ, Brucker-Davis F, Doppman JL, Skarulis MC. MRI-demonstrable regression of a pituitary mass in a case of primary hypothyroidism after a week of acute thyroid hormone therapy. *J Clin Endocrinol Metab.* 1997;82:808-811.

189. Sawin CT, Geller A, Kaplan MM, Bacharach P, Wilson PW, Hershman JM. Low serum thyrotropin (thyroid-stimulating hormone) in older persons without hyperthyroidism. *Arch Intern Med.* 1991;151:165-168.

190. Sawin CT, Geller A, Wolf PA, et al. Low serum thyrotropin concentrations as a risk factor for atrial fibrillation in older persons. *N Engl J Med.* 1994;331:1249-1252.

191. Schimmelpfennig B, Baumgartner A. Manifestations of possible trophic changes in the corneal epithelium due to decreased trigeminal function. *Klin Monatsbl Augenheilkd.* 1988;192:149-153.

192. Schlienger JL, Sapin R, Gasser F, Chabrier G, Simon C, Imler M. Ultrasensitive determination of thyrotropin: improvement in the performance and reduction of the cost of thyroid function tests. *Presse Medicale.* 1987;16:15-18.

193. Scott-Moncrieff JC, Nelson RW, Bruner JM, Williams DA. Comparison of serum concentrations of thyroid-stimulating hormone in healthy dogs, hypothyroid dogs, and euthyroid dogs with concurrent disease. *J Am Vet Med Assoc.* 1998;212:387-391.

194. Serri O, Somma M, Beauregard H, et al. The treatment of prolactinoma. *Union Med Can.* 1993;122:496-499.

195. Simons LA, McCallum J, Friedlander Y, Simons J. Risk factors for ischemic stroke: Dubbo Study of the elderly. *Stroke.* 1998;29:1341-1346.

196. Skyler JS, Marks JB. Type I (insulin-dependent) diabetes mellitus. In: Hurst JW, ed. *Medicine for the Practicing Physician.* 4th ed. Stamford, CT: Appleton & Lange; 1996:628-635.

197. Sparks PB, Mond HG, Kalman JM, Jayaprakash S, Lewis MA, Grigg LE. Atrial fibrillation and anticoagulation in patients with permanent pacemakers: implications for stroke prevention. *Pacing Clin Electrophysiol.* 1998;21:1258-1267.

198. Sriussadaporn S, Ploybutr S, Peerapatdit T, et al. Nocturnal 8 mg dexamethasone suppression test: a practical and accurate test for identification of the cause of endogenous Cushing's syndrome. *Br J Clin Pract.* 1996;50:9-13.

199. Staub JJ, Althaus B, Wiggli U, Gratzl O. [Drug therapy of hyperprolactinemia and acromegaly]. *Schweiz Med Wochenschr.* 1983;113:733-738.

200. Stevens A, Pleet AB. Neuroendocrine disorders. In: Brandt T, Caplan LR, Dichgans J, Diener HC, Kennard C, eds. *Neurological Disorders: Course and Treatment.* San Diego: Academic Press; 1998:1017-1033.

201. Stockigt JR, Essex WB, West RH, Murray RM, Breidahl HD. Visual failure during replacement therapy in primary hypothyroidism with pituitary enlargement. *J Clin Endocrinol Metab.* 1976;43:1094-1100.

202. Stolinsky DC. Paraneoplastic syndromes. *West J Med.* 1980;132:189-208.

203. Strebel PM, Zacur HA, Gold EB. Headache, hyperprolactinemia, and prolactinomas. *Obstet Gynecol.* 1986;68:195-199.

204. Swanson J, Kelly J Jr, McConnley W. Neurologic aspects of thyroid dysfunction. *Mayo Clin Proc.* 1981;56:504-512.

205. Szabolcs I, Ploenes C, Bernard W, Herrmann J. Screening of geriatric patients for thyroid dysfunction with thyrotropin-releasing-hormone test, sensitive thyrotropin and free thyroxine estimation. *Horm Metab Res.* 1990;22:298-302.

206. Teramoto A, Takakura K, Kitahara S, Fukushima T. Pneumocephalus induced by bromocriptine treatment in male prolactinoma: a case report. *No Shinkei Geka.* 1983;11:1305-1310.

207. Theodorakis SP, Tedesco VE, Sutherland CM. Breast cancer in a patient with prolactinoma. *Surgery.* 1985;98:367-369.

208. Timperley WR, Boulton AJ, Davies-Jones GA, Jarratt JA, Ward JD. Small vessel disease in progressive diabetic neuropathy associated with good metabolic control. *J Clin Pathol.* 1985;38:1030-1038.

209. Tokunaga T, Hayashi T, Honda E, Kikuchi N, Utsunomiya H. [A case of male acromegaly with galactorrhea]. *No Shinkei Geka.* 1988;16:1101-1105.

210. Tyrrell JB, Findling JW, Aron DC, Fitzgerald PA, Forsham PH. An overnight high-dose dexamethasone suppression test for rapid differential diagnosis of Cushing's syndrome. *Ann Intern Med.* 1986;104:180-186.

211. Umpierrez GE. Hypocalcemia and hypoparathyroidism. In: Hurst JW, ed. *Medicine for the Practicing Physician.* 4th ed. Stamford, CT: Appleton & Lange; 1996:662-666.

212. Ura S, Araki E, Kishikawa H, et al. Molecular scanning of the insulin receptor substrate-1 (IRS-1) gene in Japanese patients with NIDDM: identification of five novel polymorphisms. *Diabetologia.* 1996;39:600-608.

213. Vagenakis AG, Dole K, Braverman LE. Pituitary enlargement, pituitary failure, and primary hypothyroidism. *Ann Intern Med.* 1976;85:195-198.

214. Vaidya RA, Aloorkar SD, Raikar RS, et al. Functional pituitary hyperplasia in primary hypothyroidism: normalisation of visual field defects on thyroid replacement in a girl with galactorrhoea-amenorrhoea. *J Assoc Physicians India.* 1977;25:923-928.

215. Van Camp G, Bourdoux PP, Bonnyns MA. Age influence on clinical features in hospitalized thyroid patients: dissimilarity between clinical and laboratory findings in adulthood—a retrospective study. *Thyroidology.* 1992;4:75-82.

216. Vanderpump MP, Neary RH, Manning K, Clayton RN. Does an increase in the sensitivity of serum thyrotropin assays reduce diagnostic costs for thyroid disease in the community? *J R Soc Med.* 1997;90:547-550.

217. Volpe R. Rational use of thyroid function tests. *Crit Rev Clin Lab Sci.* 1997;34:405-438.

218. von Herrath MG, Holz A, Homann D, Oldstone MB. Role of viruses in type I diabetes. *Semin Immunol.* 1998;10:87-100.

219. Wakai S, Fukushima T, Teramoto A, Sano K. Pituitary apoplexy: its incidence and clinical significance. *No To Shinkei.* 1981;33:561-568.

220. Walsh JP, Pullan PT. Hyperprolactinaemia in males: a heterogeneous disorder. *Aust N Z J Med.* 1997;27:385-390.

221. Watanabe K, Hagura R, Akanuma Y, et al. Characteristics of cranial nerve palsies in diabetic patients. *Diabetes Res Clin Pract.* 1990;10:19-27.

222. Watts NB. Use of a sensitive thyrotropin assay for monitoring treatment with levothyroxine. *Arch Intern Med.* 1989;149:309-312.

223. Watts NB. Cushing's syndrome. In: Hurst JW, ed. *Medicine for the Practicing Physician.* 4th ed. Stamford, CT: Appleton & Lange; 1996:558-563.

224. Watts NB, Tindall GT. Acromegaly. In: Hurst JW, ed. *Medicine for the Practicing Physician.* 4th ed. Stamford, CT: Appleton & Lange; 1996:549-552.

225. Weisberg LA. Asymptomatic enlargement of the sella turcica. *Arch Neurol.* 1975;32:483-485.

226. Wiener K, Roberts NB. The relative merits of haemoglobin $A_{1c}$ and fasting plasma glucose as first-line diagnostic tests for diabetes mellitus in non-pregnant subjects. *Diabet Med.* 1998;15:558-563.

227. Wilber J. Hypothyroidism. In: Hurst JW, ed. *Medicine for the Practicing Physician.* 4th ed. Stamford, CT: Appleton & Lange; 1996:599-602.

228. Wong J, Oh V, Chia B, Rauff A, Tan L. Adrenal phaeochromocytoma and neurofibromatosis presenting with hypotension. *Ann Acad Med Singapore.* 1986;15:127-131.

229. Wright H, Hansotia P. Isolated fourth cranial nerve palsies: etiology and prognosis. *Wis Med J.* 1977;76:S-8.

230. Yamakita N, Ikeda T, Murai T, Komaki T, Hirata T, Miura K. Thyrotropin-producing pituitary adenoma discovered as a pituitary incidentaloma. *Intern Med.* 1995;34:1055-1060.

231. Yamamoto K, Saito K, Takai T, Naito M, Yoshida S. Visual field defects and pituitary enlargement in primary hypothyroidism. *J Clin Endocrinol Metab.* 1983;57:283-287.

232. Yamamoto K, Saito K, Takai T, Yoshida S. Unusual manifestations in primary hypothyroidism. *Prog Clin Biol Res.* 1983;116:169-187.

233. Yamaura K, Kao B, Iimori E, Urakami H, Takahashi S. Recurrent ventricular tachyarrhythmias associated with QT prolongation following hydrofluoric acid burns. *J Toxicol Clin Toxicol.* 1997;35:311-313.

234. Zabalgoitia M, Halperin JL, Pearce LA, Blackshear JL, Asinger RW, Hart RG. Transesophageal echocardiographic correlates of clinical risk of thromboembolism in nonvalvular atrial fibrillation. Stroke Prevention in Atrial Fibrillation III Investigators. *J Am Coll Cardiol.* 1998;31:1622-1626.

# 27

# Rheumatologic Disorders

*Russell Bartt and Kathleen M. Shannon*

Rheumatologic disorders include a variety of conditions that may affect any part of the nervous system, usually as part of a systemic illness. Many rheumatologic disorders are autoimmune in nature. Ehrlich used the term *horror autotoxicus* in the early 1900s to describe this disturbing phenomenon of inflammation directed against host tissues.[8] Despite subsequent advances in the field of autoimmunity, the etiologies of many of the rheumatologic syndromes remain obscure, and their definitions rely on clinical and pathologic criteria. Because there are pathophysiologic similarities among these disorders, their neurologic manifestations generally take the form of one or more relatively discreet syndromes. A given neurologic syndrome may have a number of potential rheumatologic causes. A basic understanding of the scope and underlying pathophysiology of the rheumatologic diseases makes the differential diagnosis and evaluation of these syndromes more straightforward.

In general, rheumatologic syndromes can be categorized as those that cause tissue injury by affecting the blood vessels (e.g., vasculitis) and those that directly damage tissue itself (e.g., connective tissue diseases). Vasculitis, regardless of cause, is inflammation of the vessel wall. The lesions that result from this inflammation are ischemic or, more rarely, hemorrhagic. Neurologic syndromes occur when blood vessels in the nervous system are involved. The nosologic classification of the vasculitides is often by vessel size, as shown in Figure 27–1 and Table 27–1. Connective tissue diseases are those conditions in which there is inflammation directed against tissue components (i.e., synovial tissue in arthritis). Involvement of the nervous system results either from the occurrence of this inflammation in nervous tissue itself or from secondary damage related to inflammation in adjacent skeletal or other tissues. Some syndromes, such as systemic lupus erythematosus (SLE), may simultaneously cause vascular and connective tissue injury. Immune reactions to infectious, toxic, and neoplastic diseases that damage vessels and connective tissues are not considered rheumatologic by definition and will not be discussed in this chapter.

## PERIPHERAL NERVOUS SYSTEM

### CRANIAL NEUROPATHY

Ischemic cranial neuropathies secondary to disease of the vasa nervorum are seen in the vasculitides, particularly giant cell (temporal) arteritis (GCA), primary angiitis of the central nervous system (PACNS), rheumatoid vasculitis, and Wegener's granulomatosis. The presence of isolated trigeminal neuropathy is particularly suggestive of progressive systemic sclerosis or mixed connective tissue disease.

### MONONEURITIS MULTIPLEX

The typical peripheral neuropathy seen with vasculitis is an ischemic mononeuritis multiplex. In several series of vasculitic disorders, it is the most common neurologic manifestation of the disease.[15,21,25] The small- to medium-vessel vasculitides affect the extrinsic or intrinsic vessels of the vasa nervorum, resulting in nerve ischemia and dysfunction. Ten to 15% of patients present with unilateral or bilateral wrist or foot drop due to involvement of the radial or peroneal nerves.[25] In 50% to 60% of patients, multiple nerves are involved at initial clinical presentation. Widespread and severe mononeuritis multiplex, seen in about 30% of patients, may obscure individual nerve involvement, and the clinical syndrome more closely resembles a distal sensorimotor "stocking-glove" neuropathy.[20,25] At the time most patients present with neuropathy, they have obvious systemic disease. In a review of 34 patients with vasculitic neuropathy by Hawke et al,[15] two patients (<5%) had only mononeuritis multiplex without systemic evidence of vasculitis.

### SENSORY, SENSORIMOTOR, AND MOTOR NEUROPATHY

Some patients with Sjögren's syndrome present with a pansensory neuropathy and gait ataxia due to inflammation of the dorsal root ganglion.[13] This presentation is striking and often includes autonomic features.[13] Sensory neuropathy also occurs in thromboangiitis obliterans secondary to peripheral nerve ischemia or fibrous encasement of distal neurovascular bundles.[33] An ischemic sensory or sensorimotor neuropathy is associated with rheumatoid vasculitis and SLE.[16,34] The clini-

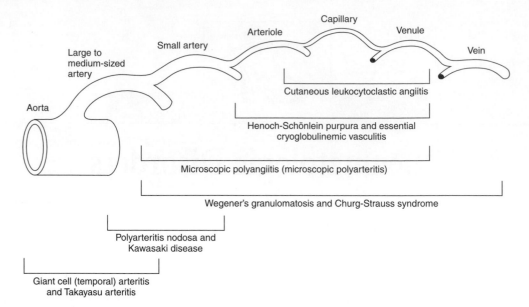

**FIGURE 27–1.** Predominant range of vascular involvement by vasculitides as defined by the Chapel Hill Consensus Conference on the Nomenclature of Systemic Vasculitis. Note substantial overlap among diseases. *Large artery* refers to aorta and largest branches directed toward major body regions (e.g., to extremities and head and neck); *medium-sized artery* refers to main visceral arteries (e.g., renal, hepatic, coronary, and mesenteric arteries), and *small artery* refers to distal intraparenchymal arterial radicals that connect with arterioles. (From Jennette JC, Falk RJ, Andrassay K, et al. Nomenclature of the systemic vasculitides. *Arthritis Rheum.* 1994;37:187-192.)

---

**TABLE 27–1. Names and Definitions of Vasculitides Adopted by the Chapel Hill Consensus Conference on the Nomenclature of Systemic Vasculitis\***

**Large Vessel Vasculitis**

| | |
|---|---|
| Giant cell (temporal) arteritis | Granulomatous arteritis of the aorta and its major branches, with a predilection for the extracranial branches of the carotid artery. *Often involves the temporal artery. Usually occurs in patients older than 50 and often is associated with polymyalgia rheumatica.* |
| Takayasu's arteritis | Granulomatous inflammation of the aorta and its major branches. *Usually occurs in patients younger than 50.* |

**Medium-Sized Vessel Vasculitis**

| | |
|---|---|
| Polyarteritis nodosa[†] (classic polyarteritis nodosa) | Necrotizing inflammation of medium-sized or small arteries without glomerulonephritis or vasculitis in arterioles, capillaries, or venules. |
| Kawasaki disease | Arteritis involving large, medium-sized, and small arteries, and associated with mucocutaneous lymph node syndrome. *Coronary arteries are often involved. Aorta and veins may be involved. Usually occurs in children.* |

**Small Vessel Vasculitis**

| | |
|---|---|
| Wegener's granulomatosis[‡] | Granulomatous inflammation involving the respiratory tract, and necrotizing vasculitis affecting small to medium-sized vessels (e.g., capillaries, venules, arterioles, and arteries). *Necrotizing glomerulonephritis is common.* |
| Churg-Strauss syndrome[‡] | Eosinophil-rich and granulomatous inflammation involving the respiratory tract, and necrotizing vasculitis affecting small to medium-sized vessels, and associated with asthma and eosinophilia. |
| Microscopic polyangiitis[†] (microscopic polyarteritis)[‡] | Necrotizing vasculitis, with few or no immune deposits, affecting small vessels (i.e., capillaries, venules, or arterioles). *Necrotizing arteritis involving small and medium-sized arteries may be present. Necrotizing glomerulonephritis is very common. Pulmonary capillaritis often occurs.* |
| Henoch-Schönlein purpura | Vasculitis, with IgA-dominant immune deposits, affecting small vessels (i.e., capillaries, venules, or arterioles). *Typically involves skin, gut, and glomeruli, and is associated with arthralgias or arthritis.* |
| Essential cryoglobulinemic vasculitis | Vasculitis, with cryoglobulin immune deposits, affecting small vessels (i.e., capillaries, venules, or arterioles), and associated with cryoglobulins in serum. *Skin and glomeruli are often involved.* |
| Cutaneous leukocytoclastic angiitis | Isolated cutaneous leukocytoclastic angiitis without systemic vasculitis or glomerulonephritis. |

\*Large vessel refers to the aorta and the largest branches directed toward major body regions (e.g., to the extremities and the head and neck); medium-sized vessel refers to the main visceral arteries (e.g., renal, hepatic, coronary, and mesenteric arteries); small vessel refers to venules, capillaries, arterioles, and the intraparenchymal distal arterial radicals that connect with arterioles. Some small and large-vessel vasculitides may involve medium-sized arteries, but large and medium-sized vessel vasculitides do not involve vessels smaller than arteries. Essential components are represented by normal type; italicized type represents usual, but not essential, components.

[†]Preferred term.

[‡]Strongly associated with antineutrophil cytoplasmic autoantibodies.

From Jennette JC, Falk RJ, Andrassay K, et al. Nomenclature of the systemic vasculitides. *Arthritis Rheum.* 1994;37:187-192.

cal syndrome of Guillain-Barré syndrome has been seen with the antiphospholipid antibody syndrome.[26]

### ENTRAPMENT NEUROPATHY

Rheumatoid arthritis and other arthritides can often be complicated by mononeuropathies secondary to involvement of nerve trunks in proximity to inflamed joints. For example, carpal tunnel involvement with median nerve entrapment is common.[29] Entrapment neuropathies are also common in progressive systemic sclerosis and mixed connective tissue disease.[35] Compression can also cause nerve root dysfunction in rheumatoid arthritis. The facet joints of the vertebrae may be inflamed with secondary panus formation or osteophyte formation, or there may be subluxation of the vertebral bodies, particularly in the cervical spine.[7]

### MYOPATHY

Myopathy that clinically or histologically resembles dermatomyositis or polymyositis may occur in the context of a rheumatologic syndrome. These "overlap syndromes" may include scleroderma, Sjögren's syndrome, SLE, mixed connective tissue disease, and rheumatoid arthritis and can be defined by their extramuscular manifestations.[8,9] If patients have been receiving treatment of the rheumatologic syndrome with corticosteroids, a steroid myopathy needs to be considered in the differential diagnosis.[9]

## CENTRAL NERVOUS SYSTEM

### DISORDERS OF THE BRAIN COVERINGS

Meningoencephalitis or aseptic meningitis has been reported in patients with Sjögren's syndrome or mixed connective tissue disease. Meningitis or sagittal sinus thrombosis can occur in Behçet's disease and although neurologic involvement is not required for diagnosis, such involvement often leads to the proper diagnosis of the patient's syndrome.[10]

### DIFFUSE HEMISPHERIC DYSFUNCTION

Signs of diffuse hemispheric dysfunction in patients with vasculitis or connective tissue disease include delirium, encephalopathy, and dementia. All have been described in PACNS, Churg-Strauss syndrome, rheumatoid vasculitis, SLE, and progressive systemic sclerosis.[4,5,28] Generalized seizures have been reported in all the vasculitides as well as in progressive systemic sclerosis.[28] It can be difficult to ascertain from published material whether these seizures are primarily or secondarily generalized.

### FOCAL BRAIN LESIONS

Stroke and transient ischemic attack may occur with vasculitides; in particular, evaluation of "stroke in the young" should include evaluation of these entities. In general the larger the vessels involved (i.e., aorta and cervicocephalic branches) in the vasculitis, the more likely the central nervous system (CNS) will be involved.[6,24,28] However, stroke and transient ischemic attack are also seen in diseases with involvement of smaller vessels, such as SLE and periarteritis nodosa (PAN).

Anterior ischemic optic neuropathy, or granulomatous involvement of the optic nerve, may complicate several of the rheumatologic syndromes associated with vasculitis, most notably GCA but also Wegener's granulomatosis, Churg-Strauss syndrome, and other small- to medium-sized vasculitides.[18,23,25]

### MYELOPATHY

Spinal cord disease may be the result of ischemic, inflammatory, or compressive mechanisms. The systemic vasculitides can involve spinal arteries, and neurosarcoidosis may cause granulomas in the spinal cord. Rheumatoid arthritis of the atlantoaxial area with panus formation may cause a devastating basilar impression.[7]

## EVALUATION

### SEROLOGIC TESTING

Erythrocyte sedimentation rate (ESR), although not specific, is often used as a screening test in patients with suspected or possible rheumatologic disease. Hepatic synthesis of several plasma proteins in response to an inflammatory state will neutralize the negative charge on erythrocytes and in vitro will cause them to "fall" more quickly as a "clump." The distance these "clumps" of erythrocytes fall in 1 hour is measured in millimeters. These plasma proteins are collectively referred to as "acute-phase reactants," and one that can be measured directly is C-reactive protein (CRP), which is discussed later.[19] ESR values span a wide range, may vary among laboratories and by technique (Westergren or Wintrobe), and tend to be slightly higher in women and with advancing age. The ESR is useful when values are very elevated or to monitor disease activity after disease-modifying treatment (e.g., GCA characterized by a very high ESR). In one series of 42 patients, the mean ESR value was 96 mm/h with a range of 50 to 132 mm/h.[18] By contrast, in PACNS the ESR was normal in 34% of the cases, with the highest value being 116 mm/h and the mean only 44 mm/h.[5] The CRP more closely approximates ongoing tissue damage than ESR in most rheumatic diseases, but interestingly the CRP is only slightly elevated in SLE and its elevation should raise one's suspicion of infection.[19] The ESR and CRP are often used to follow relative disease activity in a given patient. However, serologic testing does not correlate well with disease activity by pathologic criteria in several of the autoimmune diseases. Therefore determining disease activity may require biopsy.

Autoantibodies and some nonspecific antibodies define some of the rheumatic syndromes or participate in the pathogenesis of the conditions. Rheumatoid factors are immunoglobulins directed against the Fc portion of immunoglobulin G (IgG).[19] Present in 70% to 80% of patients with rheumatoid arthritis, rheumatoid factors may also be seen in other diseases, such as Sjögren's syndrome, cryoglobulinemia, and SLE; when used alone, they are not specific.[19] Various rheumatic diseases (SLE in particular) are associated with the presence of circulating antinuclear antibodies (ANAs). As diagnostic tests, these have varying degrees of utility. The staining pattern by immunofluorescence or immunoenzyme assays may be associated with certain ANAs and therefore certain diseases[8] (Table 27–2).

Since 1985 the presence of antineutrophil cytoplasmic antibodies (ANCAs) has been of interest in the pathogenesis

**TABLE 27–2. Antinuclear Antibodies***

| STAINING PATTERN | ANTIGEN | ASSOCIATED DISEASE | CLINICAL SIGNIFICANCE |
|---|---|---|---|
| I Peripheral | Double-stranded DNA | SLE | Active SLE, renal disease |
| | Single-stranded DNA | Nonspecific | None |
| II Homogeneous | DNA-histone complex | SLE, drug-induced LE | When antihistone Ab is the only Ab, it supports diagnosis of drug-induced LE |
| III Speckled | Sm (Smith antigen) protein complexed with U1–U6 RNA (spliceosome) | SLE | Renal, CNS diseases |
| | RNP (ribonucleoproteins) complexed with U/a, U/b (spliceosome) | SLE, Sjögren's syndrome, scleroderma, polymyositis, UCTD | A low incidence of severe nephritis and CNS disease |
| | Ro (Robert) SS-A proteins complexed with hy, hy3, hy4, hy5 | SLE, Sjögren's syndrome | Subacute cutaneous LE, photosensitive skin disease, keratoconjunctivitis sicca, neonatal LE |
| | Lane SS-B phosphorylate protein complexed with small RNA polymerase III transcripts | SLE, Sjögren's syndrome | Keratoconjunctivitis sicca |
| | Jo-1 histidyl-T-RNA synthetase | Polymyositis, dermatomyositis | In polymyositis associated with interstitial lung disease |
| | Sc1-70 DNA Topoisomerase I | Scleroderma | Diffuse skin involvement, more frequent internal organ involvement |
| | Centromere proteins in kinetochore | CREST syndrome, variant scleroderma | Characterized by calcinosis cutis, Raynaud's phenomenon, esophageal hypomotility, telangiectasia |
| IV Nucleolar | RNA polymerase I, PM-Sc1, periribosomal particle | Scleroderma, polymyositis scleroderma, overlap syndrome | Diffuse systemic scleroderma, especially cardiac and skin involvement in scleroderma associated with muscle and renal involvement |

*SLE indicates systemic lupus erythematosus; LE, lupus erythematosus; CNS, central nervous system; UCTD, undifferentiated connective tissue disease; SS-A, soluble substance–A antigen; hy, cytoplasmic RNA; SS-B, soluble substance–B antigen; and CREST, calcinosis, Raynaud's (phenomenon), esophageal (dysfunction), sclerodactyly, telangiectasia.

From Condemi JJ. The autoimmune diseases. *JAMA*. 1992;268:2882-2892. Copyrighted 1992, American Medical Association.

of Wegener's granulomatosis and also in clinical testing.[22] The test uses an indirect immunofluorescence method, and a crucial distinction is made between cytoplasmic (c-ANCA) and perinuclear (p-ANCA) staining of neutrophils.[38] Although ANCAs were initially thought to be unique to Wegener's granulomatosis, reports of ANCAs in other inflammatory diseases have widened the scope of ANCA-associated conditions[22] (Table 27–3). The specificity of c-ANCA with Wegener's granulomatosis or similar syndromes (e.g., microscopic polyangiitis) is 98%.[22] The specificity of p-ANCA for the necrotizing vasculitides is 94% to 99%.[22]

**TABLE 27–3. Disease Associations of c-ANCA and p-ANCA**

| DISEASE ENTITY | c-ANCA % (ANTIPROTEINASE-3) | P-ANCA % (ANTIMYELOPEROXIDASE) |
|---|---|---|
| Idiopathic crescentic glomerulonephritis | 30 | 70 |
| Microscopic polyarteritis | 50 | 50 |
| Wegener's granulomatosis | 80 | 20 |
| Churg-Strauss syndrome | 10 | 70 |
| Classic polyarteritis nodosa | 10 | 20 |
| Polyangiitis overlap syndrome | 40 | 20 |

ANCA, Antineutrophil cytoplasmic antibody.
Modified from Kallenberg CGM, Mulder AHL, Teravert JWC. Antineutrophil cytoplasmic antibodies: a still growing class of autoantibodies in inflammatory disorders. *Am J Med*. 1992;93:675-682 with permission from Excerpta Medica Inc.

Hepatitis B or C antigenemia may be found in association with PAN in as many as 30% of cases.[14,25] Therefore in cases of possible PAN it is important to evaluate for hepatitis B and C, since antigenemia may have additional treatment implications for the patient.

### SPINAL FLUID TESTING

Lumbar puncture is often performed in patients with CNS signs and symptoms. In PACNS the cerebrospinal fluid (CSF) is abnormal in 81% of those examined.[2] There is usually a lymphocytic or mixed pleocytosis and mild to moderate elevation of protein. Serial tests in the same patient may have spontaneous fluctuations in the degree of pleocytosis or protein concentration.[5] In a retrospective comparison of spinal fluid findings the frequency of intrathecal synthesis of immunoglobulins was 51% for SLE, 25% for sarcoidosis, and 8% for Behçet's disease.[27] Serum-to-albumin ratios were also used to define blood-brain barrier dysfunction, which was present in 30% to 50% of subjects with each of the earlier mentioned conditions. Although these studies cannot be used to differentiate among these diseases, two of the patients in that series had loss of oligoclonal bands, which may help separate these conditions from multiple sclerosis.[27]

### ELECTROMYOGRAPHY

Electromyography (EMG) and nerve conduction studies are important in defining the localization, nature, and severity of peripheral nervous system disease. Multifocal axonal loss due to ischemic lesions of the central fascicles of peripheral nerves is the "classic" pattern of mononeuropathy multiplex.[15] Chronic partial denervation, impaired motor and sensory nerve conductions, and sometimes focal conduction block may also occur.[15] Patients with a more symmetrical polyneuropathy syndrome will likely demonstrate a length-dependent pattern of denervation without clear predominance in particular nerves.[3]

Clinically suspected myopathy can be evaluated by needle EMG of affected muscles; this method can also be used to help select muscles appropriate for diagnostic biopsy. Biopsy of a muscle area studied by EMG should be avoided so that tissue damaged by the EMG needle will not be used.

## NEUROIMAGING

Magnetic resonance imaging (MRI) is the neuroimaging procedure of choice for patients with CNS signs. Computerized tomography (CT) scanning remains valuable mainly for the evaluation of acute intracranial hemorrhage or detection of calcific changes. Otherwise the role of CT in evaluating autoimmune conditions of the CNS is limited. The mechanism of injury to CNS structures in rheumatologic conditions is vasculitic. Therefore the neuroimaging characteristics visualized are most often related to vascular dynamics. Normal flow in large cerebral vessels produces an absence of magnetic signal or a "flow void." The replacement of this flow void with an isointense signal or enhancement after administering contrast is a helpful sign of slow arterial flow.[17] Flow changes or occlusion can be detected in the venous sinuses, where occlusion may occur with venous inflammation (i.e., Behçet's disease) or any of the hypercoagulable states (i.e., lupus anticoagulant).

Strokes can result from arterial or venous ischemia. The location of the stroke determines the likely vessel involved. By the same reasoning, determining the size of the vessel involved can narrow the differential of possible diagnoses (see Fig. 27–1).

Meningeal enhancement may be the only abnormality in PACNS due to inflammation of pachymeningeal vessels. This situation may be expected if one considers that a meningeal biopsy increases the sensitivity of CNS biopsy in this condition.

MRI is more sensitive for detecting SLE, sarcoidosis, or Behçet's disease than CSF analysis for oligoclonal bands or serum/CSF albumin ratios.[27] Although patients with normal MRIs have been reported to have abnormal angiograms and biopsy-proven vasculitis,[17] a positive angiogram is unlikely in the presence of a normal MRI.

Magnetic resonance angiography (MRA) is readily available in most centers and is often obtained in patients with suspected vascular disease. The tendency of MRA to overestimate stenoses is known from cases of atherosclerotic disease in the carotid circulation. Also, the resolution of MRA is still somewhat limited, and medium- to small-sized arteries are not easily visualized. It is important to realize that the flow patterns seen in some normal vessels can give the appearance of stenosis. Overall, the usefulness of MRA in most vasculitic conditions is limited.[17]

Angiography remains the "gold standard" for diagnosis of vasculitis and should be pursued based on clinical impression even in the face of normal MRI scanning. Neurologic complications occur in 2% to 3% of patients and are permanent in 0.3%.[17] Risks of complications are higher with other medical conditions, advanced age, previous stroke, and a less experienced radiologist.[17] Despite angiography's being the "gold standard," there are limitations that need to be considered in the interpretation of an angiogram. The resolution of

angiography is down to vessels several hundred micrometers in size.[17] Therefore small-vessel vasculitides (e.g., Wegener's granulomatosis) may not be detected by angiogram. Angiography may still be useful in such cases to exclude larger vessel vasculitides and nonvasculitic vascular diseases.[2] The diagnosis of PACNS depends on angiography because of the absence of symptoms of systemic vasculitis. PACNS demonstrates "classic" arteritis in 65% of cases.[4] Abnormalities may be less specific, and 13% of patients may even appear normal.[4] Overall, except for biopsy, angiography is the most helpful method of diagnosis in PACNS. Angiography is the main method of diagnosis in Takayasu's arteritis, a large-vessel vasculitis, but it carries the risk of rupture of diseased vessels. Unfortunately, angiogram cannot distinguish between chronic or recent lesions. In one series of patients with GCA, angiographic involvement of cerebral vasculature was 58% of carotid arteries and 35% of vertebral arteries.[24] Angiography of the external carotid arteries may show alternating stenotic segments or occlusion, but it is generally less reliable than biopsy.[6] Color duplex ultrasonography of the temporal arteries also may show abnormalities.[37]

## NUCLEAR IMAGING

Gallium scanning in evaluation of sarcoidosis can help delineate the sites of involvement, and it can raise the diagnostic sensitivity of angiotensin-converting enzyme alone from 83% to 99% when the tests are combined.[1] This method may provide extracranial sites for biopsy in patients with intracranial disease and suspected sarcoidosis.

## PATHOLOGY

In those conditions not defined by serologic criteria or a constellation of findings, tissue diagnosis is needed to define the disease. Therapy may have serious side effects, particularly with cytotoxic agents, and this further supports the need for accurate diagnosis in these disorders.

In patients with cutaneous manifestations of a systemic disease the skin provides an easy method of diagnosis with minimal risk. This is frequently the case in cutaneous leukocytoclastic angiitis, for example. A unique dermatologic manifestation of Behçet's disease is the appearance of a 3 to 10 mm subcutaneous nodule 24 to 48 hours after a needle stick. This response, known as *pathergy,* is present in most patients with the disease and provides a helpful clue.[32]

Biopsy of the sural, superficial peroneal, or occasionally the superficial radial nerve(s) may be done if involvement is suggested by electrophysiologic studies. Electrically normal nerves occasionally may also show pathology.[25] Simultaneous muscle biopsy provides a greater sample of vessels and raises the diagnostic yield. In a review of nerve biopsy samples the vessels involved were 30 to 240 μm in size, and almost all were epineurial vessels by location.[15] Acute axonal degeneration may be seen in nerves biopsied relatively early in the course of the illness, with those more heavily involved showing nearly complete axonal loss, fibrotic changes, and scant inflammation.[15]

Vasculitic lesions of PAN, Churg-Strauss syndrome, and microscopic polyangiitis show necrotizing lesions of the preferentially medium to small arteries and arterioles. In Churg-Strauss syndrome eosinophils are present in the lesion, as might be expected based on the increased number of circulating eosinophils in the syndrome.[15]

Muscle biopsy is often revealing and provides a low-risk way to obtain tissue for diagnosis of rheumatologic conditions. The features of involvement are similar among the disorders, showing varying degrees of fiber swelling, necrosis, degeneration, or connective tissue replacement, depending on the severity and duration of the process. Features of the individual disorders can be explained by their pathophysiology. For example, SLE, a syndrome of multiple autoantibodies, demonstrates IgG deposits in the vessels of more than 90% of the biopsy samples.[11] In sarcoidosis, skeletal muscle is frequently involved, and a "blind" muscle biopsy can often establish the diagnosis, even in cases without muscle symptoms or pain.[1] The lesions seen are noncaseating granulomas with clusters of epithelioid cells, lymphocytes, and giant cells. These lesions are often focal, and serial sections of the biopsy sample will increase the yield. Other vasculitides tend to share the features of dermatomyositis. The prominent involvement of intramuscular vessels results in ischemia of the perifascicular region with secondary atrophy of those fibers. Inflammatory cells then invade the degenerating fibers with perivascular collections of lymphocytes, plasma cells, and histiocytes.[11] The type of inflammation and vascular involvement seen in the systemic disorders is not significantly different than the changes seen in the other organs that may be involved.[11]

Temporal artery biopsy is well known as the diagnostic test to confirm the diagnosis of GCA. Of the cases reviewed in one study, 61% had active arteritis with giant cells, 22% had arteritis without giant cells, and the remaining 17% had healing or healed vasculitis.[18] Of historical note, as the annual incidence of GCA rose because of increased case surveillance, the proportion of positive biopsies decreased from 82% to 31%.[18] GCA is not the only vasculitis to involve the temporal artery. Wegener's granulomatosis has presented similarly to GCA, including vasculitis on temporal artery biopsy, with the later development of lung and kidney lesions more typical of Wegener's granulomatosis.[30] Patients with Wegener's granulomatosis should demonstrate necrosis and granulomatous inflammation, although the clear identification of granulomas may not be seen in tissue biopsies in the head and neck region. Cases of PAN have also been described.

Brain biopsy can usually be avoided in systemic vasculitides because other sites are available for tissue sample. PACNS is the disease for which this option does not exist, and brain biopsy should be considered if cytotoxic therapy is likely.[36] Leptomeningeal and cortical biopsy should be done in possible cases of PACNS after a nondiagnostic or atypical angiogram. There is a significant risk of sampling error, and in a review of 108 cases the yield of leptomeningeal and cortical tissue, at biopsy or autopsy, was 71% and 77%, respectively.[5] Some cases with normal meningeal sample had diagnostic changes in the cortex, so both tissues should be pursued. In pathologically confirmed cases with premortem biopsies the diagnostic sensitivity of biopsy was 74%.[5]

## SUMMARY

Rheumatologic disorders may affect the nervous system at any level and produce a wide variety of clinical presentations. Understanding the pathophysiologic mechanisms involved serves to simplify the approach to diagnosis of these conditions. With clinical identification of the organ systems involved in a given patient and a stepwise approach to evaluation used, the diagnostic possibilities can be limited. Realizing the benefits and limitations of the diagnostic tools available enables a clinician to minimize the risks of diagnosis and subsequent treatment.

## REFERENCES

1. Banker BQ. Other inflammatory myopathies. In: Engel AG, Franzini-Armstrong C, eds. *Myology.* 2nd ed. New York: McGraw-Hill; 1994: 1461-1486.
2. Bartt R, Shannon KM. Autoimmune and inflammatory disorders. In: Goetz CG, Pappert EJ, eds. *Textbook of Clinical Neurology.* Philadelphia: WB Saunders; 1998:1007-1034.
3. Bouche P, Leger JM, Travers MA, Cathala HP, Castigne P. Peripheral neuropathy in systemic vasculitis: clinical and electrophysiologic study of 22 patients. *Neurology.* 1986;36:1598-1602.
4. Calabrese LH, Furlan AJ, Gragg LA, Ropos TJ. Primary angiitis of the central nervous system: diagnostic criteria and clinical approach. *Cleve Clin J Med.* 1992;59:293-306.
5. Calabrese LH, Mallek JA. Primary angiitis of the central nervous system. *Medicine.* 1987;67:20-39.
6. Caselli RJ, Hunder GG. Neurologic complications of giant cell (temporal) arteritis. *Semin Neurol.* 1994;14:349-353.
7. Castro S, Verstraete K, Mielants H, Vanderstraeten D, de Reuck J, Veys EM. Cervical spine involvement in rheumatoid arthritis: a clinical, neurological and radiological evaluation. *Clin Exp Rheumatol.* 1994;12:369-374.
8. Condemi JJ. The autoimmune diseases. *JAMA.* 1992;268:2882-2892.
9. Dalakas MC. How to diagnose and treat the inflammatory myopathies. *Semin Neurol.* 1994;14:137-145.
10. Devlin T, Gray L, Allen NB, Friedman AH, Tien R, Morgenlander JC. Neuro-Behçet's disease: factors hampering proper diagnosis. *Neurology.* 1995;45:1754-1757.
11. Engel AG, Hohlfeld R, Banker BQ. The polymyositis and dermatomyositis syndromes. In: Engel AG, Franzini-Armstrong C, eds. *Myology.* 2nd ed. New York: McGraw-Hill; 1994:1335-1383.
12. Fort JG, Griffin R, Tahmoush A, Abruzzo J. Muscle involvement in polyarteritis nodosa. *J Rheumatol.* 1994;21:945-948.
13. Griffin JW, Cornblath DR, Alexander E, Campbell J, Low PA, Bird S, Feldman EL. Ataxic sensory neuropathy and dorsal root ganglionitis associated with Sjögren's syndrome. *Ann Neurol.* 1990;27:304-315.
14. Guillevin L, Lhote F. Polyarteritis nodosa and microscopic polyangiitis. *Clin Exp Immunol.* 1995;101:22-23.
15. Hawke SHB, Davies L, Pamphlett R, Guo Y-P, Pollard JD, McLeod JG. Vasculitic neuropathy: a clinical and pathological study. *Brain.* 1991; 114:2175-2190.
16. Hietaharju A, Jantii V, Korpela M, Frey H. Nervous system involvement in systemic lupus erythematosus, Sjögren syndrome and scleroderma. *Acta Neurol Scand.* 1993;88:299-308.
17. Hurst RW, Grossman RI. Neuroradiology of central nervous system vasculitis. *Semin Neurol.* 1994;14:320-340.
18. Huston KA, Hunder GG, Lie JT. Temporal arteritis: a 25-year epidemiologic, clinical and pathologic study. *Ann Intern Med.* 1978;88:162-167.
19. Ike RW, Arnold WJ. Specialized procedures in the management of patients with rheumatic diseases. In: Bennett JC, Plum F, eds. *Cecil Textbook of Medicine.* 20th ed. Philadelphia: WB Saunders; 1996:1455-1459.
20. Jennette JC, Falk RJ, Milling DM. Pathogenesis of vasculitis. *Semin Neurol.* 1994;14:291-299.
21. Kafka SP, Condemi JJ, Marsh DO, Leddy JP. Mononeuritis multiplex and vasculitis. *Arch Neurol.* 1994;51:565-568.
22. Kallenberg CGM, Mulder AH, Tervaert JWC. Antineutrophil cytoplasmic antibodies: a still-growing class of autoantibodies in inflammatory disorders. *Am J Med.* 1992;93:675-682.
23. Kattah JC, Chrousos GA, Katz PA, McCasland B, Kolsky MP. Anterior ischemic optic neuropathy in Churg-Strauss syndrome. *Neurology.* 1994; 44:2200-2202.
24. Kerr GS, Hallahan CW, Giordano J, Leavitt RY, Fauci AS, Rottem M, Hoffman GS. Takayasu arteritis. *Ann Intern Med.* 1994;120:919-929.
25. Kissel JT. Vasculitis of the peripheral nervous system. *Semin Neurol.* 1994;14:361-369.
26. Levine SR, Brey RL. Neurologic aspects of antiphospholipid antibody syndrome. *Lupus.* 1996;5:347-353.
27. McLean BN, Miller D, Thompson EJ. Oligoclonal banding of IgG in CSF, blood-brain barrier function, and MRI findings in patients with

sarcoidosis, systemic lupus erythematosus, and Behçet's disease involving the nervous system. *J Neurol Neurosurg Psychiatry.* 1995;58:548-554.

28. Moore PM, Calabrese LH. Neurologic manifestations of systemic vasculitides. *Semin Neurol.* 1994;14:300-306.

29. Nakano KK. The entrapment neuropathies of rheumatoid neuropathies. *Orthop Clin North Am.* 1975;6:837.

30. Nishino H, DeRemee RA, Rubino FA, Parisi JE. Wegener's granulomatosis associated with vasculitis of the temporal artery: report of five cases. *Mayo Clin Proc.* 1993;68:115-121.

31. Nishino H, Rubino F, Parisi J. The spectrum of involvement in Wegener's granulomatosis. *Neurology.* 1993;43:1334-1337.

32. O'Duffy JD. Vasculitis in Behçet's disease. *Rheum Dis Clin North Am.* 1990;16:423-431.

33. Olin JW. Thromboangiitis obliterans. *Curr Opin Rheumatol.* 1994;6:44-49.

34. Puechal X, Said G, Hilliquin P, et al. Peripheral neuropathy with necrotizing vasculitis in rheumatoid arthritis: a clinicopathologic and prognostic study of thirty-two patients. *Arthritis Rheum.* 1995;38:1618-1629.

35. Schady W, Sheard A, Hassel A, Holt L, Jayson MI, Klimiuk P. Peripheral nerve dysfunction in scleroderma. *Q J Med.* 1991;80:661-675.

36. Schmidley JW. Central nervous system vasculitis. In: Bradley WG, et al., eds. *Neurology in Clinical Practice: Principles of Diagnosis and Management.* 2nd ed. Boston: Butterworth-Heinemann; 1995:1086-1088.

37. Schmidt WA, Kraft HE, Vorpahl K, Volker L, Gromnica-Ihle EJ. Color duplex ultrasonography in the diagnosis of temporal arteritis. *N Engl J Med.* 1997;337:1336-1342.

38. Specks U, Homburger H. Anti-neutrophil cytoplasmic antibodies. *Mayo Clin Proc.* 1994;69:1197-1198.

# MOLECULAR GENETIC TESTING

## 28

# Molecular Diagnostic Testing

*Seth Haplea, Victoria S. Pelak, and David R. Lynch*

In the past 10 years the use of molecular diagnostic testing for neurogenetic disease has expanded more than any other area of diagnostic evaluation. As the specific genetic abnormalities for different diseases have been identified, clinical tests for these abnormalities have been developed with applications to all subspecialties of neurology. Although a new subdivision of neurology called neurogenetics has grown up around the use and interpretation of these diagnostic tests, essentially all neurologists and neurologic subspecialists must understand the general basis of these tests and the issues they raise for the practice of their area of interest.

Although the discovery of the exact abnormality in many neurogenetic diseases has advanced the understanding of these diseases, the clinical use of molecular genetic testing derived from these discoveries is frequently an area of misunderstanding. This chapter concentrates on the clinical utility of these tests rather than the basic science advances themselves. It begins with some background on the mechanisms of genetic disease and proceeds to general and specific situations in which diagnostic testing can be useful.

## MECHANISMS OF GENETIC DISEASE

The most important guide for diagnostic testing for genetic disease is the clinical evaluation. Although specific tests may confirm the diagnosis, one cannot be directed toward those tests without a detailed history and physical examination. Much time and money can be wasted if genetic testing is attempted before a thorough clinical evaluation is done, and premature testing may lead to misinterpretation of results.

### HISTORICAL FEATURES: PATTERN OF INHERITANCE

The concept of genetic disease implies that the disorder results from an abnormality inherited through the genome. Classically, one views the genome as consisting of the nuclear DNA, which encodes approximately 100,000 genes in humans. In recent years it has become apparent that diseases may also be caused by abnormalities of the mitochondrial genome, which contains only 16,500 bases and 13 genes. The location of the genetic abnormality determines the pattern of inheritance. Abnormalities of the mitochondrial genome (if genetically transmitted) are passed in a pattern of maternal inheritance, whereas nuclear abnormalities will show X-linked inheritance (if the mutation is on the X chromosome) or autosomal inheritance (dominant or recessive) (if the mutation is on one of the 22 pairs of autosomes).

Understanding the pattern of inheritance is always crucial to diagnostic testing because it directs the clinician toward specific diseases and thus prioritizes genetic inquiries. It is also crucial in the process of genetic counseling. However, in evaluating pedigrees, it is important to remember several limitations. First, when disease is seen only in one member of a family (Fig. 28–1A), one usually thinks of an autosomal recessive disease or a nongenetic illness. Unfortunately, in many individuals the family history cannot be evaluated completely. Some family members may have manifested only subtle signs of disease and may have never sought medical care for them, whereas others may have died before the expected age of onset. The pedigree is also complicated by the concept of variable expressivity, in which manifestations of the same disease vary in different family members. Thus the family history must be viewed as a component of the history that is

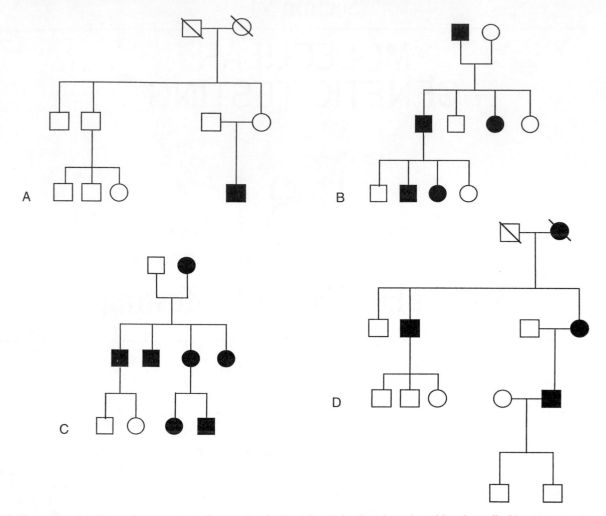

**FIGURE 28–1.** Sample pedigrees for neurogenetic diseases. **A,** A family with a single affected member. Although usually this represents autosomal recessive or sporadic disease, it is impossible to rule out any form of inheritance. **B,** A family with male-to-male and male-to-female transmission. This pedigree can only be autosomal dominant. **C,** A family with passage of the abnormality only through females. This pedigree is likely to represent maternal inheritance, but the absence of passage through males does not rule out an autosomal dominant pattern. **D,** A pedigree similar to that of **C** in which either autosomal dominant or maternal inheritance could be present.

subject to critical appraisal, as are the other parts of the history. In addition, many autosomal dominant diseases may arise de novo in a family, leading to an apparent autosomal recessive or sporadic case. The frequency of de novo mutations varies between different diseases, and this concept can be used in evaluating a patient for a particular disease. For example, since new mutations occur in approximately 50% of patients with neurofibromatosis type 1, patients with no family history of this disorder are not unusual.[157] In contrast, new mutations in Huntington's disease occur but are uncommon.[1,129] Thus one must interpret the pedigree within the overall clinical picture of the patient.

Critically assessing a pedigree also requires an understanding of several other limitations. In many cases, pedigrees must be viewed not by what mode of inheritance is present but by what modes are ruled out. X-linked inheritance is ruled out by male-to-male transmission, whereas maternal inheritance is ruled out by transmission from a male to any offspring. In a multigenerational family such as Family B (Fig. 28–1B), these concepts rule out X-linked and maternal inheritance, leaving this pedigree as an example of autosomal dominant inheritance. However, other pedigrees frequently exist with the converse pattern. Family C (Fig. 28–1C) shows a family with seeming maternal inheritance. However, this family might also be interpreted as having an autosomal dominant pedigree with the chance event that only females have passed the abnormal gene. Although this seems obvious in this simple scenario, when disease expression is influenced by other factors (e.g., variable expressivity, incomplete penetrance, sex-linked expressivity), interpretation of pedigrees can be quite complex.

Why detail the pedigree and other clinical features of the patient if genetic testing defines the diagnosis? There are at least three reasons. First, as mentioned earlier, clinical analysis directs one to specific tests so a knowledgeable clinician can avoid an expensive search for different disease-causing mutations. Second, patients with genetic disease may also have other diagnoses. This may be revealed by unusual features in the history or examination. Finally, even though genetic testing is in many cases the most specific and sensitive test available, in no case are the theoretical specificity and sensitivity equal to 100%. Since most of these tests are new, the epidemiologic characteristics of these tests, when applied to specific patient populations, are continually changing. Thus the result must be interpreted in the context of the appropriate clinical scenario.

## TECHNIQUES IN MOLECULAR BIOLOGY

The advances in genetic testing depend on recent advances in molecular biology. A variety of techniques are used in genetic testing, of which only a few will be discussed here. The newest technique is that of polymerase chain reaction (PCR). PCR allows the amplification of selective pieces of deoxyribonucleic acid (DNA) from the nuclear or mitochondrial genome. These pieces can then be studied by the techniques described here. The major advantage of PCR is that a specific piece of genome can be selected from the whole genome without the necessity of purifying it from the whole DNA. This allows specific pieces of DNA to be studied from very small amounts of tissue. PCR relies on the specificity of single-stranded oligonucleotide primers flanking a region of interest. These primers only anneal to the region flanking the portion to be amplified. When these primers are used, a new strand of DNA is made across the region of interest with DNA polymerase. The strands are separated, new primer strands are allowed to anneal to the single strands, and the process is repeated. This gives rise to exponential amplification of the DNA region between the primers. This amplified DNA may be sequenced or studied by using other testing methods.

Several mechanisms are available for assessing DNA for abnormalities (Fig. 28–2). Some tests involve direct sequencing of DNA, in which the actual nucleotide sequence is determined. Although this is particularly useful for finding new mutations, it is a relatively time-consuming procedure. Many clinical tests use other methods to assess for the presence of single-base changes. DNA also may be assessed by its ability to be hydrolyzed by specific enzymes called restriction endonucleases. Abnormalities in DNA may introduce or eliminate these sites. Other abnormalities may change the size of a specific region of DNA and thus alter the distance between restriction sites on a piece of DNA. These abnormalities also may be detected by the assessment of the size of an amplified piece of DNA. Hybridization tests also may be used to search DNA for abnormalities. In these tests a labeled piece of nucleic acid is allowed to bind to DNA based on the complementary nature of the bases. The hybridization signal is detected by a variety of methods. The DNA to be analyzed can be a PCR-amplified piece, a larger fragment of the genome (as in a Southern blot), or a whole chromosome (such as in fluorescence in situ hybridization). Varying the probe determines the particular sequence that is tested for by the hybridization.

Although the abnormality in a genetic disease always exists in the DNA, it is sometimes easier to test for the abnormal protein that is produced. This is particularly true if different mutations in DNA produce similar effects at the level of protein. In such cases the abnormal protein (frequently a truncated form) may be assayed.

## TYPES OF GENETIC ABNORMALITIES

Since the nuclear and mitochondrial DNA represent the genetic material of the cell, all genetic disease must reflect abnormalities of DNA, typically called mutations. However, the changes in the DNA that mediate disease vary greatly. These include differences in size and location. The nature of these changes influences the course of the disease and the characteristics of the tests that are used to detect such disease.

The size of the abnormality of DNA can vary greatly among different diseases. One characteristic change is the deletion or duplication of a region of DNA. The deletion or duplication may be as large as an entire chromosome, as is seen in Down syndrome, in which one copy of chromosome 22 is duplicated, or Turner's syndrome, in which one X chromosome is absent in phenotypic females. Smaller deletions or duplications of pieces of chromosomes, such as the interstitial deletion of chromosome 22q11.2, which gives rise to DiGeorge syndrome, are also seen.[31] In all cases these deletions may frequently be detected by studies of whole chromosomes with high-resolution banding. In addition, specific probes are available for the more common deletions, which hybridize directly to the missing or extra piece of DNA. In such cases, fluorescence in situ hybridization (FISH) may detect the missing or extra piece of DNA.

Smaller deletions or triplications also may produce neurologic diseases. CMT 1a is caused by duplication of a specific 1.5 mB piece of chromosome 17, whereas hereditary neuropathy with disposition to pressure palsies is caused by a deletion of the same region.[20] In these cases, testing is performed by using hybridization with probes specific for this region and for the particular breakpoint involved in producing the deletion.

A more common mechanism of disease production is associated with single-base changes in the DNA called point mutations. These base changes may occur in the region coding for protein or outside the region coding for protein. In some cases they occur in regions that affect messenger RNA (mRNA) splicing. Missense mutations change a single amino acid, and nonsense mutations produce a truncated protein. Insertion or deletion of single bases changes the

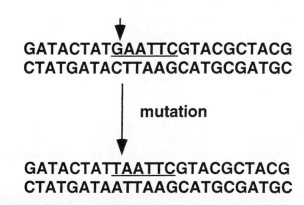

**FIGURE 28–2.** Methods of mutation detection. This base change (G to T) may be detected in many different ways:

1. Direct sequencing would reveal the base change.
2. This change removes a restriction enzyme site for the enzyme Eco RI (underlined). This could be assessed by tests with this enzyme to detect the presence or absence of this restriction site.
3. A hybridization test would assess the ability of the original complementary strand to bind to the mutated strand. This single base disruption would prevent this annealing.
4. This mutation also would create a potential termination codon in the messenger RNA made from this gene if it is in the same reading frame. This could be tested by examining the protein produced.

The best test used for a given disease would depend on the clinical questions asked for that disease and on the number of different mutations that produce a specific disease.

DNA reading frame and thus produces abnormal amino acids and frequently a truncation of the protein.

Another type of genetic abnormality is the expanded triplet repeat. The genetic abnormality in these diseases is an expansion of a naturally occurring series of three bases (triplet repeat). When the expansion reaches a defined level, diseases occur. In subsequent generations the triplet repeat may expand further, giving rise to an earlier age of onset in subsequent generations. This is the phenomenon of anticipation. The triplet repeat disorders may subdivided into two types: those in which the expanded repeat is a CAG and all others[129] (Table 28–1). The pathology in the CAG repeat diseases is limited to the nervous system, and the triplet repeat is in the coding region for the protein, thus leading to long glutamine sequences in the protein. Non-CAG repeat diseases frequently have non-nervous-system disease and may have the triplet repeats placed outside the region of the mRNA that codes for protein.

Another genetic characteristic, polymorphisms, may at times be linked to disease. Polymorphisms are naturally occurring genetic differences within the population that have no specific pathologic significance, which differentiates them from mutations. However, in selected situations they may be useful for diagnostic testing or may alter the course of human disease. Differences in the ApoE4 locus may constitute risk factors for Alzheimer's disease.[110] However, these polymorphisms do not cause disease but are merely risk factors.

Polymorphisms also may be useful for diagnostic testing. Although they are not pathologic for any disease, these polymorphisms may be located very close to the disease-producing mutation on a chromosome. Within a family a polymorphism thus may be linked to the pathologic mutation, giving rise to "linkage tests." In linkage analysis, testing for a disease is done by examining a family for linked polymorphisms and assessing the proband for their presence. Linkage analysis is used less today because of the availability of direct tests for many mutations. It requires the presence of a large family with affected and unaffected members, and the answers obtained may be less accurate than those from direct tests. The error rate is approximately 2%.[47] Nevertheless, linkage tests are still used for predictive purposes and may be the only test available for diseases in which many distinct mutations cause disease.

---

### TABLE 28–1.  Triplet Repeat Diseases*

**CAG Repeat Diseases**
Kennedy's syndrome (X-linked spinobulbar muscular atrophy)
Dentatorubropallidoluysian atrophy
Spinocerebellar ataxia
   SCA 1
   SCA 2
   SCA 3 (Machado-Joseph disease)
   SCA 6
   SCA 7
Huntington's disease

**Non-CAG Disorders**
Friedreich's ataxia
Myotonic dystrophy
Fragile X syndrome

*These disorders are caused by expanded triplet repeats. All show variable expressivity and anticipation.

---

## MODIFICATIONS FOR MITOCHONDRIAL DISEASE

Mitochondrial DNA (mtDNA) analysis requires a slightly different interpretation than that for nuclear DNA analysis. All mtDNA is derived from one's mother, with no paternal contribution classically. However, because not all the mother's mitochondria necessarily have identical mtDNA, one may have various amounts of a given mutation in mtDNA distributed through the body. This difference, called heteroplasmy, may be amplified by differing amounts of specific mtDNA molecules being distributed to different tissues. Consequently, the relative amount of heteroplasmy for a given mutation may influence the phenotype of the disorder. Heteroplasmy also may influence the detectability of a disorder as mutations present in some tissues at a high frequency may not be detectable in DNA from tissues with low levels of a specific mutation.[86]

In addition, mtDNA differs from nuclear DNA in its mutation rate. The mutation rate of mtDNA is believed to be higher than of nuclear DNA, which gives rise not only to frequent new mutations but also to silent polymorphisms.[97] Thus it is important to have solid evidence to confirm that a new change in DNA represents a mutation rather than a polymorphism unconnected to the disease being studied. Such evidence must include the absence of the base change in individuals lacking a particular syndrome and its presence in many individuals with a specific syndrome. However, this evidence is purely correlative; it is difficult to develop causal evidence owing to the difficulty of introducing mtDNA mutations into controlled experimental systems. Once techniques for this become readily available, it is possible that some of the less common of the many mtDNA base changes associated with disease may be found to be polymorphisms.

## SITUATIONS FOR GENETIC TESTING

Genetic tests must be interpreted in the context of the entire clinical evaluation. Although they are useful for confirming the diagnosis of a genetic disease in a typical genetic case, they are probably more useful in other situations. For example, in patients with an unknown cause of demyelinative neuropathy without a family history of the disease, the diagnostic test for demyelinating Charcot-Marie-Tooth disease (CMT) can confirm the diagnosis without the need for nerve biopsy or a therapeutic trial of medication to rule out acquired causes. Genetic tests are also useful in patients with a family history who present with atypical manifestations or who present early in the disease, before all the clinical signs may be apparent.

However, there are certain situations in which use of genetic testing is controversial. One in particular is presymptomatic testing. There are valid reasons for patients needing to know in advance of developing symptoms. In any disease in which a preventive therapy is available, presymptomatic testing is obviously appropriate. Presymptomatic testing is also useful if there are specific changes in life that patients would make based on knowing that they have inherited a gene. Such changes would include decisions about reproducing and other matters. However, presymptomatic testing comes with a price. Patients must to be able to understand the implications of testing. Once patients are tested, the test becomes part of their medical record, which may impede their ability to apply for life, health, or disability insurance. In addition, many patients may already have altered their life on the presumption that they will acquire disease. In such cases the trauma of not having the disease can be quite severe. Thus obtaining presymptomatic testing is a personal decision and usually requires psychologic assessments before testing. With these considerations, presymptomatic testing is not appropriate in at least one scenario. It is considered unethical to test children at risk for a disease who are asymptomatic and for whom no preventive therapy is available if they carry the gene for that disease.

# MOLECULAR DIAGNOSIS OF GENETIC NEUROPATHIC DISORDERS

Recent advances in the field of molecular biology have had a major impact on the evaluation of patients with inherited neuromuscular disorders. However, because the majority of these inherited disorders have no specific therapy at present, the clinical value of knowing the exact cause of a genetic neuromuscular disorder is not always clear. Because of the time and cost involved in performing full molecular screening for genetic neuromuscular disorders, clinical and electrophysiologic examinations should be used as mechanisms for directing molecular testing. In conjunction with the physical examination and electrophysiologic testing, molecular testing is an important tool in separating patients with genetic and usually untreatable neuromuscular disorders from those with acquired neuromuscular disorders, which may be treatable. For those patients with inherited peripheral neuropathies, it may soon be possible to correlate specific genotypic abnormalities with phenotypic differences and thus understand how the variable natural history of disease is attributable to specific mutations. Such understanding facilitates the investigation of modifiable, nongenetic factors that influence the course of the neuropathy and thus account for the highly variable phenotype seen in many genetic neuromuscular disorders.

## DEMYELINATIVE NEUROPATHIES

Charcot-Marie-Tooth neuropathy type 1 (CMT 1) is the most common autosomal dominant sensorimotor neuropathy, with a prevalence of about 1 in 2500 people. When all family members are examined and interviewed in detail, sporadic cases are uncommon.[115,116] Several genetic abnormalities are associated with CMT 1. Most patients are genetically linked to chromosome 17, and these patients are designated CMT 1a. Most of these patients (70% to 80%) have a specific duplication of 1.5 megabases of chromosome 17 in the region of the band 17p11.2-12. The size and location of the duplication is similar, if not identical, for virtually all individuals with CMT 1a, including most sporadic patients with de novo CMT 1a.[61,71,104,176,182] The 17p11.2-12 region contains the gene coding for the peripheral nerve myelin protein PMP22, a specific integral membrane protein component of myelin in the peripheral nervous system but not in the central nervous system.[108,127] Presumably, this duplication gives rise to an abnormality of myelin synthesis as a result of excess transcription or translation of PMP22. The importance of PMP22 in CMT 1 is also suggested by other patients whose disease maps to the same region of chromosome 17 but who lack the CMT 1a duplication. These patients usually have point mutations in the PMP22 gene, which could lead to abnormal myelin assembly and demyelination.[100,139] Some PMP22 mutations seem to be

dominant at the cellular level, but others are recessive and have no clinical effect in the absence of a deletion of the other PMP22 allele in a given patient.[140]

Other patients with CMT 1 have genetic abnormalities that map to chromosome 1, and they are designated CMT 1b. These patients carry mutations in another myelin protein called myelin protein zero, $P_0$.[64,96] Like PMP22, $P_0$ is an integral membrane protein of myelin. Mutations in $P_0$ may cause disease in a manner similar to that seen in patients with point mutations in PMP22.

Genetic abnormalities in other patients with CMT 1 map to other genomic locations, which suggests that other less common genetic abnormalities may produce the phenotype of CMT 1. Although occasional patients may have autosomal recessive demyelinating CMT, most sporadic cases harbor new duplications of chromosome 17p11.2-12.[104] A few other families with autosomal dominant disease map to sites distinct from those of CMT 1a and 1b and have been designated CMT 1c.[21]

Molecular testing for the CMT 1a duplication is available in commercial laboratories. Although this test is valuable in confirming the disease in patients with a positive family history, it is most useful in sporadic cases. The frequency of the CMT 1a duplication is about 70% to 80% in both familial and sporadic cases.[116,194] The CMT 1a test thus can be useful in differentiating de novo CMT 1a from a slowly progressive acquired demyelinating neuropathy. Such distinction may be difficult clinically in patients with slowly progressive or mild disease. In such cases, genetic confirmation may eliminate the need for nerve biopsy. This is particularly important because differentiation between CMT 1 and chronic inflammatory demyelinating polyneuropathy may not be easy using morphologic criteria only.[46] Although the duplication is specific for CMT 1a, it does not detect patients who have point mutations in PMP22. Thus the molecular assay for the duplication provides a powerful biologic marker for screening suspected patients and family members at risk, but a negative result does not rule out the diagnosis of CMT 1 or even CMT 1a. Unlike most instances of CMT 1a, no specific or frequently occurring mutations have been identified for CMT 1b. For patients with CMT 1b, sequencing the $P_0$ gene is required to make the molecular diagnosis. Unfortunately, this molecular evaluation currently is not available commercially.

Although not a form of CMT 1, hereditary neuropathy with liability to pressure palsy (HNPP) is a disorder of multiple mononeuropathies with the genetic abnormality of a deletion on chromosome 17 that is identical in size and location to the duplication seen in CMT 1a.[20] The link to this region of chromosome 17 suggests that the absence of PMP22 is a contributing factor to the pathology of HNPP. Molecular testing for the deletion in HNPP is commercially available.

Dejerine-Sottas disease (DSD), also known as CMT 3, is a severe autosomal recessive neuropathy with onset in infancy or early childhood. Motor nerve conduction velocities are <10 m/s. Although the phenotypic definition of DSD is narrow, detailed genetic analysis confirms heterogeneity of this disorder. DSD has been associated with point mutations in the PMP22 gene or the $P_0$ gene.[63,74,78,135,141] Therefore the PMP22 and $P_0$ genes can be sequenced to make a specific molecular diagnosis of DSD. Different mutations in the $P_0$

## TABLE 28–2. Abnormalities Found in Many Neurogenetic Diseases*

| DISORDER | INHERITANCE | LOCATION | GENE | COMMON ABNORMALITIES | AVAILABLE TESTS |
|---|---|---|---|---|---|
| **Myopathy** | | | | | |
| Duchenne's muscular dystrophy | X-linked | Xp22 | Dystrophin | Deletion, pm, truncation | 1. DNA testing<br>2. Muscle biopsy for dystrophin |
| Becker's muscular dystrophy | X-linked | Xp22 | Dystrophin | Deletion, pm, truncation | 1. DNA testing<br>2. Muscle biopsy for dystrophin |
| Facioscapulohumeral muscular dystrophy | AD | 4q35 | ? | ? | Linkage analysis to a known 3.3 kB repeat |
| Limb-girdle muscular dystrophy | AD (type 1) or AR (type 2) | 1. 5q22.3-31.3<br>2B. 2p16-13 | 1. ?<br>2A. Calpain deficiency<br>2C. γ sarcoglycan<br>2D. α sarcoglycan<br>2E. β sarcoglycan | pm | Muscle biopsy; limited genetic linkage |
| Myotonic dystrophy | AD | 19q13.3 | Myotonin protein kinase | CTG triplet repeat expansion | Direct testing for triplet repeat |
| Emery-Dreifuss muscular dystrophy | X-linked | Xq28 | Emerin | pm, truncation | DNA sequencing |
| **Metabolic Myopathies** | | | | | |
| McArdle's disease | AD | 11 | Myophosphorylase | pm | Direct test for most common pm; muscle biopsy |
| **Myotonic Disorders** | | | | | |
| Myotonia congenita | AD (Thomsen's disease) or AR (Becker's muscular dystrophy) | 7q35 | Chloride channel | pm | Direct sequencing |
| Paramyotonia congenita | AD | 17q23 | Sodium channel alpha 4 | pm | Direct sequencing |
| Hyperkalemic periodic paralysis | AD | 17q23 | Sodium channel alpha 4 | pm | Direct sequencing |
| Hypokalemic periodic paralysis | AD | 1q31 | Calcium channel | pm | Direct sequencing |
| **Neuropathy** | | | | | |
| CMT 1a | AD | 17p11.2 | *PMP22* | 1. Duplication of *PMP22* gene<br>2. pm in *PMP22* gene | 1. Direct DNA test for duplication<br>2. DNA sequencing |
| CMT 1b | AD | 1q21.2 | *P(0)* | pm | DNA sequencing |
| CMT 1c | AD | ? | ? | ? | ? |
| CMT 2A | AD | 1p35-36 | ? | ? | ? |
| Hereditary neuropathy with disposition to pressure palsies | AD | 17p11.2 | *PMP22* | 1. Deletion of *PMP22* gene<br>2. pm in *PMP22* gene | 1. Direct DNA test for duplication<br>2. DNA sequencing |
| CMT 3 | AD/AR/sporadic | 1, 17, 8, other | *PMP22, P(0)* | pm in *PMP22, P(0)*, other | Nerve conduction; nerve biopsy |
| CMT 4 | AR | 8q13-21.1 | ? | ? | Linkage |
| CMT 5 | AR/AD | ? | ? | ? | Linkage |
| CMT 6 | AR/AD | ? | ? | ? | Linkage |
| CMT-X | X-linked (X1, X2, X3) | 1. Xq13<br>2. Xq22.2<br>3. Xq26 | Connexin 32 | pm | DNA sequencing; other direct tests |
| Refsum's disease | AR | 10 | Phytanoyl CoA hydroxylase | pm | Phytanic acid level; DNA sequencing |
| Familial amyloidosis | AD | 1. 18<br>2. 9 | 1. Transthyretin<br>2. Gelsolin | 1. pm<br>2. pm | Direct testing; DNA sequencing |

*Basic inheritance and testing characteristics for many neurologic illnesses. This list represents only some of the disorders seen in neurogenetics. References used but not included in the text are those for optic atrophy,[16] ataxia telangiectasia,[23] adrenoleukodystrophy,[28,105,145] parkinsonism,[62a] and Refsum's disease.[77,110]

AD, Autosomal dominant; AR, autosomal recessive; AVED, ataxia with vitamin E deficiency; CADASIL, cerebral autosomal dominant arteriopathy with subcortical infarcts and leukoencephalopathy; CMT, Charcot-Marie-Tooth disease; CSF, cerebrospinal fluid; EM, electron microscopy; HERNS, hereditary endotheliopathy with retinopathy, nephropathy, and stroke; mtDNA, mitochondrial DNA; NAIP, neuronal apoptosis inhibitory protein; NF, neurofibromatosis; pm, point mutation; SCA, spinocerebellar ataxia.

gene may produce CMT 1, DSD, or congenital hypomyelinating neuropathy, depending on the exact mutation and on the number of copies of the abnormal mutation. Thus, in patients with $P_0$ or PMP22 abnormalities and the clinical phenotype of DSD, the disease may be viewed both clinically and pathophysiologically as the extreme end of the CMT 1 phenotype. However, other families with DSD do not fit this

simple scheme. In some families the genetic basis of DSD is not known but is distinct from simple PMP22 or $P_0$ mutations.[79,101] In still other cases, DSD has arisen as a result of homozygosity for CMT 2.[156] Thus DSD is a heterogeneous disorder that is defined by clinical criteria and cannot be ruled out by molecular testing alone.

Approximately 10% of patients with CMT have X-

## TABLE 28–2.  Abnormalities Found in Many Neurogenetic Diseases *Continued*

| DISORDER | INHERITANCE | LOCATION | GENE | COMMON ABNORMALITIES | AVAILABLE TESTS |
|---|---|---|---|---|---|
| **Ataxias** | | | | | |
| Friedreich's ataxia | AR | 9 | Frataxin | GAA repeat expansion in intronic DNA | Direct DNA test for expanded repeat |
| AVED | AR | 8 | Tocopherol transfer protein | pm | DNA sequencing |
| SCA 1 | AD | 6p21.3 | Ataxin 1 | CAG repeat expansion | Direct DNA test for expanded repeat |
| SCA 2 | AD | 12q23 | Ataxin 2 | CAG repeat expansion | Direct DNA test for expanded repeat |
| SCA 3 (Machado-Joseph disease) | AD | 14q24 | Ataxin 3 | CAG repeat expansion | Direct DNA test for expanded repeat |
| SCA 4 | AD | 16q22.1 | ? | ? | ? |
| SCA 5 | AD | 11p11-q11 | ? | ? | ? |
| SCA 6 | AD | 19 | Calcium channel, subunit alpha 1A | CAG repeat expansion | Direct DNA test for expanded repeat |
| SCA 7 | AD | 3p14-21.1 | Novel protein | CAG repeat expansion | Direct DNA test for expanded repeat |
| Paroxysmal ataxia with myokymia | AD | 12p13 | Potassium channel, alpha 1 | pm | Direct sequencing |
| Paroxysmal ataxia | AD | 19 | Calcium channel, subunit alpha 1A | pm | Direct sequencing |
| **Paraparesis** | | | | | |
| Hereditary (familial) spastic paraparesis | AD (types 1 and 2) or AR | (1) 14q (2) 2p24 | ? | ? | Clinical examination |
| **Motor Neuron Diseases** | | | | | |
| Amyotrophic lateral sclerosis | AD | 21q22 | Superoxide dismutase 1 | pm (multiple) | Direct sequencing |
| Spinal muscular atrophy | AR (all types) | 5q11.2-13.3 | NAIP, SMN | Deletion | Direct DNA test by hybridization |
| Spinal bulbar muscular atrophy | X-linked | Xq13-22 | Androgen receptor gene | CAG repeat expansion | Direct DNA test for expanded repeat |
| Adrenomyeloneuropathy | X-linked | Xq28 | Peroxisomal membrane transporter | pm (multiple) | DNA sequencing; long chain fatty acids |
| **Movement Disorders** | | | | | |
| Wilson's disease | AR | 13q14.1 | *ATP7B* | pm, deletion | Ceruloplasmin; urine copper/liver biopsy |
| Huntington's disease | AD | 4p16.3 | Huntingtin | CAG repeat expansion | Direct DNA test for expanded repeat |
| Dentatorubro-pallidoluysian atrophy | AD | 12pter-p12 | Atrophin 1 | CAG repeat expansion | Direct DNA test for expanded repeat |
| Dopa-responsive dystonia | AD (1) or AR (2) | (1) 14q22 (2) | (1) GTP cyclohydrolase I (2) Tyrosine hydroxylase | (1) pm (2) pm | L-dopa challenge; CSF biopterin; phenylalanine loading |
| Neuroacanthocytosis | AR (rarely AD) | ? | ? | ? | Blood smear |
| Lubag dystonia | X-linked | Xq11.2 | ? | ? | Linkage |
| Idiopathic torsion dystonia | AD | 9q34 | Torsin | Three-base deletion | DNA sequencing |
| Juvenile parkinsonism | AR | 6q25-27 | Parkin | Deletions | DNA sequencing |
| Familial parkinsonism | AD | 4q21-23 | Alpha synuclein | pm | DNA sequencing |

*Table continued on following page*

linked inheritance, and this disorder has been designated CMT X. Many of these individuals have a similar phenotype, and female carriers may manifest symptoms and signs without significant functional disability.[45,131] The characterization of the molecular deficits in CMT X demonstrates the true demyelinating nature of this disorder. In most families CMT X maps to chromosome Xq12-13 and is associated with point mutations in the connexin-32 gene.[10,42,45,80,123] This protein is important in gap junction formation and is localized in the Schwann cell at the nodes of Ranvier and the Schmidt-Lanterman clefts.[128,167] Because of the lack of specific and frequently occurring mutations in patients with CMT X, this disorder must also be diagnosed by sequencing of the abnormal gene (connexin-32 gene). Commercial testing is available for CMT X based on DNA sequencing.

## AXONAL NEUROPATHIES

CMT 2 designates a group of autosomal dominant sensorimotor axonal neuropathies. The variability of clinical phenotypes seen in CMT 2 is reflected in the findings from studies that have attempted to map the genes in patients with CMT 2. Several different loci have been detected, but no single locus presently accounts for the majority of patients with CMT 2.[195] Because of this marked genetic heterogeneity, molecular testing is of limited value in patients with CMT 2. Linkage testing is available through selected laboratories working on the mechanisms of this disorder.

**TABLE 28–2. Abnormalities Found in Many Neurogenetic Diseases** *Continued*

| DISORDER | INHERITANCE | LOCATION | GENE | COMMON ABNORMALITIES | AVAILABLE TESTS |
|---|---|---|---|---|---|
| **Dementia** | | | | | |
| Alzheimer's disease | AD | (1) 21q21<br>(2) 14q24.3<br>(3) 1q42 | (1) Amyloid precursor protein<br>(2) Presenilin 1<br>(3) Presenilin 2 | pm | DNA sequencing |
| Creutzfeldt-Jakob disease; fatal familial insomnia; Gerstman-Straussler syndrome | AD | 20p.12 | Prion protein | Distinct pm for each syndrome | DNA sequencing |
| **Stroke Syndromes** | | | | | |
| CADASIL | AD | 19p | Notch 3 gene | pm | DNA sequencing; EM of skin biopsy |
| HERNS | AD | ? | ? | ? | EM of skin biopsy |
| Familial hemiplegic migraine | AD | 19 | Calcium channel, subunit alpha 1A | pm | DNA sequencing |
| Optic neuropathy | | | | | |
|   Leber's neuropathy | Maternal | mtDNA | Multiple | pm | DNA sequencing |
|   Kjer | AD | 3q28 | ? | ? | Linkage |
| Phakomatoses | | | | | |
|   NF 1 | AD | 15 | Neurofibromin | Many distinct pm/deletions | Clinical diagnosis; DNA sequencing; protein truncation test |
|   NF 2 | AD | 22 | Merlin | Many distinct pm/deletions | Clinical diagnosis; DNA sequencing; protein truncation test |
| Tuberous sclerosis | AD | 9q34<br>16p13.3 | Hamartin<br>Tuberin | Multiple distinct mutation | Clinical diagnosis; DNA sequencing; protein truncation test |
| Ataxia-telangiectasia | AR | 11q23 | *ATN* gene | pm | DNA sequencing |
| **Epilepsy Syndromes** | | | | | |
| Hyperexplexia | AD | 5q31 | Glycine receptor | pm | DNA sequencing |
| Benign neonatal epilepsy | AD | (1) 20q23.3<br><br>(2) 8q | Acetylcholine receptor<br>? | pm | DNA sequencing |
| Progressive myoclonic epilepsy | AR | 21q23 | Cystatin B gene | pm | DNA sequencing |
| Fragile X syndrome | X-linked | X chromosome | FRAXA locus<br>FRAX B | Triplet repeat | Direct assay for triplet repeat |

The familial amyloidotic polyneuropathies (FAPs) are a group of autosomal dominantly inherited disorders associated most commonly with mutations in the transthyretin protein and frequently resulting in an axonal neuropathy with amyloid deposition in various tissues, including peripheral nerve. More than 50 specific mutations have been found, and all produce different phenotypes, including neuropathy, cardiomyopathy, nephropathy, meningovascular amyloidosis, and vitreous disease.[14,143,148,186] DNA analysis of the transthyretin mutation is usually performed by PCR methods. Genetic testing is now commercially available for the most common transthyretin mutation and may be performed by more detailed single-stranded confirmation polymorphism testing for other mutations.[177] With the use of various molecular methods, all the known transthyretin mutations can be sought and detected in a sample of genomic DNA. Prenatal diagnosis also has been performed successfully by using chorionic villous samples or amniotic fluid cell cultures.

The diagnosis of amyloid neuropathy (familial and acquired) also can be established by nerve biopsy. Therefore genetic testing may be a confirmatory test in the evaluation of a symptomatic individual with a positive family history who already has been diagnosed with an amyloid neuropathy based on nerve pathology. Genetic testing is particularly helpful in the evaluation of symptomatic relatives of affected individuals. Genotype/phenotype correlation does not always hold across different families, and individuals in certain ethnic populations carry the genetic abnormality without expressing the disease.[62,137] Thus, although FAP genetic testing is useful in symptomatic individuals, it must be applied cautiously to asymptomatic persons or those with atypical phenotypes.

## MOTOR NEURONOPATHIES

There are several hereditary neuromuscular disorders that result in motor neuron degeneration, including the childhood-onset spinal muscular atrophies, X-linked spinal bulbar muscular atrophy, and familial amyotrophic lateral sclerosis (ALS). These motor neuronopathies were previously defined by their time of onset and their clinical phenotype. Recently, specific genetic disturbances have been discovered for each of these disorders, and this has allowed physicians to test for these specific disorders when there is clinical ambiguity or uncertain familial inheritance.

Childhood-onset spinal muscular atrophy (SMA) is an autosomal recessive motor neuron disorder. The gene(s) for the three types of SMA have been mapped to a single locus on chromosome 5q13 by linkage analysis. The survival motor neuron (SMN) gene exists as two highly homologous copies, a centromeric and a telomeric form. The telomeric copy is homozygously missing in more than 90% of patients with all forms of childhood-onset SMA.[163] Another multicopy gene, the neuronal apoptosis inhibitory protein (NAIP), also is homozygously absent in patients with SMA. Only one copy of NAIP contains the full complement of exons in an individual, and it is this copy that is deleted in about 50% of the patients with SMA type 1 (infantile onset) and to a lesser extent in the later childhood-onset forms, SMA type 2 and SMA type 3.[142] PCR testing for the telomeric form of SMN is available, and the homozygous loss of this gene occurs in a predicted 95% of individuals with SMA type 1. The low percentage of false-positive and false-negative results make this molecular test highly sensitive and specific. In the rare ambiguous case, DNA sequencing of the SMN and NAIP genes can be used to render an accurate answer.

Although the molecular diagnosis of SMA may be established with these tests, the variability in phenotype does not correlate well with the more uniform genetic disturbance found in most or all affected individuals within a family. Even within families with several affected individuals of the same generation, different clinical severities may exist.[161,163,193] No genetic marker clearly explains this phenomenon. Most likely, it represents modification of the phenotype by other alleles distinct from the disease-causing allele on chromosome 5. This phenomenon demonstrates that although we may detect SMA with certainty, predicting the severity of the phenotype is not yet possible.

X-linked spinal bulbar muscular atrophy (Kennedy's disease) is a disorder caused by an expanded trinucleotide repeat (CAG repeats of between 30 to 60 in this disorder) within the first exon of the androgen receptor gene.[95] In contrast to myotonic dystrophy, another trinucleotide repeat disorder, this CAG repeat is in a coding region and leads to an expanded polyglutamine tract within the receptor. As with other trinucleotide repeat disorders, PCR testing is commercially available and can detect with great accuracy the length of the expansion, which usually correlates with the severity of the phenotype and the age of onset.

Although most cases of ALS are sporadic, about 10% of cases arise as a dominantly inherited trait.[117] Clinically and pathologically sporadic ALS and inherited ALS are virtually identical. Genetic linkage was established to chromosome 21q in a fraction of ALS pedigrees.[159] Subsequently the gene product that was encoded at the familial ALS locus was discovered as the cytosolic copper–zinc superoxide dismutase (SOD).[147] Unfortunately only about 20% of familial ALS clans have shown mutations in this gene, which significantly limits the molecular testing for this disorder at present. However, if a family has shown a specific mutation in this region, DNA sequencing in this region of other family members could be used to establish the presence or absence of that familial genotype.

In what groups of patients are tests for the different motor neuronopathies most helpful? The phenotype of familial ALS is identical to that seen in sporadic disease; therefore familial ALS testing is useful only in that group of individuals who have a strong family history. In addition, the absence of a mutation in SOD does not rule out inherited ALS if no other affected family member has been shown to carry such a mutation. In contrast, SMA types 1, 2, and 3 and Kennedy's disease may present with proximal weakness and resemble a myopathic disorder. Thus, although testing for SMA and Kennedy's disease is useful for confirmation in people with family histories and typical clinical features, it also must be considered in patients who may appear clinically to have a myopathy but have evidence of denervation on electromyography or muscle biopsy. In these rare patients, molecular testing may alter the approach to a given patient. On occasion, genetic testing for Kennedy's disease has been diagnostic in patients with predominantly proximal weakness who have carried the diagnosis of ALS.[126] This distinction is important since Kennedy's disease generally carries a more favorable prognosis than does ALS.

## MUSCULAR DYSTROPHIES

The muscular dystrophies are a group of inherited muscle disorders that show skeletal muscle deterioration as the primary pathologic abnormality on muscle biopsy. This group of disorders includes the congenital muscular dystrophies, Duchenne's muscular dystrophy, Becker's muscular dystrophy, Emery-Dreifuss muscular dystrophy, facioscapulohumeral muscular dystrophy, limb-girdle muscular dystrophy, myotonic dystrophy, and others. The specific genetic and biochemical defects in many of these disorders have been identified, although only a few of these disorders can be reliably diagnosed with molecular testing.

The majority of cases of muscular dystrophy are caused by disorders associated with abnormal dystrophin protein, such as the X-linked recessive disorders Duchenne muscular dystrophy (DMD) and Becker muscular dystrophy (BMD) (collectively called dystrophinopathies). The molecular tests that are available for routine diagnostic purposes include analysis of the dystrophin protein in muscle tissue from a biopsy and analysis of the dystrophin gene by using lymphocyte DNA from a peripheral blood sample.[111] The protein tests involve detecting dystrophin from muscle with immunohistochemical or immunofluorescent staining methods using monoclonal or polyclonal antibodies.[30] Skeletal muscle from patients with DMD shows a marked dystrophin deficiency with these methods, whereas tissue from patients with BMD typically shows a mild-to-moderate reduction in dystrophin staining when compared to normal samples. This interpretation can be difficult if the biopsy is processed poorly. Therefore these immunologic methods are suboptimal as the sole test to diagnose patients with the milder dystrophinopathy, BMD. Dystrophin immunoblotting, which allows accurate analysis of the small differences in the molecular weight of the abnormal dystrophin protein in patients with BMD as compared to normal dystrophin protein, is a better method for determining the diagnosis of BMD. Hoffman et al[68] have suggested that patients with BMD could be subdivided into mild-to-moderate disease (dystrophin levels of at least 20% of normal) and severe disease (dystrophin levels of 5% to 15% of normal). Dystrophin levels of <3% of normal on immunoblot testing are diagnostic of DMD. The limitation to immunoblot testing is in the patients who have BMD with normal-molecular-weight dystrophin protein that is reduced in quantity. This may lead to false-negative results in some cases. Another limitation is in patients with primary deficiencies of other dystrophin-associated proteins, such as $\alpha$-sarcoglycan, $\beta$-sarcoglycan, or $\gamma$-sarcoglycan, who also have abnormal dystrophin levels and could be diagnosed as having DMD or BMD instead of a sarcoglycanopathy.

Because of the limitations of dystrophin immunoreactivity testing and the desire to avoid muscle biopsy in some cases, direct testing of the dystrophin gene from lymphocytic DNA is another valuable tool in the diagnosis of DMD or BMD. Analysis of the abnormal dystrophin gene commonly involves the commercially available dystrophin gene deletion test with use of the 18 exon multiplex PCR.[7] The dystrophin gene contains almost 80 exons, and this test evaluates the presence or absence of the commonly deleted exons. About 98% of deletions are detected by the 18-exon assay.[7] The test is positive if one or more exons are deleted and defines the patient as having a primary dystrophinopathy. If the exon deletion is in-frame and simply causes the omission of several amino acids, the resultant phenotype is BMD. In contrast, if the exon deletion is out-of-frame and results in the production of many incorrect amino acids and a truncated protein, the resultant phenotype is typically DMD. These predictions hold true with about 90% accuracy. Unfortunately, the reading frame is difficult to predict with this multiplex PCR testing, which leaves the distinction of DMD vs. BMD to phenotypic and morphologic criteria. If all 18 exons are intact (a negative test result), the patient still may have a dystrophinopathy and should undergo muscle biopsy and immunohistochemical and immunoblot testing. About 45% of DMD patients and 30% of BMD patients have duplications or point mutations in the dystrophin gene, resulting in abnormal dystrophin protein.[68] These patients may not have a positive 18-exon deletion test and therefore require additional testing (e.g., muscle biopsy) to make the diagnosis of a dystrophinopathy.

Southern blot analysis with the entire dystrophin cDNA sequence as a probe can detect all deletion mutations; however, it is more time consuming and costly. Although this method is no longer used commonly for diagnostic purposes, Southern blot analysis still is used for detection of female carriers of deletion mutations. Another type of DNA analysis is through gene linkage, which typically is done only after a dystrophinopathy has been diagnosed on muscle biopsy or by family history. As with Southern blot analysis, this analysis is costly and time consuming, which makes the 18-exon multiplex PCR a good screening test. Although all these DNA tests face several obstacles for use in DMD and BMD, including the high sporadic mutation rate (new mutations and gonadal mosaicism) and the large size of the gene (resulting in an increased frequency of intragenic recombination events), these are relatively noninvasive methods of diagnosis for the most common types of muscular dystrophy.

Even females who clinically appear to be affected by one of the muscular dystrophies should not be excluded from molecular testing for one of the more common X-linked dystrophinopathies since about 10% of women with muscular dystrophy show an underlying dystrophinopathy as the cause of their disease.[69] The muscle pathology from female carriers varies between patients and even within an individual patient on different regions of the specimen. This variability is presumably the result of different X-chromosome inactivation patterns and can manifest clinically by a carrier exhibiting localized weakness in one limb and not another, presumably because of variations in the increased percentage of mutant dystrophin genes being expressed in that limb. Therefore the muscle biopsy of a female carrier may or may not show dystrophic areas even if the sample is from a weak muscle. Muscle biopsy can be of limited value in carrier evaluation because these regional dystrophic areas may be missed in sampling.

Prenatal diagnosis for DMD and BMD typically is done by DNA testing of amniocytes or chorionic villous cells. If the results show a deletion mutation, the fetus has one of these two disorders. If there is no deletion detected, a fetal muscle biopsy may be necessary for the diagnosis. Under ultrasound guidance a biopsy is obtained from the gluteal or quadriceps muscle between 18 and 24 weeks' gestation. Accurate diagnosis by fetal muscle protein testing has been reported by several groups.[40,92]

The X-linked Emery-Dreifuss muscular dystrophy (EDMD) is clinically distinct from DMD and BMD. Typically these patients have the phenotype of childhood muscular dystrophy along with the development of contractures at the elbows and ankles, slow progression of weakness, and early cardiac conduction disturbances. Although the abnormal gene and protein have been identified in a series of patients,[12] molecular diagnostic testing is not commercially available and exists only in a few research laboratories. Recently one group used a test for altered expression of the protein emerin in lymphocytes and skin cells by using a monoclonal antibody to the protein.[105] This method also has enabled identification of a female carrier of the disease by showing reduced levels of the protein on the lymphocyte Western blot test and a mosaic pattern of expression by immunofluorescence microscopy of the skin biopsy.

The limb-girdle muscular dystrophies (LGMD) are a subset of the muscular dystrophies that typically do not show abnormal dystrophin on muscle biopsy. There is a substantial overlap in their clinical features.[184] With the exception of the dominantly inherited LGMD type 1a, the other LGMDs are autosomal recessive and have been designated LGMD type 2; they are subtyped based on the protein component that is deficient (2a = calpain 3 deficiency; 2c = γ-sarcoglycan deficiency; 2d = α-sarcoglycan deficiency; and 2e = β-sarcoglycan deficiency).[33,34,181] All these LGMDs map to different chromosomes. Although the location of these genes has been determined for these disorders, molecular testing is not commercially available. Many of the mutations identified for these disorders have been missense mutations, which require direct sequencing for identification. Also, patients with any of the primary sarcoglycan deficiencies can show secondary deficiencies of other sarcoglycans. In particular, a patient with a deficiency of α-sarcoglycan on muscle biopsy could show a mutation in any of the sarcoglycan genes or in the dystrophin gene on DNA analysis. Thus biochemical screening is not diagnostic, and it is necessary to identify patient gene mutations in the specific sarcoglycan gene for a definitive diagnosis.

Facioscapulohumeral muscular dystrophy (FSHD), an autosomal dominant disorder, remains largely a clinical diagnosis. FSHD has marked clinical heterogeneity, even in the same family, and patients with familial FSHD may present at different ages. Muscle biopsy and electromyographic evaluation can be quite confusing with both neuropathic and myopathic features. Consequently, gene testing is helpful for sporadic cases. After the discovery that FSHD localized to the distal part of chromosome 4q35, a 3.3 kB repeat sequence of variable size was found to be truncated in patients with the disorder. About 80% of kindreds with familial FSHD have a small repeat fragment, as do most sporadic cases,[51] but no candidate gene has been discovered in this fragment or in the local vicinity. It is possible that a reduction in the number of repeat units brings the FSHD gene closer to the telomeric DNA, which interferes with gene expression.[189,192] This has been termed position effect variegation. There are several limitations to DNA testing for FSHD at present. On chromosome 10q26 and 1q, similar restriction enzyme (EcoRI) fragments to those on 4q have been detected.[189] In addition, there is evidence of locus heterogeneity in FSHD.[51] In certain cases the molecular testing that is available presently can be used to determine if an individual has the truncated repeat sequence. In well-defined familial cases of FSHD with the 4q35 abnormality, molecular testing is helpful to evaluate other at-risk family members as long as one recognizes the risk of recombination (about 10%). In a sporadic case a small repeat fragment in an affected individual but not in the patient's parents establishes a new mutation and the diagnosis of FSHD.[57] Until specific FSHD-associated mutations can be detected, the diagnostic utility of DNA testing for this disorder will remain limited.

The congenital muscular dystrophies are rare disorders of muscle weakness with early onset. About half of patients with congenital muscular dystrophy have shown merosin deficiency on muscle biopsy with localization to chromosome 6q2.[87,121,171] Unfortunately these disorders are characterized by genetic heterogeneity, making molecular diagnosis less than adequate at present. Therefore diagnosis is based on clinical and pathologic grounds, with the muscle biopsy changes being quite similar to those seen in other muscular dystrophies.

Myotonic dystrophy is one of a growing number of autosomal dominant neurologic disorders caused by a variable trinucleotide repeat sequence.[129] The genetic error for myotonic dystrophy is a CTG repeat sequence located in the 3′ untranslated region of a gene with protein kinase domains on chromosome 19. Normal individuals have a polymorphic CTG repeat varying in length up to about 40 repeats. Affected individuals have a repeat varying from 50 to several thousand repeats. The length of repeated sequences may increase during inheritance, usually resulting in a more severe phenotype with a longer repeat (anticipation). Also, each tissue of an individual can have different-sized repeat sequences, depending on the expression of the gene in that tissue; however, lymphocyte DNA from a blood sample usually is adequate for routine evaluation. Commonly, PCR amplification of the allele can detect with great accuracy the length of the repeat in the sample analyzed, but it may miss extraordinarily long repeats seen in the neonatal form of myotonic dystrophy. Southern blot analysis also may be used to detect this trinucleotide expansion, although the smaller expansions may not be large enough to be detected by this method. These tests are available commercially and together are highly sensitive and specific for the diagnosis of myotonic dystrophy.

## OTHER MUSCLE DISORDERS

The congenital myopathies (i.e., central core disease, nemaline myopathy, and centronuclear or myotubular myopathy) are relatively rare disorders of muscle weakness that may present in childhood or, uncommonly, in adulthood. Muscle biopsy still is the test of choice for diagnosis of the congenital myopathies, since they are defined by their morphologic appearance, which is quite different from that of the muscular dystrophies. Unfortunately, these disorders are characterized by genetic heterogeneity, making molecular diagnosis less than adequate at present.

Myophosphorylase deficiency (McArdle's disease) is an autosomal recessive disorder of glycogenosis. The gene has been localized on chromosome 11.[178] By far the most common genetic error in Caucasian patients is a nonsense mutation at codon 49, which was observed in about 75% of patients in one series[5,38] and in 100% in another series.[5] This mutation was less common (about 55%) in northern Italian patients.[106] This mutation has not yet been encountered in the Japanese population.[179] Because of the high prevalence of the codon 49 mutation in Caucasians (Americans and British), this disorder can be diagnosed with molecular genetic analysis of lymphocytic DNA, thereby avoiding muscle biopsy in this subset of patients. In other patients, muscle biopsy must be performed to assess phosphorylase activity to make this diagnosis. At present many of the other disorders of glycogen storage (glycogenoses) are diagnosed by biochemical documentation of a specific enzyme defect in muscle and not by genetic analysis.[25]

## MITOCHONDRIAL ILLNESSES

The mitochondrial disorders are characterized by the unusual signs of myopathy, neuropathy, sensorineural hearing loss, cardiac and gastrointestinal dysfunction, optic neuropathy, dystonia, external ophthalmoplegia myoclonic seizures, and recurrent encephalopathy. Although they can be separated into separate disorders clinically, the phenotype frequently overlaps (see Table 28–3).[41,53,67,86,97,151,180] These disorders may be subgrouped according to the molecular abnormality found: mtDNA point mutations vs. multiple DNA deletions. The mtDNA point mutations are inherited in a maternal inheritance pattern, whereas multiple deletion syndromes are either sporadic or inherited in an autosomal dominant fashion, demonstrating that the actual mutation is present in a nuclear gene that regulates mitochondrial DNA replication. Mitochondrial neurogastrointestinal encephalopathy (MNGIE) may be inherited in a recessive manner.[67] This demonstrates an interesting difference between these disorders: For point mutation syndromes molecular testing demonstrates the genetic abnormality, but in mtDNA deletion syndromes molecular testing shows a marker of disease produced by another cause, most likely a nuclear gene.

Each of the point mutation syndromes is associated with a particular mtDNA mutation (Table 28–3). However, at times there may be overlap between these syndromes. Thus, when testing for particular mtDNA mutations, it may be necessary to test for a series of mutations before the diagnosis is made. Since there are few disorders that resemble mitochondrial disease when many of the disease manifestations are present, DNA testing is an excellent mechanism for confirming the diagnosis. It is also helpful when patients manifest incomplete syndromes. However, care must be taken in some situations.[41,67] First, if the patient has a syndrome that is atypical for mitochondrial illness, it may be difficult to determine if the genetic abnormality causes a

**TABLE 28–3. Maternally Inherited Mitochondrial Disorders in Neurology***

| SYNDROME | FEATURES | POSITIONS OF BASE CHANGES |
|---|---|---|
| MELAS | Mitochondrial encephalopathy with lactic acidosis and stroke-like episodes | 3243, 3271 |
| MERRF | Myoclonic epilepsy with ragged-red fibers | 8344, 8356 |
| Leber's hereditary optic neuropathy (LHON) | Optic neuropathy | 11778, 3460, 15257, 14484 |
| NARP | Neuropathy, ataxia, retinitis pigmentosa | 8993 |

*These disorders are all associated with point mutations in the mitochondrial genome. Diagnosis may be made by clinical phenotype in association with DNA analysis of the appropriate tissue.

particular symptom. One must also conduct a complete search for other disease entities if the clinical phenotype is unusual for mitochondrial disease.

## CENTRAL NERVOUS SYSTEM DISORDERS

### HEREDITARY ATAXIAS

The inherited ataxias include Friedreich's ataxia, ataxia with vitamin E deficiency, spinocerebellar ataxia (types 1–7), paroxysmal ataxia with myokymia, paroxysmal ataxia with nystagmus, dentatorubral-pallidoluysian atrophy, and other less defined syndromes. Because features of many of these diseases overlap, they are often difficult to diagnose accurately on the basis of phenotype despite the existence of several classification schemes. However, recent genetic data have made it possible to characterize the inherited ataxias on the basis of genotype, and a precise diagnosis frequently can now be made. The molecular basis for many of these disorders is frequently expansion of unstable triplet repeat sequences, and ataxia can be found in autosomal dominant, autosomal recessive, and on occasion X-linked inheritance patterns.[166]

In isolated cases it would be easy to perform an exhausting search for a cause of ataxia. The key directive for such a search must be the history and physical examination. For example, the major autosomal recessive ataxias (Friedreich's ataxia and ataxia with vitamin E deficiency) have a phenotype that is the same as that of a dorsal column disease and may be associated with abnormalities outside the nervous system, including diabetes and cardiomyopathy. In contrast, the autosomal dominant ataxias will not have manifestations outside the central nervous system, and the ataxia is usually of a cerebellar origin, although dorsal column disease may be present.

### AUTOSOMAL RECESSIVE DISEASES

The most common early-onset ataxia is Friedreich's ataxia (FA), an autosomal recessive disorder with an estimated European prevalence of 1 in 50,000. The responsible gene has been mapped to chromosome 9, and mutations in the form of expanded GAA repeats within the gene are responsible for the disorder.[18] The protein encoded by this gene is designated "frataxin," but the function of this protein and how the expansion of GAA repeats causes disease is unclear. Homozygosity for the expansion confers the disease, but heterozygotes with point mutations on nonexpanded alleles have been discovered in as many as 6% of patients with FA.[18] The typical number of repeats present in a normal frataxin gene ranges from 7 to 29,[39] and an expansion of up to 34 repeats has been found in a normal allele.[26] Individuals meeting the criteria for FA usually have repeats in the range of 120 to more than 1000, with most alleles containing 700 to 800.[17] The shortest known expansion in a patient with FA is 66 GAA repeats.[39] As with most other triplet repeat diseases, earlier age of onset and poorer prognosis correspond with larger expansions.[35,43] The presence and severity of left ventricular hypertrophy also corresponds with the number of repeats.[82,112] Genetic testing in individuals meeting the criteria for, or suspected of having, FA can be useful in diagnosis and prognosis. When one is attempting to determine carrier status in asymptomatic individuals for purposes of genetic counseling, it is important to note that in cases of intermediate size alleles, one cannot accurately predict whether an expansion will result in affected offspring. For example, a carrier with only 38 GAA repeats has been identified.[26]

Ataxia with vitamin E deficiency (AVED) is a recessive disorder with a phenotype similar to, if not identical to that of FA. Neurologic symptoms improve with vitamin E supplementation. Thus genetic testing would be extremely useful for diagnosis of patients with ataxia and low serum vitamin E levels and could be used to identify preclinical individuals with inherited vitamin E deficiency. The molecular basis for this disorder is a defective (alpha)-tocopherol-transfer protein, which is responsible for hepatic incorporation of the biologically active form of vitamin E into very low density lipoproteins. Point mutations in the gene, located on chromosome 8, are responsible for the disease in more than 18 families with ataxia with vitamin E deficiency.[54,124] Because the disease is relatively rare and the genetic abnormalities vary among families, direct genetic testing is not yet commercially available. The appropriate test for this disorder is a vitamin E level, not only because of the difficulty of genetic testing but also because it detects the nongenetic causes of vitamin E deficiency.

In what type of patients is testing for the autosomal recessive causes of ataxia appropriate? Testing for inherited vitamin E deficiency is needed in any patient with an unexplained ataxia because this represents a treatable syndrome. The progression of the disorder stops with treatment, and some improvement may occur. In addition, the use of FA testing has demonstrated that some people who do not meet the defined criteria for FA carry two copies of an abnormal "frataxin" gene. These include people with later onset, patients with retained tendon reflexes (thought at one time to be a distinct disease), and people without dysarthria.[9,27,48] This is particularly important in recognition of the many individuals with later-onset ataxia for whom a cause is never found. If such an individual has any dorsal column signs, testing for FA may disclose the diagnosis.

### AUTOSOMAL DOMINANT DISEASE

Spinocerebellar ataxia (SCA) types 1 through 7 and dentatorubral-pallidoluysian atrophy (DRPLA) are dominantly inherited disorders with many overlapping clinical characteristics, but they are now distinguishable on the basis of their distinct genotypes. Unstable trinucleotide repeat expansions are responsible for SCA 1, 2, 3, 6, and 7 and DRPLA.[129] The genetic basis for SCA 4 and SCA 5 remains unknown at this time, although the genes have been mapped to chromosomes 16 and 11, respectively.[44] SCA 1 and SCA 2, which are considered "olivopontocerebellar atrophy" phenotypes, have been mapped to chromosomes 6 and 12, and their gene products are denoted ataxin 1 and ataxin 2, respectively.[17,76,133,138,146] SCA 3, or Machado-Joseph disease (MJD), has been mapped to chromosome 14, and its gene product is ataxin 3.[65] The length of the repeat in MJD ranges from 67 to 80,[153] but an atypical case of MJD with only 56 repeats has been reported.[170] DRPLA, which shares some features of MJD, has been mapped to chromosome 12, and the defective protein is atrophin 1.[75] SCA 6 has been mapped to chromosome 19, and the protein is an alpha 1A calcium channel subunit.[109] This SCA has been found in a large number of sporadic patients.[109] SCA 7, also referred to as autosomal dominant ataxia with retinal degeneration, has been mapped to chromosome 3.[85] Its gene product is a novel protein in which disease is associated with an expansion of a novel triplet repeat.[28] SCA 7 differs from other SCAs in that it is associated with retinal degeneration.

In patients with autosomal dominant cerebellar ataxia without retinal degeneration, SCA 1, 2, and 3 account for more than 40% of the cases. In most series, MJD is the most common, accounting for 18% to 41%; SCA 1 represents 3% to 10%, and SCA 2 accounts for 10% to 18%.[19,98,134,153,160] SCA 6 represents 2% to 38% of autosomal dominant ataxias in different series.[50,168] DRPLA is a relatively rare disorder. However, the relative frequency of these disorders varies greatly among different populations. The number of repeats inversely correlates with age of onset in these disorders and in SCA 7.[28,32,50,138]

Have the various genetic tests suggested a clinical differentiation? MJD is classically viewed as having four different phenotypes. However, with genetic testing it is clear that (except for retinal degeneration in SCA 7) no phenotype is perfectly demonstrative of any disease, nor is any clinical sign found in only one disorder.[17,36,47,56,138,149] Thus, if genetic testing is done for any of these disorders, rationally it should be performed for all of them. It is possible to make educated guesses based on clinical presentation to direct genetic testing within these groups.[153] For example, the phenotype of SCA 6 is a purer cerebellar ataxia, which might direct a test for SCA 6 first in a patient with pure cerebellar disease. Slow saccades are a feature of SCA 2 but also may be seen in SCA 1 and SCA 3.[17,149] In these cases it is possible to prioritize testing, but it is frequently necessary to test for all SCAs to make a firm diagnosis.

Another observation directly relevant to clinical practice is the observed new mutation rate. Although an exact rate has not yet been determined, new cases of SCAs are infrequent (with the exception of SCA 6).[138] In almost all cases a history of some related neurologic abnormality can be found in the parents or siblings of the proband. Patients with sporadic disease typically fit the phenotype of "olivopontocerebellar atrophy." In the absence of a family history of the condition, almost all of these persons will have disease that is a variant of the nongenetic disorder multisystem atrophy. However, since SCA 6 and SCA 2 have been reported in patients with no family history of the disease, a search for all SCA types in patients without a family history may, on occasion, provide a diagnosis.[19,138,153]

Paroxysmal ataxia with myokymia and paroxysmal ataxia are rare autosomal dominant disorders also known as episodic ataxia with myokymia (EA-M or EA-1) and episodic ataxia with nystagmus (EA-N or EA-2).[23,55,122] They have been mapped to chromosome 12 and 19, respectively. The molecular basis for EA-M is a defect in the alpha 1 potassium channel subunit caused by several recognized point mutations. The alpha 1A calcium channel subunit is affected in EA-N. Thus EA-N, SCA 6, and familial hemiplegic migraine all represent distinct disorders from the same gene. However, although they are distinct disorders, a few patients with SCA 6 develop paroxysmal features, and patients with EA-N eventually develop residual cerebellar dysfunction. Thus they may eventually blend into the phenotype of other cerebellar atrophies with less obvious paroxysmal components. To date, molecular testing for EA-N is not available except through research laboratories.

## DYSTONIA

Dystonia may describe either a symptom of a more diffuse neurogenetic disease or its own defined genetic illness. A large number of genetic diseases have dystonia as a symptom, including Wilson's disease, spinocerebellar ataxias, genetic Parkinson's disease, mitochondrial illness, or genetic dementias. The crucial one of these to note is Wilson's disease because it is a treatable entity.

Dystonia also may be present in isolation as an inherited disease. Inherited dystonia is distinguishable into at least three types. Autosomal dominant torsion dystonia (DYT 1) is a disorder that is most common in the Ashkenazi Jewish population. It is variably expressive and has variable penetrance. Not all affected individuals are identically affected, and some obligate gene carriers manifest no symptoms. A mutation in a novel gene has recently been found that causes the disorder in the Ashkenazi Jewish population and other ethnic groups. It is a 3-base deletion in an ATP-binding protein gene.[125] The mechanism by which it causes disease is not clear. To this point no other mutation has been found in this gene. Testing is available, but studies do not yet indicate what percent of people with autosomal dominant dystonia have mutations in this gene. Initial estimates suggest that approximately 80% of people with early-onset generalized dystonia have this specific mutation. However, this mutation is not commonly found in people with sporadic, late-onset, focal dystonia.[15] Other loci for dystonia have been suggested based on other studies, usually involving single families.[8,70]

A second form of autosomal dominant dystonia is referred to as dopa-responsive dystonia or hereditary dystonia with diurnal fluctuations. This disorder also may begin in childhood and affects women more severely than men. It frequently has a strong diurnal variation, with patients feeling much better in the morning. This disorder is readily responsive to L-dopa, which is explained by the known genetic defects. In most families it is associated with mutations in the GTP cyclohydrolase I gene, which is passed in a dominant manner.[72] This enzyme synthesizes biopterin, the cofactor for tyrosine hydroxylase. This genetic defect is thus directly linked to catecholamine synthesis, explaining the exquisite response to dopamine. The mutations are almost all different point mutations, making simple genetic testing difficult.[66,84]

A far easier diagnostic test is administration of oral L-dopa, which produces a dramatic response in most patients.

A few patients with dopa-responsive dystonia inherit the disorder in an autosomal recessive pattern. In these cases the disorder results from point mutations in the tyrosine hydroxylase gene.[4] This may be diagnosed by sequencing, but the easiest approach is usually a therapeutic trial of L-dopa.

A final form of dystonia is the X-linked disorder known as Lubag. Found most commonly in people of Filipino background, the disorder presents with a mixture of dystonia and parkinsonian symptoms. Although mapped to the X chromosome, the exact gene is not yet known.[190]

## WILSON'S DISEASE

Wilson's disease, also known as hepatolenticular degeneration, is an autosomal recessive disorder of copper metabolism. This disease most commonly presents as hepatic dysfunction in children or as neurologic or psychiatric disease in adults. The neurologic presentation may be any movement disorder, and effective treatment in the form of oral D-penicillamine is available.[187] Thus the identification of symptomatic and presymptomatic patients is extremely important. The gene responsible encodes a copper-transporting P-type ATPase (a family of enzymes involved in cation transport) that is located on chromosome 13 and denoted as ATP7B.[130] Unfortunately, Wilson's disease is genetically heterogeneous and has been associated with more than 50 mutations in the *ATP7B* gene.[173,174] Several types of mutations have been identified, including point mutations and frameshift mutations, which account for 30% of the mutations identified in patients in the United States.[173] One particular point mutation, His1069Gln, is found in 61% of Austrian patients with Wilson's disease.[102] Interestingly, some genotypes correlate with specific phenotypes; for example, mutations that cause complete disruption of the gene may result in presentation with liver disease in early childhood, whereas missense mutations are more likely to present with neurologic or psychiatric disease later in life.[173] DNA linkage analysis or other DNA testing may be useful to perform in presymptomatic siblings of patients in whom the diagnosis is made to initiate early therapeutic intervention.[103] Identification of presymptomatic individuals is important in this disorder because of the available treatments. For this purpose, measurement of serum ceruloplasmin levels is impractical because heterozygous carriers may have low ceruloplasmin levels, and patients with Wilson's disease may not have lowered ceruloplasmin levels. Urinary copper excretion may be used to screen people, but this measure may be normal in early presymptomatic individuals. Thus genetic confirmation directed by linkage or direct testing for the known mutations in a given family should be an excellent method for presymptomatic evaluation. However, because of the genetic heterogeneity of Wilson's disease, genetic testing remains impractical as a widespread screening test in sporadic patients. Currently, the clinical history, presence of Kayser-Fleischer rings, low serum ceruloplasmin levels, increased urinary copper excretion, and liver biopsy (in appropriate cases) are the criteria used to make the diagnosis in the isolated patient.

## PARKINSON'S DISEASE

A variety of genetic disorders may present with a phenotype that resembles or even matches Parkinson's disease (PD). Although most of these disorders are not responsive to L-dopa, this is not always the case. A subset of persons with SCA 3 (Machado-Joseph disease) will present with parkinsonism, which is responsive to L-dopa. In addition, a few patients, particularly men, who carry the gene for dopa-responsive dystonia, present in adult life with PD.[169] Thus it is crucial to check for these diseases in a person with parkinsonism and a family history of neurologic dysfunction.

In addition, a very few families with highly penetrant autosomal dominant forms of PD have been reported. A gene defect in the alpha synuclein gene has been reported in four large kindreds, and highly penetrant families may be assessed for this mutation on a research basis.[132] This mutation has not been found in any patients with sporadic PD. Unfortunately, evaluation for this mutation is not generally applicable to most patients with PD and a family history. Many patients with PD have a family history of one or more affected relatives, but a clear pattern of inheritance is not usually present. Consequently, other inherited forms of L-dopa-responsive PD are poorly characterized and have been reported to be autosomally recessive (possibly linked to chromosome 6), maternally inherited, or polygenic in various studies.[107,196]

## HUNTINGTON'S DISEASE

Huntington's disease (HD) is an autosomal dominant disorder associated with an unstable CAG trinucleotide repeat. The gene has been identified on chromosome 4 and encodes a protein called huntingtin. The function of the normal protein and the mechanism leading to disease in patients with the mutated protein are unknown. A direct CAG repeat test is commercially available and is highly sensitive and specific. There are numerous ethical, financial, and psychologic issues to consider when testing asymptomatic relatives of patients with HD. Pretest and posttest counseling are important and necessary steps in this process. Guidelines and recommendations for HD testing have been formulated by the World Federation of Neurology Research Group on Huntington's Chorea.[77] Testing of asymptomatic children is generally considered unethical, and restraint is appropriate when testing symptomatic children with atypical features.[120]

The normal length of the repeat ranges from as few as 9 to as many as 39.[91,162] In affected individuals, typically one allele is of normal length and the other allele has 36 to 121 repeats, although homozygotes have been identified.[91] Rarely, asymptomatic individuals who never develop signs or symptoms of HD carry intermediate expansions (35–39) that expand in subsequent generations to lengths that cause HD. In addition, de novo expansions can occur in up to 3% of patients, and this new expansion seems to arise from the paternal allele.[145] These observations further emphasize the instability of the triplet repeat associated with HD. The length of the repeat and age of onset are inversely correlated, as in most diseases associated with triplet repeats, and very large CAG repeats have been identified in children with juvenile HD. Interestingly, paternal inheritance accounts for most cases of juvenile onset, presumably because of marked expansion of the CAG repeat during spermatogenesis. In general, the test is considered "positive" for the Huntington's gene if the triplet repeat is greater than 38, although "normal" alleles with 39 repeats have been identified.[37,91]

## ALZHEIMER'S DISEASE

Familial Alzheimer's disease (AD) accounts for <5% of all cases of AD. Four genetic abnormalities have been associated with familial AD, and mutations in three of these genes convey a high disease penetrance inherited in an autosomal dominant pattern. These include beta-amyloid precursor protein (APP) on chromosome 21, presenilin-1 (PS1) on chromosome 14, and presenilin-2 (PS2) on chromosome 1.[22,94,158] In patients with AD, each of these altered genes, all caused by point mutations, increase production or deposition of amyloid beta protein (A beta), which is the major constituent of the neuritic plaques found in the brains of patients with AD.[154,172] It has been estimated that 50% to 70%[172] of familial AD cases have mutations in one of the three identified genes—APP, PS1, or PS2. More than half of the cases are mutations of the PS1 gene, and only two reported families have been found to carry PS2 mutations thus far. More than 40 point mutations have been identified, and diagnostic genetic testing for the known mutations is available. However, it is clear that a negative screen does not rule out the possibility of the existence of an unknown mutation. Penetrance has only rarely been found to be incomplete, but the true predictive value of a positive test has not been determined.[13]

A fourth gene, the epsilon 4 allele of apolipoprotein E (apoE4) on chromosome 19, has been associated with increased risk for the development of familial and sporadic AD.[110,150] However, the presence of this allele does not guarantee the disease, nor does its absence prevent a person from having the illness. It thus is a risk factor for the disease, and consequently issues concerning testing for the apoE4 allele are much more complicated. The apoE4 allele is present in 34% to 65% of patients with AD and in 24% to 31% of nonaffected adults (JAMA consensus, 1995). Homozygosity for apoE4 increases the risk for AD, which has been estimated to carry a cumulative risk of 50% by 80 years (JAMA consensus, 1995). Thus the presence of one or two apoE4 alleles is neither sensitive nor specific for the diagnosis of AD. At this time genetic testing for the presence of apoE4 is not recommended for predictive use in asymptomatic individuals. Although some groups are in favor of its use as an adjunctive test in patients suspected of having AD, its role in the diagnosis of AD is unclear at this time.[110]

## INHERITED EPILEPSIES

Inherited epilepsies can be associated with symptomatic epilepsies (in which diffuse brain dysfunction exists) and with idiopathic epilepsy (in which seizure disorder is the main neurologic manifestation). More than 200 symptomatic genetic epilepsies have been described.[11] One example is progressive myoclonus epilepsy, which includes Lafora type, Unverricht-Lundborg disease and related syndromes, ceroid lipofuscinosis, sialidosis type 1, and myoclonic epilepsy with ragged-red fibers. Another example is fragile X syndrome, a triplet repeat disorder in which epilepsy is a portion of the overall syndrome. Genetic testing is available and may be useful in the diagnosis of many of these disorders. The idiopathic inherited epilepsies include benign familial neonatal convulsion, juvenile myoclonic epilepsy, childhood absence epilepsy, benign rolandic epilepsy, autosomal dominant nocturnal frontal lobe epilepsy (ADNFLE), and several others.[11] The first idiopathic genetic epilepsy for which a gene has been identified is ADNFLE. The gene is located on chromosome 20 and codes for the alpha 4 subunit of the nicotinic acetylcholine receptor. A nonsense mutation in this gene has also been associated with benign neonatal familial convulsions.[6] Many of the genes for the other idiopathic epilepsies have not been identified beyond location of the chromosome. Despite the advances in genotypic characterization of these disorders, genetic testing for the idiopathic epilepsies is not clinically available, and these epilepsies must be diagnosed clinically in association with characteristic electroencephalographic findings.

## STROKE

Genetic testing is rarely used in stroke because well-identified risk factors for stroke are usually present. However, there are many genetic disorders that predispose patients to thromboembolic events, including specifically identified stroke syndromes. These include sickle cell anemia, homocystinuria, mitochondrial myopathy encephalopathy lactic acidosis and strokelike episodes (MELAS), and the inherited disorders that cause hypercoagulability, including protein C deficiency, protein S deficiency, antithrombin III deficiency, and factor V Leiden.[53,88,136,175] In addition, there is a series of genetic disorders in which the primary manifestation is stroke or other vascular abnormalities. For these disorders there is no useful genetic screening tests, and they are presently best characterized by clinical evaluation with the use of genetic testing as a research tool.[55,88,122]

## NEUROCUTANEOUS SYNDROMES

The neurocutaneous syndromes (neurofibromatosis [NF 1, NF 2], tuberous sclerosis [TS], VHL) represent an area where reliable molecular testing could substantially improve the evaluation of patients at risk. These disorders have substantial variation in expressivity; therefore clinical evaluation in combination with other diagnostic testing may still not find all the individuals who carry the disorder.[58] The genes for these disorders have been cloned, and many distinct molecular abnormalities have been found. Unfortunately, the diversity of the molecular abnormalities in these disorders limits the value of the tests derived from this information.[59]

NF 1 is associated with mutations in a large protein called neurofibromin. New mutations are present in approximately 50% of all individuals, which agrees with clinical observations of the absence of a family history in 50% of new families.[157] However, the mutations in the protein are quite diverse. No single mutation accounts for a majority of the mutations, and the NF 1 gene product is large and contains 60 exons. Thus screening for mutations is extraordinarily difficult. Many mutations truncate protein; therefore testing for the presence of truncated proteins (premature truncation test [PTT]) can detect 60% to 70% of the cases when combined with DNA sequencing to confirm the mutation.[58] However, in clinical practice this test (which is relatively expensive by typical standards) is not helpful for most clinical situations. NF 1 can usually be diagnosed by clinical criteria; in fact, it is defined by clinical criteria. However, the more difficult question is how to rule out NF 1 in a patient with insufficient clinical criteria. For this situation a test that misses 30% of patients is suboptimal. Thus current PTT testing is usually of limited value. The testing can be valuable within a family with an appropriate question. If one person in the family has an abnormality detected by PTT, the test will detect the same abnormality in all patients in that family who have NF and thus will be useful for prenatal and asymptomatic testing. Linkage analysis is also quite useful within families having multiple affected family members. However, a single molecular diagnostic test for NF 1 with high sensitivity and specificity does not yet exist for isolated cases.

Diagnostic testing for NF 2 is similar at the present time. NF 2 is caused by mutation in another protein called merlin. As in NF 1, most of the mutations produce truncated proteins, but no mutation accounts for a substantial percentage of the total. As a result, tests that examine the presence of truncated protein again have a false-negative rate of >30%.[58] Again, linkage analysis is effective in families with more than one affected member, and if a mutation is found in one family member, it should be found in all members of that family who have the disease. It appears that in NF 2 the specific mutations may correlate with more severe phenotypes.[58] However, use of the exact mutation for phenotypic prediction and its extrapolation to asymptomatic individuals must be done cautiously.

With TS, the situation is even more complex. New mutations occur in approximately two thirds of all patients in one of two separate genetic loci for TS.[93,144,185] As a result, no efficacious molecular test is yet available for TS.

## CONCLUSION

The use of diagnostic tests is complicated and depends greatly on the clinical characteristics of the disease being assessed. Although genetic testing may be useful for diagnosis, counseling, and selection of therapy, it is not the only clinical tool for assessing genetic disease. Advances in clinical evaluation of genetic disease will reflect advances in all clinical tools and always will depend heavily on a reliable history and physical examination in all patients.

## REFERENCES

1. Alford RL, Ashizawa T, Jankovic J, et al. Molecular detection of new mutations, resolution of ambiguous results and complex genetic counseling issues in Huntington disease. *Am J Med Genet.* 1996;66:281.
2. Almasy L, Bressman SB, Raymond D, et al. Idiopathic torsion dystonia linked to chromosome 8 in two Mennonite families. *Ann Neurol.* 1997; 42:670.
3. Apolipoprotein E genotype in familial Parkinson's disease. The French Parkinson's Disease Genetics Study Group. *J Neurol Neurosurg Psychiatry.* 1997;63:384.
4. Bartholome K, Ludecke B. Mutations in the tyrosine hydroxylase gene cause various forms of L-dopa–responsive dystonia. *Adv Pharmacol.* 1998;42:48.
5. Bartram C, Edwards RHT, Clague J, et al. McArdle's disease: a nonsense mutation in exon 1 of the muscle glycogen phosphorylase gene explains some but not all the cases. *Hum Mol Genet.* 1993;2:1291.
6. Beck C, Moulard B, Steinlein O, et al. A nonsense mutation in the alpha 4 subunit of the nicotinic acetylcholine receptor (CHRNA4) cosegregates with 20q-linked benign neonatal familial convulsions (EBNI). *Neurobiol Dis.* 1994;1:95.
7. Beggs AH, Koenig M, Boyce FM, et al. Detection of 98% of Duchenne muscular dystrophy/Becker muscular dystrophy gene deletions by polymerase chain reaction. *Hum Genet.* 1990;86:45.
8. Bentivoglio AR, Del Grosso N, Albanese A, et al. Non-DYT1 dystonia in a large Italian family. *J Neurol Neurosurg Psychiatry.* 1997;62:357.
9. Berciano J, Combarros O, De Castro M, et al. Intronic GAA triplet repeat expansion in Friedreich's ataxia presenting with pure sensory ataxia. *J Neurol.* 1997;244:390.

10. Bergoffen J, Scherer SS, Wang S, et al. Connexin mutations in X-linked Charcot-Marie-Tooth disease. *Science.* 1993;262:2039.
11. Berkovic SF, Scheffer IE. Epilepsies with single gene inheritance. *Brain Dev.* 1997;19:13.
12. Bione S, Maestrini E, Rivella S. Identification of a novel X-linked gene responsible for Emery-Dreifuss muscular dystrophy. *Nat Genet.* 1994; 8:323.
13. Bird TD, Levy-Lahad E, Poorkaj T, et al. Wide range in age of onset for chromosome 1–related familial Alzheimer's disease. *Ann Neurol.* 1996; 40:932.
14. Booth DR, Tan SY, Hawkins PN, et al. A novel variant of transthyretin, 59Thr→Lys, associated with autosomal dominant cardiac amyloidosis in an Italian family. *Circulation.* 1995;91:962.
15. Bressman SB, de Leon D, Raymond D, et al. Secondary dystonia and the *DYT1* gene. *Neurology.* 1997;48:1571.
16. Brown J Jr, Fingert JH, Taylor CM, et al. Clinical and genetic analysis of a family affected with dominant optic atrophy (OPA1). *Arch Ophthal.* 1997;115:95.
17. Burk K, Abele M, Fetter M, et al. Autosomal dominant cerebellar ataxia type I clinical features and MRI in families with SCA1, SCA2 and SCA3. *Brain.* 1996;119:1497.
18. Campuzano V, Montermini L, Molto MD, et al. Friedreich's ataxia: autosomal recessive disease caused by an intronic GAA triplet repeat expansion. *Science.* 1996;271:1423.
19. Cancel G, Durr A, Didierjean O, et al. Molecular and clinical correlations in spinocerebellar ataxia 2: a study of 32 families. *Hum Mol Genet.* 1997;6:709.
20. Chance PF, Alderson MK, Leppig KA, et al. DNA deletion associated with hereditary neuropathy with liability to pressure palsies. *Cell.* 1993;72:143.
21. Chance PF, Matsunami N, Lensch W, et al. Analysis of the DNA duplication 17p11.2 in Charcot-Marie-Tooth neuropathy type 1 pedigrees: additional evidence for a third autosomal CMT1 locus. *Neurology.* 1992;42:2037.
22. Citron M, Oltersdorf T, Haass C, et al. Mutation of the beta-amyloid precursor protein in familial Alzheimer's disease increases beta-protein production. *Nature.* 1992;360:672.
23. Comu S, Giuliani M, Narayanan V. Episodic ataxia and myokymia syndrome: a new mutation of potassium channel gene *Kv1.1. Ann Neurol.* 1996;40:684.
24. Concannon P, Gatti RA. Diversity of ATM gene mutations detected in patients with ataxia-telangiectasia. *Hum Mutat.* 1997;10:100.
25. Cornelio F, Bresolin N, DiMauro S, et al. Congenital myopathy due to phosphorylase deficiency. *Neurology.* 1983;33:1383.
26. Cossee M, Schmitt M, Campuzano V, et al. Evolution of the Friedreich's ataxia trinucleotide repeat expansion: founder effect and permutations. *Proc Nat Acad Sci U S A.* 1997;94:7452.
27. Cruz-Martinez A, Anciones B, Palau F. GAA trinucleotide repeat expansion in variant Friedreich's ataxia families. *Muscle Nerve.* 1997;20: 1121.
28. David G, Abbas N, Stevanin G, et al. Cloning of the *SCA7* gene reveals a highly unstable CAG repeat expansion. *Nat Genet.* 1997;17:65.
29. Dodd A, Rowland SA, Hawkes SL, Kennedy MA, Love DR. Mutations in the adrenoleukodystrophy gene. *Hum Mutat.* 1997;9:500.
30. Doriguzzi C, Palmucci L, Mongini T, et al. Systematic use of dystrophin testing in muscle biopsies: results in 201 cases. *Eur J Clin Invest.* 1997;27:352.
31. Driscoll DA, Salvin J, Sellinger B, et al. Prevalence of 22q11 microdeletions in DiGeorge and velocardiofacial syndromes: implications for genetic counseling and prenatal diagnosis. *J Med Genet.* 1993;30:813.
32. Dubourg O, Durr A, Cancel G, et al. Analysis of the *SCA1* CAG repeat in a large number of families with dominant ataxia: clinical and molecular correlations. *Ann Neurol.* 1995;37:176.
33. Duggan DJ, Gorospe JR, Fanin M, et al. Mutations in the sarcoglycan genes in patients with myopathy. *N Engl J Med.* 1997;336:618.
34. Duggan DJ, Hoffman EP. Autosomal recessive muscular dystrophy and mutations of the sarcoglycan complex. *Neuromuscul Dis.* 1996;6:475.
35. Dürr A, Cossee M, Agid Y, et al. Clinical and genetic abnormalities in patients with Friedreich's ataxia. *N Engl J Med.* 1996;335:1169.
36. Durr A, Stevanin G, Cancel G, et al. Spinocerebellar ataxia 3 and Machado-Joseph disease: clinical, molecular, and neuropathological features. *Ann Neurol.* 1996;39:490.
37. Duyao M, Ambrose C, Myers R, et al. Trinucleotide repeat length instability and age of onset in Huntington's disease. *Nat Genet.* 1993; 4:387.

38. El-Schahawi M, Tsujino S, Shanske S, et al. Diagnosis of McArdle's disease by molecular genetic analysis of blood. *Neurology.* 1996;47:579.

39. Epplen C, Epplen JT, Frank G, et al. Differential stability of the (GAA)n tract in the Friedreich ataxia (*STM7*) gene. *Hum Genet.* 1997; 99:834.

40. Evans MI, Greb A, Kunkel LM, et al. In utero fetal muscle biopsy for the diagnosis of Duchenne muscular dystrophy. *Am J Obstet Gynecol.* 1991;165:728.

41. Fadic R, Johns DR. Clinical spectrum of mitochondrial diseases. *Semin Neurol.* 1996;16:11.

42. Fairweather N, Bell C, Cochrane S, et al. Mutations in the connexin 32 gene in X-linked dominant Charcot-Marie-Tooth disease (CMTX1). *Hum Mol Genet.* 1994;3:29.

43. Filla A, De Michele G, Cavalcanti F, et al. The relationship between trinucleotide (GAA) repeat length and clinical features in Friedreich ataxia. *Am J Hum Genet.* 1996;59:554.

44. Flanigan K, Gardner K, Alderson K, et al. Autosomal dominant spinocerebellar ataxia with sensory axonal neuropathy (SCA4): clinical description and genetic localization to chromosome 16q22.1. *Am J Hum Genet.* 1996;59:392.

45. Fryns JP, Van Den Berghe H. Sex linked recessive inheritance in Charcot-Marie-Tooth disease with partial manifestations in female carriers. *Hum Genet.* 1980;55:413.

46. Gabreels-Festen AA, Gabreels FJ, Hoogendijk JE, et al. Chronic inflammatory demyelinating polyneuropathy or hereditary motor and sensory neuropathy? Diagnostic value of morphological criteria. *Acta Neuropathol.* 1993;86:630.

47. Gasser T, Harding AE. Molecular genetic diagnosis of neurological diseases. In: Brandt T, Caplan LR, Dichgans J, Diener HC, Kennard C, eds. Neurological Disorders: Course and Treatment. New York: Academic Press; 1996:1085.

48. Gellera C, Pareyson D, Castellotti B, et al. Very late onset Friedreich's ataxia without cardiomyopathy is associated with limited GAA expansion in the *X25* gene. *Neurology.* 1997;49:1153.

49. Geschwind DH, Perlman S, Figueroa CP, et al. The prevalence and wide clinical spectrum of the spinocerebellar ataxia type 2 trinucleotide repeat in patients with autosomal dominant cerebellar ataxia. *Am J Genet.* 1997;60:842.

50. Geschwind DH, Perlman S, Figueroa KP, et al. Spinocerebellar ataxia type 6: frequency of the mutation and genotype phenotype correlations. *Neurology.* 1997;49:1196.

51. Gilbert JR, Stajich JM, Wall S, et al. Evidence for heterogeneity in facioscapulohumeral muscular dystrophy (FSHD). *Am J Hum Genet.* 1993;53:401.

52. Goldfarb LG, Vasconcelos O, Platonov FA, et al. Unstable triplet repeat and phenotypic variability of spinocerebellar ataxia type 1. *Ann Neurol.* 1996;39:500.

53. Goto Y. MELAS (mitochondrial myopathy, encephalopathy lactic acidosis, and stroke-like episodes): clinical features and mitochondrial DNA mutations. *Nippon Rinsho.* 1993;51:2373.

54. Gotoda T, Arita M, Arai H, et al. Adult-onset spinocerebellar dysfunction caused by a mutation in the gene for the (alpha)-tocopherol-transfer protein. *N Engl J Med.* 1995;333:1313.

55. Greenberg DA. Calcium channels in neurological disease. *Ann Neurol.* 1997;42:275.

56. Greenstein PE, Moore D, Levy-Lohad E, et al. Nine families with the SCA3/Machado-Joseph disease type of inherited ataxia. *Neurology.* 1996;47:1106.

57. Griggs RC, Tawil R, Storvick D, et al. Genetics of facioscapulohumeral muscular dystrophy: new mutations in sporadic cases. *Neurology.* 1993;43:2369.

58. Gutmann DH, Aylsworth A, Carey JC, et al. The diagnostic evaluation and multidisciplinary management of neurofibromatosis 1 and neurofibromatosis 2. *JAMA.* 1997;278:51.

59. Haass C, Hung AY, Selkoe DJ, et al. Mutations associated with a locus for familial Alzheimer's disease result in alternative processing of amyloid beta-protein precursor. *J Biol Chem.* 1994;269:17741.

60. Hahnen E, Schonling J, Rudnik-Schoneborn S, et al. Missense mutations in exon 6 of the survival motor neuron gene in patients with spinal muscular atrophy (SMA). *Hum Mol Genet.* 1997;6:821.

61. Hallam PJ, Harding AE, Berciano J, et al. Duplication of part of chromosome 17 is commonly associated with hereditary motor and sensory neuropathy type 1 (Charcot-Marie-Tooth disease type 1). *Ann Neurol.* 1992;31:570.

62. Hardell L, Holmgren G, Steen L, Fredrikson M, Axelson O. Occupational and other risk factors for clinically overt familial amyloid polyneuropathy. *Epidemiology.* 1995;6:598.

62a. Hattori N, Kitada T, Matsumine H, et al. Molecular genetic analysis of a novel parkin gene in Japanese families with autosomal recessive parkinsonism: evidence for variable homozygous deletions in the parkin gene in affected individuals. *Ann Neurol.* 1998;44:935.

63. Hayasaka K, Himoro M, Sawaishi Y, et al. De novo mutation of the myelin $P_0$ gene in Dejerine-Sottas disease (hereditary motor and sensory neuropathy type III). *Nat Genet.* 1993;5:266.

64. Hayasaka K, Himoro M, Sato W, et al. Charcot-Marie-Tooth neuropathy type 1B is associated with mutations of the myelin $P_0$ gene. *Nat Genet.* 1993;5:31.

65. Higgins JJ, Nee LE, Vasconcelos O, et al. Mutations in American families with spinocerebellar ataxia (SCA) type 3: SCA3 is allelic to Machado-Joseph disease. *Neurology.* 1996;46:208.

66. Hirano M, Imaiso Y, Ueno S. Differential splicing of the GTP cyclohydrolase I RNA in dopa-responsive dystonia. *Biochem Biophys Res Commun.* 1997;234:316.

67. Hirano M, Silvestri G, Blake DM, et al. Mitochondrial neurogastrointestinal encephalomyopathy (MNGIE): clinical, biochemical, and genetic features of an autosomal recessive mitochondrial disorder. *Neurology.* 1994;44:721.

68. Hoffman EP, Kunkel LM, Angelini C, et al. Improved diagnosis of Becker muscular dystrophy by dystrophin testing. *Neurology.* 1989;39:1011.

69. Hoffman EP, Pegoraro E, Scacheri P, et al. Genetic counseling of isolated carriers of Duchenne muscular dystrophy. *Am J Med Genet.* 1996;63:573.

70. Holmgren G, Ozelius L, Forsgren L, et al. Adult onset idiopathic torsion dystonia is excluded from the DYT 1 region (9q34) in a Swedish family. *J Neurol Neurosurg Psychiatry.* 1995;59:178.

71. Hoogendijk JE, Hensels GW, Gabreels-Festen AA, et al. De novo mutation in hereditary motor and sensory neuropathy type 1. *Lancet.* 1992;339:1081.

72. Ichinose H, Nagatsu T. Molecular genetics of hereditary dystonia: mutations in the *GTP* cyclohydrolase I gene. *Brain Res Bull.* 1997;43:35.

73. Ikeda S, Nakano T, Yanagisawa N, Nakazato M, Tsukagoshi H. Asymptomatic homozygous gene carrier in a family with type I familial amyloid polyneuropathy. *Eur Neurol.* 1992;32:308.

74. Ikegami T, Nicholson G, Ikeda H, et al. A novel homozygous mutation of the myelin $P_0$ gene producing Dejerine-Sottas disease (hereditary motor and sensory neuropathy type III). *Biochem Biophys Res Commun.* 1996;222:107.

75. Ikeuchi T, Koide R, Onodera O, et al. Dentatorubral-pallidoluysian atrophy (DRPLA): molecular basis for wide clinical features of DRPLA. *Clin Neurosci.* 1995;3:23.

76. Imbert G, Saudou F, Yvert G, et al. Cloning of the gene for spinocerebellar ataxia 2 reveals a locus with high sensitivity to expanded CAG/glutamine repeats. *Nat Genet.* 1996;14:285.

77. International Huntington's Association (IHA) and the World Federation of Neurology (WFN) Research Group on Huntington's Chorea. Guidelines for the molecular genetics predictive test in HD. *Neurology.* 1994;44:1533.

78. Ionasescu VV, Ionasescu R, Searby CC, et al. Dejerine-Sottas disease with de novo dominant point mutation of *PMP 22* gene. *Neurology.* 1995;45:1766.

79. Ionasescu VV, Kimura J, Searby CC, Smith WL, Ross M, Ionasescu RA. Dejerine-Sottas neuropathy family with a gene mapped on chromosome 8. *Muscle Nerve.* 1996;19:319.

80. Ionasescu V, Searby C, Ionasescu R. Point mutations of the connexin 32. (GJB1) gene in X-linked dominant Charcot-Marie-Tooth neuropathy. *Hum Mol Genet.* 1994;3:355.

81. Ionasescu V, Searby C, Ionasescu R, et al. New point mutations and deletions of the connexin 32 gene in X-linked Charcot-Marie-Tooth neuropathy. *Neuromuscul Dis.* 1995;5:297.

82. Isnard R, Kalotka H, Dürr A, et al. Correlation between left ventricular hypertrophy and GAA trinucleotide repeat length in Friedreich's ataxia. *Circulation.* 1997;95:2247.

83. Jansen GA, Ofman R, Ferdinandusse S, et al. Refsum disease is caused by mutations in the phytanoyl-CoA hydroxylase gene. *Nat Genet.* 1997;17:190.

84. Jarman PR, Bandmann O, Marsden CD, et al. GTP cyclohydrolase I mutations in patients with dystonia responsive to anticholinergic drugs. *J Neurol Neurosurg Psychiatry.* 1997;63:304.

85. Jobsis GJ, Weber JW, Barth PG, et al. Autosomal dominant cerebellar

ataxia with retinal degeneration (ADCA II): clinical and neuropathological findings in two pedigrees and genetic linkage to 3p12-p21.1. *J Neurol Neurosurg Psychiatry*. 1997;62:367.

86. Johns DR. Seminars in medicine of the Beth Israel Hospital, Boston. Mitochondrial DNA and disease. *N Engl J Med*. 1995;333:638.

87. Jones KJ, North KN. Recent advances in diagnosis of the childhood muscular dystrophies. *J Paediatr Child Health*. 1997;33:195.

88. Joutel A, Corpechot C, Ducros A, et al. Notch 3 mutations in cerebral autosomal dominant arteriopathy with subcortical infarcts and leukoencephalopathy (CADASIL), a mendelian condition causing stroke and vascular dementia. *Ann N Y Acad Sci*. 1997;826:213.

89. Kiechle FL, Kaul KL, Farkas DH. Mitochondrial disorders: methods and specimen selection for diagnostic molecular pathology. *Arch Pathol Lab Med*. 1996;120:597.

90. Kraus JP. Komrower Lecture: molecular basis of phenotype expression in homocystinuria. *J Inherit Metab Dis*. 1994;17:383.

91. Kremer B, Goldberg P, Andrew SE, et al. A worldwide study of the Huntington's disease mutation: the sensitivity and specificity of measuring CAG repeats. *N Engl J Med*. 1994;330:1402.

92. Kuller JA, Hoffman EP, Fries MH, Golbus MS. Prenatal diagnosis of Duchenne muscular dystrophy by fetal muscle biopsy. *Hum Genet*. 1992;90:34.

93. Kwiatkowska J, Slomski R, Jozwiak S, et al. Human XPMC2H: cDNA cloning, mapping to 9q34, genomic structure, and evaluation as TSC1. *Genomics*. 1997;44:350.

94. Lampe TH, Bird TD, Nochlin D, et al. Phenotype of chromosome 14-linked familial Alzheimer's disease in a large kindred. *Ann Neurol*. 1994;36:368.

95. LaSpada AR, Wilson EM, Lubahn DB, et al. Androgen receptor gene mutations in X-linked spinal and bulbar muscular atrophy. *Nature*. 1991;352:77.

96. Latour P, Blanquet F, Nelis E, et al. Mutations in the myelin protein zero associated with Charcot-Marie-Tooth disease type 1B. *Hum Mutat*. 1995;6:50.

97. Lestienne P, Bataille N. Mitochondrial DNA alterations and genetic diseases: a review. *Biomed Pharmacother*. 1994;48:199.

98. Lorenzetti D, Bohlega S, Zoghbi HY. The expansion of the CAG repeat in ataxin-2 is a frequent cause of autosomal dominant spinocerebellar ataxia. *Neurology*. 1997;49:1009.

99. Lossos A, Cohen O, Meiner V, et al. Intrafamilial heterogeneity of movement disorders: report of three cases in one family. *J Neurol*. 1997;244:426.

100. Lynch DR, Chance PF. Inherited peripheral neuropathies. *Neurologist*. 1997;3:277.

101. Lynch DR, Hara H, Yum S, et al. Autosomal dominant transmission of Dejerine-Sottas disease (HMSN III). *Neurology*. 1997;49:601.

102. Maier-Dobersberger T, Ferenci P, Polli C, et al. Detection of the His1069Gln mutation in Wilson disease by rapid polymerase chain reaction. *Ann Intern Med*. 1997;127:21.

103. Maier-Dobersberger T, Mannhalter C, Rack S, et al. Diagnosis of Wilson's disease in an asymptomatic sibling by DNA linkage analysis. *Gastroenterology*. 1996;109:2015.

104. Mancardi GL, Uccelli A, Bellone E, et al. 17p11.2 duplication is a common finding in sporadic cases of Charcot-Marie-Tooth type 1. *Eur Neurol*. 1994;34:135.

105. Manilal S, Sewry CA, Man N, et al. Diagnosis of X-linked Emery-Dreifuss muscular dystrophy by protein analysis of leukocytes and skin with monoclonal antibodies. *Neuromuscul Dis*. 1997;7:63.

106. Martinuzzi A, Tsujino S, Vergani L, et al. Molecular characterization of myophosphorylase deficiency in a group of patients from Northern Italy. *J Neurol Sci*. 1996;137:14.

107. Matsumine H, Saito M, Shimoda-Matsubayashi S, et al. Localization of a gene for an autosomal recessive form of juvenile Parkinsonism to chromosome 6q25.2-27. *Am J Hum Genet*. 1997;60:588.

108. Matsunami N, Smith B, Ballard L, et al. Peripheral myelin protein-22 gene maps in the duplication in chromosome 17p11.2 associated with Charcot-Marie-Tooth 1A. *Nat Genet*. 1992;1:176.

109. Matsuyama Z, Kawakami H, Maruyama H, et al. Molecular features of the CAG repeats of spinocerebellar ataxia 6 (SCA6). *Hum Mol Genet*. 1997;6:1283.

110. Mayeaux R, Saunders AN, Shea S, et al. Utility of apolipoprotein E genotype in the diagnosis of Alzheimer's disease. *N Engl J Med*. 1998; 338:506.

111. Miller RG, Hoffman EP. Molecular diagnosis and modern management of muscular dystrophy. *Neurol Clin*. 1994;12:699.

112. Monros E, Molto MD, Martinez F, et al. Phenotype correlation and intergenerational dynamics of the Friedreich ataxia GAA trinucleotide repeat. *Am J Hum Genet*. 1997;61:101.

113. Montermini L, Richter A, Morgan K, et al. Phenotypic variability in Friedreich ataxia: role of the associated GAA repeat expansion. *Ann Neurol*. 1997;41:675.

114. Moser HW. Adrenoleukodystrophy: phenotype, genetics, pathogenesis and therapy. *Brain*. 1997;120:1485.

115. Mostacciuolo ML, Micaglio G, Fardin P, et al. Genetic epidemiology of hereditary motor and sensory neuropathies (type 1). *Am J Med Genet*. 1991;39:479.

116. Mostacciuolo ML, Schiavon F, Angelini C, et al. Frequency of duplication at 17p11.2 in families of northeast Italy with Charcot-Marie-Tooth disease type 1. *Neuroepidemiology*. 1995;14:49.

117. Mulder DW, Kurland LT, Offord KP, et al. Familial adult motor neuron disease: amyotrophic lateral sclerosis. *Neurology*. 1986;36:511.

118. Nadal N, Rolland MO, Tranchant C, et al. Localization of Refsum disease with increased pipecolic acidaemia to chromosome 10p by homozygosity mapping and carrier testing in a single nuclear family. *Hum Mol Genet*. 1995;4:1963.

119. Nagatsu T, Ichinose H. Genetic basis of dominant dystonia. *Adv Pharmacol*. 1998;42:44.

120. Nance MA. Genetic testing of children at risk for Huntington's disease. U.S. Huntington Disease Genetic Testing Group. *Neurology*. 1997;49: 1048.

121. Nonaka I, Kobayashi O, Osari S. Nondystrophinopathic muscular dystrophies including myotonic dystrophy. *Semin Pediatr Neurol*. 1996; 3:110.

122. Ophoff RA, Terwindt GM, Vergouwe MN, et al. Familial hemiplegic migraine and episodic ataxia type-2 are caused by mutations in the $Ca^{2+}$ channel gene CACNL1A4. *Cell*. 1996;87:543.

123. Orth U, Fairweather N, Exler MC, et al. X-linked dominant Charcot-Marie-Tooth neuropathy: valine-38-methionine substitution of connexin 32. *Hum Mol Genet*. 1994;3:1699.

124. Ouahchi K, Arita M, Kayden H, et al. Ataxia with isolated vitamin E deficiency is caused by mutations in the (alpha)-tocopherol transfer protein. *Nat Genet*. 1995;9:141.

125. Ozelius LJ, Hewett JW, Page CE, et al. The early-onset torsion dystonia gene (DYT1) encodes an ATP-binding protein. *Nat Genet*. 1997; 17:40.

126. Parboosingh JS, Figlewicz DA, Krizus A, et al. Spinobulbar muscular atrophy can mimic ALS: the importance of genetic testing in male patients with atypical ALS. *Neurology*. 1997;49:568.

127. Patel PI, Roa BB, Welcher AA, et al. The gene for the peripheral myelin protein PMP-22 is a candidate for Charcot-Marie-Tooth disease type 1A. *Nat Genet*. 1992;1:159.

128. Paul DL. New functions for gap junctions. *Curr Opin Cell Biol*. 1995; 7:665.

129. Paulson HL, Fischbeck KH. Trinucleotide repeats in neurogenetic disorders. *Ann Rev Neurosci*. 1996;19:79.

130. Petrukhin K, Fisher SG, Pirastu M, et al. Mapping, cloning and genetic characterization of the region containing the Wilson's disease gene. *Nat Genet*. 1993;5:338.

131. Phillips LH, Kelly TE, Schnatterly P, et al. Hereditary motor-sensory neuropathy (HMSN): possible X-linked dominant inheritance. *Neurology*. 1985;35:498.

132. Polymeropoulos MH, Lavedan C, Leroy E, et al. Mutation in the alpha-synuclein gene identified in families with Parkinson's disease. *Science*. 1997;276:2045.

133. Pulst SM, Nechiporuk A, Nechiporuk T, et al. Moderate expansion of a normally biallelic trinucleotide repeat in spinocerebellar ataxia type 2. *Nat Genet*. 1996;14:269.

134. Ranum LP, Lundgren JK, Schut LJ, et al. Spinocerebellar ataxia type 1 and Machado-Joseph disease: incidence of CAG expansions among adult-onset ataxia patients from 311 families with dominant, recessive, or sporadic ataxia. *Am J Hum Genet*. 1995;57:603.

135. Rautenstrauss B, Nelis E, Grehl H, et al. Identification of a de novo insertional mutation in $P_0$ in a patient with a Dejerine-Sottas syndrome (DSS) phenotype. *Hum Mol Genet*. 1994;3:1701.

136. Rees D. The population genetics of factor V Leiden (Arg 506 Gln). *Br J Haematol*. 1996;95:579.

137. Reilly MM, Staunton H, Harding AE. Familial amyloid polyneuropathy (TTR ala 60) in northwest Ireland: a clinical, genetic, and epidemiological study. *J Neurol Neurosurg Psychiatry*. 1995;59:45.

138. Riess O, Schols L, Bottger H, et al. SCA6 is caused by moderate CAG

expansion in the alpha 1A-voltage-dependent calcium channel gene. *Hum Mol Genet.* 1997;6:1289.

139. Roa BB, Dyck PJ, Marks HG, et al. Dejerine-Sottas syndrome associated with point mutation in the peripheral myelin protein 22 (PMP22) gene. *Nat Genet.* 1993;5:269.

140. Roa BB, Garcia CA, Pentao L, et al. Evidence for a recessive PMP22 point mutation in Charcot-Marie-Tooth disease type 1A. *Nat Genet.* 1993;5:189.

141. Roa BB, Garcia CA, Suter U, et al. Charcot-Marie-Tooth disease type 1A: association with a spontaneous point mutation in the PMP22 gene. *N Engl J Med.* 1993;329:96.

142. Roy N, Mahadevan MS, McLean M, et al. The gene for neuronal apoptosis inhibitory protein is partially deleted in individuals with spinal muscular atrophy. *Cell.* 1995;80:167.

143. Salvi F, Salvi G, Volpe R, et al. Transthyretin-related TTR hereditary amyloidosis of the vitreous body: clinical and molecular characterization in two Italian families. *Ophthalmol Paediatr Genet.* 1993;14:9.

144. Sampson JR, Harris PC. The molecular genetics of tuberous sclerosis. *Hum Mol Genet.* 1994;3(Spec No):1477.

145. Sanchez M, Mila M, Castellvi S, et al. Maternal transmission in sporadic Huntington's disease. *J Neurol Neurosurg Psychiatry.* 1997;62:535.

146. Sanpei K, Takano H, Igarashi S, et al. Identification of the spinocerebellar ataxia type 2 gene using a direct identification of repeat expansion and cloning technique, DIRECT. *Nat Genet.* 1996;14:277.

147. Sapp R, Rosen D, Hosler B, et al. Identification of three novel mutations in the gene for Cu/Zn superoxide dismutase in patients with familial amyotrophic lateral sclerosis. *Neuromuscul Dis.* 1995;5:353.

148. Saraiva MJ. Transthyretin mutations in health and disease. *Hum Mutat.* 1995;5:191.

149. Sasaki H, Fukazawa T, Wakisaka A, et al. Central phenotype and related varieties of spinocerebellar ataxia 2 (SCA2): a clinical and genetic study with a pedigree in Japan. *J Neurol Sci.* 1996;144:176.

150. Saunders AM, Strittmatter WJ, Schmechel D, et al. Association of apolipoprotein E allele epsilon 4 with late-onset familial and sporadic Alzheimer's disease. *Neurology.* 1993;43:1467.

151. Schapira AH. Mitochondrial disorders. *Curr Opin Neurol.* 1997;10:43.

152. Scheuner D, Eckman C, Jensen M, et al. Secreted amyloid beta-protein similar to that in the senile plaques of Alzheimer's disease is increased in vivo by the presenilin 1 and 2 and APP mutations linked to familial Alzheimer's disease. *Nat Med.* 1996;2:864.

153. Schols L, Amoiridis G, Epplen JT, et al. Relations between genotype and phenotype in German patients with Machado-Joseph disease mutation. *J Neurol Neurosurg Psychiatry.* 1996;61:466.

154. Selkoe DJ. Alzheimer's disease: genotypes, phenotypes, and treatments. *Science.* 1997;275:630.

155. Seneca S, Lissens W. DNA diagnosis of X-linked adrenoleukodystrophy. *J Inherit Metab Dis.* 1995;18(suppl 1):34.

156. Sghirlanzoni A, Pareyson D, Balestrini MR, et al. HMSN III phenotype due to homozygous expression of a dominant HMSN II gene. *Neurology.* 1992;42:2201.

157. Shen MH, Harper PS, Upadhyaya M. Molecular genetics of neurofibromatosis type 1 (NF1). *J Med Genet.* 1996;33:2.

158. Sherrington R, Froelich S, Sorbi S, et al. Alzheimer's disease associated with mutations in presenilin 2 is rare and variably penetrant. *Hum Mol Genet.* 1996;5:985.

159. Siddique TS, Figlewicz DA, Pericak-Vance M, et al. Linkage of a gene causing familial amyotrophic lateral sclerosis to chromosome 21 and evidence of genetic locus heterogeneity. *N Engl J Med.* 1991;324:1381.

160. Silveira I, Lopes-Cendes I, Kish S, et al. Frequency of spinocerebellar ataxia type 1, dentatorubropallidoluysian atrophy, and Machado-Joseph disease mutations in a large group of spinocerebellar ataxia patients. *Neurology.* 1996;46:214.

161. Simard LR, Rochette C, Semionov A, et al. SMN(T) and NAIP mutations in Canadian families with spinal muscular atrophy (SMA): genotype/phenotype correlations with disease severity. *Am J Med Genet.* 1997;72:51.

162. Snell RG, MacMillan JC, Cheadle JP, et al. Relationship between trinucleotide repeat expansion and phenotypic variation in Huntington's disease. *Nat Genet.* 1993;4:393.

163. Somerville MJ, Hunter AG, Aubry HL, et al. Clinical application of the molecular diagnosis of spinal muscular atrophy: deletions of neuronal apoptosis inhibitor protein and survival motor neuron genes. *Am J Med Genet.* 1997;69:159.

164. Sousa A, Andersson R, Drugge U, Holmgren G, Sandgren O. Familial amyloidotic polyneuropathy in Sweden: geographical distribution, age of onset, and prevalence. *Hum Hered.* 1993;43:288.

165. Spencer MJ, Tidball JG, Anderson LV, et al. Absence of calpain 3 in a form of limb-girdle muscular dystrophy (LGMD2A). *J Neurol Sci.* 1997;146:173.

166. Spira PJ, McLeod JG, Evans WA. A spinocerebellar degeneration with X-linked inheritance. *Brain.* 1979;102:27.

167. Spray DC, Dermietzel R. X-linked dominant Charcot-Marie-Tooth disease and other potential gap-junction diseases of the nervous system. *Trends Neurosci.* 1995;18:256.

168. Stevanin G, Durr A, David G, et al. Clinical and molecular features of spinocerebellar ataxia type 6. *Neurology.* 1997;49:1243.

169. Takahashi H, Snow BJ, Nygaard TG, Calne DB. Clinical heterogeneity of dopa-responsive dystonia: PET observations. *Adv Neurol.* 1993;60:586.

170. Takiyama Y, Sakoe K, Nakano I, et al. Machado-Joseph disease: cerebellar ataxia and autonomic dysfunction in a patient with the shortest known expanded allele (56 CAG repeat units) of the MJD1 gene. *Neurology.* 1997;49:604.

171. Tan E, Topaloglu H, Sewry C, et al. Late onset muscular dystrophy with cerebral white matter changes due to partial merosin deficiency. *Neuromuscul Dis.* 1997;7:85.

172. Tanzi RE, Kovacs DM, Kim TW, et al. The gene defects responsible for familial Alzheimer's disease. *Neurobiol Dis.* 1996;3:159.

173. Thomas GR, Forbes JR, Roberts EA, et al. The Wilson disease gene: spectrum of mutations and their consequences. *Nat Genet.* 1996;9:210.

174. Thomas GR, Roberts EA, Walshe JM, et al. Haplotypes and mutations in Wilson disease. *Am J Hum Genet.* 1995;56:1325.

175. Thorarensen O, Ryan S, Hunter J, et al. Factor V Leiden mutation: an unrecognized cause of hemiplegic cerebral palsy, neonatal stroke, and placental thrombosis. *Ann Neurol.* 1997;42:372.

176. Timmerman V, Nelis E, Van Hul W, et al. The peripheral myelin protein gene PMP-22 is contained within the Charcot-Marie-Tooth disease type 1A duplication. *Nat Genet.* 1992;1:171.

177. Torres MF, Almeida MR, Saraiva MJ. TTR exon scanning in peripheral neuropathies. *Neuromuscul Dis.* 1995;5:187.

178. Tsujino S, Shanske S, DiMauro S. Molecular genetic heterogeneity of myophosphorylase deficiency (McArdle's disease). *N Engl J Med.* 1993;329:241.

179. Tsujino S, Shanske S, Goto Y, et al. Two mutations, one novel and one frequently observed, in Japanese patients with McArdle's disease. *Hum Mol Genet.* 1994;3:1005.

180. Uziel G, Moroni I, Lamantea E, Fratta GM, Ciceri E, Carrara F, Zeviani M. Mitochondrial disease associated with the T8993G mutation of the mitochondrial ATPase 6 gene: a clinical, biochemical, and molecular study in six families. *J Neurol Neurosurg Psychiatry.* 1997;63:16.

181. Vainzof M, Passos-Bueno MR, Canovas M, et al. The sarcoglycan complex in the six autosomal recessive limb-girdle muscular dystrophies. *Hum Mol Genet.* 1996;5:1963.

182. Valentijn LJ, Baas F, Wolterman RA, et al. Identical point mutations of PMP-22 in Trembler-J mouse and Charcot-Marie-Tooth disease type 1A. *Nat Genet.* 1992;2:288.

183. Valentijn LJ, Baas F, Zorn I, et al. Alternatively sized duplication in Charcot-Marie-Tooth disease type 1A. *Hum Mol Genet.* 1993;2:2143.

184. van der Kooi AJ, Barth PG, Busch HF, et al. The clinical spectrum of limb girdle muscular dystrophy: a survey in The Netherlands. *Brain.* 1996;119:1471.

185. van Slegtenhorst M, de Hoogt R, Hermans C, et al. Identification of the tuberous sclerosis gene TSC1 on chromosome 9q34. *Science.* 1997;277:805.

186. Vidal R, Garzuly F, Budka H, et al. Meningocerebrovascular amyloidosis associated with a transthyretin mis-sense mutation at codon 18 (TTRD 18G). *Am J Pathol.* 1996;148:361.

187. Walshe JM. Treatment of Wilson's disease: the historical background. *QJM.* 1996;89:553.

188. Warner TT, Schapira AH. Genetic counseling in mitochondrial diseases. *Curr Opin Neurol.* 1997;10:408.

189. Weiffenbach B, Dubois J, Storvick D, et al. Mapping the facioscapulohumeral muscular dystrophy gene is complicated by chromosome 4q35 recombination. *Nat Genet.* 1993;4:165.

190. Wilhelmsen KC, Weeks DE, Nygaard TG, et al. Genetic mapping of "Lubag" (X-linked dystonia-parkinsonism) in a Filipino kindred to the pericentromeric region of the X chromosome. *Ann Neurol.* 1991;29:124.

191. Winane S, Bergoffen J, Fairweather ND, et al. X-linked Charcot-Marie-Tooth disease (CMTX1): a study of 15 families with 12 highly informative polymorphisms. *J Med Genet.* 1994;31:193.

192. Winokur ST, Bengtsson U, Feddersen J, et al. The DNA rearrangement associated with facioscapulohumeral muscular dystrophy involves a heterochromatin-chromatin structure in the pathogenesis of the disease. *Chromosome Res.* 1994;2:225.

193. Wirth B, Tessarolo D, Hahnen E, et al. Different entities of proximal spinal muscular atrophy within one family. *Hum Genet.* 1997;100:676.

194. Wise CA, Garci CA, Davis SN, et al. Molecular analyses of unrelated Charcot-Marie-Tooth (CMT) disease patients suggest a high frequency of the CMT1A duplication. *Am J Hum Genet.* 1993;53:853.

195. Yoshioka R, Dyck PJ, Chance PF. Genetic heterogeneity in Charcot-Marie-Tooth neuropathy type 2. *Neurology.* 1996;46:569.

196. Prusiner SB. The prion diseases. *Brain Pathol.* 1998;8:499.

197. Kobayashi H, Garcia CA, Alfonso G, et al. Molecular genetics of familial spastic paraplegia: a multitude of responsible genes. *J Neurol Sci.* 1996;137:131.

198. Ptacek L. The familial periodic paralyses and nondystrophic myotonias. *Am J Med.* 1998;105:58.

# DIAGNOSTIC REASONING, MEDICOLEGAL ASPECTS, AND PRACTICE PARAMETERS

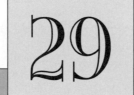

# Decision Making and Diagnostic Reasoning

*David R. Gifford, Brian S. Mittman, and Barbara G. Vickrey*

Physicians' decisions about diagnostic tests, procedures, hospitalization, referrals, and treatments affect patient outcomes and also drive many health care costs. A number of studies have shown that physicians, including neurologists, often differ in their use of diagnostic tests to evaluate similar patients[2,8,20,53,90,105] and in their use of treatments for similar clinical presentations.[2,10,39,69,78,105] The variation in physicians' clinical decisions is hypothesized to be greater when evidenced-based practice standards are lacking.[108,109] Because of concerns about the provision of high-quality care and because of the link between the costs of health care and physicians' clinical decision making, there have been efforts to reduce variation by improving decision making through greater adherence to standards of care.[14,15,32] Within the neurology community, the American Academy of Neurology (ANN) has supported efforts to improve clinical decision

making through continuing medical education (CME) programs such as CONTINUUM[77] and the development of practice parameters.[92] Despite these and other efforts, the impact on physicians' decisions, when assessed, is often modest.[15,27,32] To design more effective strategies to improve clinical decision making, others have examined the factors influencing the process and outcomes of decision making by physicians, including the diagnostic reasoning process.

This chapter focuses on the clinical decision making process and the role that diagnostic reasoning plays in it, particularly as it applies to neurologists. The principles and characteristics of clinical decision making are discussed along with the diagnostic reasoning process and several of the more important factors influencing the decision-making process. Strategies to improve decision making and diagnostic reasoning are also highlighted. Even though this chapter focuses on diagnostic decisions about the use of tests, most of the principles and concepts discussed also apply to management decisions.

## CLINICAL DECISION MAKING AND UNCERTAINTY

Clinical decision making embodies the complex processes by which physicians assess information, make judg-

This chapter is based on "Diagnostic Reasoning in Neurology," published in *Neurologic Clinics,* February 1996, and was supported in part by the Office of Research and Development, Health Services Research and Development Service, Department of Veterans Affairs, through the Sepulveda HSR&D Field Program (Center for the Study of Heathcare Provider Behavior). In addition, this work was conducted while Dr. Gifford was a Pfizer/American Geriatrics Society Postdoctoral Fellow.

**TABLE 29–1. Types of Clinical Decisions Made by Physicians**

**Diagnostic Decisions**
Assigning diagnosis
Ordering test(s)
Ordering procedures
Referring to specialist
Gathering additional information (e.g., review old records)

**Management Decisions**
Initiating treatments
Providing patient counseling or education
Referring to specialist
Arranging for follow-up
Adjusting medications
Admitting or discharging from hospital
Ordering therapeutic procedure(s)
Ordering test(s) for monitoring purposes

Modified from Gifford DR, Mittman BS, Vickrey BG. Diagnostic reasoning in neurology. *Neurol Clin.* 1996;14:224.

ments, and reach decisions. Physicians make many different types of clinical decisions, most of which can be categorized as either diagnostic or management (Table 29–1). Intrinsic to all types of decision making, and at the heart of diagnostic reasoning, is some degree of uncertainty. Uncertainty is pervasive in medicine. Uncertainty is present when a physician is defining a disease, making a diagnosis, selecting a procedure or treatment, and considering possible outcomes.[16] Therefore, at each step in the decision-making process, physicians experience some level of uncertainty.

In general, physicians use diagnostic reasoning to reduce uncertainty to a level at which they feel comfortable making a decision. Since absolute certainty is rarely achieved in clinical decision making, physicians usually must make decisions with at least some degree of uncertainty (i.e., a probability <100%). In most cases physicians make a decision or change their management at some threshold of uncertainty (or certainty about the patient's diagnosis or condition): above some probability threshold for the diagnosis, a physician will take one course of action (e.g., initiate treatment without ordering a diagnostic test), whereas below that threshold the physician would take a different course of action (e.g., withhold treatment until results of diagnostic tests become available).[18,110] This has been described as a threshold approach to decision making.[18,83,98] Implicit in the threshold approach to decision making is the concept that, although a diagnosis has a greater or lesser degree of uncertainty, this uncertainty should not impede the clinician from making a testing or treatment decision.[99]

When a threshold approach is applied to diagnostic testing, physicians must determine whether the result of the test will change their estimated probability of disease to a sufficient degree that the threshold to initiate treatment or withhold treatment is crossed. There are three thresholds with respect to treatment and testing. At one threshold, when the probability of disease is low (indicated by *P1* in Fig. 29–1), the physician does not order tests or initiate treatment. At the other extreme, when the probability of disease is high, the physician is confident of the diagnosis and initiates treatment without further diagnostic testing (*P3* in Fig. 29–1). Between these two thresholds (*P1* and *P3*) lies the no-treatment–treatment threshold (*P2* in Fig. 29–1). The levels

of these thresholds depend on many factors, including the operating characteristics of the diagnostic test (e.g., sensitivity and specificity), the prevalence of disease, and the risks and benefits associated with treatment.[83]

The range of probabilities of disease in which testing could potentially affect the decision about whether or not to initiate treatment is between *P1* and *P3* in Figure 29–1. For testing to be of value, the change in estimated probability of disease that a positive or negative test result would generate would need to cross the no-treatment–treatment threshold (*P2*). If the prior probability of disease lies below the no-treatment–treatment threshold (but above *P1*), the physician must determine whether a positive test result will sufficiently increase the probability estimate so that the treatment threshold (*P2*) is crossed. Conversely, if the prior probability estimate is above the no-treatment–treatment threshold (but below *P3*), the physician must determine whether a negative test result would lower the probability estimate so that the threshold to withhold treatment is crossed.

The failure to incorporate prognostic information provided by a diagnostic test is a limitation of the threshold approach to decision making. The change in probability of having a disease or disorder given either a positive or negative test result can change a patient's expectations and understanding about his or her condition, even if the threshold to change or initiate treatment is not crossed.[3] This may explain why women with a normal pregnancy are willing to pay for ultrasounds even though their management is unlikely to change regardless of the test's results.[6] The threshold approach therefore may not apply when patients or physicians use tests to obtain prognostic information rather than to decide if treatment should be started or altered.[3]

The threshold approach can be a powerful tool to guide physicians about when to stop further diagnostic testing and start treatment. However, physicians' tolerance or comfort with uncertainty may bias their decision making despite reaching their stated threshold since some diagnostic uncertainty will always remain. For example, in one report all physicians who ordered a liver-spleen scan to evaluate patients for suspected metastatic colon cancer were asked to state the threshold at which they would initiate treatment without ordering any further diagnostic tests.[1] However, half of the physicians were observed to continue to order additional diagnostic tests to rule out metastatic colon cancer to the liver despite reaching that previously stated threshold to initiate treatment without any additional tests.

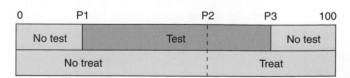

**FIGURE 29–1.** Test-treatment thresholds for a hypothetical condition. *P1* depicts the probability threshold below which no testing or treatment is initiated. *P2* depicts the threshold at which treatment is begun. *P3* depicts the threshold above which treatment is initiated without testing. Between *P1* and *P3* the results of a positive or negative test may change the probability estimate so that the treatment threshold *P2* is crossed. When the prior probability estimate is within the test region (*P1* to *P2*), a diagnostic test should be performed to determine if treatment should be withheld or initiated. (Modified from Sox HC, Blatt MA, Higgens MC, et al. *Medical Decision Making.* Boston: Butterworth-Heinemann; 1988:288.)

There are other studies that have examined the role of physicians' tolerance or comfort with uncertainty in decision making.[26,30,85] For example, emergency department physicians who were more comfortable with uncertainty, as measured by their risk-taking scores (and hence less discomfort with uncertainty), admitted 31% of patients presenting with chest pain, compared to physicians with low risk-taking scores, who admitted 51% of the patients seen with chest pain.[85] In general, studies have shown that individuals feel more comfortable with any given level of uncertainty when they are provided with more information, even when this information is irrelevant or does not reduce the uncertainty of an event.[55] The excessive use of testing that has little diagnostic benefit has been hypothesized as a mechanism by which physicians increase the amount of information available and thereby increase their comfort with uncertainty, especially when making decisions in the presence of high levels of uncertainty.[58]

Among neurologists, tolerance or comfort with uncertainty also appears to affect test ordering and treatment decisions.[105] In a national sample of neurologists who were presented with a clinical scenario depicting a typical presentation of Parkinson's disease, approximately half of the neurologists indicated they would order a neuroimaging study and start a medication to treat Parkinson's disease, despite being extremely certain of the diagnosis.[105] In addition, neurologists having higher levels of anxiety from uncertainty and less tolerance for ambiguity indicated they would order a neuroimaging study to evaluate a typical presentation of Parkinson's disease more often than neurologists who had less anxiety from uncertainty and more tolerance for ambiguity.[28] Similarly, neurologists with less reluctance to disclose uncertainty to patients were significantly more likely to discontinue antiepileptic medication that had been initiated by another physician in a patient with a single unprovoked seizure (and normal clinical imaging and electroencephalographic [EEG] studies) than neurologists having greater reluctance to disclose uncertainty to patients.[105]

Uncertainty about the outcome of a decision can also influence a physician's decisions, particularly when bad or unfavorable outcomes might occur. The regret associated with a decision that can result in an unfavorable outcome may alter a physician's decision making if the regret over such an outcome is great.[21,46] For example, studies have shown that physicians first identify a result that would, in retrospect, cause them the greatest regret and then make decisions that would minimize the chance that the result may occur.[40,76] In one study, physicians who had higher levels of regret over missing pneumonia in patients presenting to the emergency department with a fever and cold symptoms were more likely to order an unnecessary chest x-ray examination to rule out pneumonia, compared to physicians with lower levels of regret about missing pneumonia.[40]

## ASSESSING THE CHARACTERISTICS OF A DIAGNOSTIC TEST

When faced with the decision of whether to order a diagnostic test, physicians need to know how the information obtained from the test will change their uncertainty (or certainty) about a patient's condition or diagnosis.[36] To estimate the change in uncertainty about the diagnosis given a

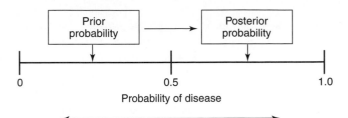

**FIGURE 29–2.** Bayes' theorem tells a physician how much to adjust the probability of disease to account for new diagnostic information. The probability of disease before new diagnostic information is interpreted is referred to as the *prior probability*. The probability of disease that results from using Bayes' theorem to interpret new diagnostic information is called the *posterior probability*. (From Sox HC, Blatt MA, Higgens MC, et al. *Medical Decision Making.* Boston: Butterworth-Heinemann; 1988:5.)

test result, physicians need to estimate the probability that the patient has the condition prior to ordering the diagnostic test, commonly referred to as the "prior probability" (Fig. 29–2). The new probability estimate of the diagnosis given the results of a diagnostic test is referred to as the "posttest" or "posterior" probability (see Fig. 29–2). If the results of a diagnostic test—positive or negative—will change the physician's "prior probability" to such a degree that the "posttest" probability crosses their threshold to assign a diagnosis or to initiate treatment, then the test provides useful information and should be ordered. On the other hand, if a negative or positive test result will have little effect on the probability estimate of disease, the test may be of little clinical value and, in general, should not be performed.[36] Instead of guessing what the change in probability will be, Bayes' theorem allows physicians to estimate more accurately the change in probability that will occur, given the results of a diagnostic test.

To apply Bayes' theorem, physicians need to estimate the prior probability and know the sensitivity and specificity of the diagnostic test. They estimate the prior probability of disease by using all available data (i.e., patient's history and physical findings), or they use the prevalence of disease (i.e., base rate probability) for their patient population. However, physicians often do not know the prevalence in their population, or they do not accurately estimate the prior probability from the information at hand (see discussion of decision heuristics).

To apply Bayes' theorem to determine the usefulness of a diagnostic test, physicians also need to know the accuracy of the diagnostic test (e.g., sensitivity and specificity). Sensitivity is a measure of the proportion of patients with the disease of interest who have a positive test result. Specificity represents the proportion of patients without the disease of interest who have a negative test (Fig. 29–3). Depending on the reason a physician orders a diagnostic test, he or she may want to select a diagnostic test with high sensitivity, high specificity, or both. For example, screening tests should have a high sensitivity to maximize the detection of patients with the target condition or disease, whereas tests used to select individuals for a high-risk procedure should have a high specificity—to minimize the number of false-positive results.[93] However, knowing the sensitivity or specificity alone does not tell a physician how useful a diagnostic test will be in most circumstances. Rather, physicians usually want to know the predictive value of a test. The predictive value is

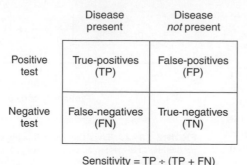

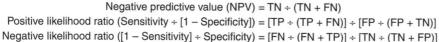

**FIGURE 29–3.** The $2 \times 2$ table method to calculate operating characteristics and utility of diagnostic tests.

Sensitivity = TP ÷ (TP + FN)

Specificity = TN ÷ (TN + FP)

Positive predictive value (PPV) = TP ÷ (TP + FP)

Negative predictive value (NPV) = TN ÷ (TN + FN)

Positive likelihood ratio (Sensitivity ÷ [1 − Specificity]) = [TP ÷ (TP + FN)] ÷ [FP ÷ (FP + TN)]

Negative likelihood ratio ([1 − Sensitivity] ÷ Specificity) = [FN ÷ (FN + TP)] ÷ [TN ÷ (TN + FP)]

Accuracy or agreement = (TP + TN) ÷ (TP + FP + FN + TN)

the probability that a patient with a positive or negative test result has the disease or does not have the disease.

By using the diagnostic test's sensitivity and specificity in conjunction with the prevalence of disease in the base population, the positive and negative predictive value of a test (in that population) can be calculated (see Fig. 29–3). The *positive predictive value* (PPV) is the proportion of patients with a positive test result (TP) who *have* disease [PPV = TP/(TP + FP)] and the *negative predictive value* (NPV) is the proportion of patients with a negative test result (TN) who *do not have* disease [NPV = TN/(TN + FN)].[24] For interpreting the results of a diagnostic test, the PPV and NPV values are more informative than the sensitivity and specificity of a diagnostic test. For example, without changing the test's sensitivity or specificity, the prevalence of disease can significantly influence the PPV and NPV and, consequently, the decision to use and the interpretation of the result of a diagnostic test.[98] Imagine a diagnostic test with both a 90% sensitivity and 90% specificity that is applied to three different populations of patients, each with a different disease prevalence: 1%, 10%, and 90% (Table 29–2). The PPV varied from 8% to 98%, and the NPV varied from 50% to 99.8%, depending on the disease prevalence. Thus, depending on the disease prevalence (or prior probability), the information that a diagnostic test provides can vary tremendously. It is also interesting to note that even when sensitivity and specificity are relatively high (i.e., 90%), the PPV can be <50% when the prevalence of disease is low (see Table 29–2).

The PPV and NPV will also vary as the sensitivity and specificity vary. Figure 29–4 demonstrates the posterior probability for a positive and negative diagnostic test result for differing prior probabilities and differing sensitivities and specificities. In general, when the prior probability is low, a positive test result will not aid in the diagnosis (i.e., will not change the pretest probability significantly) unless the test's specificity is very close to 100%.[58,99] When the prior probability is high, a negative test result only rarely substantially lowers the pretest probability (i.e., rules out the diagnosis), unless the test's sensitivity is very close to 100%.[58,99]

Once the PPV and NPV are known, Bayes' theorem can be used to estimate the change in probability, given either a positive or negative test. The PPV is equivalent to the posttest probability of disease when a test result is positive, and 1-NPV is equivalent to the posttest probability of disease when a test result is negative. Thus all one needs to know is the sensitivity and specificity of a diagnostic test and the prevalence of disease in the patient population to construct a $2 \times 2$ table and calculate the PPV and 1-NPV. For example, we can use the sensitivity and specificity of the apoE genotype test for Alzheimer's disease (AD) and the reported prevalence of AD among all patients with dementia to construct a $2 \times 2$ table in a hypothetical cohort of 100 patients with dementia (Fig. 29–5). The sensitivity of the apoE test is estimated to be 60%[79,95] and the specificity to be 68%.[68] The prevalence of AD in patients with dementia is estimated to be 57%.[9] With these estimates used, the PPV and NPV can

**TABLE 29–2. Effect of Disease Prevalence on Positive Predictive Value (PPV) and Negative Predictive Value (NPV)**

| Test Result* | Prevalence = 1% Disease† Present | Absent | Prevalence = 10% Disease† Present | Absent | Prevalence = 90% Disease† Present | Absent |
|---|---|---|---|---|---|---|
| Positive | 9 | 99 | 90 | 90 | 810 | 10 |
| Negative | 1 | 891 | 10 | 810 | 90 | 90 |
| TOTAL | 10 | 990 | 100 | 900 | 900 | 100 |
| PPV | 9/108 = 8% | | 90/180 = 50% | | 810/820 = 98.8% | |
| NPV | 891/892 = 99.8% | | 810/820 = 98.7% | | 90/180 = 50% | |

*Test sensitivity and specificity = 90%.

†Population size = 1000.

Modified from Woolf SH, Kamerow DB. Testing for uncommon conditions: the heroic search for positive test results. *Arch Intern Med.* 1990;150:2452.

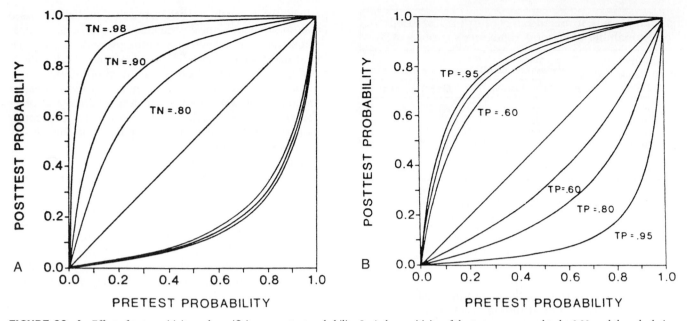

**FIGURE 29–4.** Effect of test sensitivity and specificity on posttest probability. In **A** the sensitivity of the test was assumed to be 0.90, and the calculations were repeated for several values of test specificity (TN, true negative rate). In **B** the specificity of the test was assumed to be 0.90, and the calculations were repeated for several values of sensitivity (TP, true positive rate). In both figures the top family of curves corresponds to positive test results, and the bottom family of curves corresponds to negative test results. (From Sox HC. Probability theory in the use of diagnostic tests. *Ann Intern Med.* 1986;104:60-65. Reprinted with permission from the American College of Physicians.)

be calculated from the 2 × 2 table (see Fig. 29–5). If Bayes' theorem is used, the change in probability of having AD would be from 57% to 71% for a positive apoE test and from 57% to 44% for a negative apoE test when the test is performed on a patient selected from a population of patients with dementia in which the prevalence of AD is 57%. The change in probability of having AD, given a positive or negative apoE test result, applied to patients with different prior probabilities of having AD is shown in Table 29–3.

Physicians can also estimate the change in probability of a diagnostic test by calculating the likelihood ratio of a diagnostic test. This ratio expresses the odds that a test result

would occur in a patient with the disease as opposed to a patient without the disease.[93] A positive likelihood ratio (LR) represents the ratio of those who test positive with disease (i.e., sensitivity) to those who test positive without disease (i.e., 1-specificity) or [{TP/(TP + FN)} / {FP/(FP + TN)}] (see Fig. 29–3). The negative LR represents the ratio of those who test negative with disease (i.e., sensitivity) to those who test negative without disease (i.e., specificity) or [{FN/(TP + FN)} / {TN/(FP + TN)}] (Fig. 29–3). For example, with the sensitivity and specificity for the apoE test used, the positive LR equals 1.86, and the negative LR equals 0.59 (see Fig. 29–5). To demonstrate this difference, use the nomogram in

|  | AD<br>present | AD<br>*not* present |
|---|---|---|
| ApoE test<br>positive | 34<br>True-positives<br>(TP) | 14<br>False-positives<br>(FP) |
| ApoE test<br>negative | 23<br>False-negatives<br>(FN) | 29<br>True-negatives<br>(TN) |
| Total | 57 | 43 |

**FIGURE 29–5.** Calculating utility of apoE genotype test for Alzheimer's disease (AD).

The table is constructed in a hypothetical cohort of 100 patients with dementia with a 57% prevalence of AD using a sensitivity of 60% and specificity of 68% for ApoE genotype test to diagnose AD [Prevalence 0.57 = 57/(57 + 43); Sensitivity 0.60 = TP ÷ (TP + FN) or 34/(34 + 23); Specificity 0.68 = TN ÷ (TN + FP) or 29/(29 +23)]

Positive predictive value (PPV) = TP ÷ (TP + FP) or 34/(34 + 14) = 0.708
Negative predictive value (NPV) = TN ÷ (TN + FN) or 29/(29 + 23) = 0.588
Positive likelihood ratio [Sensitivity/(1 − Specificity)] = 0.60/(1 − 0.68) or 1.86
Negative likelihood ratio [(1 − Sensitivity)/Specificity] = (1.0 − 0.60)/0.68 or 0.59

**TABLE 29–3.  Estimated Effect of ApoE Test Result on Probability of Having Alzheimer's Disease (AD)**

| PROBABILITY OF AD BEFORE ApoE TESTING | PROBABILITY OF AD AFTER ApoE TESTING* | |
|---|---|---|
| | ApoE TEST POSITIVE | ApoE TEST NEGATIVE |
| 40 | 56 | 28 |
| 50 | 65 | 37 |
| 60 | 74 | 53 |
| 70 | 81 | 58 |
| 80 | 88 | 70 |
| 90 | 94 | 84 |

*Numbers were calculated with assumption of a sensitivity of 0.60 and a specificity of 0.68. They represent the pooled estimate of reported sensitivities and specificities for AD of having at least an apoE 4 genotype. Presence of either the 3/4 or 4/4 apoE 4 allele was considered a positive test for AD.

Modified from Kosik KS, Gifford DR, Greenberg SM, et al. *Dementia Care CONTINUUM: a program of the American Academy of Neurology.* Baltimore: Williams & Wilkins; 1996;2:133.)

Figure 29–6. Place a ruler on the pretest probability of 60%, and rotate the ruler until it intersects the middle line at a likelihood ratio of 1.86. The posttest probability is the value where the ruler intersects the right-hand margin of the nomogram, or 72% in this case. The same procedure can be repeated by using the negative LR to estimate the probability of having AD given a negative apoE test. Thus, if the sensitivity and specificity are known, the LR is easy to calculate, and physicians can use Figure 29–6 to quickly estimate the posttest probability and thus decide if the diagnostic test will be helpful.

## DIAGNOSTIC REASONING

Diagnostic reasoning is an integral component of the physician's decision making process. It includes the sequence of cognitive activities during which the physician generates and evaluates different diagnostic hypotheses.[58] This activity requires the integration of multiple sources of information obtained from a patient's clinical history, physical findings, and laboratory data, along with the physician's understanding of the current scientific evidence. As the diagnostic reasoning process proceeds, some initial broad hypotheses are made more specific, other hypotheses are deleted, and new ones may be added.[58] These hypotheses form the framework for subsequent clinical decisions regarding further diagnostic testing or treatment. In general, a physician reduces uncertainty about his or her primary hypothesis to an acceptable level or threshold through the diagnostic reasoning process. This allows the physician to feel comfortable in making subsequent clinical decisions.

Physicians may employ several different approaches to diagnostic reasoning, including probabilistic, causal, and deductive approaches.[58] Each approach has advantages and disadvantages, and physicians may use one or more approaches to varying degrees in different situations.

*Probabilistic reasoning* uses probabilities that describe the association between clinical variables to generate and test hypotheses. By using probabilities, a physician expresses uncertainty in a standard form, allowing testing and evaluation of hypotheses by using mathematical principles of clinical decision making (discussed earlier). However, to employ a probabilistic approach optimally, a physician must estimate

probabilities correctly and calculate a final probability based on a multitude of clinical variables. This can be difficult, as demonstrated by research in cognitive psychology which has found that humans have difficulty performing calculations based upon more than six or seven pieces of information—a number often exceeded when physicians must consider symptoms, laboratory results, physical findings, and other information.[55,73] Research has also shown that probability estimates are subject to many biases, possibly limiting the accuracy of such estimates.[55,103]

Probabilistic reasoning can be flawed as a result of biased estimation of the prior probability of disease or because of ignoring the prevalence of disease, which leads to an incorrect calculation of the PPV and the NPV or to a biased estimate of the degree to which the test result (positive or negative) will significantly change the probability estimate. Because the clinician's perception of the value of the test is inaccurate, the physician may make an inappropriate decision about whether or not to order a diagnostic test in a given situation.

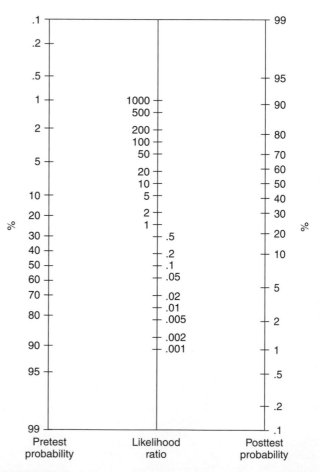

**FIGURE 29–6.** Nomogram for calculating the posterior probability of disease given the likelihood ratio of a diagnostic test. The middle scale represents the likelihood ratio of a diagnostic test (defined in Fig. 29–3). Place a ruler on the right-hand scale, which corresponds to the prior probability of disease; then adjust the ruler so that it intersects the likelihood ratio calculated for a *positive* diagnostic test. Read the posterior probability of disease for a *positive* diagnostic test on the left-hand scale. Repeat with the *negative* likelihood ratio to estimate the posterior probability of disease if the diagnostic test is *negative*. (Modified from Sackett DL. A primer on the precision and accuracy of the clinical examination. *JAMA.* 1992;267:2638. Copyrighted 1992, American Medical Association.)

*Causal reasoning* relies upon a physician's belief and knowledge of causality to test and refine hypotheses. Kassirer notes that "the process of testing, validation, verifying, and falsifying causal connections is a fundamental aspect of medical practice."[58] Causal reasoning examines the physiologic cause-and-effect relationship between clinical variables and requires a complete understanding of the scientific evidence about pathophysiology. In diagnostic decision making, causal reasoning allows a physician to determine if a patient's clinical findings are consistent with known pathophysiologic manifestations of disease and to assess alternate explanations. This process is helpful when two findings have a strong statistical relationship but no causal relationship. In this manner, causal reasoning helps to identify discrepancies among competing diagnostic hypotheses and allows the physician to gain confidence (i.e., reduce uncertainty) regarding a diagnosis.[58] When the scientific evidence is unknown or the physician's comprehension of the scientific literature is incomplete, reliance upon this process may lead to variations in decisions and practices.

*Deductive reasoning* follows a defined strategy or set of rules to generate and evaluate hypotheses. It has often been represented by branching algorithms or flow charts that follow an if-then format.[58] Many of the recently developed clinical practice guidelines and critical pathways are examples of decision support tools that rely on deductive reasoning.[37,86] However, deductive reasoning is not always applicable to all clinical conditions and decisions; for example, it is difficult to apply to patients with multiple complaints or complex clinical problems such as multiple diseases.[86]

## DECISION HEURISTICS

Decision heuristics are frequently used by physicians to assist with diagnostic reasoning. Heuristics are exemplified by unconscious cognitive processes or shortcuts, such as "rules of thumb," that are systematic and consistent and are used when arguing, recalling, or processing information.[55,98] This method is frequently used to assess probabilities and predict future events. Heuristics often improve the efficiency of diagnostic reasoning, but it also may lead to biases and errors (e.g., in probability estimation) that can result in poor decision making. Three common heuristic approaches are representativeness, availability, and anchoring and adjustment. Each plays a role in the assessment of probabilities and evaluation of diagnostic hypotheses. Physicians use each (although not consciously) in the decision making process. Each heuristic may lead to errors—particularly when used with the probabilistic reasoning approach.

The *representativeness* heuristic is the process by which an individual estimates the probability of an event (e.g., a diagnosis) based on how closely the situation resembles (or represents) the event for the entire population.[55,98] Pattern recognition is an example of physicians' use of the representativeness heuristic in medicine. For example, physicians using this approach ask how closely a patient's presentation or characteristics associated with Parkinson's disease resemble the symptoms for all patients with Parkinson's disease. This heuristic, when employed correctly, can be a powerful tool to estimate probabilities and improve diagnostic reasoning. When used incorrectly, however, the representativeness heuristic can lead to biased probability estimates and

errors in decision making.[103] Improper use of the representativeness heuristic occurs when physicians (1) use clinical cues that do not accurately predict disease, (2) rely upon clinical characteristics that are highly correlated and therefore not independent predictors of disease, and (3) compare patients to a small unrepresentative population (e.g., the patients in their own practice setting).

Physicians often rely upon previous experience with similar patients when making decisions. Unfortunately, when physicians rely heavily upon personal experience alone, they ignore base rates in favor of representativeness of personal experience. Because participants in any single practice rarely represent all patients in the relevant population, this use of the representativeness heuristic frequently leads to errors in probability estimations. As noted previously, correctly estimating the prior probability is crucial to understanding the potential value of results of a diagnostic test and thus to deciding whether to order the test.

The *availability* (recall) heuristic refers to the ease with which instances or associations come to mind in order to estimate the frequency or probability of an event.[55] In general, more frequent events are easier to remember than rare or infrequent events. Therefore frequent events should be assigned higher probabilities than infrequent events, and use of the availability heuristic should improve probabilistic reasoning. However, characteristics other than the frequency of past events can affect recall. The vividness, familiarity, salience, and distinctiveness of past events will also increase their availability for recall.[98] For example, seeing a case of a rare disease such as neuroacanthocytoses is more distinctive than reading about the disorder. Similarly, recent patients are more vividly remembered than patients seen in the distant past.

The occurrence of prior bad outcomes or the severity of the consequences associated with a decision may also increase the likelihood that a past event will be selectively or preferentially recalled. For example, the patient with atrial fibrillation who is taking coumadin and suffers a hemorrhagic stroke may be remembered more easily than the majority of other patients with atrial fibrillation taking coumadin who did not have this adverse event. Therefore use of the availability heuristic may lead to an overestimation of the probability of hemorrhagic stroke for patients with atrial fibrillation who are taking coumadin, and it may cause the physician to withhold coumadin for the next patient seen with atrial fibrillation. A survey of neurologists and cardiologists about the use of coumadin in patients with atrial fibrillation found that a perception of an increased risk of hemorrhage was the leading reason that coumadin was not recommended for a clinical scenario in which coumadin should be prescribed based upon the published risks and benefits of coumadin use in atrial fibrillation.[69] Use of the availability heuristic by surgeons and cardiologists has also been shown to lead to poor clinical decisions.[63,94] Surgeons who reported previous adverse patient outcomes that may have been prevented by a blood transfusion gave inappropriately high estimates of future bad outcomes if blood transfusions were withheld.[94] Similarly, cardiologists who chose to use tissue plasminogen activator (tPA) instead of streptokinase reported having significantly more previous adverse outcomes with streptokinase than did cardiologists who chose streptokinase.[63]

The *anchoring and adjusting* heuristic is the process by which a probability estimate is made by starting from an initial estimate (the anchor) and adjusting to take account of new information.[99] Several common errors in probability estimation can result in biased estimates when this heuristic is used because physicians generally anchor their probability estimates near the extremes (i.e., near 0% or 100%), regardless of the problem at hand, and they fail to adjust these estimates properly based upon new information.[99] Individuals also tend to overestimate small probabilities (i.e., <1%) and underestimate large probabilities (i.e., >90%). Physicians commonly base their initial probability estimates on patient age, gender, and chief complaint before gathering any additional information to adjust the initial estimate.[98] These initial estimates may be inaccurate if the anchoring and adjustment heuristic is used. As already shown, varying the prior probability significantly influences the PPV and NPV of a diagnostic test.

## FACTORS INFLUENCING CLINICAL DECISIONS

Many other factors besides uncertainty may influence physicians' clinical decisions. Studies have demonstrated that various nonclinical characteristics of a patient, characteristics of the physician, and characteristics of the practice environment contribute to variation in physicians' decisions.[17,43,57,65] These findings and corresponding theory are summarized in a conceptual model of the factors influencing clinical decision making shown in Figure 29–7. This model provides a general framework for summarizing the various factors influencing clinical decision making. The influence of any one variable on a given clinical decision depends on the type of decision in question and the interaction between the various factors present. To date, there are no published studies evaluating the relative importance of patient, physician, and practice environment characteristics—taken together—on decision making. A few studies have si-

multaneously measured and examined the relative impacts of physician and practice environment characteristics. These studies have shown that characteristics of the practice environment tend to exert greater influence on clinical decisions than do physician characteristics.[51,63]

### PHYSICIAN CHARACTERISTICS

Physician characteristics that influence decision making can be categorized into three areas: (1) demographic traits, including age and gender; (2) experience and training, including medical school training, residency, and fellowship training and prior work experience; and (3) attitudes, beliefs, and other psychologic traits, including tolerance for uncertainty and ambiguity and attitudes toward risk. All these characteristics have been shown or hypothesized to influence physician decision making. Among these numerous factors, two in particular—fear of malpractice and cost-consciousness—are especially important in a discussion of diagnostic test ordering.

Defensive medicine resulting from fear of malpractice frequently has been suggested as a cause of excessive test ordering. Few studies have evaluated this hypothesis,[17] and the results of those studies have generally not supported the hypothesis.[31] Studies of sued vs. nonsued physicians found differences in physician record keeping, avoidance of certain patients, and limitations in the scope of practice but no differences in clinical decisions or practice patterns.[96,102,107] Studies specifically examining the relationship between fear of malpractice and diagnostic test use generally have found little or no association.[4,29,31] For example, when physicians in 58 different practices recorded the reasons why they were ordering a head CT scan in 369 patients with a headache, only 5% were ordered for medicolegal concerns.[4] However, another study found that obstetricians who practiced in areas with higher rates of malpractice and who expected that more of their colleagues would be sued in the next year performed

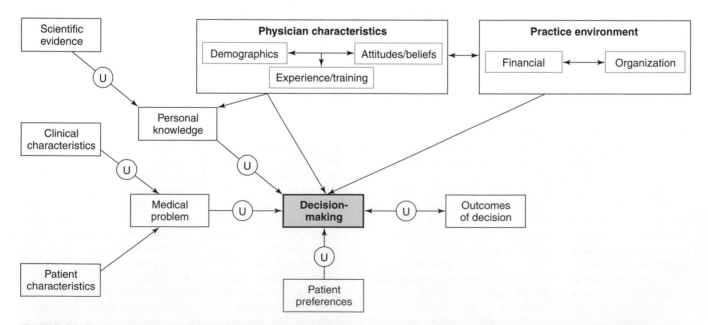

**FIGURE 29–7.** Conceptual model showing the various factors influencing clinical decision making. *Decision making* in the shaded box refers to all types of clinical decisions. Bidirectional arrows demonstrate the potential interaction between variables. Areas where uncertainty may affect decision making or modify the effect of a characteristic on decision making are depicted by a circled U. (From Gifford DR, Mittman BS, Vickrey BG. Diagnostic reasoning in neurology. *Neurol Clin.* 1996;14:231.)

more cesarean section deliveries than their counterparts with less fear of malpractice.[64]

In contrast to the evidence regarding malpractice fear, physicians' *cost-consciousness* has consistently been found to be related to test ordering. Most studies of programs that provide physicians with cost information show an approximately 30% reduction in test utilization.[17] Many of these studies are conducted on house staff or physicians who receive no financial gains or losses from test utilization, suggesting that physician attitudes toward cost containment may be independent of the financial incentives or penalties associated with use of tests. A recent study of test ordering patterns by neurologists found that neurologists with higher cost-consciousness were significantly less likely than neurologists having lower cost consciousness to indicate they would (1) order a neuroimaging study when given a clinical presentation typical for early idiopathic Parkinson's disease or (2) order an EEG when given a clinical presentation typical of Alzheimer's disease.[105]

### PRACTICE ENVIRONMENT

Practice environment characteristics can be divided into two broad categories: (1) financial (e.g., insurance mix of patients, physician's salary structure) and (2) practice organization (e.g., solo, group, or multispecialty practice or hospital- vs. non-hospital-based practice). The associations of these factors with decision making have been reviewed elsewhere[17,84]; however, a brief discussion of physician payment mechanisms is warranted in light of recent changes in the U.S. health care system.

The ways in which physicians are paid appears to have a significant effect on clinical decision making.[38,49,50] There are essentially three types of physician payment mechanisms: fee-for-service, capitation, and fixed salary.[48] Capitation is defined as "a method of payment by which the physician receives a periodic fee for each enrollee to cover all care required"; salary is "a method of payment by which the physician is remunerated at a constant rate on a regular basis."[48] Fee-for-service (FFS) is defined as a fee paid to the physician for every service rendered. In clinical situations where there are no clear standards for appropriate care, the incentives operating under FFS reimbursement are likely to induce higher utilization, whereas the incentives under capitation are for lower utilization.[13,17,48] A study examining this hypothesis found that physicians made different clinical decisions for patients in the intensive care unit (ICU) based on the patients' mechanism of reimbursement: physicians ordered fewer tests and discharged patients sooner from the ICU for patients with capitated insurance relative to comparable patients with FFS insurance.[87] Salaried physicians may experience financial incentives to overuse when bonuses are present. For example, Hemenway et al[42] found that salaried physicians significantly increased their use of tests when they received bonuses linked to increased test utilization. However, bonuses associated with capitated payments may have the opposite effect and may result in underutilization since the bonus is more often linked to lower use of resources.[47]

In relevant situations, financial incentives and disincentives do appear to exert measurable influences on physician decision making. This effect may be greater for medical care in which there is a lack of evidence or consensus about the appropriate decision. Eisenberg has suggested that "uncer-tain clinical situations may well be the ones in which the economic, sociologic, and psychological factors most influence [doctors'] decisions."[17(p 65)]

## STRATEGIES FOR IMPROVING DIAGNOSTIC REASONING AND DECISION MAKING

This chapter highlights many key challenges facing neurologists when they are attempting to make effective and efficient diagnostic and treatment decisions in the face of uncertainty, limited information, and multiple (often conflicting) objectives. In recent years the research and practitioner communities have developed and applied a broad range of strategies and tools designed to overcome these challenges and improve medical decision making. Many of these strategies aim to summarize recommended clinical decisions and practices in user-friendly formats (e.g., evidence-based reviews and clinical practice guidelines) and encourage physicians to use these resources to improve their decisions. Other strategies incorporate specific decision support tools or corrective procedures designed to eliminate or counteract adverse effects of decision biases and errors resulting from use of simplified decision heuristics. The remainder of this chapter reviews selected examples of these strategies and tools, describing applications in neurology, where available, and other specialties where applications in neurology are unknown.

### EVIDENCE-BASED MEDICINE AND CLINICAL PRACTICE GUIDELINES

The health care "outcomes" and "effectiveness" research movement of the late 1980s and 1990s and the accompanying focus on accountability and assessment in health care have been accompanied by development of a broad range of approaches for improving clinical decisions and quality. Much of this work is designed to supplement (or replace) the traditional reliance that physicians have placed on individual knowledge, judgment, and experience with more consistent and reliable bases for clinical decisions, including systematic reviews of research evidence and explicit clinical policies and practice guidelines.[11]

Clinical practice guidelines are designed to summarize and facilitate application of evidence and expert opinion regarding use of a specific clinical intervention or care for a specific medical condition.[22] Guidelines are particularly valuable for complex decisions in which the relevant evidence is extensive but not well integrated and where evidence exists regarding some of the relevant clinical decisions but not others. Guidelines are intended to substitute evidence and evidence-based expert opinion for individual clinician judgment and experience, both of which are subject to biases and errors. To ensure this foundation for evidence, many guidelines and algorithms, including the AAN's practice parameters, are developed by using an explicit evidence-based approach.[92] The expert opinion foundations of guidelines, however, are subject to decision biases and errors inherent in human judgment. For this reason, guidelines typically rely on expert consensus opinion only when research evidence is unavailable or insufficient. Furthermore, when expert opinion is incorporated into guidelines, developers of guidelines often apply methods to elicit and summarize these opinions that minimize bias and error. Methods such as the Delphi technique[82] and other tools specifically designed to avoid or compensate for individual and group decision biases (e.g., Groupthink[41]) are often used for developing practice guidelines. Guideline panels generally include individuals with a broad range of backgrounds and expertise to compensate for individual biases. Finally, many guidelines include information regarding the quality and source of evidence underlying each recommendation, using ratings that range from randomized trial data (highest rating) to weaker research designs, to case reports and informal group consensus or opinion (lowest rating).

Guidelines may be presented in many formats, including unstructured text, bulleted lists of formal clinical recommendation statements, and clinical algorithms.[37,62] The algorithms are usually highly specific and directive; they include flowcharts and decision diagrams that provide a specific sequence of points where information is needed and individual decisions must be made. By dividing a complex decision into a series of simpler individual decisions, an algorithm may reduce the tendency for a physician to make a global judgment based on a limited number of clinical variables or past experience, which may be nonrepresentative, rather than on relevant evidence and logic. However, algorithms do not always simplify nor improve complex decisions sufficiently. As Kassirer notes, "Algorithms frequently become so complicated that they cannot be represented readily in a printed figure or retained in one's conscious."[59] Algorithms have other flaws. If conditions and branch points within an algorithm are ambiguous or poorly defined, physicians may easily follow the wrong path, resulting in a careful but incorrect decision. For example, if a branch point in an algorithm for the treatment of Parkinson's disease requires an assessment of functional impairment and functional impairment is not clearly defined, two physicians using different criteria to judge functional impairment would be likely to make different decisions for the same patient. Similar problems may arise when guidelines are written in unstructured text or use a less-than-explicit format. In general, however, clinical practice guidelines, including evidence- and consensus-based guidelines, facilitate greater consistency in judgments and decisions.[106]

The benefits of clinical practice guidelines, however, are rarely achieved simply on the basis of appropriate development and content. Research and applied efforts to encourage use of guidelines in health care have shown consistently that physician acceptance and use of guidelines (i.e., guideline implementation) rarely occurs routinely and is difficult to achieve, even when targeted efforts are applied.[67] The failure of the health care practitioner communities to adopt published guidelines or to modify their practice patterns to conform to guidelines is well known and documented extensively.[17,57,74] Among the many barriers that have been identified are distrust of guidelines developed by unknown organizations or groups of experts and the perception that guidelines represent "cookbook" or "one-size-fits-all" medicine, which fails to account for unique and critical patient differences, concerns about medical malpractice, and fear of loss of autonomy.[101] Although these factors may represent barriers to acceptance of guidelines, the challenge of guideline implementation is more likely to rest on the more general problem of extreme stability and typically slow rates of change in clinical practice demonstrated by physicians.[33]

This stability has many benefits, most notably in avoiding premature responses to new evidence that has not yet been confirmed broadly or evidence whose significance, relative to existing evidence, has not yet been appropriately weighted. Its adverse consequences, however, include the extreme difficulty of incorporating evidence and other new information that *is* known to be valid into routine practices. Reviews of applicable behavioral theory[33,74] and of empirical studies[32,35,81] have identified a number of strategies that seem more consistently effective than traditional methods for changing physicians' clinical practices. Often referred to as intensive behavioral strategies or social influence strategies,[75] these methods include academic detailing,[97] opinion leaders,[66] study groups,[60] and group process quality improvement methods (e.g., Continuous Quality Improvement).[7,54] These methods operate on the "sociologic and psychological" factors that Eisenberg and Hershey cited as important influences on clinical decision making.[18]

## DECISION SUPPORT TOOLS

Complementing clinical practice guidelines and other broad strategies for improving medical decision making are tools and techniques designed as specific responses to the decision heuristics and biases discovered through research on human judgment and decision processes. They are often operationalized as computer-aided decision support tools; however, very few applications of such tools have been documented in clinical decision making—and even fewer in neurology. Yet these tools offer potential benefit in many decision situations, particularly as clinical decisions and medical practice become more dependent on computerized support (e.g., electronic charting, test ordering, and diagnostic work). Embedding these tools in the computer systems that clinicians must use to perform routine activities (e.g., reading and adding notes to charts; ordering tests or drugs) offers a valuable means of providing decision support in a transparent, nonintrusive manner.[19]

## DEBIASING AND OTHER CORRECTIVE PROCEDURES

Studies analyzing the origins and consequences of decision heuristics have stimulated development of a broad range of debiasing tools and other corrective techniques intended to reduce the adverse consequences of decision heuristics.[23,80] Many of these tools have direct applicability to problems in diagnostic reasoning and clinical decision making. For example, overconfidence in a diagnosis may result from reliance on availability and representativeness heuristics: when improperly used, these heuristics may lead to insufficient sensitivity to nonrandomness in small samples, resulting in inflated estimates of disease probability. Overconfidence in a diagnosis may be reduced through a number of de-biasing methods. For example, requiring a clinician to identify and document alternative diagnoses, a form of the "devil's advocate" approach,[61] tends to increase the clinician's subjective uncertainty regarding a diagnosis by highlighting other possibilities. Another technique, based on the Socratic approach,[56] involves leading physicians through a series of questions designed to demonstrate clearly the implications of small sample sizes and other sampling issues. For example, by asking a clinician to compute the NPV and PPV of a test, given certain sensitivity and specificity values and prior probabilities, the implications of low disease prevalence become more obvious and are more likely to be considered appropriately.

Although use of de-biasing and other corrective tools is rare, Hershberger et al[45] offer a seminar focusing on cognitive bias in medical decision making; through the use of a test of such bias,[44] the seminar leaders have observed significant decreases in rates of bias in decision making regarding clinical scenarios.[45]

## DECISION ANALYSIS

Formal decision analysis methods use a threshold approach to decision making to reduce or eliminate the influences of nonclinical factors, variable tolerance for uncertainty and risk, and biased probability estimates and other errors arising from use of decision heuristics. Decision analysis provides an objective means of factoring new information into a clinical decision.[99] Since new information (e.g., a test result) often changes the probability of disease, the threshold to treat is often crossed. For neurologic conditions, decision analysis has only rarely been applied,[104] but it should have an increasing presence in the neurology literature.[52] For an introduction to the clinician's use and interpretation of decision analysis studies, the reader is referred to two articles.[88,89]

## EVIDENCE TABLES, OUTCOMES TABLES

Tables summarizing the results of clinical trials or providing summarized outcomes data may also be used to counter biases associated with use of decision heuristics. Evidence from large samples and properly designed clinical trials provides a superior basis for clinical decision making than data accumulated from a clinician's own (small and nonrepresentative) patient population.[12,25,91] Outcomes data presented with demographic stratification further helps to ensure that proper inferences are drawn. For many conditions such tables provide striking evidence of the large variations in disease prevalence among various demographic groups, clearly demonstrating the need for sensitivity to this factor in estimating probabilities and selecting diagnostic testing strategies. Although clinical practice guidelines can be developed to provide equivalent decision support, the less directive nature of evidence tables may increase the likelihood of their acceptance over established guidelines or other means of providing outcome evidence. Since evidence tables can be created by incorporating the physician's (and the physician's local peers) own patient outcomes data (in addition to sufficient samples of other physicians' patients to produce statistically reliable estimates), the evidence might also be seen as more relevant and credible than nationally developed guidelines or evidence tables. This method, given its heavy reliance on data and quantitative analysis, must be supported with appropriate computing technology. It will also be more likely to be accepted and used if it is incorporated into an existing computer-based patient care system that clinicians routinely use for all aspects of patient care.

## COMPUTER-ASSISTED DIAGNOSIS, ANALYSIS, AND INTERPRETATION AND COMPUTERIZED REMINDER SYSTEMS

Computer-based diagnostic aides and other decision support tools have been developed in several areas to assist clinicians in selecting, interpreting, and using diagnostic tests and for other clinical decisions (e.g., diagnostic image interpretation and evaluation of pathogen etiology). These systems are designed to support clinician judgment with objective analysis in areas where complex calculations and manipulation of probabilities are necessary. They often rely on software development methods such as expert systems, neural nets, and other techniques associated with artificial intelligence.[34] Most of these systems remain as research or teaching tools and are not in routine clinical use; several studies examining currently available systems have produced mixed reviews of their value and their potential role in routine clinical decision making.[5,70]

Other computer-based tools for decision support include trials of computerized reminder systems.[71,100] Reminder systems provide suggestions and prompts (usually based on explicit clinical practice guidelines) regarding necessary services and actions that are frequently neglected because of limitations in physicians' ability to store and process large quantities of information or to recall and apply complex rules to a diverse patient population. Reminder systems may improve physicians' ability to determine (and remember) which preventive services are appropriate for a patient at a given time, and they may also serve to ensure that appropriate follow-up occurs after use of a diagnostic test.[72] As with evidence tables, computerized reminder systems are more likely to be accepted and successful if they are incorporated and smoothly integrated into computing systems that clinicians routinely use for other purposes.

## SUMMARY

Studies examining physicians' clinical decisions have demonstrated considerable variation in decisions and practices and have identified numerous challenges to effective, efficient, and accurate decision making. Although use of the decision aids and tools described in this chapter may help to overcome many of these challenges, greater awareness of one's own diagnostic reasoning process and the factors influencing one's decisions will also help improve clinical decisions and reduce variation, irrespective of the use of these tools. Continued research into the determinants and nature of the diagnostic reasoning process will provide additional insights that can be used to develop and apply improved decision aids and corrective procedures to facilitate more accurate and effective clinical decision making and higher quality of care.

## REFERENCES

1. Allman RM, Steinberg E, Keruly J. Physician tolerance for uncertainty: use of liver spleen scans to detect metastases. *JAMA*. 1985;254:246.
2. Anderson DC. How twin cities neurologists treat ischemic stroke. *Arch Neurol*. 1993;50:1098-1103.
3. Asch DA, Patton JP, Hershey JC. Knowing for the sake of knowing. *Med Decis Making*. 1990;10:47-57.
4. Becker LA, Green LA, Beaufait D, Kirk J, Froom J, Freeman WL. Use of CT scans for the investigation of headache: a report from ASPN (pt 1). *J Fam Pract*. 1993;37:129-134.
5. Bermer ES, Webster GD, Shugerman AA, et al. Performance of four computer-based diagnostic systems. *N Engl J Med*. 1994;330:1792-1796.
6. Berwick DM, Weinstein MC. What do patients value? Willingness to pay for ultrasound in normal pregnancy. *Med Care*. 1985;23:881-893.
7. Burns LR, Denton M, Goldfein S, Warrick L, Morenz B, Sales B. The use of Continuous Quality Improvement methods in the development and dissemination of medical practice guidelines. *Q Rev Bull*. 1992;18:434-439.

8. Chassin MR, Brook R, Park R. Variations in the use of medical and surgical services by the Medicare population. *N Engl J Med.* 1986;314:285-290.

9. Clarfield AM. The reversible dementias: do they reverse. *Ann Intern Med.* 1988;109:476-486.

10. Colenda CC, Rapp SR, Leist JC, Poses RM. Clinical variables influencing treatment decisions for agitated dementia patients: survey of physician judgments. *J Am Geriatr Soc.* 1996;44:1375-1379.

11. Cook DJ, Greengold NL, Ellrodt AG, Weingarten SR. The relation between systematic reviews and practice guidelines. *Ann Intern Med.* 1997;127:210-216.

12. Counsell CE, Fraser H, Sandercock PAG. Archie Cochrane's challenge: can periodically updated reviews of all randomised controlled trials relevant to neurology and neurosurgery be produced? *J Neurol Neurosurg Psychiatry.* 1994;57:529-533.

13. Danzon PM, Manning W, Marquis M. Factors affecting laboratory test use and price. *Health Care Finan Rev.* 1984;5:23-30.

14. Davis DA, Thomson MA, Oxman AD, Haynes RB. Evidence for the effectiveness of CME: a review of 50 randomized controlled trials. *JAMA.* 1992;268:1111-1117.

15. Davis DA, Thomson MA, Oxman AD, Haynes RB. Changing physician performance: a systematic review of the effect of continuing medical education strategies. *JAMA.* 1995;274:700-705.

16. Eddy DM. Variations in physician practice: the role of uncertainty. *Health Aff (Milwood).* 1984;3:74-89.

17. Eisenberg JM. *Doctors' Decisions and the Cost of Medical Care: The Reasons for Doctors' Practice Patterns and Ways to Change Them.* Ann Arbor, Mich: Health Administration Press Perspectives; 1986.

18. Eisenberg JM, Hershey JC. Thresholds. *Med Decis Making.* 1983;3:155-168.

19. Elson RB, Connelley DP. Computerized decision support systems in primary care. *Prim Care.* 1995;22:365-384.

20. Evans RW, Evans RI, Sharp MJ. The physician survey on the post-concussion and whiplash syndromes. *Headache.* 1994;34:268-274.

21. Feinstein AR. The "chagrin factor" and qualitative decision analysis. *Arch Intern Med.* 1985;145:1257-1259.

22. Field MJ, Lohr KH, eds. *Clinical Practice Guidelines: Directions for a New Program.* Washington, DC: National Academy Press; 1990.

23. Fischoff B, Debiasig I, Kaheman D, Slovic P, Tversky A, eds. *Judgment Under Uncertainty: Heuristics and Biases.* Cambridge, England: Cambridge University Press; 1982.

24. Fletcher RH, Fletcher SW, Wagner EH. Diagnostic test. In: *Clinical Epidemiology: The Essentials.* Baltimore: Williams & Wilkins; 1982:41-58.

25. Freemantle N, Grilli R, Grimshaw J, Oxman A (for the Cochrane Collaboration on Effective Professional Practice). Implementing findings of medical research: the Cochrane Collaboration on Effective Professional Practice. *Qual Health Care.* 1995;4:45-47.

26. Gerrity MS, Earp JL, DeVellis RF, Light DW. Uncertainty and professional work: perceptions of physicians in clinical practice. *Am J Surg.* 1992;97:1022-1051.

27. Gifford DR, Mittman B, Fink A, Lanto A, Lee M, Vickrey B. Can a specialty society educate its members to think differently about clinical decisions? *J Gen Intern Med.* 1996;11:664-672.

28. Gifford DR, Vickrey BG, Mittman BS, et al. How physician uncertainty influences clinical decision-making: a study of the evaluation and management of early Parkinson's disease. *J Gen Intern Med.* 1995;10(suppl):66.

29. Glassman PA, Kravtz RL, Petersen LP, Rolph JE. Differences in clinical decision making between internists and cardiologists. Arch Intern Med 1997;157:506-512.

30. Glassman P, Kravitz RL, Peterson L, et al. The effect of malpractice experience on clinical decision making. *J Gen Intern Med.* 1994;9(suppl 2):54.

31. Glassman PA, Rolph JE, Petersen LP, Bradley MA, Kravitz RL. Physicians' personal malpractice experiences are not related to defensive clinical practices. *J Health Polit Law.* 1996;21:219-241.

32. Greco PJ, Eisenberg JM. Changing physicians' practices. *N Engl J Med.* 1993;329:1271-1273.

33. Greer AL. The state of the art versus the state of the science: the diffusion of new medical technologies into practice. *Int J Technol Assess Health Care.* 1988;4(1):5-26.

34. Grigsby J, Kramer R, Schneiders J, Gates J, Smith W. Predicting outcome of anterior temporal lobectomy using simulated neural networks. *Epilepsia.* 1998;39:61-66.

35. Grimshaw J, Freemantle N, Wallace S, et al. Developing and implementing clinical practice guidelines. *Qual Health Care.* 1995;4:55-64.

36. Griner PF, Mayewski RJ, Mushlin AI, et al. Selection and interpretation of diagnostic tests and procedures. *Ann Intern Med.* 1981;94(pt 2):559-592.

37. Hadorn DC, McCormick K, Diokno A. An annotated algorithm approach to clinical guidelines development. *JAMA.* 1992;267:3311-3314.

38. Harris SJ. Why doctors do what they do: determinants of physician behavior. *J Occup Med.* 1990;32:1207-1220.

39. Hays RM, Hackworth SR, Speltz ML, Weinstein P. Physicians' practice patterns in pediatric electrodiagnosis. *Arch Phys Med Rehabil.* 1993;74:494-496.

40. Heckerling PS, Tape TG, Wigton RS. Relation of physicians' predicted probabilities of pneumonia to their utilities for ordering chest x-rays to detect pneumonia. *Med Decis Making.* 1992;12:32-38.

41. Heinemann GD, Farrell MP, Schmitt MH. Groupthink theory and research: implications for decision making in geriatric health care teams. *Educ Gerontol.* 1994;20:71-85.

42. Hemenway D, Killen A, Cashman SB, et al. Physicians' responses to financial incentives: evidence from a for-profit ambulatory care center. *N Engl J Med.* 1990;322:1059-1063.

43. Hemminki E. Review of literature on the factors affecting drug prescribing. *Soc Sci Med.* 1975;9:111-115.

44. Hershberger PJ, Part HM, Markert RJ, Cohen SM, Finger WW. Development of a test of cognitive bias in medical decision making. *Acad Med.* 1994;69:839-842.

45. Hershberger PJ, Part HM, Markert RJ, Cohen SM, Finger WW. Teaching awareness of cognitive bias in medical decision making. *Acad Med.* 1995;70:661.

46. Hershey JC, Baron J. Clinical reasoning and cognitive processes. *Med Decis Making.* 1987;7:203-211.

47. Hillman AL. Financial incentives for physicians in HMOs: is there a conflict of interest? *N Engl J Med.* 1987;317:1743-1748.

48. Hillman AL, Pauly M, Kerstein J. How do financial incentives affect physicians' clinical decisions and the financial performance of health maintenance organizations? *N Engl J Med.* 1989;321:86-92.

49. Hillman AL, Welch W, Pauly M. Contractual arrangements between HMOs and primary care physicians: three-tiered HMOs and risk pools. *Med Care.* 1992;30:136-148.

50. Hillman BJ, Joseph C, Mabry M. Frequency and costs of diagnostic imaging in office practice: a comparison of self-referring and radiologist-referring physicians. *N Engl J Med.* 1990;323:1605-1608.

51. Hlatky MA, Lee K, Botvinick E. Diagnostic test use in different practice settings: a controlled comparison. *Arch Intern Med.* 1983;143:1886-1889.

52. Holloway RG, Mushlin AI, Mooney C. Intracranial mass lesions in patients with AIDS: outcomes of a decision analysis compared with the expectations of health care professionals. *Med Decis Making.* 1994;14:432. Abstract.

53. Hopkins A, Menken M, DeFriese GH, et al. Differences in strategies for the diagnosis and treatment of neurologic disease among British and American neurologists. *Arch Neurol.* 1989;46:1142-1148.

54. Horowitz CR, Goldberg HI, Martin DP, et al. Conducting a randomized controlled trial of CQI and academic detailing to implement clinical guidelines. *Joint Commiss J Qual Improv.* 1996;22:734-750.

55. Kahneman D, Slovic P, Tversky A, eds. *Judgement Under Uncertainty: Heuristics and Biases.* New York: Cambridge University Press; 1991.

56. Kahneman D, Tversky A. Variants of uncertainty. *Postscript.* 1982;11:143-157.

57. Kanouse D, Brook RH, et al. *Changing Medical Practice Through Technology Assessment: An Evaluation of the NIH Consensus Development Program Publication.* (RAND) R-3452-NIH. Santa Monica, Calif: The RAND Corp; 1989.

58. Kassirer JP. Diagnostic reasoning. *Ann Intern Med.* 1989;110:893-900.

59. Kassirer JP. Our stubborn quest for diagnostic certainty. *N Engl J Med.* 1989;320:1489-1491.

60. Keller RB, Chapin AM, Soule DN. Informed inquiry into practice variations: the Maine Medical Assessment Foundation. *Qual Assur Health Care.* 1990;2:69-75.

61. Kiriat A, Lichtenstein S, Fischoff B. Reasons for confidence. *J Exp Psychol Learn Mem Cogn.* 1980;6:107-118.

62. Koller WC, Silver DE, Lieberman A. An algorithm for the management of Parkinson's disease. *Neurology.* 1994;44(suppl 10):S1-S52.

63. Lessler DS, Avins AL. Cost, uncertainty, and doctors decisions: the case of thrombolytic therapy. *Arch Intern Med.* 1992;152:1665-1672.

64. Localio AR, Lawthers AG, Bengston JM, et al. Relationship between malpractice claims and cesarean delivery. *JAMA.* 1993;269:366-373.

65. Lohr KN, Brook RH, Kaufman MA. Quality of care in the New Mexico Medicaid program (1971–1975). *Med Care.* 1980;18:i-vi, 1-129.

66. Lomas J, Enkin M, Anderson GM, Hannah WJ, Vayda E, Singer J. Opinion leaders vs audit and feedback to implement practice guidelines: delivery after previous cesarean section. *JAMA.* 1991;265:2202-2207.

67. Lomas J, Haynes RB. A taxonomy and critical review of tested strategies for the application of clinical practice recommendations: from "official" to "individual" clinical policy. *Am J Prevent Med.* 1988; 4(suppl 4):77-94.

68. Mayeux R, Saunders AM, Shea S, Mirra S, Evans D, Roses AD, et al. Utility of the apolipoprotein e genotype in the diagnosis of Alzheimer's disease. *N Engl J Med.* 1998;338:506-511.

69. McCrory DC, Matchar DB, Samsa G, Sanders LL, Pritchett C. Physician attitudes about anticoagulation for nonvalvular atrial fibrillation in the elderly. *Arch Intern Med.* 1995;155:277-281.

70. McDonald CJ. Protocol-based computer reminders: the quality of care and the nonperfectability of man. *N Engl J Med.* 1976;295:1351-1355.

71. McDonald CJ, Hui SL, Smith DM, et al. Reminders to physicians from an introspective computer medical record: a two-year randomized trial. *Ann Intern Med.* 1984;100:130-138.

72. McDowell I, Newell C, Rosser W. A randomized trial of computerized reminders for blood pressure screening in primary care. *Med Care.* 1989;27:297-305.

73. Miller GA. The magical number seven, plus or minus two: some limits on the capacity for processing information. *Psychol Rev.* 1956;63: 91-97.

74. Mittman BS, Siu AL. Changing provider behavior: applying research on outcomes and effectiveness in health care. In: Shortell S, Reinhardt U, eds. *Improving Health Policy and Management: Nine Critical Research Issues for the 1990's.* Ann Arbor, Mich: Health Administration Press; 1992:195-226.

75. Mittman BS, Tonesk X, Jacobson PD. Implementing clinical practice guidelines: social influence strategies and practitioner behavior change. *Qual Rev Bull.* 1992;18:413-422.

76. Moskowitz AJ, Kuipers BJ, Kassirer JP. Dealing with uncertainty, risks, and tradeoffs in clinical decisions. *Ann Intern Med.* 1988;108:435-449.

77. Munsat TL, Mancall EL, DesLauriers MP. The AAN launches a new education program: CONTINUUM lifelong learning in neurology. *Neurology.* 1994;44:771-772.

78. Munschauer FE, Priore RL, Hens M, Castilone A. Thromboembolism prophylaxis in chronic atrial fibrillation. *Stroke.* 1997;28:72-76.

79. Nalbantoglu J, Gilfix BM, Bertrand P, et al. Predictive value of apolipoprotein E genotyping in Alzheimer's disease: results of an autopsy series and an analysis of several combined studies. *Ann Neurol.* 1994; 36:889-895.

80. Nisbett RE, Krantz DH, Jepson C, et al. Improving inductive inference. In: Kahneman D, Slovic P, Tversky A, eds. *Judgment Under Uncertainty: Heuristics and Biases.* Cambridge, England: Cambridge University Press; 1982.

81. Oxman AD, Thomson MA, Davis DA, Haynes RB. No magic bullets: a systematic review of 102 trials of interventions to improve professional practice. *Can Med Assoc J.* 1995;153:1423-1431.

82. Park RE, Fink A, Brook RH, et al. Physician ratings of appropriate indications for six medical and surgical procedures. *Am J Public Health.* 1986;76:766-772.

83. Pauker SG, Kassirer JP. The threshold approach to clinical decision making. *N Engl J Med.* 1980;302:1109-1117.

84. Pauly MV, Eisenberg JM, Radany MH, Erder MH, Feldman R, Schawtz JS. *Paying Physicians: Options for Controlling Cost, Volume, and Intensity of Services.* Ann Arbor, Mich: Health Administration Press; 1992.

85. Pearson SD, Goldman L, Orav EJ, Guadagnoli E, Garcia TB. Triage decisions for emergency department patients with chest pain: do physicians' risk attitudes make the difference? *J Gen Intern Med.* 1995;10: 557-564.

86. Pearson SD, Goulart-Fisher D, Lee TH. Critical pathways as a strategy for improving care: problems and potential. *Ann Intern Med.* 1995; 123:941-948.

87. Rapoport J, Gehlbach S, Lemeshow S. Resource utilization among intensive care patients: managed care vs. traditional insurance. *Arch Intern Med.* 1992;152:2207-2212.

88. Richardson WS, Detsky AS (for the Evidence-Based Medicine Working Group). Users' guides to the medical literature. VII. How to use a clinical decision analysis. A. Are the results of the study valid? *JAMA.* 1995; 273:1292-1295.

89. Richardson WS, Detsky AS (for the Evidence-Based Medicine Working Group). Users' guides to the medical literature. VII. How to use a clinical decision analysis. B. What are the results and will they help me in caring for my patients? *JAMA.* 1995;273:1610-1613.

90. Ringel SP, Franklin GM, DeLapp HC, et al. A cross-sectional comparative study of outpatient neurologic practices in Colorado. *Neurology.* 1988;38:1308-1314.

91. Rosenberg W, Donald A. Evidence based medicine: an approach to clinical problem-solving. *BMJ.* 1995;310:1122-1125.

92. Rosenberg J, Greenberg MK. Practice parameters: strategies for survival into the nineties. *Neurology.* 1992;42:1110-1115.

93. Sackett DL. A primer on the precision and accuracy of the clinical examination. *JAMA.* 1992;267:2638.

94. Salem-Schatz SR, Avorn J, Soumerai SB. Influence of clinical knowledge, organizational context, and practice style on transfusion decision making: implications for practice change strategies. *JAMA.* 1990; 264:476-483.

95. Seshadri S, Drachman DA, Lippa CF. Apolipoprotein E e4 allele and the lifetime risk of Alzheimer's disease: what physicians know, and what they should know. *Arch Neurol.* 1995;52:1074-1079.

96. Shapiro RS, Simpson D, Lawrence S. A survey of sued and nonsued physicians and suing patients. *Arch Intern Med.* 1989;149:2190-2196.

97. Soumerai SB, Avorn J. Principles of educational outreach ('academic detailing') to improve clinical decision making. *JAMA.* 1990;263:549-556.

98. Sox HC. Probability theory in the use of diagnostic tests. *Ann Intern Med.* 1986;104:60-66.

99. Sox HC, Blatt MA, Higgins MC, et al. *Medical Decision Making.* Boston: Butterworth-Heinemann; 1988.

100. Tierney WM, Hui SL, McDonald CJ. Delayed feedback of physician performance versus immediate reminders to perform preventive care: effects on physician compliance. *Med Care.* 1986;24:659-666.

101. Tunis SR, Hayward RS, Wilson MC, et al. Internists' attitudes about clinical practice guidelines. *Ann Intern Med.* 1994;120:956-963.

102. Tussing AD, Wojtowyez MA. The cesarean decision in New York State, 1986: economic and noneconomic aspects. *Medicare Care.* 1992;30: 529-540.

103. Tversky AD, et al. Judgement under uncertainty: heuristics and biases. *Science.* 1974;185;1124-1131.

104. van Crevel H, Habbema JDF, Braakman R. Decision analysis of the management of incidental intracranial saccular aneurysms. *Neurology.* 1986;36:1335-1339.

105. Vickrey BG, Gifford DR, Belin TR, et al. Practice styles of US compared to UK neurologists. *Neurology.* 1998;50:1661-1668.

106. Weisberg LA, Strub RL, Garcia CA. *Decision Making in Adult Neurology.* St. Louis: Mosby; 1987.

107. Weisman C, Morlock L, Teitelbaum M. Practice changes in response to the malpractice litigation climate. *Med Care.* 1989;27:16-24.

108. Wennberg JE, Barnes, Zubkoff M. Professional uncertainty and the problem of supplier induced demand. *Soc Sci Med.* 1982;16:811-824.

109. Wennberg J, Gestelsohn. Small area variations in health care delivery. *Science.* 1973;182:1102-1108.

110. Winkenwerder W, Levy BD, Eisenberg JM, Williams SV, Young MJ, Hershey JC. Variation in physicians' decision making thresholds in management of a sexually transmitted disease. *J Gen Intern Med.* 1993; 8:369-373.

# 30

# Medicolegal Aspects

*H. Richard Beresford*

The benefits of advances in neurodiagnostic testing are plain to see. Quick and precise diagnoses enable timely and relevant treatments. Even if prompt diagnoses open no therapeutic windows, test data may enhance prognostication and counseling. Clinicians can also be more efficient and productive if they know they can depend on results of tests performed by technicians or nonclinical specialists. In addition, biomedical researchers rely on newer tests to monitor responses to experimental therapies systematically and to gain insights into the pathophysiology of disease.

Against this roseate backdrop, the raising of legal concerns may seem churlish. Yet these concerns are unavoidable. Some testing methodologies are invasive and thus potentially harmful. Other, less physically risky tests may still be misapplied or misinterpreted in ways that produce psychosocial or economic harm. In our legal system, which entitles injured persons to recover monetary damages from wrongdoers, claims for test-related harms are utterly predictable. Claimants may assert that the test itself caused harm, either because of significant intrinsic danger or because it was carelessly conducted. Or they may assert that the choice of a particular test was inappropriate or that the clinician mishandled test data in a harmful way.

Legal challenge to a decision to perform a particular test is improbable unless there is a plausible link between the test and an adverse outcome. For example, failure to order a brain computed tomography (CT) scan or magnetic resonance imaging (MRI) for a patient with a history of increasing headache will generate a plausible malpractice claim if the patient is later found to have a lesion that was treatable when the test allegedly should have been ordered.[13] Other claims may allege negligent performance of a test, failure to obtain informed consent to testing, or negligent mishandling of data obtained through testing.

This chapter briefly reviews the legal issues that may arise with respect to neurodiagnostic testing. The focus will be on applications of malpractice law. The impact of the doctrine of informed consent will be explored in this context. The chapter will close with a consideration of so-called enterprise liability, a concept that has special relevance to test-related claims arising in the setting of managed care.

## NEGLIGENCE IN TESTING

### NEGLIGENCE DOCTRINE

In law, negligence implies a careless breach of a lawful duty. The breach can take the form of *nonfeasance,* the failure to act when one should have acted, or *misfeasance,* the failure to act carefully enough. But before liability will attach, a claimant must establish that the breach of duty caused measurable harm. In other words, nonfeasance or misfeasance ordinarily is not actionable unless it results in provable injury. Thus, even if a physician carelessly fails to inform a patient that stroke is a risk of angiography, the physician would be liable for negligence only if the angiogram indeed caused a stroke. The physician could, in theory, be vulnerable to a charge of battery (unlawful touching) for not disclosing a significant risk before testing. But the costs of litigating such a claim would ordinarily far outstrip what a claimant could recover in damages.

When the core of a negligence claim is medical malpractice, a claimant must produce medical expert testimony to establish standard of care, breach of duty, and causal relationship between breach of duty and harm. Although the large volume of medical malpractice litigation may lead physicians to believe otherwise, the requirement of substantiating expert testimony offers considerable protection against medically baseless charges.

Before an expert's opinion is admissible as evidence in a malpractice case, the expert must testify that "with reasonable medical certainty" (or words to that effect) a defendant physician acted negligently. A less definite opinion will be excluded or can be grounds for reversal on appeal if it is admitted into evidence at a trial. Moreover, even if a court hears an expert's opinion that lacks medical or scientific support, a defendant can attack it on cross-examination or produce other experts to refute it. Compelling claimants to substantiate their cases with testimony from medical professionals does not ensure a just outcome in every case. Some experts will testify ignorantly or unconscionably, and some courts will misinterpret what they hear.[2,10] Yet the requirement averts the turmoil that could emerge if courts decided malpractice cases without benefit of informed opinions from medical professionals.

## NEGLIGENT FAILURE TO TEST

As more and better neurodiagnostic tests become available, it is foreseeable that some clinicians will fail to use them to an optimal degree. They may not know the tests exist, what the tests can achieve, or the proper indications for ordering them. They may view the tests as insufficiently precise or too costly in light of the expected benefits. Or they may respond to pressures to contain health care costs by withholding testing they might choose if price were irrelevant. In any of these circumstances, claims may arise in which physicians are charged with negligent failure to conduct medically indicated testing.

Few such claims will raise novel legal issues, no matter how exotic the test. The focus will remain on whether a physician violated accepted standards of medical practice by not testing. That a particular new diagnostic technology is complex, extraordinarily powerful, or costly is not in itself legally significant. What is significant is the existing state of medical practice with respect to conducting the test.[9,14] If the average practitioner in the relevant specialty would have ordered the test under the clinical circumstances at issue, then a defendant who failed to order the test would be at legal risk. However, if the test is used only at large academic medical centers or is seldom ordered by most clinical practitioners, the legal risk of withholding it is considerably less, even if the test is clearly useful.

Tests that only slowly or haltingly gain general acceptance may be especially problematic. During the shakedown period in which knowledge about the utility of a new test is accumulating, some clinicians may forego ordering it because of honest uncertainty about its value. But suppose the test ultimately proves highly reliable for diagnosing a treatable disorder and a patient in fact had that disorder at the time when the physician chose not to perform the test. In an ensuing malpractice suit the claimant could argue that the physician was negligent in not performing a test that the claimant's experts testify was medically indicated. The defendant would then need to overcome the inference, derived from hindsight, that it was careless to omit what is now regarded as a clinically valuable test. In this situation the most fruitful tactic would be to locate experts who are willing to testify that at the relevant time it was uncertain whether the test was medically indicated. The defendant could then argue that omitting the test did not violate the temporally relevant standard of care.

The preceding hypothetical situation underscores why it is important for clinicians to inform themselves about new diagnostic tests, especially those that may enable detection of treatable disorders. Foregoing such tests may have substantial adverse consequences for some patients, leading inevitably to lawsuits. Moreover, physicians' reputations, and perhaps referrals, may suffer if it becomes widely known that they lack current knowledge about diagnostic technologies. Obvious as these pitfalls of incomplete knowledge are, the fact remains that it may be difficult for physicians to achieve fully up-to-date knowledge about new modalities of testing. This is especially true for physicians with large practices that include patients with a wide range of diagnoses and problems. Even specialists in neurology may be hard-put to stay informed about such diverse technologies as functional neuroimaging, transcranial Doppler ultrasonography, magnetoencephalography, immunologic tests for autoimmune neurologic disorders, and molecular genetic diagnostic tests, despite the fact that these technologies may be quite relevant for evaluating some patients in their practices.

Law does not, of course, require physicians to know everything about all tests that may pertain to their patients. It only requires that physicians know what the average or "reasonable" practitioner in a comparable environment knows about such tests.[9,10] This means, for example, that if failure to perform functional neuroimaging is at issue, the relevant standard of care is that of similarly situated practitioners, not that of the university-based specialist in functional neuroimaging. A claimant's lawyer might produce such a specialist as an expert witness because he or she has impressive credentials and may—so the lawyer hopes—awe the jury. Nevertheless, a defendant neurologist is not chargeable with the knowledge of such a specialist unless the claimant can prove that the defendant's clinical peers also possess such knowledge.

## NEGLIGENT CHOICE OF TEST

Rather than failing to test, a clinician may choose what is allegedly the wrong test. For example, suppose a neurologist orders an MRI of the cervical and thoracic spine for a patient with lower limb weakness, spasticity, and hyperreflexia and then tells the patient, after the MRI is found to be normal, that she probably has a degenerative or demyelinating spinal cord disease. If the patient is subsequently found to have a parasagittal meningioma after further progression of spastic paraparesis and appearance of severe headache, the stage would be set for a lawsuit alleging negligent misdiagnosis.

The hypothesized claimant would probably have little difficulty finding expert witnesses to support two linked theories of liability. One theory would be that the initial evaluation should have included brain imaging since the differential diagnosis of lower limb weakness with corticospinal signs includes parasagittal or bifrontal lesions, regardless of the fact that the claimant did not complain of headaches when evaluated by the defendant. The second theory is that the defendant should have ordered brain imaging when the spine MRI was found to be normal rather than presuming that the claimant had an untreatable myelopathy. In other words, the defendant arguably either chose the wrong test initially or, even if the initial choice of test was reasonable, negligently failed to order additional testing.

The defendant clinician might try to justify the alleged misfeasance or nonfeasance by emphasizing that a spinal cord disorder was a more likely cause of the claimant's presenting signs than a brain tumor and that the spine MRI was the most appropriate and reliable way to exclude spinal cord disease. Although the defendant could probably secure expert witnesses who would support these propositions, they might be reluctant to support the choice not to perform brain imaging, especially after spine imaging was negative. However, they might be willing to testify that the decision not to do brain imaging was reasonable under the clinical circumstances, even though it turned out to be an unwise choice in retrospect. They might also be willing to weigh in with something about the probabilistic nature of medical diagnoses and the unjustifiable extravagance of performing every available test when confronting certain clinical problems.

Cases of this sort accent the more general question of the extent to which clinicians should try to be discriminating in their use of costly diagnostic technologies. One might conclude that the easy answer is that they should not try. Inevitably, it might be argued, a highly selective approach to testing will result in missing a few improbable but important diagnoses. Equally inevitably, this would result in lawsuits. The counterpoint is that the social costs of nonselective testing outweigh the benefits of a few more correct diagnoses and a few less malpractice suits. Adjusting these conflicting viewpoints is ultimately a political problem, one that society must eventually confront as more and more expensive diagnostic technologies appear. In the meantime, individual clinicians will need to balance their desire to achieve as much diagnostic certainty as possible against the practical constraints on employing the full range of available tests.

### NEGLIGENT PERFORMANCE OF TESTING

Some neurologic clinicians conduct their own diagnostic tests (e.g., electromyography, muscle biopsy, lumbar puncture, carotid artery and transcranial Doppler ultrasonography). In this role they are vulnerable to claims of negligent technical error. There are two variants of such claims. One is that the claimant sustained direct physical injury because the test was carelessly done (e.g., excessive bleeding from muscle biopsy, spinal nerve root injury during lumbar puncture). The other variant is that the unskillful performance of the test produced inaccurate or misleading data to the detriment of the patient (e.g., failure to detect a high-grade carotid artery stenosis on an ultrasound study).

Proof of negligence in these cases would require testimony from clinicians with expertise in performing the procedures in question. The role of these experts would be to define what is an acceptable standard of technical competence and to express an opinion as to whether a defendant met that standard while testing the claimant. Mere proof that a claimant sustained a complication or that the test yielded inaccurate or misleading data would not alone sustain a claim of negligence. There must also be a showing that it is more probable than not that the testing was both carelessly done and that this carelessness caused the asserted harm, whether direct physical injury or generation of consequentially wrong data.

For the tests that neurologists commonly perform themselves, the legal risks seem small. The greater risk would seem to lie in the generation of inaccurate data. Significant direct injury from the minimally invasive tests most neurologists conduct must be rare. But a carelessly done carotid artery Doppler study could result in missing or delaying an opportunity to perform a protective carotid endarterectomy. Given the emerging evidence for the benefits of carotid endarterectomy when significant carotid stenosis exists, it is easy to envision a claim by a patient with stroke and such a stenosis against a neurologist whose carotid artery Doppler study had failed to identify the stenosis.

### NEGLIGENT INTERPRETATION OF TEST

If it is assumed that a test yields valid data, a physician may, nonetheless, misinterpret the data. A neurologist, for example, might erroneously interpret localized spiking on an electroencephalographic recording as artifact when in fact it is a focal epileptiform discharge; or he or she might in-correctly conclude that a nonenhancing cerebral lesion is an infarct rather than a neoplasm. Errors of this sort may or may not be negligent. However, if they prove consequential, they may fuel malpractice claims. The outcome of such claims ordinarily rests on the testimony of neurologic expert witnesses. For claimants to prevail, the preponderance of expert opinion must be that the defendants violated accepted or prevailing standards of neurologic practice in interpreting the data in question.

More subtle questions about interpretation of tests may arise with respect to data that have important psychosocial dimensions. For example, neurologists may elect to perform molecular genetic testing to diagnose a suspected hereditary disorder (e.g., Huntington's disease) or to determine if a patient is at heightened risk of developing a neurologic disorder because of a particular genotype (e.g., apoE4). The information gleaned from such testing can have a powerful impact on patients. Unless they have been appropriately informed about the implications of testing or appropriately counseled about the significance of test results, considerable harm may result. This could include suicide triggered by learning that one has, or is at significant risk for, an incurable neurologic disease and by stigmatization and loss of employment or insurance if the test results are wrongfully or thoughtlessly disseminated.

Neurologists who fail to anticipate such outcomes or who fail to ensure appropriate genetic testing may be vulnerable to a charge of negligent nonfeasance. The argument might be that neurologists have a duty to prepare their patients for the foreseeable consequences of testing and that failure to provide or ensure medically appropriate genetic counseling violates this duty. Claimants might find it difficult to sustain such an argument in court. One barrier may be to prove that appropriate counseling would have averted an adverse outcome. Also, a defendant might argue that genetic tests are qualitatively similar to other tests that may yield diagnoses of lethal or untreatable diseases and that physicians cannot reasonably be expected to shield patients from the psychologic suffering that positive test results may inflict. Legal nuances aside, however, the potential for claims of this sort should encourage neurologists and other physicians who order genetic testing to prepare their patients carefully for the possibility of a result that confirms or foretells a terrible disease.

## CONSENT-BASED LIABILITY

### INFORMED CONSENT DOCTRINE

Most claims that allege failure by physicians to obtain informed consent to testing are essentially malpractice claims. The core of the claim is that a physician violated a professional duty to tell the patient enough.[4,5] Defining what is enough virtually always requires expert medical testimony to describe the test and its indications, risks, benefits, and alternatives. Medical testimony is also needed to determine whether a claimant sustained measurable injury as a result of an allegedly inadequate disclosure. Moreover, in some states the law tests adequacy of disclosure by what the average or reasonable physician tells patients, not by reference to what average or reasonable patients expect to hear.

Focus on the question of whether a physician violated a lawful professional duty protects physicians in an important way. Claimants cannot establish lack of informed consent simply by proving that physicians failed to disclose certain facts about tests. They must also show that the nondisclosure violated prevailing professional norms, largely as defined by physicians. For example, suppose a neurologist admittedly failed to tell a patient who underwent a medically appropriate lumbar puncture that diplopia due to cranial nerve VI palsy is a rare complication of the procedure. If the patient then charges the physician with failure to obtain informed consent, he or she does not win a lawsuit merely by proving that the neurologist did not tell the patient about a rare complication that materialized. The claimant must also prove that the nondisclosure of this remote risk violated professional standards, as depicted by his medical experts. If it is assumed that the claimant could find physicians who would testify that the defendant should have disclosed the remote risk of diplopia, this testimony would be subject to rebuttal by testimony from other neurologists to the effect that disclosure of such remote risks is not standard practice.

Even if this claimant satisfies a legal decision maker that the risk of diplopia was so material that the neurologist should have disclosed it, the claimant does not necessarily win. The claimant must also prove that, had the remote risk of diplopia been disclosed, he or she would have refused lumbar puncture. In other words, the claimant must show somehow that the minuscule risk of transient diplopia would have led him or her to decline a test that was medically indicated. The law of most states would require such a claimant to show that the average or reasonable patient would have declined the test in those circumstances.[4,5] Standing alone, the claimant's hindsight-based assertion of what he or she would have done if told of the remote risk would not suffice. Indeed, the legal requirement that claimants prove that they would have declined testing if an omitted disclosure had been made does much to explain why claimants rarely win suits against physicians based solely on lack of informed consent.

## CONSENT TO NEWLY DEVELOPED TESTS

When a new diagnostic testing technology is introduced, a measure of uncertainty may exist about both its safety and utility. To the extent that the technology has been subject to regulatory oversight (as with new medical devices that require premarketing approval by the Food and Drug Administration), the most important safety issues will have been resolved, as well as many issues relating to validity and reliability. Physicians who use the technology nevertheless have a legal obligation to secure informed consent to its use.

Suppose, for example, that the new testing technology is an arterial catheter that facilitates angiographic study of intracranial vascular occlusive disease. As with any potentially risky diagnostic test, a neurologist who employs the new catheter must explain the technology to the patient or lawful surrogate, describe the indications for its use, and disclose expected benefits, risks, and alternatives. Because it is new technology, however, its full risk profile may not be known. In this instance the legally prudent approach is to be overinclusive, rather than underinclusive, in disclosing potential risks and to stress that unforeseen risks may materialize. This sort of broad disclosure will alert patients to the fact that the test is new and that an unexpected adverse event is possible.

## TESTING IN RESEARCH

Clinical investigators may employ generally accepted diagnostic technologies in their studies of human subjects, or they may use human subjects to study the safety and efficacy of new diagnostic technologies. In either context they must obtain informed consent to testing.

In many instances, the requirements for securing informed consent will be spelled out in institutional review board (IRB)–approved research protocols, which, in turn, are subject to federal[6] or state[15] regulations pertaining to human research. Generally speaking, experimental protocols of this sort mandate expansive disclosures. Moreover, when the research offers little or no prospect of directly benefiting the experimental subjects, clinical investigators should be especially sensitive to the need for exhaustive disclosure of potential risks and for disabusing subjects of beliefs that the research might somehow benefit them. In other words, clinical investigators ought to view themselves as fiduciaries with respect to research subjects, invariably placing the well-being of experimental subjects ahead of their own interests in gaining scientific knowledge.[15]

At times the line between clinical testing and research may be indistinct. In one sense this is immaterial since testers must obtain informed consent to testing in both circumstances. Still, how the testing is characterized may be significant. Suppose, for example, that a patient with parkinsonism who has had little response to levodopa is asked by the attending neurologist to undergo positron emission tomography (PET). Suppose, further, that the neurologist is also engaged in a study of dopamine metabolism in "Parkinson look-alike" disorders. The PET study may be useful in clarifying why the patient has not responded to levodopa and in suggesting alternative therapeutic strategies. However, it will also yield data for the neurologist's scientific study.

If the neurologist fully explains and discloses the risks of PET and the potential utility of the study in explaining the poor response to levodopa, the patient arguably has enough information to decide about PET. Nevertheless, if a disclosed risk of PET materializes (e.g., vascular thrombosis), the patient might claim that the neurologist did not disclose her conflict of interest with respect to the PET study and that, if she had, the patient would have declined the test. How this claim would play out might depend on whether the claimant could persuade a legal decision maker that a reasonable person would have declined the test if the neurologist had disclosed her conflict of interest. Obviously the neurologist could have easily avoided such a claim by honoring an ethical obligation to disclose the conflict.

When a test is itself the focus of research, experimenters should be aware of a potential obligation to disclose more than the foreseeable risks of the test itself. They should also consider disclosing any financial or other gains they anticipate realizing if the test proves to be valid and useful. Thus the California Supreme Court recently decided that investigators who seek cells and tissues of research subjects for developing biotechnology products must inform the research subjects of their commercial expectations.[11] One rationale for this decision is that experimental subjects should be given the opportunity to bargain with researchers for a share of any profits that might be realized from use of their cells and tissues. As more and more clinical investigators establish links with biotechnology companies, issues of this sort may become more than rare curiosities.

## UNAVOIDABLY DANGEROUS TECHNOLOGIES

Under the law of product liability, manufacturers of certain products may be held liable even if claimants injured by the products do not prove that the products are defective. Thus, if a product is useful but unavoidably dangerous despite careful manufacture (e.g., some prescription drugs), the manufacturers can be held liable if they do not provide adequate warnings to users of the products. However, if such products are prescribed or used by physicians, manufacturers can shift the liability for injuries caused by the products to the physicians if the manufacturers can establish that they adequately warned physicians of materialized risks, even if the manufacturers did not warn patients or the public directly.

A simple example relates to penicillin. Manufacturers of various forms of this antibiotic are careful to advise physicians that penicillins may trigger anaphylactic reactions. If a patient incurs such a reaction after receiving a penicillin from a physician who did not warn him or her of this risk, the liability is that of the physician, not the manufacturer. An exception to this "learned intermediary" doctrine is a situation in which the claimant can show that the penicillin itself was defectively made.

One impact of the "learned intermediary" doctrine is to reinforce the obligation of physicians to disclose risks of medical products or devices that they employ for diagnostic purposes. Physicians can escape liability by showing that manufacturers did not in fact warn them about materialized risks. But as any careful reader of package inserts for pharmaceuticals or materials that accompany medical devices knows, some disclosed risks are indeed remote. Although a physician might try to argue that such disclosures obfuscate more than they inform, if a risk of a testing device or product is clearly stated and the physician did not communicate that risk to an injured patient, the manufacturer is likely to escape liability. The physician might still prevail by showing that the risk in question was so remote that virtually no physician would disclose it or that, even if the physician did, patients would generally accept it.[5]

# ENTERPRISE LIABILITY AND DIAGNOSTIC TESTS

## CONCEPT OF ENTERPRISE LIABILITY

Calls for medical malpractice reform have grown in recent years, and many states have enacted laws that aim to reduce the financial and social costs of medical liability litigation. By and large, the reforms have amounted to modifications of existing tort laws rather than bold changes. Proposals to shift to a "no-fault" system or an administrative system akin to workers' compensation have been largely rejected. However, a proposal that has attracted more attention, as managed care has expanded, is "enterprise liability."[1] The concept seems particularly well adapted to the increasingly corporate dominance of contemporary health care.

The essence of enterprise liability is to shift liability for medical maloccurrences from individual physicians to the corporate entities to which they are linked. In such a paradigm the presumption is that the firm will have a powerful incentive to oversee the performance of its physicians and that this oversight will compensate for any tendency of physicians to behave less carefully because of their insulation from personal liability. In short, if a firm becomes the "deep pocket" with respect to claims by injured patients, it is likely to deploy intrusive measures to prevent such claims from arising. The ensuing micromanagement could be considerable, and some physicians might find the trade-off for freedom from personal liability intolerable. But as more and more physicians become involved in corporate medicine, their antipathy toward close oversight may lessen.

## DIAGNOSTIC TESTING IN MANAGED CARE

A gnawing concern of physicians and much of the public is that pressure to contain health care costs through managed care will lead to underutilization of testing. It is difficult to deny that some tests, including neuroimaging and electrophysiologic studies, have been overused in the past. But this does not in itself justify draconian efforts to constrain use of certain costly but valuable tests—be they existing ones, such as MRI, or evolving new technologies. Such tests may be eminently cost-effective when used by discerning clinicians. In addition, rules that inflexibly restrict their use are unlikely to either save money or enhance the quality of care.

The challenge is thus to ensure that firms are held legally accountable for policies or conduct that compels physicians to delay or forego demonstrably beneficial testing. Accountability of this sort should lead managers to adapt testing policies to the medical needs of their enrollees rather than to sheer fiscal concerns. On the other hand, corporate accountability would not relieve physicians of their obligation to advocate for testing in the face of constraining rules. Existing legal precedent indicates that physicians cannot successfully invoke managed care policies to justify their own personal failures to actively promote the best medical interests of their patients.[14,16]

## ENTERPRISE LIABILITY AND DIAGNOSTIC TESTS

If enterprise liability were to become the dominant model for processing medical injury claims, targets of most claims would be firms that hold contract-based power over physicians whose conduct generated the claims. For diagnostic tests, this would mean that claims based on allegedly wrongful selection, performance, interpretation, or omission of diagnostic tests for enrollees of the enterprise would be brought against the enterprise rather than the offending physicians. Presumably claims based on lack of informed consent to testing would also be brought against the enterprise, even though it might be argued that informed consent claims should be treated differently because of the personal or fiduciary nature of the transactions involved. However, since most informed consent claims are treated by courts as malpractice claims, the rationale for enterprise liability should apply to them as well.

A firm might attempt to defeat enterprise liability claims by asserting that the conduct of physicians accused of wrongdoing violated norms or rules of the firm and that therefore the physicians themselves should bear full legal responsibility for resulting harms to patients. Whether this type of defense succeeds would depend in part on the nature of the contract between the physician and the enterprise and the state laws of agency. If, for example, the contract provided that physicians must obtain informed consent (as defined in the contract) before performing risky diagnostic tests and the physician failed to disclose a known and materialized risk of a test, the enterprise might escape liability. But unless a physician is in clear violation of the firm's rules, the logic of the enterprise liability doctrine is that ambiguities of contract or circumstance should be resolved in favor of targeting the firm rather than the physician.

The case for enterprise liability is particularly strong where a claimant asserts that indicated testing was omitted because of a firm's inappropriate cost-containment policies. This is arguably a form of corporate negligence, a doctrine that courts have invoked to hold hospitals liable for some actions of physicians who hold staff privileges but are not employees.[1] The rationale is that a hospital corporation that has assumed credentialing responsibilities with respect to physicians should take reasonable steps to determine their competence and to oversee their clinical activities in the hospital, including the conduct of diagnostic testing. Similarly, a managed care firm that has undertaken to credential and manage physicians should bear legal responsibility for test-related acts or omissions occurring within the framework of its managed care contracts with physicians. Formal acceptance of the enterprise liability principle would eliminate the need for directly involving physicians in claims stemming from these acts or omissions.

### In Default of Enterprise Liability

The existing reality is, of course, that the corporate entities that dominate managed care have largely escaped legal accountability for much of the harm that their cost-containment policies have occasioned. Two explanations for this situation come to mind. One is that managed care firms have shifted blame away from themselves by successfully arguing that it was the conduct of physicians—not that of managers or firm policies—that caused harm.[14,16] A second explanation is the "ERISA (Employee Retirement Income Security Act) shield," which permits managed care firms acting on behalf of self-insuring employers to escape application of state medical malpractice laws and to limit their liability essentially to payment for the health care services they wrongfully refused to cover.[8] A few courts recently have cracked the ERISA shield,[7,12] and there is considerable political support for legislation that would either remove the shield entirely or at least make it easier for injured enrollees to mount meaningful damage claims against managed care firms.[3] How these developments proceed will clearly influence how far managed care firms are likely to go in trying to restrict access to demonstrably useful neurodiagnostic tests.

## SUMMARY

Legal issues that may arise in neurodiagnostic testing are briefly explored. The focus is on applications of medical malpractice law with respect to negligence in selection, conduct, and interpretation of tests. The impact of the doctrine of informed consent is considered, both in the context of malpractice law and human subjects research. The chapter closes with a discussion of enterprise liability and diagnostic tests, indicating how the growing role of managed care firms in health care delivery may evoke shifts in how claims for test-related harms are processed. The goal is to convey an appreciation of the law's role in reducing test-related harms by making individuals and firms accountable for the consequences of their conduct.

## REFERENCES

1. Abraham KS, Weiler PC. Enterprise medical liability and the evolution of the American health care system. *Harvard Law Rev.* 1994;108:381-436.
2. Beresford HR. Neurologist as expert witness. *Neurol Clin.* 1992;10:1059-1071.
3. Bodenheimer T. The managed care backlash: righteous or reactionary? *N Engl J Med.* 1996;335:1601-1604.
4. *Canterbury v Spence*, 464 F2d 772 (DC Cir 1972), *cert denied*, 93 Sup Ct 560.
5. *Cobbs v Grant*, 502 P2d 1 (Sup Ct CA 1972).
6. *Code Fed Regs 45*, 46:405-407 (1983).
7. *Dukes v US Health Care*, 57 F3d 350 (3rd Cir 1993).
8. *Employee Retirement Income Security Act of 1988*, 29 USC §1140.
9. *Hall v Hilbun*, 466 So2d 856 (Sup Ct MS 1985).
10. Imwinkelried EJ. *The Methods of Attacking Scientific Evidence.* 3d ed. Charlottesville, Va: Lexis Law Publishing; 1997:235-260.
11. *Moore v Regents of Univ of California*, 271 CA Rptr 146, 793 Pac2d 479 (1990).
12. *Pappas v Asbel et al*, 675 A2d 711 (PA Sup Ct 1996).
13. *Richter v Northwestern Memorial Hosp*, 177 Ill App3d 247, 532 NE2d 269 (1988).
14. Siliciano J. Wealth, equity, and the Unitary Medical Malpractice Standard. *Virginia Law Rev.* 1991;77:439-484.
15. *T.D. v NY State Office of Mental Health*, 650 NYS2d 173 (Sup Ct App Div, 1st Dept 1996).
16. *Wickline v State of California*, 228 CA Rptr 661 (CA App 1986), *petition for review dismissed*, 741 Pac2d 613 (1987).

# 31

# Practice Parameters

*Michael K. Greenberg and Gary M. Franklin*

The Quality Standards Subcommittee (QSS) of the American Academy of Neurology (AAN) is responsible for the development of practice parameters. Practice parameters are evidence based documents developed to answer specific questions concerning the diagnosis or management of selected clinical conditions. The use of diagnostic testing has been included in some disease-specific practice parameters or has been the primary subject of others. This chapter discusses the methods used by QSS in the AAN practice parameters program to evaluate the relevance of diagnostic technologies.

## WHICH TESTS TO EVALUATE?

A diagnostic test is performed (1) for a specific clinical diagnosis when there is uncertainty as to its existence, (2) to exclude a confounding clinical entity, (3) to quantify the degree of affliction, (4) to estimate risk (or likelihood) of developing a specific disorder, or (5) to measure a treatment effect (or if a treatment modality is to be used). A test is useful to the physician or the patient when the performance of the test effects clinical decision making or affects patient outcome. As part of the QSS process of practice parameter development, the committee may evaluate a diagnostic technology for a document on the global management of a specific condition or as a stand-alone document to focus on the test itself and its use in specific clinical circumstances. Evaluation is performed when a new diagnostic tool for a specific entity becomes available, a new indication for a known technology emerges, or a technology is on the wane (because of advances in competing methods or limited usefulness in clinical practice). The evidence needed to perform an assessment or make recommendations may not be readily available. As magnetic resonance imaging was introduced into clinical practice, in the first 5 years <28% of literature citations compared this technology to alternative methods.[15]

The QSS process requires a justification for pursuing the development of a practice parameter. In this justification statement a list of attributes about the topic are considered. These include frequency of use, controversy regarding validity, potential for improving health outcomes, potential for reducing practice variation, economic impact, and external constraints. In addition, resources required for document preparation and the adequacy of available evidence are considered. Practice parameter topics may be suggested by any member of the AAN, the AAN practice committee, the AAN executive board, or outside organizations that deal with neurologically related disciplines.

Specific tasks are needed for practice parameter development. The health outcomes of the target condition need to be identified, in particular, those that are important patient outcomes. The evidence of the effect of a practice intervention on those outcomes is analyzed. Estimates of the magnitude on the outcomes and the costs of the intervention must be considered. The benefits and harms of the intervention are disclosed. Finally, a comparison is made between the intervention and alternative clinical practices to determine priority of use.

## PRACTICE VARIATION AND PARAMETERS

Practice variation is studied by examining the occurrence of activities in relation to the size of the population served. Quality is usually questioned when there is perceived variation among practitioners. Systems have been built into most medical organizations to identify the "outliers." But is the outlier providing suboptimal care, or are those who follow "standard and accepted" methods providing care that may not be best for their individual patients? It follows that when there is variation in practice, some patients will be receiving suboptimal (or even harmful) care.

Variation is found in practice

1. Where there is interobserver and intraobserver variability
2. Between geographic regions
3. When there are multiple levels of clinical certainty
4. By variation of efficacy of available interventions
5. When there are competing agendas among providers, patients, and payers
6. When there is conflicting evidence (or opinion)
7. When there is variable access to information and time (or ability) to interpret the information
8. Because of patient characteristics

Observer variability is the phenomenon in which different observers look at the same thing (or a single observer looks at the same thing twice) and there is disagreement (10% to 50% of the time).[3] For example, in a prospective study of patients with transient ischemic attacks, the patients' angiograms were submitted to three radiologists to assess agreement on the degree of bifurcation stenosis. The mean interobserver variation was 9.5%, and the intraobserver variation was 8.5%. Clinically important differences (e.g., surgery vs. no surgery) were found in 3.4%, 3.9%, and 6.1% of the comparisons.[20]

Regional variation can occur between one country and another or from one region of a country to another. Working with appropriateness panels has shown that the composition of the panel affects the assessment. For example, the mix of physician specialties represented on the panel and the nationality of the panel members affects panel results.[4]

The personal characteristics of physicians can lead to variation in delivery of care. In the treatment of breast cancer, breast-conserving procedures were significantly correlated to the number of female surgeons on a hospital's staff.[5] When the treatment of unstable angina was compared between a group of cardiologists and a group of internists, the internists were more likely to use exercise tests and less likely to use catheterization and angioplasty. The infarction rate was similar between the two groups, but the death rate was higher in the internist group (4% vs. 1.8%).[18]

Clinical decision making requires that the clinician make an estimate of the consequences (outcomes) of the available options. The ability of individual clinicians to make accurate assessments is impaired by a lack of time to review relevant studies or to process the information in a way that is meaningful to the patient affected. The uncertainty hypothesis is the assumption that when variation cannot be explained by differences in disease prevalence, access to and availability of services, or enabling factors (e.g., insurance), it reflects differences in physicians' beliefs about the value of the variable procedures and practices for meeting patients' needs.[19] Often, physicians will rely on their perception of the problem and use their own judgment and intuition to estimate outcomes. Variation in these perceptions can be demonstrated between different physician groups as well as within a single specialty. Given the same information, physicians may draw different conclusions and make different decisions. The result is that some of these decisions will be wrong in the sense that they are based on mistaken perceptions of the facts and are not in the patient's best interest. This decision making will spill over to informed consent, expert testimony, consensus development, and malpractice adjudication.

The problem of practice variation is hardly corrected by preguessing or second-guessing clinician decisions. The basic assumption in these strategies (i.e., quality assurance, utilization review, cost containment) is that there is accuracy in numbers. It is based on the idea that the individual physician's decision cannot be independently trusted and that the collective decisions or actions of a larger number can. The problem is that the "check" is not against reality but simply the perceptions of others. The second opinion cannot be assumed to be closer to the truth, nor can the precertification manual of a patient's HMO. Since utilization review programs are driven by concerns about cost control, the carrier's actual review process relies on aggregate utilization and spending targets that have little to do with clinical concerns. The carrier's medical review rhetoric ("medically necessary," "fraud," "abuse") highlights the carrier's focus on cost control rather than concern about why services are used.[6]

Physicians are forced to make decisions about complex problems under difficult conditions, often with little support. Frequently they must act without knowing the range of outcomes for their possible actions. The position of the physician requires that decisions be made in the midst of an exponentially enlarging database of information along with the pressure of patient expectations, personal goals, changing reimbursement systems, competition, malpractice threat, peer pressure, and politics.

## DIMENSIONS OF DIAGNOSTIC TEST EVALUATION

The implementation of a diagnostic test begins with innovation and ends with a generally usable and effective clinical instrument. The literature in support of the test must establish the scientific basis for its performance and demonstrate its capability to identify a target condition in a population of patients. A sequenced systematic evaluation of a proposed diagnostic test should consist of the following:

1. A study of the basic performance of the test
2. Determination if the test can distinguish obvious cases of disease from healthy controls
3. Testing its use on a broad spectrum of disease cases
4. Studies that broaden the challenge for disease and control subjects
5. "Clinical trial" format on a relatively unselected cohort of consecutive patients[13]

If these methods are used, the technical capacity of the test can be determined along with calculations of sensitivity, specificity, and predictive values.

Kent and Larson[12] have provided an overview of diagnostic test evaluation that serves as a conceptual framework and includes (1) technical capacity, (2) test accuracy (reliability, validity), (3) diagnostic value or cost compared to existing (or competing) tests, and (4) ability to improve outcome.

The first dimension, technical capacity, includes (1) adequate description of the technical specifications of the test so that replication is possible, (2) demonstrated reproducibility (test-retest reliability) and minimal variation in interpretation (interobserver and intraobserver variation), and (3) a clear demonstration of how a normal test (or value) is defined. In general, an emerging literature on a new technology should demonstrate all three technical capacity points. A minimum criterion for an established technology is that its technical specifications be clearly defined in each paper (e.g., which instruments, what calibration, or setting). An additional criterion for tests for which normal values are critical is a clear description of the population from which normal values were derived and how such values were derived.

Second, the accuracy of the test is the key to determining the quality of the literature. It is in this dimension that the reliability and validity of the test are evaluated. Methods have been described by Kent et al[11] and by Sackett et al[17] in which the answer to each of a series of questions defines a separate methodologic domain to be evaluated in each paper reviewed. These include the following:

1. Has the diagnostic test been evaluated in a patient sample that included an appropriate spectrum of disease severity (mild and severe, treated and untreated individuals with different but commonly confused disorders)?
2. Are the persons applying or interpreting the test independent of and blind to disease status or patient outcome?
3. Has the sample of patients, after the diagnostic test is applied, then been followed prospectively for the development of disease?
4. Has disease status been identified by a "gold standard" (e.g., another well-accepted test or valid case definition)?

The third dimension of evaluation is an extension of accuracy and clinical value to the determination of the relative or marginal contribution of the test in question compared to existing tests.

Last, the fourth dimension of evaluation is whether the application of diagnostic test improves outcomes; if there is improvement, a determination of the magnitude of the improvement and how it is achieved is needed. It is in this dimension alone that the randomized controlled clinical trial becomes relevant. The outcomes in question could be related to health services (e.g., reduced hospitalizations) or patient centered (e.g., improved function, reduced morbidity). These kinds of studies, although badly needed, are rarely available. Figure 31–1 presents an ideal study design that allows for determination of clinically important patient outcomes.

The reviewer must be aware of biases that can contaminate or corrupt a study's results. These may include verification bias,[2] workup bias, diagnostic review bias, test-review bias, and incorporation bias.[16] Attention must be directed to how the cohort population of disease patients and controls are assembled to ensure that the estimates of accuracy are meaningful and generalizable for the practicing clinician.

In the body of available clinical studies and the supporting literature, there is wide variation in the rigor of study design and methods of reporting.[14] Although there may be general agreement about what criteria are important for evaluation, the subsets of criteria actually applied are at times quite varied or inconsistent.

Approaches to actual grading of articles is illustrated by several examples. The American Association of Electrodiagnostic Medicine (AAEM) performed a review on the useful nerve conduction studies for carpal tunnel syndrome.[1] The authors applied six study criteria to the literature reviewed, four dealing with technical capacity and two with diagnostic accuracy. The technical capacity elements included the following:

1. Electrodiagnostic procedure described in sufficient detail to permit duplication
2. Limb temperature monitored and reference values reported (for nerve conduction velocity)
3. Description of the method for determining reference values
4. Criteria for abnormal values clearly stated

Elements of diagnostic accuracy included (1) prospective study and (2) conduct of electrodiagnostic studies independent of determination of carpal tunnel syndrome status.

Only articles meeting at least four of the six criteria were considered without additional weighting for which of the criteria were met. However, only articles meeting all six criteria were displayed in the evidence tables. An additional post hoc criterion was applied to those articles meeting all six criteria: if ≥90% of patients with carpal tunnel syndrome demonstrated abnormalities on any one electrodiagnostic test, the study was excluded from the evidence tables. The justification for such exclusion was the assumption that such prevalent abnormalities likely reflect a very biased referral population.

Gronseth and Greenberg,[7] in their review of the literature of the utility of the electroencephalogram in evaluating headache, used six criteria adapted from Sackett et al.[17] Five of the criteria were related to diagnostic accuracy, and one was related to technical capacity.

Hoffman et al,[9] in an evaluation of the literature on thermography for lumbar radiculopathy, used two criteria for technical capacity and five criteria for diagnostic accuracy. They decided on a scheme to aggregate all the criteria into a grade for each paper. Independence of test and diagnosis interpretation and adequacy of the gold standard were required for a paper to receive a "high" rating.

These examples illustrate that general agreement about important criteria may exist; however, the set of criteria actually used and their relative importance for purposes of grading journal articles has been inconsistent. In addition, a method by which article grading would be incorporated into practice parameter recommendations for the use of the test remains unclear.

Meta-analyses are potentially useful in health services research, including the evaluation of diagnostic tests. This can provide a summary of accuracy, help determine study validity, distinguish variability in accuracy from variability in patient characteristics or test performance, and help define research deficiencies and guide future research.[10]

## EVIDENCE INTO PRACTICE

There are three steps for taking empiric evidence to practice: (1) getting the evidence straight; (2) developing clinical practice parameters that are faithful to both the evidence and the clinical and personal situations of patients; and (3) applying these parameters to the right patient at the right time in the right way. Problems in getting the evidence straight stem from difficulties in finding sound evidence. Lack of agreement on evidence standards undermines the effectiveness of authoritative practice parameters. Applying

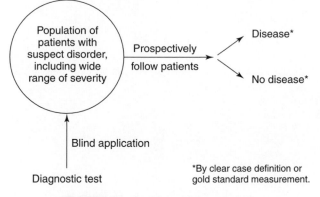

**FIGURE 31–1.** Diagnostic test accuracy.

evidence and practice parameters effectively and efficiently is often thwarted by mismatches between evidence and usual practice circumstances. Time pressures undermine interpretation and application of evidence at every step.[8]

## WHAT IS THE GOAL OF PRACTICE PARAMETERS?

A degree of uncertainty exists in most areas of clinical practice. With respect to the use of diagnostic technologies, uncertainty about the capability of the test to answer specific clinical questions must be kept in mind when ordered. Many questions about the value of testing can be answered with competent appraisal of the supporting literature. QSS anticipates and attempts to simplify decisions that would otherwise be made by clinicians individually. Once such an appraisal is completed, a clinician will have a frame of reference in which to interpret the results for an individual patient. Most clinicians (and patients) have neither the time nor the expertise to perform such an appraisal. Practice parameters provide an assessment of the relevance of testing for a specific disorder and serve as a vehicle to disseminate that appraisal in a form that can assist in reducing clinical uncertainty and may narrow practice variation.

If established correctly, practice parameters will allow for an estimate of the effect of a practice intervention on outcomes that are important to patients. The comparison of the benefits of the outcomes to the harms and costs of the intervention will similarly be enhanced for clinicians. The principal goal is to reduce uncertainty and improve patient outcomes. The benefits of this effort include consistent patient care, improved efficiency, and, possibly, cost reduction (although some costs may rise). The risks from the process include restrictions on practice, limitations on patient preference, and effects on liability.

## REFERENCES

1. AAEM Quality Assurance Committee, Jablecki CK, et al. Literature review of the usefulness of nerve conduction studies and electromyography for the evaluation of patients with carpal tunnel syndrome. *Muscle Nerve.* 1993;16:1392-1414.
2. Begg CB. Advances in statistical methodology for diagnostic medicine in the 1980's. *Stat Med.* 1991;10:1887-1895.
3. Feinstein A. A bibliography of publications on observer variations. *Chronic Dis.* 1985;38:619-632.
4. Fraser GM, Pilpel D, Kosecoff J, Brook RH. Effect of panel composition on appropriateness ratings. *Int J Qual Health Care.* 1994;6:251-255.
5. Grilli R, Scorpiglione N, Nicolucci A, et al. Variation in use of breast surgery and characteristics of hospitals' surgical staff. *Int J Qual Health Care.* 1994;6:233-238.
6. Grogan CM, Feldman RD, Nyman JA, et al. How will we use clinical guidelines? The experience of Medicare carriers. *J Health Polit Policy Law.* 1994;19:7-26.
7. Gronseth GS, Greenberg MK. The utility of the electroencephalogram in the evaluation of patients presenting with headache: a review of the literature. *Neurology.* 1995;45:1263-1267.
8. Haynes RB. Some problems in applying evidence in clinical practice. *Ann N Y Acad Sci.* 1993;703:210-224.
9. Hoffman RM, Kent DL, Deyo RA. Diagnostic accuracy and clinical utility of thermography for lumbar radiculopathy: a meta-analysis. *Spine.* 1991;16:623-628.
10. Irwig L, Tosteson ANA, Gatsonis C, et al. Guidelines for meta-analyses evaluating diagnostic tests. *Ann Intern Med.* 1994;120:667-676.
11. Kent DL, Haynor DR, Lonstreth WT, et al. The clinical efficacy of magnetic resonance imaging in neuroimaging. *Ann Int Med.* 1994;120:856-871.
12. Kent DL, Larson EB. Health policy in radiology: disease, level of impact, and quality of research methods—three dimensions of clinical efficacy applied to magnetic resonance imaging. *Invest Radiol.* 1992;27:245-254.
13. Nierenberg AA, Feinstein AR. How to evaluate a diagnostic test. *JAMA.* 1988;259:1699-1702.
14. Nuwer MR. On the process for evaluating proposed new diagnostic EEG tests. *Brain Topogr.* 1992;4:243-247.
15. Ramsey SD, Hillman AL, Renshaw LR, et al. How important is the scientific literature in guiding clinical decisions? *Intl J Technol Assess Health Care.* 1993;9:253-262.
16. Ransohoff DF, Feinstein AR. Problems of spectrum and bias in evaluating the efficacy of diagnostic tests. *N Engl J Med.* 1978;299:926-930.
17. Sackett DL, Haynes RB, Guyatt GH, Tugwell P. *Clinical Epidemiology: A Basic Science for Clinical Medicine.* 2nd ed. Boston: Little, Brown; 1991: 51-152.
18. Schreiber TL, Elkhatib A, Grines CL, et al. Cardiologist versus internist management of patients with unstable angina: treatment patterns and outcomes. *J Am Coll Cardiol.* 1995;26:577-582.
19. Wennberg JE, Barnes BA, Zubkoff M. Professional uncertainty and the problem of supplier-induced demand. *Soc Sci Med.* 1982;16:811-824.
20. Young GR, Sandercock PAG, Slattery J, et al. Observer variation in the interpretation of intra-arterial angiograms and the risk of inappropriate decisions about carotid endarterectomy. *J Neurol Neurosurg Psychiatry.* 1996;60:152-157.

# Index

Note: Page numbers in *italics* refer to illustrations; page numbers followed by t refer to tables.

ISBN 0-7216-7603-0